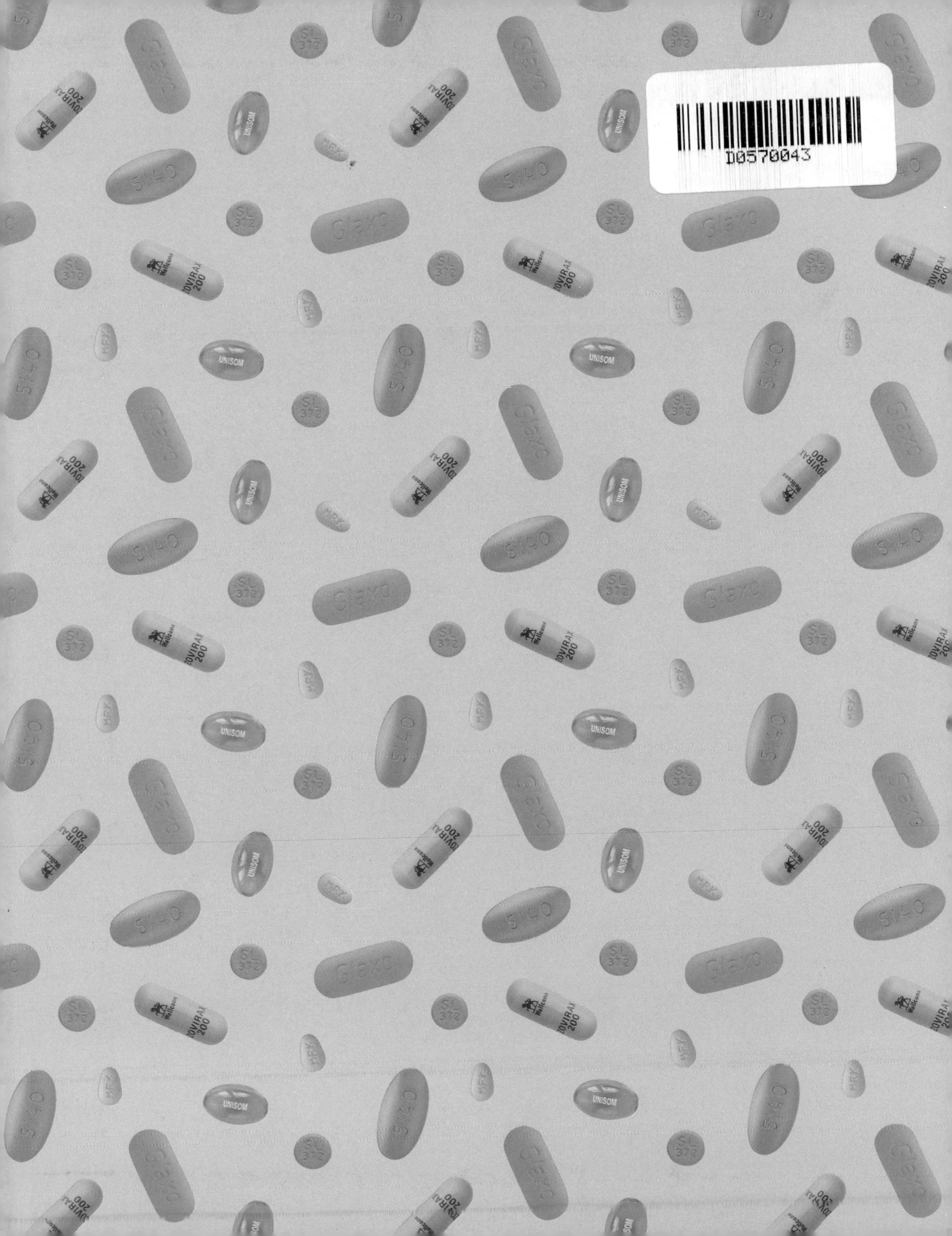

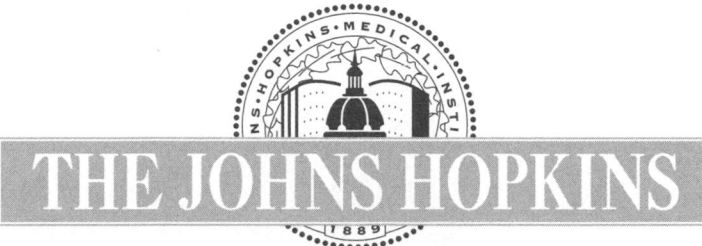

THE JOHNS HOPKINS

CONSUMER GUIDE TO

DRUGS

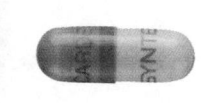 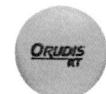 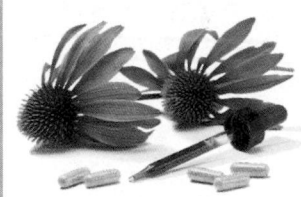 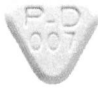 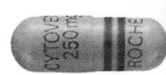

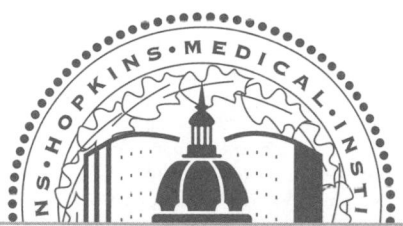

THE JOHNS HOPKINS

CONSUMER GUIDE TO
DRUGS

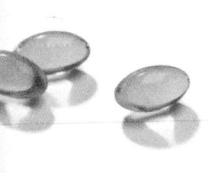 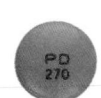 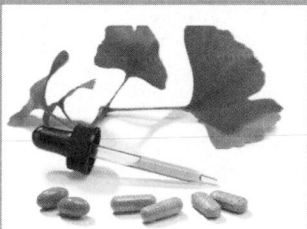 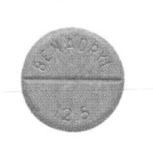 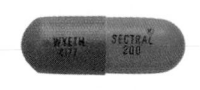

Medical Editor
SIMEON MARGOLIS, M.D., PH.D.

Prepared by the Editors of
THE JOHNS HOPKINS MEDICAL LETTER HEALTH AFTER 50

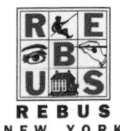

REBUS
NEW YORK

JOHNS HOPKINS HEALTH AFTER 50 PUBLICATIONS

www.HopkinsAfter50.com

The Johns Hopkins Consumer Guide to Drugs is one of many indispensable medical publications for consumers from America's leading health center. We publish comprehensive reference encyclopedias, including *The Johns Hopkins Consumer Guide to Medical Tests* and *Johns Hopkins Symptoms & Remedies;* White Papers providing in-depth information on specific disorders such as coronary heart disease, arthritis, and diabetes; and *The Johns Hopkins Medical Letter HEALTH AFTER 50,* our monthly 8-page newsletter that presents recommendations from Hopkins experts on current medical issues that affect you.

All of our publications provide timely information for everyone concerned with taking control of his or her own health and medical care, using clear, nontechnical language that is easy to understand. And, they all come from the century-old tradition of Johns Hopkins excellence.

Visit us online at www.HopkinsAfter50.com for health and medical updates as well as information on our publications. For a trial subscription to our newsletter, you can call 386-447-6313 or write to Subscription Dept., Health After 50, P.O.Box 420179, Palm Coast, FL 32142.

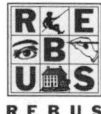

REBUS

This book is not intended as a substitute
for the advice and expertise of a physician or a pharmacist. Readers who suspect they may
have specific medical problems should consult a physician about any suggestions made in this book.

Library of Congress Cataloging-in-Publication Data

The Johns Hopkins consumer guide to drugs / medical editor, Simeon Margolis ;
prepared by the editors of the Johns Hopkins medical letter health after 50.
    p. cm.
  Includes index.
  ISBN 0-929661-66-4
  1. Drugs–Handbooks, manuals, etc. 2. Drugs–Popular works I. Margolis, Simeon,
1931 – II. Johns Hopkins medical health letter health after 50.

RM301.12.J636 2002
615'.1–dc21

                                                              2001048754

Printed in the United States of America
10 9 8 7 6 5 4 3 2

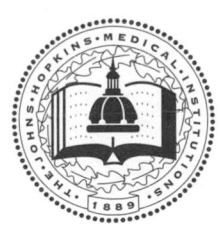

The Johns Hopkins Consumer Guide to Drugs

RODNEY FRIEDMAN
Publisher

THOMAS DICKEY
Executive Editor

JEREMY D. BIRCH
Managing Editor

EVAN HANSEN
Contributing Editor

CARNEY W. MIMMS III
Production Database Designer

JOHN VASILIADIS
Production Database Programmer

TIMOTHY JEFFS
Art Director

ROBERT DUCKWALL
Medical Illustrator

BARBARA MAXWELL O'NEILL
Associate Publisher

Johns Hopkins Medical Books are published under the auspices of The Johns Hopkins Medical Letter HEALTH AFTER 50

RODNEY FRIEDMAN
Editor and Publisher

PATRICE BENNEWARD
Executive Editor

DEVON SCHUYLER
Senior Editor

SUZANNE R. UNDY
Senior Writer

KIMBERLY FLYNN
Writer

ELIZABETH CURRY
Associate Editor

DAVID DeVELLIS, M.D.
Medical Consultant

BARBARA MAXWELL O'NEILL
Associate Publisher

HELEN MULLEN
Circulation Director

DAVID ALEXANDER
Circulation Manager

JERRY LOO
Product Manager

ALLISON HORDOS
Promotion Coordinator

Special Acknowledgment

GIGA COMMUNICATIONS, INC.
Digital Production

**DEBORAH WIBLE AND THE STAFF OF
THE DEPARTMENT OF PHARMACY,
BETH ISRAEL MEDICAL CENTER, NEW YORK, NY
MT. SINAI HOSPITAL MEDICAL CENTER, CHICAGO, IL**
Pharmacological Resources

HOW TO USE THIS BOOK

The Johns Hopkins Consumer Guide to Drugs contains the most essential information regarding nearly every major medication available for consumers—both prescription and over-the-counter (OTC) drugs. It presents the facts about medications in plain, easy-to-understand language so that everyone, and particularly older adults (the largest group of people using medications), can achieve the maximum therapeutic benefit from taking drugs, while keeping side effects and adverse reactions to a minimum.

Each drug is covered in a succinct one- or two-page profile. These profiles appear in alphabetical order according to the generic name of the drug (e.g., acetaminophen). If you do not know the generic name, you can look up the drug's brand name (e.g., Tylenol) in the general index starting on page 830, and it will guide you to the appropriate page. You can also look up a specific ailment in the disorder index (page 16) and see the various drugs used to treat it.

Following the drug profiles are two additional sections. The first is devoted to color photographs of many of the pills described in the book. The second section is an overview of herbs and other dietary supplements, which are widely used to self-treat health problems. The overview focuses on issues of efficacy and safety concerning supplements, including their potential for interactions with conventional medications. Following the overview are profiles of 10 of the most popular supplements.

Important Note Regarding the Color Pill Photographs in This Book: The physical appearance of a particular drug may vary considerably from one manufacturer to another, or from one dosage strength to another even when made by the same manufacturer. The pictures that appear with the drug profiles (and in the color pill section on pages 797-808) of this book represent but one dosage strength of one brand of a drug made by one manufacturer. If the pill you take looks different from the one you see in the photograph, do not be alarmed. However, if you have any doubts, concerns, or questions whatsoever about the medication you take, consult your doctor or pharmacist.

DRUGS AND AGING

If you're over 50, chances are you're taking more kinds of medications and in greater quantities than you ever did in previous decades. Indeed, people between the ages of 55 and 64 are given an average of eight different prescriptions during the course of a year. And those over age 70 take an average of 6.5 medications per day. It's only logical that the more medications you take concurrently, the more likely it is that an adverse drug reaction could occur. And for older people, such risks are further compounded by physiological changes that make the body more sensitive to the effects of drugs (see below). Consequently, adverse reactions to drugs are seven times more common in older people than younger ones and account for approximately 20 percent of all hospitalizations among older adults. If you fall into this age group, knowledge about the medications you take can help ensure that your drug therapy is effective—and as safe as possible.

HOW AGING AFFECTS THE BODY'S RESPONSE TO DRUGS

Beginning sometime during our middle thirties and continuing throughout life, measurements of functional capacity of most major organ systems show a gradual decline. Such changes, which are natural and inevitable, do not necessarily have any noticeable effect on one's quality of life. But they can affect the way that our bodies respond to drugs, and make us more susceptible to untoward reactions and side effects. For one thing, there is an overall decrease in body fluid volume. This results in proportionally higher concentrations of drugs or other substances in the bloodstream, thus increasing the risk of toxicity. This effect may be further compounded by an age-related decline in liver and kidney function. These organs are primarily responsible for metabolizing drugs and eliminating toxins. Therefore, a decrease in their function means chemical substances remain in the body longer and are more likely to build up to potentially hazardous levels. Conversely, a sluggish digestive system can slow the rate that drugs are absorbed into the bloodstream, meaning that less of the drug is available to produce the desired therapeutic effect.

Diminished blood flow to the brain may boost the likelihood that certain drugs will cause dizziness, fainting, loss of coordination, forgetfulness, confusion, or other signs of cognitive impairment. In some people the heart functions less efficiently with age, which in turn may deprive other organs of an adequate blood supply, causing further disruptions in how drugs are distributed in the body.

SOME WAYS THE BODY CHANGES WITH AGE

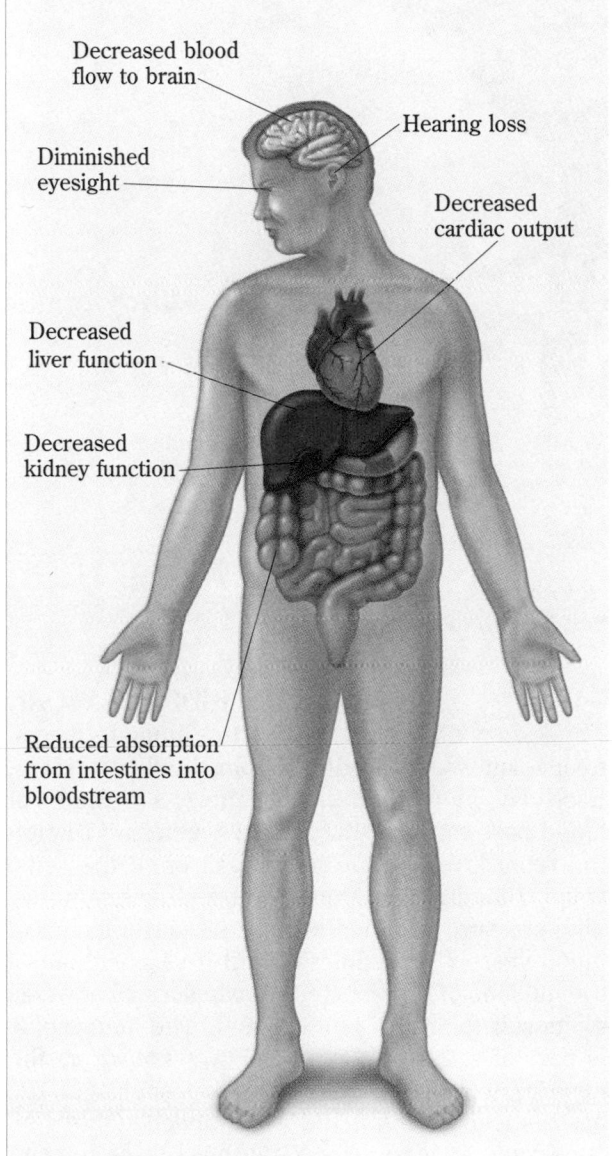

Decreased blood flow to brain

Hearing loss

Diminished eyesight

Decreased cardiac output

Decreased liver function

Decreased kidney function

Reduced absorption from intestines into bloodstream

The physiological changes that occur with age can affect the way our bodies react to drugs.

Finally, age-associated decrements in vision, hearing, and memory may affect an older person's ability to properly understand prescription labels, package inserts, or doctors' instructions. Bear in mind, however, that chronological age alone is not necessarily a good predictor of the degree of functional decline; there is considerable variability from one person to another in the rate at which such changes occur. For example, approximately one-third of healthy elderly people exhibit no significant decrease in kidney function.

DRUGS AND THE DIGESTIVE SYSTEM

Drugs are absorbed primarily in the stomach and small intestine. As we age, these organs may not absorb food and medications as well as they once did, resulting in reduced therapeutic levels of the drug in the bloodstream. A larger dose may be needed to compensate for this phenomenon. A more common problem is that some drugs are not metabolized as efficiently as we age. As a result, greater amounts of the drug circulate in the bloodstream for longer periods of time; thus smaller dosages may be warranted for older patients.

HOW THE LIVER BREAKS DOWN DRUGS AND TOXINS

One of the primary functions of the liver is to cleanse and detoxify the blood of drugs (including alcohol) and poisonous substances that would otherwise build up in the bloodstream. How does it do this? First, nutrient-rich blood passes from the stomach and small intestine through the portal vein into the liver (see illustration, page 10). This blood is then exposed to the many thousands of cells (hepatocytes) within the liver. Here, the nutrients are extracted and chemically broken down (metabolized) into their smallest useful components, and then either stored in the liver for future use or returned to the bloodstream via the hepatic vein to become available for use by cells throughout the body. Many drugs and toxins are also chemically modified (most often inactivated) in the liver. Most of the byproducts of the metabolism of nutrients, toxins, and drugs are also returned to the bloodstream and travel to the kidneys where they are eliminated in the urine. The substances that cannot

THE ROUTE OF BLOOD THROUGH THE LIVER

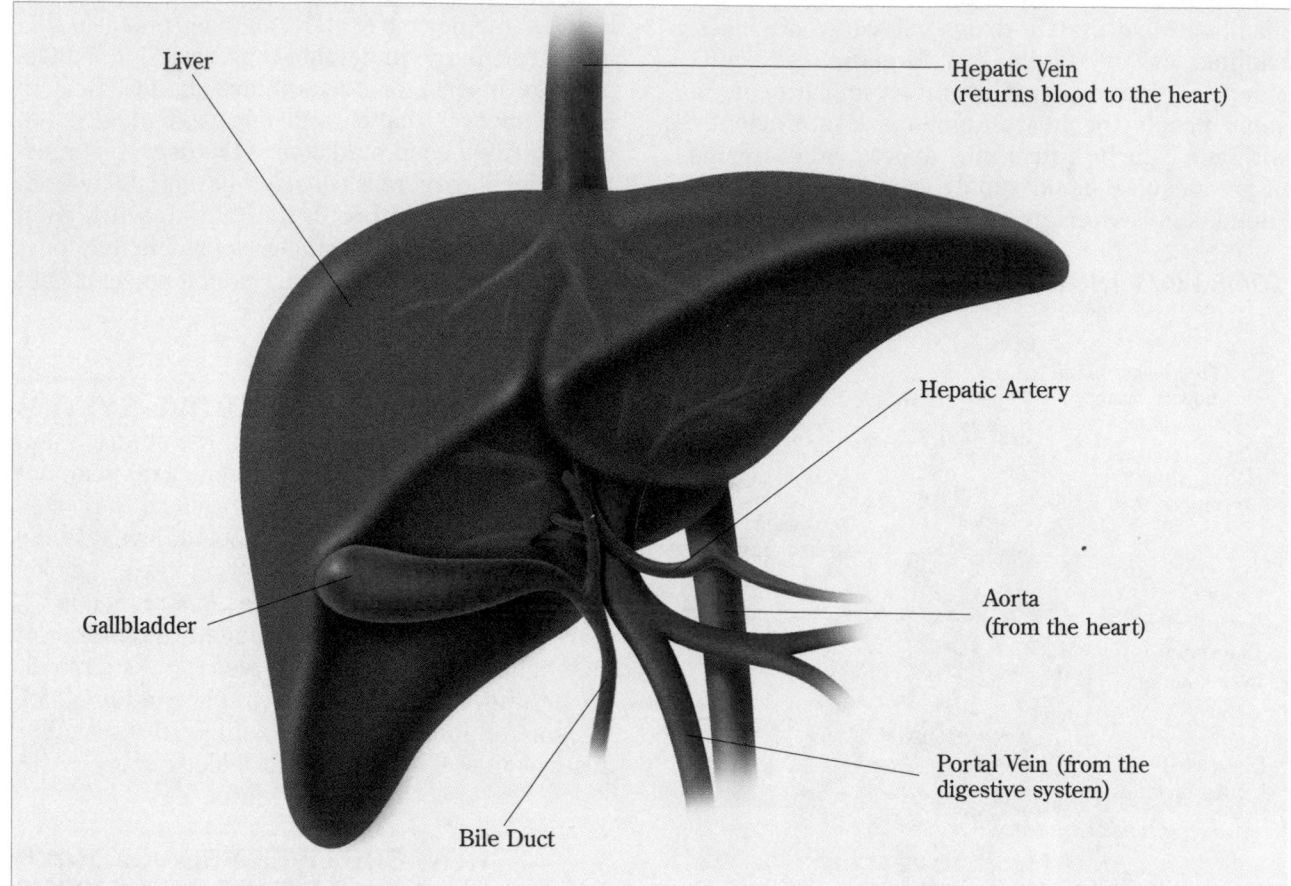

Liver

Hepatic Vein
(returns blood to the heart)

Hepatic Artery

Aorta
(from the heart)

Gallbladder

Portal Vein (from the
digestive system)

Bile Duct

Blood passes through the spongelike channels of the liver where liver cells extract nutrients and metabolize them for use by the rest of the body, and neutralize most toxins and many drugs.

be eliminated by the kidneys are incorporated into the bile, a digestive fluid produced by liver cells and stored in the gallbladder. Bile is released via the common bile duct to help absorb fats in the small intestine, and its constituents are mostly excreted in the feces. Liver cells themselves are nourished by fresh blood coming in through the hepatic artery, a branch of the aorta—the heart's primary artery.

The liver is composed of 50,000 to 100,000 individual clusters of cells known as lobules. At the core of each lobule is a centrilobar vein, from which radiate hundreds of hepatocytes. Each lobule is served by a network of minuscule branches of the bile ducts, the hepatic artery, and the portal vein. This structure is suggestive of a liver lobule's function as a minuscule chemical processing plant.

HOW THE KIDNEYS WORK

The kidney's primary task is to eliminate drugs, toxins, and waste products from the bloodstream. Each day, more than 2,500 pints (1,175 liters) of blood pass through the kidneys, entering though the renal arteries and leaving through the renal veins. Blood pours from the renal artery under high pressure into increasingly narrow branches of blood vessels (arterioles), until it reaches one of the millions of tiny clusters of capillaries known as glomeruli (plural of glomerulus). The glomerulus is part of a microscopic structure known as the nephron (see illustration on the opposite page), the basic functional unit of the kidney. Each kidney contains roughly one million nephrons. At the top end of the nephron is Bowman's capsule, which surrounds the glomerulus. Water, salts, wastes, and

THE KIDNEYS

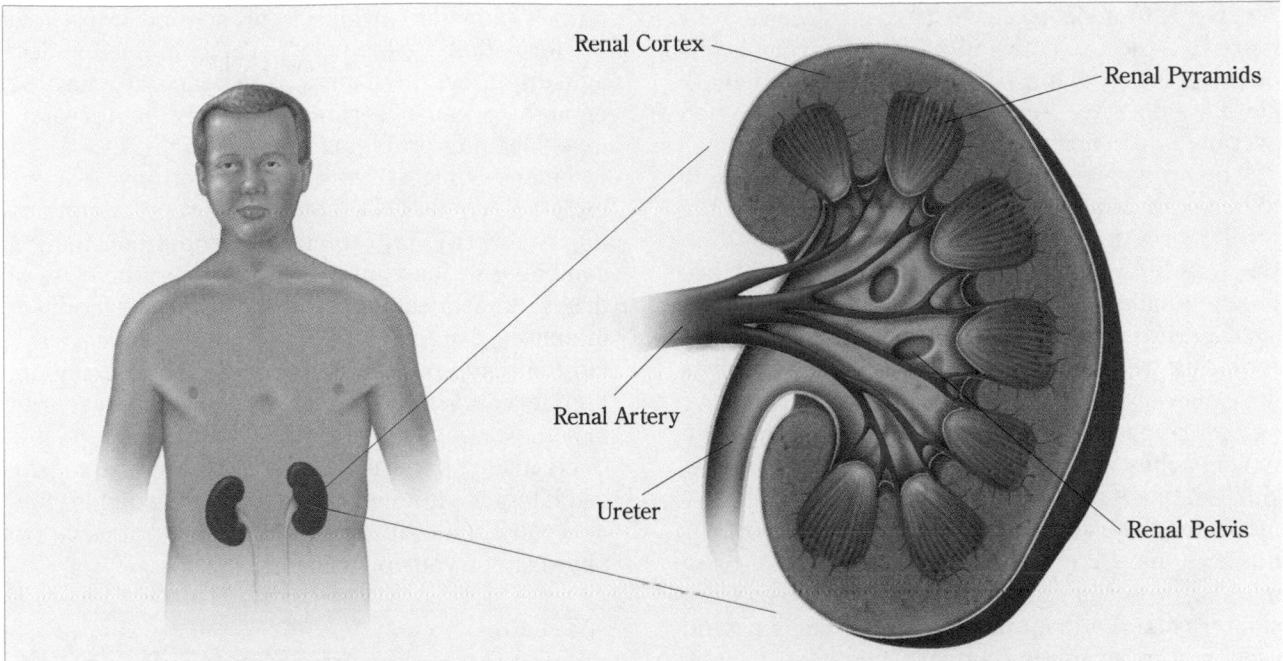

In conjunction with the liver, the kidney is responsible for cleansing the blood of drugs and toxins.

toxins filter through the tiny blood vessels of the glomerulus and enter Bowman's capsule. This filtrate, which will become urine, passes from Bowman's capsule through the nephron's convoluted tubule, which has a hairpin turn known as the loop of Henle (the structure affected by so-called loop diuretics). Next it travels back out to the renal cortex (the outer region of the kidney), down through the collecting tubule, and out the renal pelvis, where it flows into the ureter, the conduit through which urine reaches the bladder. Meanwhile, the purified portion of the filtrate (containing almost all the salts and water entering the kidney) is conserved and returned to the bloodstream via the renal vein. Indeed, for all of the many quarts of fluid the kidney processes per day, only one quart or so is eliminated as urine.

AGING AND THE RISKS OF MULTIPLE DRUG USE

Two-thirds of all people over 65 take medications on a daily basis, and many of those in this population take more than one medication at a time. Among persons ages 65 to 84, 61 percent receive 3

A NEPHRON

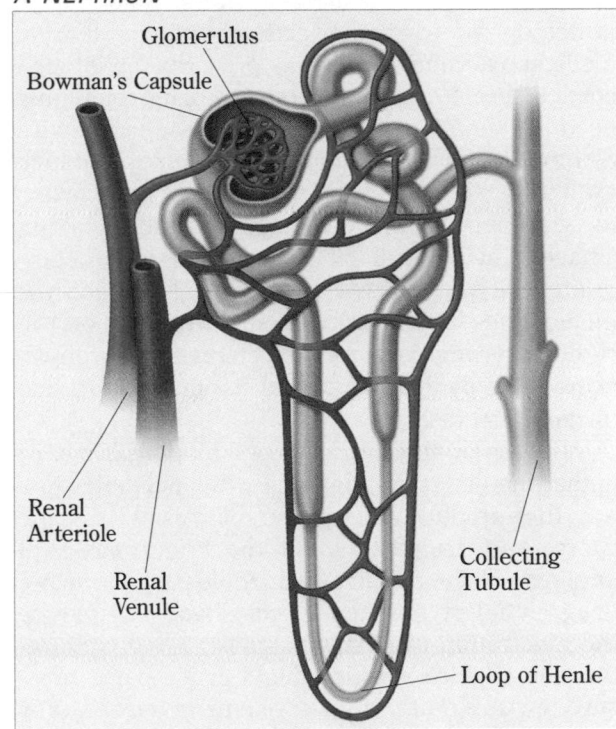

In the tiny capillaries of the nephron, wastes are filtered out of the blood to be excreted in the urine.

or more different drugs in a year; 37 percent receive 5 or more; and 19 percent receive 7 or more. (At the extreme end of the spectrum, it has been reported that a portion of Medicare beneficiaries who rate their health as poor receive an average of 31 separate prescriptions per year.)

The primary reason older people are more likely to be taking multiple drugs is simply that they often have more than one chronic medical condition (such as high blood pressure, glaucoma, or arthritis) simultaneously. In fact, elderly people have, on average, five separate coexisting medical conditions requiring treatment, which almost always involves drug therapy.

Unfortunately, in some instances relief from the typical aches and pains of aging—rather than specific treatment of illness or restoration of function—motivates the use of multiple prescription and OTC medications. Or oftentimes, an unnecessary drug may be prescribed merely to help counteract the side effects of a drug initially prescribed for good reason. For example, suppose you take a beta-blocker (such as propranolol) for high blood pressure and you begin to experience wheezing, a known side effect of beta-blockers. Rather than switching you to another class of antihypertensive medication, your doctor may prescribe an inhaled corticosteroid, a powerful type of drug commonly used to suppress the wheezing associated with asthma. In turn, the corticosteroid may produce even more side effects that require yet more drugs to treat them. Ultimately, you may wind up taking a handful of medications when a single more appropriate one would have sufficed. Taking multiple medications at the same time—whether for the right or wrong reasons—is referred to by physicians as "polypharmacy," and it can be a formula for potential disaster.

Another significant risk posed by polypharmacy is that the drugs may interact with each other in a way that produces an undesirable result. In some cases, one drug can blunt the effectiveness of another. For example, two cholesterol-lowering drugs (cholestyramine and colestipol) can reduce the absorption of diuretics such as hydrochlorothiazide (Esidrix), which could cause blood pressure to rise. In other cases, one drug may actually enhance the effects of another drug so that dangerous adverse effects may occur, as when aspirin, which has an anticlotting effect, is taken with warfarin (Coumadin), which is prescribed to prevent the formation of blood clots. The combined anticoagulant effect of aspirin and warfarin may be enough to cause serious—possibly life-threatening—bleeding problems (hemorrhaging).

Finally, some drugs simply do not mix. A seemingly innocuous OTC cough suppressant containing the active ingredient dextromethorphan, if combined with an antidepressant from the class of drugs known as MAO (monoamine oxidase) inhibitors, can result in a dangerous chemical cocktail that can produce extreme nervous excitation, high fever, a sharp increase in blood pressure, and in some cases, death. In light of such dangers, it is imperative to know if any new drug you plan to take can interact with one you are already using; to find out, you should always consult your primary-care physician or your pharmacist.

ASSESSING THE RISKS

Broadly defined as any unwanted response to a drug, adverse drug reactions (ADRs) occur with considerable frequency in persons over the age of 60. At least 17 percent—but as many as 30 percent by some estimates—of all hospital admissions and one in a thousand hospital deaths of older Americans are a direct result of drug toxicity or ADRs. The Inspector General of the U.S. Department of Health and Human Services estimates that 32,000 hip fractures, 163,000 cases of mental impairment, and 61,000 cases of drug-induced parkinsonism occur annually as a result of ADRs in the elderly. Women are generally at greater risk for ADRs because more drugs are prescribed for them on average than for men; and women lose significantly more muscle mass as they age, which increases their sensitivity to drugs. Yet the single most important contributing factor to ADRs is the number of medications taken. Susceptibility to ADRs increases with each drug added to the therapeutic regimen. Recent findings indicate that the presence of coexisting disease is equally important in determining the risk of ADRs. Individual health status, rather than chronological age alone, becomes a key predictor in assessing risk for ADRs.

It must be noted, however, that not all multiple drug combinations are undesirable or unnecessary.

Appropriate drug therapy can be vastly beneficial for older persons by providing symptom relief, improved functional capacities, pain management, reduced complications of chronic disease, and even prolongation of life. Naturally, every drug has the potential for adverse effects. But minor or irritating side effects, or even more problematic ones, must be weighed against benefits that could make a pronounced difference in terms of the quality and length of a person's life

PREVENTING ADVERSE DRUG REACTIONS

Considering the age-related physiological changes that can affect the body's response to drugs, as well as the alarming statistics regarding polypharmacy and adverse drug reactions, the message is clear that extra caution is in order when older people take medications. The first step is simply to put all of your medicines into a paper bag and bring them to your doctor for a review of everything you are currently taking. Include all of your over-the-

Drugs That Don't Mix with Grapefruit Juice

While doctors, pharmacists, and the package inserts that come with medications provide clear warnings against adverse interactions between one drug and another, patients are considerably less likely to be warned of potential bad reactions caused by taking a drug with a particular food. In recent years it has come to light that grapefruit may cause potentially serious interactions when taken with a number of drugs. A compound found in grapefruit (but not other citrus fruits) can block an enzyme in the small intestine which helps to metabolize certain drugs. As a result, more of the drug is absorbed and the level of the drug is increased in the bloodstream. However, this enhancement of the drug occurs only if the drug and grapefruit juice are taken close together.

In some situations, the effect may be beneficial. Those taking a calcium channel blocker such as felodipine (Plendil) for hypertension may suddenly acquire better, more stable control of their blood pressure, or be able to take a lower—and thus safer—dose while obtaining the same therapeutic benefit. On the other hand, for some patients, excessive quantities of felodipine may build up in the blood and cause blood pressure to drop precipitously and cause dizziness or fainting. (Interestingly, medical researchers are currently looking for ways to harness the natural effect of grapefruit juice on drug metabolism, so that one day it could be incorporated into the formulation of certain medications to achieve optimal results while using less of the primary active ingredient. Because individual responses vary so widely, however, many experts are skeptical that such an approach would work reliably from patient to patient.)

The following is a list of the medications known to interact adversely with grapefruit juice. If you take any of these drugs and you also regularly eat grapefruit or drink its juice, you don't need to suddenly change your dietary habits. Rather, you should consult your doctor for advice.

- **Calcium channel blockers**, especially felodipine (Plendil), nifedipine (Adalat, Procardia), and nimodipine (Nimotop). Also affects verapamil (Calan, Isoptin, Verelan), but to a lesser degree. No apparent affect on diltiazem (Cardizem, Dilacor, Tiazac).
- **Cilostazol** (Pletal).
- **Cyclosporine** (Sandimmune).
- **Tacrolimus** (Prograf).
- **Midazolam** (a short-acting benzodiazepine marketed only in injectable form in the US). Grapefruit juice may also increase elimination times of other benzodiazepine tranquilizers, such as alprazolam (Xanax) and triazolam (Halcion).
- **Statins**, such as atorvastatin (Lipitor) and simvastatin (Zocor).
- **Estrogens**.
- **Caffeine**.
- **Saquinavir** (Invirase), an antiviral drug used against HIV. (Curiously, grapefruit juice actually decreases elimination times for indinavir, a similar drug.)

counter medicines as well. Your doctor can evaluate whether any of the drugs might interact badly with one another, or determine which ones may not be appropriate at all for you (see box below, for example). Repeat this "brown-bag review" once every year. In addition, the following tips can help you use your medications more safely.

YOU AND YOUR MEDICATIONS
▶ Keep a record of all your medications. Note the name of the drug, the doctor who prescribed it, the amount you take, and the times of day you take it, along with comments on any allergies or other reactions you have had to medications. If for some reason you need to see a new doctor, take your medication record with you, so the new doctor can see the drugs you are currently taking. If your pharmacist does not keep a medications record for you, take your record to the drugstore each time you purchase a medication.

Drugs Not Recommended for Older Patients

According to a report published several years ago in the *Journal of the American Medical Association* by a panel of experts in the field of geriatrics and pharmacology, 24 drugs commonly prescribed to older adults may be potentially inappropriate for them. These drugs are regarded as either ineffective in older people or generally more toxic than equally effective alternatives. Some of these drugs have a strong anticholinergic effect, meaning they block the neurotransmitter acetylcholine, which in turn blocks the transmission of certain nerve impulses. Since the amount of acetylcholine in the body decreases with age, older people are especially sensitive to the effects of anticholinergic agents and are prone to experiencing side effects from them. These include daytime drowsiness, mental confusion, dizziness, and loss of coordination. Such effects may precipitate falls or traffic accidents. A conservative estimate indicates that 25 percent of patients over the age of 65 are prescribed one or more of these inappropriate and potentially dangerous drugs.

It is important to point out, however, that just because a drug appears on this list does not completely rule out its use by older patients. While some drugs such as chlorpropamide and phenylbutazone should probably always be avoided, others—particularly the antihypertensives—can and have been used successfully by many patients for years with no adverse consequences. There's no reason such patients should change their drug regimens. If you are alarmed because one of the medications you take is cited in the list here, talk to your doctor. There may be good reasons why the drug is needed. On the other hand, perhaps another drug that has a similar therapeutic effect, but is safer to use in older people, can be prescribed instead. Above all, you should never stop taking any prescription drug without first consulting your doctor. Many medications need to be tapered off gradually; dangerous reactions could occur if they are discontinued abruptly.

Sedative or Hypnotic Drugs
Chlordiazepoxide (Librium)
Diazepam (Valium)
Flurazepam (Dalmane)
Meprobamate (Equanil, Miltown)
Pentobarbital (Nembutal)
Secobarbital (Seconal)

Antidepressants
Amitriptyline (Elavil)
Amitriptyline + Perfenazine (Trilafon, Etrafon)

Nonsteroidal Anti-inflammatory Drugs (NSAIDs)
Indomethacin (Indocin)
Phenylbutazone (Butazolidin)

Oral Antidiabetics
Chlorpropamide (Diabinese)

Dementia Treatments
Cyclandelate (Cyclospasmol)
Isoxsuprine (Vasodilan)

Platelet Inhibitors
Dipyridamole (Persantine)

Muscle Relaxants/ Antispasmodics
Carisoprodol (Rela, Soma)
Cyclobenzaprine (Flexeril)
Methocarbamol (Robaxin)
Orphenadrine Citrate (Norflex)

Antiemetic (Antinausea) Drugs
Trimethobenzamide (Tigan)

Antihypertensives
Methyldopa (Aldomet)
Propranolol (Inderal)
Reserpine (Serpasil)

Analgesics
Pentazocine (Talwin)
Propoxyphene (Darvon)

- Know what each drug is intended to treat.
- Know what side effects to expect, and which ones warrant medical treatment. Virtually all drugs can produce side effects in addition to their desired therapeutic effects, even when taken exactly as prescribed. You can find this information in the drug profiles in this book. Although the profiles for most drugs carry a long list of possible side effects, any one or more of these reactions usually affect only a small number of the patients taking the medication. Any unfavorable change that occurs after you begin taking a new medication—whether listed in the drug profile or not—should be reported to your physician.
- Do not stop taking a prescribed drug without first consulting your doctor.
- If you take a drug at night, turn on a light, and if you need glasses for reading, put them on to make certain you are taking the right medicine.
- If you transfer your medication from its original container to another bottle, make sure you label the new bottle thoroughly and accurately.
- Never take drugs prescribed for someone else or share your prescription medications with others.
- Store your medication in a cool, dry place—not in the bathroom medicine cabinet where steam might affect it.
- Discard any drugs that have become discolored or begun to give off an unusual odor, or whose expiration dates have passed. Do not save medication (such as antibiotics) with the intent to treat or ward off future illnesses.

YOU AND YOUR PHARMACIST

- Try to use one pharmacy for all your drug purchases. When buying any new drug, ask the pharmacist how it might interact with other drugs you take, including over-the-counter drugs, and if there are any special instructions about when or how it should be taken. Be sure to read any written instructions included with your prescription.
- Many pharmacies can provide labels in foreign languages. If it would help you to have a label in another language, ask your pharmacist.
- If you have trouble opening a medicine's bottle or container, ask your pharmacist for an easy-to-open container.

AVOIDING INTERACTIONS

- Know which foods or drugs to avoid while taking your medication. For example, grapefruit is dangerous when taken with various types of medication (see box, page 13), while patients taking monoamine oxidase (MAO) inhibitors for depression must avoid foods containing tyramines (aged cheeses; sauerkraut; organ meats; pickled or smoked meat, poultry, or fish; and processed meats such as bologna and salami). Likewise, people taking anticoagulants such as warfarin (Coumadin) should avoid liver, green leafy vegetables, and other foods high in vitamin K, which can counteract the effect of the drug.
- Do not drink alcoholic beverages while taking a medication unless your physician okays it. According to the FDA, "of the 100 medicines most commonly prescribed, over half contain at least one substance that reacts badly with alcohol."

This section is designed to help guide you to information about the drugs that appear in this book as they are classified for use to treat specific disorders. Beneath each major category (for example, the Heart and Blood Vessels), you will find the various disorders (such as hypertension) that belong to that category, followed by a list of the drugs used to treat that disorder. (If you want to find information about a particular drug directly, look it up in the general index in the back of the book, page 830, or, if you know the drug's generic name, you can find it simply by flipping through the book, which is organized in alphabetical order by generic drug name.) The disorders featured in this index are grouped under the following general categories:

1. *Cancer*
2. *The Blood*
3. *The Brain and Nervous System*
4. *Dental and Oral Disorders*
5. *The Digestive System*
6. *The Ears, Nose, and Throat*
7. *The Endocrine System*
8. *The Eyes*
9. *The Heart and Blood Vessels*
10. *The Genitourinary Tract*
11. *The Lungs and Respiratory System*
12. *The Muscles and Bones*
13. *Infectious Disease*
14. *The Skin*
15. *Health Concerns of Men*
16. *Health Concerns of Women*
17. *Mental Health*

3
The Brain and Nervous System

ALZHEIMER'S DISEASE
Donepezil
Galantamine Hydrobromide
Rivastigmine Tartrate
Tacrine

CHRONIC OR MODERATE TO SEVERE PAIN
Acetaminophen with Codeine Phosphate
Amitriptyline Hydrochloride
Bromfenac Sodium
Butorphanol Tartrate
Clomipramine Hydrochloride
Codeine
Diclofenac Systemic
Diflunisal
Fentanyl Transdermal
Fentanyl Transmucosal
Fluoxetine Hydrochloride
Hydrocodone Bitartrate/ Acetaminophen
Hydrocodone Bitartrate/Ibuprofen
Hydromorphone Hydrochloride
Ketorolac Tromethamine Systemic
Meperidine Hydrochloride
Methadone Hydrochloride
Morphine
Nalbuphine Hydrochloride
Nortriptyline Hydrochloride
Oxycodone Hydrochloride
Oxycodone/Acetaminophen
Oxycodone/Aspirin
Pentazocine
Propoxyphene
Propoxyphene/Acetaminophen
Tramadol Hydrochloride

DEMENTIA
Ergoloid Mesylates

DIZZINESS/MOTION SICKNESS
Dimenhydrinate
Diphenhydramine Hydrochloride
Meclizine
Promethazine Hydrochloride
Scopolamine Systemic
Trimethobenzamide Hydrochloride

EPILEPSY/SEIZURE DISORDER
Carbamazepine
Clonazepam
Diazepam
Ethosuximide
Felbamate
Gabapentin
Lamotrigine
Levetiracetam
Mephenytoin
Oxcarbazine
Pentobarbital Sodium
Phenobarbital
Phenytoin
Primidone
Tiagabine Hydrochloride
Topiramate
Valproic Acid

HEADACHE/MIGRAINE
Acetaminophen
Acetaminophen/Aspirin/Caffeine
Almotriptan Malate
Butalbital/Acetaminophen/ Caffeine
Butalbital/Acetaminophen/ Caffeine/Codeine
Butalbital/Aspirin/Caffeine
Butalbital/Aspirin/Caffeine/ Codeine Phosphate
Butorphanol Tartrate
Diclofenac Systemic
Diflunisal

Dihydroergotamine Mesylate
Ergotamine/Belladonna Alkaloids/Phenobarbital
Etodolac
Fenoprofen Calcium
Flurbiprofen Oral
Ibuprofen
Indomethacin
Ketoprofen
Meclofenamate Sodium
Mefenamic Acid
Methysergide Maleate
Nabumetone
Naproxen
Naratriptan Hydrochloride
Oxaprozin
Piroxicam
Propranolol Hydrochloride
Rizatriptan Benzoate
Sulindac
Sumatriptan Succinate
Timolol Maleate Oral
Tolmetin Sodium
Zolmitriptan

MULTIPLE SCLEROSIS
Betamethasone Systemic
Cortisone Oral
Dexamethasone Systemic
Glatiramer Acetate (Copolymer-1)
Hydrocortisone Systemic
Interferon Beta-1a
Interferon Beta-1b (rIFN-B)
Methylprednisolone
Prednisolone Systemic
Prednisone
Tizanidine Hydrochloride
Triamcinolone Systemic

PARKINSON'S DISEASE
Amantadine Hydrochloride
Benztropine Mesylate
Biperiden
Bromocriptine Mesylate

Diphenhydramine Hydrochloride
Entacapone
Levodopa
Levodopa/Carbidopa
Orphenadrine Citrate
Pergolide Mesylate
Pramipexole Dihydrochloride
Procyclidine
Ropinirole Hydrochloride
Selegiline Hydrochloride
    (L-Deprenyl)
Tolcapone
Trihexyphenidyl Hydrochloride

SHINGLES
Acyclovir
Amitriptyline Hydrochloride
Capsaicin
Famciclovir
Valacyclovir Hydrochloride

TOURETTE'S SYNDROME
Haloperidol

TREMOR
Trihexyphenidyl Hydrochloride
Propranolol Hydrochloride

—— 4 ——
*Dental and Oral
Disorders*

**CANKER SORES AND COLD
    SORES**
Amlexanox
Benzocaine
Lidocaine Hydrochloride Topical
Penciclovir

PERIODONTAL DISEASE
Chlorhexidine Gluconate

TOOTHACHE/DENTAL PAIN
Benzocaine

—— 5 ——
The Digestive System

CIRRHOSIS OF THE LIVER
Ethacrynic Acid
Furosemide
Torsemide
Triamterene

CONSTIPATION
Bisacodyl
Castor Oil
Docusate
Glycerin Rectal
Lactulose
Magnesium Citrate
Milk of Magnesia
Psyllium
Senna
Sodium Phosphate/Sodium
    Biphosphate

DIARRHEA
Attapulgite
Bismuth Subsalicylate
Charcoal, Activated
Diphenoxylate Hydrochloride/
    Atropine Sulfate
Kaolin with Pectin
Loperamide Hydrochloride
Loperamide/Simethicone
Psyllium
Trimethoprim/Sulfamethoxazole

ESOPHAGITIS
Aluminum Salts
Cimetidine
Esomeprazole Magnesium
Magaldrate

Omeprazole
Pantoprazole
Rabeprazole
Ranitidine

FLATULENCE/GAS
Charcoal, Activated
Simethicone

GALLSTONES
Ursodiol

**GASTROESOPHAGEAL REFLUX
    DISEASE**
Aluminum Salts
Cimetidine
Esomeprazole Magnesium
Famotidine
Lansoprazole
Magaldrate
Nizatidine
Omeprazole
Ranitidine

HEARTBURN/INDIGESTION
Aluminum Salts
Bismuth Subsalicylate
Famotidine
Magaldrate
Magnesium Oxide
Metoclopramide Hydrochloride
Milk of Magnesia
Nizatidine
Ranitidine
Simethicone
Sodium Bicarbonate

HEMORRHOIDS
Benzocaine
Hydrocortisone Topical

IRRITABLE BOWEL SYNDROME
Atropine Sulfate Oral
Atropine Sulfate/Scopolamine
    Hydrobromide/ Hyoscyamine
    Sulfate/Phenobarbital

Dicyclomine Hydrochloride

PANCREATIC ENZYME DEFICIENCY
Pancrelipase

ULCERATIVE COLITIS
Mesalamine
Olsalazine Sodium
Sulfasalazine

ULCERS, STOMACH AND DUODENAL
Aluminum Salts
Bismuth Subsalicylate
Cimetidine
Clarithromycin
Esomeprazole Magnesium
Famotidine
Glycopyrrolate
Lansoprazole
Magaldrate
Magnesium Oxide
Milk of Magnesia
Misoprostol
Nizatidine
Omeprazole
Propantheline Bromide
Rabeprazole
Ranitidine
Ranitidine Bismuth Citrate
Sucralfate

VIRAL HEPATITIS
Interferon Alfacon-1

6
The Ears, Nose, and Throat

EAR INFECTION
Azithromycin
Bacampicillin Hydrochloride

Cefepime
Cefpodoxime Proxetil
Cefprozil
Cefuroxime
Cephalexin
Cephradine
Chloramphenicol Otic
Clarithromycin
Colistin/Neomycin/Hydrocortisone
Neomycin/Polymyxin B/ Hydrocortisone Otic
Ofloxacin Otic
Penicillin G
Penicillin V
Phenylephrine Hydrochloride Systemic
Sulfisoxazole Systemic
Trimethoprim/Sulfamethoxazole

NASAL CONGESTION
Ephedrine
Epinephrine Hydrochloride
Oxymetazoline Nasal
Phenylephrine Hydrochloride
Phenylpropanolamine Hydrochloride
Phenylpropanolamine Hydrochloride/Guaifenesin
Pseudoephedrine
Pseudoephedrine/Guaifenesin

SINUSITIS
Amoxicillin/Potassium Clavulanate
Ampicillin
Azithromycin
Phenylephrine Hydrochloride Systemic
Phenylpropanolamine Hydrochloride/Guaifenesin
Pseudoephedrine

THROAT INFECTION
Amoxicillin
Cefaclor
Cefadroxil

Cefamandole Nafate
Cefepime
Cefpodoxime Proxetil
Cefprozil
Cefuroxime
Cephalexin
Cephradine
Dirithromycin
Loracarbef
Penicillin G
Penicillin V
Phenylpropanolamine Hydrochloride/Guaifenesin

7
The Endocrine System

DIABETES MELLITUS
Acarbose
Acetohexamide
Chlorpropamide
Glimepiride
Glipizide
Glucagon
Glyburide
Insulin
Insulin Glargine (rDNA origin)
Metformin
Miglitol
Nateglinide
Pioglitazone
Repaglinide
Rosiglitazone
Tolazamide
Tolbutamide

HYPOPARATHYROIDISM
Calcium
Vitamin D

OBESITY
Benzphetamine

Diethylpropion Hydrochloride
Orlistat
Phentermine
Sibutramine Hydrochloride
  Monohydrate

PITUITARY TUMORS
Bromocriptine Mesylate

THYROID DISEASE
Iodine, Strong
Levothyroxine Sodium
Liothyronine Sodium
Methimazole
Propylthiouracil

8
The Eyes

GLAUCOMA
Acetazolamide
Betaxolol Ophthalmic
Brimonidine Tartrate
Brinzolamide
Carteolol Hydrochloride
  Ophthalmic
Dipivefrin
Dorzolamide Hydrochloride
Glycerin Oral
Latanoprost
Levobunolol
Pilocarpine Ophthalmic
Timolol Maleate Ophthalmic

EYE INFECTION OR
   INFLAMMATION
Bacitracin
Chloramphenicol Ophthalmic
Cidofovir Intravenous
Ciprofloxacin Ophthalmic
Cromolyn Sodium Ophthalmic
Dexamethasone Ophthalmic

Emedastine Difumarate
Erythromycin Ophthalmic
Fluorometholone
Homatropine Hydrobromide
Hydrocortisone Ophthalmic
Idoxuridine
Ketorolac Tromethamine
  Ophthalmic
Ketotifen Fumarate
Levocabastine
Loteprednol Etabonate
Medrysone
Natamycin
Nedocromil Sodium Ophthalmic
Neomycin/Polymyxin B/Bacitracin
  Ophthalmic
Neomycin/Polymyxin B/
  Hydrocortisone Ophthalmic
Ofloxacin Ophthalmic
Olopatadine
Oxymetazoline Ophthalmic
Phenylephrine Hydrochloride
  Ophthalmic
Prednisolone Ophthalmic
Rimexolone
Scopolamine Ophthalmic
Sulfacetamide
Sulfisoxazole Ophthalmic
Tobramycin
Zinc Sulfate Ophthalmic

9
The Heart and Blood
Vessels

ANGINA/HEART DISEASE
Amlodipine
Amyl Nitrite
Aspirin
Atenolol
Clopidogrel Bisulfate

Diltiazem Hydrochloride
Dipyridamole
Isosorbide Dinitrate
Isosorbide Mononitrate
Metoprolol
Mibefradil Dihydrochloride
Nadolol
Nicardipine Hydrochloride Oral
Nifedipine
Nitroglycerin
Propranolol Hydrochloride
Torsemide
Triamterene
Verapamil Hydrochloride
Warfarin

CARDIAC ARRHYTHMIAS
Acebutolol Hydrochloride
Amiodarone
Atenolol
Digitoxin
Digoxin
Diltiazem Hydrochloride
Disopyramide
Flecainide Acetate
Metoprolol
Mexiletine Hydrochloride
Nadolol
Procainamide Hydrochloride
Propafenone
Propranolol Hydrochloride
Quinidine
Sotalol Hydrochloride
Verapamil Hydrochloride

CONGESTIVE HEART FAILURE
Benazepril Hydrochloride
Captopril
Carvedilol
Chlorothiazide
Chlorthalidone
Digitoxin
Digoxin

Enalapril Maleate
Enalapril/Hydrochlorothiazide
Ethacrynic Acid
Fosinopril Sodium
Furosemide
Hydralazine Hydrochloride
Hydrochlorothiazide
Hydrochlorothiazide/Triamterene
Indapamide
Lisinopril
Metolazone
Moexipril Hydrochloride
Quinapril Hydrochloride
Ramipril
Spironolactone/
  Hydrochlorothiazide
Torsemide
Trandolapril

HIGH CHOLESTEROL

Atorvastatin
Cholestyramine
Colesevelam Hydrochloride
Colestipol Hydrochloride
Fluvastatin
Lovastatin
Niacin (Vitamin B3)
Pravastatin
Simvastatin

HIGH TRIGLYCERIDES

Atorvastatin
Fenofibrate
Gemfibrozil
Simvastatin

HYPERTENSION

Acebutolol Hydrochloride
Atenolol
Atenolol/Chlorthalidone
Benazepril Hydrochloride
Betaxolol Oral
Bisoprolol Fumarate
Bisoprolol Fumarate/

Hydrochlorothiazide
Capecitabine
Captopril
Carteolol Hydrochloride Oral
Carvedilol
Chlorothiazide
Chlorthalidone
Clonidine Hydrochloride
Diltiazem Hydrochloride
Doxazosin Mesylate
Enalapril
Enalapril/Diltiazem
Enalapril/Felodipine
Enalapril/Hydrochlorothiazide
Felodipine
Fosinopril Sodium
Furosemide
Guanabenz Acetate
Guanadrel Sulfate
Guanethidine Monosulfate
Guanfacine Hydrochloride
Hydralazine Hydrochloride
Hydrochlorothiazide
Hydrochlorothiazide/Triamterene
Irbesartan
Isradipine
Labetalol Hydrochloride
Lisinopril
Lisinopril/Hydrochlorothiazide
Losartan Potassium
Methyldopa
Metoprolol
Mibefradil Dihydrochloride
Minoxidil Oral
Moexipril Hydrochloride
Moexipril Hydrochloride/
  Hydrochlorothiazide
Nadolol
Nicardipine Hydrochloride Oral
Nifedipine
Penbutolol Sulfate
Perindopril Erbumine

Pindolol
Prazosin
Propranolol Hydrochloride
Propranolol/Hydrochlorothiazide
Quinapril Hydrochloride
Quinapril Hydrochloride/
  Hydrochlorothiazide
Ramipril
Spironolactone/
  Hydrochlorothiazide
Telmisartan
Terazosin
Timolol Maleate Oral
Torsemide
Trandolapril
Trandolapril/Verapamil
  Hydrochloride
Valsartan
Valsartan/Hydrochlorothiazide
Verapamil Hydrochloride

PERIPHERAL VASCULAR DISEASE

Cilostazol
Isoxsuprine Hydrochloride
Papaverine Hydrochloride
Pentoxifylline

STROKE

Isoxsuprine Hydrochloride
Nimodipine
Warfarin

—————— *10* ——————
The Genitourinary Tract

DIABETES INSIPIDUS

Desmopressin Acetate
Vasopressin

GENITAL HERPES

Acyclovir
Famciclovir

11
The Lungs and Respiratory System

Salmeterol Xinafoate
Terbutaline Sulfate
Theophylline
Triamcinolone Inhalant and Nasal
Triamcinolone Systemic
Zafirlukast
Zileuton

BRONCHITIS, ACUTE

Azithromycin
Clarithromycin
Loracarbef
Tobramycin
Trovafloxacin

COUGH/COLD

Codeine
Dextromethorphan
Diphenhydramine Hydrochloride
Guaifenesin
Phenylephrine Hydrochloride
    Systemic
Pseudoephedrine
Pseudoephedrine/Guaifenesin

CHRONIC OBSTRUCTIVE PULMONARY DISEASE (EMPHYSEMA; CHRONIC BRONCHITIS)

Acetylcysteine
Albuterol
Aminophylline
Bitolterol Mesylate
Dyphylline
Epinephrine Hydrochloride
Ipratropium Bromide
Isoetharine
Isoproterenol
Levofloxacin
Metaproterenol Sulfate
Pirbuterol Acetate
Salmeterol Xinafoate
Sparfloxacin
Terbutaline Sulfate

Theophylline
Trimethoprim/Sulfamethoxazole

INFLUENZA

Amantadine Hydrochloride
Aspirin
Ibuprofen
Influenza Virus Vaccine
Oseltamivir Phosphate
Pseudoephedrine/Guaifenesin
Rimantadine Hydrochloride
Zanamivir

PNEUMONIA

Acetylcysteine
Atovaquone
Azithromycin
Clarithromycin
Dirithromycin
Erythromycin Systemic
Levofloxacin
Linezolid
Loracarbef
Metronidazole
Pentamidine Isethionate
Pneumococcal Vaccine
Sparfloxacin
Trimethoprim/Sulfamethoxazole
Trovafloxacin

12
The Muscles and Bones

BURSITIS

Acetaminophen
Aspirin
Diclofenac Systemic
Diflunisal
Etodolac
Fenoprofen Calcium
Flurbiprofen Oral

Ibuprofen
Indomethacin
Ketoprofen
Meclofenamate Sodium
Mefenamic Acid
Nabumetone
Naproxen
Oxaprozin
Piroxicam
Sulindac
Tolmetin Sodium

GOUT

Allopurinol
Colchicine
Diclofenac Systemic
Flurbiprofen Oral
Indomethacin
Meclofenamate Sodium
Mefenamic Acid
Nabumetone
Naproxen
Oxaprozin
Piroxicam
Probenecid
Sulfinpyrazone
Sulindac
Tolmetin Sodium

MUSCLE SPASMS

Baclofen
Carisoprodol
Chlordiazepoxide
Chlorzoxazone
Cyclobenzaprine
Dantrolene Sodium
Diazepam
Methocarbamol
Orphenadrine Citrate

OSTEOARTHRITIS

Acetaminophen/Aspirin/Caffeine
Aspirin

Aspirin/Caffeine
Betamethasone Systemic
Capsaicin
Celecoxib
Cortisone Oral
Dexamethasone Systemic
Diclofenac Systemic
Diclofenac/Misoprostol
Diflunisal
Etodolac
Fenoprofen Calcium
Flurbiprofen Oral
Hydrocortisone Systemic
Ibuprofen
Indomethacin
Ketoprofen
Meclofenamate Sodium
Mefenamic Acid
Meloxicam
Methylprednisolone
Nabumetone
Naproxen
Oxaprozin
Piroxicam
Prednisolone Systemic
Prednisone
Rofecoxib
Salsalate
Sulindac
Tolmetin Sodium
Triamcinolone Systemic

OSTEOPOROSIS

Alendronate Sodium
Calcitonin — Salmon
Calcium
Etidronate Disodium
Raloxifene Hydrochloride
Vitamin D

PAGET'S DISEASE

Alendronate Sodium
Calcitonin — Salmon

Calcium
Etidronate Disodium
Risedronate Sodium
Tiludronate Disodium
Vitamin D

RHEUMATOID ARTHRITIS

Auranofin
Azathioprine
Celecoxib
Diclofenac/Misoprostol
Etanercept
Gold Sodium Thiomalate
Indomethacin
Leflunomide
Methotrexate
Penicillamine
Salsalate

TENDINITIS

Acetaminophen
Aspirin
Diclofenac Systemic
Diflunisal
Etodolac
Fenoprofen Calcium
Flurbiprofen Oral
Ibuprofen
Indomethacin
Ketoprofen
Meclofenamate Sodium
Mefenamic Acid
Nabumetone
Naproxen
Oxaprozin
Piroxicam
Sulindac
Tolmetin Sodium

====== *13* ======
Infectious Disease

AIDS/HIV

Abacavir Sulfate

Amprenavir
Delavirdine
Didanosine (ddI)
Efavirenz
Indinavir
Lamivudine (3TC)
Lamivudine/Zidovudine
Nelfinavir
Nevirapine
Ritonavir
Saquinavir
Stavudine (d4T)
Zalcitabine (ddC)
Zidovudine (AZT)

BACTERIAL INFECTION

Amoxicillin
Amoxicillin/Potassium Clavulanate
Ampicillin
Ampicillin Sodium/Sulbactam
  Sodium
Azithromycin
Bacampicillin Hydrochloride
Bacitracin
Carbenicillin Indanyl Sodium
Cefaclor
Cefadroxil
Cefamandole Nafate
Cefazolin Sodium
Cefepime
Cefixime
Cefotetan Disodium
Cefpodoxime Proxetil
Cefprozil
Cefuroxime
Cephalexin
Cephradine
Chloramphenicol (Oral and
  Topical)
Ciprofloxacin Systemic
Clarithromycin
Clindamycin
Dicloxacillin Sodium

—————— 14 ——————
The Skin

Gentamicin Topical
Haloprogin
Ketoconazole Topical
Lindane
Mupirocin
Neomycin/Polymyxin B/Bacitracin Topical
Nystatin
Ofloxacin Oral
Penicillin G
Penicillin V
Tobramycin
Triamcinolone Topical

SKIN LESIONS

Acitretin
Adapalene
Alitretinoin
Becaplermin
Benzoyl Peroxide
Calcipotriene
Clindamycin
Doxycycline
Interferon Gamma-1b
Isotretinoin
Masoprocol
Methotrexate
Minocycline
Resorcinol
Sulfur Topical
Tazarotene
Tetracycline Hydrochloride
Tretinoin

----- *15* -----
Health Concerns of Men

BENIGN PROSTATIC HYPERPLASIA

Finasteride
Tamsulosin Hydrochloride
Terazosin

ERECTILE DYSFUNCTION

Alprostadil Injection
Papaverine Hydrochloride
Sildenafil Citrate
Yohimbine

HAIR LOSS (ALOPECIA)

Finasteride
Minoxidil Topical

----- *16* -----
Health Concerns of Women

BENIGN BREAST CONDITIONS

Danazol

MENOPAUSE

Estradiol
Estrogens, Conjugated
Estropipate
Medroxyprogesterone Acetate

BLEEDING, ABNORMAL UTERINE

Estradiol
Estrogens, Conjugated
Estropipate
Ethinyl Estradiol
Medroxyprogesterone Acetate
Norethindrone
Progesterone Systemic

URINARY INCONTINENCE

Dicyclomine Hydrochloride
Flavoxate
Oxybutynin Chloride

YEAST INFECTION

Butoconazole Nitrate
Clotrimazole

Fluconazole
Nystatin
Terconazole
Tioconazole

----- *17* -----
Mental Health

ALCOHOLISM

Chlordiazepoxide
Disulfiram
Hydroxyzine
Naltrexone
Oxazepam

ANXIETY DISORDERS

Alprazolam
Buspirone Hydrochloride
Chlordiazepoxide
Chlordiazepoxide/Amitriptyline
Clomipramine Hydrochloride
Clonazepam
Clorazepate Dipotassium
Diazepam
Fluoxetine Hydrochloride
Lorazepam
Meprobamate
Nortriptyline Hydrochloride
Oxazepam
Sertraline Hydrochloride

BIPOLAR (MANIC-DEPRESSIVE) DISORDER

Lithium
Valproic Acid

DEPRESSION

Amitriptyline Hydrochloride
Amoxapine
Bupropion Hydrochloride
Clomipramine Hydrochloride
Citalopram

Desipramine Hydrochloride
Doxepin Hydrochloride
Fluoxetine Hydrochloride
Imipramine
Maprotiline Hydrochloride
Mirtazapine
Nefazodone Hydrochloride
Nortriptyline Hydrochloride
Paroxetine Hydrochloride
Phenelzine Sulfate
Protriptyline Hydrochloride
Sertraline Hydrochloride
Tranylcypromine Sulfate
Trazodone
Venlafaxine

NARCOLEPSY/ATTENTION-DEFICIT HYPERACTIVITY DISORDER (ADHD)

Amphetamine
Amphetamine/
   Dextroamphetamine
Dextroamphetamine Sulfate
Methamphetamine Hydrochloride

Methylphenidate Hydrochloride

OBSESSIVE-COMPULSIVE DISORDER

Fluvoxamine Maleate

SCHIZOPHRENIA/PSYCHOSIS

Chlorpromazine Hydrochloride
Clozapine
Fluphenazine
Haloperidol
Loxapine
Molindone
Olanzapine
Perphenazine
Quetiapine Fumarate
Risperidone
Thioridazine Hydrochloride
Thiothixene
Trifluoperazine Hydrochloride

SLEEP DISORDERS/INSOMNIA

Chloral Hydrate
Diphenhydramine Hydrochloride

Estazolam
Ethchlorvynol
Flurazepam Hydrochloride
Hydroxyzine
Lorazepam
Quazepam
Temazepam
Triazolam
Zaleplon
Zolpidem

SMOKING CESSATION

Bupropion Hydrochloride
Nicotine

A to Z
Drug Profiles

Abacavir Sulfate

▶ Drug Class: Antiviral/reverse transcriptase inhibitor

▶ Available in: Tablets, oral solution

▶ Available OTC? No

▶ As Generic? No

Side Effects

SERIOUS
Uncommon (in approximately 5% of patients) and possibly fatal hypersensitivity reactions have been reported. Symptoms may include fever, skin rash, fatigue, nausea, vomiting, diarrhea, abdominal pain, weakness, lethargy, muscle and joint pain, swelling, shortness of breath, numbness, tingling, or prickling sensations, conjunctivitis, and mouth sores. Stop taking the drug and call your doctor immediately. Rarely, abacavir can also cause lactic acidosis (which is often fatal) and a greatly enlarged liver.

COMMON
Nausea, vomiting, weakness, fatigue, headache, loss of appetite, and diarrhea.

LESS COMMON
Insomnia and other sleep disorders.

PRINCIPAL USES
To treat human immunodeficiency virus (HIV) infection in combination with other drugs. While not a cure for HIV, such drugs may suppress the replication of the virus and delay the progression of the disease.

HOW THE DRUG WORKS
Abacavir prevents HIV from reproducing in two ways. A metabolite of the drug inhibits the activity of an enzyme needed for the replication of DNA in viral cells. The metabolite is also incorporated into viral DNA and terminates the formation of the complete DNA.

DOSAGE
Adults: To start, 300 mg 2 times a day. The drug must be taken in combination with other drugs for HIV to delay the development of resistant strains of the virus. Children 3 months to 16 years: 8 mg per 2.2 lbs (1 kg) of body weight 2 times a day in combination with other drugs for HIV. Children should take no more than 300 mg twice a day.

ONSET OF EFFECT
Unknown. With most antiretroviral drugs, an early response can be seen within the first few days of therapy, but the maximum effect may take 12 to 16 weeks.

DURATION OF ACTION
Unknown. Effects of the drug may be prolonged when abacavir is used in combination with other effective drugs and the virus is maximally suppressed.

DIETARY ADVICE
Abacavir can be taken with or without food.

STORAGE
Store at room temperature in a tightly sealed container away from heat, moisture, and direct light. The oral solution may be refrigerated, but should not be allowed to freeze.

IF YOU MISS A DOSE
Take it as soon as you remember. If it is near the time for the next dose, skip the missed dose and resume your regular dosage schedule. Do not double the next dose. It is especially important to take abacavir on schedule, to assure constant, proper blood levels of the drug.

STOPPING THE DRUG
The decision to stop taking the drug should be made in consultation with your physician.

PROLONGED USE
See your doctor regularly for tests and examinations.

PRECAUTIONS
Over 60: It is not known whether abacavir causes different or more severe side effects in older patients.

Driving and Hazardous Work: Do not drive or engage in hazardous work until you determine how the medicine affects you.

Alcohol: Alcohol may raise the blood concentration of the drug.

Pregnancy: Abacavir has been shown to cause birth defects in animals. Human studies have not been done. This medication should be given during pregnancy only if potential benefits outweigh the risks to the unborn child.

Breast Feeding: Women infected with HIV should not breast feed, to avoid transmitting the virus to an uninfected child.

Infants and Children: Your pediatrician will determine the appropriate dosage based on your child's weight. Call your doctor immediately if you notice rash or any other side effects while your child is taking abacavir. The drug has not been tested in infants less than 3 months of age.

Special Concerns: If, while taking abacavir, you have a skin rash or two or more of the following sets of symptoms, you may be having a serious, possibly fatal, allergic reaction: fever; nausea, vomiting, diarrhea, or abdominal pain; severe tiredness, achiness, or general feeling of illness; sore throat, shortness of breath, or cough. Use of abacavir does not eliminate the risk of passing the AIDS virus to other persons. You should take appropriate preventive measures.

OVERDOSE
Symptoms: No cases of overdose have been reported.

What to Do: If you suspect an overdose or if someone takes a much larger dose than prescribed, call your doctor, emergency medical services (EMS), or the nearest poison control center immediately.

DRUG INTERACTIONS
Currently, there are no clinically significant drug interactions. Further studies are being conducted.

FOOD INTERACTIONS
No known food interactions.

DISEASE INTERACTIONS
Currently, there are no clinically significant disease interactions. Further studies are being conducted.

Acarbose

BRAND NAME
Precose

Precose 50 mg
(BAYER)

▶ Drug Class: Antidiabetic agent

▶ Available in: Tablets

▶ Available OTC? No

▶ As Generic? No

Side Effects

SERIOUS
There are no serious side effects associated with acarbose.

COMMON
Feelings of bloating, gas, abdominal discomfort, diarrhea. These symptoms tend to decrease over time.

LESS COMMON
Rise in liver enzymes, causing yellowish tinge to eyes or skin (jaundice), when maximal dose is exceeded. When used in combination with sulfonylureas, may cause symptoms of low blood sugar, which include sweating, tremor, anxiety, hunger, confusion, seizures, rapid heartbeat, vision changes, dizziness, headache, loss of consciousness. Hypoglycemia must be treated by ingestion of glucose (dextrose). Sucrose (table sugar) and foods or drinks containing sugars or starches are ineffective because acarbose prevents their breakdown and absorption.

PRINCIPAL USES
As an adjunct (supplemental) therapy in patients with diabetes who do not require insulin injections yet are unable to control their blood glucose levels with diet alone or with other medications.

HOW THE DRUG WORKS
Acarbose inhibits the activity of enzymes required to break carbohydrates down into simple sugars within the intestine. This effect delays the digestion of carbohydrates and thus reduces the rise in blood sugar that typically occurs after meals.

DOSAGE
Initially, 25 mg, 1 to 3 times a day. The dose may be increased (at 4- to 8-week intervals) to a maximum of 100 mg, 3 times daily.

ONSET OF EFFECT
Within 1 hour.

DURATION OF ACTION
Up to 2 hours.

DIETARY ADVICE
This medicine should be taken with the first bite of breakfast, lunch, and dinner. Follow your doctor's advice regarding diet, weight loss, and exercise.

STORAGE
Keep in a tightly sealed container away from heat and direct light.

IF YOU MISS A DOSE
If you have finished a meal without taking the medication, skip the missed dose and resume your regular dosing schedule with the next meal. Do not double the next dose.

STOPPING THE DRUG
Take it as prescribed for the full treatment period.

PROLONGED USE
Since non-insulin-dependent diabetes is a chronic condition, use of acarbose will be ongoing. Blood glucose levels should be checked regularly during treatment so that the dosage may be adjusted if necessary.

PRECAUTIONS
Over 60: No special precautions required.

Driving and Hazardous Work: Acarbose should not impair your ability to perform such tasks safely.

Alcohol: Drink only in moderation when taking acarbose.

Pregnancy: Consult your doctor for advice. Insulin is usually the treatment of choice for pregnant diabetic patients.

Breast Feeding: Trace amounts of acarbose can be found in breast milk; however, adverse effects in infants have not been documented. Consult your doctor for advice.

Infants and Children: Safety and effectiveness have not been established for patients under 18 years of age. Consult your doctor for specific advice.

Special Concerns: You should not take acarbose if you've had an allergic reaction to it previously or if you are taking, or took within the past 14 days, a monoamine oxidase (MAO) inhibitor (a class of antidepressant drugs).

OVERDOSE
Symptoms: Increased gas, diarrhea, and stomach pain.

What to Do: These symptoms usually subside on their own within a short period of time. If not, consult your doctor for advice. Symptoms of hypoglycemia should not occur when taking acarbose alone, but may occur if a patient is also taking sulfonylurea or insulin for diabetes.

DRUG INTERACTIONS
Do not take acarbose if you are taking, or took within the past 14 days, an MAO inhibitor. Consult your doctor for specific advice if you are taking any of the following drugs that may interact with acarbose: digestive enzyme preparations containing amylase or pancreatin, intestinal absorbents (such as charcoal), insulin, or sulfonylureas (oral antidiabetic agents).

FOOD INTERACTIONS
Avoid foods that contain large amounts of sugar (for example, cake, cookies, candy, acidic fruits). Closely follow the diet your doctor has prescribed.

DISEASE INTERACTIONS
This drug should not be taken by patients with a history of diabetic ketoacidosis, intestinal disorders (including malabsorption or obstruction), inflammatory bowel disease (for example, Crohn's disease or ulcerative colitis), liver or kidney disease, or gastric ulcers.

Acebutolol Hydrochloride

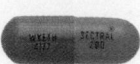

Sectral 200 mg
(WYETH-AYERST)

▶ Drug Class: Beta-blocker

▶ Available in: Capsules

▶ Available OTC? No

▶ As Generic? Yes

Side Effects

SERIOUS
Severe shortness of breath and rapid heartbeat (symptoms of congestive heart failure), worsening of asthma, severe allergic reaction (skin rash, itching, wheezing, swelling of lips, tongue, and throat). If any of these symptoms develop, seek medical attention immediately.

COMMON
Cough, diarrhea, decreased sexual ability, depression, drowsiness, dizziness, fatigue, frequent urination, gas, indigestion, nausea, trouble sleeping, cold hands and feet, numbness or tingling in fingers or toes.

LESS COMMON
Fever, sore throat, abdominal pain, headache, anxiety, joint or back pain, dry or burning eyes, unusual bleeding or bruising, dark urine, nightmares or unusually vivid dreams.

PRINCIPAL USES
To treat mild to moderate high blood pressure; also used to prevent or control heartbeat irregularities (cardiac arrhythmias).

HOW THE DRUG WORKS
Acebutolol slows the rate and force of contraction of the heart by blocking certain nerve impulses, thus reducing blood pressure. By modifying nerve impulses to the heart, the drug also helps to stabilize heart rhythm.

DOSAGE
Adults: Initially, 400 mg a day, either as a single dose in the morning or as two 200 mg doses taken in the morning and evening (12 hours apart). Maximum daily dose is 1,200 mg; for those over 65, daily dose should not exceed 800 mg.

ONSET OF EFFECT
1 to 1 ½ hours.

DURATION OF ACTION
Up to 24 hours.

DIETARY ADVICE
Follow your doctor's dietary recommendations to improve control over high blood pressure and heart disease.

STORAGE
Store away from heat, moisture, and direct light.

IF YOU MISS A DOSE
Take it as soon as you remember. If it is within 4 hours of the next scheduled dose, skip the missed dose and resume your regular dosage schedule. Do not double the next dose.

STOPPING THE DRUG
Suddenly stopping acebutolol may cause blood pressure to rise (rebound) to high or even dangerous levels, possibly triggering angina or a heart attack in patients with advanced heart disease. Slow reduction of the dose over a period of 2 to 3 weeks is advised, under careful supervision by your doctor.

PROLONGED USE
Regular visits to your doctor are needed to evaluate the drug's ongoing, long-term effectiveness.

PRECAUTIONS
Over 60: Many elderly patients are more sensitive to the drug than younger persons. Smaller doses and frequent blood pressure checks may be advised.

Driving and Hazardous Work: Use caution until you determine how the medication affects you.

Alcohol: Drink in careful moderation, if at all. Alcohol may interact with the drug and cause a dangerous drop in blood pressure.

Pregnancy: Discuss with your doctor the relative risks and benefits of using this drug while pregnant.

Breast Feeding: Trace amounts of this drug can be found in breast milk, though adverse effects in infants have not been documented. Consult your doctor for advice.

Infants and Children: Not recommended.

Special Concerns: Use of the drug should be considered but one element of a comprehensive therapeutic program that includes weight control, smoking cessation, regular exercise, and a healthy low-salt, low-fat diet.

OVERDOSE
Symptoms: Unusually slow or rapid heartbeat, severe dizziness or fainting, poor circulation in the hands (bluish skin), breathing difficulty, seizures.

What to Do: Contact your doctor immediately.

DRUG INTERACTIONS
Consult your doctor for specific advice if you are taking amphetamines, oral antidiabetic agents, asthma medication (such as aminophylline or theophylline), calcium channel blockers, clonidine, guanabenz, halothane, allergy shots, insulin, MAO inhibitors, reserpine, or other beta-blockers.

FOOD INTERACTIONS
None reported.

DISEASE INTERACTIONS
Acebutolol should be used with caution in people with diabetes, especially insulin-dependent diabetes, since the drug may mask symptoms of hypoglycemia. Consult your doctor for specific advice if you have a history of allergies or asthma, heart or blood vessel disease (including congestive heart failure and peripheral vascular disease), hyperthyroidism, irregular (slow) heartbeat, myasthenia gravis, psoriasis, respiratory problems such as bronchitis or emphysema, kidney or liver disease, or mental depression.

Acetaminophen

Tylenol Regular Strength 325 mg
(**McNeil**)

Additional photographs

▶ Drug Class: Analgesic; antipyretic (fever reducer)

▶ Available in: Capsules, caplets, tablets, powder, liquid, suppositories

▶ Available OTC? Yes

▶ As Generic? Yes

Side Effects

SERIOUS
Allergic reaction causing rash, itching, hives, swelling, or breathing difficulty; yellow-tinged skin and eyes (indicating liver damage). Seek medical assistance immediately.

COMMON
No common side effects have been reported.

LESS COMMON
Sore throat and fever (not present before treatment and not caused by the condition being treated), extreme fatigue or weakness, unexplained bleeding or bruising, blood in urine, painful, decreased, or frequent urination.

PRINCIPAL USES
To treat mild to moderate pain and fever, including simple headaches, muscle aches, and mild forms of arthritis. Acetaminophen is useful for patients who cannot take aspirin, such as those taking anticoagulants or suffering from gastro-intestinal ulcers or bleeding disorders.

HOW THE DRUG WORKS
Acetaminophen appears to interfere with the action of prostaglandins, substances in the body that cause inflammation and make nerves more sensitive to pain impulses. It also relieves fever, probably by acting on the heat-regulating center of the brain.

DOSAGE
For adults and teenagers: 325 to 650 mg every 4 to 6 hours, or 1 g, 3 to 4 times a day, as needed. Extended-release caplets: Take 2 every 8 hours. Maximum dosage with short-term therapy should not exceed 4 g a day; with long-term therapy it should not exceed 2.6 g a day unless otherwise prescribed by your doctor. For children 12 years and under: Consult a pediatrician for proper dose. Liquid form may be recommended for young children.

ONSET OF EFFECT
Within 15 to 30 minutes.

DURATION OF ACTION
3 to 4 hours; 8 hours for extended-release form.

DIETARY ADVICE
Take it with water 30 minutes before or 2 hours after meals. It may be taken with milk to minimize stomach upset. If you are on a salt-restricted diet, be sure to account for the sodium present in the powder form of acetaminophen.

STORAGE
Store in a tightly sealed container away from heat and direct light. Refrigerate liquid forms (to make them more palatable) and rectal suppositories. Do not allow the medication to freeze.

IF YOU MISS A DOSE
Take it as soon as you remember. If it is near the time for the next dose, skip the missed dose and resume your regular dosage schedule. Do not double the next dose.

STOPPING THE DRUG
Unless directed otherwise by your doctor, limit use to 5 days for children under 12 and 10 days for adults.

PROLONGED USE
Prolonged use may lead to liver problems, kidney problems, or anemia in some patients. Talk to your doctor about the need for periodic physical examinations and laboratory tests.

PRECAUTIONS
Over 60: Adverse reactions may be more likely and more severe in older patients; lower doses may be warranted.

Driving and Hazardous Work: No problems are expected.

Alcohol: Avoid alcohol; combining the two can cause serious liver problems. Patients with a history of alcohol abuse should not use acetaminophen except under close supervision by a doctor.

Pregnancy: No problems have been reported. Consult your doctor if you are or plan to become pregnant.

Breast Feeding: No problems have been reported.

Infants and Children: No problems are expected; however, some formulations are sweetened with aspartame, which should not be consumed by children with phenylketonuria.

OVERDOSE
Symptoms: Nausea, vomiting, appetite loss, abdominal pain, excessive sweating, confusion, drowsiness or exhaustion, stomach tenderness, heartbeat irregularities, yellowing of the skin and eyes.

What to Do: If you suspect an overdose, seek medical aid immediately, even if no symptoms are present. Steps must be taken promptly to avoid potentially fatal liver damage.

DRUG INTERACTIONS
Consult your doctor for specific advice if you are taking anticoagulants (such as warfarin), aspirin, an NSAID, barbiturates, carbamazepine, hydantoins, rifampin, sulfinpyrazone, isoniazid, nicotine, or zidovudine.

FOOD INTERACTIONS
No known food interactions.

DISEASE INTERACTIONS
Consult your doctor if you have liver or kidney disease, diabetes mellitus, phenylketonuria, or a history of alcohol abuse.

Acetaminophen with Codeine Phosphate

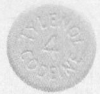

Tylenol With Codeine 300/60 mg (McNeil)

Additional photographs

▶ Drug Class: Opioid (narcotic) analgesic/antipyretic

▶ Available in: Capsules, tablets, oral solution, oral suspension

▶ Available OTC? No

▶ As Generic? Yes

Side Effects

SERIOUS
See Overdose and Special Concerns.

COMMON
Dizziness, lightheadedness, nausea or vomiting, drowsiness, constipation, unusual fatigue.

LESS COMMON
Stomach pain, allergic reaction, false sense of well-being (euphoria), depression, loss of appetite, blurring or change in vision, nightmares or unusual dreams, dry mouth, general feeling of illness, headache, nervousness, insomnia.

PRINCIPAL USES
To relieve mild to severe pain when nonprescription pain relievers prove inadequate. A narcotic analgesic such as codeine, in combination with acetaminophen, may provide better pain relief than either medicine used alone. Used together, pain relief may be achieved at lower doses of the two medications.

HOW THE DRUG WORKS
Acetaminophen appears to interfere with the action of prostaglandins, naturally occurring substances in the body that cause inflammation and make nerves more sensitive to pain impulses. It also relieves fever, probably by acting on the heat-regulating center of the brain. Unlike aspirin, however, acetaminophen does not reduce inflammation. Codeine, a narcotic analgesic, is believed to relieve pain by acting on specific areas in the spinal cord and brain that process pain signals from nerves throughout the body.

DOSAGE
Adults— Capsules or tablets: 1 or 2 capsules containing 15 or 30 mg of codeine with acetaminophen or 1 capsule containing 60 mg of codeine with acetaminophen, every 4 hours as needed. Oral solution or suspension: 1 tablespoon every 4 hours as needed. Children— Oral solution or suspension: Ages 3 to 6: 1 teaspoon 3 or 4 times a day as needed. Ages 7 to 12: 2 teaspoons 3 or 4 times a day as needed.

ONSET OF EFFECT
Acetaminophen: Rapid. Codeine: Within 2 hours.

DURATION OF ACTION
Up to 4 hours.

DIETARY ADVICE
Take it with meals or milk to avoid stomach upset, unless doctor directs you to do otherwise.

STORAGE
Store in a tightly sealed container away from heat, moisture, and direct light. Keep liquid forms from freezing.

IF YOU MISS A DOSE
If you are taking acetaminophen with codeine on a fixed schedule, take it as soon as you remember. If it is near the time for the next dose, skip the missed dose and resume your regular dosage schedule. Do not double the next dose.

STOPPING THE DRUG
You should take the medication as prescribed for the full treatment period, but you may stop taking it if you are feeling better before the scheduled end of therapy. This drug should never be stopped abruptly after long-term regular use.

PROLONGED USE
Narcotic drugs such as codeine may cause physical dependence. Taking too much acetaminophen may cause liver damage. Therapy with acetaminophen and codeine should not continue for more than 2 weeks and may actually cease to be effective before then.

PRECAUTIONS
Over 60: Adverse reactions may be more likely and more severe in older patients.

Driving and Hazardous Work: Acetaminophen with codeine can cause dizziness or drowsiness; proceed with caution.

Alcohol: Avoid alcohol. The combination of alcohol and this drug may increase the depressant effects of the medicine. Drinking alcohol-containing beverages while taking acetaminophen greatly increases the risk of liver damage.

Pregnancy: Use of this drug during pregnancy can cause fetal addiction and may cause breathing problems in the newborn infant if taken during or just before delivery. Consult your doctor for specific guidelines and advice and discuss the relative risks and benefits of using this drug while pregnant.

Breast Feeding: Acetaminophen with codeine passes into breast milk; avoid or discontinue nursing while taking this drug.

Infants and Children: This medicine should not be given to infants. The drug may be used by children over the age of 3, but only with extreme caution and under the careful supervision of your doctor. Children are generally prescribed the oral solution or suspension instead of the capsule or tablet.

Special Concerns: Taking a narcotic such as codeine for an extended period of time can lead to physical dependence. When discontinuing the drug after using it for an extended period, it is important to decrease the dosage gradually under the supervision of your doctor to reduce the risk of suffering from withdrawal symptoms. Call your doctor if you notice these symptoms after discontinuing the drug: shivering or trembling; insomnia; gooseflesh; nausea or vomiting; body aches; loss of appetite; stomach cramps; weakness; diarrhea; restlessness, nervousness, or irritability;

Acetaminophen with Codeine Phosphate (continued)

rapid heartbeat; runny nose, sneezing, or fever; increased yawning; or increased sweating. Overuse of acetaminophen with codeine may also lead to anemia, liver problems, or central nervous system disorders. Contact your doctor as soon as possible if you experience any of the following symptoms during or after the use of this drug: bloody, dark, or cloudy urine; severe pain in the lower back or side; frequent urge to urinate; painful or difficult urination; sudden decrease in urine output; pale or black, tarry stools; yellow discoloration of the eyes or skin (jaundice); hal-lucinations; unusual bleeding or bruising; skin rash, hives, or itching; pinpoint red spots on skin; sore throat and fever; unusual excitability; trembling or uncontrolled muscle movements; redness, flushing, or swelling of the face.

OVERDOSE

Symptoms: Severe dizziness or drowsiness; cold, clammy skin; difficult or slow breathing or shortness of breath; severe confusion; seizures; stomach cramps or pain; diarrhea; low blood pressure; increased sweating; constricted pupils; nausea or vomiting; irregular heartbeat; severe weakness.

What to Do: Call your doctor, emergency medical services (EMS), or the nearest poison control center immediately.

DRUG INTERACTIONS

Some drugs may interact with acetaminophen and codeine. Consult your doctor for specific advice if you are taking any prescription or over-the-counter drugs, especially if they contain acetaminophen; central nervous system depressants such as antihistamines or medicine for hay fever, allergies, or colds; barbiturates; seizure medicine; muscle relaxants; anesthetics; or tranquilizers, sedatives, or sleep medications.

FOOD INTERACTIONS

No significant food interactions have been reported.

DISEASE INTERACTIONS

Consult your doctor if you have a head injury or brain disease, an underactive thyroid, an enlarged prostate, seizures, kidney or liver disease, gallbladder problems, a blood disorder, or a history of alcohol or drug abuse. These conditions may increase the likelihood of side effects from acetaminophen and codeine.

Acetaminophen/Aspirin/Caffeine

▶ Drug Class: Analgesic

▶ Available in: Tablets, caplets, oral powder

▶ Available OTC? Yes

▶ As Generic? No

Side Effects

SERIOUS
Difficulty swallowing; dizziness, lightheadedness, or fainting; flushing, redness, or change in color of skin; difficulty breathing, shortness of breath, tightness in the chest, or wheezing; sudden decrease in urine output; swelling of face, eyelids, or lips; black or tarry stools; unusual bleeding or bruising; yellow discoloration of the skin and eyes (indicating liver damage). Call your doctor immediately.

COMMON
Indigestion, nausea and vomiting, stomach pain.

LESS COMMON
Sleeping difficulty, nervousness, irritability.

PRINCIPAL USES
For the temporary relief of mild to moderate pain associated with arthritis or migraine headache.

HOW THE DRUG WORKS
Acetaminophen and aspirin both appear to interfere with the production of prostaglandins, naturally occurring substances in the body that cause inflammation and make nerves more sensitive to pain impulses. Caffeine is believed to enhance the effectiveness of pain relievers.

DOSAGE
Because the amount of each of the components varies with different brands, consult your doctor for the appropriate dose. The following are general guidelines. Adults and teenagers— Tablets and caplets: 1 to 2 tablets or caplets every 3 to 6 hours, as needed and depending on the strength of the product. Do not take more than 8 pills in a 24-hour period. If migraine pain persists for more than 48 hours or joint pain lasts for more than 10 days, stop taking the medication and call your doctor. Oral powder: 1 packet of powder followed immediately by a full glass of water every 6 hours. Children— Generally not recommended for children.

ONSET OF EFFECT
Unknown.

DURATION OF ACTION
Unknown.

DIETARY ADVICE
Should be taken with food or a full glass of water to minimize stomach upset.

STORAGE
Store in a tightly sealed container away from heat, moisture, and direct light.

IF YOU MISS A DOSE
Skip the missed dose and then resume your regular dosage schedule. Do not double the next dose.

STOPPING THE DRUG
You may stop taking the drug whenever you choose.

PROLONGED USE
This combination is indicated for short-term use only. Side effects are more likely with prolonged use.

PRECAUTIONS
Over 60: Adverse reactions may be more likely and more severe.

Driving and Hazardous Work: May cause drowsiness or vision difficulties.

Alcohol: Do not consume more than 2 alcohol-containing beverages a day.

Pregnancy: Discuss with your doctor the relative risks and benefits of using this drug while pregnant. This drug should not be used during the last 3 months of pregnancy.

Breast Feeding: This drug may pass into breast milk; consult your doctor for specific advice.

Infants and Children: Consult your pediatrician. This drug is not recommended for children under 16, since the aspirin component may cause a rare but life-threatening condition known as Reye's syndrome.

Special Concerns: Be sure your doctor knows you are taking this medication; it can interfere with the results of some blood and urine tests. Patients allergic to aspirin should not take this medication.

OVERDOSE
Symptoms: Nausea and vomiting, disorientation, seizures, rapid breathing, ringing or buzzing in the ears, fever, appetite loss, abdominal pain, excessive sweating, drowsiness or exhaustion, stomach tenderness, heartbeat irregularities, yellow discoloration of the skin and eyes, agitation, anxiety, excitement, restlessness, delirium.

What to Do: Call your doctor, emergency medical services (EMS), or the nearest poison control center immediately.

DRUG INTERACTIONS
Consult your doctor before taking this drug if you are currently taking any of the following: blood pressure medication, gout or arthritis drugs, anticoagulants such as warfarin, antidiabetic agents, steroids, seizure medication, NSAIDs, barbiturates, nicotine, zidovudine (AZT), isoniazid, any central nervous system stimulant, a MAO inhibitor, amantadine, over-the-counter cold and allergy medications, or asthma medicine.

FOOD INTERACTIONS
Do not drink large amounts of caffeine-containing beverages like coffee, tea, cola, cocoa, or chocolate milk.

DISEASE INTERACTIONS
Consult your doctor if you have liver or kidney disease, diabetes mellitus, phenylketonuria, a history of alcohol abuse, asthma, a bleeding disorder, congestive heart failure, gout, hemophilia, high blood pressure, thyroid disease, a peptic ulcer, anxiety, panic attacks, agoraphobia, or insomnia.

Acetazolamide

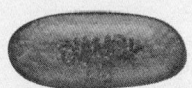

Diamox 500 mg
(STORZ)

Additional photographs

▶ Drug Class: Carbonic anhydrase inhibitor; anticonvulsant

▶ Available in: Tablets, extended-release capsules, injection

▶ Available OTC? No

▶ As Generic? Yes

Side Effects

SERIOUS
Breathing difficulty, seizures, serious allergic reaction (hives, itching, swelling of eyes, lips, and throat).

COMMON
Unusual fatigue; diarrhea; increase in volume and frequency of urination; loss of appetite and weight; metallic taste in mouth; numbness, tingling, or prickling sensations in hands, feet, fingers, toes, lips, and elsewhere.

LESS COMMON
Worsening nearsightedness, dark or bloody urine, painful urination, depression, lower back or flank pain, sudden decrease in urine output, unusual bruising or bleeding, bloody, black, pale, or tarry stools, confusion, clumsiness.

PRINCIPAL USES
To treat glaucoma, seizures, familial periodic paralysis; to prevent or treat mountain (altitude) sickness; to prevent one type of kidney stones.

HOW THE DRUG WORKS
For glaucoma: Blocks the enzyme carbonic anhydrase, thus decreasing the normal secretion of fluid inside the eyeball. For seizures: Appears to reduce the firing of neurons in the brain. For paralysis: Stabilizes muscle membranes. For mountain sickness: Stimulates greater oxygen intake, improves blood flow to the brain, and improves release of oxygen from red blood cells. For kidney stones: Increases alkalinity of urine, which reduces stone formation.

DOSAGE
Tablets— For glaucoma: Adults: 250 mg, 1 to 4 times a day. Children: 4.5 to 6.8 mg per lb of body weight per day in divided doses. For seizures: 4.5 mg per lb daily in divided doses. For altitude sickness: 250 mg, 2 to 4 times a day. Extended-release capsules— For glaucoma: 500 mg twice a day (morning and evening). For altitude sickness: 500 mg, 1 to 2 times a day. Injection— For glaucoma: Adults: 500 mg once a day. Children: 2.3 to 4.5 mg per lb every 6 hours.

ONSET OF EFFECT
Tablets: Within 60 to 90 minutes. Extended release capsules: 2 hours. Injection: 2 minutes.

DURATION OF ACTION
Tablets: 8 to 12 hours. Extended-release capsules: 18 to 24 hours. Injection: 4 to 5 hours.

DIETARY ADVICE
Take oral acetazolamide with food or milk to avoid stomach upset. Tablets can be crushed and mixed with sweet foods to cover taste. (Do not crush extended-release capsules.) Eat foods high in potassium.

STORAGE
Store in a tightly sealed container away from heat, moisture, and direct light.

IF YOU MISS A DOSE
Take it as soon as you remember. If it is near the time for the next dose, skip the missed dose and resume your regular dosage schedule. Do not double the next dose.

STOPPING THE DRUG
The decision to stop taking the drug should be made by your doctor. Do not stop taking the drug abruptly.

PROLONGED USE
Prolonged use of this drug may require increased potassium intake.

PRECAUTIONS
Over 60: Adverse reactions may be more likely and more severe in older patients.

Driving and Hazardous Work: Do not drive or engage in hazardous work until you determine how the medicine affects you.

Alcohol: Alcohol may interfere with seizure control.

Pregnancy: Adequate studies have not been done; discuss the relative risks and benefits with your doctor.

Breast Feeding: It may be necessary to switch medications or discontinue breast feeding.

Infants and Children: No problems are expected.

Special Concerns: May increase urine output, especially at first, as your body adapts to the drug. To keep this condition from disrupting sleep, take a single dose after breakfast if possible; if you take multiple daily doses, take the last one before 6 pm, unless your doctor instructs otherwise.

OVERDOSE
Symptoms: Drowsiness, numbness, nausea, thirst, vomiting, seizures, coma.

What to Do: Call your doctor, emergency medical services (EMS), or the nearest poison control center immediately.

DRUG INTERACTIONS
Do not take acetazolamide with high doses of aspirin or amphetamines, as this may be toxic. Do not take it if you are allergic to sulfa-type drugs. Consult your doctor if you are taking mecamylamine, quinidine, lithium, methenamine, or oral hypoglycemia agents.

FOOD INTERACTIONS
Avoid black licorice. Include high-potassium foods such as bananas and citrus fruits in your diet.

DISEASE INTERACTIONS
Do not take acetazolamide if you have serious liver or kidney disease, Addison's disease, low blood levels of potassium or sodium, or diabetes mellitus. Consult your doctor if you have gout or a lung disease such as emphysema, or a history of kidney stones.

Acetohexamide

Generic 250 mg
(SCHEIN)

▶ Drug Class: Antidiabetic
   agent/sulfonylurea

▶ Available in: Tablets

▶ Available OTC? No

▶ As Generic? Yes

Side Effects

SERIOUS
Hypoglycemia (blood sugar levels that are too low), resulting in shakiness, headache, cold sweats, anxiety, and changes in mental state. Stop taking the drug and seek medical help immediately. Severe diarrhea, bleeding, bruising, chills, fever, stomach pain, or heartburn may also occur; stop taking the drug and notify your doctor. Other serious but less-common side effects include bone marrow suppression, hemolytic anemia, and elevation of liver-associated enzymes; these problems can be detected by your doctor.

COMMON
Increased skin sensitivity to sunlight.

LESS COMMON
Fatigue, itchy skin, sore throat, ringing in ears, weakness.

PRINCIPAL USES
Used as an adjunct (supplemental) therapy to dietary modification to help control sugar levels in patients with non-insulin-dependent (type 2) diabetes mellitus.

HOW THE DRUG WORKS
It stimulates the pancreas to produce more insulin. Increased insulin levels reduce blood glucose levels and promote the transport of glucose into muscle cells and other tissues, where it is burned for energy.

DOSAGE
Starting at 250 mg once a day, increased as needed to a maximum of 1.5 g per day. In patients receiving less than 1 g per day, sugar levels can usually be controlled with a once-a-day dose; for those receiving between 1 and 1.5 g, the drug is given in two daily doses, morning and evening.

ONSET OF EFFECT
Within 1 hour.

DURATION OF ACTION
12 to 24 hours.

DIETARY ADVICE
Take it with food or liquid to minimize stomach upset.

STORAGE
Store in a tightly sealed container away from heat, moisture, and direct light.

IF YOU MISS A DOSE
If you miss a dose, take it as soon as you remember unless it is almost time for the next dose. In that case, skip the missed dose and return to your regular schedule. Do not double the next dose.

STOPPING THE DRUG
Do not stop taking acetohexamide without consulting your doctor.

PROLONGED USE
The dosage may need to be adjusted with prolonged use. Over time, many patients become resistant to the effects of the medication and may require treatment with insulin instead.

PRECAUTIONS
Over 60: A smaller dosage is usually warranted for older patients.

Driving and Hazardous Work: No problems are expected.

Alcohol: Drink in moderation only. Small amounts of alcohol at mealtimes usually cause no problems with blood sugar; however, alcohol may cause unpleasant flushing in the face, arms, and neck, up to 12 hours after ingestion.

Pregnancy: Acetohexamide is not usually given during pregnancy. Insulin is generally the treatment of choice for pregnant diabetic patients.

Breast Feeding: Acetohexamide may pass into breast milk; caution is advised. Consult your doctor if you are considering breast feeding.

Infants and Children: Safety and effectiveness have not been established for young patients.

Special Concerns: Follow your doctor's advice about diet, exercise, and weight control carefully. These aspects of treatment are just as essential to the proper control of diabetes as taking the medication. Be sure to carry at all times some form of medical identification that indicates you have diabetes and that lists all of the drugs you are taking.

OVERDOSE
Symptoms: Excessive hunger, nausea, anxiety, cold sweats, drowsiness, rapid heartbeat, weakness, changes in mental state, loss of consciousness (indications of hypoglycemia). Overdose is most likely to occur after you have delayed or missed a meal, have exercised more than usual, or have consumed more than a small amount of alcohol.

What to Do: Call your doctor, emergency medical services (EMS), or local hospital immediately.

DRUG INTERACTIONS
The effects of acetohexamide can be altered by anticoagulants, antidepressants, aspirin, over-the-counter cold preparations containing aspirin, some diuretics, glucagon, beta-blockers, steroids, phenylbutazone, probenecid, rifampin, nonprescription drugs for colds, hay fever, and appetite control, and sulfa-containing antibiotics.

FOOD INTERACTIONS
A special diet is essential for proper control of blood glucose levels. Avoid foods high in sugar.

DISEASE INTERACTIONS
Liver disease, overactive or underactive thyroid, and kidney disease can affect the activity of the drug.

Acetylcysteine

BRAND NAMES
Mucomyst, Mucosil

▶ Drug Class: Decongestant/ cough drug

▶ Available in: Inhalant solution

▶ Available OTC? No

▶ As Generic? Yes

Side Effects

SERIOUS
Wheezing, tightness in the chest, and breathing difficulty (especially among patients with asthma); spitting up of blood. Contact your doctor immediately if any such symptoms arise.

COMMON
Acetylcysteine does not commonly cause side effects.

LESS COMMON
Clammy skin, fever, increased mucus production in the lungs, pain or irritation around the mouth or throat, nausea and vomiting, runny nose, drowsiness. Such symptoms are likely to diminish as your body adjusts to the medication.

PRINCIPAL USES
To relieve congestion and make breathing easier in lung conditions associated with the production of large amounts of thick mucus, such as bronchiectasis (irreversible destruction of the bronchial walls), bronchitis, pneumonia, and cystic fibrosis. It may also be used in patients who have undergone tracheostomy (surgical opening in the neck to establish an airway when the throat is obstructed), or who have a collapsed lobe of the lung due to a plug of mucus blocking an airway.

HOW THE DRUG WORKS
Acetylcysteine liquefies and thins mucus so that it may be coughed up (or removed with suction if necessary).

DOSAGE
3 to 5 ml of 20% solution, or 6 to 10 ml of 10% solution by nebulizer every 2 to 6 hours. (The medicine may be inhaled through a face mask, mouthpiece, or via tracheostomy.) Or, 1 to 2 ml of 10% or 20% solution placed directly into the trachea via catheter every hour. The dosage differs from patient to patient; follow your doctor's directions carefully.

ONSET OF EFFECT
Within 1 minute.

DURATION OF ACTION
Up to several hours.

DIETARY ADVICE
This drug should not be taken with meals. Be sure to drink plenty of fluids.

STORAGE
Before opening, store container away from heat and direct light. After opening, store it in the refrigerator, but do not allow it to freeze. Discard the container 96 hours after opening.

IF YOU MISS A DOSE
Take it as soon as you remember. Take the rest of the day's doses at evenly spaced intervals.

STOPPING THE DRUG
The decision to stop taking the drug should be made by your doctor.

PROLONGED USE
No special problems are expected.

PRECAUTIONS
Over 60: No special problems are expected.

Driving and Hazardous Work: Be cautious if acetylcysteine makes you drowsy.

Alcohol: Alcohol intake should be limited.

Pregnancy: The effects of acetylcysteine on the human fetus have not been documented; consult your doctor or OB/GYN for specific advice if your are pregnant or plan to become pregnant.

Breast Feeding: It is not known whether acetylcysteine passes into breast milk; problems have not been documented. Consult your doctor for specific advice before deciding to nurse while using this drug.

Infants and Children: No special problems are expected.

Special Concerns: Be sure to tell your doctor if you have ever had any unusual or allergic reaction to acetylcysteine, or if you are allergic to any other substances including foods, preservatives, latex, or dyes. If you use a nebulizer to administer the medication, it should be cleaned immediately after use, since residues of the medicine can be sticky and may clog the apparatus. Nebulized solution may be inhaled directly from the nebulizer, or the nebulizer may be fitted with a plastic face mask or mouthpiece. When acetylcysteine is used by patients with asthma or other types of hypersensitivity of the airways, a bronchodilator should be administered first to prevent bronchospasm.

OVERDOSE
Symptoms: Unusual breathing difficulties.

What to Do: Call your doctor, emergency medical services (EMS), or local hospital immediately.

DRUG INTERACTIONS
Simultaneous use of acetylcysteine with tetracycline, erythromycin, lactobionate, amphotericin B, ampicillin, chymotrypsin, or hydrogen peroxide in the same solution should be avoided. Such medications should be taken at another time.

FOOD INTERACTIONS
No known food interactions.

DISEASE INTERACTIONS
Acetylcysteine can aggravate asthma or other respiratory diseases.

Acitretin

BRAND NAME
Soriatane

▶ Drug Class: Retinoid

▶ Available in: Capsules

▶ Available OTC? No

▶ As Generic? No

Side Effects

SERIOUS
Severe headache, liver damage, eye lesions, joint pain, abnormal spinal bone growth, rigidity, violent shivering associated with chills and fever. Call your doctor as soon as possible.

COMMON
Dry mouth, dryness and cracking of the lips, runny nose, nosebleeds, skin peeling, hair loss, dry skin, nail problems, itching, rash, increased sensitivity to touch, numbness or tingling, inflammation of fingers or toes, sticky skin, dry eyes, irritation of eyes, loss of eyebrows and eyelashes.

LESS COMMON
Bleeding gums, increased saliva, thirst, inflammation of the mouth, abnormal skin odor, blisters, cold and clammy skin, increased sweating, skin infection, ulcerations, sunburn, abnormal or blurred vision, reduced night vision, joint pain, back pain, muscle pain, mild headache, abdominal pain, diarrhea, nausea, odd taste in mouth, ringing in ears, depression, insomnia.

PRINCIPAL USES
To treat severe psoriasis. Acitretin is used only when other medications to treat psoriasis prove ineffective.

HOW THE DRUG WORKS
The exact mechanism of action of acitretin is unknown. It appears to establish a more normal pattern of growth and shedding of skin cells.

DOSAGE
To start, 25 mg once a day. A maintenance dose, given after the initial response to therapy, is 25 to 50 mg once a day. If the response to the drug is unsatisfactory after 4 weeks and there are minimal side effects, the dose may be increased by your doctor, depending on your condition and body weight.

ONSET OF EFFECT
It may take 2 or 3 months to attain the full therapeutic benefit of acitretin.

DURATION OF ACTION
Unknown.

DIETARY ADVICE
Acitretin is best taken with the main meal of the day.

STORAGE
Store in a tightly sealed container away from heat, moisture, and direct light.

IF YOU MISS A DOSE
Take it as soon as you remember. If it is near the time for the next dose, skip the missed dose and resume your regular dosage schedule. Do not double the next dose.

STOPPING THE DRUG
You should take it as prescribed for the full treatment period, but you may stop taking the drug before the scheduled end of therapy if the symptoms have

sufficiently resolved. Consult your doctor.

PROLONGED USE
Acitretin is generally prescribed for 1-month periods. See your doctor regularly for tests and examinations to assess the effectiveness and safety of the drug.

PRECAUTIONS
Over 60: Adverse reactions may be more likely and more severe in older patients.

Driving and Hazardous Work: Do not drive or engage in hazardous work until you determine how the medicine affects you.

Alcohol: Avoid alcohol during and for two months after completing therapy.

Pregnancy: Acitretin can cause serious birth defects. Before your doctor will prescribe it, you must sign a waiver agreeing to use contraceptive measures for one month prior to therapy and three years afterward. You must receive a negative result on a pregnancy test within one week of beginning treatment.

Breast Feeding: Acitretin may pass into breast milk and cause serious harm. Do not nurse while taking this medication.

Infants and Children: No studies have been done with children, although it is believed that acitretin could adversely affect growth.

Special Concerns: You may experience increased sensitivity to contact lenses while taking acitretin. If it causes increased sensitivity to sunlight, wear protective clothing, use a sun block, and try to avoid exposure to sunlight. Do not donate

blood while you take acitretin and for three years afterward. Many patients will experience a relapse and require further treatment after they stop taking acitretin.

OVERDOSE
Symptoms: No cases of overdose have been reported.

What to Do: An overdose of acitretin is unlikely to be life-threatening. However, if someone takes a much larger dose than prescribed, call your doctor, emergency medical services (EMS), or the nearest poison control center immediately.

DRUG INTERACTIONS
Other drugs may interact with acitretin. Consult your doctor if you are taking vitamin A, any other retinoid, or methotrexate. Also tell your doctor if you are taking any other prescription or over-the-counter drug.

FOOD INTERACTIONS
No known food interactions.

DISEASE INTERACTIONS
Consult your doctor for advice if you have diabetes mellitus, liver disease, or any other medical condition.

Acyclovir

BRAND NAME
Zovirax

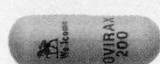

Zovirax 200 mg
(**GLAXO WELLCOME**)

▶ Drug Class: Antiviral

▶ Available in: Capsules, tablets, liquid, ointment, injection

▶ Available OTC? No

▶ As Generic? Yes

Side Effects

SERIOUS
No known serious side effects are associated with the use of acyclovir.

COMMON
Rash, nausea and vomiting. Ointment can cause pain, burning, or itching at the site where it is applied. Should such adverse symptoms persist, notify your doctor. Injection can cause inflammation of the vein (phlebitis); call your doctor if this occurs.

LESS COMMON
Diarrhea, stomach pain, lightheadedness, dizziness, confusion, tremor. In rare cases kidney function may be altered when the drug is given by injection, causing such symptoms as decreased urine output.

PRINCIPAL USES
To treat herpes virus infections such as genital herpes, shingles, herpes simplex, and chicken pox.

HOW THE DRUG WORKS
Acyclovir interferes with the activity of enzymes needed for the replication of viral DNA in cells. This prevents the virus from multiplying.

DOSAGE
Oral forms— For genital herpes: Up to 1,200 mg a day in evenly distributed doses, every 4 or 8 hours. For shingles: Up to 4,000 mg a day in evenly distributed doses every 4 hours. For chicken pox: Up to 800 mg, 4 times a day, not to exceed 3,200 mg a day. Topical form— To relieve herpes symptoms: Apply a small amount to lesions every 3 hours (6 times a day) for 7 days. Use a glove or finger cot when applying medication.

ONSET OF EFFECT
2 hours or more.

DURATION OF ACTION
Up to 5 hours following the final dose.

DIETARY ADVICE
Capsule, tablet, and liquid forms should all be taken with food and with a full (8 oz) glass of water.

STORAGE
Store in a dry place at room temperature, away from direct sunlight. Refrigerate any liquid form of acyclovir, but do not allow it to freeze.

IF YOU MISS A DOSE
If you miss a tablet, capsule, or liquid dose, take it as soon as you remember, up to 2 hours late. If more than 2 hours, wait for the next scheduled dose. Do not double the next dose. For ointment, apply dose as soon as you remember, then return to your regular dosing schedule.

STOPPING THE DRUG
Take the drug as prescribed for the full treatment period, even if you begin to feel better before the scheduled end of therapy, but do not take it for longer than the recommended period.

PROLONGED USE
Women with genital herpes are at increased risk of developing cervical cancer; annual Pap smears are recommended for these patients.

PRECAUTIONS
Over 60: Adverse reactions and side effects may be more common in older persons. Such effects can be minimized by drinking at least 2 to 3 quarts of liquid per day.

Driving and Hazardous Work: The use of acyclovir should not impair your ability to perform such tasks safely.

Alcohol: Alcohol may accentuate the side effects of lightheadedness and dizziness.

Pregnancy: Acyclovir has been used by pregnant women and no birth defects or other related problems have been reported; however, studies in humans have been limited and inconclusive. Consult your doctor about using acyclovir if you are pregnant or plan to become pregnant.

Breast Feeding: Acyclovir may pass into breast milk. Breast feeding should be avoided while taking any oral form of the drug. No problems are expected with the topical form.

Infants and Children: Acyclovir should not be used for children under 2 years of age. Its use for children under 12 should be carefully supervised by a physician.

Special Concerns: Be sure to tell your doctor if you have ever had any unusual or allergic reaction to acyclovir. It is important to remember that the use of acyclovir is not a cure and will not help prevent you from spreading herpes infections to others.

OVERDOSE
Symptoms: No specific ones have been reported.

What to Do: An overdose of acyclovir is unlikely to be life-threatening. However, if someone takes a much larger dose than prescribed, call your doctor, emergency medical services (EMS), or the nearest poison control center right away for advice. Prolonged overdose may lead to kidney damage.

DRUG INTERACTIONS
Consult your doctor for specific advice if you are taking cyclosporine, probenecid, meperidine, or zidovudine.

FOOD INTERACTIONS
No significant food interactions have been reported.

DISEASE INTERACTIONS
Use of acyclovir may cause complications in patients with liver or kidney disease, since these organs work together to remove the medication from the body.

Adapalene

▶ Drug Class: Acne drug

▶ Available in: Topical gel

▶ Available OTC? No

▶ As Generic? No

Side Effects

SERIOUS
No serious side effects are associated with adapalene.

COMMON
Redness, dryness, and scaling of skin; itching or burning immediately after application.

LESS COMMON
Skin irritation, sunburn, flareups of acne. These usually occur during the first month of treatment and then decrease in severity and frequency.

PRINCIPAL USES
To treat acne.

HOW THE DRUG WORKS
Its exact mechanism of action is unclear, but adapalene appears to bind with specific receptors in skin cells in a way that encourages the formation of normal skin cells and discourages the formation of acne lesions.

DOSAGE
After washing affected areas, apply a thin film of adapalene once a day to affected skin areas before bedtime.

ONSET OF EFFECT
Becomes noticeable after 8 to 12 weeks. During the first few weeks of therapy, acne may actually get worse before it begins to get better. This is because the drug is affecting previously unseen lesions, and it should not be considered a reason to stop using the medication.

DURATION OF ACTION
Unknown.

DIETARY ADVICE
Adapalene can be used without regard to diet.

STORAGE
Store in a tightly sealed container away from heat and direct light.

IF YOU MISS A DOSE
Apply it as soon as you remember. If it is near the time for the next dose, skip the missed dose and resume your regular dosage schedule. Do not double the next dose.

STOPPING THE DRUG
The decision to stop using the drug should be made by your doctor.

PROLONGED USE
No problems are expected with prolonged use.

PRECAUTIONS
Over 60: No special precautions are required.

Driving and Hazardous Work: No special precautions are required.

Alcohol: No special precautions are required.

Pregnancy: In some tests, large doses of adapalene caused minor birth defects (an excess number of ribs) in animals, and theoretically could cause major birth defects. Human tests have not been done. Generally, adapalene should not be used during pregnancy. Consult your doctor for specific advice.

Breast Feeding: Adapalene may pass into breast milk; caution is advised. Consult your doctor for specific advice.

Infants and Children: The safety and effectiveness of adapalene in children under the age of 12 have not been established.

Special Concerns: Anyone with a history of allergy to adapalene or any ingredients in the gel should not use this medication. Acne may appear to worsen temporarily during the first weeks of adapalene therapy; cosmetic improvement should become apparent after 8 to 12 weeks. The medicine should be kept away from the eyes, lips, nostrils, and mucous membranes. It should not be applied to cuts, abrasions, scaly or flaky skin, or patches of sunburned skin. The extremes of winter weather, including high winds and cold temperatures, can cause extra skin irritation and dryness. In sunny conditions, protect the treated area with sunscreen products (with a minimum sun protection factor, or SPF, of 15) and adequate clothing; keep exposure to sunlight to a minimum. If you get a sunburn, adapalene therapy should be stopped or delayed until the sunburned areas return to normal. Use of skin products containing alcohol, astringents, spices, or lime should be avoided.

OVERDOSE
Symptoms: Excessive application of adapalene may lead to redness, pain, and peeling of the skin.

What to Do: Discontinue the drug and consult your doctor. If accidentally ingested, seek emergency medical aid right away.

DRUG INTERACTIONS
Some drugs may interact with adapalene. Consult your doctor for specific advice if you are taking other products that can irritate the skin, such as medicated or abrasive soaps and cleansers and products containing sulfur, resorcinol, or salicylic acid. They generally should not be used during adapalene therapy unless otherwise recommended by your doctor.

FOOD INTERACTIONS
No food interactions have been documented.

DISEASE INTERACTIONS
Caution is advised when using adapalene. Consult your doctor if you have any other skin condition.

Albendazole

BRAND NAME
Albenza

▶ Drug Class: Anthelmintic

▶ Available in: Tablets

▶ Available OTC? No

▶ As Generic? No

Side Effects

SERIOUS
Neutropenia (low white blood cell count), thrombocytopenia (low platelet count), and hepatitis can occur during prolonged therapy, but are reversible by discontinuing the drug. If fever, sore throat, abdominal pain, loss of appetite, unusual fatigue, skin rash, or itching occur, call your doctor immediately.

COMMON
No common side effects are associated with albendazole.

LESS COMMON
Nausea, vomiting, dizziness, stomach upset, diarrhea, headache. Alopecia (thinning or loss of hair), a rare side effect, can occur, but is reversible by stopping the drug.

PRINCIPAL USES
To treat hydatid disease and neurocysticercosis. Hydatid disease is a parasitic infection, usually of the liver, caused by echinococcus (dog tapeworm) larvae. Humans can become infected through ingestion of tapeworm eggs in dog feces. Neurocysticercosis is a parasitic infection of the nervous system, caused by taenia solium (pork tapeworm) larvae. It can be contracted by ingesting egg-containing feces from an infected person, owing to food mishandling. Albendazole may be used to treat a variety of other roundworm infections and may be useful in treating a type of intestinal protozoan common in AIDS patients, but it is not licensed for such uses in the United States.

HOW THE DRUG WORKS
Albendazole interferes with various energy-producing processes of helminths (worms), including impairing the uptake of glucose (sugar) for energy.

DOSAGE
For hydatid disease—Patients weighing more than 132 lbs (60 kg): 1 cycle consisting of 400 mg twice a day for 28 days followed by a 14-day albendazole-free period; repeat for at least 3 cycles. Patients weighing less than 132 lbs (60 kg): 1 cycle consisting of 7.5 mg per 2.2 lbs (1 kg) of body weight twice a day for 28 days followed by a 14-day albendazole-free period; repeat for at least 3 cycles. For neurocysticercosis—Patients weighing more than 132 lbs (60 kg): 400 mg twice a day for 8 to 30 days. Patients weighing less than 132 lbs (60 kg): 7.5 mg per 2.2 lbs twice a day for 8 to 30 days. Corticosteroids are often administered con-

currently for therapy of neurocysticercosis to control the inflammation caused by dying larvae.

ONSET OF EFFECT
Unknown.

DURATION OF ACTION
Unknown.

DIETARY ADVICE
Take it with meals high in fat content to help the body better absorb the drug.

STORAGE
Store in a tightly sealed container away from heat, moisture, and direct light.

IF YOU MISS A DOSE
Take it as soon as you remember. If it is near the time for the next dose, skip the missed dose and resume your regular dosage schedule. Do not double the next dose.

STOPPING THE DRUG
Take it as prescribed for the full treatment period even if you begin to feel better before the scheduled end of therapy. The decision to stop taking the drug should be made by your doctor.

PROLONGED USE
See your doctor regularly for tests and examinations every 2 weeks if you must take this medicine for a prolonged period of time.

PRECAUTIONS
Over 60: No studies have been done specifically on older patients; adverse reactions may be more likely or more severe.

Driving and Hazardous Work: Do not drive or engage in hazardous work until you determine how the medicine affects you.

Alcohol: No special precautions are necessary.

Pregnancy: Pregnant women should not use albendazole except when no other alternative is available. Discuss with your doctor the relative risks and benefits of using this drug while pregnant.

Breast Feeding: Albendazole may pass into breast milk; caution is advised. Consult your doctor for specific advice.

Infants and Children: No special problems are expected.

OVERDOSE
Symptoms: No cases of overdose have been reported.

What to Do: If someone takes a much larger dose than prescribed, call your doctor, emergency medical services (EMS), or the nearest poison control center right away.

DRUG INTERACTIONS
Other drugs may interact with albendazole. Consult your doctor for specific advice if you are taking dexamethasone, praziquantel, cimetidine, theophylline, or any other prescription or over-the-counter medication.

FOOD INTERACTIONS
No known food interactions.

DISEASE INTERACTIONS
Dosage may need to be adjusted in patients with cirrhosis. Consult your doctor for specific advice if you have any other medical condition.

Albuterol

Generic 2 mg
(BIOCRAFT)

▶ Drug Class: Bronchodilator/sympathomimetic

▶ Available in: Inhaler, solution, capsules, tablets, syrup

▶ Available OTC? No

▶ As Generic? Yes

Side Effects

SERIOUS
Inhaled form: May become ineffective if used too often, resulting in more-severe breathing difficulty that does not improve. Signs include persistent wheezing, coughing, or shortness of breath; confusion; bluish color to lips or fingernails; inability to speak. Ingested form: Chest pain or heaviness; irregular, racing, fluttering, or pounding heartbeat; lightheadedness; fainting; severe weakness; severe headache.

COMMON
Nervousness, tremor, dizziness, headache, insomnia.

LESS COMMON
Dryness and irritation of the nose, mouth, and throat; heartburn; nausea; muscle cramps.

PRINCIPAL USES
To dilate air passages in the lungs that have become narrowed as a result of disease or inflammation. It is used in the treatment of asthma and chronic obstructive pulmonary disease (COPD).

HOW THE DRUG WORKS
Albuterol widens constricted airways by relaxing the smooth muscles that surround the bronchial passages in the lungs.

DOSAGE
Use it when needed to relieve breathing difficulty. For bronchospasm: 1 to 2 puffs of aerosol inhaler every 4 to 6 hours; or 2.5 mg of solution delivered via nebulizer 3 to 4 times a day; or 200 micrograms (mcg) of capsules for inhalation using Rotahaler every 4 to 6 hours; or 2 to 4 mg of tablets 3 or 4 times a day, not to exceed 32 mg per day. Children may require a smaller dose, and the syrup form of the drug may be preferable to young patients. For prevention of exercise-induced asthma: 1 or 2 inhalations (at least 1 full minute apart), 15 minutes prior to exercise.

ONSET OF EFFECT
Inhalant: Within 5 minutes. Oral forms: Within 15 to 30 minutes.

DURATION OF ACTION
Inhalant: 3 to 6 hours. Oral forms: 8 hours.

DIETARY ADVICE
Albuterol can be taken on an empty stomach or with food or milk.

STORAGE
Contents of aerosol canisters are under pressure; do not puncture. Store canister away from heat, open flame, and direct light.

IF YOU MISS A DOSE
Skip the missed dose and resume your regular dosage schedule. Do not double the next dose.

STOPPING THE DRUG
It may not be necessary to finish the recommended course of therapy. Consult your doctor.

PROLONGED USE
Therapy may require months or years. Excessive use may result in temporary loss of effectiveness.

PRECAUTIONS
Over 60: Adverse reactions may be more likely and more severe.

Driving and Hazardous Work: Avoid such activities until you determine how the medicine affects you.

Alcohol: No special precautions are necessary.

Pregnancy: Studies have indicated that albuterol may cause birth defects in mice when given in extremely large doses; effects from normal doses have not been established. Consult your doctor for advice.

Breast Feeding: Albuterol may pass into breast milk; caution is advised. Consult your doctor for advice.

Infants and Children: Not recommended for use by children under age 2.

Special Concerns: Be sure to tell your doctor if you have ever had any unusual or allergic reaction to albuterol. The inhaler should be primed prior to the first use and in cases when it has not been used for more than four days. Prime it by releasing four test sprays in the air away from the face. You should

wash your rotahaler (once every two weeks) and inhaler (once a week) to prevent medication build-up and blockage. Wash the two halves of the rotahaler or the mouthpiece of the inhaler (with the canister removed) with warm water and shake to remove excess water. Both the rotahaler and the inhaler should be air-dried thoroughly.

OVERDOSE
Symptoms: Confusion, delirium, severe anxiety, seizures, nervousness, headache, nausea, dry mouth, dizziness, insomnia, chest pain, muscle tremors, profound weakness, rapid and irregular pulse.

What to Do: Call your doctor, emergency medical services (EMS), or your local hospital immediately.

DRUG INTERACTIONS
Albuterol should not be used within 14 days of using an MAO inhibitor or tricyclic antidepressants. Consult your doctor for specific advice if you are taking beta-blockers, loop or thiazide diuretics, high blood pressure medication, digitalis drugs, epinephrine, ergot, finasteride, furazolidone, guanadrel, guanethidine, maprotiline, methyldopa, any nitrate, a phenothiazine, pseudo-ephedrine-containing products, rauwolfia alkaloids, terazosin, theophylline or other asthma medications, or thyroid hormone.

FOOD INTERACTIONS
No known food interactions.

DISEASE INTERACTIONS
Consult your doctor if you have an overactive thyroid, diabetes mellitus, a history of seizures, heart problems, high blood pressure, or blood vessel disease.

Alclometasone

▶ Drug Class: Topical corticosteroid

▶ Available in: Cream, ointment

▶ Available OTC? No

▶ As Generic? No

Side Effects

SERIOUS
Failure of skin to heal; severe burning and continued itching of skin. Seek medical assistance immediately.

COMMON
Burning, itching, irritation, redness, dryness, acne, stinging and cracking of skin.

LESS COMMON
Prolonged use, especially in covered areas, may produce blistering and pus near hair follicles, unusual bleeding or easy bruising, darkening or prominence of small surface veins, or increased susceptibility to infection.

PRINCIPAL USES
To relieve swelling, itching, redness, and other kinds of discomfort associated with certain skin conditions.

HOW THE DRUG WORKS
Alclometasone appears to interfere with the formation of natural substances within the body that are directly responsible for the process of inflammation, which produces swelling, redness, and itching.

DOSAGE
Apply sparingly (as a thin film), 2 or 3 times a day, only to the specific areas of skin where it is needed. Prior to application, wash or soak the affected area and allow it to dry; this may improve the absorption of the medication.

ONSET OF EFFECT
Rapid, but may take 24 to 48 hours to see the effect.

DURATION OF ACTION
Unknown.

DIETARY ADVICE
No special precautions.

STORAGE
Store in a tightly sealed container away from heat and direct light.

IF YOU MISS A DOSE
Apply it as soon as you remember. If it is close to the next application, skip the missed dose and resume your regular dosage schedule as prescribed.

STOPPING THE DRUG
Take it as prescribed for the full treatment period, even if you begin to feel better before the scheduled end of therapy. For some conditions, you may be directed to taper off the medication if symptoms and rash abate.

PROLONGED USE
See your doctor regularly for tests and examinations if you must use this drug for a prolonged period; use of this drug for more than 14 days is generally not recommended unless your doctor advises otherwise. Avoid prolonged use, particularly near the eyes, on the face in general, on genital or rectal areas, or in the folds of the skin.

PRECAUTIONS
Over 60: Side effects may be more likely and more severe in elderly patients; therapy with topical corticosteroids should therefore be brief and infrequent.

Driving and Hazardous Work: Use of alclometasone should not impair your ability to perform such tasks safely.

Alcohol: No special precautions are necessary.

Pregnancy: Should not be used for prolonged periods by pregnant women or by women trying to become pregnant.

Breast Feeding: Although problems have not been documented, caution is advised. Do not apply to breasts prior to nursing.

Infants and Children: Should not be used for more than 2 weeks on children and adolescents, unless otherwise directed by your doctor. Do not use tight-fitting diapers or plastic pants on children when treating skin irritation in the diaper area.

Special Concerns: Do not use alclometasone longer or more frequently than recommended by your doctor. Do not use it for other skin problems without a doctor's approval. Do not bandage or otherwise wrap the skin unless directed by your doctor. Wash the skin gently and allow it to dry and cool before applying. Be careful not to get the medicine in your eyes; if you do, flush your eyes with water. Wash hands after applying it with your fingers. Do not apply it to the face, mucous membranes, armpits, groin, or under breasts unless your doctor so directs. When treating a hairy site, part the hair and apply directly to the lesion.

OVERDOSE
Symptoms: No cases of overdose have been reported.

What to Do: An overdose of alclometasone is unlikely. However, in the event of accidental ingestion, call your doctor, emergency medical services (EMS), or the nearest poison control center immediately.

DRUG INTERACTIONS
Do not mix topical alclometasone with other products, especially alcohol-containing preparations (which include colognes, aftershave, and many moisturizer lotions), since this may cause dryness and irritation, or increase the risk of an allergic reaction. Consult your doctor if you are taking antifungal agents or antibiotics.

FOOD INTERACTIONS
No known food interactions.

DISEASE INTERACTIONS
Consult your doctor if you have cataracts; diabetes mellitus; glaucoma; infection, sores, or ulcerations of the skin; infection elsewhere in your body; or tuberculosis.

Alendronate Sodium

Fosamax 10 mg
(MERCK)

▶ Drug Class: Bisphosphonate inhibitor of bone resorption

▶ Available in: Tablets

▶ Available OTC? No

▶ As Generic? No

Side Effects

SERIOUS
No serious side effects have been reported in association with alendronate.

COMMON
Abdominal pain or bloating (persistent abdominal pain should be reported to your doctor), indigestion, heartburn, nausea.

LESS COMMON
Headache, constipation, diarrhea, gas, swallowing difficulty, throat irritation, abdominal swelling or tightness, muscle or bone pain, changes in taste perception.

PRINCIPAL USES
To prevent and treat osteoporosis by increasing bone mass. Alendronate also treats glucocorticoid-induced osteoporosis in those receiving corticosteroids. Also used to treat Paget's disease, a disorder characterized by rapid breakdown and reformation of bone, which can lead to fragility and malformation of bones.

HOW THE DRUG WORKS
Healthy bones are continuously remodeled (broken down and then reformed); the minerals and other components of bones are reabsorbed by one set of cells (osteoclasts) and replaced by another set of cells to form new bone. Alendronate suppresses the activity of osteoclasts; consequently, the breakdown of bone tissue occurs more slowly than the laying down of new bone. This action preserves bone density and strength.

DOSAGE
For prevention of osteoporosis: 5 mg once a day or 35 mg once a week. For treatment of osteoporosis: 10 mg once a day or 70 mg once a week. For glucocorticoid-induced osteoporosis in men and women: 5 mg once a day; postmenopausal women not receiving estrogen should take 10 mg once a day. For Paget's disease: 40 mg once a day. The dose is taken in the morning. Swallow tablets whole; do not suck or chew them. Do not lie down for 30 minutes following your dosage. The tablet must be taken with an 8 oz glass of water at least 30 minutes before any food or other medication.

ONSET OF EFFECT
Within 2 hours.

DURATION OF ACTION
24 hours to 7 days.

DIETARY ADVICE
Take alendronate at least 30 minutes before your first food or beverage of the day, with a full glass of water. Some patients may be advised to take calcium or vitamin D supplements to aid in the formation of new bone tissue.

STORAGE
Store in a tightly sealed container away from heat, moisture, and direct light.

IF YOU MISS A DOSE
Take it as soon as you remember. If it is near the time for the next dose, skip the missed dose and resume your regular dosage schedule. Do not double the next dose.

STOPPING THE DRUG
The decision to stop taking the drug should be made by your doctor. In most cases, patients with Paget's disease are treated for 6 months; the drug is then stopped. Retreatment may be necessary if such patients show signs of relapse after a subsequent 6-month observation period.

PROLONGED USE
No special precautions.

PRECAUTIONS
Over 60: No special problems are expected.

Driving and Hazardous Work: No special warnings.

Alcohol: Alcohol should be restricted in high-risk women because it is a risk factor for osteoporosis.

Pregnancy: Alendronate is normally not used in premenopausal women. The drug should not be given to pregnant women because animal studies have shown adverse effects in the fetus.

Breast Feeding: Alendronate may pass into breast milk; consult your doctor for specific advice.

Infants and Children: Not recommended.

Special Concerns: Patients taking alendronate are encouraged to engage in regular weight-bearing exercise and should avoid cigarettes and limit alcohol, which inhibit healthy bone production.

OVERDOSE
Symptoms: Severe heartburn, stomach cramps, or throat irritation might occur if an overdose disturbs the body's normal mineral (electrolyte) balance.

What to Do: Few alendronate overdoses have been reported. However, if someone takes a much larger dose than prescribed, call your doctor or the nearest poison control center.

DRUG INTERACTIONS
Consult your doctor for specific advice if you are taking antacids, calcium supplements, aspirin or other non-steroidal anti-inflammatory drugs (NSAIDs), or hormone replacement therapy. Wait at least 30 minutes after taking alendronate before taking any other drugs.

FOOD INTERACTIONS
Any food eaten within 30 minutes of taking alendronate decreases its effect. Mineral water, coffee, tea, and fruit juice can interfere with the drug's absorption.

DISEASE INTERACTIONS
Kidney impairment or a gastrointestinal disease may increase the risk of side effects. Low blood calcium levels and vitamin D deficiency must be treated before using alendronate.

Alitretinoin

▶ Drug Class: Retinoid

▶ Available in: Topical gel

▶ Available OTC? No

▶ As Generic? No

Side Effects

SERIOUS
No serious side effects are associated with alitretinoin.

COMMON
Redness, rash, itching, numbness and tingling, skin cracking, scabbing, swelling, burning sensation, and pain at application site.

LESS COMMON
No less common side effects are associated with alitretinoin.

PRINCIPAL USES
To treat skin lesions topically in patients with AIDS-related Kaposi's sarcoma (a type of skin cancer that commonly affects immuno-compromised patients). Not for use when systemic anti-Kaposi's sarcoma therapy is required.

HOW THE DRUG WORKS
Alitretinoin, a vitamin A-related retinoid found naturally in the body, inhibits the growth of Kaposi's sarcoma cells.

DOSAGE
To start, apply a generous layer of gel to the skin lesions twice a day. Frequency of application may be gradually increased by your doctor to 3 to 4 times a day.

ONSET OF EFFECT
A response to the gel may be seen as soon as 2 weeks after the initiation of therapy. However, some patients require up to 14 weeks of therapy before a response is noted.

DURATION OF ACTION
Unknown.

DIETARY ADVICE
No special restrictions.

STORAGE
Store in a tightly sealed container away from heat, moisture, and direct light.

IF YOU MISS A DOSE
If you fail to apply the medication on one day, return to your regular schedule the next day; do not apply an extra amount in an attempt to compensate for the missed dose.

STOPPING THE DRUG
Use of alitretinoin should be continued as long as its benefit persists. Consult your doctor before discontinuing treatment.

PROLONGED USE
Long-term therapy with this medication is often required.

PRECAUTIONS
Over 60: Information is inadequate, but no special problems are expected.

Driving and Hazardous Work: The use of alitretinoin should not impair your ability to perform such tasks safely.

Alcohol: No special precautions are necessary.

Pregnancy: Alitretinoin should not be used if you are pregnant or plan to become pregnant. Adequate birth-control methods should be practiced when alitretinoin is used in women of child-bearing age.

Breast Feeding: Alitretinoin may pass into breast milk. However, women infected with HIV should not breast-feed, so as to avoid transmitting the virus to an uninfected child.

Infants and Children: Not recommended for use by children.

Special Concerns: Avoid applying the gel to unaffected skin, as skin irritation may result. Allow the gel to dry for 3 to 5 minutes before covering with clothing. Do not apply near mucous membranes such as the nose, eyes, and mouth. Patients with cutaneous T-cell lymphoma are less tolerant to the drug.

OVERDOSE
Symptoms: Excessive use of alitretinoin may lead to skin redness, peeling, or discomfort.

What to Do: An overdose is unlikely to occur. If someone accidentally ingests alitretinoin, call your doctor.

DRUG INTERACTIONS
If you are using alitretinoin, do not use any products containing DEET, a common ingredient in some insect repellents.

FOOD INTERACTIONS
No known food interactions.

DISEASE INTERACTIONS
Consult your doctor if you have any other skin condition before using alitretinoin.

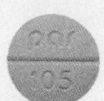

Side Effects

SERIOUS
Anemia or other blood or bone marrow disorders that may produce fatigue, bleeding, or bruising; yellowish tinge to eyes or skin (signifying hepatitis or liver damage); severe skin reactions (marked by rashes, skin ulcers, hives, intense itching); chest tightness; weakness. Call your doctor right away if such symptoms arise.

COMMON
Mild rash, drowsiness, nausea, diarrhea. The frequency of gout attacks may increase during the first weeks of use.

LESS COMMON
Headache, abdominal pain, boils on face, chills or fever, vomiting, hair loss.

PRINCIPAL USES
To treat chronic gout or excessive uric acid buildup caused by kidney disorders, cancer, or the use of chemotherapy drugs for cancer. Also prescribed to prevent recurrence of uric acid kidney stones. Allopurinol should not be used for treating acute gout attacks in progress.

HOW THE DRUG WORKS
Allopurinol blocks the enzyme xanthinc oxidase, which is required for the production of uric acid, thus reducing blood levels of uric acid.

DOSAGE
Adults: Initially 100 mg per day, increased by 100 mg per week to a maximum of 800 mg per day. 100 mg doses are administered once a day; doses of 300 mg or more are taken in 2 or 3 evenly divided portions throughout the day. Children ages 6 to 10: 300 mg per day for certain types of cancer. Children age 6 and under: 50 mg per day in 3 evenly divided portions.

ONSET OF EFFECT
Reduces uric acid levels in 2 to 3 days; may take 6 months for full effect to occur.

DURATION OF ACTION
1 to 2 weeks.

DIETARY ADVICE
Take it with food or milk to avoid stomach irritation. Drink 10 to 12 glasses (8 oz each) of water a day.

STORAGE
Store in a tightly sealed container away from heat and direct light.

IF YOU MISS A DOSE
Take it as soon as you remember. However, if it is near the time for the next dose, skip the missed dose and resume your regular dosage schedule. Do not double the next dose.

STOPPING THE DRUG
Take allopurinol as prescribed for the full treatment period, even if you begin to feel better before the scheduled end of therapy.

PROLONGED USE
Consult your doctor about the need for tests of liver function, kidney function, blood counts, and blood and urine levels of uric acid.

PRECAUTIONS
Over 60: Adverse reactions may be more likely and more severe in older patients.

Driving and Hazardous Work: Allopurinol may cause drowsiness. If possible, avoid driving and hazardous work.

Alcohol: No special precautions are necessary.

Pregnancy: Caution is advised; consult your doctor about whether the benefits outweigh potential risks to the unborn child.

Breast Feeding: Allopurinol passes into breast milk; avoid or discontinue use while nursing.

Infants and Children: Follow your doctor's instructions carefully for children.

OVERDOSE
Symptoms: No specific symptoms have been reported.

What to Do: An overdose of allopurinol is unlikely to be life-threatening. However, if someone takes a much larger dose than prescribed, contact your doctor, poison control center, or local emergency room for instructions.

DRUG INTERACTIONS
Consult your doctor for specific advice if you are taking an antibiotic (such as amoxicillin, ampicillin, or bacampicillin), an anticoagulant (warfarin, dicumarol), an anticancer (chemotherapy) drug, chlorpropamide, a diuretic, or theophylline.

FOOD INTERACTIONS
None are likely, but a low-purine diet is recommended to reduce the risk of gout attacks. Foods high in purines include anchovies, sardines, legumes, poultry, sweetbreads, liver, kidneys, and other organ meats.

DISEASE INTERACTIONS
Caution is advised when taking allopurinol. Consult your doctor if you have high blood pressure, diabetes mellitus, kidney disease, or impaired iron metabolism.

Almotriptan Malate

BRAND NAME
Axert

▶ Drug Class: Antimigraine/antiheadache drug

▶ Available in: Tablets

▶ Available OTC? No

▶ As Generic? No

Side Effects

SERIOUS
Serious side effects with almotriptan are rare. However, almotriptan may cause a heart attack, chest pain or tightness, sudden or severe abdominal pain, shortness of breath, wheezing, heartbeat irregularities, swelling of eyelids, face, or lips, skin rash, or hives. Seek emergency medical assistance immediately.

COMMON
Nausea, drowsiness, prickling or tingling sensations, dry mouth, headache.

LESS COMMON
Many less common side effects can occur; consult your doctor if you are concerned about any adverse or unusual reactions you experience while taking this drug.

PRINCIPAL USES
To treat severe, acute migraine headaches. Almotriptan is not intended as a migraine preventive or for use against any other kinds of pain or headache, including basilar and hemiplegic migraines.

HOW THE DRUG WORKS
The exact mechanism of almotriptan's action is unknown. However, it is believed that almotriptan may reduce the swelling of blood vessels in the brain that are associated with the pain of migraine, block the release of substances from nerve endings that cause more pain and other symptoms of migraine, and interrupt the transmission of specific pain signals from the brain.

DOSAGE
A single dose ranging from 6.25 to 12.5 mg is generally effective. If the migraine returns or there is only partial relief, the dose may be repeated once after 2 hours, but no more than 25 mg should be taken in a 24-hour period. Since individual response to almotriptan may vary, your doctor will determine the appropriate dosage. A general recommendation is to take one 6.25 mg tablet as the initial dose.

ONSET OF EFFECT
Within 2 hours.

DURATION OF ACTION
Unknown.

DIETARY ADVICE
The medication can be taken with or without food.

STORAGE
Store in a tightly sealed container away from heat, moisture, and direct light.

IF YOU MISS A DOSE
Not applicable, since the drug is taken only when necessary.

STOPPING THE DRUG
Consult your doctor before discontinuing almotriptan.

PROLONGED USE
No special problems are expected.

PRECAUTIONS
Over 60: This drug should not be used unless coronary heart disease has been ruled out through appropriate diagnostic tests.

Driving and Hazardous Work: Some people feel drowsy or dizzy during or following a migraine attack or after taking almotriptan. Avoid driving or other tasks requiring concentration if you have such symptoms.

Alcohol: No special warnings, although alcohol may trigger or exacerbate migraine headaches.

Pregnancy: Adequate human studies have not been done. Discuss with your doctor the relative risks and benefits of using almotriptan while pregnant.

Breast Feeding: Almotriptan may pass into breast milk; consult your doctor for specific advice.

Infants and Children: Safety and effectiveness have not been established for children under age 18.

Special Concerns: Serious, but rare, heart-related problems may occur after taking almotriptan. Almotriptan should not be used by anyone with any symptoms of coronary artery disease (chest pain or tightness, shortness of breath). Anyone at risk for unrecognized CAD—such as postmenopausal women, men over the age of 40, or those with known risk factors for heart disease (hypertension, high blood cholesterol levels, obesity, diabetes, strong family history of heart disease, or cigarette smoking)—should have the first dose of almotriptan administered in a doctor's office, and then only after tests show they are probably free of coronary artery disease.

OVERDOSE
Symptoms: No overdoses have been reported.

What to Do: Although overdose is unlikely, if you take a much larger dose than prescribed, seek medical attention immediately.

DRUG INTERACTIONS
Do not take almotriptan within 24 hours of taking naratriptan, rizatriptan, sumatriptan, zolmitriptan, ergotamine-containing medication, dihydroergotamine mesylate, or methysergide mesylate. Almotriptan and MAO inhibitors such as phenelzine, tranylcypromine, procarbazine, and selegiline should not be used within 14 days of each other. Do not take almotriptan within one week of using ketoconazole, itraconazole, or erythromycin.

FOOD INTERACTIONS
No known food interactions.

DISEASE INTERACTIONS
You should not take almotriptan if you have a history of angina, heart disease, stroke, uncontrolled hypertension, heartbeat irregularities, or peripheral vascular disease. Almotriptan should be used with caution in patients with liver disease or severely impaired kidney function.

Alprazolam

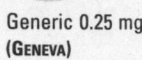

Generic 0.25 mg
(GENEVA)

▶ Drug Class: Benzodiazepine tranquilizer; antianxiety agent

▶ Available in: Tablets, oral solution

▶ Available OTC? No

▶ As Generic? Yes

Side Effects

SERIOUS
Difficulty concentrating, outbursts of anger, other behavior problems, depression, hallucinations, low blood pressure (causing faintness or confusion), memory impairment, muscle weakness, skin rash or itching, sore throat, fever and chills, sores or ulcers in throat or mouth, unusual bruising or bleeding, extreme fatigue, yellowish tinge to eyes or skin. Call your doctor immediately.

COMMON
Drowsiness, loss of coordination, unsteady gait, dizziness, lightheadedness, slurred speech.

LESS COMMON
Change in sexual desire or ability, constipation, false sense of well-being, nausea and vomiting, urinary problems, unusual fatigue.

PRINCIPAL USES
To treat anxiety and panic disorder.

HOW THE DRUG WORKS
In general, alprazolam produces mild sedation by depressing activity in the central nervous system. In particular, alprazolam appears to enhance the effect of gamma-aminobutyric acid (GABA), a natural chemical that inhibits the firing of neurons and dampens the transmission of nerve signals, thus decreasing nervous excitation.

DOSAGE
Adults: Initial dose is 1.5 mg a day, taken in 3 divided doses; may be gradually increased to a maximum dose of 4 mg a day. Older adults: Initial dose is 0.5 to 0.75 mg per day, taken in 2 or 3 divided doses; may be gradually increased to a maximum dose of 2 mg a day. Children: Not usually prescribed.

ONSET OF EFFECT
2 hours.

DURATION OF ACTION
Up to 6 hours.

DIETARY ADVICE
Alprazolam can be taken on an empty stomach or with food or milk.

STORAGE
Store in a tightly sealed container away from heat and direct light.

IF YOU MISS A DOSE
If you miss a dose, take it if you remember within 1 hour. Otherwise, skip the missed dose and take the next one at the regular time. Do not double the next dose.

STOPPING THE DRUG
Never stop taking the drug abruptly, as this can cause withdrawal symptoms (seizures, sleep disruption, nervousness, irritability, diarrhea, abdominal cramps, muscle aches, memory impairment). Dosage should be reduced gradually as directed by your doctor.

PROLONGED USE
Short-term therapy (8 weeks or less) is typical; do not take it for a longer period unless so advised by your doctor.

PRECAUTIONS
Over 60: Use with caution; side effects such as drowsiness and dizziness may be more pronounced in older patients.

Driving and Hazardous Work: Alprazolam can impair mental alertness and physical coordination. Adjust your activities accordingly.

Alcohol: Alcohol intake should be extremely moderate or stopped altogether while taking alprazolam.

Pregnancy: Use of this drug during pregnancy should be avoided if possible. Be sure to tell your doctor if you are pregnant or plan to become pregnant.

Breast Feeding: Alprazolam passes into breast milk; do not take it while nursing.

Infants and Children: Safety and effectiveness have not been established for children under age 18.

Special Concerns: Use of this drug can lead to psychological or physical dependence. Short-term therapy (8 weeks or less) is typical; patients should not take the drug for a longer period unless so advised by their doctor. Never take more than the prescribed daily dose.

OVERDOSE
Symptoms: Extreme drowsiness, confusion, slurred speech, slow reflexes, poor coordination, staggering gait, tremor, slowed breathing, loss of consciousness.

What to Do: Call your doctor, emergency medical services (EMS), or the nearest poison control center immediately.

DRUG INTERACTIONS
Other drugs may interact with alprazolam. Consult your doctor for specific advice if you are taking any drugs that depress the central nervous system; these include antihistamines, antidepressants (including nefazodone) or other psychiatric medications, barbiturates, sedatives, cough medicines, decongestants, and painkillers. Be sure your doctor knows about any over-the-counter medication you may take.

FOOD INTERACTIONS
None reported.

DISEASE INTERACTIONS
Consult your doctor if you have a history of alcohol or drug abuse, stroke or other brain disease, any chronic lung disease, hyperactivity, depression or other mental illness, myasthenia gravis, sleep apnea, epilepsy, porphyria, kidney disease, or liver disease.

Alprostadil Injection

BRAND NAMES
Caverject, Edex, Prostin
VR Pediatric

▶ Drug Class: Vasodilator

▶ Available in: Injection

▶ Available OTC? No

▶ As Generic? Yes

Side Effects

SERIOUS
Painful or prolonged erection (lasting more than 4 hours), usually as a result of excessive dosage. If erection does not resolve on its own in a reasonable amount of time, seek medical help promptly. If erection does resolve on its own, subsequent doses should be reduced; consult your doctor for specific guidelines.

COMMON
Pain, itching, or burning at site of injection.

LESS COMMON
Bruising or bleeding at site of injection.

PRINCIPAL USES
To treat erectile dysfunction (impotence) in men; also, to help maintain adequate blood flow in infants during heart surgery.

HOW THE DRUG WORKS
Alprostadil causes dilation of blood vessels, thereby increasing blood flow to the tissues supplied by the vessels affected by the drug. When injected into the penis, alprostadil causes the penile arteries to dilate, thus promoting erection.

DOSAGE
For adult men: Injection of 0.001 to 0.04 mg, self-administered at the base of the penis as needed. It should not be administered more than once a day. For infants: Injection of 0.005 to 0.01 mg before surgery.

ONSET OF EFFECT
5 to 10 minutes.

DURATION OF ACTION
30 minutes to 3 hours.

DIETARY ADVICE
Diet is not significant in alprostadil therapy.

STORAGE
Keep the liquid form of alprostadil refrigerated, but do not allow it to freeze.

IF YOU MISS A DOSE
Not applicable; the drug is taken only when the patient chooses.

STOPPING THE DRUG
Consult your doctor if you wish to discontinue therapy or if you feel alprostadil is losing its effectiveness.

PROLONGED USE
Alprostadil should not be used more frequently than a physician recommends, which is generally not more than 3 times a week, with at least 24 hours between each dose. Patients who self-administer alprostadil should visit their doctor every 3 months for evaluation; dosage adjustments or the decision to stop using the drug will be made at these times. Never increase the dosage without consulting your doctor.

PRECAUTIONS
Over 60: Information about use specifically in older persons is not available, though elderly patients are more likely to suffer from circulatory problems and thus may be less responsive to the drug than their younger counterparts. Your doctor may need to adjust the dosage.

Driving and Hazardous Work: No special precautions are necessary.

Alcohol: No special precautions are necessary.

Pregnancy: Not applicable; the drug is used only in men and infants. No problems have been reported in women who became pregnant by partners using alprostadil.

Breast Feeding: Not applicable; the drug is used only by men or in infants.

Infants and Children: Prostin VR Pediatric should be used for infants only in a hospital setting.

Special Concerns: Your doctor should instruct you on how to administer the injection of alprostadil before you attempt to do it yourself. Only men who have been diagnosed with and are being medically treated for erectile dysfunction should use this drug as a sexual aid.

OVERDOSE
Symptoms: Painful erection or an erection that persists for more than 4 hours.

What to Do: Call your doctor, emergency medical services (EMS), or your local hospital right away. Prolonged erection may result in permanent damage to the tissues of the penis and the inability to achieve subsequent erections.

DRUG INTERACTIONS
None reported in infants. Adults should notify their doctor if they are taking any other drugs.

FOOD INTERACTIONS
No significant interactions have been reported.

DISEASE INTERACTIONS
An adult who has a blood coagulation defect, liver disease, sickle cell disease, or a history of priapism (erections lasting more than 4 hours) should inform his physician before using alprostadil.

Altretamine

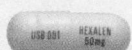

Hexalen 50 mg
(US Bioscience)

▸ Drug Class: Antineoplastic (anticancer) agent

▸ Available in: Capsules

▸ Available OTC? No

▸ As Generic? No

Side Effects

SERIOUS
Anemia or other blood problems that cause fatigue, bleeding, bruising, fever, and chills; anxiety, confusion, dizziness, weakness, and loss of balance or coordination; numbness or tingling in the arms and legs. Call your doctor right away.

COMMON
Dizziness, drowsiness, mood changes, nausea, vomiting.

LESS COMMON
Diarrhea, loss of appetite, abdominal cramps, skin rash, temporary hair loss.

PRINCIPAL USES
To treat persistent or recurrent ovarian cancer. This drug is generally used following first-line treatment with other chemotherapy agents.

HOW THE DRUG WORKS
The exact mechanism of action of altretamine is not known, but the drug appears to interfere with the synthesis of genetic material within cells, thereby inhibiting the growth of cancer cells.

DOSAGE
260 mg per square meter of body size, in 4 equally divided doses per day (at mealtimes and at bedtime), generally given 14 or 21 consecutive days out of a 28-day cycle. The actual dose will depend on how much toxicity has occurred in previous cycles of chemotherapy.

ONSET OF EFFECT
Peak blood levels are achieved within 3 hours.

DURATION OF ACTION
Up to 10 hours.

DIETARY ADVICE
Take it after meals to minimize nausea and vomiting. Maintain adequate intake of food and fluids.

STORAGE
Store in a tightly sealed container away from heat and direct light.

IF YOU MISS A DOSE
Take it as soon as you remember, unless it is almost time for the next dose. In that case, skip the missed dose and take the next one. If you miss more than one dose, call your doctor.

STOPPING THE DRUG
The decision to stop taking the drug should be made in consultation with your physician.

PROLONGED USE
Prolonged use can increase the incidence of nausea and vomiting, which can be treated by antiemetic drugs. Blood tests should be taken every 2 to 4 weeks and prior to the beginning of each new course of therapy with altretamine. Neurological exams should be performed regularly as well to determine whether altretamine is causing any nerve damage.

PRECAUTIONS
Over 60: No special problems are expected.

Driving and Hazardous Work: This drug may produce side effects such as dizziness or nausea; avoid any potentially dangerous activities until you determine how the medication affects you.

Alcohol: Alcohol intake should be limited; drink only in moderation while taking this drug.

Pregnancy: Altretamine should not be used during pregnancy because it may cause birth defects. When using this drug, a reliable method of birth control is recommended.

Breast Feeding: Breast feeding is not recommended; altretamine passes into breast milk and may harm the nursing child.

Infants and Children: No specific information on use in children is available.

Special Concerns: This drug may affect your ability to resist infections. If possible, avoid others who are sick with any sort of infection. Be careful when using a toothbrush, dental floss, or a toothpick, and check with your doctor before having any dental work done. Avoid touching your eyes, nose, or mouth, unless your hands are very clean. Be careful not to cut yourself with objects such as razors or nail clippers, and avoid contact sports or any other activities that could result in injuries.

OVERDOSE
Symptoms: The symptoms of an altretamine overdose have not been well-defined, but an overdose may be life-threatening.

What to Do: If someone takes a much larger dose than prescribed, call emergency medical services (EMS) immediately to receive evaluation and treatment in the closest emergency facility.

DRUG INTERACTIONS
Consult your doctor if you are taking amphotericin B (by injection), antithyroid drugs, azathioprine, chlorambucil, colchicine, flucytosine, ganciclovir, interferon, plicamycin, zidovudine, or an MAO inhibitor (a class of antidepressants). Do not get vaccinated against bacteria or viruses while you are taking altretamine.

FOOD INTERACTIONS
None expected.

DISEASE INTERACTIONS
Caution is advised when taking altretamine. Consult your doctor if you have any of the following conditions: bone marrow depression, chicken pox, shingles, any infection, or reduced kidney function.

Aluminum Salts

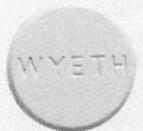

Amphojel 600 mg
(WYETH-AVERST)

▶ Drug Class: Antacid

▶ Available in: Tablets, capsules, oral suspension, gel

▶ Available OTC? Yes

▶ As Generic? Yes

Side Effects

SERIOUS
Severe and continuing constipation, dizziness, lightheadedness, and heartbeat irregularities. Bone loss may occur, especially with prolonged use in dialysis patients. Hypophosphatemia (too little phosphate in the blood) may occur with prolonged use and a low-phosphate diet; symptoms include bone pain, fractures, muscle weakness, loss of appetite, mood changes, a general feeling of discomfort, swelling of the wrists and ankles, unusual weight loss, and anemia (decreased number of red blood cells; symptoms include weakness and fatigue).

COMMON
Chalky taste.

LESS COMMON
Mild constipation, stomach cramps, speckling or whitish coloration of stools, increased thirst, nausea and vomiting.

PRINCIPAL USES
To treat heartburn, acid indigestion, sour stomach, peptic ulcers, gastritis, esophagitis, and gastro-esophageal reflux. May also be used to treat or prevent excess phosphate in the blood or to prevent urinary phosphate stones.

HOW THE DRUG WORKS
Aluminum salts neutralize stomach acid and reduce the action of pepsin, a digestive enzyme. This provides symptomatic relief from excess stomach acid.

DOSAGE
1 to 2 tablets or capsules or 5 to 30 ml suspension or gel as often as every 2 hours, up to 12 times per day. Take the dose between meals unless your doctor directs otherwise. When used as sole treatment of peptic ulcer or esophagitis, take it 1 and 3 hours after meals and at bedtime. Tablets should be chewed.

ONSET OF EFFECT
Within minutes.

DURATION OF ACTION
20 minutes to 3 hours.

DIETARY ADVICE
Avoid a low-phosphate diet during prolonged use, unless your doctor directs otherwise. Some recommended high-phosphate foods include red meat, poultry, fish, eggs, dark green leafy vegetables, dairy products, and nuts.

STORAGE
Store in a tightly sealed container away from heat, moisture, and direct light. Keep liquid forms refrigerated.

IF YOU MISS A DOSE
Take it as soon as you remember. Do not double the next dose.

STOPPING THE DRUG
Take as directed.

PROLONGED USE
Do not take it for more than 2 weeks unless your doctor recommends otherwise.

PRECAUTIONS
Over 60: Constipation or intestinal trouble is more common in older persons. Older patients who have or who are at high risk for osteoporosis or other bone disorders should avoid frequent use of this medicine.

Driving and Hazardous Work: No special precautions are necessary.

Alcohol: Alcohol decreases the effect of antacids.

Pregnancy: Consult your doctor before taking aluminum salts while pregnant.

Breast Feeding: Aluminum-containing antacids pass into breast milk. It is unknown whether this poses any risk to nursing infants. Consult your doctor for advice.

Infants and Children: Antacids should not be dispensed to children under age 6 unless otherwise instructed by a physician.

Special Concerns: Use over-the-counter antacids only occasionally unless otherwise directed by your doctor. Persistent heartburn not readily relieved by antacids may be signaling a heart attack or another serious disorder. In such cases, seek medical help promptly.

OVERDOSE
Symptoms: Shallow breathing, dry mouth, constipation or diarrhea, confusion, headache, weakness or fatigue, bone pain, stupor.

What to Do: Seek medical assistance immediately.

DRUG INTERACTIONS
Other medications may lose their effectiveness when taken within 1 hour of antacids. Consult your doctor for specific advice if you are taking amphetamines, bisacodyl, citrates, chenodiol, digoxin, enteric-coated medications, iron salts, isoniazid, ketoconazole, mecamylamine, methenamine, penicillamine, phosphates, nitrofurantoin, quinidine, salicylates, or tetracyclines.

FOOD INTERACTIONS
Taking an aluminum salt with food can decrease its activity. Wait at least 60 minutes after eating before taking it.

DISEASE INTERACTIONS
Do not take aluminum salts if you have any symptoms of appendicitis or an inflamed bowel (abdominal pain, cramps, soreness, bloating, nausea, vomiting). Aluminum salts are not recommended for Alzheimer's patients. Consult your doctor if you have chronic constipation, colitis, ileostomy, colostomy, intestinal or stomach blockage, bone fractures, diarrhea, kidney disease, hypophosphatemia, heart disease, liver disease, edema, stomach bleeding, intestinal bleeding.

Amantadine Hydrochloride

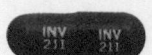

Generic 100 mg
(INVAMED)

▶ Drug Class: Antiviral/
antiparkinsonism agent

▶ Available in: Tablets, syrup

▶ Available OTC? No

▶ As Generic? Yes

Side Effects

SERIOUS
Skin rash, confusion, seizures, hallucinations, swollen feet or arms, difficulty breathing. Call your doctor at once.

COMMON
Dizziness, irritability, distractibility, difficulty sleeping. Consult your doctor if such symptoms persist.

LESS COMMON
Mild skin rash, weakness, depression, fatigue, anxiety, headache, lightheadedness, loss of appetite, nausea, constipation, dry mouth. Consult your doctor if such symptoms persist.

PRINCIPAL USES
To prevent or treat type A influenza; to treat Parkinson's disease. It may also be used to minimize stiffness and shaking caused by certain other drugs prescribed for treating nervous, mental, or emotional disorders.

HOW THE DRUG WORKS
The exact mechanism of action is unknown, though amantadine appears to prevent the influenza A virus from penetrating and entering healthy cells. In Parkinsonism, it increases the release and activity of dopamine, which plays a key role in the control of muscle movement. The increased availability of dopamine in the brain helps compensate for the reduction in the natural supply caused by the disease, and so eases symptoms of Parkinsonism.

DOSAGE
For treatment or prevention of influenza— Adults: 100 to 200 mg a day in 1 or 2 doses for 5 days. Children: Up to 150 mg once a day. For Parkinsonism— Adults: 100 mg, 2 times a day. In some cases the maximum dose may be increased to 400 mg a day. Older patients and those with a history of seizure disorders are usually given reduced doses, generally 100 mg a day.

ONSET OF EFFECT
For influenza A: 2 hours. For Parkinsonism: 48 hours.

DURATION OF ACTION
Up to 12 hours.

DIETARY ADVICE
Take it with or after meals.

STORAGE
Store in a tightly sealed container away from heat and direct light.

IF YOU MISS A DOSE
If you miss a dose, take it as soon as you remember unless it is almost time for your next dose. In that case, skip the missed dose and return to your regular schedule. Do not double the next dose.

STOPPING THE DRUG
Influenza: For prevention, take amantadine for the full treatment period as recommended by your doctor; for treatment, do not stop taking amantadine without consulting your doctor. Parkinsonism: Doses must be decreased gradually according to your doctor's instructions.

PROLONGED USE
Prolonged use requires periodic checks by your doctor.

PRECAUTIONS
Over 60: Older persons are generally more sensitive to amantadine and more likely to experience adverse side effects. Smaller doses may be warranted.

Driving and Hazardous Work: Amantadine can cause drowsiness, dizziness, blurred vision, or confusion. Avoid driving and hazardous work until you determine how the medicine affects you.

Alcohol: Avoid alcohol since it may increase side effects such as dizziness and blurred vision.

Pregnancy: In some animal studies, amantadine has been shown to cause birth defects, though human studies have not been done. Accordingly, the drug should be avoided during the first 3 months of pregnancy. Notify your doctor if you are pregnant or plan to become pregnant.

Breast Feeding: Amantadine passes into breast milk and should not be taken while breast feeding.

Infants and Children: Safety for children under the age of 1 has not been established.

Special Concerns: Individuals with kidney disease must take reduced dosages and be closely monitored.

OVERDOSE
Symptoms: Hyperactivity, disorientation, confusion, visual hallucinations, seizures, drop in blood pressure, palpitations or heart rhythm disturbances.

What to Do: Call your doctor, emergency medical services (EMS), or the nearest poison control center immediately.

DRUG INTERACTIONS
The effects of amantadine can be altered by amphetamines, diet pills, asthma and cold medicines, methylphenidate, nabilone, and pemoline. Anticholinergic drugs can increase the side effects of amantadine.

FOOD INTERACTIONS
None are expected.

DISEASE INTERACTIONS
Caution is advised when taking this medication. Consult your doctor if you have eczema, epilepsy, heart disease, circulation problems, kidney disease, or an emotional disorder.

Amiloride Hydrochloride

BRAND NAME
Midamor

Midamor 5 mg
(MERCK)

▶ Drug Class: Potassium-sparing diuretic

▶ Available in: Capsules, tablets

▶ Available OTC? No

▶ As Generic? Yes

Side Effects

SERIOUS
Heartbeat irregularities, lightheadedness (caused by high blood potassium levels). Notify your doctor at once.

COMMON
There are no common side effects associated with the use of amiloride.

LESS COMMON
Headache, nausea, loss of appetite, weight loss, diarrhea, vomiting, weakness, dizziness, drowsiness, abdominal pain, constipation, impotence, increased skin sensitivity to sunlight, nervousness, irregular heartbeat, shortness of breath, tingling in hands, feet, or lips.

PRINCIPAL USES
As adjunctive (supplementary) treatment with other diuretics to increase excretion of sodium and water in the urine, while conserving potassium.

HOW THE DRUG WORKS
Amiloride promotes loss of sodium and water from the body by altering kidney enzymes that control urine production. Unlike other types of diuretics, amiloride belongs to a class that promotes excretion of excess water but does not deplete normal levels of potassium. In conjunction with thiazide or loop diuretics, amiloride reduces the overall fluid volume in the body and helps to control symptoms of heart disease, kidney disease, and liver disease.

DOSAGE
In most cases, 5 mg a day, increased to 10 mg a day if necessary. Maximum dose is 20 mg a day. The drug is usually taken in one daily dose, preferably in the morning.

ONSET OF EFFECT
2 to 4 hours.

DURATION OF ACTION
Up to 24 hours.

DIETARY ADVICE
Amiloride can be taken with liquid or food to lessen stomach irritation. Avoid large quantities of high-potassium foods (see Food Interactions).

STORAGE
Store in a tightly sealed container away from heat and direct light.

IF YOU MISS A DOSE
Take it as soon as you remember. If it is near the time for the next dose, skip the missed dose and resume your regular dosage schedule. Do not double the next dose.

STOPPING THE DRUG
The decision to stop taking the drug should be made by your doctor.

PROLONGED USE
No apparent problems.

PRECAUTIONS
Over 60: No special precautions are warranted.

Driving and Hazardous Work: No special precautions are necessary.

Alcohol: No special precautions are necessary.

Pregnancy: Animal studies have not shown birth defects. Adequate human studies have not been done. Consult your doctor about taking amiloride during pregnancy.

Breast Feeding: It is not known whether amiloride passes into breast milk. Consult your doctor about its use while nursing.

Infants and Children: A small dose (0.625 mg per day) may be used in young children.

OVERDOSE
Symptoms: Rapid, irregular heartbeat, shortness of breath, nervousness, confusion, weakness, stupor.

What to Do: Call your doctor, emergency medical services (EMS), or the nearest poison control center immediately.

DRUG INTERACTIONS
Tell your doctor if you are taking other drugs, especially ACE inhibitors, nonsteroidal anti-inflammatory drugs (NSAIDs), digoxin, lithium, potassium supplements, or another diuretic.

FOOD INTERACTIONS
Avoid consuming large servings of high-potassium foods, which include bananas, citrus fruits and juices, melons, prunes, (and most fruits in general), avocados, potatoes, nuts, baked beans, brussels sprouts, and skim milk.

DISEASE INTERACTIONS
Caution is advised when taking amiloride. Consult your doctor if you have any of the following: diabetes mellitus, gout, kidney stones, liver disease, or kidney disease.

Aminocaproic Acid

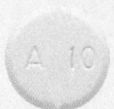

Amicar 500 mg
(IMMUNEX)

▶ Drug Class: Antifibrolytic (bleeding prevention) agent

▶ Available in: Tablets, syrup, injection

▶ Available OTC? No

▶ As Generic? Yes

Side Effects

SERIOUS
Shortness of breath; weakness or numbness of arm or leg; slurred speech; severe and sudden headache; sharp pain in the chest, upper arm, or legs; vision changes. Although the frequency is rare, such symptoms may be signaling a stroke or heart attack. Other rare, but serious side effects include: bleeding problems, seizures, and hallucinations. Discontinue the medication and seek emergency medical treatment immediately.

COMMON
Nausea, diarrhea, severe menstrual cramps, muscle cramps and aches, vomiting. Notify your doctor if such symptoms persist.

LESS COMMON
Dizziness, headache, muscle weakness and fatigue, ringing in the ears, skin rash, abdominal pain, rapid weight gain, swelling in the feet, face, and legs, nasal congestion, delirium, confusion.

PRINCIPAL USES
To treat serious bleeding that occurs after surgery or dental work or to prevent potentially life-threatening bleeding during surgery in patients with hemophilia, low blood platelet counts, or other medical problems.

HOW THE DRUG WORKS
Aminocaproic acid inhibits certain biochemical reactions that involve enzymes, including the activation of plasminogen, a natural enzyme that dissolves blood clots. As a result, blood becomes more prone to clotting, which helps to stanch episodes of uncontrolled bleeding.

DOSAGE
Adults: Initial dose is 5 g, then 1 or 1.25 g per hour, 3 or 4 times a day after the initial dose. The maximum daily dose is 30 g per day. It may be taken by mouth or intravenously. Children: Initial dose is 45.5 mg per lb of body weight, followed by 15.1 mg per lb, 3 or 4 times a day, for 2 to 8 days.

ONSET OF EFFECT
Within 1 hour.

DURATION OF ACTION
3 to 4 hours.

DIETARY ADVICE
Tablet or syrup forms may be taken with food to prevent stomach irritation.

STORAGE
Store in a tightly sealed container away from heat and direct light.

IF YOU MISS A DOSE
Take the missed dose as soon as you remember, unless it is almost time for the next dose. In that case, double the next dose. Then resume your regular dosage schedule.

STOPPING THE DRUG
Do not stop taking aminocaproic acid without your doctor's consent, unless a serious problem occurs, at which time discontinue the drug immediately. Gradual reduction of the dosage may be necessary if you have taken the drug for a long time. Consult your doctor for specific guidelines. Never take more than 30 g per day.

PROLONGED USE
Ask your doctor about the need for medical examinations or laboratory studies with prolonged use.

PRECAUTIONS
Over 60: No special problems are expected.

Driving and Hazardous Work: Do not drive or engage in hazardous work until you determine how the drug affects you.

Alcohol: Alcohol should be avoided because it decreases the therapeutic effect of aminocaproic acid.

Pregnancy: It is not known whether aminocaproic acid can cause fetal harm. It should be used during pregnancy only if clearly necessary, after a detailed discussion with your doctor.

Breast Feeding: Aminocaproic acid passes into breast milk, although it has not been reported to cause health problems in nursing infants. Consult your doctor or pediatrician for specific advice.

Infants and Children: Safety and effectiveness in young patients have not been established; this drug should be used in children only under a doctor's careful supervision.

OVERDOSE
Symptoms: Few cases of overdose have been reported. However, symptoms following high doses of injectable aminocaproic acid may include dizziness, confusion, slow heartbeat, fainting, sluggishness, fatigue, confusion, seizures, increased urination, gastrointestinal bleeding.

What to Do: Discontinue the medication and call your doctor, emergency medical services (EMS), or local hospital immediately.

DRUG INTERACTIONS
Oral contraceptives and estrogens boost the the clot-promoting effect of aminocaproic acid, which may therefore increase the risk of potentially dangerous blood clot formation. Thrombolytic (blood-clot-dissolving) agents such as streptokinase decrease the effect of aminocaproic acid.

FOOD INTERACTIONS
No significant food interactions have been reported.

DISEASE INTERACTIONS
Patients with a history of disseminated intravascular coagulation (also known as DIC, a rare disorder marked by excessive and hazardous blood coagulation) should not take aminocaproic acid. If you are pregnant or have heart disease, kidney disease, or liver disease, you may be at increased risk for side effects.

Aminophylline

Generic 100 mg
(WEST-WARD)

▶ Drug Class: Bronchodilator/
xanthine

▶ Available in: Tablets, liquid,
injection, suppositories

▶ Available OTC? No

▶ As Generic? Yes

Side Effects

SERIOUS
Although very rare,
aminophylline may lead
to heartbeat irregularities,
seizures, or extreme
breathing difficulty. Seek
emergency medical assis-
tance immediately.

COMMON
Headache, irritability, nervousness, nausea, vomit-
ing, rapid breathing or
heartbeat, restlessness,
insomnia, stomach pain,
increased urine output.

LESS COMMON
Hives or skin rash, diar-
rhea, dizziness, lightheadedness, loss of appetite,
fatigue.

PRINCIPAL USES
To widen the airways (bronchodilation) and so prevent
the wheezing and constriction of the airways associated with asthma and other
breathing disorders, such as
chronic bronchitis, emphysema, and chronic obstructive pulmonary disease
(COPD).

HOW THE DRUG WORKS
An asthma attack occurs
when the smooth muscles
in the bronchial passages of
the lungs go into a spasm
(bronchospasm). Amino-
phylline relaxes these muscles, thus helping to widen
the constricted airways and
restore normal breathing.

DOSAGE
Adults: 6 to 8 mg per day
per 2.2 lbs (1 kg) of body
weight. Children: 18 mg per
day per 2.2 lbs of body
weight. The dosage must be
adjusted for each person.
Higher doses are warranted
during an acute asthma
attack and taken as needed.
Maintenance dose is taken
every 6 to 8 hours.

ONSET OF EFFECT
15 to 60 minutes.

DURATION OF ACTION
Several hours, depending
on dosage and form.

DIETARY ADVICE
Best taken 1 hour before or
2 hours after eating. Can be
taken with meals to lessen
any stomach upset.

STORAGE
Keep in a tightly sealed container away from heat, moisture, and direct light.

IF YOU MISS A DOSE
If you miss a dose, take it
as soon as you remember
up to 2 hours late. If more
than 2 hours, wait for the
next scheduled dose. Do
not double the next dose.

STOPPING THE DRUG
Take it as long as your doctor advises. See your doctor
for regular checkups.

PROLONGED USE
If used properly, amino-
phylline can be taken safely
for a lifetime; no specific
problems are expected.

PRECAUTIONS
Over 60: Adverse reactions
may be more likely and
more severe in older
patients.

**Driving and Hazardous
Work:** Do not engage in
such activities until you
determine how the drug
affects you. If you experience side effects such as
dizziness and lightheadedness, proceed with caution.

Alcohol: No special precautions are necessary.

Pregnancy: It is unclear
whether aminophylline
causes fetal harm; discuss
the risks with your doctor.
Generally, this drug should
be used only if necessary
and if a substitute cannot be
prescribed.

Breast Feeding: Aminophylline passes into breast
milk and may be toxic to
nursing infants; avoid the
drug or discontinue breast
feeding.

Infants and Children:
Be alert for side effects
such as agitation, irritability,
fever, lethargy, rapid heartbeat and breathing, or
seizures. The liquid form of
aminophylline is often recommended for children to
make it easier to use and
ensure a more accurate
dosage.

Special Concerns: Aminophylline should not be used
by patients who have had
prior allergic reactions to it
or its components (including ethylenediamide).

OVERDOSE
Symptoms: Acute restlessness, irritability, confusion,
breathing difficulties, heart
rhythm irregularities, delirium, seizures.

What to Do: Stop taking
the drug and contact your
doctor, emergency medical
services (EMS), or the
nearest poison control center immediately.

DRUG INTERACTIONS
Consult your doctor for specific advice if you are taking
allopurinol, cimetidine,
ciprofloxacin, erythromycin,
troleandomycin, lithium,
oral contraceptives, phenytoin, propranolol, or
rifampin.

FOOD INTERACTIONS
Avoid excessive use of caffeine-containing beverages.
High-carbohydrate and
high-fat meals can decrease
the effect of aminophylline.

DISEASE INTERACTIONS
You should not take aminophylline if you have active
peptic ulcer disease or an
underlying disorder that
causes seizures (unless you
are also taking appropriate
anticonvulsant medication).
The suppository form
should not be used by people with inflammation or
infection of the rectum or
lower colon. Use caution
when taking aminophylline
if you have heart disease,
liver disease, or an underactive thyroid (hypothy-
roidism). Consult your
doctor in such cases.

Aminosalicylate Sodium

BRAND NAMES
Sodium P.A.S., Tubasal

▶ Drug Class: Anti-infective/ antitubercular agent

▶ Available in: Tablets

▶ Available OTC? No

▶ As Generic? No

Side Effects

SERIOUS
Joint pain, fever, unusual fatigue, skin rash or itching, lower back pain, yellow discoloration of the eyes or skin, severe abdominal pain, sore throat, pale skin, headache, pain or burning while urinating. Call your doctor immediately.

COMMON
Abdominal discomfort, nausea and vomiting, diarrhea, loss of weight and appetite.

LESS COMMON
Peptic ulcer disease, intestinal bleeding, lowered white and red blood cell counts.

PRINCIPAL USES
To treat active tuberculosis; must be used in conjunction with other antitubercular agents, such as isoniazid, streptomycin, and rifampin.

HOW THE DRUG WORKS
Aminosalicylate kills tuberculosis bacteria by preventing them from utilizing folic acid, a vitamin necessary for cell growth and reproduction.

DOSAGE
Adults and teenagers: 4 to 6 grams every 12 hours; usually not more than 68 to 91 mg per lb of body weight a day. Children age 12 and under: 23 to 34 mg per lb of body weight every 12 hours. Aminosalicylate is taken in conjunction with other antitubercular agents.

ONSET OF EFFECT
Unknown.

DURATION OF ACTION
Unknown.

DIETARY ADVICE
Take it with or after meals or with an antacid to minimize stomach irritation.

STORAGE
Store in a tightly sealed container away from heat, moisture, and direct light.

IF YOU MISS A DOSE
Take it as soon as you remember. This will help keep a constant level of medication in your system. If it is near the time for the next dose, skip the missed dose and resume your regular dosage schedule. Do not double the next dose.

STOPPING THE DRUG
Take it as prescribed for the full treatment period, even if you begin to feel better before the scheduled end of therapy. Treatment may continue for months or years. The decision to stop taking the drug should be made by your doctor.

PROLONGED USE
Prolonged use with high doses may cause swelling in the front of the neck, menstrual changes in women, decreased sexual ability in men, unusual weight gain, and dry, puffy skin. Consult your doctor about the need for periodic medical examinations and laboratory tests if you take this medication for a prolonged period.

PRECAUTIONS
Over 60: Adverse reactions may be more likely and more severe in older patients.

Driving and Hazardous Work: Do not drive or engage in hazardous work until you determine how the medicine affects you.

Alcohol: No special precautions are necessary.

Pregnancy: Adequate studies of aminosalicylate use during pregnancy have not been done. Consult your doctor for specific advice if you are pregnant or plan to become pregnant.

Breast Feeding: Aminosalicylate passes into breast milk, but no problems have been documented.

Infants and Children: No special warnings; children may tolerate the drug better than adults.

Special Concerns: Do not take tablets that are brown or purple in color.

OVERDOSE
Symptoms: An overdose with aminosalicylate is unlikely.

What to Do: Emergency instructions not applicable.

DRUG INTERACTIONS
Do not take rifampin within 6 hours of taking aminosalicylate. Other drugs may interact with aminosalicylate. Consult your doctor if you are taking aminobenzoates or other over-the-counter or prescription medications.

FOOD INTERACTIONS
None are anticipated, although aminosalicylate can interfere with the absorption of vitamin B12 and other nutrients; vitamin supplementation may be necessary.

DISEASE INTERACTIONS
Caution is advised when taking aminosalicylate. Consult your doctor if you have any of the following: gastric ulcers, epilepsy, heart disease, cancer, an overactive thyroid, or adrenal insufficiency. Use of aminosalicylate may cause complications in patients with liver or kidney disease, since these organs work together to remove the medication from the body.

Amiodarone

Cordarone 200 mg
(WYETH-AYERST)

▶ Drug Class: Antiarrhythmic

▶ Available in: Tablets

▶ Available OTC? No

▶ As Generic? Yes

Side Effects

SERIOUS
Cough, shortness of breath, increased palpitations, loss of voice (rare). Seek medical assistance immediately. Nausea, vomiting, and yellow-tinged skin or eyes (jaundice) may occur as an indication of serious liver problems; notify your doctor right away if such symptoms arise.

COMMON
Stomach upset, nausea, vomiting, constipation, loss of appetite, low-grade fever, heightened skin sensitivity to sun, resulting in greater predisposition to sunburn, numbness or tingling in the fingers or toes, trembling or shaking, unsteadiness when walking, headache.

LESS COMMON
Bitter or metallic taste in the mouth, blue-gray discoloration of skin, vision disturbances, dry eyes, dry, puffy skin, coldness or chills, dizziness, nervousness or restlessness, diminished sex drive in males, scrotal pain and swelling, slow heartbeat, unusual or profuse sweating, insomnia, fatigue, unexpected gain or loss of weight.

PRINCIPAL USES
To prevent and treat heartbeat irregularities, including atrial fibrillation and ventricular tachycardia. The relative risks of using this drug must be weighed carefully against its benefits, since amiodarone can be toxic, especially when taken at high doses or for long periods of time.

HOW THE DRUG WORKS
Amiodarone slows and helps regulate nerve impulses in the heart, and acts directly on the tissue of the heart, making heart muscle less responsive to abnormal stimuli.

DOSAGE
Adults: 800 to 2,400 mg per day in 3 or 4 equally divided doses at first; then 600 to 800 mg per day for one month; then 200 to 400 mg per day. Children: Dosage schedule varies according to the severity of the arrhythmia and often according to individual physician preferences.

ONSET OF EFFECT
2 or 3 days to 2 to 3 weeks.

DURATION OF ACTION
10 days to several months depending on total amount of time the drug has been prescribed and total quantity consumed.

DIETARY ADVICE
Amiodarone be taken with liquid or food to minimize the risk of stomach upset.

STORAGE
Store in a tightly sealed container away from heat, moisture, and direct light.

IF YOU MISS A DOSE
Skip the missed dose and return to your regular schedule. Do not double next dose.

STOPPING THE DRUG
The decision to stop taking the drug should be made by your doctor. Be sure to report any unusual symptoms after you discontinue the medication.

PROLONGED USE
Dosage is typically reduced (to 100 to 200 mg daily) with prolonged use.

PRECAUTIONS
Over 60: Side effects may be more likely and more severe. Thyroid problems (both hypo- and hyperthyroidism) as well as walking difficulty, and numbness, tingling, trembling, or weakness in the hands and feet are likely to develop.

Driving and Hazardous Work: Proceed with caution until you determine how the drug affects you.

Alcohol: Drink only in strict moderation if at all.

Pregnancy: Studies have indicated that amiodarone may cause thyroid and heart problems in unborn children. Nonetheless, the drug may be needed if a history of serious cardiac arrhythmia is a threat to the mother's life. Discuss the relative risks and benefits with your doctor.

Breast Feeding: Amiodarone passes into breast milk; consult your doctor for advice.

Infants and Children: Amiodarone can be used in children who have symptomatic or life-threatening arrhythmias. Discuss relative risks and benefits with your doctor.

Special Concerns: To screen for early signs of side effects, most patients should have regular blood tests for liver, thyroid, and pulmonary function, and have eye exams at least annually. Before dental work, emergency treatment, or surgery requiring general anesthesia, be sure to tell the attending doctor or dentist that you are taking amiodarone.

OVERDOSE
Symptoms: Seizures, irregular or very slow heartbeat, loss of consciousness.

What to Do: Call your doctor, emergency medical services (EMS), or the nearest poison control center immediately.

DRUG INTERACTIONS
Consult your doctor for specific advice if you are taking anticoagulants, other heart medications, theophylline, or phenytoin. The blood-thinning effect of warfarin may be drastically enhanced within days of starting amiodarone. Usually the dose of warfarin is reduced once amiodarone is prescribed; prothrombin time is monitored carefully.

FOOD INTERACTIONS
None are expected.

DISEASE INTERACTIONS
Consult your doctor if you have liver or kidney disease, or a thyroid disorder.

Amitriptyline Hydrochloride

Side Effects

SERIOUS
Confusion, heartbeat
irregularities, hallucinations, seizures, extreme
fatigue or drowsiness,
blurred or altered vision,
breathing difficulty, constipation, impaired con-
centration, difficult
urination, fever, extreme
and persistent restless-
ness, loss of coordination
and balance, difficulty
swallowing or speaking,
dilated pupils, eye pain,
fainting. Also trembling,
shaking, weakness, and
stiffness in the extremi-
ties; shuffling gait. Call
your doctor immediately.

COMMON
Drowsiness, dizziness,
or lightheadedness;
headache, dry mouth or
unpleasant taste, fatigue,
heightened sensitivity to
light, unusual weight
gain, increased appetite,
nausea.

LESS COMMON
Heartburn, insomnia,
diarrhea, increased
sweating, vomiting.

PRINCIPAL USES
To relieve symptoms of
major depression and
chronic pain.

HOW THE DRUG WORKS
Amitriptyline affects levels
of specific brain chemicals
(serotonin, norepinephrine,
and acetylcholine) that are
thought to be linked to
mood, emotions, and
mental state.

DOSAGE
Adults: To start, 25 mg, 2 to
4 times a day; may be
increased to 150 mg a day.
Teenagers: 10 mg, 3 times a
day, and 20 mg at bedtime.
Children ages 6 to 12: 10 to
30 mg a day. Older adults:
To start, 25 mg a day at
bedtime; may be increased
to 100 mg a day.

ONSET OF EFFECT
1 to 6 weeks.

DURATION OF ACTION
Unknown.

DIETARY ADVICE
To lessen stomach upset,
take with food, unless your
doctor instructs otherwise.
Increase intake of fiber
and fluids.

STORAGE
Store in a tightly sealed container away from heat, moisture, and direct light.

IF YOU MISS A DOSE
If you take a one-time daily
bedtime dose, do not take
the missed dose in the
morning; it may cause
drowsiness. Call your doctor. If you take more than 1
dose a day, take it as soon
as you remember. If it is
near the time for the next
dose, skip the missed dose
and resume your regular
dosage schedule. Do not
double the next dose.

STOPPING THE DRUG
Take it as prescribed for the
full treatment period, even if
you feel better before the
scheduled end of therapy.
The decision to stop taking
the drug should be made in
consultation with your doctor. The dosage should be
gradually tapered over 5 to
7 days when stopping.

PROLONGED USE
The usual course of therapy
lasts 6 months to 1 year;
some patients may benefit
from additional therapy.

PRECAUTIONS
Over 60: Adverse reactions
are more likely and more
severe in older patients.
Amitriptyline is generally
not recommended, as there
are safer alternatives for
older patients. A lower dose
may be warranted.

**Driving and Hazardous
Work:** Use caution when
driving and engaging in hazardous work until you determine how the medicine
affects you. Drowsiness or
lightheadedness can occur.

Alcohol: Avoid alcohol.

Pregnancy: Adequate
human studies have not
been done in pregnant
women. Consult your doctor
for advice.

Breast Feeding:
Amitriptyline passes into
breast milk; do not use it
while nursing.

Infants and Children:
Not prescribed for children
under the age of 6.

Special Concerns: This
is a potentially dangerous
drug, especially if taken in
excess. Tricyclic antidepressants should not be within
easy reach of suicidal
patients. If dry mouth

occurs, use sugarless gum
or candy.

OVERDOSE
Symptoms: Breathing difficulty, fever, severe fatigue,
impaired concentration,
mental confusion, hallucinations, dilated pupils, irregular heartbeat or palpitations,
and seizures.

What to Do: Call your
doctor, emergency medical
services (EMS), or the
nearest poison control center immediately.

DRUG INTERACTIONS
Consult your doctor for specific advice if you are taking
antithyroid agents, cimetidine, clonidine, guanadrel,
guanethidine, metrizamide,
appetite suppressants, isoproterenol, ephedrine, epinephrine, amphetamines,
phenyl-ephrine, antipsy-
chotic drugs, pimozide,
methyldopa, metyrosine,
metoclopramide, pemoline,
promethazine, trimeprazine,
rauwolfia alkaloids, MAO
inhibitors, or any drugs that
depress the central nervous
system.

FOOD INTERACTIONS
No known food interactions.

DISEASE INTERACTIONS
Consult your doctor if you
have any of the following:
a history of alcohol abuse,
difficulty urinating, asthma,
bipolar disorder, high blood
pressure, stomach or intestinal problems, glaucoma,
overactive thyroid, enlarged
prostate, schizophrenia,
seizures, a blood disorder,
or kidney, heart, or liver
disease.

Amlexanox

▶ Drug Class: Antiaphthous ulcer drug

▶ Available in: Adhesive oral paste

▶ Available OTC? No

▶ As Generic? No

Side Effects

SERIOUS
No serious side effects are associated with amlexanox.

COMMON
Transient pain, stinging, or burning at site of application.

LESS COMMON
Nausea, diarrhea, inflammation of the mucous membranes.

PRINCIPAL USES
To help heal aphthous ulcers (canker sores) of the mouth. Amlexanox works best if it is taken as soon as such ulcers are diagnosed.

HOW THE DRUG WORKS
The exact way in which amlexanox works is unknown. Studies have suggested that it inhibits the formation and release of substances in the body associated with allergic reactions and inflammation.

DOSAGE
Apply ¼ inch of paste on each lesion (mouth ulcer), 4 times a day.

ONSET OF EFFECT
Unknown.

DURATION OF ACTION
Unknown.

DIETARY ADVICE
The paste is best applied after each meal and at bedtime.

STORAGE
Store in a tightly sealed container away from heat and direct light.

IF YOU MISS A DOSE
Apply it as soon as you remember. If it is near the time for the next dose, skip the missed dose and resume your regular dosage schedule. Do not double the next dose.

STOPPING THE DRUG
Use this drug as prescribed for the full treatment period, even if you begin to feel better before the scheduled end of therapy.

PROLONGED USE
You should see your doctor regularly for tests and examinations if you take this medicine for a prolonged period. If ulcers have not healed significantly or pain has not been reduced after 10 days, consult your doctor.

PRECAUTIONS
Over 60: It is not known whether amlexanox causes side effects in older patients different from or more severe than those in younger persons.

Driving and Hazardous Work: No special warnings.

Alcohol: No special precautions are necessary.

Pregnancy: In animal studies, amlexanox has not caused birth defects or other problems. Human studies have not been done. Before you take amlexanox, tell your doctor if you are pregnant or plan to become pregnant.

Breast Feeding: Amlexanox may pass into breast milk; caution is advised. Consult your doctor for specific advice.

Infants and Children: The safety and effectiveness of amlexanox in children have not been established.

Special Concerns: Wash your hands immediately after applying amlexanox. Flush your eyes with water promptly if they come in contact with the paste. If a rash or inflammation of the mucous membranes develops, discontinue use of amlexanox and contact your doctor.

OVERDOSE
Symptoms: None have been reported.

What to Do: An overdose of amlexanox is very unlikely to occur. Emergency instructions are not applicable.

DRUG INTERACTIONS
Consult your doctor for specific advice if you are taking any other prescription or over-the-counter drug.

FOOD INTERACTIONS
No known food interactions.

DISEASE INTERACTIONS
Caution is advised when taking amlexanox. Consult your doctor for specific advice if you have any other medical condition, especially a weakened immune system, which is prevalent in people receiving immunosuppressant drugs or chemotherapy, as well as those with acquired immunodeficiency syndrome (AIDS). The safety and effectiveness of amlexanox in persons with a weakened immune system have not been established. In addition, amlexanox should not be used by anyone who has had a previous allergic reaction to the medication or any other ingredient in the formulation.

Amlodipine

▶ Drug Class: Calcium channel blocker

▶ Available in: Tablets, capsules

▶ Available OTC? No

▶ As Generic? No

Side Effects

SERIOUS
Increased angina attacks, dizziness upon arising from a sitting or lying position, shortness of breath, weakness, very slow heartbeat. Call your doctor immediately.

COMMON
Headache; flushing in the face and body; water retention causing decreased urination, swelling of the feet and ankles, weight gain.

LESS COMMON
Fatigue, dizziness, drowsiness, palpitations, nausea, abdominal pain.

PRINCIPAL USES
To relieve angina (chest pain associated with heart disease) and to treat hypertension.

HOW THE DRUG WORKS
Amlodipine interferes with the movement of calcium into heart muscle cells and the smooth muscle cells in the walls of the arteries. This action relaxes blood vessels (causing them to widen), which lowers blood pressure, increases the blood supply to the heart, and decreases the heart's overall workload.

DOSAGE
2.5 to 10 mg per day in one daily dose (usually in the morning, with breakfast).

ONSET OF EFFECT
1 to 2 hours.

DURATION OF ACTION
24 hours.

DIETARY ADVICE
It can be taken with or after meals to minimize stomach irritation. Be sure to follow a low-sodium, low-fat diet if your doctor so advises.

STORAGE
Store in a tightly sealed container away from heat and direct light.

IF YOU MISS A DOSE
If you miss a dose, take it as soon as you remember, unless the next dose is less than 4 hours away. In that case, skip the missed dose and go back to your regular schedule. Do not double the next dose.

STOPPING THE DRUG
Take as prescribed for the full treatment period. Do not stop taking this drug suddenly, as this may cause potentially serious health problems. If therapy is to be discontinued, dosage should be reduced gradually, according to doctor's instructions.

PROLONGED USE
In some cases amlodipine therapy may be required for years or even a lifetime. Consult your doctor about the need for medical or laboratory tests of heart activity, blood pressure, kidney function, and liver function.

PRECAUTIONS
Over 60: Adverse reactions may be more likely and more severe in older patients. Smaller doses (2.5 mg per day) are generally prescribed.

Driving and Hazardous Work: Avoid driving or engaging in hazardous work until you determine how this medication affects you. Be cautious if it causes dizziness.

Alcohol: Alcohol should be used with caution because it may increase the effect of the drug and cause an excessive drop in blood pressure.

Pregnancy: Amlodipine should not be taken during the first 3 months of pregnancy and should be used in the last 6 months only if your doctor so advises.

Breast Feeding: Amlodipine should not be taken by nursing mothers.

Infants and Children: Amlodipine is not usually prescribed for patients under the age of 12.

Special Concerns: Amlodipine should not be taken by anyone who has had a prior adverse reaction to it. When taking amlodipine, avoid sudden changes in position, especially standing up quickly after sitting or lying down; such movements may cause dizziness.

OVERDOSE
Symptoms: Severe drop in blood pressure resulting in weakness, dizziness, drowsiness, confusion, or slurred speech.

What to Do: Call your doctor, emergency medical services (EMS), or your local hospital immediately.

DRUG INTERACTIONS
Other heart drugs taken with amlodipine can cause heart rate and rhythm problems. In general, consult your doctor if you are taking any other prescription or nonprescription drugs.

FOOD INTERACTIONS
Avoid excessive intake of foods high in sodium.

DISEASE INTERACTIONS
Consult your doctor if you have kidney disease, liver disease, high blood pressure, or any heart disease other than coronary artery disease.

Amobarbital/Secobarbital

▶ Drug Class: Barbiturate; central nervous system depressant

▶ Available in: Capsules

▶ Available OTC? No

▶ As Generic? No

Side Effects

SERIOUS
Extreme confusion, severe drowsiness, shortness of breath, wheezing or difficulty breathing, fever, bleeding, rash, hives, hallucinations. Stop taking the drug and call your doctor immediately if you experience any of these side effects.

COMMON
Clumsiness or unsteadiness; dizziness or lightheadedness; drowsiness; hangover-like feelings.

LESS COMMON
Nausea, vomiting, constipation, headache, irritability, sleep disturbances including nightmares and difficulty falling asleep.

PRINCIPAL USES
Amobarbital/secobarbital was previously used for the short-term treatment of insomnia. It is now prescribed only rarely by doctors, usually for the purpose of sedation.

HOW THE DRUG WORKS
This medication is actually two barbiturates, amobarbital and secobarbital, in combination. These drugs act on the central nervous system as a powerful sedative.

DOSAGE
100 or 200 mg at bedtime.

ONSET OF EFFECT
Within 15 minutes.

DURATION OF ACTION
From 3 to 8 hours.

DIETARY ADVICE
The capsules may be crushed and taken with food or liquids.

STORAGE
Store in a tightly sealed container away from heat, moisture, and direct light.

IF YOU MISS A DOSE
Amobarbital/secobarbital is prescribed for once-daily use at bedtime only. If you are unable to take this medication on a particular night, resume only your regularly scheduled dose the following night. Do not double the next dose.

STOPPING THE DRUG
Never stop taking the drug abruptly, as this can cause withdrawal symptoms (seizures, sleep disruption, nervousness, irritability, diarrhea, abdominal cramps, muscle aches, memory impairment). Dosage should be reduced gradually, as directed by your doctor.

PROLONGED USE
Barbiturates are habit-forming. Prolonged use of amobarbital/secobarbital increases the risk of dependency. Amobarbital/secobarbital should not be prescribed for long-term therapy because safer and more effective drugs are available.

PRECAUTIONS
Over 60: Adverse reactions may be more likely and more severe in older patients.

Driving and Hazardous Work: The use of amobarbital/secobarbital may impair your ability to perform such tasks safely.

Alcohol: Avoid alcohol completely; the combination of alcohol and barbiturates is potentially lethal.

Pregnancy: Discuss with your doctor the relative risks and benefits of using this drug while pregnant.

Breast Feeding: Do not use this drug while nursing.

Infants and Children: This drug is not recommended for children.

Special Concerns: Amobarbital/secobarbital is a potentially dangerous drug. Barbiturates should not be used for the treatment of anxiety or stress.

OVERDOSE
Symptoms: Lethargy, excessive sleepiness, slurred speech, severe clumsiness, difficulty walking, confusion, extremely slow, noisy breathing, loss of consciousness. Some patients may become agitated and unusually excited (paradoxical excitation). Pupils may become very tiny, although with severe overdose the pupils may become very dilated.

What to Do: Contact emergency medical services (EMS) immediately.

DRUG INTERACTIONS
The risk of an undesirable interaction is increased when amobarbital/secobarbital is used with any or all of the following drugs: alcohol-containing medicines, antihistamines, allergy medications, sedatives, antiseizure medications, pain medications (especially prescription pain relievers and narcotics), muscle relaxants, and antidepressants. Use of amobarbital/secobarbital may cause the following to be less effective: blood thinners, birth control pills, and medications similar to cortisone.

FOOD INTERACTIONS
No known food interactions.

DISEASE INTERACTIONS
Patients with kidney or liver disease should avoid amobarbital/secobarbital. The drug may make the following conditions worse: asthma, emphysema, and other respiratory diseases; mental depression; porphyria; and diabetes mellitus.

Amoxapine

Asendin 50 mg
(LEDERLE)

▶ Drug Class: Tricyclic antidepressant

▶ Available in: Tablets

▶ Available OTC? No

▶ As Generic? Yes

Side Effects

SERIOUS
Confusion; sexual dysfunction; heartbeat irregularities; hallucinations; seizures; extreme fatigue or drowsiness; blurred or altered vision; breathing difficulty; constipation; staring and absence of facial expression; impaired concentration; difficult urination; fever; extreme and persistent restlessness; loss of coordination and balance; difficulty swallowing or speaking; dilated pupils; eye pain; fainting; trembling, shaking, weakness, and stiffness in the extremities; shuffling gait; persistent, uncontrolled chewing, lip-smacking, or tongue movements; uncontrolled movements, including tics, twitching, twisting movements, and muscle spasms in the face, arms hands, and legs. Call your doctor immediately.

COMMON
Drowsiness or dizziness, headache, dry mouth or unpleasant taste, fatigue, heightened sensitivity to light, nausea, weight gain, increased appetite.

LESS COMMON
Heartburn, insomnia, diarrhea, sweating, vomiting.

PRINCIPAL USES
To relieve symptoms of major depression.

HOW THE DRUG WORKS
Amoxapine affects levels of norepinephrine, a brain chemical that is thought to be linked to mood, emotions, and mental state.

DOSAGE
Adults: To start, 50 mg, 2 to 3 times a day. Older adults: To start, 25 mg, 2 to 3 times a day. Dosages may be gradually increased, as determined by your doctor.

ONSET OF EFFECT
1 to 6 weeks.

DURATION OF ACTION
Unknown.

DIETARY ADVICE
To lessen stomach upset, take with food, unless your doctor instructs otherwise. Increase intake of fiber and fluids.

STORAGE
Store in a tightly sealed container away from heat, moisture, and direct light.

IF YOU MISS A DOSE
If you take a one-time daily bedtime dose, do not take a missed dose in the morning because it may cause drowsiness. Call your doctor. If you take more than 1 dose a day, take it as soon as you remember. If it is near the time for the next dose, skip the missed dose and resume your regular dosage schedule. Do not double the next dose.

STOPPING THE DRUG
Take it as prescribed for the full treatment period, even if you feel better before the scheduled end of therapy. The decision to stop taking the drug should be made in consultation with your doctor. The dosage should be gradually tapered over several days when stopping.

PROLONGED USE
The usual course of therapy lasts 6 months to 1 year; some patients may benefit from additional therapy. There is increased risk of movement disorders with prolonged use.

PRECAUTIONS
Over 60: Adverse reactions may be more likely and more severe in older patients. A lower dose may be warranted.

Driving and Hazardous Work: Use caution when driving or engaging in hazardous work until you determine how the medication affects you. Drowsiness and lightheadedness can occur.

Alcohol: Avoid alcohol.

Pregnancy: Adequate human studies have not been done. Consult your doctor.

Breast Feeding: Amoxapine passes into breast milk; do not use it while nursing.

Infants and Children: Not prescribed for children under the age of 6.

Special Concerns: This is a potentially dangerous drug, especially if taken in excess. Tricyclic antidepressants should not be within easy reach of suicidal patients. If dry mouth occurs, use sugarless gum or candy for relief.

OVERDOSE
Symptoms: Difficulty breathing, severe fatigue, seizures, confusion, hallucinations, dilated pupils, irregular heartbeat, heart palpitations, fever, difficulty concentrating.

What to Do: Call your doctor, emergency medical services (EMS), or the nearest poison control center immediately.

DRUG INTERACTIONS
Consult your doctor for specific advice if you are taking antithyroid agents, cimetidine, clonidine, guanadrel, guanethidine, metrizamide, appetite suppressants, isoproterenol, ephedrine, epinephrine, amphetamines, phenylephrine, antipsychotic drugs, pimozide, methyldopa, metyrosine, metoclopramide, pemoline, promethazine, trimeprazine, rauwolfia alkaloids, MAO inhibitors, or central nervous system depressants.

FOOD INTERACTIONS
No known food interactions.

DISEASE INTERACTIONS
Consult your doctor if you have any of the following: a history of alcohol abuse, difficulty urinating, asthma, bipolar disorder, high blood pressure, stomach or intestinal problems, glaucoma, overactive thyroid, enlarged prostate, schizophrenia, seizures, a blood disorder, or kidney, heart, or liver disease.

Amoxicillin

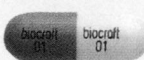

Generic 250 mg
(BIOCRAFT)

797

Additional photographs

▶ Drug Class: Penicillin antibiotic

▶ Available in: Capsules, oral suspension, chewable tablets, liquid drops

▶ Available OTC? No

▶ As Generic? Yes

Side Effects

SERIOUS
Irregular, rapid, or labored breathing, light-headedness or sudden fainting, joint pain, fever, severe abdominal pain and cramping with watery or bloody stools, severe allergic reaction (marked by sudden swelling of the lips, tongue, face, or throat; breathing difficulty; skin rash, itching, or hives), unusual bleeding or bruising, yellowish tinge to eyes or skin. Call your doctor immediately.

COMMON
Rash, mild diarrhea, nausea, vomiting, headache, vaginal discharge and itching, pain or white patches in the mouth or on the tongue.

LESS COMMON
Diminished urine output, chills, weakness, fatigue.

PRINCIPAL USES
To treat bacterial infections of the ear, nose, and throat, genitourinary tract, skin and soft tissues, and the lower respiratory tract. It is used, often with other drugs, to treat uncomplicated gonorrhea. It is also prescribed preventively before surgery or dental work to patients at risk for endocarditis (infection of the interior lining of the heart). It is also used to treat some stages of Lyme disease and, along with other drugs, to treat *H. pylori* infection (the cause of stomach ulcers). Amoxicillin is also approved for prophylactic use following known exposure to anthrax bacteria and for treating anthrax infections.

HOW THE DRUG WORKS
Amoxicillin blocks the formation of bacterial cell walls, rendering bacteria unable to multiply and spread.

DOSAGE
For infections— Adults: 250 to 500 mg every 8 hours (3 doses per day). Children: 3 to 6 mg per lb of body weight every 8 hours (3 doses per day). To treat gonorrhea— 3 g in a single oral dose.

ONSET OF EFFECT
Rapid; within 2 hours.

DURATION OF ACTION
8 hours.

DIETARY ADVICE
Best taken on an empty stomach, but may be taken with food to minimize stomach irritation or diarrhea.

STORAGE
Store in a tightly sealed container away from heat and direct light. Keep any liquid form refrigerated, but do not allow it to freeze, and discard after 14 days.

IF YOU MISS A DOSE
Take it as soon as you remember. If it is near the time for the next dose, skip the missed dose and resume your regular dosage schedule. Do not double the next dose.

STOPPING THE DRUG
Take as prescribed for the full treatment period, even if you begin to feel better before the scheduled end of therapy. Stopping the drug prematurely may slow your recovery or lead to a rebound infection, also known as superinfection, in which the heartier strains of bacteria survive and multiply, leading to a more serious and drug-resistant infection.

PROLONGED USE
Prolonged use of any antibiotic increases the risk of superinfection; caution is advised.

PRECAUTIONS
Over 60: No special problems are expected.

Driving and Hazardous Work: The use of amoxicillin should not impair your ability to perform such tasks safely.

Alcohol: No special precautions are necessary.

Pregnancy: Adequate studies of the use of this drug during pregnancy have not been done; however, no problems have been reported.

Breast Feeding: Amoxicillin passes into breast milk and may cause diarrhea, fungal infections, and allergic reactions in nursing infants; avoid use while nursing.

Infants and Children: No special problems are expected.

Special Concerns: Amoxicillin can cause false results on some urine sugar tests for diabetics. Those who are prone to asthma, hay fever, hives, or allergies may be more likely to have an allergic reaction to a penicillin antibiotic. Oral contraceptives may not be effective while you are taking amoxicillin; use other methods of contraception to avoid unplanned pregnancy.

OVERDOSE
Symptoms: Severe nausea, vomiting, diarrhea, muscle spasticity, seizures.

What to Do: Call your doctor, emergency medical services (EMS), or the nearest poison control center immediately.

DRUG INTERACTIONS
Consult your doctor for specific advice if you are taking: aminoglycosides, ACE inhibitors, diuretics, potassium supplements or potassium-containing medications, anticoagulants or other anticlotting drugs, nonsteroidal anti-inflammatory drugs (NSAIDS), sulfinpyrazone, cholestyramine, colestipol, oral contraceptives, methotrexate, probenecid, allopurinol, or rifampin.

FOOD INTERACTIONS
No known food interactions.

DISEASE INTERACTIONS
Consult your doctor if you have a history of allergies, asthma, congestive heart failure, gastrointestinal disorders (especially colitis associated with the use of antibiotics), or impaired kidney function.

Amoxicillin/Potassium Clavulanate

BRAND NAME
Augmentin

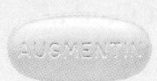

Augmentin 500/125 mg
(SMITHKLINE BEECHAM)

▶ Drug Class: Penicillin antibiotic combination

▶ Available in: Tablets, chewable tablets, oral suspension

▶ Available OTC? No

▶ As Generic? No

Side Effects

SERIOUS
Irregular, rapid, or labored breathing, lightheadedness or sudden fainting, seizures, joint pain, fever, severe abdominal pain and cramping with watery or bloody stools, severe allergic reaction (marked by sudden swelling of the lips, tongue, face, or throat; breathing difficulty; skin rash, itching, or hives), unusual bleeding or bruising, yellowish tinge to eyes or skin. Call your doctor immediately.

COMMON
Rash, mild diarrhea, nausea, vomiting, headache, vaginal discharge and itching, pain or white patches in the mouth or on the tongue.

LESS COMMON
Weakness, fatigue.

PRINCIPAL USES
To treat a variety of bacterial infections, including those of the sinuses and middle ear, skin and soft tissues, genitourinary tract, and the respiratory tract. The medication is effective only against infections caused by bacteria, not against those caused by viruses, fungi, or other microorganisms.

HOW THE DRUG WORKS
Amoxicillin blocks the formation of bacterial cell walls, rendering bacteria unable to multiply and spread. Clavulanate enhances the effectiveness of amoxicillin by inhibiting the activity of a specific enzyme (beta-lactamase) produced by certain drug-resistant strains of bacteria.

DOSAGE
Tablets— Adults and children more than 88 lbs: 250 to 500 mg of amoxicillin with 125 mg of clavulanate every 8 hours. Children up to 88 lbs: 6.7 to 13.3 mg of amoxicillin with 1.7 to 3.3 mg of clavulanate per 2.2 lbs (1 kg) of body weight every 8 hours. Chewable tablets and oral suspension— Adults and children more than 88 lbs: 250 to 500 mg of amoxicillin with 62.5 to 125 mg of clavulanate every 8 hours. Children up to 88 lbs: 6.7 to 13.3 mg of amoxicillin with 1.7 to 3.3 mg of clavulanate per 2.2 lbs (1 kg) of body weight every 8 hours. Newer dosage for adults: 875 mg of amoxicillin with 125 mg of clavulanate twice a day.

ONSET OF EFFECT
1 to 2 hours.

DURATION OF ACTION
6 to 8 hours.

DIETARY ADVICE
Best taken on an empty stomach, but may be taken with food to minimize stomach irritation or diarrhea.

STORAGE
Store in a tightly sealed container away from heat and direct light. Keep the liquid form refrigerated, but do not allow it to freeze.

IF YOU MISS A DOSE
Take it as soon as you remember unless it is almost time for the next dose. In that case, skip the missed dose and take the next one. Do not double the next dose.

STOPPING THE DRUG
Take this medication as prescribed for the full treatment period, even if you begin to feel better before the scheduled end of therapy.

PROLONGED USE
Prolonged use can make you more susceptible to bacterial or fungal infections (such as yeast infections).

PRECAUTIONS
Over 60: No special problems are expected.

Driving and Hazardous Work: Do not drive or engage in hazardous work until you determine how the medicine affects you.

Alcohol: No special precautions are necessary.

Pregnancy: Limited studies have found no evidence of birth defects. Consult your doctor if you are pregnant or plan to become pregnant.

Breast Feeding: Amoxicillin/clavulanate may pass into breast milk and cause problems in the nursing infant; avoid use while breast feeding.

Infants and Children: No special problems are expected.

Special Concerns: Those who are prone to asthma, hay fever, hives, or allergies may be more likely to have an allergic reaction to a penicillin antibiotic. If severe diarrhea occurs as a side effect of this drug, do not take antidiarrheal medications; call your doctor for advice instead. This drug can cause false results on some urine sugar tests for patients who have diabetes.

OVERDOSE
Symptoms: Severe diarrhea, nausea, unusual excitability, seizures, or vomiting.

What to Do: Call your doctor, emergency medical services (EMS), or the nearest poison control center immediately.

DRUG INTERACTIONS
Consult your doctor for advice if you are taking erythromycins, disulfiram, anticoagulants, tetracyclines, oral contraceptives, or gout drugs.

FOOD INTERACTIONS
None expected.

DISEASE INTERACTIONS
Consult your doctor if you have a history of allergies, asthma, congestive heart failure, gastrointestinal disorders (especially colitis associated with the use of antibiotics), or impaired kidney function.

Amphetamine

BRAND NAME
Amphetamine is available in generic form only.

▶ Drug Class: Central nervous system stimulant/ amphetamine

▶ Available in: Tablets

▶ Available OTC? No

▶ As Generic? Yes

Side Effects

SERIOUS
Irregular heartbeat, chest pain, increased blood pressure, skin rash, uncontrollable movements of arms and legs, mental changes, unusual weakness, very high fever. Call your doctor immediately.

COMMON
Mood changes, insomnia, drowsiness, restlessness.

LESS COMMON
Blurred vision, constipation, diarrhea, loss of appetite, headache, increased sweating, stomach cramps or pain, nausea or vomiting, changes in sexual desire or decreased sexual ability.

PRINCIPAL USES
To treat narcolepsy and attention-deficit hyperactivity disorder (ADHD) in children and adults.

HOW THE DRUG WORKS
Amphetamine activates nerve cells in the brain and spinal cord to increase motor activity and alertness and lessen drowsiness and fatigue.

DOSAGE
For narcolepsy— Adults: 5 to 60 mg a day, 1 to 3 times a day; not to exceed 60 mg a day. Teenagers: 5 mg twice a day. Children ages 6 to 12: 2.5 mg twice a day. For ADHD— Adults and children age 6 and older: 5 to 40 mg a day, 1 to 3 times a day; not to exceed 40 mg a day. Children ages 3 to 6: 2.5 mg once a day.

ONSET OF EFFECT
Variable.

DURATION OF ACTION
Variable.

DIETARY ADVICE
Swallow with liquid. May be taken with or without food. Avoid caffeine-containing beverages like tea, coffee, and some carbonated colas. Avoid acidic foods rich in vitamin C, such as fruit juices and other citrus products. Avoid vitamin C tablets.

STORAGE
Store in a tightly sealed container away from heat, moisture, and direct light.

IF YOU MISS A DOSE
If dosage is once daily, take your missed dose as soon as you remember, unless your bedtime is within the next 6 hours. If so, do not take the missed dose. Take your next dose at the proper time and resume your regular schedule. Do not double the next dose. If dosage is more than once daily, take your missed dose as soon as you remember, unless the time for your next scheduled dose is within the next 2 hours. If so, do not take the missed dose. Take your next dose at the proper time and resume your regular schedule. Do not double the next dose.

STOPPING THE DRUG
Take amphetamine as prescribed for the full treatment period, even if you begin to feel better before the scheduled end of therapy. The decision to stop taking the drug should be made by your doctor. The doctor may decrease your dosage gradually to reduce the possibility of withdrawal symptoms.

PROLONGED USE
Amphetamines may be habit-forming, and prolonged use may increase the risk of dependency.

PRECAUTIONS
Over 60: Adverse reactions may be more likely and more severe in older patients.

Driving and Hazardous Work: Do not drive or engage in hazardous work until you determine how the medicine affects you.

Alcohol: Avoid alcohol.

Pregnancy: Amphetamine taken during pregnancy may cause premature delivery, low birth weight, and birth defects. Discuss with your doctor the relative risks and benefits of using this drug while pregnant.

Breast Feeding: Amphetamine passes into breast milk; avoid or discontinue use while nursing. Consult your doctor for specific advice.

Infants and Children: Long-term amphetamine use by children can affect behavior and growth. Discuss the use of the drug and its relative risks and benefits with your doctor.

OVERDOSE
Symptoms: Extreme degrees of restlessness, agitation, bizarre behavior; panic; rapid breathing; confusion; high fever; hallucinations; seizures; coma.

What to Do: Call your doctor, emergency medical services (EMS), or the nearest poison control center immediately.

DRUG INTERACTIONS
The following drugs may interact with amphetamine. Consult your doctor for specific advice if you are taking tricyclic antidepressants, caffeine, beta-blockers, digitalis drugs, central nervous system stimulants, meperidine, MAO inhibitors, sympathomimetic agents, or thyroid hormones.

FOOD INTERACTIONS
Citrus juices and caffeinated beverages and foods may interact with amphetamine.

DISEASE INTERACTIONS
Caution is advised when taking amphetamine. Consult your doctor if you have any of the following: advanced blood vessel disease, heart disease, hyperthyroidism, high blood pressure, severe anxiety, Tourette's syndrome, glaucoma, or a history of drug abuse.

Amphetamine/Dextroamphetamine

BRAND NAME
Adderall

▶ Drug Class: Central nervous system stimulant/ amphetamine

▶ Available in: Tablets

▶ Available OTC? No

▶ As Generic? No

Side Effects

SERIOUS
Irregular heartbeat, chest pain, increased blood pressure, skin rash, uncontrollable movements of arms and legs, mental changes, unusual weakness, very high fever. Call your doctor immediately.

COMMON
Mood changes, insomnia, drowsiness, restlessness.

LESS COMMON
Blurred vision, constipation, diarrhea, loss of appetite, headache, increased sweating, stomach cramps or pain, nausea or vomiting, changes in sexual desire or decreased sexual ability.

PRINCIPAL USES
To treat narcolepsy and attention-deficit hyperactivity disorder (ADHD) in children and adults.

HOW THE DRUG WORKS
Amphetamine and dextro-amphetamine activate nerve cells in the brain and spinal cord to increase motor activity and alertness and lessen drowsiness and fatigue. In hyperactivity disorders and narcolepsy, amphetamines improve mental focus and the ability to stay awake or concentrate.

DOSAGE
For narcolepsy— Adults: 5 to 60 mg a day, 1 to 3 times a day; not to exceed 60 mg a day. Teenagers: To start, 10 mg a day. Children ages 6 to 12: To start, 5 mg a day. To treat ADHD— Children age 6 and older: To start, 5 mg, 1 or 2 times a day. Children ages 3 to 6: To start, 2.5 mg a day.

ONSET OF EFFECT
Within 30 to 45 minutes.

DURATION OF ACTION
Adults: 8 to 12 hours. Children: 6 to 10 hours.

DIETARY ADVICE
Take it with liquid 30 to 45 minutes before meals. Avoid caffeine-containing beverages like tea, coffee, and some carbonated colas. Avoid acidic foods rich in vitamin C, such as fruit juices and other citrus products. Avoid vitamin C tablets.

STORAGE
Store in a tightly sealed container away from heat, moisture, and direct light.

IF YOU MISS A DOSE
If dosage is once daily, take your missed dose as soon as you remember, unless your bedtime is within the next 6 hours. If so, do not take the missed dose. Take your next dose at the proper time and resume your regular schedule. Do not double the next dose. If dosage is more than once daily, take your missed dose as soon as you remember, unless the time for your next scheduled dose is within the next 2 hours. If so, do not take the missed dose. Take your next dose at the proper time and resume your regular schedule. Do not double the next dose.

STOPPING THE DRUG
The decision to stop taking the drug should be made in consultation with your doctor. The doctor may decrease your dosage gradually to reduce the possibility of withdrawal symptoms.

PROLONGED USE
Amphetamines may be habit-forming, and prolonged use may increase the risk of dependency.

PRECAUTIONS
Over 60: Adverse reactions may be more likely and more severe.

Driving and Hazardous Work: Do not drive or engage in hazardous work until you determine how the medicine affects you.

Alcohol: Avoid alcohol.

Pregnancy: Amphetamines taken during pregnancy may cause premature delivery, low birth weight, and birth defects. Discuss with your doctor the relative risks and benefits of using this drug while pregnant.

Breast Feeding: Amphetamine passes into breast milk; avoid or discontinue use while nursing.

Infants and Children: Not recommended for use by children under age 3.

Special Concerns: Take only as directed and do not increase the dose on your own. Remember that fatigue, excessive drowsiness, sleepiness, or depression while taking stimulants may mean an emergency situation is developing. Difficulty sleeping may be improved by taking the last scheduled dose several hours before bedtime.

OVERDOSE
Symptoms: Extreme restlessness, agitation, or bizarre behavior; panic; rapid breathing; confusion; high fever; hallucinations; seizures; coma.

What to Do: Call your doctor, emergency medical services (EMS), or the nearest poison control center immediately.

DRUG INTERACTIONS
The following drugs may interact with amphetamines. Consult your doctor for specific advice if you are taking tricyclic antidepressants, caffeine, beta-blockers, digitalis drugs, central nervous system stimulants, meperidine, MAO inhibitors, sympathomimetic agents (such as ephedrine, phenylephrine, and diethylpropion), or thyroid hormones.

FOOD INTERACTIONS
Citrus juices and caffeinated beverages and foods may interact with this drug.

DISEASE INTERACTIONS
Consult your doctor if you have any of the following: advanced blood vessel disease, heart disease, hyperthyroidism, high blood pressure, severe anxiety, Tourette's syndrome, glaucoma, or a history of drug abuse.

Amphotericin B

BRAND NAMES
Abelcet, AmBisome, Amphocin, Fungizone, Fungizone Intravenous

▶ Drug Class: Antifungal

▶ Available in: Cream, lotion, ointment, injection

▶ Available OTC? No

▶ As Generic? Yes

Side Effects

SERIOUS
Topical: Redness, burning, itching, or irritation not present prior to therapy. Injection into a vein: Headache, fever, muscle pain or cramps, fatigue, chills, heartbeat irregularities, seizures, increased or decreased urine output, nausea, vomiting, pain at site of injection, change in or blurred vision, skin rash or itching, breathing difficulties, tightness in chest, unusual bleeding or bruising, sore throat. Injection into the spinal column: Urination difficulties, change in or blurred vision, numbness, tingling, fatigue, or weakness.

COMMON
Topical: None reported. Injection: Mild headache, diarrhea, indigestion, stomach pain, loss of appetite, mild nausea or vomiting.

LESS COMMON
Topical (cream only): Dry skin. Injection into the spinal column: Severe nausea or vomiting, dizziness or lightheadedness, headache, pain in the back, leg, or neck.

PRINCIPAL USES
To treat serious and potentially life-threatening fungal infections.

HOW THE DRUG WORKS
Amphotericin B prevents fungal organisms from producing vital substances required for growth and function. This drug is effective only for infections caused by fungal organisms. It will not work for bacterial or viral infections.

DOSAGE
Topical forms: Apply a liberal amount to the affected area 2 to 4 times a day, according to doctor's instructions. It should be applied externally only. Injection: Dose is determined by your doctor based on many factors.

ONSET OF EFFECT
Topical: Not applicable. Injection: Immediate.

DURATION OF ACTION
Injection and topical: Unknown.

DIETARY ADVICE
Increase fluid intake to 2 to 3 quarts a day.

STORAGE
Can be stored at room temperature for 24 hours or in the refrigerator for 7 days in a tightly sealed container away from heat, moisture, and direct light. Keep it from freezing.

IF YOU MISS A DOSE
Tell your doctor if you miss an injected dose. If you miss a topical dose, apply it as soon as you remember, then resume your regular dosage schedule.

STOPPING THE DRUG
Take it as prescribed for the full treatment period, even if you begin to feel better before the scheduled end of therapy. The decision to stop taking the drug should be made by your doctor.

PROLONGED USE
Topical forms are generally prescribed for short-term therapy (1 to 4 weeks). Consult your doctor if your condition does not improve, or worsens, within 1 to 2 weeks. The injection may be prescribed for up to 12 months. Your doctor will determine the proper length of therapy.

PRECAUTIONS
Over 60: Adverse reactions may be more likely and more severe in older patients.

Driving and Hazardous Work: Avoid such activities until you determine how the medicine affects you.

Alcohol: Avoid alcohol.

Pregnancy: Adequate studies of the use of amphotericin B use during pregnancy have not been done. Consult your doctor for specific advice if you are pregnant or plan to become pregnant.

Breast Feeding: Amphotericin B may pass into breast milk; caution is advised. Consult your doctor for advice.

Infants and Children: No special problems are expected.

Special Concerns: Use gloves when applying the topical form of amphotericin B, as it can stain or discolor skin and clothing. The stain may be removed by hand washing with warm water and soap. Do not use an airtight dressing to cover the topical form, since this may increase the risk of infection.

OVERDOSE
Symptoms: Heartbeat irregularities; breathing difficulty.

What to Do: Treatment should be discontinued. Call your doctor, emergency medical services (EMS), or the nearest poison control center immediately.

DRUG INTERACTIONS
Consult your doctor for specific advice if you are taking corticosteroids, corticotropin, digitalis drugs, potassium-sparing diuretics, bone marrow depressants, nephrotoxic medications, or other topical prescription or over-the-counter medications. Also consult your doctor if you are undergoing radiation therapy.

FOOD INTERACTIONS
No known food interactions.

DISEASE INTERACTIONS
Caution is advised when taking amphotericin B. Consult your doctor if you have any other medical problem, especially kidney disease.

Ampicillin

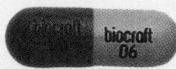

Generic 500 mg
(BIOCRAFT)

Additional photographs

▶ Drug Class: Penicillin antibiotic

▶ Available in: Capsules, oral suspension, injection (available only in hospitals)

▶ Available OTC? No

▶ As Generic? Yes

Side Effects

SERIOUS
Irregular, rapid, or labored breathing, light-headedness or sudden fainting, joint pain, fever, severe abdominal pain and cramping with watery or bloody stools, severe allergic reaction (marked by sudden swelling of the lips, tongue, face, or throat; breathing difficulty; skin rash, itching, or hives), unusual bleeding or bruising, yellowish tinge to eyes or skin. Call your doctor immediately.

COMMON
Mild rash, mild diarrhea, nausea, vomiting, headache, vaginal discharge and itching, pain or white patches in the mouth or on the tongue.

LESS COMMON
Diminished urine output, chills, weakness, fatigue, seizures.

PRINCIPAL USES
Oral ampicillin is used to treat infections of the skin, urinary tract, and respiratory tract (sinuses, tonsils, and lung) caused by certain bacteria known to be susceptible to this antibiotic. Injectable ampicillin is used to treat more serious infections in hospitalized patients.

HOW THE DRUG WORKS
Ampicillin blocks the formation of bacterial cell walls, rendering bacteria unable to multiply and spread.

DOSAGE
Adults or children weighing more than 44 lbs (20 kg): 250 to 500 mg, 4 times a day. The dosage for smaller children must be adjusted according to weight.

ONSET OF EFFECT
Within 2 hours of oral dose.

DURATION OF ACTION
6 to 8 hours with oral dose.

DIETARY ADVICE
Should be taken on an empty stomach with plenty of water.

STORAGE
Store in a tightly sealed container away from heat and direct light. Keep the suspension refrigerated, but do not allow it to freeze.

IF YOU MISS A DOSE
Take it as soon as you remember. If it is within 60 to 90 minutes of the next dose, skip the missed dose and resume your regular dosage schedule. Do not double the next dose.

STOPPING THE DRUG
Take it as prescribed for the full treatment period, even if you begin to feel better before the scheduled end of therapy. Stopping the drug prematurely may slow your recovery or lead to a rebound infection, also known as superinfection, in which the heartier strains of bacteria survive and multiply, leading to a more serious and drug-resistant infection.

PROLONGED USE
Therapy with ampicillin is usually completed within 7 to 10 days. Prolonged use may promote infection by bacteria resistant to the medication's effects (superinfection).

PRECAUTIONS
Over 60: No special problems are expected.

Driving and Hazardous Work: No problems are expected.

Alcohol: No interactions are expected, but alcohol may dampen the immune system's response against infection and may increase the risk of stomach upset when taking this drug.

Pregnancy: Ampicillin may be used during pregnancy under certain conditions. Consult your doctor for guidelines.

Breast Feeding: Ampicillin may pass into breast milk and cause problems in the nursing infant; avoid use while nursing.

Infants and Children: No special problems are expected.

Special Concerns: If severe diarrhea occurs as a side effect of this drug, do not take antidiarrheal medications; call your doctor. Oral contraceptives may not be effective while you are taking ampicillin; consider other methods of birth control. Those who are prone to asthma, hay fever, hives, or allergies may be more likely to have an allergic reaction to a penicillin antibiotic.

OVERDOSE
Symptoms: Severe nausea, vomiting, diarrhea, muscle spasticity, seizures.

What to Do: Call your doctor, emergency medical services (EMS), or the nearest poison control center immediately.

DRUG INTERACTIONS
Consult your doctor for specific advice if you are taking aminoglycosides, ACE inhibitors, diuretics, potassium supplements or potassium-containing medications, anticoagulants or other anticlotting drugs, nonsteroidal anti-inflammatory drugs, sulfinpyrazone, cholestyramine, colestipol, oral contraceptives, methotrexate, probenecid, allopurinol, or rifampin.

FOOD INTERACTIONS
Acidic fruits or juices can interfere with this drug's therapeutic effect.

DISEASE INTERACTIONS
Consult your doctor if you have a history of allergies, asthma, congestive heart failure, gastrointestinal disorders (especially colitis associated with the use of antibiotics), infectious mononucleosis, or impaired kidney function.

Ampicillin Sodium/Sulbactam Sodium

BRAND NAME
Unasyn

▶ Drug Class: Penicillin antibiotic

▶ Available in: Injection (available primarily in hospitals and nursing facilities)

▶ Available OTC? No

▶ As Generic? No

Side Effects

SERIOUS
Irregular, rapid, or labored breathing, lightheadedness or sudden fainting, joint pain, fever, severe abdominal pain and cramping with watery or bloody stools, severe allergic reaction (marked by sudden swelling of the lips, tongue, face, or throat; breathing difficulty; skin rash, itching, or hives), unusual bleeding or bruising, yellowish tinge to eyes or skin. Call your doctor immediately.

COMMON
Mild rash, mild diarrhea, nausea, vomiting, headache, vaginal discharge and itching, pain or white patches in the mouth or on the tongue, pain at the site of injection.

LESS COMMON
Diminished urine output, chills, weakness, fatigue.

PRINCIPAL USES
Ampicillin sodium/sulbactam sodium is used to treat moderately severe bacterial infections requiring hospitalization. These infections are frequently caused by bacteria that are likely to be resistant to penicillin and not treatable with oral antibiotics alone.

HOW THE DRUG WORKS
Ampicillin blocks the formation of bacterial cell walls, rendering bacteria unable to multiply and spread; sulbactam is added to protect ampicillin from the effects of a destructive enzyme (betalactamase) produced by certain drug-resistant strains of bacteria.

DOSAGE
Adults: 1.5 to 3 g injected into a muscle or vein every 6 hours. Children age 1 and older: 300 mg per 2.2 lbs (1 kg) of body weight per day into a vein in divided doses every 6 hours.

ONSET OF EFFECT
Immediate with intravenous injection; unknown for intramuscular injection.

DURATION OF ACTION
Unknown.

DIETARY ADVICE
No special restrictions.

STORAGE
Not applicable.

IF YOU MISS A DOSE
Not applicable; the dosage schedule is determined by a doctor or other health care professional.

STOPPING THE DRUG
The decision to stop treatment with this drug will be made by your doctor.

PROLONGED USE
Therapy with ampicillin sodium/sulbactam sodium is usually completed within 7 to 14 days. Infections in hospitalized patients may be more serious and can respond unpredictably to treatment. But treatment may also result in rapid improvement, and your doctor may stop intravenous or intramuscular ampicillin sodium/sulbactam sodium earlier than 7 to 14 days and begin oral therapy with another appropriate antibiotic in preparation for your discharge.

PRECAUTIONS
Over 60: Adverse reactions may be more likely and more severe in older patients.

Driving and Hazardous Work: Not applicable; therapy with this drug generally requires hospitalization.

Alcohol: Avoid alcohol.

Pregnancy: Adequate studies of the use of penicillin antibiotics during pregnancy have not been done. Consult your doctor concerning the use of ampicillin sodium/sulbactam sodium if you are pregnant.

Breast Feeding: Avoid or discontinue the use of ampicillin sodium/sulbactam sodium while nursing.

Infants and Children: This drug is not recommended for infants and children under age 1.

Special Concerns: Anyone who has had a prior allergic reaction to penicillin or any penicillin antibiotic should not take this drug. Those who are prone to asthma, hay fever, hives, or allergies are at increased risk of having an allergic reaction to it.

OVERDOSE
Symptoms: Seizures may occur with very high doses; overdose is nonetheless unlikely.

What to Do: Call your doctor or emergency medical services (EMS) immediately if you suspect an overdose.

DRUG INTERACTIONS
Consult your doctor for specific advice if you are taking aminoglycosides, ACE inhibitors, diuretics, potassium supplements or potassium-containing medications, anticoagulants or other anticlotting drugs, nonsteroidal anti-inflammatory drugs, sulfinpyrazone, cholestyramine, colestipol, oral contraceptives, methotrexate, probenecid, allopurinol, or rifampin.

FOOD INTERACTIONS
No known food interactions.

DISEASE INTERACTIONS
Consult your doctor if you have a history of allergies, asthma, bleeding disorders (such as hemophilia), congestive heart failure, gastrointestinal disorders (especially colitis associated with the use of antibiotics), infectious mononucleosis, or impaired kidney function.

Amprenavir

▶ Drug Class: Antiviral/protease inhibitor

▶ Available in: Capsules, oral solution

▶ Available OTC? No

▶ As Generic? No

Side Effects

SERIOUS
Severe rash or moderate rash with other symptoms. Call your doctor immediately. High blood sugar (diabetes) has occurred in patients taking drugs of this class, although a cause-and-effect relationship has not been established. Call your doctor if you develop increased thirst or excessive urination.

COMMON
Nausea, vomiting, abdominal pain, rash, diarrhea.

LESS COMMON
Taste disorders, numbness, tingling, prickling sensation, depression.

PRINCIPAL USES
To treat advanced HIV (human immunodeficiency virus) infection and AIDS (acquired immunodeficiency syndrome), usually in combination with other drugs. While not a cure for HIV infection, this drug may suppress the replication of the virus and delay the progression of the disease.

HOW THE DRUG WORKS
Amprenavir blocks the activity of a viral protease, an enzyme that is needed by HIV to reproduce. Blocking the protease causes HIV to make copies that cannot infect new cells.

DOSAGE
Capsules— Adults and children age 13 to 16: 1200 mg (8 capsules) 2 times a day, in combination with other antiretroviral drugs. Oral solution— Recommended for children age 4 and older: Consult pediatrician for appropriate dosage. The capsules and the oral solution are not interchangeable. Do not change forms without consulting your doctor.

ONSET OF EFFECT
Unknown. With most antiretroviral drugs, an early response can be seen within the first few days of therapy, but the maximum effect may take 12 to 16 weeks.

DURATION OF ACTION
Unknown.

DIETARY ADVICE
Amprenavir can be taken with or without food. However, taking it with a meal high in fat could reduce the absorption of the drug from the intestine.

STORAGE
Store in a tightly sealed container away from heat, moisture, and direct light. Do not refrigerate.

IF YOU MISS A DOSE
If you miss a dose, take it as soon as you remember up to 4 hours late. If more than 4 hours, wait for the next scheduled dose. Do not double the next dose.

STOPPING THE DRUG
The decision to stop taking the drug should be made in consultation with your physician.

PROLONGED USE
See your doctor regularly for tests and examinations.

PRECAUTIONS
Over 60: It is not known whether amprenavir causes different or more severe side effects in older patients.

Driving and Hazardous Work: Do not drive or engage in hazardous work until you determine how the medicine affects you.

Alcohol: Avoid alcohol if liver function is impaired.

Pregnancy: Adequate studies of amprenavir use during pregnancy have not been done. There is no evidence that the drug will reduce the risk of transmitting the virus from the mother to the fetus.

Breast Feeding: It is unknown whether amprenavir passes into breast milk; however, to avoid transmitting the virus to an uninfected child, women infected with HIV should not breast feed.

Infants and Children: The safety and effectiveness of amprenavir have not been established for children under 4 years of age.

Special Concerns: Do not switch between the capsules and solution without consulting your doctor; the body

absorbs them at different rates. Taking amprenavir does not eliminate the risk of passing the AIDS virus to other persons. Take appropriate preventive measures.

OVERDOSE
Symptoms: No overdoses have been reported.

What to Do: If you suspect an overdose or if someone takes a much larger dose than prescribed, seek medical attention immediately.

DRUG INTERACTIONS
Amprenavir should not be used at the same time as astemizole, bepridil, dihydroergotamine, ergotamine, midazolam, triazolam, rifampin, oral contraceptives, and vitamin E supplements. Use extreme caution if you are taking amiodarone, systemic lidocaine, tricyclic antidepressants, quinidine, warfarin, sildenafil, phenobarbital, phenytoin, carbamazepine, statin (cholesterol-lowering) drugs, and the herb St. John's wort. Patients taking antacids or didanosine should take them at least one hour before or after amprenavir. Rifabutin dosage may have to be adjusted by your doctor. Consult your doctor if you are taking any other prescription or over-the-counter medications.

FOOD INTERACTIONS
Meals high in fat could reduce the absorption of amprenavir.

DISEASE INTERACTIONS
Consult your doctor for advice if you have any other medical condition, especially hemophilia. Use of amprenavir can cause complications in patients with diseases of the liver, which works to remove the drug from the body.

Amyl Nitrite

BRAND NAME
Amyl nitrite is available in generic form only.

▶ Drug Class: Nitrate

▶ Available in: Glass capsule

▶ Available OTC? No

▶ As Generic? Yes

Side Effects

SERIOUS
Shortness of breath, extreme dizziness or fainting, bluish appearance of lips, fingernails, and palms of hands, irregular heartbeat.

COMMON
Dizziness or lightheadedness, especially upon arising from a seated or lying position, rapid heartbeat and pulse, headache, restlessness, flushing in the face and neck. Such side effects tend to occur less frequently as your body adjusts to the medication. Contact your doctor if such symptoms do not subside quickly or if they interfere with your daily activities.

LESS COMMON
Unusual tiredness or weakness, skin rash.

PRINCIPAL USES
To prevent or relieve attacks of angina (chest pain associated with heart disease).

HOW THE DRUG WORKS
Amyl nitrite relaxes the smooth muscle of the blood vessels and increases the supply of blood and oxygen to the heart. It also reduces the heart's workload and demand for oxygen.

DOSAGE
No fixed schedule; take as needed. When angina attack occurs, break the protective cloth-covered glass capsule between your fingers and inhale 1 to 6 times while seated. If inhaling 2 capsules in 10 minutes does not bring relief, seek medical assistance immediately. When inhaling 2 capsules, wait 3 to 5 minutes between capsules.

ONSET OF EFFECT
30 seconds to 5 minutes.

DURATION OF ACTION
3 to 5 minutes.

DIETARY ADVICE
Amyl nitrite can be taken without regard to diet.

STORAGE
Store away from direct light and heat. Heat may cause the medicine to break down. Do not store it in the kitchen, because amyl nitrite is flammable. Keep refrigerated, but do not allow it to freeze.

IF YOU MISS A DOSE
Not applicable.

STOPPING THE DRUG
Consult your doctor before stopping use.

PROLONGED USE
Prolonged, too-frequent use can lead to tolerance of the drug, reducing its effectiveness. Notify your doctor if you experience an increase in angina attacks.

PRECAUTIONS
Over 60: Adverse reactions and side effects may be more common and severe in older persons.

Driving and Hazardous Work: The use of amyl nitrite may impair your ability to perform such tasks safely.

Alcohol: Alcohol can increase the lightheadedness caused by amyl nitrite and may cause a serious drop in blood pressure. Consult your doctor for specific advice.

Pregnancy: Use is not recommended during pregnancy because of the danger to the unborn baby.

Breast Feeding: Amyl nitrite may pass into breast milk; caution is advised. Consult your doctor for advice.

Infants and Children: Safety and effectiveness have not been determined. Consult your pediatrician.

Special Concerns: Before use, extinguish all tobacco products and stay away from open flames, since amyl nitrite is highly flammable. Since dizziness is common after taking amyl nitrite, it is advisable to sit or lie down rather than remain standing while taking the medication. For relief of headache (very common following use of amyl nitrate), take acetaminophen.

OVERDOSE
Symptoms: Blue lips, palms of hands, or fingernails; extreme dizziness, extreme headache or feeling of intense pressure in the head; fainting; shortness of breath; unusual weakness; weak and rapid heartbeat.

What to Do: Call your doctor, emergency medical services (EMS), or the nearest poison control center immediately.

DRUG INTERACTIONS
Consult your doctor for specific advice if you are taking drugs for high blood pressure, norepinephrine, or sympathomimetic drugs (such as ephedrine, phenylephrine, or epinephrine).

FOOD INTERACTIONS
No known food interactions.

DISEASE INTERACTIONS
Caution is advised when taking amyl nitrite. Consult your doctor if you have any of the following: severe anemia, recent head trauma, recent heart attack or brain hemorrhage, glaucoma, hyperthyroidism, or prior allergic reaction to nitrates.

BRAND NAME
Arimidex

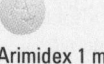

Arimidex 1 mg
(**AstraZeneca**)

▶ Drug Class: Antiestrogen;
antineoplastic (anticancer)
agent

▶ Available in: Tablets

▶ Available OTC? No

▶ As Generic? No

Side Effects

SERIOUS
No serious side effects
from therapy with anas-
trozole have been
reported.

COMMON
Headache, diarrhea, nau-
sea, hot flashes, back
pain, weakness, and a
feeling of reduced energy
(asthenia).

LESS COMMON
Dizziness; chest pain; tingling or numbness in the
extremities (paresthesia);
weight gain; abdominal
pain; vaginal itching, dryness, and occasionally
bleeding; swelling of fingers and skin around the
eyes; rash; formation of
blood clots.

PRINCIPAL USES
Anastrozole is given for
breast cancer chemotherapy.

HOW THE DRUG WORKS
The growth of some breast
tumors is stimulated by
estradiol, a hormone that is
produced by adult females.
Anastrozole is not directly
toxic to cancer cells but
rather reduces blood levels
of estradiol in the body and
thus inhibits the growth of
such tumors.

DOSAGE
1 mg once a day.

ONSET OF EFFECT
Unknown.

DURATION OF ACTION
Unknown.

DIETARY ADVICE
Maintain adequate food and
fluid intake. Calorie, protein,
and vitamin needs increase
in patients with cancer.
Good nutrition is essential
to cope with the demands of
chemotherapy.

STORAGE
Store safely and securely
away from heat and light.

IF YOU MISS A DOSE
Anastrozole is prescribed
for once-daily use only. If
you are unable to take this
medication on a particular
day, skip the missed dose
and resume your regularly
scheduled dose the following day. Do not double the
next dose.

STOPPING THE DRUG
This medication is used to
treat a chronic condition.
You may need to remain on
this medication for an
extended period, and you
should take the drug
exactly as prescribed
throughout the course of
treatment. The decision to
stop the drug must be made
in consultation with your

doctor. Do not stop taking
anastrozole on your own,
even if you are feeling better. Contact your doctor if
you have any questions
about the way you feel
while taking anastrozole, or
if you think that you are
experiencing a side effect
that would require discontinuation of the drug.

PROLONGED USE
There is no standard duration of therapy with anastrozole, although you can
expect to remain on it for
several weeks in order to
determine if it is effective.
Your doctor will determine
whether your response to
the drug is satisfactory or
not, and will recommend
the continuation or discontinuation of therapy.

PRECAUTIONS
Over 60: Adverse reactions
may be more likely and
more severe in older
patients.

**Driving and Hazardous
Work:** The use of anastrozole may impair your ability
to drive or operate machinery safely or perform hazardous work.

Alcohol: Avoid alcohol
while taking this drug.

Pregnancy: Anastrozole
must not be used in preg-
nant women. Although anastrozole is not generally
prescribed for premeno-
pausal women, it is important that patients be sure
they are not pregnant
before starting treatment
with this drug.

Breast Feeding: Use of
this drug is not recom-
mended while breast feed-
ing; the benefits must
clearly outweigh potential
risks. Consult your doctor
for advice.

Infants and Children:
Use of anastrozole is not
approved for infants and
children.

Special Concerns:
Patients with cancer are
very often weakened by
their illness, by poor nutrition, and by the effects of
chemotherapy, radiation,
and surgery. Such patients
are more likely to experience undesirable side
effects of a medication. In
addition, these side effects
may be more pronounced.
Follow all medication directions carefully.

OVERDOSE
Symptoms: No cases of
overdose with anastrozole
have been reported.

What to Do: An overdose
is unlikely; however, if you
have any reason to suspect
that one has occurred, call
emergency medical services
(EMS) to receive evaluation
and treatment in the closest
emergency facility.

DRUG INTERACTIONS
No significant interactions.

FOOD INTERACTIONS
No significant interactions.

DISEASE INTERACTIONS
No significant interactions.

Aspirin

Generic 325 mg
(LNK)

Additional photographs

▶ Drug Class: Nonsteroidal
anti-inflammatory drug
(NSAID); analgesic;
anticoagulant

▶ Available in: Tablets,
capsules

▶ Available OTC? Yes

▶ As Generic? Yes

Side Effects

SERIOUS
Vomiting, agitation,
extreme fatigue, confu-
sion; allergic reaction
causing troubled breath-
ing, redness of face, itching, swelling of face, lips,
or eyelids. These are
symptoms of Reye's syn-
drome, a rare but serious
disorder that is most
likely to affect patients
under the age of 16. Seek
emergency medical atten-
tion immediately.

COMMON
Stomach upset, rash,
nausea, ringing in the
ears.

LESS COMMON
Insomnia.

PRINCIPAL USES
For mild to moderate everyday pain and inflammation;
to reduce fever; to prevent
the formation of blood clots,
a primary cause of heart
attack, stroke, and other circulatory problems; to ease
the inflammation, joint pain,
and stiffness associated with
arthritis.

HOW THE DRUG WORKS
Nonsteroidal anti-inflammatory drugs (NSAIDs) such
as aspirin inhibit the release
of chemicals in the body
called prostaglandins, which
play a role in inflammation,
though it is unknown
exactly how they exert their
pain-relieving, fever-reduc-
ing, and anti-inflammatory
effects.

DOSAGE
For pain or fever: 325 to
650 mg every 4 hours as
needed. For prevention of
blood clots: 80 to 100 mg
daily or every other day.
For arthritis: 3,600 to 5,400
mg daily in divided doses.

ONSET OF EFFECT
30 minutes.

DURATION OF ACTION
For pain relief, up to 4
hours.

DIETARY ADVICE
Swallow aspirin with food or
a full glass of water to
lessen stomach irritation.

STORAGE
Store in a tightly sealed container away from heat and
direct light.

IF YOU MISS A DOSE
For pain and fever, take a
missed dose as soon as you
remember, then wait 4
hours for your next dose.
For arthritis, take the
aspirin as soon as you
remember up to 2 hours
late, then return to your
regular schedule.

STOPPING THE DRUG
For pain and fever, stop
when relief is achieved. For
arthritis and blood clotting,
consult your doctor about
stopping.

PROLONGED USE
Talk to your doctor about
the need for medical examinations or laboratory tests if
you must take aspirin regularly for a prolonged period.

PRECAUTIONS
Over 60: Gastrointestinal
bleeding and irritation are
more likely to occur in
older persons.

**Driving and Hazardous
Work:** The use of aspirin
should not impair your ability to perform such tasks
safely.

Alcohol: Alcohol intake
should be limited because it
increases the risk of stomach irritation and bleeding.

Pregnancy: Do not use
aspirin during the last 3
months of pregnancy unless
prescribed by your doctor.

Breast Feeding: Aspirin
passes into breast milk.
Avoid it or do not nurse.

Infants and Children:
Do not give aspirin to children under age 16 unless
your doctor instructs otherwise, since it may cause a
very rare but life-threatening condition known as
Reye's syndrome.

OVERDOSE
Symptoms: Nausea, disorientation, seizures, vomiting,
rapid breathing, fever.

What to Do: Call your
doctor, emergency medical
services (EMS), or the
nearest poison control center immediately.

DRUG INTERACTIONS
Consult your doctor before
taking aspirin if you currently take a blood pressure
medication, a medication for
gout, an arthritis drug, an
anticoagulant such as warfarin, a diabetes medication,
a steroid, or an antiseizure
medication.

FOOD INTERACTIONS
No known adverse food
interactions. Taking aspirin
with caffeine-containing
foods or beverages may
actually enhance the medicine's pain-relieving effects.

DISEASE INTERACTIONS
Consult your doctor about
taking aspirin if you have
asthma, a bleeding disorder,
congestive heart failure, diabetes mellitus, gout, hemophilia, high blood pressure,
kidney disease, liver disease, thyroid disease, or a
peptic ulcer.

▶ Drug Class: Nonsteroidal anti-inflammatory drug (NSAID); analgesic; antirheumatic

▶ Available in: Tablets

▶ Available OTC? Yes

▶ As Generic? No

Side Effects

SERIOUS
Vomiting, agitation, extreme fatigue, confusion; allergic reaction causing troubled breathing, redness of face, itching, swelling of face, lips, or eyelids. These are symptoms of Reye's syndrome, a rare but serious disorder that is most likely to affect patients under the age of 16. Seek emergency medical attention immediately.

COMMON
Stomach upset, rash, nausea, ringing in the ears.

LESS COMMON
Insomnia.

PRINCIPAL USES
For mild to moderate everyday pain and inflammation; to reduce fever; to ease the inflammation, joint pain, and stiffness associated with arthritis.

HOW THE DRUG WORKS
Aspirin appears to interfere with the production of prostaglandins, naturally occurring substances in the body that cause inflammation and make nerves more sensitive to pain impulses. Caffeine may enhance the effectiveness of pain relievers.

DOSAGE
Adults— For pain or fever: 325 to 650 mg every 4 hours as needed. For arthritis: 3,600 to 5,400 mg daily in divided doses. Children 9 years of age and older— For pain or fever: 325 to 400 mg every 4 hours as needed. For arthritis: 80 to 100 mg per 2.2 lbs (1 kg) of body weight a day in divided doses.

ONSET OF EFFECT
For pain, inflammation, or fever: within 30 minutes. For arthritis: May take 2 to 3 weeks to achieve maximum effect.

DURATION OF ACTION
For pain relief, up to 4 hours.

DIETARY ADVICE
Take with food or a full glass of water to lessen stomach irritation.

STORAGE
Store in a tightly sealed container away from heat, moisture, and direct light.

IF YOU MISS A DOSE
For pain and fever, take a missed dose as soon as you remember, then wait 4 hours for your next dose. For arthritis, take as soon as you remember up to 2 hours late, then return to your regular schedule.

STOPPING THE DRUG
For pain and fever, stop when relief is achieved. For arthritis, consult your doctor about stopping.

PROLONGED USE
Talk to your doctor about the need for medical examinations or laboratory tests if you must take this medication regularly for a prolonged period.

PRECAUTIONS
Over 60: Gastrointestinal bleeding and irritation are more likely to occur in older persons.

Driving and Hazardous Work: No special precautions are necessary.

Alcohol: Alcohol intake should be limited because it increases the risk of stomach irritation and bleeding.

Pregnancy: Do not use this drug during the last 3 months of pregnancy unless prescribed by your doctor.

Breast Feeding: Aspirin passes into breast milk. Avoid it or do not nurse.

Infants and Children: Do not give products that contain aspirin to children under age 16 unless your doctor instructs otherwise, since it may cause a very rare but life-threatening condition known as Reye's syndrome.

OVERDOSE
Symptoms: Nausea, disorientation, seizures, vomiting, rapid breathing, fever.

What to Do: Call your doctor, emergency medical services (EMS), or the nearest poison control center immediately.

DRUG INTERACTIONS
Consult your doctor before taking this drug if you currently take a blood pressure medication, a medication for gout, an arthritis drug, an anticoagulant such as warfarin, a diabetes medication, a steroid, or an antiseizure medication.

FOOD INTERACTIONS
No known interactions.

DISEASE INTERACTIONS
Consult your doctor about taking this drug if you have asthma, a bleeding disorder, congestive heart failure, diabetes mellitus, gout, hemophilia, high blood pressure, kidney disease, liver disease, thyroid disease, or a peptic ulcer.

Atenolol

BRAND NAME
Tenormin

Generic 100 mg
(MYLAN)

Additional photographs

▶ Drug Class: Beta-blocker

▶ Available in: Tablets (Injection is for hospital use only.)

▶ Available OTC? No

▶ As Generic? Yes

Side Effects

SERIOUS
Depression, shortness of breath, wheezing, slow heartbeat (especially less than 50 beats per minute), chest pain or tightness, swelling of the ankles, feet, and lower legs. If you experience such symptoms, stop taking atenolol and call your doctor immediately.

COMMON
Decreased sexual ability; decreased ability to engage in usual physical activities or exercise; dizziness or lightheadedness, especially when rising suddenly from a sitting or lying position; drowsiness, fatigue, or weakness; insomnia.

LESS COMMON
Anxiety, irritability; constipation; diarrhea; dry eyes; itching; nausea or vomiting; nightmares or intensely vivid dreams; numbness, tingling, or other unusual sensations in the fingers and toes; abdominal pain; nasal congestion.

PRINCIPAL USES
To treat mild to moderate high blood pressure and to treat angina; also used to prevent or control heartbeat irregularities (cardiac arrhythmias). The injectable form is used in hospitals to treat heart attack.

HOW THE DRUG WORKS
Atenolol slows the rate and force of contraction of the heart by blocking certain nerve impulses, thus reducing blood pressure. By modifying nerve impulses to the heart, the drug also helps to stabilize heart rhythm.

DOSAGE
50 to 100 mg, once a day. Smaller doses may be recommended for elderly patients or for those with impaired kidney function.

ONSET OF EFFECT
Oral: 1 to 2 hours; the full therapeutic effect may take 1 to 2 weeks. Injectable: Within 10 minutes.

DURATION OF ACTION
Up to 24 hours.

DIETARY ADVICE
Take atenolol on an empty stomach. Avoid alcohol and caffeine.

STORAGE
Store in a tightly sealed container away from heat and direct light.

IF YOU MISS A DOSE
Take it as soon as you remember. If it is within 4 hours of the next scheduled dose, skip the missed dose and resume your regular schedule. Do not double the next dose.

STOPPING THE DRUG
Suddenly stopping atenolol may cause serious health problems. Slow reduction of the dose over a period of 2 to 3 weeks is advised, under doctor's careful supervision.

PROLONGED USE
Therapy with atenolol may be lifelong; prolonged use may be associated with an increased risk of side effects.

PRECAUTIONS
Over 60: Adverse reactions may be more likely and more severe in older patients; a reduction in dosage may be warranted.

Driving and Hazardous Work: In rare cases atenolol may impair your ability to drive or operate machinery safely or perform hazardous work. Use caution, especially soon after beginning therapy.

Alcohol: Drink in careful moderation if at all. Alcohol may interact with the drug and cause a dangerous drop in blood pressure.

Pregnancy: Discuss with your doctor the relative risks and benefits of using this drug while pregnant.

Breast Feeding: Avoid or discontinue the use of atenolol while nursing.

Infants and Children: Proper dose will be determined by pediatrician.

Special Concerns: Use of the drug should be considered but one element of a comprehensive therapeutic program that includes weight control, smoking cessation, regular exercise, and a healthy low-salt, low-fat diet.

OVERDOSE
Symptoms: Slow heartbeat; severe dizziness, lightheadedness or fainting; rapid or irregular heartbeat; difficulty breathing; extreme weakness; seizures; confusion; coma.

What to Do: Call your doctor, emergency medical services (EMS), or the nearest poison control center immediately.

DRUG INTERACTIONS
Consult your doctor if you are taking amphetamines, oral antidiabetic agents, asthma medication (such as aminophylline or theophylline), calcium channel blockers, clonidine, guanabenz, halothane, allergy shots, insulin, MAO inhibitors, reserpine, or other beta-blockers.

FOOD INTERACTIONS
None known.

DISEASE INTERACTIONS
Atenolol should be used with caution in people with diabetes, especially insulin-dependent diabetes, since the drug may mask symptoms of hypoglycemia. Consult your doctor for specific advice if you have allergies or asthma, heart or blood vessel disease (including congestive heart failure and peripheral vascular disease), irregular (slow) heartbeat, hyperthyroidism, myasthenia gravis, psoriasis, respiratory problems such as bronchitis or emphysema, kidney or liver disease, or a history of mental depression.

Atenolol/Chlorthalidone

▶ Drug Class: Beta-blocker/diuretic

▶ Available in: Tablets

▶ Available OTC? No

▶ As Generic? Yes

Side Effects

SERIOUS
Mental depression; shortness of breath, wheezing; slow heartbeat (especially less than 50 beats per minute); chest pain or tightness; swelling of the ankles, feet, and lower legs. If you experience such symptoms, stop taking this drug and call your doctor immediately.

COMMON
Decreased sexual ability; decreased ability to engage in usual physical activities or exercise; dizziness or lightheadedness, especially when rising suddenly from a sitting or lying position; drowsiness, fatigue, or weakness; insomnia.

LESS COMMON
Anxiety, irritability; constipation; diarrhea; dry eyes; itching; nausea or vomiting; nightmares or intensely vivid dreams; numbness, tingling, or other unusual sensations in the fingers and toes; abdominal pain; visual disturbances.

PRINCIPAL USES
To treat high blood pressure with or without concurrent angina.

HOW THE DRUG WORKS
Atenolol slows the rate and force of contraction of the heart by blocking certain nerve impulses, thus reducing blood pressure. Chlorthalidone (a diuretic) increases the elimination of urine from the body. By reducing the overall fluid volume and excess sodium in the body, diuretics reduce blood volume and so reduce pressure within the blood vessels.

DOSAGE
Initial dose is 1 tablet a day (each tablet contains 50 mg atenolol and 25 mg chlorthalidone). The dose can be increased to 2 tablets a day.

ONSET OF EFFECT
Within 1 hour.

DURATION OF ACTION
24 hours.

DIETARY ADVICE
This drug can be taken with or without food, as instructed by your doctor.

STORAGE
Store in a tightly sealed container away from heat and direct light.

IF YOU MISS A DOSE
If you miss a dose, take it as soon as you remember unless the next dose is less than 8 hours away. In that case, skip the missed dose and go back to your regular schedule. Do not double the next dose.

STOPPING THE DRUG
Suddenly stopping this drug may cause blood pressure to rise dangerously high, possibly triggering angina or heart attack in patients with advanced heart disease. Slow reduction of the dose over a period of 2 to 3 weeks is advised, under careful supervision by your doctor.

PROLONGED USE
No special problems are expected, although prolonged use may increase the chance of side effects. Regular visits to your doctor are needed to evaluate the drug's ongoing, long-term effectiveness.

PRECAUTIONS
Over 60: Older persons with reduced kidney function may require a lower dosage.

Driving and Hazardous Work: Be cautious about any activity that requires acuity since this medication may cause drowsiness and impaired alertness.

Alcohol: Drink in careful moderation if at all. Alcohol may interact with the drug and cause a dangerous drop in blood pressure.

Pregnancy: This drug may harm the developing child. Inform your doctor if you are pregnant or plan to become pregnant.

Breast Feeding: This drug passes into breast milk; avoid breast feeding while taking it.

Infants and Children: Not usually prescribed for infants or children.

Special Concerns: Use of the drug should be considered but one element of a comprehensive therapeutic program that includes weight control, smoking cessation, regular exercise, and a healthy low-salt, low-fat diet.

OVERDOSE
Symptoms: Breathing difficulties, slow heartbeat, sluggishness, extremely low blood pressure.

What to Do: Call your doctor, emergency medical services (EMS), or the nearest poison control center immediately.

DRUG INTERACTIONS
Consult your doctor for specific advice if you are taking amphetamines, oral antidiabetic agents, asthma medication (such as aminophylline or theophylline), calcium channel blockers, clonidine, guanabenz, halothane, allergy shots, insulin, MAO inhibitors, reserpine, or other beta-blockers.

FOOD INTERACTIONS
None expected.

DISEASE INTERACTIONS
Atenolol/chlorthalidone should be used with caution in people with diabetes, especially insulin-dependent diabetes, since atenolol can mask the symptoms of hypoglycemia. Consult your doctor if you have allergies or asthma, heart or blood vessel disease (including congestive heart failure and peripheral vascular disease), irregular (slow) heartbeat, hyperthyroidism, myasthenia gravis, psoriasis, respiratory problems such as bronchitis or emphysema, kidney or liver disease, or a history of mental depression.

Atorvastatin

Lipitor 20 mg
(PARKE-DAVIS)

▶ Drug Class: Antilipidemic (cholesterol-lowering agent)

▶ Available in: Tablets

▶ Available OTC? No

▶ As Generic? No

Side Effects

SERIOUS
Fever, chest pain, unusual or unexplained muscle aches and tenderness. Call your doctor right away.

COMMON
Side effects occur in only 1% to 2% of patients. These include constipation or diarrhea, dizziness or lightheadedness, bloating or gas, heartburn, nausea, allergic reaction, stomach pain, rise in liver enzymes.

LESS COMMON
Sleeping difficulty, skin rash.

PRINCIPAL USES
To treat high cholesterol. Usually prescribed after the first lines of treatment—including diet changes, weight loss, and exercise—fail to reduce to acceptable levels the amounts of total and low-density lipoprotein (LDL) cholesterol in the blood.

HOW THE DRUG WORKS
Atorvastatin blocks the action of an enzyme required for the manufacture of cholesterol, thereby interfering with its formation. By lowering the amount of cholesterol in the liver cells, atorvastatin increases the formation of receptors for LDL, and thereby reduces blood levels of total and LDL cholesterol. In addition to lowering LDL cholesterol, atorvastatin also modestly reduces triglyceride levels and raises HDL (the so-called "good") cholesterol.

DOSAGE
Initial dose is 10 mg a day, taken once daily. It may be increased by your doctor as needed up to a maximum dose of 80 mg per day. Unlike other "-statin" cholesterol-lowering drugs, atorvastatin does not have to be taken in the evening to be maximally effective.

ONSET OF EFFECT
2 to 4 weeks.

DURATION OF ACTION
The effect persists for the duration of therapy.

DIETARY ADVICE
Cholesterol-lowering drugs are only one part of a total program that should include regular exercise and a healthy diet. The American Heart Association publishes a "Healthy Heart" diet, which is recommended.

STORAGE
Store in a tightly sealed container in a dry place away from heat and direct light.

IF YOU MISS A DOSE
Take it as soon as you remember. Take your next scheduled dose at the proper time and resume your regular dosage schedule. Do not double your next dose.

STOPPING THE DRUG
The decision to stop taking the drug should be made in consultation with your doctor. Once the medication is discontinued, blood cholesterol is likely to return to original elevated levels.

PROLONGED USE
Side effects are more likely with prolonged use. As you continue with atorvastatin, your doctor will periodically order blood tests to evaluate liver function.

PRECAUTIONS
Over 60: No special problems are expected in older patients.

Driving and Hazardous Work: The use of atorvastatin should not impair your ability to perform such tasks safely.

Alcohol: No special precautions are necessary.

Pregnancy: Should not be used during pregnancy or by women who plan to become pregnant in the near future.

Breast Feeding: This drug is not recommended for women who are nursing.

Infants and Children: Safety and effectiveness are not known; this drug is rarely used in children. Consult your pediatrician.

Special Concerns: Important elements of treatment for high cholesterol include proper diet, weight loss, regular moderate exercise, and avoidance of certain medications that may increase cholesterol levels. Because atorvastatin has potential side effects, it is important that you maintain a recommended healthy diet and cooperate with other treatments your doctor may suggest.

OVERDOSE
Symptoms: An overdose of atorvastatin is unlikely.

What to Do: Emergency instructions not applicable.

DRUG INTERACTIONS
Consult your doctor if you are taking cyclosporine, gemfibrozil, niacin, antibiotics, especially erythromycin, or medications for fungus infections. All of these drugs may increase the risk of myositis (muscle inflammation) when taken with atorvastatin and may lead to kidney failure.

FOOD INTERACTIONS
No known food interactions.

DISEASE INTERACTIONS
Consult your doctor if you have any of the following problems: liver, kidney, or muscle disease, or a medical history involving organ transplant or recent surgery.

Atovaquone

BRAND NAME
Mepron

▶ Drug Class: Anti-infective/antiprotozoal

▶ Available in: Oral suspension, tablets

▶ Available OTC? No

▶ As Generic? No

Side Effects

SERIOUS
Skin rash, fever. Call your doctor immediately.

COMMON
Insomnia, diarrhea, cough, headache, nausea or vomiting.

LESS COMMON
Lack of energy, fatigue, itching, stomach upset or abdominal pain, constipation, dizziness.

PRINCIPAL USES
To treat mild to moderately severe *Pneumocystis carinii* pneumonia (PCP) in patients who cannot take the antibiotic trimethoprim/sulfamethoxazole (the standard therapy for PCP). This serious type of pneumonia is prevalent among patients with AIDS.

HOW THE DRUG WORKS
Atovaquone prevents infecting cells from manufacturing DNA and other substances necessary for growth and reproduction.

DOSAGE
Adults and teenagers— Oral suspension: 750 mg twice a day, with meals, for 21 days. Tablets: 750 mg, 3 times a day, with meals, for 21 days.

ONSET OF EFFECT
Unknown.

DURATION OF ACTION
Unknown.

DIETARY ADVICE
Take it with meals high in fat content to help the body absorb the medication.

STORAGE
Store in a tightly sealed container away from heat, moisture, and direct light. Do not allow to freeze. Keep away from extreme temperatures.

IF YOU MISS A DOSE
Take it as soon as you remember. This will help keep a constant level of medication in your system. However, if it is near the time for the next dose, skip the missed dose and resume your regular dosage schedule. Do not double the next dose.

STOPPING THE DRUG
Take it as prescribed for the full treatment period, even if you begin to feel better before the scheduled end of therapy. The decision to stop taking the drug should be made in consultation with your doctor. Stopping the drug prematurely may slow your recovery or lead to a rebound infection.

PROLONGED USE
Therapy with atovaquone requires 21 days. Prolonged use of atovaquone beyond this period may be associated with an increased chance of side effects.

PRECAUTIONS
Over 60: No studies have been done specifically on older patients; adverse reactions may be more likely or more severe.

Driving and Hazardous Work: Do not drive or engage in hazardous work until you determine how the medicine affects you.

Alcohol: No special precautions are necessary.

Pregnancy: Adequate human studies on the use of this drug in pregnant women have not been done. Before taking atovaquone, tell your doctor if you are pregnant or plan to become pregnant. Discuss with your doctor the relative risks and benefits of using this drug while pregnant.

Breast Feeding: Atovaquone may pass into breast milk; caution is advised. Consult your doctor for advice.

Infants and Children: Adequate studies of the use of atovaquone in children have not been done. Consult your pediatrician for advice.

Special Concerns: A regular teaspoon may not hold the correct amount of medication. Use a specially marked measuring spoon or other device to dispense each dose.

OVERDOSE
Symptoms: No cases of atovaquone overdose have been reported.

What to Do: If someone takes a much larger dose than prescribed, call your doctor, emergency medical services (EMS), or the nearest poison control center as soon as possible.

DRUG INTERACTIONS
Other drugs may interact with atovaquone. Consult your doctor for specific advice if you are taking rifampin, rifabutin, sulfamethoxazole and trimethoprim combination, or zidovudine.

FOOD INTERACTIONS
No known food interactions.

DISEASE INTERACTIONS
Atovaquone may not work properly in patients with a stomach or an intestinal condition (such as colitis) that limits drug absorption. Consult your doctor for more information.

Atropine Sulfate Ophthalmic

BRAND NAMES
Atropair, Atropine Sulfate
S.O.P., Atropine-Care,
Atropisol, Atrosulf,
I-Tropine, Isopto Atropine,
Ocu-Tropine

▶ Drug Class: Eye muscle relaxant, pupil enlarger

▶ Available in: Ophthalmic solution, ointment

▶ Available OTC? No

▶ As Generic? Yes

Side Effects

SERIOUS
Hallucinations, confusion, extreme sleepiness, heart palpitations. Call your doctor immediately.

COMMON
Blurred vision, increased sensitivity of eyes to light.

LESS COMMON
Eye crusting or drainage, itching and redness of the eye, swelling within the eye, eye pain, dry eyes, dry skin, dry mouth, irritability, agitation, flushing, fever.

PRINCIPAL USES
Used for eye examinations, before and after eye surgery, and to treat certain types of eye conditions, including uveitis (inflammation of the uvea, or the central portion of the eye) and posterior synechiae (a potentially blinding eye disorder). May also be used to help determine the proper prescription for eyeglasses in young children.

HOW THE DRUG WORKS
Atropine sulfate relaxes the ciliary muscle, which controls the shape of the eye's lens as it focuses, and another eye muscle called the sphincter, which controls the narrowing and widening of the pupil. Relaxation of these muscles prevents the lens from focusing and widens the pupil. This allows the doctor to view the interior structures of the eye during an ophthalmologic procedure. And, by immobilizing the tiny structures within the eye, the drug prevents scarring of eye tissue and may also alleviate pain somewhat.

DOSAGE
For eye examination—Adults: Dose to be determined by your doctor. Children: Ophthalmic solution: 1 drop in the eye twice a day for 2 days before the examination. Ointment: A thin strip of ointment applied to the eye 3 times a day for up to 3 days before the examination. For uveitis— Adults: 1 drop in the eye or a thin strip of ointment applied to the eye 1 to 4 times a day. Children: 1 drop in the eye or a thin strip of ointment applied to the eye up to 3 times a day.

ONSET OF EFFECT
Unknown.

DURATION OF ACTION
From 6 to 12 days. The drug's effect on the lens's ability to focus may last longer than its effect on the size of the pupil.

DIETARY ADVICE
No special restrictions.

STORAGE
Store in a tightly sealed container away from heat, moisture, and direct light.

IF YOU MISS A DOSE
If you miss a dose, apply the missed dose as soon as possible unless it is almost time for the next dose. In that case, skip the missed dose and go back to your regular schedule. Do not double the next dose.

STOPPING THE DRUG
The decision to stop using the drug should be made by your doctor.

PROLONGED USE
Call your doctor if symptoms persist for more than 14 days.

PRECAUTIONS
Over 60: Sleepiness and agitation are more likely.

Driving and Hazardous Work: Avoid such activities until temporary blurring of vision goes away.

Alcohol: No special precautions are necessary.

Pregnancy: Adequate human studies have not been done. Tell your doctor if you are pregnant or are planning a pregnancy.

Breast Feeding: Small amounts of this drug may pass into breast milk; extreme caution is advised. Infants exposed to atropine may exhibit a rapid pulse, fever, or dry skin.

Infants and Children: Infants, young children, and children with blond hair or blue eyes may be more sensitive to the effects of this drug and may have an increased risk of side effects. Use with extreme caution in these groups.

Special Concerns: Before administering the drug, wash your hands. Tilt your head back. Gently apply pressure to the inside corner of the eyelid and pull downward on the lower eyelid to make a space. Drop the medicine or put about ⅓ inch of ointment into this space and close your eye. Apply pressure for 1 or 2 minutes while the eye is closed. Wash your hands again. Make sure the tip of the applicator does not touch any other surface.

OVERDOSE
Symptoms: Impaired vision, extreme sensitivity to light, confusion, clumsiness, dizziness, hallucinations, irregular heartbeat, extreme drowsiness or weakness, unusual dry skin or mouth.

What to Do: Call your doctor, emergency medical services (EMS), or the nearest poison control center immediately.

DRUG INTERACTIONS
Consult your doctor if you use tranquilizers, drugs for glaucoma or myasthenia gravis, or any other eye drops or medications.

FOOD INTERACTIONS
None expected.

DISEASE INTERACTIONS
Do not use if you have glaucoma, especially closed-angle glaucoma, without consulting your doctor. The drug may increase abdominal pain in gastrointestinal disorders.

Atropine Sulfate Oral

Generic 0.4 mg
(LILLY)

▶ Drug Class: Anticholinergic; antispasmodic

▶ Available in: Tablets

▶ Available OTC? No

▶ As Generic? Yes

Side Effects

SERIOUS
Blurring or changes in vision; large, dilated pupils; eye pain; hot, dry, or flushed skin; high fever; heartbeat irregularities; seizures; fainting; coma; unusual agitation; bizarre behavior; hallucinations. Call your doctor immediately.

COMMON
Dry mouth, nose, throat, or skin; constipation; decreased sweating.

LESS COMMON
Difficult urination, decreased breast milk production, difficulty swallowing, headache, memory loss, increased sensitivity of eyes to light, nausea or vomiting, unusual fatigue.

PRINCIPAL USES
To relieve painful cramps and spasms due to irritable bowel syndrome. It is also used in rare cases to treat stomach ulcers in conjunction with other drugs such as cimetidine, and as an antidote to poisoning with certain pesticides.

HOW THE DRUG WORKS
Nerve impulses are transmitted to muscles and glands throughout the body by the action of specialized, naturally occurring chemicals known as neurotransmitters. Atropine blocks the ability of the neurotransmitter acetylcholine to stimulate certain muscles and glands. This produces effects ranging from drying of secretions (saliva, perspiration) to changing the size of the pupils and relief of intestinal muscle spasms.

DOSAGE
Adults and teenagers: 300 to 1,200 micrograms (mcg) every 4 to 6 hours. Children: 4.5 mcg per lb of body weight every 4 to 6 hours, not exceeding 400 mcg per dose.

ONSET OF EFFECT
Within 30 to 60 minutes.

DURATION OF ACTION
From 4 to 6 hours.

DIETARY ADVICE
Take it 30 to 60 minutes before meals and at bedtime.

STORAGE
Store in a tightly sealed container away from heat, moisture, and direct light.

IF YOU MISS A DOSE
Take it as soon as you remember. However, if it is near the time for the next dose, skip the missed dose and resume your regular dosage schedule. Do not double the next dose.

STOPPING THE DRUG
Take it as prescribed for the full treatment period, even if you feel better before the scheduled end of therapy.

PROLONGED USE
Therapy with this medication may require a period of several days to weeks. Prolonged use may increase the risk of an undesirable side effect.

PRECAUTIONS
Over 60: Common side effects may be more likely and more severe in older patients, who may also develop confusion and drowsiness.

Driving and Hazardous Work: The use of atropine may impair your ability to perform such tasks safely.

Alcohol: Use alcohol only in moderation.

Pregnancy: Although studies have been limited, atropine crosses the placenta and is not recommended during pregnancy. Before taking atropine, tell your doctor if you are pregnant or plan to become pregnant.

Breast Feeding: Atropine passes into breast milk and should not be used during breast feeding. This medication may also inhibit milk formation.

Infants and Children: Not recommended for use by children unless under close medical supervision. Infants and very young children are very susceptible to the effects of atropine.

Special Concerns: Atropine must be used with care; it is potentially a very dangerous drug. Use caution when exercising, especially when physical activity is sustained or carried out in hot weather. By inhibiting perspiration, atropine may impair your ability to cool down; heat stroke may result.

OVERDOSE
Symptoms: Blurred or altered vision, dilated pupils, eye pain, hot, dry, or flushed skin, high fever, heartbeat irregularities, seizures, unusual agitation, bizarre behavior, hallucinations, fainting, coma.

What to Do: Call your doctor, emergency medical services (EMS), or the nearest poison control center immediately.

DRUG INTERACTIONS
Consult your doctor for specific advice if you are taking antacids or diarrhea medication; decongestants, antihistamines, and other medications for allergies or colds; ketoconazole; medicines that cause drowsiness, such as barbiturates, sedatives, and cough medicines; psychiatric medications, including antidepressants; alcohol-containing medicines; or painkillers.

FOOD INTERACTIONS
No known food interactions.

DISEASE INTERACTIONS
Consult your doctor if you have heart disease or a history of heart rhythm irregularities, pacemaker usage, or fainting; esophagitis or hiatal hernia; glaucoma; a history of intestinal obstruction, intestinal inflammation (colitis), or other gastrointestinal problems; myasthenia gravis; prostate enlargement or other urinary problems.

Atropine Sulfate/Scopolamine Hydrobromide/Hyoscyamine Sulfate/Phenobarbital

▶ Drug Class: Anticholinergic; antispasmodic

▶ Available in: Tablets, elixir, capsules, extended-release tablets

▶ Available OTC? No

▶ As Generic? Yes

Side Effects

SERIOUS
Yellow-tinged eyes or skin, skin rash or hives, eye pain, unusual bruising or bleeding, sore throat and fever. Call your doctor immediately.

COMMON
Constipation; dry mouth, nose, skin, or throat; decreased sweating; dizziness; drowsiness.

LESS COMMON
Loss of memory, difficult urination, blurred vision, nausea or vomiting, bloated feeling, unusual weakness or tiredness, difficulty swallowing, decreased flow of breast milk.

PRINCIPAL USES
To relieve symptoms of irritable bowel syndrome, peptic and duodenal ulcers, and gastrointestinal cramps.

HOW THE DRUG WORKS
Acetylcholine is a naturally occurring chemical in the body that is involved in the activity of nerves, muscles, glands, and other physiological processes. This drug interferes with the action of acetylcholine, leading to a variety of effects including the drying of secretions (saliva, perspiration), relief of muscle spasms in the intestines, and changing the size of the pupils.

DOSAGE
Capsules or tablets— Adults and teenagers: 1 or 2 capsules, 2 to 4 times a day. Children ages 2 to 12: ½ to 1 chewable tablet, 3 or 4 times a day. Elixir— Adults: 5 to 10 ml, 3 to 4 times a day. Children: 0.5 to 7.5 ml every 4 to 6 hours. Extended-release tablets— Adults and teenagers: 1 tablet every 8 to 12 hours. Children: Not recommended for use in patients under the age of 13.

ONSET OF EFFECT
Unknown.

DURATION OF ACTION
Unknown.

DIETARY ADVICE
Take this medication 30 to 60 minutes before meals unless your doctor orders otherwise.

STORAGE
Store in a tightly sealed container away from heat, moisture, and direct light. Keep the liquid form refrigerated, but do not allow it to freeze.

IF YOU MISS A DOSE
Take it as soon as you remember. If it is near the time for the next dose, skip the missed dose and resume your regular dosage schedule. Do not double the next dose.

STOPPING THE DRUG
The decision to stop taking the drug should be made by your doctor.

PROLONGED USE
No special problems are expected.

PRECAUTIONS
Over 60: Adverse reactions may be more likely and more severe in older patients.

Driving and Hazardous Work: Do not drive or engage in hazardous work until you determine how the medicine affects you.

Alcohol: Avoid alcohol when using this medication.

Pregnancy: Tell your doctor if you are pregnant or plan to become pregnant before taking this medicine.

Breast Feeding: This drug may pass into breast milk; caution is advised. Consult your doctor for advice.

Infants and Children: The drug should not be prescribed for children under age 2. Adverse reactions may be more likely and more severe in infants and young children, especially those suffering from brain damage or spastic paralysis.

OVERDOSE
Symptoms: Nausea, vomiting, headache, blurred vision, dilated pupils, weak pulse, fever, hallucinations, seizures, unconsciousness, confusion, dry skin and mouth.

What to Do: Call your doctor, emergency medical services (EMS), or the nearest poison control center immediately.

DRUG INTERACTIONS
Other drugs may interact with this medication. Consult your doctor for specific advice if you are taking an anticholinergic (such as belladonna), an adrenocorticoid, an antacid, an antidiarrheal medicine containing kaolin or attapulgite, ketoconazole, an anticoagulant (blood thinner), central nervous system depressants (such as antihistamines, cold medicines, sleep aids, or tranquilizers), an MAO inhibitor, haloperidol, or potassium chloride.

FOOD INTERACTIONS
No known food interactions.

DISEASE INTERACTIONS
Caution is advised when taking this drug. Consult your doctor if you have any of the following: a nerve disorder, asthma or other lung problems, an enlarged prostate, severe and continuing dry mouth, liver disease, kidney disease, Down's syndrome, intestinal blockage or other intestinal problems, an overactive thyroid gland, heart disease, high blood pressure, glaucoma, or ulcerative colitis.

Attapulgite

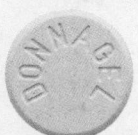

Donnagel 600 mg
(WYETH-AYERST)

▶ Drug Class: Antidiarrheal

▶ Available in: Oral suspension, tablets, chewable tablets

▶ Available OTC? Yes

▶ As Generic? Yes

Side Effects

SERIOUS
No serious side effects are associated with attapulgite. However, loss of body water due to diarrhea can cause dry mouth, increased thirst, dizziness, lightheadedness, decreased urination, and wrinkling of skin. Call your doctor immediately.

COMMON
Constipation.

LESS COMMON
There are no less-common side effects associated with the use of attapulgite.

PRINCIPAL USES
To treat diarrhea.

HOW THE DRUG WORKS
Attapulgite is believed to bind to and remove large volumes of bacteria and toxins from the digestive tract. It may also reduce the fluidity of the stool associated with diarrhea. There is some debate regarding attapulgite's effectiveness.

DOSAGE
Adults and teenagers— Suspension and tablets: 1,200 to 1,500 mg taken after each loose bowel movement; take no more than 9,000 mg in 24 hours. Chewable tablets: 1,200 mg after each loose bowel movement; take no more than 8,400 mg in 24 hours. Children ages 6 to 12— Suspension and chewable tablets: 600 mg after each loose bowel movement; take no more than 4,200 mg in 24 hours. Tablets: 750 mg after each loose bowel movement; take no more than 4,500 mg in 24 hours. Children ages 3 to 6— Suspension and chewable tablets: 300 mg after each loose bowel movement; take no more than 2,100 mg in 24 hours. Tablets: Should not be taken by children in this age group.

ONSET OF EFFECT
Unknown.

DURATION OF ACTION
Unknown.

DIETARY ADVICE
A mild diet is recommended when recovering from diarrhea. Bananas, rice, applesauce, and plain toast are good choices. Be sure to get plenty of fluids.

STORAGE
Store in a tightly sealed container away from heat, moisture, and direct light.

IF YOU MISS A DOSE
Take it as soon as you remember. However, if it is near the time for the next dose, skip the missed dose and resume your regular dosage schedule. Do not double the next dose.

STOPPING THE DRUG
You may stop taking the drug if you feel better before the scheduled end of therapy.

PROLONGED USE
If diarrhea has not improved or has gotten worse in 2 days, or if you develop a fever, call your doctor.

PRECAUTIONS
Over 60: Older persons are more likely to experience excessive loss of body fluid and therefore are advised to increase fluid intake accordingly.

Driving and Hazardous Work: The use of attapulgite should not impair your ability to perform such tasks safely.

Alcohol: Avoid alcohol.

Pregnancy: Attapulgite is not absorbed by the body and is not expected to cause problems during pregnancy.

Breast Feeding: Attapulgite is not absorbed by the body and is not expected to cause problems while nursing.

Infants and Children: Should not be given to children under the age of 3 without consulting your doctor. Be sure your child drinks a sufficient amount of fluids.

Special Concerns: In addition to taking attapulgite, it is important to replace the body fluids lost because of diarrhea. During the first day you should drink ample amounts of clear liquids, like decaffeinated colas, ginger ale, and decaffeinated tea, and eat gelatin. On the following day you should continue your fluid intake and eat bland foods, such as applesauce, cooked cereals, and bread. Do not take attapulgite if your diarrhea is accompanied by blood or mucus in the stools.

OVERDOSE
Symptoms: No cases of overdose have been reported.

What to Do: An overdose of attapulgite is unlikely to be life-threatening. However, if someone takes a much larger dose than prescribed, seek medical assistance immediately.

DRUG INTERACTIONS
Other drugs may interact with attapulgite. If you are taking any other medication, do not take it within 2 to 3 hours before or after taking attapulgite.

FOOD INTERACTIONS
Eating fried or spicy foods, bran, fruits, vegetables, or drinking caffeinated or alcoholic beverages can make diarrhea worse.

DISEASE INTERACTIONS
Consult your doctor if you have dysentery or any other medical condition.

Auranofin

BRAND NAME
Ridaura

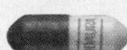

Generic 3 mg
(SMITHKLINE BEECHAM)

▶ Drug Class: Antirheumatic

▶ Available in: Capsules

▶ Available OTC? No

▶ As Generic? No

Side Effects

SERIOUS
Severe abdominal pain, widespread rash, neurological disturbances causing confusion or seizures.

COMMON
Itching, hives, sores or spots in mouth or throat, poor appetite, diarrhea, nausea, vomiting, rashes, fever, stomach pains, indigestion, heartburn, constipation.

LESS COMMON
Coughing, hoarseness, breathing difficulty, or wheezing; dark urine or reduced urine output; impaired vision; difficulty swallowing; sore throat; fever and chills; hair loss; hallucinations; painful urination; low back pain or flank pain; red, painful, itching eyes; unusual bleeding or bruising; red, thickened, or scaly patches on skin; swelling of face, legs, or feet; swollen or painful glands; excessive fatigue or weakness; yellow discoloration of the eyes or skin (jaundice).

PRINCIPAL USES
To treat rheumatoid arthritis. Because of the risk of highly unpleasant side effects, auranofin is generally prescribed for patients who have not responded adequately to other more conservative arthritis treatments, such as non-steroidal anti-inflammatory drugs, corticosteroids, and aspirin. (Auranofin is not appropriate for the treatment of osteoarthritis, which is much more common.)

HOW THE DRUG WORKS
Auranofin contains gold. It is not precisely known how gold compounds work, but evidently they reduce some of the painful joint inflammation associated with arthritis. Auranofin can halt the progress of severe rheumatoid arthritis, preventing further joint damage, and in some cases it may bring about a remission from the disease.

DOSAGE
Adults: 6 mg once a day, or 3 mg twice a day. After 6 months of therapy, your doctor may increase the dose to 3 mg, 3 times a day. Children: Consult your pediatrician for proper dosage.

ONSET OF EFFECT
Within 3 to 4 months.

DURATION OF ACTION
Unknown.

DIETARY ADVICE
Maintain your usual food and fluid intake.

STORAGE
Store in a tightly sealed container away from heat and direct light.

IF YOU MISS A DOSE
Take the missed dose as soon as you remember. If you are within 2 hours of your next scheduled dose, skip the missed dose. Take your next scheduled dose at the proper time, then resume your regular dosage schedule. Do not double the next dose.

STOPPING THE DRUG
This medication should be taken as prescribed for the full treatment period. Do not stop taking it on your own if you are feeling better before the scheduled end of drug therapy unless you are experiencing a serious side effect.

PROLONGED USE
Several months of therapy may be necessary to determine whether this medication is helping you. Prolonged use of auranofin may increase the risk of side effects.

PRECAUTIONS
Over 60: Adverse reactions may be more likely and more severe in older patients.

Driving and Hazardous Work: The use of auranofin may impair your ability to perform such tasks safely.

Alcohol: Avoid alcohol while taking this drug.

Pregnancy: Do not use this drug during pregnancy.

Breast Feeding: Auranofin passes into breast milk; avoid or discontinue use while nursing.

Infants and Children: Not recommended.

Special Concerns: Gold compounds may have many adverse effects resulting from gold toxicity. Your doctor will order periodic blood tests to determine if you are having any undesirable reactions to auranofin, such as anemia or low white blood cell count. Always contact your doctor if you have any concerns about the way you feel while taking auranofin. Auranofin may cause heightened sensitivity to sunlight. Avoid direct sunlight during peak hours, and wear protective clothing. Use sunscreens if possible.

OVERDOSE
Symptoms: No cases of overdose have been reported.

What to Do: If you are concerned about the possibility of an overdose, contact your doctor, emergency medical services (EMS), or the nearest poison control center immediately.

DRUG INTERACTIONS
Consult your doctor for specific advice if you are taking penicillamine.

FOOD INTERACTIONS
No known food interactions.

DISEASE INTERACTIONS
Consult your doctor if you have anemia or any other blood disease, skin disease, colitis or any other intestinal disease, ulcers or heartburn, kidney disease, or systemic lupus erythematosus (SLE).

BRAND NAME
Imuran

Generic 50 mg
(ROXANE)

▶ Drug Class: Immunosuppressant

▶ Available in: Tablets, injection

▶ Available OTC? No

▶ As Generic? Yes

Side Effects

SERIOUS
Rapid heartbeat; sudden fever or chills; back, side, muscle, or joint pain; unusual tiredness or weakness; cough or hoarseness; shortness of breath; black, tarry stools; blood in urine or stools; difficult or painful urination; severe or sudden stomach pain with nausea, vomiting, or diarrhea; red spots, red patches, or blisters on skin; unusual bleeding or bruising; abrupt or sudden, unusual feeling of discomfort or illness. These may be signs of serious infection, bleeding emergencies, or gastrointestinal problems. Seek immediate medical assistance.

COMMON
Moderate nausea and vomiting; loss of appetite.

LESS COMMON
Liver problems, skin rash, sores in mouth, stomach pain, swelling of feet or lower legs, shortness of breath.

PRINCIPAL USES
To slow down or reduce the natural tendency of the immune system to reject organ transplants, and to treat rheumatoid arthritis and other conditions.

HOW THE DRUG WORKS
Azathioprine prevents the immune system from attacking transplanted organs and slows down immune cells that cause inflammation in joints and elsewhere.

DOSAGE
For transplant rejection— Tablet and injection: Initially, 3 to 5 mg per 2.2 lbs (1 kg) of body weight daily. With improvement the dose may be reduced to 1 to 2 mg per 2.2 lbs daily. For rheumatoid arthritis— Tablet: 1 mg per 2.2 lbs daily. This may be increased to not more than 2.5 mg per 2.2 lbs daily.

ONSET OF EFFECT
4 to 8 weeks.

DURATION OF ACTION
Suppression of the immune system may persist long after the drug is completely eliminated.

DIETARY ADVICE
Take it with food or immediately following a meal to reduce stomach irritation.

STORAGE
Store in a tightly sealed container in a dry place away from heat and direct light. Keep liquid form refrigerated, but do not allow it to freeze.

IF YOU MISS A DOSE
For once-daily schedules: Do not take the missed dose. Take your next scheduled dose at the proper time and resume your regular dosage schedule. Do not double the next dose. For multiple-dose daily schedules: Take your missed dose as soon as you remember. If it is time for your next scheduled dose, take the two doses together and resume your regular dosage schedule. If you miss more than one dose in a day, call your doctor.

STOPPING THE DRUG
Take this drug as prescribed for the full length of treatment, even if you begin to feel better before the scheduled end of therapy.

PROLONGED USE
Prolonged use increases the risk of side effects and the possibility of cancer.

PRECAUTIONS
Over 60: Adverse reactions may be more likely and more severe in older patients.

Driving and Hazardous Work: The use of azathioprine may impair your ability to perform such tasks safely.

Alcohol: Avoid alcohol.

Pregnancy: Do not use this drug if you are pregnant. It should not be used by either the male or the female partners if you are trying to become pregnant.

Breast Feeding: Azathioprine passes into breast milk; avoid or discontinue use while nursing.

Infants and Children: Azathioprine has not been shown to affect children differently than adults. Consult your pediatrician for advice.

Special Concerns: Infection is a great threat to people with suppressed immune systems. Azathioprine may lower your ability to resist infection by lowering the number of white blood cells in the blood. Do not receive any vaccinations without approval from your doctor. Avoid people with infections. Azathioprine may also suppress platelets (the blood components that control blood coagulation), and thus cause bleeding problems. Use care with scissors, nail clippers, nail files, razors, toothbrushes, dental floss, or toothpicks. Inform your dentist that you are taking azathioprine.

OVERDOSE
Symptoms: Unusual bleeding, increased susceptibility to infection.

What to Do: Call your doctor, emergency medical services (EMS), or the nearest poison control center immediately.

DRUG INTERACTIONS
Inform your doctor if you are taking allopurinol, ACE inhibitors, chlorambucil, corticosteroids, cotrimoxazole, cyclophosphamide, cyclosporine, mercaptopurine, or muromonab-CD3.

FOOD INTERACTIONS
No known food interactions.

DISEASE INTERACTIONS
Caution is advised when taking azathioprine. Consult your doctor if you have any of the following: chicken pox, shingles, gout, infection, kidney or liver disease, or pancreatitis.

Azelastine

▶ Drug Class: Histamine (H1) blocker

▶ Available in: Nasal spray

▶ Available OTC? No

▶ As Generic? No

Side Effects

SERIOUS
No serious side effects are associated with the use of azelastine.

COMMON
Bitter taste in the mouth, drowsiness, headache, unexpected weight gain.

LESS COMMON
Nasal burning, sore throat, dry mouth, sneezing, nausea, fatigue, dizziness, nosebleeds.

PRINCIPAL USES
To treat or relieve symptoms of hay fever (allergic rhinitis) and chronic nasal inflammation and obstruction (vasomotor rhinitis).

HOW THE DRUG WORKS
Azelastine blocks the effects of histamine, a naturally occurring substance within the body that causes swelling, itching, sneezing, watery eyes, hives, and other symptoms of allergic reaction.

DOSAGE
Adults and teenagers: 2 sprays per nostril, not to exceed 2 times per day. Children ages 5 to 11 (allergic rhinitis only): 1 spray per nostril twice a day.

ONSET OF EFFECT
Within 1 to 3 hours.

DURATION OF ACTION
12 hours.

DIETARY ADVICE
No special restrictions.

STORAGE
Store upright in a tightly sealed container away from heat, moisture, and direct light. Do not allow the medication to freeze.

IF YOU MISS A DOSE
Take it as soon as you remember. If it is near the time for the next dose, skip the missed dose and resume your regular dosage schedule. Do not double the next dose.

STOPPING THE DRUG
Take it as prescribed for the full treatment period, even if you start to feel better before the scheduled end of therapy.

PROLONGED USE
Safety and effectiveness during prolonged use have yet to be established.

PRECAUTIONS
Over 60: No special problems are expected.

Driving and Hazardous Work: Azelastine may cause drowsiness. Do not drive or engage in hazardous work until you determine how the medication affects you.

Alcohol: No specific restrictions, though alcohol may increase the drug's sedative effects in some patients.

Pregnancy: Adequate studies of azelastine use during pregnancy have not been done. Before taking it, tell your doctor if you are pregnant or plan to become pregnant. Discuss with your doctor the relative risks and benefits of using this drug.

Breast Feeding: Azelastine may pass into breast milk; caution is advised. Consult your doctor for specific advice.

Infants and Children: The safety and effectiveness of azelastine use by children under the age of 5 have not been determined.

Special Concerns: If the pump has not been used for 3 days or more, it should be reprimed with at least 2 sprays or until a fine mist appears. To avoid the possible spread of infection, this medicine should be used by one person only. Before using this medication, blow your nose gently. When inhaling the nasal spray, keep your head upright and sniff briskly while spraying.

OVERDOSE
Symptoms: No cases of overdose have been reported.

What to Do: An overdose of azelastine is unlikely to occur or to be life-threatening. However, if someone takes a much larger dose than prescribed or accidentally ingests the medication, you should seek medical assistance immediately.

DRUG INTERACTIONS
No drug interactions have been reported. Azelastine may, however, increase the depressant effects of alcohol, sedatives, tranquilizers, pain-killers, barbiturates, or other antihistamines on the central nervous system. Consult your doctor for specific advice.

FOOD INTERACTIONS
No food interactions have been reported.

DISEASE INTERACTIONS
No disease interactions have been reported.

Azithromycin

PRINCIPAL USES
To treat various bacterial infections, particularly of the sinuses, throat, and respiratory tract (such as bronchitis and pneumonia); infections of the ear; venereal disease due to chlamydial and chancroid infection; skin infections; and diarrhea associated with campylobacter and other bacteria that cause food poisoning. Also used to prevent and treat a tuberculosis-like disease known as Mycobacterium avium complex (MAC), which is common in people with advanced AIDS.

HOW THE DRUG WORKS
Azithromycin prevents bacterial cells from manufacturing specific proteins necessary for their survival.

DOSAGE
For bronchitis, strep throat, pneumonia, and skin infections: 500 mg (2 pills) taken in a single dose on the first day of treatment; then, 250 mg (1 pill) per day on days 2 through 5. For chlamydia and chancroid: 1,000 mg (4 pills) taken in a single one-time dose. To prevent MAC: 1,200 mg weekly. To treat MAC: 500 mg, twice a day.

ONSET OF EFFECT
Unknown.

DURATION OF ACTION
Unknown.

DIETARY ADVICE
Take capsules on an empty stomach, at least 1 hour before or 2 hours after eating. Tablets may be taken with or without food. Drink plenty of fluids (at least 2 to 3 quarts of water per day).

STORAGE
Store in a tightly sealed container away from heat and direct light.

IF YOU MISS A DOSE
Take it as soon as you remember. If you miss a day entirely, skip the missed dose and resume your regular dosage schedule the next day. Do not double the next dose.

STOPPING THE DRUG
It is very important to take this drug as prescribed for the full treatment period, even if you begin to feel better before the scheduled end of therapy.

PROLONGED USE
For acute infections, treatment is usually complete after 5 days with capsules, and 1 day with the powdered form. For MAC prevention and treatment, therapy may be lifelong. Prolonged use may be associated with an increased risk of side effects.

PRECAUTIONS
Over 60: Adverse reactions may be more likely and more severe.

Driving and Hazardous Work: The use of azithromycin should not impair your ability to perform such tasks safely.

Alcohol: Avoid alcohol while taking this drug.

Pregnancy: Adequate studies of the use of azithromycin during pregnancy have not been done; consult your doctor for advice.

Breast Feeding: It is not known if azithromycin passes into breast milk; consult your doctor for advice.

Infants and Children: The safety and effectiveness of azithromycin use in patients under 16 years of age have not been established, although no special problems are expected.

Special Concerns: Before taking any antibiotic, make sure you tell your doctor about allergies that you might have. If you are allergic to erythromycin, you are likely to be allergic to azithromycin. Azithromycin is useful only against bacteria that are susceptible to its effects. Therefore, it is important to tell your doctor if your condition has not improved, or instead has worsened, within a few days of starting the drug. The particular bacteria causing your illness may be resistant to azithromycin.

OVERDOSE
Symptoms: No cases of overdose have been reported.

What to Do: Emergency instructions not applicable.

DRUG INTERACTIONS
Other drugs may interact with azithromycin. Consult your doctor for specific advice if you are taking anticoagulants (such as warfarin), anticonvulsants (such as phenytoin and carbamazepine), antihistamines (especially terfenadine), and theophylline. Antacids that contain aluminum or magnesium can interfere with the absorption of azithromycin; separate the use of azithromycin and an antacid by at least 2 hours.

FOOD INTERACTIONS
Azithromycin capsules should be taken on an empty stomach.

DISEASE INTERACTIONS
Consult your doctor if you have a medical history that includes liver disease.

Bacampicillin Hydrochloride

BRAND NAME
Spectrobid

▶ Drug Class: Penicillin antibiotic

▶ Available in: Capsules, oral suspension

▶ Available OTC? No

▶ As Generic? No

Side Effects

SERIOUS
Irregular, rapid, or labored breathing, light-headedness or sudden fainting, joint pain, fever, severe abdominal pain and cramping with watery or bloody stools, severe allergic reaction (marked by sudden swelling of the lips, tongue, face, or throat; breathing difficulty; severe rash, itching, or hives, unusual bleeding or bruising, yellowish tinge to eyes or skin. Call your doctor immediately.

COMMON
Rash, mild diarrhea, headache, sore tongue, sore mouth, vaginal discharge and itching, white patches in mouth.

LESS COMMON
Diminished urine output, chills, weakness, fatigue.

PRINCIPAL USES

To treat a variety of bacterial infections, including those of the respiratory tract, gastrointestinal tract, urinary tract, and middle ear. Bacampicillin is effective only against infections caused by bacteria; it is ineffective against those caused by viruses, fungi, or other microorganisms.

HOW THE DRUG WORKS

Bacampicillin blocks the formation of bacterial cell walls, rendering bacteria unable to multiply and spread.

DOSAGE

Adults and children weighing 55 lbs or more: 400 to 800 mg every 12 hours (2 times a day). Children weighing less than 55 lbs: 5.7 to 11.4 mg per lb of body weight every 12 hours.

ONSET OF EFFECT

Unknown.

DURATION OF ACTION

Unknown.

DIETARY ADVICE

Tablets can be taken with or without food. The oral suspension should be taken on an empty stomach, at least 1 hour before or 2 hours after meals, with plenty of water.

STORAGE

Store in a tightly sealed container away from heat and direct light. The suspension can be refrigerated but should not be frozen.

IF YOU MISS A DOSE

Take it as soon as you remember. If it is near the time for the next dose, skip the missed dose and resume your regular dosage schedule. Do not double the next dose.

STOPPING THE DRUG

Take it as prescribed for the full treatment period, even if you begin to feel better before the scheduled end of therapy. Stopping the drug prematurely may slow your recovery or lead to a rebound infection, also known as superinfection, in which the heartier strains of bacteria survive and multiply, leading to a more serious and drug-resistant infection.

PROLONGED USE

The prolonged use of any antibiotic will increase the risk of superinfection; caution is advised.

PRECAUTIONS

Over 60: No special problems are expected.

Driving and Hazardous Work: Do not drive or engage in hazardous work until you determine how the medicine affects you.

Alcohol: No special precautions are necessary.

Pregnancy: Adequate studies of the use of penicillin antibiotics during pregnancy have not been done; however, no problems have been reported.

Breast Feeding: Bacampicillin may pass into breast milk and cause problems in the nursing infant; avoid use of this drug while nursing.

Infants and Children: No special problems are expected.

Special Concerns: Bacampicillin can cause false results on some urine sugar tests for patients with diabetes. Those who are prone to asthma, hay fever, hives, or allergies may be more likely to have an allergic reaction to a penicillin antibiotic. If severe diarrhea occurs as a side effect of this drug, do not take antidiarrheal medications; call your doctor.

OVERDOSE

Symptoms: Severe nausea, vomiting, diarrhea, muscle spasticity, seizures.

What to Do: Call your doctor, emergency medical services (EMS), or the nearest poison control center immediately.

DRUG INTERACTIONS

Consult your doctor for specific advice if you are taking aminoglycosides, ACE inhibitors, diuretics, potassium supplements or potassium-containing drugs, anticoagulants or other anti-clotting drugs, nonsteroidal anti-inflammatory drugs, sulfinpyrazone, cholestyramine, colestipol, oral contraceptives, methotrexate, probenecid, allopurinol, or disulfiram.

FOOD INTERACTIONS

No known food interactions.

DISEASE INTERACTIONS

Consult your doctor if you have a history of allergies, asthma, congestive heart failure, gastrointestinal disorders (especially colitis associated with the use of antibiotics), infectious mononucleosis, or impaired kidney function.

Bacitracin

BRAND NAMES
Baciguent ointment (dermatologic), Baciguent ophthalmic ointment, Bactine Triple Antibiotic ointment (dermatologic combining polymyxin, neomycin, and bacitracin), Polysporin ointment (dermatologic combining polymyxin and bacitracin), Polysporin ophthalmic ointment (combination of polymyxin and bacitracin)

▶ Drug Class: Antibiotic

▶ Available in: Ophthalmic ointment and solution; dermatologic (skin) ointment

▶ Available OTC? Yes

▶ As Generic? Yes

Side Effects

SERIOUS
Dermatologic and ophthalmic ointment: Rare severe allergic reaction that may cause hives, breathing difficulty, or at the extreme, total closure of the airways with potentially fatal anaphylactic shock. Contact emergency medical services (EMS) immediately. Ophthalmic preparations only: Severe eye pain, headache, rapid change in vision, sudden appearance of floating spots, acute redness of eye, pain on exposure to light, double vision, itching, burning, inflammation. Call your doctor or ophthalmologist immediately.

COMMON
No common side effects have been reported.

LESS COMMON
Dermatologic ointment: Irritation or skin allergy at the site of application, marked by redness, burning, itching, or the development of a rash.

PRINCIPAL USES
Dermatologic (skin) ointment is available over the counter for application to minor cuts and abrasions to prevent infection. Ophthalmic preparations are prescribed by a doctor for application to the eyelids or into the eye to treat early minor bacterial infections of the eyelids or conjunctiva (the mucous membranes that line the inner surface of the eyelids).

HOW THE DRUG WORKS
Hinders the ability of bacteria to manufacture cell walls, which causes cell death.

DOSAGE
Dermatologic ointment: Apply to a small cut or abrasion 2 times daily. Ophthalmic preparations: Apply to the eye 1 or more times daily.

ONSET OF EFFECT
Unknown.

DURATION OF ACTION
Unknown.

DIETARY ADVICE
No special restrictions.

STORAGE
Store in a tightly sealed container away from heat and direct light.

IF YOU MISS A DOSE
Apply it as soon as you remember and resume your regular dosage schedule.

STOPPING THE DRUG
You can stop using the dermatologic ointment as soon as the cut or abrasion is sufficiently healed. The decision to stop using the ophthalmic preparation should be made by your doctor.

PROLONGED USE
Ongoing observation is needed when the ointment is used, to detect any possible overgrowth of bacterial organisms that are not susceptible to the drug (known as superinfection).

PRECAUTIONS
Over 60: No special problems are expected.

Driving and Hazardous Work: Ophthalmic ointment may cloud vision; caution is advised.

Alcohol: No special precautions required.

Pregnancy: Before using bacitracin, tell your doctor if you are pregnant or plan to become pregnant.

Breast Feeding: Bacitracin may pass into breast milk. Consult your doctor for specific advice.

Infants and Children: No special problems are expected.

Special Concerns: Bacitracin preparations should not be used if you have a history of sensitivity or allergy to bacitracin or any of the other components in the ointment. To use the eye drops or the ointment, first wash your hands. Tilt your head back. Gently apply pressure to the inside corner of the eyelid and with the index finger of the same hand, pull downward on the lower eyelid to make a space. Drop the medicine or put a short strip of ointment (about ⅓ inch long) into this space and close your eye. Apply gentle pressure for 1 or 2 minutes while keeping the eye closed without blinking. Then wash your hands again. Make sure the tip of the dropper or the applica-tor does not touch your eye, finger, or any other surface. If your symptoms do not improve in a few days or if they become worse, check with your doctor.

OVERDOSE
Symptoms: Severe eye pain, headache, rapid change in vision, sudden appearance of floating spots, acute redness of eye, pain on exposure to light, double vision, itching, burning, inflammation.

What to Do: Call your doctor, emergency medical services (EMS), or the nearest poison control center immediately.

DRUG INTERACTIONS
No other drugs should be applied topically when using bacitracin unless otherwise instructed by your doctor. Bacitracin has not been shown to have any significant interactions with orally taken medications.

FOOD INTERACTIONS
No known food interactions.

DISEASE INTERACTIONS
Caution is advised when using bacitracin. Consult your doctor if superinfection (see Prolonged Use) with nonsusceptible bacteria occurs during therapy, so appropriate treatment can be started immediately.

Baclofen

Generic 10 mg
(ZENITH)

▶ Drug Class: Muscle relaxant

▶ Available in: Tablets

▶ Available OTC? No

▶ As Generic? Yes

Side Effects

SERIOUS
Chest pain, bloody or dark urine, skin rash or itching, hallucinations, fainting, depression or changes in mood, ringing or buzzing in the ears. Call your doctor.

COMMON
Dizziness, drowsiness, weakness (especially muscle weakness), fatigue, nausea, headache, insomnia.

LESS COMMON
Muscle or joint pain; numbness or tingling in hands or feet; unsteadiness, clumsiness, trembling, or other muscle control problems; stomach pain or discomfort; diarrhea; constipation; false sense of well-being (euphoria); loss of appetite; sexual problems in males; swelling of ankles; frequent urge to urinate or uncontrolled urination; difficult or painful urination or decreased urine output; unexpected weight gain; unusual excitability.

PRINCIPAL USES
To relax muscles and relieve the pain of muscle spasms and cramping. Chronic muscle spasms may be associated with disorders such as multiple sclerosis or spinal injuries. Baclofen has also been shown to improve urinary or fecal incontinence in patients with spinal cord injuries.

HOW THE DRUG WORKS
Baclofen appears to reduce the transmission of nerve impulses from the spinal cord to muscle tissue.

DOSAGE
To start, 5 mg, 3 times a day for 3 days. The dose may then increase 5 mg every 3 days until the desired response is attained. The maximum dose is 80 mg a day.

ONSET OF EFFECT
Varies from hours to weeks.

DURATION OF ACTION
Unknown.

DIETARY ADVICE
Take it with milk or food to reduce stomach upset.

STORAGE
Store in a tightly sealed container away from heat, moisture, and direct light.

IF YOU MISS A DOSE
Take it as soon as you remember if it is within an hour of the scheduled dose. If more than an hour has passed, do not take the missed dose. Take your next scheduled dose at the proper time, and resume your regular dosage schedule. Do not double the next dose.

STOPPING THE DRUG
Do not stop taking this medication suddenly. Consult your doctor about reducing the doses gradually to avoid suffering from withdrawal symptoms such as hallucinations or seizures.

PROLONGED USE
Consult your doctor about reducing doses gradually after prolonged use.

PRECAUTIONS
Over 60: Central nervous system side effects such as confusion, dizziness, and drowsiness are more likely in older persons.

Driving and Hazardous Work: This drug may cause drowsiness; avoid driving or engaging in hazardous work until you determine how the medicine affects you.

Alcohol: Avoid alcohol while taking this drug.

Pregnancy: Some animal studies have found that very large doses of baclofen can cause birth defects. Human studies have not been done. Before taking baclofen, tell your doctor if you are pregnant or are planning to become pregnant.

Breast Feeding: Baclofen passes into breast milk; caution is advised. Consult your doctor for specific advice.

Infants and Children: The safety and effectiveness of baclofen in children under age 12 have not been determined.

Special Concerns: Baclofen may cause dizziness, lightheadedness, or faintness when you rise from a sitting or lying position; avoid any sudden position changes. Some side effects may appear after stopping baclofen; if any of the following develop, call your doctor immediately: hallucinations; seizures; confusion or changes in mental state; increase in muscle spasms, cramping, or tightness; unusual restlessness or nervousness.

OVERDOSE
Symptoms: Blurred or loss of vision, drowsiness, loss of consciousness, muscle weakness, twitching, seizures, slowed breathing, vomiting.

What to Do: Call your doctor, emergency medical services (EMS), or the nearest poison control center immediately.

DRUG INTERACTIONS
Consult your doctor for specific advice if you are taking an antidepressant, an MAO inhibitor, a tranquilizer, a sedative, a barbiturate, another muscle relaxant, or a narcotic pain reliever.

FOOD INTERACTIONS
No known food interactions.

DISEASE INTERACTIONS
Caution is advised when taking baclofen. Consult your doctor if you have a history of any of the following: stroke, diabetes mellitus, a mental or emotional problem, epilepsy, or kidney disease.

Becaplermin

▶ Drug Class: Topical recombinant human growth factor

▶ Available in: Topical gel

▶ Available OTC? No

▶ As Generic? No

Side Effects

SERIOUS
No serious side effects are associated with the use of becaplermin.

COMMON
Irritation at the site of application.

LESS COMMON
No less-common side effects are associated with becaplermin.

PRINCIPAL USES
To treat diabetic ulcers that develop on the lower legs.

HOW THE DRUG WORKS
Becaplermin is a genetically engineered form of a naturally occurring human platelet-derived growth factor. It helps heal ulcers by attracting and promoting the growth of cells involved in wound repair and the formation of new tissue.

DOSAGE
Apply a thin, continuous layer (approximately 1/16th of an inch in thickness) of becaplermin, as directed by your doctor, to the affected area once a day. Cover the treated area with a saline-moistened dressing and leave in place for 12 hours. The dressing should then be removed and the area rinsed with water or saline to remove any residual gel. Cover the area again with a second saline-moistened dressing (without the gel) for the rest of the day. Your doctor will tell you how much becaplermin to apply to the affected area and how to apply it.

ONSET OF EFFECT
Unknown.

DURATION OF ACTION
Unknown.

DIETARY ADVICE
Becaplermin can be applied without regard to meals.

STORAGE
Keep refrigerated, but do not allow it to freeze. Discard unused portions after the expiration date.

IF YOU MISS A DOSE
If you miss a dose on one day, resume your regular treatment regimen the next day, following your doctor's instructions on the amount of gel to apply.

STOPPING THE DRUG
The decision to stop taking the drug should be made in consultation with your physician.

PROLONGED USE
Consult your doctor if the ulcer does not shrink in size by 30% after 10 weeks or complete healing has not occurred after 20 weeks.

PRECAUTIONS
Over 60: No special problems are expected.

Driving and Hazardous Work: The use of becaplermin should not impair your ability to perform such tasks safely.

Alcohol: No special precautions are necessary.

Pregnancy: Adequate human studies have not been done. Before using becaplermin, tell your doctor if you are pregnant or plan to become pregnant.

Breast Feeding: Becaplermin may be absorbed into the bloodstream and pass into breast milk; caution is advised. Consult your doctor for specific advice.

Infants and Children: Not recommended for use by children under age 16.

Special Concerns: Wash your hands thoroughly before and after applying becaplermin. Do not allow the tip of the tube to touch the ulcer, your finger, or any other surface. Becaplermin should be applied in a carefully measured quantity each day. Your doctor will teach you how to determine the correct amount based on the size of the ulcer area. The calculated amount of gel should be squeezed onto a clean measuring surface (for example, wax paper). Becaplermin should then be transferred to the affected area using an applicator such as a clean cotton swab or a tongue depressor. The amount of becaplermin to be applied should be recalculated at weekly or biweekly intervals by your doctor. Becaplermin should be used together with a good ulcer-care program, including a strict non-weight-bearing program.

OVERDOSE
Symptoms: No cases of overdose have been reported.

What to Do: An overdose with becaplermin is unlikely. If someone applies a much larger dose than prescribed or accidentally ingests the gel, call your doctor.

DRUG INTERACTIONS
Consult your doctor if you are applying any other topical medication to the affected area.

FOOD INTERACTIONS
No known food interactions.

DISEASE INTERACTIONS
You should not apply becaplermin if you have any cancerous or other unusual growths at the affected area. Consult your doctor for specific advice.

Beclomethasone Inhalant and Nasal

BRAND NAMES
Beclovent, Beconase AQ Nasal Spray, Beconase Nasal Inhaler, Vancenase AQ Nasal Spray, Vancenase Nasal Inhaler, Vanceril

▶ Drug Class: Respiratory corticosteroid

▶ Available in: Nasal inhaler, oral inhalation

▶ Available OTC? No

▶ As Generic? No

Side Effects

SERIOUS
No serious side effects are associated with beclomethasone.

COMMON
Nasal form: Nosebleeds or bloody nasal secretions, nasal burning or irritation, sore throat. Oral inhalation: Sore throat, white patches in the mouth or throat, hoarseness.

LESS COMMON
Eye pain, watering eyes, gradual decrease of vision, stomach pain and digestive disturbances.

PRINCIPAL USES
To treat bronchial asthma; to treat allergic rhinitis (seasonal and perennial allergies such as hay fever); to prevent recurrence of nasal polyps after they have been removed surgically.

HOW THE DRUG WORKS
Respiratory corticosteroids such as beclomethasone primarily reduce or prevent inflammation of the lining of the airways (the underlying cause of asthma), reduce the allergic response to inhaled allergens, and inhibit secretion of mucus within airways.

DOSAGE
Adults and teenagers—Nasal inhaler: 1 or 2 inhalations in each nostril, 1 or 2 times a day. Oral inhalation: 2 inhalations, 3 or 4 times a day. For severe asthma: 12 to 16 inhalations daily (maximum of 20 inhalations per day). Children ages 6 to 12— Nasal inhaler: 1 inhalation in each nostril, 1 to 3 times a day. Oral inhalation: 1 to 2 inhalations, 3 or 4 times a day. Maximum of 10 inhalations per day.

ONSET OF EFFECT
Within 5 to 7 days; it may take 3 weeks for the full effect to occur.

DURATION OF ACTION
6 hours or more.

DIETARY ADVICE
Use it before or after meals.

STORAGE
Store away from fire and direct light.

IF YOU MISS A DOSE
Take it as soon as you remember. However, if it is near the time for the next dose, skip the missed dose and resume your regular dosage schedule. Do not double the next dose.

STOPPING THE DRUG
Take it as prescribed for the full treatment period, even if you begin to feel better before the scheduled end of the therapy.

PROLONGED USE
Consult your doctor about the need for periodic medical examinations and laboratory tests if you must take this drug for a prolonged period.

PRECAUTIONS
Over 60: No special problems are expected.

Driving and Hazardous Work: The use of beclomethasone should not impair your ability to perform such tasks safely.

Alcohol: No special precautions are necessary.

Pregnancy: Nasal or inhaled steroids have not been reported to cause birth defects if taken during pregnancy. Before using such drugs, tell your doctor if you are pregnant or plan to become pregnant.

Breast Feeding: Beclomethasone may pass into breast milk; caution is advised. Consult your doctor for advice.

Infants and Children: It has not been established whether beclomethasone is safe and effective in young children.

Special Concerns: Inhaled steroids will not help an asthma attack in progress. Inhaled steroids can lower resistance to yeast infections of the mouth, throat, or voice box. To prevent yeast infections, gargle or rinse your mouth with water after each use; do not swallow the water. Know how to use the inhaler effectively; read and follow the directions that come with the device. Before you have surgery, tell the doctor or dentist that you are using a steroid.

OVERDOSE
Symptoms: No specific ones have been reported.

What to Do: An overdose of beclomethasone is unlikely to be life-threatening. However, if someone takes a much larger dose than prescribed, call your doctor, emergency medical services (EMS), or the nearest poison control center immediately.

DRUG INTERACTIONS
Consult your doctor for specific advice if you are taking systemic corticosteroids, other inhaled corticosteroids, or any drugs that suppress the immune system.

FOOD INTERACTIONS
No known food interactions.

DISEASE INTERACTIONS
Consult your doctor if you have any of the following: a lung disease such as tuberculosis; an infection of the mouth, nose, sinuses, throat, or lungs; a herpes infection of the eye; or any other untreated infection.

Lotensin 20 mg
(NOVARTIS)

▶ Drug Class: Angiotensin-converting enzyme (ACE) inhibitor

▶ Available in: Tablets

▶ Available OTC? No

▶ As Generic? No

Side Effects

SERIOUS
Fever and chills, sore throat and hoarseness, sudden difficulty breathing or swallowing, swelling of the face, mouth, or extremities, impaired kidney function (ankle swelling, decreased urination), confusion, yellow discoloration of the eyes or skin (indicating liver disorder), intense itching, chest pain or palpitations, abdominal pain. Serious side effects are very rare; contact your doctor immediately.

COMMON
Dry, persistent cough.

LESS COMMON
Dizziness or fainting, skin rash, numbness or tingling in the hands, feet, or lips, unusual fatigue or muscle weakness, nausea, drowsiness, loss of taste, headache.

PRINCIPAL USES
To control high blood pressure; to treat congestive heart failure; to treat patients with left ventricular dysfunction (damage to the pumping chamber of the heart); and to minimize further kidney damage in diabetics with mild kidney disease.

HOW THE DRUG WORKS
Angiotensin-converting enzyme (ACE) inhibitors block an enzyme that produces angiotensin, a naturally occurring substance that causes blood vessels to constrict and stimulates production of the adrenal hormone, aldosterone, which promotes sodium retention in the body. As a result, ACE inhibitors relax blood vessels (causing them to widen) and reduces sodium retention, which lowers blood pressure and so decreases the workload of the heart.

DOSAGE
If you are not also taking a diuretic (water pill), 10 mg once a day to start, increased to 20 to 80 mg a day in 1 or 2 doses. If you are taking a diuretic, 5 mg per day.

ONSET OF EFFECT
60 to 90 minutes.

DURATION OF ACTION
Up to 24 hours.

DIETARY ADVICE
Take it on an empty stomach, about 1 hour before mealtime. Follow your doctor's dietary advice to improve control over high blood pressure and heart disease. Avoid high-potassium foods like bananas and citrus fruits and juices, unless you are also taking medications, such as diuretics, that lower potassium levels.

STORAGE
Store in a tightly sealed container away from heat and direct light.

IF YOU MISS A DOSE
Take it as soon as you remember. If it is near the time for the next dose, skip the missed dose and resume your regular dosage schedule. Do not double the next dose.

STOPPING THE DRUG
Do not stop taking this drug abruptly, as this may cause potentially serious health problems. Dosage should be reduced gradually, according to your doctor's instructions.

PROLONGED USE
See your doctor regularly for examinations and tests if you must take this medicine for a prolonged period. Remember that benazepril helps control high blood pressure but does not cure it. Lifelong therapy may be necessary.

PRECAUTIONS
Over 60: Adverse reactions may be more likely and more severe in older patients.

Driving and Hazardous Work: Avoid such activities until you determine how the medication affects you.

Alcohol: Consume alcohol only in moderation since it may increase the effect of the drug and cause an excessive drop in blood pressure.

Pregnancy: Tell your doctor before taking this medication if you are pregnant or plan to become pregnant. Use of this drug during the last 6 months of pregnancy may cause severe defects, even death, in the fetus.

Breast Feeding:
Benazepril passes into breast milk; if possible, avoid using the drug while nursing.

Infants and Children:
Benazepril is generally not prescribed for children; benefits must be weighed against risks. Consult your pediatrician for specific advice.

OVERDOSE
Symptoms: None reported.

What to Do: While overdose is unlikely, call your doctor, emergency medical services (EMS), or the nearest poison control center immediately if you suspect that someone has taken a much larger dose than prescribed.

DRUG INTERACTIONS
Consult your doctor if you are taking diuretics (especially potassium-sparing diuretics), potassium supplements or drugs containing potassium (check ingredient labels), lithium, anticoagulants (such as warfarin), indomethacin or other anti-inflammatory drugs, or any over-the-counter drugs (especially cold remedies and diet pills).

FOOD INTERACTIONS
Avoid low-salt milk and salt substitutes. Many of these products contain potassium.

DISEASE INTERACTIONS
Consult your doctor if you have systemic lupus erythematosus or if you have had a prior allergic reaction to ACE inhibitors. This medication should be used with caution by patients with severe kidney disease or renal artery stenosis (narrowing of one or both of the arteries that supply blood to the kidneys).

Benzocaine

Americaine Topical Anesthetic First Aid Ointment, Anbesol, Baby Orabase, Baby Orajel, Benzodent, Children's Chloraseptic Lozenges, Dent-Zel-Ite, Dentapaine, Hurricaine, Num-Zit Lotion or Gel, Numzident, Orabase-B with Benzocaine, Orajel, Oratect Gel, Rid-A-Pain, SensoGARD Canker Sore Relief, Spec-T Sore Throat Anesthetic

▶ Drug Class: Anesthetic

▶ Available in: Cream, ointment, aerosol spray, dental paste, lozenges, solution

▶ Available OTC? Yes

▶ As Generic? No

Side Effects

SERIOUS
Skin: Severe allergic reaction, producing large, red, hive-like swellings on the skin. Dental use: Large swellings in the mouth or throat. Call your doctor immediately.

COMMON
No common side effects are associated with the skin product or the dental product.

LESS COMMON
Contact dermatitis (skin irritation), causing mild burning, stinging, swelling, itching, redness, or tenderness not present before treatment; hives in or around the mouth.

PRINCIPAL USES
To relieve minor pain and itching of the skin caused by mild burns, bites, cuts, abrasions, and contact dermatitis (skin inflammation caused by contact with an irritant such as poison ivy, or by an allergic response to certain metals or other substances). Dental forms of benzocaine are used to treat pain caused by toothache, teething, cold sores, canker sores, dentures, or other dental appliances.

HOW THE DRUG WORKS
Benzocaine interferes with the ability of certain nerves to conduct electrical signals, which blocks the transmission of nerve impulses that carry pain messages.

DOSAGE
Skin cream, ointment, aerosol spray: Apply to affected area 3 or 4 times a day as needed. Dental paste: Apply as needed. Lozenges: 1 lozenge dissolved in the mouth every 2 hours as needed. Aerosol dental solution: 1 or 2 sprays of at least 1 second each, taken as needed.

ONSET OF EFFECT
Within minutes.

DURATION OF ACTION
Unknown.

DIETARY ADVICE
Forms applied to skin: Can be taken without regard to diet. Oral and dental forms: Do not eat or drink anything for 1 hour after using medicine.

STORAGE
Store in a tightly sealed container away from heat and direct light.

IF YOU MISS A DOSE
Take it as soon as you remember. If it is near the time for the next dose, skip the missed dose and resume your regular dosage schedule. Do not double the next dose.

STOPPING THE DRUG
It is advisable to take the medication as prescribed for the full treatment period. However, you may stop taking the drug before the scheduled end of therapy if you are feeling better.

PROLONGED USE
For skin pain or discomfort: Check with your doctor if the condition does not improve within 7 days. For dental pain: If used temporarily for a toothache, arrange for proper dental treatment as soon as possible. For sore throat: Check with your doctor if pain lasts more than 2 days.

PRECAUTIONS
Over 60: Skin: No information is available. Dental use: Adverse reactions may be more likely and more severe in older patients.

Driving and Hazardous Work: No special precautions are necessary.

Alcohol: No special precautions are necessary.

Pregnancy: Benzocaine has not been reported to cause problems during pregnancy.

Breast Feeding: No problems are expected.

Infants and Children: Dental paste can be used in teething babies 4 months and older. Use of other forms of benzocaine is not recommended for children under 2 unless prescribed by your doctor.

Special Concerns: Do not swallow the dental form unless your doctor has instructed you to do so.

OVERDOSE
Symptoms: Both skin and dental forms: Blurred or double vision; confusion; convulsions; dizziness or lightheadedness; drowsiness; feeling hot, cold, or numb; headache; increased sweating; ringing or buzzing in ears; shivering or trembling; slow or irregular heartbeat; trouble breathing; anxiety, nervousness, or restlessness; pale skin; unusual fatigue.

What to Do: Call your doctor, emergency medical services (EMS), or the nearest poison control center immediately.

DRUG INTERACTIONS
With dental benzocaine, consult your doctor for specific advice if you are taking cholinesterase inhibitors or sulfonamides.

FOOD INTERACTIONS
No known food interactions.

DISEASE INTERACTIONS
Consult your doctor if you have any other condition affecting the mouth or skin.

Benzoyl Peroxide

▶ Drug Class: Acne drug

▶ Available in: Lotion, cream, gel, pads, cleansing bar, facial mask, stick

▶ Available OTC? Yes

▶ As Generic? Yes

Side Effects

SERIOUS
Allergic reaction causing burning, blistering, crusting, itching, severe redness, and swelling of skin. Contact your doctor right away.

COMMON
Mild dryness and peeling of skin.

LESS COMMON
Excessive dryness, unusual feeling of warmth or heat, mild stinging, redness, irritation. This medicine may cause a rash or intensify sunburn in areas of the skin exposed to sunlight or ultraviolet light; avoid excessive sun exposure and tell your doctor if a skin reaction occurs.

PRINCIPAL USES
To treat mild to moderate acne. In more severe cases benzoyl peroxide may be used in conjunction with other acne treatments, such as antibiotics, retinoic acid preparations, and sulfur- or salicylic-acid-containing medications. It may also be used to treat pressure sores and other skin disorders.

HOW THE DRUG WORKS
Benzoyl peroxide slowly releases oxygen, which has an antibacterial effect (bacteria are a primary cause of acne). It also causes peeling and drying of skin, which helps to eliminate blackheads and whiteheads.

DOSAGE
For the cream, gel, lotion or stick form of benzoyl, first wash the affected area of skin with medicated soap and water. Pat dry gently with a towel; apply enough medicine to cover the affected area and rub in gently once or twice a day. For the shave cream form, wet the area to be shaved, apply a small amount of the cream, rub over the entire area, shave, then rinse the area and pat it dry. Check with your doctor about using aftershave lotions. If you have a fair complexion, start with a single daily application at bedtime. Keep the medicine away from eyes, nose, and mouth.

ONSET OF EFFECT
1 to several weeks.

DURATION OF ACTION
Up to 24 hours.

DIETARY ADVICE
This medication may be used without regard to diet.

STORAGE
Store in a tightly sealed container away from heat and direct light.

IF YOU MISS A DOSE
If you miss an application, apply it as soon as you remember.

STOPPING THE DRUG
Although benzoyl peroxide can be discontinued when acne improves, stopping usually leads to a recurrence of acne.

PROLONGED USE
Check with your doctor if you do not see improvement within 4 to 6 weeks. Other medications may be necessary to control acne and to prevent permanent scarring.

PRECAUTIONS
Over 60: No special problems are expected.

Driving and Hazardous Work: No special precautions are necessary.

Alcohol: No special precautions are necessary.

Pregnancy: Problems in pregnancy have not been documented, but the manufacturer recommends that the medicine should not be used by pregnant women unless it is considered essential.

Breast Feeding: Benzoyl peroxide may pass into breast milk. Ask your doctor about its use during breast feeding.

Infants and Children: Studies on this medicine have been done only with teenagers and adults, so there is no specific information about its use with other age groups. Nonetheless, no special side effects or problems are expected in children over 12. No studies have been done in children under 12. Use and dose must be determined by a doctor.

OVERDOSE
Symptoms: Overapplication to the skin may cause burning, itching, scaling, swelling, or redness.

What to Do: Discontinue the drug and consult your doctor. If this drug is accidentally ingested, call your doctor, emergency medical services (EMS), or the nearest poison control center immediately.

DRUG INTERACTIONS
Use of this medicine with skin-peeling agents such as salicylic acid, sulfur, tretinoin, or resorcinol can cause excessive skin irritation. Consult your doctor if you take an oral contraceptive, or if you are using any other prescription or nonprescription medication for acne, or if you use medicated cosmetics or abrasive skin cleaners.

FOOD INTERACTIONS
See below.

DISEASE INTERACTIONS
A history of allergy to cinnamon and foods containing benzoic acid increases the chances of developing an allergic skin rash to benzoyl peroxide. Be sure to notify your doctor if you have either of these allergies. Consult your doctor if you have any skin condition other than acne before using benzoyl peroxide.

Benzphetamine

BRAND NAME
Didrex

▶ Drug Class: Appetite suppressant

▶ Available in: Tablets

▶ Available OTC? No

▶ As Generic? Yes

Side Effects

SERIOUS
Mental depression, nausea or vomiting, abdominal pain, trembling, overactivity, rapid heartbeat, confusion, hallucinations, convulsions, coma, highly elevated blood pressure. Call your doctor at once.

COMMON
Irritability, nervousness, insomnia, mood changes including elation, euphoria, or a false sense of well-being.

LESS COMMON
Irregular or pounding heartbeat, difficulties with urination; call your doctor at once. Blurred vision, dry mouth, unpleasant or metallic taste in the mouth, decreased sexual ability, increased sweating, diarrhea, headache. Notify your doctor if such symptoms persist.

PRINCIPAL USES
For short-term use in a weight reduction program.

HOW THE DRUG WORKS
Benzphetamine reduces appetite by acting on the satiety center in the brain.

DOSAGE
To start, 25 to 50 mg once a day. Usually taken in mid-morning or midafternoon. The dose can be increased up to 150 mg per day, taken in 3 doses, if necessary and if the patient can tolerate this dosage without severe side effects. The magnitude of the increased weight loss associated with benzphetamine is a fraction of a pound a week, with the weight loss greatest in the first weeks of therapy.

ONSET OF EFFECT
Within 1 to 2 hours.

DURATION OF ACTION
Up to 4 hours.

DIETARY ADVICE
Take the drug 1 hour before or 2 hours after meals, in midmorning or midafternoon. The last dose should be taken at least 4 to 6 hours before bedtime, since this medicine may cause insomnia.

STORAGE
Store in a tightly sealed container away from heat, moisture, and direct light.

IF YOU MISS A DOSE
If you miss a dose, take it if you remember within 2 hours. However, if more than 2 hours have passed, skip the missed dose and return to your regular schedule. Do not double the next dose.

STOPPING THE DRUG
Take it as prescribed for the full treatment period. The decision to stop taking the drug should be made in consultation with your physician.

PROLONGED USE
The dose should be reduced with prolonged use. Prolonged use may cause drug dependence. The maximum recommended duration of therapy is 8 to 12 weeks.

PRECAUTIONS
Over 60: Adverse reactions and side effects may be more common in older persons.

Driving and Hazardous Work: Don't drive or engage in hazardous work until you determine how the medicine affects you. It may cause dizziness or blurred vision.

Alcohol: Drink in strict moderation if at all while using this drug.

Pregnancy: Benzphetamine should not be taken during pregnancy because it may harm the fetus. A reliable form of birth control should be used while taking this medicine.

Breast Feeding: Benzphetamine passes into breast milk. It should not be taken while breast feeding.

Infants and Children: Benzphetamine should not be used in children under the age of 12.

OVERDOSE
Symptoms: Overactivity, irritability, trembling, insomnia, rapid heartbeat, confusion, hallucinations, convulsions, coma.

What to Do: Call your doctor, emergency medical services (EMS), or the nearest poison control center immediately.

DRUG INTERACTIONS
Benzphetamine should not be used with any other central nervous stimulant drug. It may decrease the effect of drugs for high blood pressure and increase the effect of antidepressants. Caution is necessary when urinary acidifiers or alkalizers are taken with benzphetamine. Avoid MAO inhibitors. Vitamin C supplements increase excretion and therefore decrease the effectiveness of this drug.

FOOD INTERACTIONS
Avoid beverages containing caffeine since they may increase the drug's effect of stimulating the central nervous system.

DISEASE INTERACTIONS
This medicine should not be taken by persons with advanced arteriosclerosis, moderate to severe high blood pressure, hyperthyroidism, or glaucoma. It should not be given to persons with a history of drug abuse. For people with diabetes, taking this medicine may affect the amount of insulin or oral antidiabetic medicines that must be taken.

Benztropine Mesylate

▶ Drug Class: Antiparkinsonism drug

▶ Available in: Capsules, injection

▶ Available OTC? No

▶ As Generic? Yes

Side Effects

SERIOUS
Unusually rapid or slow heartbeat, heart palpitations, abnormal behavior, confusion, bowel obstruction. Call your doctor immediately.

COMMON
Constipation. It can be reduced by drinking more fluids and eating high-fiber foods.

LESS COMMON
Restlessness, irritability, disorientation, headache, sleepiness, depression, muscle weakness, eye sensitivity to light, dry mouth, heartburn, nausea, vomiting, difficulty swallowing, increased body temperature, decreased sweating.

PRINCIPAL USES
To treat Parkinson's disease or the adverse effects of some central nervous system drugs, which produce Parkinson-like symptoms or affect muscle control.

HOW THE DRUG WORKS
The exact mechanism of action is unknown, but it is believed to help increase the release of certain neurological chemicals that improve control over muscle movement.

DOSAGE
For Parkinson's disease: 0.5 to 6 mg per day in 1 dose at bedtime. For drug-induced Parkinson reactions: 1 to 4 mg per day either in 1 dose or 2 to 3 doses. For drug-induced nervous system effects: 1 to 4 mg per day in 1 to 3 doses.

ONSET OF EFFECT
Within 1 to 2 hours.

DURATION OF ACTION
Up to 24 hours.

DIETARY ADVICE
Benztropine can be taken with food to reduce stomach irritation.

STORAGE
Store this medicine in a tightly sealed container away from heat and direct light.

IF YOU MISS A DOSE
If you miss a dose, take it as soon as you remember unless the next scheduled dose is to be taken within 2 hours. In that case, skip the missed dose and resume your normal schedule. Do not double the next dose.

STOPPING THE DRUG
Do not stop taking benztropine suddenly. If therapy is to be discontinued, dosage should be reduced gradually, according to your doctor's instructions.

PROLONGED USE
Prolonged use of this drug may increase pressure in the eye and thus increase the risk of glaucoma, especially in older persons.

PRECAUTIONS
Over 60: Side effects may be more common in older persons. Smaller starting doses are advisable.

Driving and Hazardous Work: Avoid driving and hazardous work until you determine if the drug causes drowsiness.

Alcohol: Alcohol should be avoided or used with caution because it may increase the sedative effects of this medication.

Pregnancy: Benztropine may affect the unborn child's intestinal tract. Do not use the drug while pregnant.

Breast Feeding: It is not known whether benztropine passes into breast milk. Do not use the drug while breast feeding.

Infants and Children: Not generally prescribed for children under the age of 3. Your doctor must determine the exact dosage for older children.

Special Concerns: Eye pressure should be measured regularly because of the risk of glaucoma. Limit physical activity in hot weather.

OVERDOSE
Symptoms: Clumsiness, drowsiness, fast or slow heartbeat, flushed skin, breathing difficulty, seizures, loss of consciousness, muscle weakness, inability to sweat, uncoordinated movement.

What to Do: Call your doctor, emergency medical services (EMS), or the nearest poison control center immediately.

DRUG INTERACTIONS
The activity of benztropine can affect or be affected by many drugs. Talk to your doctor about any drug you are taking, especially phenothiazines, tricyclic antidepressants, and amantadine.

FOOD INTERACTIONS
None are expected.

DISEASE INTERACTIONS
Consult your doctor if you have glaucoma, high blood pressure, heart disease, impaired liver function, kidney disease, or myasthenia gravis.

Beta-Carotene

BRAND NAMES
Max-Caro, Provatene,
Solatene

▶ Drug Class: Dietary
supplement

▶ Available in: Capsules,
tablets

▶ Available OTC? Yes

▶ As Generic? Yes

Side Effects

SERIOUS
No serious side effects
are associated with beta-
carotene.

COMMON
Yellowing of the palms,
hands, or soles of feet,
and, in some cases, the
face.

LESS COMMON
No less common side
effects are associated
with the use of beta-
carotene.

PRINCIPAL USES
Beta-carotene is a natural source of vitamin A. While most Americans get sufficient amounts of vitamin A in their diet, beta-carotene may be prescribed as a dietary supplement for people with certain medical conditions that increase the need for the vitamin. Such conditions include cystic fibrosis, long-term chronic illness, chronic diarrhea, and intestinal malabsorption. A profound deficiency of vitamin A (which occurs very rarely) can lead to night blindness. It may also lead to skin problems, dry eyes and eye infections, and slowed growth. Beta-carotene may also be prescribed in larger doses to reduce the severity of photosensitive reactions (heightened sensitivity to sunlight) that occur in patients with a rare inherited disorder known as erythopoietic protoporphyria. Beta-carotene is an antioxidant that has been prescribed to prevent atherosclerosis and coronary heart disease, but beta-carotene supplements did not reduce the incidence of heart attacks in three large clinical trials.

HOW THE DRUG WORKS
Approximately half of ingested beta-carotene is converted to vitamin A in the intestine. The rest is absorbed unchanged and is stored in various tissues, especially fat.

DOSAGE
As a dietary supplement—Adults and teenagers: 6 to 15 mg a day. Children: 3 to 6 mg a day. To treat erythopoietic porphyria— 30 to 300 mg a day.

ONSET OF EFFECT
Unknown.

DURATION OF ACTION
Unknown.

DIETARY ADVICE
It is best taken with meals.

STORAGE
Store in a tightly sealed container away from heat, moisture, and direct light. Do not refrigerate beta-carotene, and keep it from freezing.

IF YOU MISS A DOSE
There is no danger in doubling the next dose if you miss a scheduled dose.

STOPPING THE DRUG
Take it as prescribed. If beta-carotene is prescribed for a specific medical condition, the decision to stop taking it should be made in consultation with your physician.

PROLONGED USE
No known problems.

PRECAUTIONS
Over 60: No special precautions are warranted.

Driving and Hazardous Work: No precautions are necessary.

Alcohol: No special precautions are necessary.

Pregnancy: Beta-carotene has not been studied in pregnant women, but no problems with fertility or pregnancy have been reported in women taking up to 30 mg of beta-carotene a day. The effects of higher daily doses are unknown.

Breast Feeding: Beta-carotene may pass into breast milk, although problems have not been documented with the intake of normal recommended amounts. Consult your doctor for advice.

Infants and Children: No problems have been reported with the intake of recommended amounts of beta-carotene.

Special Concerns: Beta-carotene is found in carrots, dark-green leafy vegetables such as spinach and lettuce, tomatoes, sweet potatoes, broccoli, cantaloupe, and winter squash. Be sure to eat a proper, balanced diet to obtain adequate amounts of beta-carotene from foods. Some fat is needed so that the body can absorb beta-carotene. Beta-carotene is safer than vitamin A because high doses of vitamin A can be harmful. If high levels of vitamin A are present, less beta-carotene is converted to vitamin A by the body.

OVERDOSE
Symptoms: None have been reported.

What to Do: An overdose of beta-carotene is unlikely to be dangerous. Emergency instructions do not apply.

DRUG INTERACTIONS
Consult your doctor for specific advice if you are taking cholestyramine or colestipol (cholesterol-lowering drugs), mineral oil, neomycin (an antibiotic), or vitamin E.

FOOD INTERACTIONS
No known food interactions.

DISEASE INTERACTIONS
If you have any medical problems, consult your doctor before taking beta-carotene. Large doses of beta-carotene may cause complications in patients with liver disease or kidney disease.

BRAND NAME
Celestone

▶ Drug Class: Corticosteroid

▶ Available in: Syrup, tablets, extended-release tablets, injection, rectal solution

▶ Available OTC? No

▶ As Generic? Yes

Side Effects

SERIOUS
Vision problems, frequent urination, increased thirst, rectal bleeding, blistering skin, confusion, hallucinations, paranoia, euphoria, depression, mood swings, redness and swelling at injection site. Call your doctor immediately.

COMMON
Increased appetite, indigestion, nervousness, insomnia, greater susceptibility to infections, increased blood pressure, slowed healing of wounds, unusual weight gain, easy bruising, fluid retention.

LESS COMMON
Change in skin color, dizziness, headache, increased sweating, unusual growth of body or facial hair, increased blood sugar, peptic ulcers, adrenal insufficiency, muscle weakness, cataracts, glaucoma, osteoporosis.

PRINCIPAL USES
To treat numerous conditions that involve inflammation (a response by body tissues, producing redness, warmth, swelling, and pain). Such conditions include arthritis, allergic reactions, asthma, some skin diseases, multiple sclerosis flare-ups, and other autoimmune diseases. Also prescribed to treat deficiency of natural steroid hormones.

HOW THE DRUG WORKS
Betamethasone mimics the effects of the body's corticosteroids. It depresses the synthesis, release, and activity of inflammation-producing chemicals. It also suppresses immune system activity.

DOSAGE
Adults— Syrup or tablets: 600 micrograms (mcg) to 7.2 mg a day, as a single dose or in divided doses. Extended-release tablets: 2 to 6 mg a day to start, then as ordered by your doctor. Injection: Up to 9 mg a day. Rectal solution: 5 mg, given as an enema at night. Consult pediatrician for children's dosage.

ONSET OF EFFECT
Within 1 hour. It may take 2 to 4 days for full effect.

DURATION OF ACTION
More than 3 days for oral forms; 24 hours or more for other forms.

DIETARY ADVICE
Take it with food or milk to minimize stomach upset. Your doctor may recommend a special diet.

STORAGE
Store in a tightly sealed container away from heat, moisture, and direct light.

IF YOU MISS A DOSE
Take it as soon as you remember. If you take several doses a day and it is close to the next dose, double the next dose. If you take 1 dose a day and you do not remember until the next day, skip the missed dose and do not double the next dose.

STOPPING THE DRUG
With long-term therapy, do not stop taking the drug abruptly; the dosage should be decreased gradually.

PROLONGED USE
See your doctor regularly for tests and examinations. Long-term use may lead to cataracts, diabetes, hypertension, or osteoporosis.

PRECAUTIONS
Over 60: Adverse reactions may be more likely and more severe in older patients.

Driving and Hazardous Work: Do not drive or engage in hazardous work until you determine how the medicine affects you.

Alcohol: May cause stomach problems; avoid alcohol unless your doctor approves occasional moderate drinking.

Pregnancy: Overuse during pregnancy can retard the child's growth and cause other developmental problems. Consult your physician.

Breast Feeding: Do not use while nursing.

Infants and Children: Betamethasone may retard the normal growth and development of bone and other tissues. Consult your doctor for advice.

Special Concerns: Avoid immunizations with live vaccines if possible. This drug can lower your resistance to infection. Patients undergoing long-term therapy should wear a medical-alert bracelet. Call your doctor if you develop a fever.

OVERDOSE
Symptoms: Fever, muscle or joint pain, nausea, dizziness, fainting, difficulty breathing. Prolonged overuse: Moonface, obesity, unusual hair growth, acne, loss of sexual function, muscle wasting.

What to Do: Seek medical assistance immediately.

DRUG INTERACTIONS
Consult your doctor for specific advice if you are taking aminoglutethimide, antacids, barbiturates, carbamazepine, griseofulvin, mitotane, phenylbutazone, phenytoin, primidone, rifampin, injectable amphotericin B, oral antidiabetes agents, insulin, digitalis drugs, diuretics, or medications that contain potassium or sodium.

FOOD INTERACTIONS
Avoid excess sodium.

DISEASE INTERACTIONS
Consult your doctor if you have a history of bone disease, chicken pox, measles, gastrointestinal disorders, diabetes, recent serious infection, tuberculosis, glaucoma, heart disease, hypertension, liver or kidney disorders, high blood cholesterol, overactive or underactive thyroid, myasthenia gravis, or lupus.

Betamethasone Topical

BRAND NAMES
Alphatrex, Beta-Val, Betatrex, Dermabet, Diprolene, Diprosone, Luxiq, Maxivate, Teladar, Uticort, Valisone, Valnac

▶ Drug Class: Topical corticosteroid

▶ Available in: Cream, gel, lotion, ointment, aerosol, foam

▶ Available OTC? **No**

▶ As Generic? **Yes**

Side Effects

SERIOUS
Serious side effects from the use of topical betamethasone are rare.

COMMON
Burning, itching, irritation, redness, dryness, acne, stinging and cracking of skin, numbness or tingling in the extremities in 0.5% to 1% of patients. Risk of such reactions is higher with lotion and gel and lower in ointment and cream. (Products vary in potency from one brand to another; higher-potency products are more likely to cause side effects.)

LESS COMMON
Blistering and pus near hair follicles, unusual bleeding or easy bruising, darkening or prominence of small surface veins, increased susceptibility to infection.

PRINCIPAL USES
To treat skin rashes and inflammation.

HOW THE DRUG WORKS
Topical betamethasone appears to interfere with the formation of natural substances within the body that are directly responsible for the process of inflammation, which produces swelling, redness, and itching.

DOSAGE
Apply sparingly as a thin film, 2 (sometimes 3) times a day, only to the specific areas of skin where needed. Wash or soak the affected area prior to application, as this may improve the absorption of the drug. Foam is for use on the scalp.

ONSET OF EFFECT
Rapid, but may take 24 to 48 hours to see effect.

DURATION OF ACTION
Unknown.

DIETARY ADVICE
No special restrictions.

STORAGE
Store in a tightly sealed container away from heat and direct light.

IF YOU MISS A DOSE
Apply it as soon as you remember. If it is near the time for the next dose, skip the missed dose and resume your regular dosage schedule as prescribed.

STOPPING THE DRUG
Take as prescribed for the full treatment period, even if you begin to feel better before the scheduled end of therapy.

PROLONGED USE
Avoid prolonged use, particularly near the eyes, on the face in general, on the genital or rectal regions, or in the folds of the skin (for example, underneath the breasts).

PRECAUTIONS
Over 60: Side effects may be more likely and more severe; therapy with topical corticosteroids should be limited.

Driving and Hazardous Work: The use of topical betamethasone should not impair your ability to perform such tasks safely.

Alcohol: No special precautions are necessary.

Pregnancy: Should not be used for prolonged periods in pregnant women or in women trying to become pregnant.

Breast Feeding: Although problems have not been documented, caution is advised. Do not apply to breasts prior to nursing. Consult your doctor for specific advice.

Infants and Children: It should not be used for more than 2 weeks on children and adolescents, unless otherwise directed by your doctor. Do not use tight-fitting diapers or plastic pants on children when treating skin irritation in the diaper area.

Special Concerns: Wash your hands thoroughly after application. Do not wrap the treated area with bandages or tight-fitting clothing unless otherwise instructed by your doctor. Doing so may cause skin infections to worsen; corticosteroid treatment may need to be discontinued to treat infections, then resumed later. Note that topical betamethasone is not a treatment for acne, burns, infections, or disorders of pigmentation.

OVERDOSE
Symptoms: No specific ones have been reported.

What to Do: An overdose of a topical corticosteroid is unlikely to be life-threatening. However, in the event of accidental ingestion or an apparent overdose, call a doctor, emergency medical services (EMS), or the nearest poison control center right away.

DRUG INTERACTIONS
Do not mix topical betamethasone with other products, especially alcohol-containing preparations (which include colognes, aftershave, and many moisturizer lotions), since this may cause dryness and irritation, or increase the risk of an allergic reaction.

FOOD INTERACTIONS
Potassium supplements may decrease this drug's effects. Avoid foods high in sodium.

DISEASE INTERACTIONS
Caution is advised when taking this drug. Consult your doctor if you have any of the following: cataracts; diabetes mellitus; glaucoma; infection, sores, or ulcerations of the skin; infection at another site in your body; or tuberculosis.

Betamethasone/Clotrimazole

BRAND NAME
Lotrisone

▶ Drug Class: Topical antifungal

▶ Available in: Cream

▶ Available OTC? No

▶ As Generic? Yes

Side Effects

SERIOUS
Blistering or ulceration of the skin; blistering of the lips, nose, and mouth.

COMMON
Brief burning or irritation after application; peeling.

LESS COMMON
Severe burning, itching, swelling, increased redness, or any increased discomfort developing at the application site that was not present prior to therapy; dry skin; pus or inflammation at base of hair follicles; change in skin color at site of application; acne.

PRINCIPAL USES
To treat fungal infections of the skin.

HOW THE DRUG WORKS
Clotrimazole prevents fungal organisms from manufacturing the vital proteins they require for growth and function. Betamethasone dipropionate is a steroid; it interferes with the formation of natural substances within the body that are directly responsible for the process of inflammation, which produces swelling, redness, and pain. The use of these two effective medications in combination for skin infections appears to hasten recovery sooner than use of clotrimazole alone. This medication is only effective for infections caused by fungal organisms. It will not work for bacterial or viral infections.

DOSAGE
Adults and children older than 12 years of age: Apply and massage a sufficient amount of cream to the affected site twice daily for 2 to 4 weeks. This combination drug contains a high-potency topical steroid that should not be used in skin creases or with bandages (occlusive dressing) unless closely supervised by your doctor.

ONSET OF EFFECT
Clotrimazole begins killing susceptible fungi shortly after contact. The effects may not be noticeable for several days or weeks.

DURATION OF ACTION
Unknown.

DIETARY ADVICE
Drink plenty of fluids.

STORAGE
Store in a tightly sealed container away from heat and direct light. Keep away from moisture and extremes in temperature.

IF YOU MISS A DOSE
Apply it as soon as you remember. If it is near the time for the next dose, skip the missed dose and resume your regular dosage schedule. Do not double the next dose or apply an excessively thick film of topical medication to compensate for a missed dose.

STOPPING THE DRUG
Apply as prescribed for the full treatment period, even if the fungal infection appears to be eradicated before the scheduled end of therapy. Unfortunately, it can be difficult to assess when the drug has achieved its desired effect since it suppresses redness and inflammation of the skin before the infection is completely clear; recurrence of fungal infection owing to inadequate length of therapy is a significant risk.

PROLONGED USE
Therapy with this medication should not exceed 4 weeks.

PRECAUTIONS
Over 60: Adverse reactions may be more likely and more severe in older patients.

Driving and Hazardous Work: No special precautions are necessary.

Alcohol: No special precautions are necessary.

Pregnancy: Not recommended during pregnancy.

Breast Feeding: Betamethasone dipropionate/clotrimazole may pass into breast milk; caution is advised. Consult your doctor for advice.

Infants and Children: Not recommended for use by children under age 12.

Special Concerns: Avoid contact with eyes. Wash hands thoroughly after application. Tell your doctor if your condition has not improved within a few days of starting the medication. As with any other antifungal, betamethasone dipropionate/clotrimazole is useful only against organisms that are vulnerable to its effects. Therefore, it is important to tell your doctor if your condition has not improved—or has worsened—within a few days of starting betamethasone dipropionate/clotrimazole. The particular organism causing your illness may be resistant to this medication.

OVERDOSE
Symptoms: No specific ones have been reported.

What to Do: An overdose is unlikely to be life-threatening. However, if someone applies a much larger dose than prescribed or ingests the medication, call your doctor, emergency medical services (EMS), or the nearest poison control center immediately.

DRUG INTERACTIONS
No specific drug interactions have been documented.

FOOD INTERACTIONS
No known food interactions.

DISEASE INTERACTIONS
Consult your physician if you have ever experienced an allergic reaction to any topical medication, or undesirable reactions to any steroid or steroid-containing preparation.

Betaxolol Ophthalmic

BRAND NAMES
Betoptic, Betoptic Pilo,
Betoptic S

▶ Drug Class: Antiglaucoma
drug; ophthalmic beta-blocker

▶ Available in: Ophthalmic
solution, suspension

▶ Available OTC? No

▶ As Generic? No

Side Effects

SERIOUS
Palpitations, trouble
breathing, dizziness and
weakness caused by low
blood pressure. Call your
doctor right away.

COMMON
Temporary eye irritation,
tearing, eye inflamma-
tion, burning, swelling.

LESS COMMON
Blurred vision, poor night
vision, and increased
sensitivity to light;
headache; insomnia;
sinus irritation; odd or
bitter taste in the mouth.

PRINCIPAL USES
To treat glaucoma.

HOW THE DRUG WORKS
Glaucoma, a sight-threatening disorder, occurs when
aqueous humor (the fluid
inside the eye) cannot drain
properly, resulting in an
increase in pressure within
the eyeball (known as
intraocular pressure).
Increased intraocular pressure can damage the optic
nerve and lead to a gradually progressive loss of
vision. Betaxolol decreases
the production of aqueous
humor, thereby reducing
intraocular pressure.

DOSAGE
1 or 2 drops of 0.5% solution
or 0.25% suspension twice
a day.

ONSET OF EFFECT
30 minutes.

DURATION OF ACTION
12 hours or more.

DIETARY ADVICE
No special restrictions or
recommendations.

STORAGE
Store in a tightly sealed container away from heat, moisture, and direct light. Do
not allow the medicine to
freeze.

IF YOU MISS A DOSE
Apply the missed dose as
soon as you remember. If it
is near the time for the next
dose, skip the missed dose
and resume your regular
dosage schedule. Do not
double the next dose.

STOPPING THE DRUG
The decision to stop taking
the drug should be made by
your doctor. Gradual discontinuation rather than a sudden stop may be required.

PROLONGED USE
Consult your doctor about
the need for periodic oph-
thalmological examinations
to check intraocular pressure (the pressure within
the eyeball).

PRECAUTIONS
Over 60: Adverse reactions
may be more likely and
more severe in older
patients.

**Driving and Hazardous
Work:** Exercise caution
until you determine how the
drug affects your vision.

Alcohol: Alcohol should be
used with caution.

Pregnancy: Ophthalmic
betaxolol has not been
shown to cause birth
defects in animals; human
studies have not been done.
Before taking it, tell your
doctor if you are pregnant
or planning a pregnancy.

Breast Feeding: Oph-
thalmic betaxolol may pass
into breast milk; caution is
advised. Consult your doctor for specific advice.

Infants and Children:
Not recommended for use
by children under age 12.

Special Concerns: To use
the eye drops, first wash
your hands. Tilt your head
back. Gently apply pressure
to the inside corner of the
eyelid and with the index
finger of the same hand,
pull downward on the lower
eyelid to make a space.
Drop the medicine into this
space and close your eye.
Apply pressure for 1 or 2
minutes while keeping the
eye closed without blinking.
Then wash your hands
again. Make sure the tip of
the dropper does not touch
your eye, finger, or any
other surface. Betaxolol
may make your eyes more

sensitive to sunlight. If this
occurs, wear sunglasses or
avoid bright light as necessary. Shake the suspension
well before using.

OVERDOSE
Symptoms: Double vision,
slow pulse, dizziness and
weakness caused by low
blood pressure, unusual
fatigue, drowsiness,
seizures, hallucinations,
loss of consciousness.

What to Do: An overdose
of this drug is unlikely to be
life-threatening. If a large
volume of the medicine
enters the eyes, flush with
water. If someone accidentally ingests it, seek medical
assistance immediately.

DRUG INTERACTIONS
It is not recommended to
use two ophthalmic beta-
blockers at the same time.
Special concern is war-
ranted in people taking
antidiabetic drugs, since
ophthalmic betaxolol may
mask symptoms of low
blood sugar. Other drugs
may interact with oph-
thalmic betaxolol. Tell your
doctor if you are using any
other prescription or over-
the-counter medication.

FOOD INTERACTIONS
No known food interactions.

DISEASE INTERACTIONS
Caution is advised when
taking ophthalmic betaxolol.
Consult your doctor if you
have any of the following
conditions: diabetes, hypoglycemia, heart disease,
high blood pressure, lung
disorders, irregular heartbeat, or an overactive thyroid gland.

Betaxolol Oral

BRAND NAME
Kerlone

▶ Drug Class: Beta-blocker

▶ Available in: Tablets

▶ Available OTC? No

▶ As Generic? No

Side Effects

SERIOUS
Shortness of breath, wheezing; irregular or slow heartbeat (50 beats per minute or less); pain or feelings of tightness or pressure in the chest; swelling of the ankles, feet, and lower legs; mental depression. If you experience such symptoms, stop taking betaxolol and call your doctor immediately.

COMMON
Dizziness or lightheadedness, especially when rising suddenly to a standing position, rapid heartbeat or palpitations, decreased sexual ability, frequent headaches.

LESS COMMON
Anxiety, irritability, nervousness; constipation; diarrhea; dry, sore eyes; itching; nausea or vomiting; nightmares or intensely vivid dreams; numbness, tingling, or other unusual sensations in the fingers, toes, or scalp.

PRINCIPAL USES
To treat high blood pressure (hypertension).

HOW THE DRUG WORKS
Betaxolol slows the rate and force of contraction of the heart by blocking certain nerve impulses, thus reducing blood pressure.

DOSAGE
To start, 10 mg, once a day. Dose may be increased to a maximum of 20 mg per day.

ONSET OF EFFECT
Within 1 hour.

DURATION OF ACTION
24 hours or more.

DIETARY ADVICE
This medication can be used without regard to diet.

STORAGE
Store in a tightly sealed container away from heat and direct light.

IF YOU MISS A DOSE
Take the missed dose as soon as possible. If it is within 8 hours of the next dose, skip the missed dose and resume your regular dosage schedule. Do not double the next dose.

STOPPING THE DRUG
Take it as prescribed for the full treatment period even if you begin to feel better before the scheduled end of therapy. Lifelong therapy with betaxolol may be necessary. Do not stop taking the medication suddenly, as this may result in potentially serious medical consequences. Dose must be tapered gradually.

PROLONGED USE
Consult your doctor about the need for periodic examinations or laboratory studies to check blood pressure, heart function, kidney function, and blood sugar levels.

PRECAUTIONS
Over 60: Adverse reactions may be more likely and more severe in older patients. Lower doses may be warranted, and frequent measurement of blood pressure is important.

Driving and Hazardous Work: Use caution when driving or engaging in hazardous work until you determine how the medication affects you.

Alcohol: Drink in careful moderation if at all. Alcohol may interact with the drug and cause a dangerous drop in blood pressure.

Pregnancy: Betaxolol has caused birth defects in animals; adequate human studies have not been done. Use of this drug should be avoided during the first three months of pregnancy if possible, and during labor and delivery, because of possible damaging effects on the newborn baby.

Breast Feeding: Betaxolol may pass into breast milk; caution is advised. Consult your doctor for advice.

Infants and Children: The safety and effectiveness of this drug for children under the age of 12 have not been established. If it is used, the child should have periodic tests for low blood glucose (sugar) levels.

OVERDOSE
Symptoms: Double vision, unusually slow or rapid heartbeat, severe dizziness or fainting, poor circulation in the hands (bluish skin), breathing difficulty, seizures.

What to Do: Call your doctor, emergency medical services (EMS), or the nearest poison control center immediately.

DRUG INTERACTIONS
Consult your doctor for specific advice if you are taking calcium channel blockers, ACE inhibitors, insulin or any other diabetes drug, antihistamines, other drugs for high blood pressure, nonsteroidal anti-inflammatory drugs, barbiturates, or clonidine.

FOOD INTERACTIONS
No known food interactions.

DISEASE INTERACTIONS
Betaxolol should be used with caution in people with diabetes, especially insulin-dependent diabetes, since the drug may mask symptoms of hypoglycemia. Consult your doctor if you have any of the following: heart disease, hay fever, asthma, chronic bronchitis, hypoglycemia, an overactive thyroid gland, impaired liver function, or impaired kidney function.

Bethanechol Chloride

Generic 5 mg
(SIDMAK)

▶ Drug Class: Cholinergic

▶ Available in: Tablets, injection

▶ Available OTC? No

▶ As Generic? Yes

Side Effects

SERIOUS
Difficulty breathing, wheezing, severe or persistent abdominal cramps, diarrhea. Call your doctor at once.

COMMON
Dizziness or lightheadedness. This can be minimized by getting up slowly from a sitting or lying position.

LESS COMMON
Headache, blurred vision, nausea, stomach discomfort, excessive urge to urinate.

PRINCIPAL USES
To treat bladder or urinary tract disorders that make urination difficult. To help initiate urination after surgery.

HOW THE DRUG WORKS
Bethanechol strengthens the ability of bladder muscles to contract, facilitating urination.

DOSAGE
Tablets— Adults: 10 to 50 mg, 3 or 4 times a day. Children: 0.6 mg per 2.2 lbs (1 kg) of body weight, in 3 to 4 doses a day. Injection— Adults: 2.5 to 5 mg injected under the skin 3 or 4 times a day. Children: 0.2 mg per 2.2 lbs of body weight per day, injected 3 to 4 times a day, as determined by your pediatrician.

ONSET OF EFFECT
30 to 90 minutes.

DURATION OF ACTION
Up to 6 hours.

DIETARY ADVICE
Take this medicine on an empty stomach with liquid 1 hour before or 2 hours after meals to avoid nausea and vomiting.

STORAGE
Store in a tightly sealed container away from heat and direct light.

IF YOU MISS A DOSE
Take it as soon as you remember. If it is near the time for the next dose, skip the missed dose and resume your regular dosage schedule. Do not double the next dose.

STOPPING THE DRUG
It may not be necessary to take this drug for the entire prescribed course of treatment. Follow your doctor's instructions about discontinuing the medicine.

PROLONGED USE
No problems expected.

PRECAUTIONS
Over 60: Adverse reactions and side effects may be more severe in older persons.

Driving and Hazardous Work: Determine if the drug causes dizziness, lightheadedness or blurred vision before driving or doing hazardous work. Danger increases if you drink alcohol or take a medicine that affects alertness, such as an antihistamine, a tranquilizer, a pain medicine, a sedative, or a narcotic.

Alcohol: Alcohol intake should be limited to 1 or 2 drinks a day because it can add to the diminished alertness caused by this medicine. Consult your doctor about the exact amount of alcohol you can consume.

Pregnancy: Animal and human studies have not been done. Consult your doctor about taking bethanechol if you are pregnant or plan to become pregnant.

Breast Feeding: It is not known whether bethanechol passes into breast milk. Consult your doctor about taking it if you are nursing.

Infants and Children: Use of bethanechol by infants and children requires close medical supervision.

Special Concerns: Bethanechol interferes with diagnostic laboratory studies of pancreas and liver function. While undergoing treatment with this drug, be cautious when standing up suddenly, as dizziness and lightheadedness are common side effects.

OVERDOSE
Symptoms: Abdominal discomfort, salivation, flushing of the skin, sweating, nausea, vomiting.

What to Do: Call your doctor, emergency medical services (EMS), or the nearest poison control center immediately.

DRUG INTERACTIONS
Consult your doctor if you are taking bethanechol at the same time that you are taking any prescription or nonprescription drugs, especially anticholinergics, ganglionic blockers, nitrates, procainamide, quinidine, or other cholinergic drugs.

FOOD INTERACTIONS
None expected.

DISEASE INTERACTIONS
Consult your doctor if you have low blood pressure, any blood vessel problem, a weakened bladder wall, any urinary tract problem, any digestive problem, an overactive thyroid (hyperthyroidism), asthma, seizures, or Parkinson's disease.

Biotin

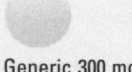

Generic 300 mcg
(TISHCON)

▶ Drug Class: Vitamin

▶ Available in: Capsules, tablets

▶ Available OTC? Yes

▶ As Generic? Yes

Side Effects

SERIOUS
No serious side effects are associated with recommended doses of biotin. However, check with your doctor if you notice anything unusual while you are taking it.

COMMON
No common side effects are associated with recommended doses.

LESS COMMON
No less-common side effects have been reported.

PRINCIPAL USES
Biotin is a vitamin found naturally in various foods (see Dietary Advice for more information). While most people get sufficient amounts of it in their diet, biotin may be prescribed as a dietary supplement for people on inadequate or unusual diets or with medical conditions that increase the need for it. Such conditions include a genetic deficiency of the enzyme (biotinidase) needed by the body to utilize biotin, intestinal malabsorption, seborrheic dermatitis in infancy, and an inability to absorb biotin as a result of surgical removal of the stomach. Biotin deficiency may lead to dermatitis, hair loss, high blood cholesterol levels, and heart problems.

HOW THE DRUG WORKS
Biotin is one of the B vitamins necessary for the formation of glucose and fatty acids, and for the metabolism of amino acids and carbohydrates. B vitamins are particularly crucial to the proper functioning of the cardiovascular and nervous systems.

DOSAGE
No recommended daily allowances (RDAs) have been established for biotin. The following daily intakes are advised. Adults and teenagers: 30 (mcg). Children ages 7 to 10 years: 30 mcg. Children ages 4 to 6 years: 25 mcg daily. Birth to 3 years: 10 to 20 mcg.

ONSET OF EFFECT
Unknown.

DURATION OF ACTION
Unknown.

DIETARY ADVICE
Biotin can be taken with or between meals. Foods that contain biotin include cauliflower, liver, salmon, carrots, bananas, cereals, yeast, and soy flour. Biotin content is reduced when food is cooked or preserved.

STORAGE
Store in a tightly sealed container away from heat, moisture, and direct light.

IF YOU MISS A DOSE
Take it as soon as you remember.

STOPPING THE DRUG
If you are taking biotin for a vitamin deficiency or medical problem, take it as prescribed for the full treatment period.

PROLONGED USE
When biotin is prescribed to overcome a deficiency, periodic monitoring of biotin levels in the blood may be required.

PRECAUTIONS
Over 60: No problems are expected in older persons taking recommended doses of biotin.

Driving and Hazardous Work: The use of biotin should not impair your ability to perform such tasks safely.

Alcohol: No special precautions are necessary.

Pregnancy: No problems are expected with the intake of recommended doses of biotin during pregnancy.

Breast Feeding: No problems are expected with the intake of recommended doses of biotin during breast feeding.

Infants and Children: No problems are expected with recommended doses.

Special Concerns: Some drastic weight-reducing diets may may not supply enough biotin. Consult your doctor for specific advice. Biotin is generally available as part of a multivitamin complex.

OVERDOSE
Symptoms: None. (No cases of biotin overdose have been documented.)

What to Do: Emergency instructions not applicable.

DRUG INTERACTIONS
There are no known drug interactions associated with biotin.

FOOD INTERACTIONS
No known food interactions.

DISEASE INTERACTIONS
None reported.

Biperiden

BRAND NAME
Akineton

Akineton 2 mg
(KNOLL)

▶ Drug Class: Antiparkinsonism drug

▶ Available in: Tablets, injection

▶ Available OTC? No

▶ As Generic? Yes

Side Effects

SERIOUS
Retention of urine (decreased urine output), confusion, disorientation.

COMMON
Blurred vision, drowsiness, agitation, dry mouth, constipation, urine retention. Constipation can be avoided by increasing the intake of fluids and high-fiber foods. Dry mouth can be relieved by cool drinks, sugarless gum, or hard candy.

LESS COMMON
Restlessness, irritability or unusual feeling of well-being, dizziness, tremor, stomach upset, nausea.

PRINCIPAL USES
To treat Parkinson's disease or the side effects of certain drugs that act on the central nervous system and produce Parkinson-like symptoms, including slowed movement, stiffness, and loss of balance.

HOW THE DRUG WORKS
The exact mechanism of action is unknown, but biperiden is believed to help increase the release of certain neurological chemicals that improve control over movement.

DOSAGE
Tablets: For Parkinson's disease, 2 mg, 3 or 4 times per day, to a maximum of 16 mg per day. For side effects of other drugs, 2 mg, 1 to 3 times per day. If you have difficulty swallowing the tablet, it can be crushed. Injection: 2 mg up to 4 times per day, injected into a muscle or vein. The maximum dose should not exceed 10 mg per day.

ONSET OF EFFECT
Within 1 hour.

DURATION OF ACTION
6 to 12 hours with tablets; 1 to 8 hours after injection.

DIETARY ADVICE
Take this medicine with or immediately after meals unless your doctor orders otherwise.

STORAGE
Store in a tightly sealed container away from heat and direct light.

IF YOU MISS A DOSE
If you miss a dose, take it as soon as you remember unless it is within 2 hours of the next dose. In that case, skip the missed dose and return to your regular schedule. Do not double the next dose.

STOPPING THE DRUG
Do not stop taking the drug suddenly. If therapy is to be discontinued, the dosage should be reduced gradually, according to your doctor's instructions, to avoid a withdrawal reaction.

PROLONGED USE
Your doctor should test your progress regularly so that the dose can be adjusted if necessary.

PRECAUTIONS
Over 60: Side effects may be more common in older persons. A reduced dose may be necessary. This medicine can aggravate symptoms of an enlarged prostate gland and cause impaired thinking, hallucinations, and nightmares in older persons.

Driving and Hazardous Work: Determine how this medicine affects you before driving or engaging in hazardous work.

Alcohol: Alcohol intake should be avoided because this medicine increases its effects.

Pregnancy: Do not use this drug while pregnant.

Breast Feeding: Do not use this drug while breast feeding.

Infants and Children: Safety and effectiveness have not been established for infants and children.

Special Concerns: Pay careful attention to dental hygiene, since biperiden tends to decrease salivation, which can promote the development of cavities and other dental problems.

OVERDOSE
Symptoms: Agitation, anxiety, restlessness, disorientation, hallucinations, blurred vision, fast pulse, difficulty swallowing, and difficulty urinating.

What to Do: Call your doctor, emergency medical services (EMS), or the nearest poison control center immediately.

DRUG INTERACTIONS
Tell your doctor about any other drugs you are taking, especially amantadine, digoxin, any drug for mental illness, antidepressants, or antacids. This medicine can decrease the activity of phenothiazines (mood-altering drugs used in the treatment of psychiatric disorders).

FOOD INTERACTIONS
No known food interactions.

DISEASE INTERACTIONS
Glaucoma, seizures, an irregular pulse, a bowel obstruction, or an enlarged prostate may make it impossible for you to take this medicine.

Bisacodyl

Correctol 5 mg
(SCHERING-PLOUGH)

Additional photographs

▶ Drug Class: Stimulant
laxative

▶ Available in: Tablets, powder,
suppositories

▶ Available OTC? Yes

▶ As Generic? Yes

Side Effects

SERIOUS
Severe stomach pain, laxative dependence. Call your doctor immediately.

COMMON
Abdominal cramping, burning sensation in the rectum (with suppository), diarrhea.

LESS COMMON
Nausea; vomiting; muscle weakness; rectal pain, bleeding, burning, or itching. If you have a sudden change in bowel habits that lasts longer than 2 weeks, consult your doctor.

PRINCIPAL USES
To relieve short-term constipation or to clear the bowel before rectal or bowel examination, surgery, or childbirth.

HOW THE DRUG WORKS
Bisacodyl increases the volume of fluid in the intestines to stimulate passage of the stool. It also acts on the smooth muscle of the intestine to increase contractions.

DOSAGE
For constipation— Adults and teenagers: Tablets: 10 to 15 mg at bedtime. Children age 6 and older: 5 mg before breakfast. Swallow tablets whole; do not chew. For medical examination— Adults and teenagers: Up to 30 mg orally, or 10 mg given rectally before examination. Children age 6 and older: 5 mg orally or rectally, before breakfast.

ONSET OF EFFECT
Tablets: Within 6 to 12 hours. Suppositories: Within 15 to 60 minutes.

DURATION OF ACTION
Variable.

DIETARY ADVICE
Take the tablet on an empty stomach for rapid effect. Increase intake of fluids and dietary fiber.

STORAGE
Store in a tightly sealed container away from heat, moisture, and direct light.

IF YOU MISS A DOSE
Take the missed dose as soon as you remember, unless it is almost time for your next dose. In that case, skip the missed dose and resume your regular dosage schedule. Do not double the next dose.

STOPPING THE DRUG
Take it as prescribed for the full treatment period. However, you may stop taking the drug if you are feeling better before the scheduled end of the therapy.

PROLONGED USE
Do not use this medicine for more than one week unless your doctor prescribes it.

PRECAUTIONS
Over 60: Excessive use of this drug by an older person can cause loss of body fluid leading to weakness and lack of coordination.

Driving and Hazardous Work: Do not drive or engage in hazardous work until you determine how the medicine affects you.

Alcohol: Avoid alcohol while taking this drug.

Pregnancy: Bisacodyl is not usually used during pregnancy, except immediately before delivery. Consult your doctor for advice.

Breast Feeding: Bisacodyl may pass into breast milk. Consult your doctor for specific advice.

Infants and Children: Do not give this medicine to a child under 6 without your doctor's approval. Do not give this medicine to a child who refuses to have a bowel movement. It may result in a painful bowel movement, which will make the child resist even more.

Special Concerns: Remember that chronic use of bisacodyl or any laxative can lead to laxative dependence. You should consume adequate amounts of fiber in your diet, sources of which include bran or whole-grain cereals, fruit, and vegetables.

OVERDOSE
Symptoms: Weakness, increased sweating, lower abdominal pain, muscle cramps, irregular heartbeat.

What to Do: An overdose of bisacodyl is unlikely to be life-threatening. However, if someone takes a much larger dose than prescribed, seek medical assistance immediately.

DRUG INTERACTIONS
Be sure to tell your doctor about any other drugs you are taking, especially antacids. Do not take an antacid within 2 hours of taking this drug.

FOOD INTERACTIONS
Do not drink milk within 2 hours of taking this drug.

DISEASE INTERACTIONS
Caution is advised when taking bisacodyl. Consult your doctor if you have very severe constipation, severe pain in the stomach or lower abdomen, cramping, bloating, nausea, or unexplained rectal bleeding. Failure to produce a bowel movement or the presence of rectal bleeding may indicate a serious medical condition.

Bismuth Subsalicylate

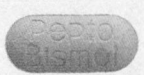

Pepto-Bismol Caplets 262 mg
(PROCTER & GAMBLE)

Additional photographs

▶ Drug Class: Antidiarrheal/
antacid

▶ Available in: Tablets, oral
suspension

▶ Available OTC? Yes

▶ As Generic? Yes

Side Effects

SERIOUS
Ringing in the ears. Call
your doctor immediately.

COMMON
Black stools, darkening of
the tongue.

LESS COMMON
Nausea, vomiting (with
high doses), abdominal
pain, increased sweating,
muscle weakness, hear-
ing loss, thirst, confusion,
dizziness, vision prob-
lems, trouble breathing.
Discontinue the medicine
and call your physician
right away.

PRINCIPAL USES
To treat heartburn, acid
indigestion, diarrhea, and
duodenal ulcers, and to help
prevent traveler's diarrhea.

HOW THE DRUG WORKS
Bismuth subsalicylate stimulates the passage of fluid
and electrolytes across the
wall of the intestinal tract,
and binds or neutralizes the
toxins of some bacteria, rendering them nontoxic. It
decreases intestinal inflammation and increases the
activity of intestinal muscles
and lining.

DOSAGE
Adults— For acid indiges-
tion or mild diarrhea: 2
tablets or 2 tablespoons of
liquid every 30 to 60 minutes, to a maximum of 16
doses daily of the regular-
strength drug for no more
than 2 days. Children ages
9 to 12— 1 tablet or 1 tablespoon every 30 to 60 min-
utes, to a maximum of 8
doses daily of the regular-
strength drug for no more
than 2 days. Children ages
6 to 9— 2 teaspoons every
30 to 60 minutes, to a maximum of 16 doses daily of
the regular-strength drug
for no more than 2 days.
Children under age 3—
Consult your pediatrician.
Tablets are not recom-
mended for children under
the age of 9.

ONSET OF EFFECT
Within 30 to 60 minutes.

DURATION OF ACTION
Unknown.

DIETARY ADVICE
A mild diet is recommended
when recovering from diarrhea. Bananas, rice, applesauce, and plain toast are
good choices. Be sure to
get plenty of fluids.

STORAGE
Store in a tightly sealed container away from heat and
direct light. Keep liquid
forms of bismuth subsalicylate refrigerated, but do not
allow the medicine to
freeze.

IF YOU MISS A DOSE
Take it as soon as you
remember. If it is near the
time for the next dose, skip
the missed dose and
resume your regular dosage
schedule. Do not double the
next dose.

STOPPING THE DRUG
Take it as prescribed for the
full treatment period. However, you may stop taking
the drug if you are feeling
better before the scheduled
end of the therapy.

PROLONGED USE
Prolonged use of this medicine may cause constipation.
Consult your physician if
relief is not achieved within
two days.

PRECAUTIONS
Over 60: Adverse reactions
may be more likely and
more severe in older
patients.

**Driving and Hazardous
Work:** Do not drive or
engage in hazardous work
until you determine how
this medicine affects you.

Alcohol: Alcohol intake
should be limited.

Pregnancy: Regular use of
this medicine late in pregnancy may harm the fetus
or cause delivery problems.
Consult your doctor about
taking it if you are pregnant
or plan to become pregnant.

Breast Feeding: Bismuth
subsalicylate passes into
breast milk; avoid or discontinue use while nursing.

Infants and Children:
Consult your doctor before
giving this medicine to a
child or teenager who has
or is recovering from
chicken pox or flu.

Special Concerns: Do not
take bismuth subsalicylate if
you are allergic to aspirin or
another salicylate, an anticoagulant, or a medicine for
diabetes or gout. Do not
swallow tablets whole. They
should be crushed, chewed,
or allowed to dissolve in the
mouth.

OVERDOSE
Symptoms: Seizures, confusion, rapid or deep breathing, hearing loss or ringing
or buzzing in the ears,
severe excitability or nervousness, severe drowsi-
ness, loss of consciousness.

What to Do: Call your
doctor, emergency medical
services (EMS), or the
nearest poison control center immediately.

DRUG INTERACTIONS
Consult your doctor for specific advice if you are taking
anticoagulants, aspirin and
other salicylates, oral diabetes medicine, heparin, probenecid, thrombolytic
agents, oral tetracycline,
or sulfinpyrazone.

FOOD INTERACTIONS
No known food interactions.

DISEASE INTERACTIONS
Caution is advised when
using bismuth subsalicylate.
Before taking this drug, tell
your doctor if you have a
history of allergies, diabetes, kidney disease, dehydration, stomach ulcers,
dysentery, gout, or a bleeding problem.

Bisoprolol Fumarate

BRAND NAME
Zebeta

Zebeta 5 mg
(LEDERLE)

▶ Drug Class: Beta-blocker

▶ Available in: Tablets

▶ Available OTC? No

▶ As Generic? No

Side Effects

SERIOUS
Shortness of breath, wheezing; irregular or slow heartbeat (50 beats per minute or less); pain or feelings of tightness or pressure in the chest; swelling of the ankles, feet, and lower legs; mental depression. If you experience such symptoms, stop taking bisoprolol and call your doctor immediately.

COMMON
Dizziness or lightheadedness, especially when rising suddenly to a standing position; rapid heartbeat or palpitations; decreased sexual ability; unusual fatigue, weakness, or drowsiness; insomnia.

LESS COMMON
Anxiety, irritability, nervousness; constipation; diarrhea; dry, sore eyes; itching; nausea or vomiting; nightmares or intensely vivid dreams; numbness, tingling, or other unusual sensations in the fingers, toes, or scalp.

PRINCIPAL USES
To control hypertension (high blood pressure).

HOW THE DRUG WORKS
Bisoprolol slows the rate and force of contraction of the heart by blocking certain nerve impulses, thus reducing blood pressure.

DOSAGE
Starting dose is 5 mg once a day, or 2.5 mg once a day for those with kidney or liver problems. If necessary, it may be increased gradually to 20 mg once a day. Maximum dose is 20 mg per day.

ONSET OF EFFECT
Within 1 to 4 hours.

DURATION OF ACTION
24 hours.

DIETARY ADVICE
Take this drug at mealtime or immediately afterward.

STORAGE
Store in a tightly sealed container away from heat and direct light.

IF YOU MISS A DOSE
If you miss a dose, take it as soon as you remember unless it is almost time for your next dose. In that case, skip the missed dose and return to your regular schedule. Do not double the next dose.

STOPPING THE DRUG
Do not stop taking this drug without consulting your doctor. It may be necessary to reduce the dosage gradually to prevent adverse effects.

PROLONGED USE
Ask your doctor about the need for medical examinations or laboratory studies of your heart, blood pressure, kidney function, and blood sugar. Monitor your blood pressure often.

PRECAUTIONS
Over 60: Adverse reactions and side effects may be more common in older persons.

Driving and Hazardous Work: Determine how bisoprolol affects you before driving or engaging in any hazardous activities.

Alcohol: Drink in careful moderation if at all. Alcohol may interact with the drug and cause a dangerous drop in blood pressure.

Pregnancy: Be sure to notify your doctor promptly if you are pregnant or plan to become pregnant. Use bisoprolol during pregnancy only if the expected benefits outweigh the possible risks.

Breast Feeding: Bisoprolol passes into breast milk. Do not use it while you are breast feeding.

Infants and Children: Your pediatrician must determine the correct dose for a child.

Special Concerns: Prior to any dental or medical procedure or test, be sure to tell the doctor or dentist that you are taking bisoprolol. This drug may mask exercise-induced chest pain (angina). Ask your doctor for advice on a safe exercise program. Dress warmly in cold weather.

OVERDOSE
Symptoms: Asthmalike attacks (wheezing, breathlessness), very slow pulse, extreme shortness of breath associated with congestive heart failure.

What to Do: Call your doctor, emergency medical services (EMS), or the nearest poison control center immediately.

DRUG INTERACTIONS
Consult your doctor if you are taking any other blood pressure drug or beta-blocker. Be sure to check with your doctor before taking any over-the-counter medication, especially diet aids or cold preparations, as these may contain ingredients that can interact adversely with bisoprolol.

FOOD INTERACTIONS
None are expected, unless you are allergic to certain foods, as this medicine may cause allergic reactions to be more severe.

DISEASE INTERACTIONS
Bisoprolol should be used with caution in people with diabetes, especially insulin-dependent diabetes, since the drug may mask symptoms of hypoglycemia. Consult your doctor if you have a medical history of heart disease, asthma, blood vessel (vascular) disease, or thyroid disease. Diabetic patients must monitor their blood glucose (sugar) levels closely.

Bisoprolol Fumarate/Hydrochlorothiazide

▶ Drug Class: Beta-blocker/thiazide diuretic

▶ Available in: Tablets

▶ Available OTC? No

▶ As Generic? No

Side Effects

SERIOUS
Slow heartbeat, difficulty breathing, mental depression, cold hands and feet, swelling of ankles, feet, or lower legs. Call your doctor immediately.

COMMON
Dizziness or lightheadedness, decreased sexual ability, drowsiness, insomnia, fatigue, diarrhea.

LESS COMMON
Anxiety, loss of appetite, upset stomach, nervousness or excitability, constipation, numbness and tingling in the fingers and toes, stuffy nose.

PRINCIPAL USES
To control hypertension (high blood pressure).

HOW THE DRUG WORKS
Bisoprolol, a beta-blocker, blocks certain nerve impulses to various parts of the body, which accounts for its many effects. For example, it reduces the rate and force of the heart's contractions (which helps to lower blood pressure), decreases the heart's oxygen requirement (which helps prevent angina) and helps stabilize heart rhythm. Hydrochlorothiazide (HCTZ), a diuretic, increases the excretion of salt and water in the urine. By reducing the overall amount of fluid in the body, diuretics reduce pressure within the blood vessels.

DOSAGE
Tablets contain 6.25 mg HCTZ and 2.5, 5, or 10 mg bisoprolol. Therapy is initiated with the lowest dose and may be increased at 1 week intervals to 2 tablets with 10 mg bisoprolol once a day.

ONSET OF EFFECT
Within 1 to 4 hours.

DURATION OF ACTION
Up to 24 hours.

DIETARY ADVICE
No special restrictions.

STORAGE
Store in a tightly sealed container away from heat, moisture, and direct light.

IF YOU MISS A DOSE
If you miss a dose on one day, resume your regular dosage schedule the next day. Do not double the next dose.

STOPPING THE DRUG
The decision to stop taking the drug should be made in consultation with your physician. Do not stop taking this drug abruptly; your doctor will gradually decrease your dose before stopping completely.

PROLONGED USE
Bisoprolol/hydrochlorothiazide can control high blood pressure, but cannot cure it. Lifelong therapy may be necessary. See your doctor regularly for tests and examinations if you must take this drug for a prolonged period of time.

PRECAUTIONS
Over 60: Adverse reactions, especially dizziness, lightheadedness, and reduced tolerance to cold, may be more likely and more severe in older patients.

Driving and Hazardous Work: Do not drive or engage in hazardous work until you determine how the medicine affects you.

Alcohol: Drink in careful moderation if at all. Alcohol may interact with the bisoprolol component and cause a dangerous drop in blood pressure.

Pregnancy: Beta-blockers and thiazide diuretics may cause problems during pregnancy. Before taking this medication, tell your doctor if you are pregnant or plan to become pregnant.

Breast Feeding: This drug passes into breast milk; caution is advised. Consult your doctor for specific advice.

Infants and Children: Adequate studies have not been done on the use of this drug in children. No special problems are expected. Consult your pediatrician for advice.

Special Concerns: In addition to taking this medicine, follow your doctor's instructions on weight control and diet for reduction of blood pressure.

OVERDOSE
Symptoms: Slow heartbeat, severe dizziness or fainting, difficulty breathing, bluish-colored fingernails or palms of hands, seizures.

What to Do: Call your doctor, emergency medical services (EMS), or the nearest poison control center immediately.

DRUG INTERACTIONS
Do not take with other beta-blockers. Consult your doctor for specific advice if you are taking any other antihypertensive medications, oral diabetes medications, insulin, digitalis drugs, cholestyramine, colestipol, clonidine, lithium, nonsteroidal anti-inflammatory drugs, MAO inhibitors, rifampin, narcotic analgesics, or skeletal muscle relaxants.

FOOD INTERACTIONS
Avoid foods high in sodium.

DISEASE INTERACTIONS
Do not use if you have a history of bronchospasm. Consult your doctor if you have any of the following: bronchial asthma, emphysema, slow heartbeat, heart or blood vessel disease, diabetes mellitus, congestive heart failure, gout, kidney disease, liver disease, depression, parathyroid disease, or an overactive thyroid (hyperthyroidism).

Bitolterol Mesylate

BRAND NAME
Tornalate

▶ Drug Class: Bronchodilator/ sympathomimetic

▶ Available in: Aerosol inhaler

▶ Available OTC? No

▶ As Generic? No

Side Effects

SERIOUS
This drug may become ineffective if used too often, resulting in more-severe breathing difficulty that does not improve. Signs include persistent wheezing, coughing, or shortness of breath; confusion; bluish color to lips or fingernails; inability to speak. Other side effects include chest pain or heaviness; irregular, racing, fluttering, or pounding heartbeat; lightheadedness; fainting; severe weakness; severe headache.

COMMON
Changes in blood pressure causing headache, blurred vision, weakness.

LESS COMMON
Nervousness, throat irritation, nausea.

PRINCIPAL USES
Bitolterol is used to dilate air passages in the lungs that have become narrowed as a result of disease or inflammation. It is used in the treatment of asthma and chronic obstructive pulmonary disease (COPD).

HOW THE DRUG WORKS
Bitolterol widens constricted airways in the lungs by relaxing the smooth muscles that surround the bronchial passages.

DOSAGE
To treat bronchial asthma and bronchospasm; use it when needed to relieve breathing difficulty: 1 or 2 inhalations at an interval of 1 to 3 minutes, with a third inhalation 2 to 3 minutes later if needed. To prevent bronchospasm: Usually 2 inhalations every 8 hours, with a maximum dose of 2 inhalations every 4 hours or 3 inhalations every 6 hours; actual dosage and administration schedule must be determined by a doctor for each patient. Specific written directions from your doctor should be followed carefully. Rinse your mouth after each dose. Rinse and dry inhaler after each use.

ONSET OF EFFECT
Within 5 minutes.

DURATION OF ACTION
From 5 to 8 hours.

DIETARY ADVICE
Excessive intake of coffee or other caffeine-containing beverages should be avoided.

STORAGE
Store in a tightly sealed container away from heat and direct light.

IF YOU MISS A DOSE
Skip the missed dose and resume your regular dosage schedule. Do not double the next dose.

STOPPING THE DRUG
It may not be necessary to finish the recommended course of therapy. Consult your doctor.

PROLONGED USE
Therapy may require months or years. Excessive use may result in temporary loss of effectiveness.

PRECAUTIONS
Over 60: Adverse reactions may be more likely and more severe in older patients.

Driving and Hazardous Work: Be cautious about driving or doing hazardous work until you determine if excessive nervousness or dizziness occurs.

Alcohol: No special precautions are necessary.

Pregnancy: Adequate studies have not been done; the benefits must be weighed against potential risks. Consult your doctor for specific advice.

Breast Feeding: Bitolterol can pass into breast milk; breast feeding should be avoided while taking bitolterol.

Infants and Children: Safety and effectiveness of bitolterol for children under the age of 12 have not been established.

Special Concerns: Call your doctor if you cannot breathe properly 1 hour after using bitolterol or if your breathing problem worsens. Do not let the spray from the inhaler get in your eyes. Discontinue use and contact your doctor if you notice an unusual smell or taste when using this product. Use of this medicine is a disqualification for piloting an aircraft.

OVERDOSE
Symptoms: Tremor, nausea, vomiting, rapid or irregular pulse.

What to Do: Call your doctor immediately.

DRUG INTERACTIONS
Use of MAO inhibitors may cause an excessive increase in blood pressure and heart stimulation. If you are also using a steroid inhaler, take bitolterol first and then wait about 15 minutes before using the steroid inhaler. This allows bitolterol to open air passages, increasing the effectiveness of the steroid.

FOOD INTERACTIONS
Excessive intake of coffee or other caffeine-containing beverages should be avoided.

DISEASE INTERACTIONS
Before taking bitolterol, consult your doctor if you have a circulatory disorder, heart disease, diabetes mellitus, epilepsy, or an overactive thyroid.

Brimonidine Tartrate

Side Effects

SERIOUS
Fainting. Call your doctor immediately.

COMMON
Burning or stinging of the eyes, fatigue, dry mouth, eye discomfort, drowsiness.

LESS COMMON
Excess tear production, redness of eyes or inner lining of the eyelids, headache, swelling of eye or eyelid, eye ache or pain, blurring or other changes in vision, dizziness, mental depression, insomnia, muscle pain or weakness, nausea, increased blood pressure, vomiting, anxiety, pounding heartbeat, change in taste, crusting in corner of eye or on eyelid, discoloration of eyeball, paleness of inner lining of eyelid, dry eyes, sensitivity of eyes to light.

PRINCIPAL USES
To treat glaucoma.

HOW THE DRUG WORKS
Glaucoma, a sight-threatening disorder, occurs when aqueous humor (fluid inside the eye) cannot drain properly, causing increased pressure within the eyeball (intraocular pressure). Increased eye pressure can damage the optic nerve and lead to a gradually progressive loss of vision. Brimonidine decreases the production of aqueous humor and promotes its outflow, thereby reducing intraocular pressure.

DOSAGE
1 drop of brimonidine in each eye 3 times a day at 8-hour intervals.

ONSET OF EFFECT
Within 60 minutes.

DURATION OF ACTION
8 hours or more.

DIETARY ADVICE
No special restrictions.

STORAGE
Store in a tightly sealed container away from heat, moisture, and direct light. Do not allow the medicine to freeze.

IF YOU MISS A DOSE
Apply it as soon as you remember. If it is near the time for the next dose, skip the missed dose and resume your regular dosage schedule. Do not double the next dose.

STOPPING THE DRUG
The decision to stop using the drug should be made by your doctor.

PROLONGED USE
You should see your doctor regularly for tests and examinations as part of glaucoma follow-up if you take this drug for a prolonged period.

PRECAUTIONS
Over 60: Adverse reactions may be more likely and more severe in older patients.

Driving and Hazardous Work: Do not drive or engage in hazardous work until you determine how the drug affects your vision.

Alcohol: Use alcohol with caution.

Pregnancy: In animal studies, brimonidine caused impaired fetal circulation. Human studies have not been done. Before you take brimonidine, tell your doctor if you are pregnant or are planning to become pregnant.

Breast Feeding: Brimonidine may pass into breast milk; caution is advised. Consult your doctor for specific advice.

Infants and Children: The safety and effectiveness of brimonidine in infants and children have not been established.

Special Concerns: To use the eye drops, first wash your hands. Tilt your head back. Gently apply pressure to the inside corner of the eyelid and with the index finger of the same hand, pull downward on the lower eyelid to make a space. Drop the medicine into this space and close your eye. Apply pressure for 1 or 2 minutes while keeping the eye closed without blinking. Then wash your hands again. Make sure the tip of the dropper does not touch your eye, finger, or any other surface. Bromonidine may make your eyes more sensitive to sunlight. If this occurs, wear sunglasses or avoid bright light as comfort dictates.

OVERDOSE
Symptoms: No specific ones have been reported.

What to Do: An overdose of brimonidine is unlikely to be life-threatening. However, if someone takes a much larger dose than prescribed or accidentally ingests the medicine, call your doctor, emergency medical services (EMS), or the nearest poison control center immediately.

DRUG INTERACTIONS
Consult your doctor for advice if you are taking MAO inhibitors, tricyclic antidepressants, central nervous system depressants, beta-blockers, antihypertensives, or digitalis drugs (such as digoxin).

FOOD INTERACTIONS
No known food interactions.

DISEASE INTERACTIONS
Caution is advised when taking brimonidine. Consult your doctor if you have cardiovascular disease, kidney disease, liver disease, depression, cerebral or coronary insufficiency, Raynaud's phenomenon, orthostatic hypotension, or thromboangiitis obliterans.

Brinzolamide

▶ Drug Class: Antiglaucoma agent; carbonic anhydrase inhibitor

▶ Available in: Ophthalmic suspension

▶ Available OTC? No

▶ As Generic? No

Side Effects

SERIOUS
Severe generalized reactions involving the skin, liver, and blood cells. Discontinue using the medication and call your doctor immediately if signs of serious reaction occur.

COMMON
Burning, stinging, or discomfort in the eye or blurred vision when drug is administered; bitter taste in mouth.

LESS COMMON
Eye pain, severe or continued tearing, nausea.

PRINCIPAL USES
To treat glaucoma or ocular hypertension (a glaucoma-like condition).

HOW THE DRUG WORKS
Glaucoma and ocular hypertension, both sight-threatening disorders, occur when poor drainage of aqueous humor (the fluid inside the front part of the eye) increases the pressure within the eyeball (known as intraocular pressure). Increased intraocular pressure can damage the optic nerve and lead to a gradual loss of vision. By inhibiting the activity of the enzyme carbonic anhydrase, brinzolamide decreases the production of aqueous humor, and reduces intraocular pressure.

DOSAGE
Adults and teenagers:
1 drop in affected eye(s) 3 times per day.

ONSET OF EFFECT
Unknown.

DURATION OF ACTION
Unknown.

DIETARY ADVICE
No special restrictions.

STORAGE
Store in a tightly sealed container away from heat, moisture, and direct light. Do not refrigerate or allow it to freeze.

IF YOU MISS A DOSE
Apply it as soon as you remember. If it is near the time for the next dose, skip the missed dose and resume your regular dosage schedule. Do not double the next dose.

STOPPING THE DRUG
The decision to stop using the drug should be made by your doctor.

PROLONGED USE
Schedule regular eye examinations with your doctor to be sure the drug is controlling the glaucoma or ocular hypertension.

PRECAUTIONS
Over 60: No special problems are expected.

Driving and Hazardous Work: Do not drive or engage in hazardous work until you determine how the medicine affects your vision.

Alcohol: No special precautions are necessary.

Pregnancy: One animal study found that very high doses of this drug caused birth defects. Human studies have not been done. Before using this medicine, tell your doctor if you are pregnant or plan to become pregnant.

Breast Feeding: It is not known whether brinzolamide passes into breast milk; caution is advised. Consult your doctor for specific advice about whether to use a different medicine or to stop breast feeding.

Infants and Children: Safety and dosage guidelines for children have not been established. Brinzolamide should be given to infants and children only under close medical supervision.

Special Concerns: To use the eye drops, first wash your hands. Tilt your head back. Gently apply pressure to the inside corner of the eyelid and with the index finger of the same hand, pull downward on the lower eyelid to make a space. Drop the medicine into this space and close your eye. Apply pressure for 1 or 2 minutes while keeping the eye closed without blinking. Then wash your hands again. Make sure that the tip of the dropper does not touch your eye, finger, or any other surface.

OVERDOSE
Symptoms: No specific ones have been reported.

What to Do: An overdose of brinzolamide is unlikely to be life-threatening. If a large volume enters the eye, flush with water. If someone accidentally ingests the medicine, call your doctor, emergency medical services (EMS), or the nearest poison control center.

DRUG INTERACTIONS
Wait 10 minutes before administering any other eye medicine. Brinzolamide should not be used in conjunction with oral carbonic anhydrase inhibitors. People allergic to sulfa-type drugs should not use brinzolamide.

FOOD INTERACTIONS
No known food interactions.

DISEASE INTERACTIONS
Do not use if you have severe kidney impairment. Use with caution if you have liver disease.

Bromocriptine Mesylate

Parlodel 2.5 mg
(NOVARTIS)

▶ Drug Class: Ergot alkaloid

▶ Available in: Tablets, capsules

▶ Available OTC? No

▶ As Generic? Yes

Side Effects

SERIOUS
Seizures, chest pain, severe nausea and vomiting, headache and blurred vision caused by high blood pressure, wet cough and shortness of breath caused by fluid in the lungs. Consult your doctor immediately.

COMMON
Dizziness, weakness, and fainting caused by low blood pressure; nasal congestion and headache; abdominal cramping or pain.

LESS COMMON
Confusion, fatigue, nervousness, depression, ringing in the ears, dry mouth, blurred vision, hallucinations, hair loss, anemia, impotence, constipation, or diarrhea.

PRINCIPAL USES
To treat hyperprolactinemia, a disorder caused by overproduction of the hormone prolactin. Hyperprolactinemia may occur by itself or in association with a tumor (prolactinoma) in the pituitary gland. The disorder causes abnormal production and persistent leakage of breast milk (in either men or women), infertility and cessation of menstrual periods in women, and testicular shrinkage and impotence in men. In some cases bromocriptine may be used to treat acromegaly (overproduction of growth hormone, causing enlargement of the hands, feet, jawbone, and internal organs). It is also used to treat Parkinson's disease.

HOW THE DRUG WORKS
Bromocriptine blocks the pituitary from releasing the hormone prolactin, which is involved in the regulation of the menstrual cycle, reproduction, and milk production. Similarly, it blocks the pituitary from releasing growth hormone. The drug activates certain chemical receptor sites in brain cells to reduce Parkinson's symptoms.

DOSAGE
For hyperprolactinemia: Starting with 1.25 to 2.5 mg a day, the dose is increased by 1.25 mg a day at 3- to 7-day intervals until the desired therapeutic effect is achieved. Maintenance dose is 1.25 to 15 mg in divided doses, 2 or 3 times a day. For acromegaly: 1.25 to 30 mg a day in divided doses, 2 or 3 times a day. For Parkinson's disease: Starting with 1.25 to 2.5 mg a day, the dose is increased by 2.5 mg a day at 14- to 28-day intervals, to a maximum of 100 mg a day in divided doses, 2 or 3 times a day.

ONSET OF EFFECT
From 30 to 90 minutes. Full effects become apparent after a few weeks of therapy.

DURATION OF ACTION
For hyperprolactinemia and acromegaly: 8 hours. For Parkinson's disease: 12 to 18 hours.

DIETARY ADVICE
For best results, bromocriptine should be taken with food or milk.

STORAGE
Store in a dry place away from heat and direct light. Discard the medicine if it becomes outdated.

IF YOU MISS A DOSE
If you miss a dose, take it if you remember within 2 hours. After that, wait for the next dose and return to your regular schedule. Do not double the next dose.

STOPPING THE DRUG
Complete the prescribed dose even though symptoms diminish or disappear. Consult your doctor before discontinuing this drug.

PROLONGED USE
Prolonged use at doses greater than 50 mg per day may cause uncontrolled movements of face, mouth, tongue, arms, or legs (a condition known as tardive dyskinesia). Consult your doctor if such symptoms occur.

PRECAUTIONS
Over 60: Adverse reactions and side effects may be more common in older persons.

Driving and Hazardous Work: Do not drive or engage in hazardous work until you determine how bromocriptine affects you.

Alcohol: Bromocriptine reduces the body's tolerance to alcohol.

Pregnancy: If you are pregnant or plan to become pregnant, tell your doctor before taking this drug.

Breast Feeding: Bromocriptine should not be used when nursing because it reduces breast milk production.

Infants and Children: Not recommended for anyone under the age of 15.

OVERDOSE
Symptoms: Severe dizziness and weakness, nausea, and vomiting.

What to Do: Call your doctor immediately.

DRUG INTERACTIONS
Consult your doctor for specific advice if you are taking any of the following drugs that may interact with bromocriptine: blood pressure medication, an oral contraceptive, erythromycin, a phenothiazine, an MAO inhibitor, progestin, levodopa, or a rauwolfia alkaloid.

FOOD INTERACTIONS
None are expected.

DISEASE INTERACTIONS
Consult your doctor if you have any of the following: diabetes, epilepsy, heart disease, lung disease, a peptic ulcer, or high blood pressure. Also tell your doctor if you plan to have surgery, including dental surgery, within 2 months.

Brompheniramine Maleate

▶ Drug Class: Antihistamine

▶ Available in: Capsules, tablets, extended-release tablets, elixir, injection

▶ Available OTC? Yes

▶ As Generic? Yes

Side Effects

SERIOUS
Bleeding problems; small, red pinpoints on the skin; fever; extreme fatigue; bleeding ulcers in the rectum, mouth, and vagina; reduced white blood cell count (rare).

COMMON
Drowsiness; unusual excitability; dry mouth, nose, or throat. Symptoms of drowsiness tend to subside after a few days' use as your body adjusts to the drug.

LESS COMMON
Vision changes, loss of appetite, dizziness, painful or difficult urination, less tolerance for contact lenses.

PRINCIPAL USES
To prevent or relieve symptoms of hay fever, other allergies, itching skin, or hives.

HOW THE DRUG WORKS
Brompheniramine blocks the effects of histamine, a substance in the body that causes swelling, itching, sneezing, watery eyes, hives, and other symptoms of allergic reaction.

DOSAGE
Capsules, tablets, elixir— Adults and teenagers: 4 mg every 4 to 6 hours. Children ages 6 to 12: 2 mg every 4 to 6 hours. Children ages 2 to 6: 1 mg every 4 to 6 hours. Extended-release tablets— Adults: 8 mg every 8 to 12 hours, or 12 mg every 12 hours. Children age 6 and older: 8 or 12 mg every 12 hours. Injection— Adults and teenagers: 10 mg under the skin or into a vein or muscle every 8 to 12 hours. Children younger than age 12: 0.125 mg per 2.2 lbs (1 kg) of body weight, under the skin or into a vein or muscle 3 or 4 times a day.

ONSET OF EFFECT
15 to 60 minutes.

DURATION OF ACTION
3 to 6 hours for regular form; 8 to 12 for extended-release tablets.

DIETARY ADVICE
Take it with food or milk to minimize stomach upset.

STORAGE
Store in a tightly sealed container away from heat and direct light.

IF YOU MISS A DOSE
Take it as soon as you remember. If it is near the time for the next dose, skip the missed dose and resume your regular dosage schedule. Do not double the next dose.

STOPPING THE DRUG
You should take it as prescribed for the full treatment period, but you may stop if you feel better before the scheduled end of therapy. It may be taken as needed.

PROLONGED USE
No special concerns.

PRECAUTIONS
Over 60: Older persons are more sensitive to antihistamine side effects, particularly confusion, dizziness, drowsiness, restlessness, irritability, nightmares, and dry mouth, nose, and throat.

Driving and Hazardous Work: Brompheniramine can make you feel tired and lessen your concentration. Do not drive or engage in hazardous work until you determine how the drug affects you.

Alcohol: Alcohol increases the likelihood and the severity of side effects like drowsiness and confusion.

Pregnancy: Studies in animals suggest that brompheniramine has no adverse effect on fetal development, but human studies have not been done. Before taking this drug, tell your doctor if you are pregnant or are planning to become pregnant.

Breast Feeding: Brompheniramine passes into breast milk; avoid or discontinue use while breast feeding.

Infants and Children: Brompheniramine should be given to children age 6 and under only as directed by a doctor.

Special Concerns: Do not break, crush, or chew the capsules or the extended-release tablets.

OVERDOSE
Symptoms: Seizures, loss of consciousness, hallucinations, severe drowsiness.

What to Do: The patient should be made to vomit immediately, using ipecac syrup. If he or she is unconscious, the patient should be taken to a hospital emergency room immediately.

DRUG INTERACTIONS
MAO inhibitors can increase the sedative effects of brompheniramine. Central nervous system depressants such as alcohol, sedatives, or narcotics should be taken only if approved by a doctor.

FOOD INTERACTIONS
No known food interactions.

DISEASE INTERACTIONS
Before taking brompheniramine, consult your doctor if you wear contact lenses or you have glaucoma, prostate enlargement, difficulty with urination, or dryness of the mouth or eyes.

Budesonide

BRAND NAMES
Pulmicort Turbuhaler,
Rhinocort Aqua,
Rhinocort Turbuhaler

▶ Drug Class: Respiratory corticosteroid

▶ Available in: Nasal inhalant, oral inhalation, inhalation powder

▶ Available OTC? No

▶ As Generic? No

Side Effects

SERIOUS
No serious side effects are associated with budesonide.

COMMON
Nasal inhalant: Nosebleeds or bloody nasal secretions, burning or irritation of the nasal passages, sore throat. Oral inhalation: Sore throat, white patches in mouth or throat, hoarseness.

LESS COMMON
Eye pain, watering eyes, gradual decrease of vision, stomach pain and digestive disturbances.

PRINCIPAL USES
To treat the symptoms of allergic rhinitis (seasonal and perennial allergies such as hay fever) and to prevent recurrence of nasal polyps after surgical removal.

HOW THE DRUG WORKS
Respiratory corticosteroids such as budesonide primarily reduce or prevent inflammation of the lining of the airways, reduce the allergic response to inhaled allergens, and inhibit the secretion of mucus within the airways.

DOSAGE
Nasal inhalant: 2 sprays (32 micrograms [mcg] each) in each nostril in the morning and evening or 4 sprays in each nostril in the morning. Oral inhalation: 200 to 800 mcg (1 to 4 inhalations), 2 times a day. Highest dose for children is 400 mcg (2 inhalations), 2 times a day. The dose may be increased or decreased as determined by your doctor, based on the patient's response.

ONSET OF EFFECT
Usually within several days; it may take 3 weeks for the full effect to occur.

DURATION OF ACTION
Up to 12 hours.

DIETARY ADVICE
Budesonide can be taken without regard to diet.

STORAGE
Store in a dry place away from heat and light, out of the reach of children.

IF YOU MISS A DOSE
Take the missed dose if you remember within an hour. Otherwise, skip the missed dose and return to your regular schedule. Do not double the next dose.

STOPPING THE DRUG
Nasal inhalant: No problems expected. Oral inhalation: Do not discontinue without consulting your doctor. Gradual reduction in dosage may be required.

PROLONGED USE
Consult with your doctor about the need for periodic physical examinations and laboratory tests.

PRECAUTIONS
Over 60: No special problems are expected.

Driving and Hazardous Work: Budesonide should not affect your ability to perform such tasks safely.

Alcohol: No special precautions are necessary.

Pregnancy: Nasal or inhaled steroids have not been reported to cause birth defects if taken during pregnancy. Before using such drugs, tell your doctor if you are pregnant or plan to become pregnant.

Breast Feeding: This drug may pass into breast milk. Consult your doctor about use of either form during breast feeding.

Infants and Children: Nasal form: Should be used only under close medical supervision. Oral form: Large doses may make children more susceptible to infectious disease. Long-term use may affect the adrenal glands.

Special Concerns: Inhaled steroids will not help an asthma attack in progress. Inhaled steroids can lower resistance to yeast infections of the mouth, throat, or voice box. To prevent yeast infections, gargle or rinse your mouth with water after each use; do not swallow the water. Know how to use the inhalant properly; read and follow the directions that come with the device. Before you have surgery, tell the doctor or dentist that you are using a steroid.

OVERDOSE
Symptoms: No specific symptoms.

What to Do: Call your doctor, emergency medical services (EMS), or the nearest poison control center if you have any reason to suspect an overdose.

DRUG INTERACTIONS
Consult your doctor for specific advice if you are taking systemic corticosteroids, other inhaled corticosteroids, or any medications that suppress the immune system.

FOOD INTERACTIONS
No known food interactions.

DISEASE INTERACTIONS
Consult your doctor if you have any other medical problem, particularly glaucoma, a herpes infection of the eye, a history of tuberculosis, liver disease, an underactive thyroid, or osteoporosis.

Bumetanide

BRAND NAME
Bumex

Generic 0.5 mg
(ZENITH)

▶ Drug Class: Loop diuretic

▶ Available in: Tablets, injection

▶ Available OTC? No

▶ As Generic? Yes

Side Effects

SERIOUS
Rapid or irregular heartbeat, dry mouth, increased thirst, mood or mental changes, muscle cramps or pain, nausea or vomiting, unusual fatigue, black and tarry stools, buzzing or ringing in ears, hearing loss, skin rash. Call your doctor immediately.

COMMON
Muscle cramps. Fluid depletion can cause dizziness when the patient rises from a sitting or lying position, as well as thirst and constipation. Minor potassium depletion can cause mild weakness, and rapid or irregular heartbeat.

LESS COMMON
Gout, increased blood sugar (glucose) levels, hearing loss.

PRINCIPAL USES
To reduce the accumulation of fluid (containing salts and water) that leads to edema (swelling) and breathlessness in patients with heart disease, cirrhosis of the liver, and kidney disease. Bumetanide may also be used to help control high blood levels of potassium.

HOW THE DRUG WORKS
Loop diuretics work on a specific portion of the kidney (the loop of Henle) to increase the excretion of both water and sodium in the urine.

DOSAGE
0.5 to 6 mg per day, usually taken in the morning; may be increased to 2 to 3 doses a day, as needed.

ONSET OF EFFECT
This drug begins eliminating excess water within 1 to 2 hours.

DURATION OF ACTION
Up to 4 hours.

DIETARY ADVICE
Bumetanide can be taken with or after meals to reduce stomach irritation.

STORAGE
Store in a tightly sealed container away from heat and direct light.

IF YOU MISS A DOSE
If you miss a dose, take it as soon as you remember unless it is almost time for the next dose. In that case, skip the missed dose and return to your regular schedule. Do not double the next dose.

STOPPING THE DRUG
Take it as prescribed for the full treatment period, even if you begin to feel better before the scheduled end of therapy. The decision to stop taking the drug should be made by your doctor.

PROLONGED USE
Prolonged use of bumetanide requires regular examinations by your doctor, since it may lead to imbalances of sodium, potassium, magnesium, and body fluid.

PRECAUTIONS
Over 60: No special problems are expected.

Driving and Hazardous Work: No special precautions are necessary.

Alcohol: No special precautions are necessary.

Pregnancy: Adequate studies of using this drug during pregnancy have not been done. Before taking this drug, tell your doctor if you are pregnant or plan to become pregnant. If diuretic treatment is warranted, other drugs are preferred.

Breast Feeding: This drug may pass into breast milk. Consult your doctor about its use while nursing.

Infants and Children: This drug is not generally prescribed for children. Its safety and effectiveness for anyone under the age of 18 have not been established.

Special Concerns: You may have to take a potassium supplement or consume foods or fluids high in potassium while taking this drug. To prevent disruption of sleep, avoid taking this drug in the evening.

OVERDOSE
Symptoms: Severe fatigue, weakness, lethargy, confusion, muscle cramps, nausea, vomiting, weak and rapid pulse, loss of consciousness.

What to Do: Call your doctor, emergency medical services (EMS), or the nearest poison control center immediately.

DRUG INTERACTIONS
Consult your doctor about any other drugs you are taking, particularly antibiotics, other blood pressure medications (especially ACE inhibitors), analgesics (pain relievers), lithium, cortisone-related drugs, digitalis drugs, or any nonsteroidal anti-inflammatory drug (NSAID).

FOOD INTERACTIONS
No food interactions have been documented.

DISEASE INTERACTIONS
Caution is advised when taking bumetanide. Consult your doctor if you have any of the following: diabetes, gout, a hearing problem, or a recent heart attack.

Bupropion Hydrochloride

Wellbutrin 100 mg
(GLAXO WELLCOME)

▶ Drug Class: Antidepressant/
smoking deterrent

▶ Available in: Tablets,
extended-release tablets

▶ Available OTC? No

▶ As Generic? No

Side Effects

SERIOUS
When treating depression: Hallucinations, heartbeat irregularities, confusion, skin rash, insomnia, severe headache, excitement or agitation, seizures. Call your doctor immediately. Smoking cessation: None reported.

COMMON
When treating depression: Nausea or vomiting, constipation, unusual weight loss, dry mouth, loss of appetite, dizziness, increased sweating, trembling or shaking. Smoking cessation: Dry mouth, insomnia.

LESS COMMON
When treating depression: Fever or chills, concentration difficulties, drowsiness, fatigue, change in or blurred vision, unusual feeling of euphoria, hostility or anger. Smoking cessation: Mild rash, tremor.

PRINCIPAL USES
To relieve symptoms of major depression. Bupropion is also used as a non-nicotine aid to smoking cessation. It should be used as a part of a comprehensive smoking cessation program carried out under the supervision of your doctor.

HOW THE DRUG WORKS
While the exact mechanism of action of bupropion is not known, it appears to help balance the levels of brain chemicals that are thought to be linked to mood, emotions, and mental state. Unlike other smoking cessation medications, bupropion does not contain nicotine. It is believed that bupropion's effects on brain chemistry help to curb the desire for nicotine and enhance the patient's ability to abstain from smoking.

DOSAGE
Depression (Wellbutrin)—Adults: To start, 100 mg twice a day. Dosage may be increased to 450 mg a day. No more than 150 mg should be taken within 4 hours. Older adults: To start, 75 or 100 mg twice a day. Children: Dosages must be determined by your doctor. Smoking cessation (Zyban)— Adults: For the first 3 days of treatment, 150 mg a day. Dosage may then be increased to 150 mg, 2 times a day. The doses should be taken at least 8 hours apart. Do not take more than 300 mg per day. You should not stop smoking until you have been taking Zyban for 1 week. Treatment generally lasts 7 to 12 weeks.

ONSET OF EFFECT
1 to 3 weeks.

DURATION OF ACTION
Unknown.

DIETARY ADVICE
Bupropion can be taken with food to reduce stomach irritation. The tablet should be swallowed whole, because it has a bitter taste and can produce an unpleasant numbing sensation inside of the mouth.

STORAGE
Store in a tightly sealed container away from heat, moisture, and direct light.

IF YOU MISS A DOSE
Take it as soon as you remember, unless your next scheduled dose is within the next 4 hours (8 hours for smoking cessation). If so, do not take the missed dose. Take your next scheduled dose at the proper time and resume your regular dosage schedule. Do not double the next dose.

STOPPING THE DRUG
Depression: Take it as prescribed for the full treatment period, even if you begin to feel better before the scheduled end of therapy. Discontinuing the drug abruptly may produce unpleasant withdrawal symptoms. Dosage should be reduced gradually according to your doctor's instructions. The decision to stop taking the drug should be made in consultation with your doctor. Smoking cessation: If you have not made significant progress toward abstinence by the end of the seventh week of treatment, consult your doctor. Treatment should probably be discontinued. You do not need to gradually decrease the dose before stopping.

PROLONGED USE
Depression: The usual course of therapy lasts 6 months to 1 year; some patients benefit from additional therapy. Smoking cessation: Treatment generally lasts 7 to 12 weeks.

PRECAUTIONS
Over 60: Dosage may be decreased because of age-related decline in liver or kidney function.

Driving and Hazardous Work: Use caution until you determine how the medication affects you. Drowsiness or lightheadedness can occur.

Alcohol: Alcohol increases the risk of seizures. It is recommended to abstain from alcohol or to drink very little while taking bupropion. If you regularly drink a lot of alcohol and then suddenly stop, this may also increase your chance of having a seizure; gradual tapering of alcohol is recommended.

Pregnancy: Bupropion has not caused birth defects in animals. Adequate human studies have not been done. Bupropion is not recommended while you are pregnant. Before taking it, tell your doctor if you are pregnant or plan to become pregnant.

Breast Feeding: Bupropion passes into breast milk; avoid or discontinue using it while nursing.

Infants and Children: Adequate studies in children have not been done. Bupropion is not recommended for use by children under age 18.

Special Concerns: This is a potentially dangerous drug, especially if taken in excess. Antidepressants should not be within easy reach of suicidal patients. To prevent insomnia, take the last dose several hours before bedtime. When tak-

Bupropion Hydrochloride (continued)

ing bupropion for smoking cessation, it is advised to continue smoking through the first week of treatment. Set a target date to stop smoking no later than the second week of therapy. Continuing to smokebeyond the designated date reduces your chances of successfully quitting. You may use a nicotine transdermal patch (see Nicotine) while taking Zyban, but consult your doctor before initiating such therapy. The combination of nicotine and bupropion increases the risk of hypertension; blood pressure should be monitored regularly throughout treatment. Zyban should be regarded as but one part of a compre-

hensive treatment program that includes counseling, social support, and regular contact with your doctor. The goal of therapy with Zyban is complete abstinence from cigarettes. Do not chew, divide, or crush the tablets or extended-release tablets.

OVERDOSE

Symptoms: Hallucinations, seizures, rapid heartbeat, chest pain, breathing difficulty, loss of consciousness. Few cases of overdose associated with treatment for smoking cessation have been reported. Some of the symptoms experienced include: vomiting, blurred vision, lightheadedness,

confusion, lethargy, nausea, jitteriness, hallucinations, drowsiness, and seizures.

What to Do: Call your doctor, emergency medical services (EMS), or the nearest poison control center immediately.

DRUG INTERACTIONS

Bupropion should not be taken if you are taking other medicines containing bupropion or within 14 days of taking an MAO inhibitor. Consult your doctor for advice if you are taking loxapine, tricyclic antidepressants, phenothiazines, clozapine, molindone, fluoxetine, thioxanthenes, haloperidol, lithium,

trazodone, maprotiline, levodopa, or theophylline.

FOOD INTERACTIONS

No known food interactions.

DISEASE INTERACTIONS

Bupropion should not be taken if you have a history of seizures, anorexia nervosa, or bulimia. Caution is advised when taking bupropion. Consult your doctor if you have any of the following: a tumor of the brain or spinal cord, heart disease, or head injury. Since the liver and kidneys work together to remove bupropion from the body, a lower dose may be prescribed for patients with impaired liver or kidney function.

Buspirone Hydrochloride

BuSpar 5 mg
(MEAD JOHNSON)

▶ Drug Class: Antianxiety drug

▶ Available in: Tablets

▶ Available OTC? No

▶ As Generic? No

Side Effects

SERIOUS
No serious side effects have been directly associated with the use of buspirone.

COMMON
Dizziness or lightheadedness, nausea, paradoxical increase in nervousness or excitability, restlessness, headache.

LESS COMMON
Blurred vision, impaired ability to concentrate, drowsiness, dry mouth, difficulty sleeping, muscle cramps or spasms, fatigue or weakness, ringing in the ears, dreams that are unusual, disturbing, or vivid.

PRINCIPAL USES
To treat anxiety.

HOW THE DRUG WORKS
Buspirone affects the activity of specific brain chemicals (dopamine and especially serotonin) that are profoundly linked to mood, emotions, and mental state. Unlike many other medications used to treat anxiety disorders, buspirone has no muscle relaxant or sedative effects, and does not appear to lead to physical dependence.

DOSAGE
To start, 5 mg, 3 times per day (for a total of 15 mg a day). Can be increased to 60 mg a day, taken in divided doses every 6 to 8 hours.

ONSET OF EFFECT
May take 1 to 2 weeks to attain the full therapeutic benefit of buspirone.

DURATION OF ACTION
8 hours or more.

DIETARY ADVICE
No special restrictions.

STORAGE
Store in a tightly sealed container away from heat, moisture, and direct light.

IF YOU MISS A DOSE
If you miss a dose, take it as soon as you remember. If it is near the time for your next dose, skip the missed dose and resume your regular dosage schedule. Do not double the next dose.

STOPPING THE DRUG
The decision to stop taking buspirone should be made in consultation with your physician.

PROLONGED USE
No known problems.

PRECAUTIONS
Over 60: Adverse side effects and reactions may be more common and more severe in older patients.

Driving and Hazardous Work: The use of buspirone may impair your ability to drive or perform hazardous tasks safely. The danger increases if you drink alcohol or take other medications that can affect alertness, such as antihistamines, painkillers, or mind-altering drugs.

Alcohol: Avoid alcohol while using this medication.

Pregnancy: No problems are expected, but adequate studies of buspirone use during pregnancy have not been done. Consult your doctor if you are pregnant or plan to become pregnant.

Breast Feeding: Buspirone can pass into breast milk. Avoid taking it if possible or refrain from breast feeding.

Infants and Children: The safety and effectiveness of buspirone have not been established for anyone under the age of 18.

Special Concerns: Before you undergo surgery requiring anesthesia, be sure to notify the surgeon that you take buspirone.

OVERDOSE
Symptoms: Severe drowsiness, dizziness, nausea and vomiting, constricted (pinpoint) pupils.

What to Do: Call your doctor, emergency medical services (EMS), or the nearest poison control center immediately.

DRUG INTERACTIONS
Other drugs may interact with buspirone. Consult your doctor for specific advice if you take any of the following: antihistamines, barbiturates, MAO inhibitors, muscle relaxants, narcotics, sedatives, or other tranquilizers.

FOOD INTERACTIONS
None expected.

DISEASE INTERACTIONS
Use of buspirone may cause complications in patients with liver or kidney disease, since these organs work together to remove the medication from the body.

Busulfan

Myleran 2 mg
(GLAXO WELLCOME)

▶ Drug Class: Alkylating agent

▶ Available in: Tablets

▶ Available OTC? No

▶ As Generic? No

Side Effects

SERIOUS
Signs of unusual bleeding, including black, tarry, or bloody stools; blood in the urine; bright red, pinpointlike dots on the skin; unusual bruising; excessive gum bleeding; uncontrolled bleeding. Seizures are associated with higher doses. Consult your doctor at once.

COMMON
Increased pigmentation (darkening) of the skin; menstrual irregularities or absent periods.

LESS COMMON
Joint pain, shortness of breath, dizziness, sudden, unexpected loss of weight or appetite, lip or mouth sores, swelling in legs, ankles, and feet, nausea and vomiting, diarrhea, unusual fatigue or weakness.

PRINCIPAL USES
To treat certain forms of chronic leukemia (myeloid, myelocytic, and granulocytic leukemias). Busulfan slows the progress of these cancers, eases symptoms, and generally improves the condition of the patient, but it does not cure the disease. It is also used in conjunction with the transplanting of bone marrow to treat other forms of cancer.

HOW THE DRUG WORKS
Leukemia, in its many varieties, is a cancer marked by overproduction and abnormal formation of white blood cells, which are made in the bone marrow. Busulfan interferes with the growth and function of all cells, including the cells of the bone marrow. By interfering with bone marrow function, busulfan slows the production of the abnormal white blood cells.

DOSAGE
From 4 to 8 mg a day, as ordered by your doctor, until the desired response occurs.

ONSET OF EFFECT
Begins to take effect in 1 to 2 weeks.

DURATION OF ACTION
Up to 24 hours.

DIETARY ADVICE
Swallow tablet with liquid after a light meal. Avoid sweet or fatty foods. Do not drink fluids with meals. Drink extra fluids between meals.

STORAGE
Store in a tightly sealed container away from heat and direct light.

IF YOU MISS A DOSE
Take it as soon as you remember. If it is near the time for the next dose, skip the missed dose and resume your regular dosage schedule. Do not double the next dose.

STOPPING THE DRUG
Stop taking this medicine only on your doctor's advice

PROLONGED USE
Careful, continuous patient monitoring is needed during prolonged use.

PRECAUTIONS
Over 60: No special precautions are warranted.

Driving and Hazardous Work: Determine whether this drug affects your alertness and physical abilities before you drive or engage in hazardous activities.

Alcohol: Do not consume alcohol while you take this medicine.

Pregnancy: Busulfan may cause birth defects; it is best to use some method of birth control while you are taking this medicine. Inform your doctor at once if you become pregnant during therapy.

Breast Feeding: It is not known whether this medicine passes into breast milk. Breast feeding is generally not recommended while taking busulfan.

Infants and Children: This medicine is not expected to cause problems or side effects in children that are different from those it causes in adults.

Special Concerns: Busulfan can increase the risk of infection because it reduces the number of white blood cells in your body. Try to avoid contact with people who have infections. The medicine can also reduce blood levels of platelets, cells that are necessary for clotting. Be careful when using a toothbrush, dental floss, or toothpick, and be careful to avoid cutting yourself when you use a knife, razor, or other sharp instrument.

OVERDOSE
Symptoms: Bleeding, chills, fever, collapse, loss of consciousness.

What to Do: Seek emergency medical assistance immediately; call emergency medical services (EMS) or go to a hospital emergency room.

DRUG INTERACTIONS
Avoid any OTC product that contains aspirin, since it increases the danger of bleeding; carefully read ingredient labels of nonprescription drugs. Tell your doctor about any other drug you are taking, including an anticoagulant, any other anticancer drug, antithyroid medication, antibiotics, and antiviral medication.

FOOD INTERACTIONS
Avoid sweet or fatty foods.

DISEASE INTERACTIONS
Consult your doctor if you have any other medical problem, such as a history of seizures, chicken pox (or recent exposure to someone with chicken pox), shingles, gout, kidney stones, any head injury, or any infection.

Butalbital/Acetaminophen/Caffeine

Fioricet 50/325/40 mg
(NOVARTIS)

▶ Drug Class: Nonnarcotic analgesic

▶ Available in: Capsules, tablets

▶ Available OTC? No

▶ As Generic? Yes

Side Effects

SERIOUS
Shallow breathing, dizziness, weakness, confusion, blood in urine or stools, unusual bleeding or bruising, bleeding or crusting sores on lips, hives, muscle cramps, chest pain, white spots on the tongue, sore throat, pinpoint red spots on skin, fever, itchiness, rash, persistent or recurrent pain before next scheduled dose, swollen or painful glands, vomiting, yellow discoloration of skin or gums. Also swelling of the eyelids, lips, tongue, or face; red, thickened, or scaly skin. Call your physician immediately.

COMMON
Abdominal pain, dizziness, nausea or vomiting, mild stomach pain, lightheadedness, drowsiness.

LESS COMMON
Mental depression.

PRINCIPAL USES
To treat headaches when nonprescription pain relievers are ineffective.

HOW THE DRUG WORKS
Butalbital, a barbiturate, acts on the central nervous system to cause sedation. Acetaminophen (APAP) appears to interfere with the action of prostaglandins, naturally occurring substances in the body that cause inflammation and make nerves more sensitive to pain impulses. Caffeine, a stimulant, is believed to enhance the effectiveness of pain relievers.

DOSAGE
1 or 2 tablets every 4 hours as needed. If your medication contains 325 or 500 mg of acetaminophen per capsule or tablet, do not take more than 6 pills a day. If your medication contains 650 mg of acetaminophen per capsule or tablet, do not take more than 4 pills a day.

ONSET OF EFFECT
Unknown.

DURATION OF ACTION
Up to 4 hours.

DIETARY ADVICE
Take this medicine with milk or meals to minimize stomach upset.

STORAGE
Store in a tightly sealed container away from heat, moisture, and direct light.

IF YOU MISS A DOSE
If your doctor has directed you to take this medication on a regular schedule, take it as soon as you remember. If it is near the time for the next dose, skip the missed dose and resume your regular dosage schedule. Do not double the next dose.

STOPPING THE DRUG
You should take it as prescribed for the full treatment period, but you may stop taking the drug if you are feeling better before the scheduled end of therapy. This medication should never be stopped abruptly after long-term regular use.

PROLONGED USE
Barbiturates such as butalbital can cause physical dependence. Taking too much acetaminophen may cause liver damage.

PRECAUTIONS
Over 60: Adverse reactions may be more likely and more severe in older patients.

Driving and Hazardous Work: The use of this medicine may impair your ability to perform such tasks safely.

Alcohol: Avoid alcohol.

Pregnancy: Before taking this medicine, tell your doctor if you are pregnant or plan to become pregnant.

Breast Feeding: This medicine passes into breast milk; do not use while breast feeding.

Infants and Children: Not recommended for use by children under age 12.

Special Concerns: The medicine works best if you take it at the first sign of a headache. Do not take the medicine if it has a strong vinegary odor. If you do not feel better 1 hour after taking this medication, call your doctor. Do not take a larger dose.

OVERDOSE
Symptoms: Difficulty breathing, excessive perspiration, impaired mental state, loss of consciousness, agitation or nervousness.

What to Do: Call your doctor, emergency medical services (EMS), or the nearest poison control center immediately.

DRUG INTERACTIONS
Consult your doctor for specific advice if you are taking antihistamines, antidepressants, antipsychotic drugs, muscle relaxants, other narcotic pain relievers, sleep medications, tranquilizers, or anticoagulants.

FOOD INTERACTIONS
No known food interactions.

DISEASE INTERACTIONS
Consult your doctor if you have any of the following: asthma, mental depression, heart disease, a blood disorder, an overactive thyroid gland, a kidney or liver disorder, or a history of alcoholism or drug abuse.

BRAND NAMES
Amaphen with Codeine #3, Fioricet with Codeine

▶ Drug Class: Opioid (narcotic) analgesic

▶ Available in: Capsules, tablets

▶ Available OTC? No

▶ As Generic? Yes

Side Effects

SERIOUS
Chest pains, muscle or joint pain, sores or ulcers in mouth, swelling of face, lips, or eyelids, yellow discoloration of eyes or skin, sore throat with or without fever. Call your doctor immediately.

COMMON
Drowsiness, dizziness, shortness of breath, light-headedness, constipation, confusion, nausea, and vomiting.

LESS COMMON
Skin rash or hives.

PRINCIPAL USES
To treat tension headaches when nonprescription pain relievers prove ineffective.

HOW THE DRUG WORKS
Butalbital, a barbiturate, acts on the central nervous system to cause sedation. Acetaminophen (APAP) appears to interfere with the action of prostaglandins, naturally occurring substances in the body that cause inflammation and make nerves more sensitive to pain impulses. Caffeine, a stimulant, is believed to enhance the effectiveness of pain relievers. Codeine, a narcotic, is believed to block pain signals to the brain and spinal cord.

DOSAGE
1 or 2 tablets or capsules every 4 hours. Do not take more than 6 pills a day.

ONSET OF EFFECT
Unknown.

DURATION OF ACTION
Unknown.

DIETARY ADVICE
This medication should be taken with food or water.

STORAGE
Store in a tightly sealed container away from heat, moisture, and direct light.

IF YOU MISS A DOSE
If your doctor has directed you to take this drug on a regular schedule, take it as soon as you remember. If it is near the time for the next dose, skip the missed dose and resume your regular dosage schedule. Do not double the next dose.

STOPPING THE DRUG
Take it as prescribed for the full treatment period, but you may stop taking the drug if you are feeling better before the scheduled end of therapy. This medicine should never be stopped abruptly after long-term regular use.

PROLONGED USE
Narcotic drugs, such as codeine, and barbiturates, such as butalbital, can cause physical dependence. Taking too much acetaminophen may cause liver damage.

PRECAUTIONS
Over 60: Adverse reactions may be more likely and more severe in older patients.

Driving and Hazardous Work: Do not drive or engage in hazardous work until you determine how the medicine affects you.

Alcohol: Avoid alcohol.

Pregnancy: Components of this medication have caused birth defects in animals. Taking the drug late in pregnancy may cause drug dependence in the unborn child. Tell your doctor if you are pregnant or plan to become pregnant before you take this drug.

Breast Feeding: Components of this medicine pass into breast milk; avoid or discontinue use while breast feeding.

Infants and Children: Not recommended for use by children under age 12.

Special Concerns: Tell any doctor or dentist whom you consult that you are taking this medicine. It works best if taken at the first sign of a headache. Tell your doctor if you begin having headaches more frequently than before you started using this drug. Check with your doctor if the medicine stops working as well as it did at the outset of therapy. This may be a sign of drug dependence. Do not increase the dose to attain better pain relief.

OVERDOSE
Symptoms: Drowsiness, confusion, nausea, vomiting, abnormal heartbeat, insomnia, slowed or suppressed breathing, trembling, loss of consciousness.

What to Do: Call your doctor, emergency medical services (EMS), or the nearest poison control center immediately.

DRUG INTERACTIONS
Consult your doctor for specific advice if you are taking beta-blockers, estrogens, felodipine, griseofulvin, nifedipine, theophylline, warfarin, carbamazepine, sulfinpyrazone, tranquilizers, sedatives, or tricyclic antidepressants.

FOOD INTERACTIONS
No known food interactions. A high-fiber diet is recommended because the medicine may cause constipation.

DISEASE INTERACTIONS
Consult your doctor if you have any of the following: asthma, liver disease, kidney disease, diabetes, mental depression, an overactive thyroid, porphyria, heart disease, or a history of alcohol or drug abuse.

Butalbital/Aspirin/Caffeine

▶ Drug Class: Nonnarcotic analgesic

▶ Available in: Capsules, tablets

▶ Available OTC? No

▶ As Generic? Yes

Side Effects

SERIOUS
Difficulty breathing, tightness in chest, coughing, or wheezing; sores or white spots in mouth; bluish discoloration, flushing, or redness of skin; stuffy nose; pinpoint pupils; fever; swollen eyelids, face, lips, or tongue; difficulty swallowing; crusting or bleeding sores on lips; sore throat; burning, tenderness, or peeling of skin. Call your physician immediately.

COMMON
Drowsiness, dizziness, heartburn.

LESS COMMON
Insomnia, nightmares, headache, constipation, increased sweating, unusual fatigue.

PRINCIPAL USES
To treat headaches or migraines.

HOW THE DRUG WORKS
Butalbital, a barbiturate, acts on the central nervous system to cause sedation. Aspirin appears to interfere with the action of prostaglandins, naturally occurring substances in the body that cause inflammation and make nerves more sensitive to pain impulses. Caffeine is believed to enhance the effectiveness of pain relievers.

DOSAGE
1 or 2 capsules or tablets every 4 hours. Do not take more than 6 pills a day.

ONSET OF EFFECT
Within 1 hour.

DURATION OF ACTION
4 hours.

DIETARY ADVICE
Take this drug with food or a full glass of water to avoid stomach irritation.

STORAGE
Store in a tightly sealed container away from heat, moisture, and direct light.

IF YOU MISS A DOSE
If your doctor has directed you to take this drug on a regular schedule, take it as soon as you remember. If it is near the time for the next dose, skip the missed dose and resume your regular dosage schedule. Do not double the next dose.

STOPPING THE DRUG
Take it as prescribed for the full treatment period, but you may stop taking the drug if you are feeling better before the scheduled end of therapy. This drug should never be stopped abruptly after long-term regular use.

PROLONGED USE
Prolonged use may result in physical dependence and may cause kidney damage. Periodic kidney function tests are recommended. Prolonged use may make exposure to cold weather more hazardous.

PRECAUTIONS
Over 60: Adverse reactions may be more likely and more severe in older patients.

Driving and Hazardous Work: Do not drive or engage in hazardous work until you determine how the medicine affects you.

Alcohol: Avoid alcohol.

Pregnancy: Taking this medicine late in pregnancy may cause drug dependence in the unborn child. Before you take it, tell your doctor if you are pregnant or are planning to become pregnant.

Breast Feeding: Butalbital and aspirin pass into breast milk; avoid or discontinue use while nursing.

Infants and Children: Consult your doctor before giving this medicine to anyone under age 18 who has a viral illness, especially chicken pox or influenza. The aspirin may cause a serious illness called Reye's syndrome.

Special Concerns: Tell any doctor or dentist whom you consult that you are taking this medicine. It works best if taken at the first sign of a headache. Tell your doctor if you begin having headaches more frequently than before you started using it, or if the drug stops working as well as it did at the outset of therapy. This may be a sign of drug dependence. Do not try to get better pain relief by increasing the dose. Do not take the drug if it has a strong vinegary odor.

OVERDOSE
Symptoms: Deep sleep, weak pulse, ringing in ears, nausea, vomiting, dizziness, deep and rapid breathing, convulsions, loss of consciousness.

What to Do: Call your doctor, emergency medical services (EMS), or the nearest poison control center immediately.

DRUG INTERACTIONS
Consult your doctor for advice if you are taking acetazolamide, gout medicines, beta-blockers, anticoagulants, methotrexate, narcotic pain relievers, nonsteroidal anti-inflammatory drugs, oral contraceptives, oral diabetes medicines, steroid medicines, tranquilizers, or valproic acid.

FOOD INTERACTIONS
No known food interactions.

DISEASE INTERACTIONS
Consult your doctor if you have any of the following: stomach or duodenal ulcers, asthma, epilepsy, anemia, gout, or a history of alcohol or drug abuse. Use of this drug may cause complications in patients with liver or kidney disease, since these organs work together to remove the medication from the body.

BRAND NAMES
Ascomp with Codeine No. 3, Butalbital Compound with Codeine, Butinal with Codeine No. 3, Fiorinal with Codeine, Idenal with Codeine, Isollyl with Codeine

▶ Drug Class: Opioid (narcotic) analgesic

▶ Available in: Capsules, tablets

▶ Available OTC? No

▶ As Generic? Yes

Side Effects

SERIOUS
Wheezing, tightness in chest, pinpoint pupils, yellowish discoloration of the skin and eyes, easy bruising, vomiting blood, sore throat, fever, mouth sores, difficult urination, hearing loss, blood in urine. Call your doctor immediately.

COMMON
Drowsiness, dizziness, lightheadedness, flushed face, depression, increased urination.

LESS COMMON
Insomnia, nightmares, headache, constipation, increased sweating, unusual fatigue.

PRINCIPAL USES
To treat tension headaches or migraines.

HOW THE DRUG WORKS
Butalbital, a barbiturate, acts on the central nervous system to relieve pain. Aspirin appears to interfere with the action of prostaglandins, naturally occurring substances in the body that cause inflammation and make nerves more sensitive to pain impulses. Caffeine is believed to enhance the effectiveness of pain relievers. Codeine, a narcotic, is believed to block pain signals to the brain.

DOSAGE
1 or 2 capsules or tablets every 4 hours. Do not take more than 6 pills a day.

ONSET OF EFFECT
Within 1 hour.

DURATION OF ACTION
4 hours.

DIETARY ADVICE
This medicine should be taken with food or water to minimize stomach irritation.

STORAGE
Store in a tightly sealed container away from heat, moisture, and direct light.

IF YOU MISS A DOSE
Take it as soon as you remember. If it is near the time for the next dose, skip the missed dose and resume your regular dosage schedule. Do not double the next dose.

STOPPING THE DRUG
You should take this medication as prescribed for the full treatment period, but you may stop taking it if you are feeling better before the scheduled end of therapy. This drug should never be stopped abruptly after long-term regular use.

PROLONGED USE
Narcotic drugs, such as codeine, and barbiturates, such as butalbital, can cause physical dependence. Prolonged use can cause kidney dysfunction.

PRECAUTIONS
Over 60: Adverse reactions may be more likely and more severe in older patients.

Driving and Hazardous Work: Do not drive or engage in hazardous work until you determine how the medicine affects you.

Alcohol: Avoid alcohol.

Pregnancy: Taking the medicine late in pregnancy may cause drug dependence in the unborn child. Before you take this medicine, tell your doctor if you are pregnant or plan to become pregnant.

Breast Feeding: Do not use while nursing.

Infants and Children: This medicine is generally not prescribed for children under age 12. Consult your doctor before giving it to anyone under age 18 who has a viral illness, especially chicken pox or influenza. The aspirin may cause a serious illness called Reye's syndrome.

Special Concerns: Tell any doctor or dentist whom you consult that you are taking this medicine. The drug works best if taken at the first sign of a headache. Tell your doctor if you begin having headaches more frequently than before you started using this medicine. Check with your doctor if the medicine stops working as well as it did at the outset of therapy. Do not try to get better pain relief by increasing the dose. Do not take this drug if it has a strong, vinegary odor.

OVERDOSE
Symptoms: Ringing in ears, slow and weak pulse, deep sleep, dizziness, nausea, vomiting, hallucinations, deep and rapid breathing, convulsions, loss of consciousness.

What to Do: Call your doctor, emergency medical services (EMS), or the nearest poison control center immediately.

DRUG INTERACTIONS
Consult your doctor for specific advice if you are taking acetazolamide, gout medicines, beta-blockers, anticoagulants, methotrexate, narcotic pain relievers, nonsteroidal anti-inflammatory drugs, oral contraceptives, oral diabetes medicines, steroid medicines, tranquilizers, or valproic acid.

FOOD INTERACTIONS
No known food interactions.

DISEASE INTERACTIONS
Consult your doctor if you have any of the following: stomach or duodenal ulcers, asthma, epilepsy, anemia, gout, or a history of alcohol or drug abuse. Use of this drug may cause complications in patients with liver or kidney disease, since these organs work together to remove the medication from the body.

Butenafine Hydrochloride

BRAND NAME
Mentax

▶ Drug Class: Topical antifungal

▶ Available in: Cream

▶ Available OTC? No

▶ As Generic? No

Side Effects

SERIOUS
No serious side effects are associated with the use of butenafine.

COMMON
Burning, stinging, irritation, itching, redness, swelling, or blistering at the site of application.

LESS COMMON
There are no less-common side effects associated with the use of butenafine.

PRINCIPAL USES
To treat tinea pedis (athlete's foot), a fungal infection.

HOW THE DRUG WORKS
Butenafine prevents fungal organisms from producing vital substances required for their growth and function. This drug is effective only for infections caused by fungal organisms. It will not work for bacterial or viral infections.

DOSAGE
Apply it to the affected area either twice a day for 7 days or once a day for 4 weeks, in accordance with your doctor's instructions.

ONSET OF EFFECT
Unknown.

DURATION OF ACTION
Unknown.

DIETARY ADVICE
No special restrictions.

STORAGE
Store in a tightly sealed container away from heat, moisture, and direct light. Do not allow the cream to freeze.

IF YOU MISS A DOSE
Apply butenafine as soon as you remember. If it is near the time for the next dose, skip the missed dose and resume your regular dosage schedule. Do not double the next dose or apply an excessively thick film of topical medication to compensate for a missed dose.

STOPPING THE DRUG
Apply as prescribed for the full treatment period, even if the fungal infection appears to be eradicated before the scheduled end of therapy. Unfortunately, it can be difficult to assess when the drug has achieved its desired effect since it suppresses redness and inflammation of the skin before the infection is completely clear; recurrence of fungal infection owing to inadequate length of therapy is a significant risk.

PROLONGED USE
If your skin problem does not improve or instead becomes worse after 4 weeks of treatment, consult your doctor.

PRECAUTIONS
Over 60: No special problems are expected.

Driving and Hazardous Work: The use of butenafine should not impair your ability to perform such tasks safely.

Alcohol: No special precautions are necessary.

Pregnancy: Adequate human studies have not been done. Before taking butenafine, tell your physician if you are pregnant or plan to become pregnant.

Breast Feeding: It is not known whether butenafine passes into breast milk; caution is advised. Consult your doctor for specific advice.

Infants and Children: The safety and effectiveness of butenafine use by children below the age of 12 have not been determined. Use of the medication in patients 12 to 16 years of age has not caused any problems and has been effective.

Special Concerns: Butenafine is intended for external use only. Wash your hands after butenafine is applied to the affected area. Contact with the eyes, nose, and mouth should be avoided. If you apply butenafine after bathing or showering, dry the affected area thoroughly first. Do not use a tight-fitting dressing unless your physician tells you to do so. Do not use butenafine for any condition other than the one for which it was prescribed. As with any antifungal, butenafine is useful only against organisms that are vulnerable to its effects. Therefore, it is important to tell your doctor if your condition has not improved—or instead has worsened—within a few days of starting butenafine. The particular organism causing your illness may be resistant to this drug.

OVERDOSE
Symptoms: No cases of overdose have been reported.

What to Do: An overdose of butenafine is unlikely to be life-threatening. However, if someone uses a much larger dose than prescribed or ingests the medicine, seek medical assistance immediately.

DRUG INTERACTIONS
Consult your doctor for specific advice if you are taking allylamine antifungal drugs. Also tell your doctor if you are taking any other prescription or over-the-counter medications.

FOOD INTERACTIONS
No known food interactions.

DISEASE INTERACTIONS
Caution is advised when taking butenafine. Consult your doctor if you have any other medical condition.

Butoconazole Nitrate

BRAND NAME
Femstat 3

▶ Drug Class: Antifungal

▶ Available in: Vaginal cream

▶ Available OTC? Yes

▶ As Generic? No

Side Effects

SERIOUS
Vaginal itching, burning, discharge, or irritation not present prior to treatment. Call your doctor as soon as possible.

COMMON
No common side effects are associated with the use of butoconazole.

LESS COMMON
Headache, stomach cramps or pain, irritation or burning of sexual partner's penis.

PRINCIPAL USES
To treat fungal (yeast) infections of the vagina.

HOW THE DRUG WORKS
Butoconazole prevents fungal organisms from producing vital substances required for growth and function. This drug is effective only for infections caused by fungal organisms. It will not work for bacterial or viral infections.

DOSAGE
Nonpregnant women and teenagers: 5 g (1 applicatorful) of cream inserted with an applicator into the vagina at bedtime for 3 consecutive days. Pregnant women and teenagers: After third month, 5 g (1 applicatorful) of cream inserted with an applicator into the vagina at bedtime for 6 consecutive days.

ONSET OF EFFECT
Unknown.

DURATION OF ACTION
Unknown.

DIETARY ADVICE
Butoconazole can be applied without regard to diet.

STORAGE
Store in a tightly sealed container away from heat, moisture, and direct light. Do not allow it to freeze.

IF YOU MISS A DOSE
Insert it as soon as you remember. If it is near the time for the next dose, skip the missed dose and resume your regular dosage schedule.

STOPPING THE DRUG
Take the medicine as directed for the full treatment period, even if you begin to feel better before the scheduled end of therapy. Recurrence of the infection is likely if you stop before the full treatment period is complete.

PROLONGED USE
Butoconazole is generally prescribed for short-term therapy (3 to 6 days).

PRECAUTIONS
Over 60: No special problems are expected.

Driving and Hazardous Work: The use of butoconazole should not impair your ability to perform such tasks safely.

Alcohol: No special precautions are necessary.

Pregnancy: Studies on the use of butoconazole during the first 3 months (trimester) of pregnancy have not been done. No adverse effects while using it during the second or third trimesters have been reported.

Breast Feeding: No problems are expected. Consult your doctor about using this medicine while nursing.

Infants and Children: Studies on the use of butoconazole in children have not been done. Consult your pediatrician for specific advice.

Special Concerns: The drug may be used with oral contraceptives and antibiotic therapy. Sanitary napkins should be used to prevent staining of clothing. The affected area should be kept cool and dry. The patient should wear loose-fitting cotton clothing and freshly laundered cotton underwear or pantyhose with a cotton crotch. Avoid underwear made from nonventilating materials. Do not sit for a long time in a wet bathing suit. Avoid feminine hygiene sprays. Wash daily with unscented soap and dry thoroughly with a clean towel. Tampons should not be used during therapy. The patient's sexual partner should wear a condom during intercourse and should consult a doctor if penile redness, itching, or discomfort occurs. Do not stop using this medicine during your menstrual period. After urination or a bowel movement, cleanse by wiping the area from front to back to prevent reinfection.

OVERDOSE
Symptoms: An overdose with butoconazole is unlikely.

What to Do: If someone should swallow a large amount of the medicine, call your doctor, emergency medical services (EMS), or the nearest poison control center immediately.

DRUG INTERACTIONS
Tell your doctor if you are using any other vaginal prescription or over-the-counter medication.

FOOD INTERACTIONS
No food interactions have been reported.

DISEASE INTERACTIONS
No disease interactions have been reported.

Butorphanol Tartrate

BRAND NAME
Stadol NS

▶ Drug Class: Opioid (narcotic) analgesic

▶ Available in: Nasal spray

▶ Available OTC? No

▶ As Generic? No

Side Effects

SERIOUS
Shallow or slow breathing, sinus congestion, changes in mental state, nosebleeds, fever, sneezing, runny nose, blurred or distorted vision, ear pain, bronchitis, itching, hallucinations, difficulty urinating, skin rash, fainting. Call your doctor immediately.

COMMON
Headache, sedation, dizziness, insomnia, nose irritation, confusion, dry mouth, nausea, vomiting, constipation, loss of appetite, clammy skin, unpleasant taste in mouth.

LESS COMMON
Nervousness, unusual dreams, sluggishness, agitation, euphoria, floating sensation, trembling, stomach pain.

PRINCIPAL USES
To relieve headaches, post-operative pain, or other pain for which a narcotic analgesic is necessary.

HOW THE DRUG WORKS
Butorphanol blocks pain impulses at specific sites in the brain and spinal cord.

DOSAGE
Spray once into one nostril only. Do not spray into both nostrils unless directed by physician. Dose may be repeated in 60 to 90 minutes, and every 4 to 6 hours if needed.

ONSET OF EFFECT
Within 15 minutes.

DURATION OF ACTION
4 to 5 hours.

DIETARY ADVICE
No special restrictions.

STORAGE
Store in a tightly sealed container away from heat, moisture, and direct light.

IF YOU MISS A DOSE
Not applicable; butorphanol should not be taken on a routine schedule.

STOPPING THE DRUG
You may stop taking the drug if you are feeling better, but butorphanol should never be stopped abruptly after long-term regular use.

PROLONGED USE
The effects of long-term use are unknown. This drug could be habit-forming. Consult your doctor regularly during prolonged use.

PRECAUTIONS
Over 60: Adverse reactions and side effects, particularly dizziness, may be more likely and more severe in older persons.

Driving and Hazardous Work: Do not drive or engage in hazardous work until you determine how the medicine affects you.

Alcohol: Avoid alcohol because it can further dull alertness and slow reflexes.

Pregnancy: Before taking butorphanol, discuss with your doctor the relative risks and benefits of using this drug while pregnant.

Breast Feeding: Butorphanol may pass into breast milk; caution is advised. Consult your doctor for specific advice.

Infants and Children: Butorphanol is not recommended for use by children under the age of 18.

Special Concerns: When you first use this medicine, get up slowly from a sitting or lying position to avoid dizziness. Tell any doctor or dentist whom you consult that you are using butorphanol. Do not increase or decrease the dosage without consulting your doctor. When using a new bottle of butorphanol, point the bottle away from you and pump about 3 times to start the pump. Each time you use the spray, wipe the tip with a clean tissue or cloth. Every 3 or 4 days, rinse the tip with warm water and wipe the tip for about 15 seconds, then dry. To administer a dose of butorphanol, first blow your nose gently. Hold your head forward a little, put the spray tip in the nostril, and aim for the back. Close the other nostril by pressing with one finger. After the spray, tilt your head back for a few seconds. Do not blow your nose.

OVERDOSE
Symptoms: Irregular heartbeat; difficulty breathing; seizures; cold, clammy skin; loss of consciousness; pinpoint pupils of eyes; severe drowsiness, restlessness, weakness, dizziness, or nervousness.

What to Do: Call your doctor, emergency medical services (EMS), or the nearest poison control center immediately.

DRUG INTERACTIONS
The following drugs may interact with butorphanol: tranquilizers, sleeping pills, barbiturates, antihistamines, heart drugs, oral diabetes drugs, and antidepressants. Consult your doctor for specific advice about any drug you are taking.

FOOD INTERACTIONS
None expected.

DISEASE INTERACTIONS
Tell your doctor if you have had a heart attack or a head injury or if you have heart disease, a respiratory disease, a kidney problem, a liver problem, or a history of alcohol or drug abuse.

Vivarin 200 mg
(SMITHKLINE BEECHAM)

Additional photographs

▶ Drug Class: Central nervous system stimulant

▶ Available in: Tablets, extended-release capsules

▶ Available OTC? Yes

▶ As Generic? Yes

Side Effects

SERIOUS
Diarrhea, insomnia, dizziness, rapid heartbeat, severe nausea, vomiting, irritability, unusual agitation, tremors. Call your doctor immediately.

COMMON
Mild nausea or jitters.

LESS COMMON
There are no less-common side effects associated with the use of caffeine.

PRINCIPAL USES
To restore mental alertness.

HOW THE DRUG WORKS
Caffeine acts as a stimulant to all levels of the central nervous system.

DOSAGE
Tablets: 100 to 200 mg; repeat after 3 or 4 hours if needed. Extended-release capsules: 200 to 250 mg; can be repeated after 3 or 4 hours if needed. Citrated caffeine: 65 to 325 mg, 3 times a day as needed. Take no more than 1,000 mg a day.

ONSET OF EFFECT
Unknown.

DURATION OF ACTION
Unknown.

DIETARY ADVICE
Take it with food to minimize stomach upset.

STORAGE
Store in a tightly sealed container away from heat and direct light. Keep away from moisture and extremes in temperature.

IF YOU MISS A DOSE
Take it as soon as you remember. If it is near the time for the next dose, skip the missed dose and resume your regular dosage schedule. Do not double the next dose.

STOPPING THE DRUG
The decision to stop taking the drug should be made by your doctor.

PROLONGED USE
Caffeine is not intended for prolonged use.

PRECAUTIONS
Over 60: No special problems are expected.

Driving and Hazardous Work: The use of caffeine should not impair your ability to perform such tasks safely.

Alcohol: No special precautions are necessary.

Pregnancy: Large doses can cause miscarriage, delay the growth of the fetus, or cause problems with the heart rhythm of the fetus. No more than 300 mg of caffeine (the amount in 3 cups of coffee) should be consumed daily during pregnancy.

Breast Feeding: Caffeine passes into breast milk; caution is advised. Consult your doctor for specific advice.

Infants and Children: Caffeine is not recommended for use by children under the age of 12.

Special Concerns: To prevent insomnia, do not take caffeine or caffeine-containing beverages too close to bedtime. After you stop taking caffeine, you may experience anxiety, dizziness, headache, irritability, muscle tension, nausea, nervousness, stuffy nose, and unusual fatigue. Consult your doctor if you suffer from any of these symptoms.

OVERDOSE
Symptoms: Stomach or abdominal pains, agitation, anxiety, excitement, restlessness, confusion, delirium, seizures. A very large overdose can cause an irregular heartbeat; seeing zig-zag flashes of light; frequent urination; increased sensitivity to touch; muscle twitching; nausea and vomiting, sometimes with blood; insomnia; and ringing in the ears.

What to Do: An overdose of caffeine is unlikely to be life-threatening. However, if someone takes a much larger dose than directed, call your doctor, emergency medical services (EMS), or the nearest poison control center right away.

DRUG INTERACTIONS
Call your doctor for specific advice if you are taking central nervous system stimulants; MAO inhibitors; amantadine; ciprofloxacin and norfloxacin (antibiotics); cold, sinus, hay fever, or allergy medications; asthma medicine; pemoline; amphetamines; nabilone; methylphenidate; or chlophedianol.

FOOD INTERACTIONS
Do not drink large amounts of caffeine-containing beverages like coffee, tea, soft drinks, cocoa, or chocolate milk.

DISEASE INTERACTIONS
Caution is advised when taking caffeine. Consult your doctor if you have any of the following: anxiety, panic attacks, heart disease, high blood pressure, agoraphobia (fear of open places), or insomnia. Use of caffeine may cause complications in patients with liver disease, since this organ works to remove the medication from the body.

Calamine

BRAND NAME
Calamox

▶ Drug Class: Topical anti-itching agent; astringent

▶ Available in: Lotion, ointment

▶ Available OTC? Yes

▶ As Generic? Yes

Side Effects

SERIOUS
No serious side effects are associated with calamine.

COMMON
No common side effects are associated with calamine.

LESS COMMON
Rash, irritation, or sensitivity of the treated area that was not present prior to beginning therapy. Call your doctor promptly if such symptoms persist.

PRINCIPAL USES
To relieve the itching, pain, and discomfort of skin irritations, such as those caused by poison ivy, poison oak, and poison sumac. Calamine will also dry the oozing and weeping of skin eruptions caused by poison ivy, poison oak, and poison sumac.

HOW THE DRUG WORKS
The exact mechanism of action is unknown; calamine appears to have natural soothing properties.

DOSAGE
Apply calamine to the affected area of skin as often as needed. To use the lotion, shake it well to start. Then moisten a wad of cotton with the lotion and use the cotton to apply the lotion to the affected area of skin. Allow the lotion to dry on the skin. To use the ointment, gently rub just enough ointment into the skin to lightly cover the affected area.

ONSET OF EFFECT
Within 1 hour.

DURATION OF ACTION
Unknown.

DIETARY ADVICE
Calamine can be used without regard to diet.

STORAGE
Store in a tightly sealed container away from heat and direct light. Do not refrigerate or allow medication to freeze.

IF YOU MISS A DOSE
If you are using calamine on a fixed schedule, apply the missed dose as soon as you remember. If it is close to the next dose, skip the missed dose and resume your regular dosage schedule. Do not use more lotion or ointment than necessary.

STOPPING THE DRUG
Take it as prescribed for the full treatment period. However, you may stop taking the drug if you are feeling better before the scheduled end of therapy.

PROLONGED USE
Call your doctor if your condition does not improve or gets worse after 7 days of treatment.

PRECAUTIONS
Over 60: No special problems have been documented in older patients.

Driving and Hazardous Work: Use of calamine should not impair your ability to perform such tasks safely.

Alcohol: No special precautions are necessary.

Pregnancy: No problems during pregnancy have been documented.

Breast Feeding: Calamine may be used safely while nursing; no problems that affect the baby during breast feeding have been documented.

Infants and Children: Studies on the use of calamine on infants and children have not been done; however, no pediatric-specific problems have been documented.

Special Concerns: Calamine is for external use only. Do not swallow it. Do not use calamine on the eyes or mucous membranes, such as the inside of the mouth, nose, genitals, or anal area. Ingestion of calamine has been reported to cause gastritis (inflammation of the stomach lining) and vomiting. Milk or antacids may be used to treat gastritis.

OVERDOSE
Symptoms: None.

What to Do: No emergency instructions are applicable, since no cases of overdose have been reported. However, if someone accidentally ingests calamine, seek medical assistance right away.

DRUG INTERACTIONS
No drug interactions with calamine have been reported. However, you should tell your doctor if you are using any other prescription or over-the-counter medication to treat the same area of skin as calamine.

FOOD INTERACTIONS
No known food interactions.

DISEASE INTERACTIONS
No disease interactions with calamine have been documented. However, tell your doctor if you have any other skin condition.

Calcipotriene

▶ Drug Class: Vitamin D analog

▶ Available in: Cream, ointment, scalp solution

▶ Available OTC? No

▶ As Generic? No

Side Effects

SERIOUS
No serious side effects have been reported in association with the use of calcipotriene.

COMMON
Temporary burning, tingling, and stinging; rash; peeling. Consult your doctor if these symptoms persist.

LESS COMMON
Skin irritation, dry skin, worsening of psoriasis, thinning of the skin, darkening of the skin.

PRINCIPAL USES
Cream and ointment are used to treat mild to moderate psoriasis in adults. Scalp solution is used to treat chronic, moderately severe psoriasis of the scalp.

HOW THE DRUG WORKS
Calcipotriene is a synthetic form of vitamin D. It appears to slow excessive growth of skin cells; however, the exact mechanism of action is unknown.

DOSAGE
Cream and ointment: Apply a thin layer to the affected area once or twice daily and rub in evenly. Do not apply to the face. Scalp solution: Comb through the hair to remove scaly debris. Apply calcipotriene only to the lesions and rub in evenly. Do not allow the solution to spread to the forehead or other unaffected areas. Wash hands thoroughly after use.

ONSET OF EFFECT
Within 24 hours.

DURATION OF ACTION
Unknown.

DIETARY ADVICE
Calcipotriene can be used without regard to diet.

STORAGE
Store in a tightly sealed container away from heat, moisture, and direct light. Do not allow it to freeze. Keep the scalp solution away from open flame.

IF YOU MISS A DOSE
Apply it as soon as you remember.

STOPPING THE DRUG
The decision to stop taking the drug should be made in consultation with your physician.

PROLONGED USE
Treatment periods, depending on the severity of the psoriasis, generally last 8 weeks but have been approved to continue for up to 1 year.

PRECAUTIONS
Over 60: Adverse reactions may be more likely and more severe in older patients.

Driving and Hazardous Work: The use of calcipotriene should not impair your ability to perform such tasks safely.

Alcohol: No special precautions are necessary.

Pregnancy: Adequate human studies have not been done. Before taking calcipotriene, tell your doctor if you are pregnant or plan to become pregnant.

Breast Feeding: Calcipotriene may pass into breast milk; caution is advised. Consult your doctor for specific advice.

Infants and Children: Not recommended for use by children under age 12.

OVERDOSE
Symptoms: Small amounts of the medication are absorbed through the skin. Symptoms of an overdose are due to elevated levels of blood calcium (hypercalcemia). Early symptoms of hypercalcemia: Constipation (especially in children), diarrhea, dry mouth, increased thirst and frequency of urination, persistent headache, loss of appetite, metallic taste, nausea and vomiting, unusual fatigue. Advanced symptoms: Bone and muscle pain, irregular heartbeat, persistent itching, extreme drowsiness, mental changes. Severe calcium toxicity may be fatal.

What to Do: Call your doctor, emergency medical services (EMS), or the nearest poison control center immediately.

DRUG INTERACTIONS
No known drug interactions.

FOOD INTERACTIONS
No known food interactions.

DISEASE INTERACTIONS
You should not take calcipotriene if you have high blood levels of calcium (hypercalcemia) or evidence of vitamin D toxicity.

Calcitonin — Salmon

BRAND NAMES
Calcimar, Miacalcin

▸ Drug Class: Hormone/bone resorption inhibitor

▸ Available in: Injection, nasal spray

▸ Available OTC? No

▸ As Generic? No

Side Effects

SERIOUS
Skin rash or hives. Call your doctor immediately.

COMMON
Diarrhea, loss of appetite, nausea or vomiting, stomach pain, pain and redness at injection site, flushing or redness of face, ears, hands, or feet.

LESS COMMON
Increased output of urine, headache, dizziness, pressure in the chest, breathing difficulty, stuffy nose, nasal bleeding or crusting, tingling of hands or feet, weakness, back pain, joint pain, chills.

PRINCIPAL USES
To treat Paget's disease, a disorder in which bone tissue is broken down and restored too rapidly, resulting in bone fragility and in some cases malformation; to prevent bone loss in women with postmenopausal osteoporosis; to treat abnormally high blood calcium levels; to treat osteoporosis resulting from hormonal disturbances, drug therapy, and immobilization; to relieve compression of nerves that may occur with Paget's disease of bone.

HOW THE DRUG WORKS
Calcitonin blocks the bone-mineral-absorbing activity of the osteoclasts (bone cells), increases calcium excretion by the kidneys, and slows bone resorption (the speed at which bone is broken down before it is replaced).

DOSAGE
Injection— For Paget's disease: 100 international units (IU) injected under the skin once a day to start. The dosage may be reduced depending on results. To prevent postmenopausal bone loss: 100 IU injected into muscle or under the skin once a day, once every other day, or 3 times a week. For excessive blood calcium: 1.8 IU per lb of body weight injected every 12 hours to start. Dose may be increased or decreased by your doctor. Nasal spray— 200 IU (1 spray) a day delivered in alternating nostrils, 1 spray a day.

ONSET OF EFFECT
Within 15 minutes.

DURATION OF ACTION
8 to 24 hours.

DIETARY ADVICE
If you are using this drug to lower blood calcium, your doctor may want you to follow a low-calcium diet. An injection is best administered at bedtime.

STORAGE
Store in a tightly sealed container away from heat and direct light.

IF YOU MISS A DOSE
If you take 2 doses a day: Take the missed dose if you remember within 2 hours. If not, skip the missed dose and resume your regular dosage schedule. If you take 1 dose a day: Take the missed dose if you remember it the same day, then resume your regular dosage schedule. If you remember the next day, skip the missed dose and resume your regular dosage schedule. If you take one dose every other day: Take the missed dose if you remember the same day. Otherwise, take the dose the next day, skip a day and resume your regular dosage schedule. If you take 1 dose 3 times a week: Take the missed dose the next day, set each dose back a day for the rest of the week, then resume your regular dosage schedule. In no cases should you double the next dose.

STOPPING THE DRUG
The decision to stop taking the drug should be made by your doctor.

PROLONGED USE
Development of antibodies to the medicine may diminish its effectiveness with prolonged use.

PRECAUTIONS
Over 60: Fluid balance should be monitored if the drug is given to reduce blood levels of calcium.

Driving and Hazardous Work: The use of calcitonin should not impair your ability to perform such tasks safely.

Alcohol: Avoid alcohol.

Pregnancy: In animal studies, large doses of calcitonin reduced birth weight. Before you take calcitonin, tell your doctor if you are pregnant or plan to become pregnant.

Breast Feeding: Calcitonin may pass into breast milk; caution is advised. Consult your doctor for specific advice.

Infants and Children: Studies of calcitonin use in infants and children have not been done. Consult your doctor for specific advice.

Special Concerns: You should not take calcitonin if you have a recently healed bone fracture.

OVERDOSE
Symptoms: No specific ones have been reported.

What to Do: An overdose of calcitonin is unlikely to be life-threatening. However, if someone takes a much larger dose than prescribed, call your doctor, emergency medical services (EMS), or the nearest poison control center.

DRUG INTERACTIONS
There are no known drug interactions.

FOOD INTERACTIONS
No known food interactions.

DISEASE INTERACTIONS
Caution is advised when taking calcitonin. Consult your doctor for specific advice if you have a kidney problem or a history of allergies.

Calcitriol

Rocaltrol 0.25 mcg
(ROCHE)

▶ Drug Class: Vitamin D analog

▶ Available in: Capsules, oral solution

▶ Available OTC? No

▶ As Generic? No

Side Effects

SERIOUS
Fatigue, headache, loss of appetite, metallic taste in mouth, nausea, vomiting, abdominal cramps, constipation or diarrhea, dizziness, drowsiness, dry mouth, ringing in ears, muscle pains, joint pains, irritability. Call your doctor immediately.

COMMON
No common side effects are associated with the use of calcitriol.

LESS COMMON
No less-common side effects are associated with calcitriol.

PRINCIPAL USES
To treat abnormally low blood levels of calcium (hypocalcemia) in those with chronic kidney failure who are undergoing dialysis or who have other conditions resulting in low blood calcium, such as hypoparathyroidism (underactive parathyroid gland).

HOW THE DRUG WORKS
Vitamin D must be modified by both the liver and kidneys before it is fully active. Calcitriol, a synthetic form of active vitamin D, promotes the absorption and utilization of calcium and phosphorus in the body. This ensures that blood levels of these minerals are high enough to support the constant turnover of bone and to supply cells with the calcium needed to perform essential functions.

DOSAGE
Frequent blood tests to measure levels of calcium and phosphorus are required when calcitriol is first taken to determine the proper dose. For hypocalcemia in dialysis patients: Adults and children age 6 and over start at 0.25 micrograms (mcg) once a day. Dose may be gradually increased every 4 to 8 weeks to no more than 1 mcg a day. Maintenance dose is usually 0.25 mcg every other day up to 1.25 mcg daily. Children ages 1 to 5: 0.25 to 2 mcg once a day. For hypoparathyroidism: Adults and children age 6 and over start at 0.25 mcg once a day. Dose may be gradually increased every 2 to 4 weeks to no more than 0.5 to 2 mcg a day. Children ages 1 to 5: 0.25 to 0.75 mcg per 2.2 lbs (1 kg) once a day.

ONSET OF EFFECT
2 to 6 hours.

DURATION OF ACTION
3 to 5 days.

DIETARY ADVICE
No special advice.

STORAGE
Store in a tightly sealed container away from heat, moisture, and direct light.

IF YOU MISS A DOSE
Take it as soon as you remember. If it is near the time for the next dose, skip the missed dose and resume your regular dosage schedule. Do not double the next dose.

STOPPING THE DRUG
The decision to stop taking the drug should be made by your doctor.

PROLONGED USE
See your doctor regularly for tests and examinations.

PRECAUTIONS
Over 60: Adverse reactions may be more likely and more severe in older patients.

Driving and Hazardous Work: Do not drive or engage in hazardous work until you determine how the medicine affects you.

Alcohol: Avoid excessive amounts of alcohol.

Pregnancy: No problems have been reported with the recommended daily dose. However, during pregnancy, calcitriol may cause problems in the unborn child when taken in excess of the recommended dosage, especially if the mother develops hypercalcemia (high blood levels of calcium). Before taking it, tell your doctor if you are pregnant or plan to become pregnant.

Breast Feeding: Calcitriol may pass into breast milk; extreme caution is advised. Some experts recommend that the mother not nurse while taking calcitriol. Consult your doctor.

Infants and Children: Calcitriol is not recommended for use by children under the age of 1. Consult your doctor.

OVERDOSE
Symptoms: Symptoms are due to the resulting hypercalcemia. Early symptoms: Constipation (especially in children), diarrhea, dry mouth, increased thirst and frequency of urination, persistent headache, loss of appetite, metallic taste, nausea and vomiting, unusual fatigue. Advanced symptoms: Bone and muscle pain, irregular heartbeat, persistent itching, extreme drowsiness, mental changes.

What to Do: Call your doctor if such symptoms occur. If someone accidentally ingests an extremely large dose, seek medical assistance right away.

DRUG INTERACTIONS
Consult your doctor for specific advice if you are taking antacids, cardiac glycosides, cholestyramine, colestipol, mineral oil, phenobarbital, phenytoin, primidone, thiazide diuretics, other forms of vitamin D, or calcium.

FOOD INTERACTIONS
No known food interactions.

DISEASE INTERACTIONS
Consult your doctor if you have blood vessel disease, heart disease, hypercalcemia, hypervitaminosis D, hypoparathyroidism, kidney disease, hyperphosphatemia, or sarcoidosis.

Calcium

Caltrate 600 600 mg
(LEDERLE)

Additional photographs

▶ Drug Class: Antihypocalcemic; dietary supplement; antacid

▶ Available in: Capsules, oral suspension, tablets, chewable tablets, liquid

▶ Available OTC? Yes

▶ As Generic? Yes

Side Effects

SERIOUS
Serious side effects are associated with excessively high doses (see Overdose).

COMMON
No common side effects with recommended doses of calcium.

LESS COMMON
Constipation, diarrhea, drowsiness, loss of appetite, dry mouth, and muscle weakness are some of the symptoms that could result if blood levels of calcium are too high (hypercalcemia).

PRINCIPAL USES
To ensure adequate calcium intake in those who do not get sufficient amounts by diet alone. Calcium is essential to many body functions, including the transmission of nerve impulses, the regulation of muscle contraction and relaxation (including of the heart), blood clotting, and various metabolic activities. Calcium is also necessary for maintaining strong bones and is commonly prescribed to prevent and treat postmenopausal osteoporosis (bone thinning). Vitamin D, which aids in the absorption of calcium from the intestine, is often prescribed along with calcium supplements to prevent or treat osteoporosis. (Indeed, some calcium supplement tablets contain vitamin D.) Calcium is also prescribed for individuals with persistently low blood calcium levels (hypocalcemia) caused, for example, by low levels of parathyroid hormone (hypoparathyroidism).

HOW THE DRUG WORKS
Calcium supplements compensate for inadequate dietary intake of this essential mineral. Forms of supplements available include calcium carbonate (the most common and inexpensive), calcium citrate (the best absorbed, but relatively expensive), calcium phosphate, calcium lactate, and calcium gluconate. Because calcium carbonate and phosphate supplements are difficult to absorb, other calcium products are preferable for individuals with low gastric (stomach) acid secretion.

DOSAGE
Optimal daily calcium intakes— Ages 0 to 6 months: 210 mg. Ages 6 months to 1 year: 270 mg. Ages 1 to 3 years: 500 mg. Ages 4 to 8 years: 800 mg. Ages 9 to 18 years: 1,300 mg. Ages 19 to 50 years: 1,000 mg. Age 51 and older: 1,200. For pregnant or breast-feeding women, under 19 years: 1,300 mg; ages 19 to 50 years: 1,000 mg. Be sure to include dietary calcium as well as the supplements in your total daily intake. It is important to realize that calcium itself constitutes only a fraction of any calciumcontaining pill. For example, calcium accounts for only 40% of the weight of a calcium carbonate tablet. Thus, a 500 mg tablet of calcium carbonate provides only 200 mg of calcium.

ONSET OF EFFECT
Unknown.

DURATION OF ACTION
For as long as the supplement is taken.

DIETARY ADVICE
Calcium carbonate and calcium phosphate supplements are best absorbed if taken 60 to 90 minutes after meals. Take with 1 full glass (8 oz) of water or juice. Follow all special dietary guidelines as recommended by your doctor.

STORAGE
Store in a tightly sealed container away from heat, moisture, and direct light.

IF YOU MISS A DOSE
If you are taking calcium supplements on a regular basis and miss a dose, take it as soon as you remember, then resume your regular dosage schedule.

STOPPING THE DRUG
The decision to stop taking calcium supplements should be made in consultation with your doctor.

PROLONGED USE
Adverse effects are more likely to occur if supplements are taken in doses greater than 2,000 to 2,500 mg a day for a long period of time. Your doctor should regularly check your blood calcium levels if you are taking calcium supplements to treat low blood calcium (hypocalcemia).

PRECAUTIONS
Over 60: No special problems are expected.

Driving and Hazardous Work: Calcium supplements should have no effect on your ability to perform such tasks safely.

Alcohol: To ensure proper absorption of calcium, consume alcohol in moderation only (no more than 2 drinks per day).

Pregnancy: It is crucial to receive enough calcium during pregnancy and to maintain those levels throughout pregnancy, preferably through diet alone. However, excessive calcium intake during pregnancy may be harmful to the mother or fetus and should be avoided.

Breast Feeding: Excessive amounts of this supplement taken while nursing may be harmful to the mother or infant and should be avoided.

Infants and Children: No special problems expected.

OVERDOSE
Symptoms: Early symptoms: Constipation (especially in children), diarrhea, dry mouth, increased thirst and frequency of urination, persistent headache, loss of appetite, metallic taste, nausea and vomiting, unusual

Calcium (continued)

fatigue. Advanced symptoms: Bone and muscle pain, irregular heartbeat, persistent itching, extreme drowsiness, mental changes. Severe calcium toxicity may be fatal.

What to Do: Call your doctor, emergency medical services (EMS), or the nearest poison control center immediately.

DRUG INTERACTIONS

Consult your doctor for specific advice if you are taking other calcium-containing preparations, cellulose sodium phosphate, digitalis drugs, etidronate, gallium nitrate, phenytoin, or tetracycline antibiotics. Combined use of calcium supplements with thiazide diuretics or vitamin D may lead to excessively high calcium levels.

FOOD INTERACTIONS

Excessive protein consumption can increase the excretion of calcium in the urine. In meals preceding calcium consumption, avoid spinach and rhubarb (high in oxalic acid), and bran andwhole cereals (high in phytic acid), since these substances may interfere with calcium absorption.

DISEASE INTERACTIONS

Consult your doctor if you have frequent episodes of diarrhea, any stomach or intestinal problems, heart disease, sarcoidosis, kidney disease, or kidney stones.

Candesartan Cilexetil

BRAND NAME
Atacand

▶ Drug Class: Antihypertensive/ angiotensin II antagonist

▶ Available in: Tablets

▶ Available OTC? No

▶ As Generic? No

Side Effects

SERIOUS
No serious side effects are associated with the use of candesartan. (In clinical trials, the incidence of adverse effects was not significantly greater with the medication than with a placebo.)

COMMON
No common side effects are associated with the use of candesartan.

LESS COMMON
Headache, dizziness, back pain, upper respiratory tract infection, sore throat, and nasal congestion.

PRINCIPAL USES
To control high blood pressure. This drug appears to have the same benefits as the class of antihypertensive drugs known as ACE inhibitors, without producing the common side effect (experienced by as many as 30% of patients) of a dry cough. Candesartan may be used by itself or in conjunction with other antihypertensive medications.

HOW THE DRUG WORKS
Candesartan blocks the effects of angiotensin II, a naturally occurring substance that causes blood vessels to narrow. Candesartan causes the blood vessels to dilate, thereby lowering blood pressure and decreasing the workload of the heart.

DOSAGE
To start, 16 mg once a day when used as the only drug to treat hypertension. Usual maintenance dose is 8 to 32 mg daily, taken once a day or divided into 2 doses.

ONSET OF EFFECT
Within 2 weeks.

DURATION OF ACTION
Up to 24 hours.

DIETARY ADVICE
No special restrictions, unless your doctor has advised a low-sodium diet or other dietary modifications to help you control your blood pressure.

STORAGE
Store in a tightly sealed container away from heat, moisture, and direct light.

IF YOU MISS A DOSE
Take it as soon as you remember. If it is near the time for the next dose, skip the missed dose and resume your regular dosage schedule. Do not double the next dose.

STOPPING THE DRUG
Take it as prescribed for the full treatment period. The decision to stop taking the drug should be made in consultation with your physician.

PROLONGED USE
Lifelong therapy may be necessary. However, if you do change certain health habits (for example, increasing exercise or losing weight), a reduced dose may be possible under a doctor's supervision.

PRECAUTIONS
Over 60: No special problems are expected.

Driving and Hazardous Work: Do not drive or engage in hazardous work until you determine how the medicine affects you.

Alcohol: No special precautions are necessary.

Pregnancy: Candesartan should not be used by pregnant women. Discontinue taking the drug as soon as possible when pregnancy is detected and discuss treatment alternatives with your doctor.

Breast Feeding: Candesartan may pass into breast milk; caution is advised. Consult your doctor for advice.

Infants and Children: The safety and effectiveness of use in children have not been established.

Special Concerns: Candesartan may cause excessively low blood pressure with dizziness or lightheadedness, which is most noticeable when you change position. This may lead to fainting, falls, and injury. Sit or lie down immediately if you feel dizzy or lightheaded. This side effect may be worsened by alcohol, hot weather, dehydration, salt depletion from diuretic use, fever, prolonged standing, prolonged sitting, or exercise.

OVERDOSE
Symptoms: Few cases of overdose have been reported. However, if you take a much larger dose than prescribed, you may experience fainting, dizziness, weak pulse that might be very slow or very fast.

What to Do: Call your doctor, emergency medical services (EMS), or the nearest poison control center immediately.

DRUG INTERACTIONS
No drug interactions have yet been observed with candesartan. Consult your doctor for specific advice if you are taking any other medication, especially other drugs for high blood pressure. Candesartan can be taken together with diuretics or other medications for high blood pressure, if your doctor approves.

FOOD INTERACTIONS
No known food interactions.

DISEASE INTERACTIONS
Patients with moderate to severe liver or kidney disease are advised to exercise caution when taking candesartan.

Capecitabine

BRAND NAME
Xeloda

▶ Drug Class: Antineoplastic (anticancer) agent

▶ Available in: Tablets

▶ Available OTC? No

▶ As Generic? No

Side Effects

SERIOUS
Fever greater than 100.5°F; severe diarrhea, nausea, and vomiting; loss of or decreased appetite; pain, redness, swelling and sores in the mouth and throat; pain, numbness, tingling, swelling, and redness of the palms of the hands or soles of the feet (hand-and-foot syndrome). Stop taking the drug and call your oncologist immediately.

COMMON
Abdominal pain, constipation, dehydration, rash, dry or itchy skin, weakness, headache, drowsiness, dizziness, mild fever.

LESS COMMON
Numerous less common side effects can occur; consult your doctor if you are concerned about any adverse or unusual reactions you experience while taking this drug.

PRINCIPAL USES
To treat advanced (metastatic) breast cancer. Capecitabine is used for secondary treatment when other therapies have not produced adequate results. Your oncologist will determine if capecitabine is appropriate for your condition.

HOW THE DRUG WORKS
By interfering with essential phases of cell division in cancer cells, capecitabine prevents them from multiplying. The drug may cause side effects by affecting other kinds of cells in the body.

DOSAGE
2,500 mg per square meter of body surface in 2 divided doses (12 hours apart) a day. Capecitabine is taken in 3-week cycles: 2 weeks on and 1 week off. Your oncologist will determine the proper dosage and how many cycles of treatment are needed.

ONSET OF EFFECT
Unknown.

DURATION OF ACTION
Unknown.

DIETARY ADVICE
Take with water within 30 minutes after the end of a meal (breakfast and dinner).

STORAGE
Store at room temperature in a tightly sealed container away from heat, moisture, and direct light.

IF YOU MISS A DOSE
It is imperative to try not to miss a dose of capecitabine. If you do miss a dose, skip the missed dose and resume your regular dosage schedule. Do not double the next dose. If you miss more than one dose, contact your oncologist.

STOPPING THE DRUG
Take it as prescribed for the full treatment period. The decision to stop taking the drug should be made by your oncologist.

PROLONGED USE
See your oncologist regularly if you must take this drug for a prolonged period.

PRECAUTIONS
Over 60: Severe gastrointestinal side effects may be more likely and more severe in patients 80 years of age and older.

Driving and Hazardous Work: Do not drive or engage in hazardous work until you determine how the medicine affects you.

Alcohol: No special precautions are necessary.

Pregnancy: Avoid becoming pregnant while taking this drug. Tell your doctor at once if you become pregnant while taking capecitabine.

Breast Feeding: Capecitabine may pass into breast milk; avoid nursing while taking this drug.

Infants and Children: The safety and effectiveness of the use of capecitabine in children under the age of 18 have not been determined.

Special Concerns: Take the medication in the combination prescribed by your oncologist for the morning and evening doses.

OVERDOSE
Symptoms: Nausea, vomiting, diarrhea, stomach irritation and bleeding, fatigue, and paleness.

What to Do: Call your oncologist, emergency medical services (EMS), or the nearest poison control center immediately.

DRUG INTERACTIONS
Do not take leucovorin or fluorouracil if you are taking capecitabine. Consult your oncologist for advice if you are taking folic acid or anticoagulants (such as warfarin).

FOOD INTERACTIONS
No known food interactions.

DISEASE INTERACTIONS
Patients with severe kidney impairment should not take capecitabine. Consult your oncologist if you have a history of heart disease. Patients with liver or kidney disease should be carefully monitored by their doctor while taking capecitabine.

Capsaicin

BRAND NAMES
Axsain, Zostrix

▶ Drug Class: Analgesic

▶ Available in: Cream

▶ Available OTC? Yes

▶ As Generic? Yes

Side Effects

SERIOUS
No serious side effects are associated with the use of capsaicin.

COMMON
Stinging or burning sensation when cream is applied. This should subside with regular use, as your body adjusts to the medication.

LESS COMMON
Skin redness; coughing, sneezing, or shortness of breath if dried residues of the drug are inhaled.

PRINCIPAL USES
To relieve neuralgia—pain in the nerve endings near the surface of the skin. Capsaicin is commonly prescribed for neuralgia associated with shingles, an acutely painful condition caused by infection with the varicella zoster virus, the same organism that causes chicken pox. Capsaicin is also used to relieve mild to moderate arthritis, diabetic neuropathy (pain caused by nerve cell damage that occurs as a complication of diabetes), and postoperative pain.

HOW THE DRUG WORKS
When applied topically, capsaicin (a derivative of hot peppers) appears to reduce the amount of a natural chemical known as substance P, which is present in painful joints. Substance P is believed to be involved in two processes central to arthritis: the release of enzymes that produce inflammation and the transmission of pain impulses from the joints to the central nervous system. By blocking the production and release of substance P, capsaicin can reduce the pain associated with arthritis as well as dampen the transmission of pain messages to the brain.

DOSAGE
Apply a small amount to the affected area up to 4 times a day. Do not apply to broken or irritated skin. If the use of a bandage is recommended, do not apply it too tightly.

ONSET OF EFFECT
Therapeutic pain response is usually achieved in 1 to 2 weeks but may take as long as 4 weeks.

DURATION OF ACTION
Up to 6 hours.

DIETARY ADVICE
This medication can be used without regard to diet.

STORAGE
Store in a tightly sealed container away from heat and direct light.

IF YOU MISS A DOSE
Apply it as soon as you remember. If it is near the time for the next dose, skip the missed dose and resume your regular dosage schedule. Do not double the next dose.

STOPPING THE DRUG
Pain relief will last only as long as capsaicin is used regularly. If you discontinue using the medication and the pain returns, it is safe to resume treatment.

PROLONGED USE
No special problems are expected. Burning and stinging sensations upon application frequently subside with prolonged use. If your condition worsens or does not improve after 1 month, discontinue using capsaicin and consult your doctor.

PRECAUTIONS
Over 60: No special problems are expected.

Driving and Hazardous Work: No problems are expected.

Alcohol: No special precautions are necessary.

Pregnancy: No problems have been reported.

Breast Feeding: No problems are expected.

Infants and Children: Not recommended for use on children under the age of 2. No problems are expected in older children.

Special Concerns: You may not be able to use capsaicin if you are allergic to it or if you have ever had an allergic reaction to hot peppers. Wash your hands thoroughly after applying the cream; if you are using it for arthritis of the hands, wait 30 minutes before washing. It can cause a burning sensation if even small amounts get into the eyes or on other sensitive areas of the body. If you wear contact lenses, be especially cautious. If it does get into your eyes, flush them with water. On other sensitive areas of the body, wash the area with warm (but not hot) soapy water. After applying capsaicin cream, avoid contact with children and pets until you have thoroughly washed your hands.

OVERDOSE
Symptoms: No cases of overdose have been reported.

What to Do: An overdose is unlikely to be life-threatening. However, if someone applies a much larger dose than prescribed, suffers adverse side effects, or accidentally ingests it, call your doctor or the nearest poison control center for advice.

DRUG INTERACTIONS
Capsaicin may alter the action of some drugs or trigger unwanted side effects. Consult your doctor about any other drugs that you take, including over-the-counter medications.

FOOD INTERACTIONS
None are known.

DISEASE INTERACTIONS
Consult your doctor if you have broken or irritated skin, or conditions that may result in broken skin, on the area to be treated.

Captopril

BRAND NAME
Capoten

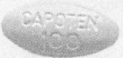

Capoten 100 mg
(BRISTOL-MYERS SQUIBB)

Additional photographs

▶ Drug Class: Angiotensin-converting enzyme (ACE) inhibitor

▶ Available in: Tablets

▶ Available OTC? No

▶ As Generic? Yes

Side Effects

SERIOUS
Fever and chills, sore throat and hoarseness, sudden difficulty breathing or swallowing, swelling of the face, mouth, or extremities, impaired kidney function (ankle swelling, decreased urination), confusion, yellow discoloration of the eyes or skin (indicating liver disorder), intense itching, chest pain or palpitations, abdominal pain. Serious side effects are very rare; contact your doctor immediately.

COMMON
Dry, persistent cough.

LESS COMMON
Dizziness or fainting, skin rash, numbness or tingling in the hands, feet, or lips, unusual fatigue or muscle weakness, nausea, drowsiness, loss of taste, headache.

PRINCIPAL USES
To control high blood pressure; to treat congestive heart failure (CHF); to treat patients with left ventricular dysfunction (damage to the pumping chamber of the heart); and to minimize further kidney damage in diabetics with mild kidney disease.

HOW THE DRUG WORKS
Angiotensin-converting enzyme (ACE) inhibitors block an enzyme that produces angiotensin, a naturally occurring substance that causes blood vessels to constrict and stimulates production of the adrenal hormone, aldosterone, which promotes sodium retention in the body. As a result, ACE inhibitors relax blood vessels (causing them to widen) and reduces sodium retention, which lowers blood pressure and so decreases the workload of the heart.

DOSAGE
Adults— For high blood pressure: 12.5 to 150 mg, 2 or 3 times a day. For CHF: 6.25 to 100 mg, 2 or 3 times a day. For left ventricular dysfunction: 6.25 to 50 mg, 3 times a day. For kidney problems associated with diabetes: 25 mg, 3 times a day. Children— Consult your pediatrician.

ONSET OF EFFECT
15 to 60 minutes.

DURATION OF ACTION
6 to 12 hours.

DIETARY ADVICE
Take it on an empty stomach, about 1 hour before mealtime. Follow your doctor's dietary advice (such as low-salt or low-cholesterol restrictions) to improve control over high blood pressure and heart disease. Avoid high-potassium foods like bananas and citrus fruits and juices, unless you are also taking medications, such as diuretics, that lower potassium levels.

STORAGE
Store in a tightly sealed container away from heat and direct light.

IF YOU MISS A DOSE
Take it as soon as you remember. If it is near the time for the next dose, skip the missed dose and resume your regular dosage schedule. Do not double the next dose.

STOPPING THE DRUG
Do not stop taking this drug abruptly, as this may cause potentially serious health problems. Dosage should be reduced gradually, according to your doctor's instructions.

PROLONGED USE
See your doctor regularly for examinations and tests if you must take this medicine for a prolonged period. Remember that captopril helps control high blood pressure but does not cure it. Lifelong therapy may be necessary.

PRECAUTIONS
Over 60: Adverse reactions may be more likely and more severe.

Driving and Hazardous Work: Avoid such activities until you determine how the medication affects you.

Alcohol: Consume alcohol only in moderation since it may increase the effect of the drug and cause an excessive drop in blood pressure.

Pregnancy: Captopril should not be used during the final 6 months of pregnancy. Notify your doctor right away if you become pregnant.

Breast Feeding: If possible, avoid using captopril while nursing.

Infants and Children: Captopril is only prescribed for children when other means of controlling hypertension fail; benefits must be weighed against risks. Consult your pediatrician for advice.

OVERDOSE
Symptoms: Dizziness or fainting; weak, rapid pulse; nausea, vomiting; chest pain.

What to Do: Call your doctor, emergency medical services (EMS), or the nearest poison control center immediately.

DRUG INTERACTIONS
Consult your doctor if you are taking diuretics (especially potassium-sparing diuretics), potassium supplements or drugs containing potassium (check ingredient labels), lithium, anticoagulants (such as warfarin), indomethacin or other anti-inflammatory drugs, or any over-the-counter drugs (especially cold remedies and diet pills).

FOOD INTERACTIONS
Avoid low-salt milk and salt substitutes. Many of these products contain potassium.

DISEASE INTERACTIONS
Consult your doctor if you have systemic lupus erythematosus or if you have had a prior allergic reaction to ACE inhibitors. This medication should be used with caution by patients with severe kidney disease or renal artery stenosis (narrowing of one or both of the arteries that supply blood to the kidneys).

Carbamazepine

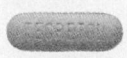

Tegretol 200 mg
(BASEL)

Additional photographs

▶ Drug Class: Anticonvulsant/
analgesic

▶ Available in: Oral suspension,
tablets, extended-release
tablets and capsules

▶ Available OTC? No

▶ As Generic? Yes

Side Effects

SERIOUS
Fever, sore throat,
swollen glands, point-like
rash, blistering or peel-
ing, easy bruising, pallor,
weakness, confusion,
lethargy, or seizures may
be a sign of a potentially
fatal blood reaction
(aplastic anemia). Call
your doctor at once.

COMMON
Drowsiness, rash, itching,
increased sensitivity of
the skin to sunlight, dizziness, blurred vision, incoordination, nausea,
vomiting, stomach pain
or upset, diarrhea, constipation, loss of appetite,
dry or inflamed mouth.

LESS COMMON
Impaired speech, involun-
tary movements of the
face, limbs, or tongue,
tingling or numbness in
the extremities, depres-
sion, agitation, psychosis,
talkativeness, abnormal
eye movements, ringing
in the ears, heart rhythm
abnormalities, impotence,
hair loss, or excessive
hair growth. There are
numerous additional
potential side effects.

PRINCIPAL USES
To control certain types of
seizures due to epilepsy.
Also to treat facial pain in
those with trigeminal neuralgia (tic douloureux).

HOW THE DRUG WORKS
Carbamazepine appears to
inhibit neurons from firing
repeatedly and uncontrol-
lably (which causes
seizures).

DOSAGE
Adults: 600 to 2,000 mg a
day, in 3 or 4 divided doses.
Children: 9 to 18 mg per lb
of body weight, in 3 or 4
divided doses. Some
patients require higher
doses. A low dose should be
used initially, then gradually
increased if needed. The
extended-release forms may
be given twice a day.

ONSET OF EFFECT
Several hours or longer.

DURATION OF ACTION
Maximum effectiveness: 12
hours or longer; effectiveness then gradually
decreases.

DIETARY ADVICE
Take with food to lessen the
chance of stomach upset.

STORAGE
Store in a tightly sealed container away from heat, moisture, and direct light.

IF YOU MISS A DOSE
Take it as soon as you
remember. If it is near the
time for the next dose, skip
the missed dose and
resume your regular dosage
schedule. Do not double the
next dose, unless advised to
do so by your doctor. Call
your doctor if you miss
more than a full day's worth
of doses.

STOPPING THE DRUG
Never stop this drug
abruptly; seizures may

occur. Your doctor will taper
the dose over many weeks.

PROLONGED USE
Therapy may last several
years or longer. Some side
effects may diminish after a
few weeks of therapy.

PRECAUTIONS
Over 60: Older patients
may require lower doses to
minimize side effects.

**Driving and Hazardous
Work:** Avoid such tasks
until you determine how the
medication affects you.

Alcohol: May contribute to
excessive drowsiness.

Pregnancy: This drug
increases the risk of birth
defects. However, seizures
during pregnancy also
increase the risks to the
fetus. Discuss potential
risks and benefits with your
doctor. Folate supplementation is advised starting 1 to
2 months before conception
and continuing throughout
pregnancy. Vitamin K1 may
be needed during the last 4
weeks of pregnancy.

Breast Feeding: This
drug passes into breast
milk, although at low levels.
Consult your doctor for
specific advice.

Infants and Children:
Behavioral side effects are
more likely to be seen in
children.

Special Concerns: The
generic form is not recommended. Do not change the
brand you are taking without consulting your doctor.
Your doctor may suggest
you carry an ID card or
bracelet saying that you
take this drug.

OVERDOSE
Symptoms: Confusion,
double vision, seizures,

extreme drowsiness, loss of
consciousness, poor muscle
control, spasms, tremors,
walking difficulty, abnormal
heartbeat, slow or irregular
breathing.

What to Do: Seek medical
assistance immediately.

DRUG INTERACTIONS
Carbamazepine may interact
with many drugs, including
other anticonvulsants (clonazepam, ethosuximide,
primidone, valproic acid,
phenytoin, and phenobarbital), anticoagulants, certain
anti-infectives (erythro-
mycin, doxycycline, troleandomycin, isoniazid), oral
contraceptives, cimetidine,
corticosteroids, danazol,
diltiazem, lithium, nicotinamide, propoxyphene,
theophylline, thyroid hormones, verapamil.

FOOD INTERACTIONS
No known food interactions.

DISEASE INTERACTIONS
Special caution is advised in
those with lupus; heart, kidney, or liver disease; diabetes; or glaucoma.

Carbenicillin Indanyl Sodium

BRAND NAMES
Geocillin, Geopen

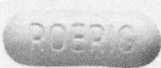

Geocillin 382 mg
(ROERIG)

▶ Drug Class: Penicillin antibiotic

▶ Available in: Tablets, injection

▶ Available OTC? No

▶ As Generic? Yes

Side Effects

SERIOUS
Irregular, rapid, or labored breathing, light-headedness or sudden fainting, joint pain, fever, severe abdominal pain and cramping with watery or bloody stools, severe allergic reaction (marked by sudden swelling of the lips, tongue, face, or throat; breathing difficulty; skin rash, itching, or hives), unusual bleeding or bruising, yellowish tinge to eyes or skin. Call your doctor immediately.

COMMON
Mild rash, mild diarrhea, nausea, vomiting, headache, vaginal discharge and itching, pain or white patches in the mouth or on the tongue.

LESS COMMON
Diminished urine output, chills, weakness, fatigue.

PRINCIPAL USES
To treat bacterial infections, especially those of the prostate and urinary tract. Carbenicillin is effective only against infections caused by bacteria; it is ineffective against those caused by viruses, fungi, or other microorganisms.

HOW THE DRUG WORKS
Carbenicillin blocks the formation of bacterial cell walls, rendering bacteria unable to multiply and spread.

DOSAGE
Tablets— Adults and teenagers: 382 to 764 mg every 6 hours. Children: Consult your pediatrician. Injection— The dose is determined by your doctor based on patient's body weight and other variables.

ONSET OF EFFECT
Unknown.

DURATION OF ACTION
Unknown.

DIETARY ADVICE
Carbenicillin should be taken on an empty stomach, at least 1 hour before or 2 hours after meals, with plenty of water. Patients with high blood pressure who follow a sodium-restricted diet should be aware that carbenicillin tablets contain a significant amount of salt.

STORAGE
Store in a tightly sealed container away from heat and direct light.

IF YOU MISS A DOSE
Take it as soon as you remember. If it is within 2 hours of the next dose, skip the missed dose and resume your regular dosage schedule. Do not double the next dose.

STOPPING THE DRUG
Take it as prescribed for the full treatment period, even if you begin to feel better before the scheduled end of therapy. Stopping the drug prematurely may slow your recovery or lead to a rebound infection, also known as superinfection, in which the heartier strains of bacteria survive and multiply, leading to a more serious and drug-resistant infection.

PROLONGED USE
Prolonged use of any antibiotic increases the risk of superinfection; caution is advised.

PRECAUTIONS
Over 60: No special problems are expected.

Driving and Hazardous Work: Do not drive or engage in hazardous work until you determine how the medicine affects you.

Alcohol: No special precautions are necessary.

Pregnancy: Adequate studies of the use of penicillin antibiotics during pregnancy have not been done; however, no problems have been reported.

Breast Feeding: Carbenicillin may pass into breast milk and cause problems in the nursing infant; avoid use while nursing.

Infants and Children: No special problems are expected.

Special Concerns: Carbenicillin can cause false results on some urine sugar tests for patients with diabetes. Those who are prone to asthma, hay fever, hives, or allergies may be more likely to have an allergic reaction to a penicillin antibiotic. If severe diarrhea occurs as a side effect of this drug, do not take antidiarrheal medications; call your doctor.

OVERDOSE
Symptoms: Seizures may occur with very high doses; overdose is nonetheless unlikely.

What to Do: If you have reason to suspect an overdose, seek medical assistance immediately.

DRUG INTERACTIONS
Consult your doctor for specific advice if you are taking aminoglycosides, ACE inhibitors, diuretics, potassium supplements or potassium-containing medications, anticoagulants or other anticlotting drugs, nonsteroidal anti-inflammatory drugs, sulfinpyrazone, cholestyramine, colestipol, oral contraceptives, methotrexate, or probenecid.

FOOD INTERACTIONS
No known food interactions.

DISEASE INTERACTIONS
Consult your doctor if you have a history of allergies, asthma, bleeding disorders (such as hemophilia), congestive heart failure, gastrointestinal disorders (especially colitis associated with the use of antibiotics), high blood pressure, or impaired kidney function.

Carisoprodol

BRAND NAMES
Rela, Soma, Vanadom

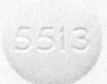

Generic 350 mg
(SCHEIN/DANBURY)

▶ Drug Class: Muscle relaxant

▶ Available in: Tablets

▶ Available OTC? No

▶ As Generic? Yes

Side Effects

SERIOUS
Fainting; palpitations or rapid heartbeat; fever; hives or severe swelling of face, lips, or tongue along with shortness of breath, chest tightness, or wheezing (indicating a potentially life-threatening allergic reaction); depression. Seek medical help immediately.

COMMON
Drowsiness, dizziness, dry mouth.

LESS COMMON
Inability to pass urine; sores on lips, ulcers in mouth; abdominal cramps or pain; clumsiness; unsteady gait; confusion; constipation; diarrhea; excitability, nervousness, restlessness, or irritability; flushing or redness of face; headache; heartburn; hiccups; muscle weakness; nausea and vomiting; trembling; insomnia or fitful sleep; burning, red eyes; stuffy nose.

PRINCIPAL USES
Skeletal muscle relaxants are used to relieve stiffness and discomfort caused by severe sprains and strains, muscle spasms, or other muscle problems. They may be prescribed in conjunction with other treatment methods, such as physical therapy.

HOW THE DRUG WORKS
Muscle relaxants such as carisoprodol depress activity in the central nervous system, which in turn interferes with the transmission of nerve impulses from the spinal cord to the muscles.

DOSAGE
Adults and teenagers: 350 mg, 3 to 4 times a day. Children ages 5 to 12: 6.25 mg per 2.2 lbs (1 kg) of body weight 4 times a day.

ONSET OF EFFECT
30 minutes.

DURATION OF ACTION
4 to 6 hours.

DIETARY ADVICE
Be sure to eat a well-balanced diet; the healing of injured tissue increases the body's protein and calorie requirements. To avoid dry mouth, maintain adequate fluid intake and suck on ice chips.

STORAGE
Store in a tightly sealed container in a dry place away from heat and direct light.

IF YOU MISS A DOSE
Take it as soon as you remember. If it is within 2 hours of the next dose, skip the missed dose and resume your regular dosage schedule. Do not double the next dose.

STOPPING THE DRUG
This medication should be taken as prescribed for the full treatment period. Do not stop taking carisoprodol abruptly.

PROLONGED USE
Therapy with carisoprodol ranges from several days to weeks. Prolonged use may be associated with an increased risk of side effects.

PRECAUTIONS
Over 60: Adverse reactions to medications such as carisoprodol may be more likely and more severe in older patients.

Driving and Hazardous Work: Carisoprodol may impair your ability to drive or perform hazardous work.

Alcohol: Avoid alcohol while taking this medication because it may compound the sedative effect and may cause liver damage.

Pregnancy: Adequate studies of carisoprodol during pregnancy have not been done; discuss the relative risks and benefits with your doctor.

Breast Feeding: Breast feeding is not recommended during therapy.

Infants and Children: No special problems have been documented; consult your pediatrician for advice.

Special Concerns: Carisoprodol will intensify the effect that alcohol, sedatives, and other central nervous system depressants have on the brain. It is not a substitute for other safe, nonmedical therapies for muscle stiffness, including rest, gentle guided exercise, and physical therapy.

OVERDOSE
Symptoms: Excessive drowsiness or difficulty awakening, even when being shaken or pinched; confusion; weakness; slowed breathing; coma.

What to Do: Call emergency medical services (EMS) or the nearest poison control center immediately.

DRUG INTERACTIONS
Consult your doctor for specific advice if you are taking antihistamines and decongestants, antidepressants, sedatives, tranquilizers, sleep aids, pain medication, barbiturates, or seizure medication.

FOOD INTERACTIONS
No known food interactions.

DISEASE INTERACTIONS
Caution is advised when taking carisoprodol. Consult your doctor if you have a history of any of the following: allergies, drug abuse or dependence, kidney disease, liver disease, porphyria, epilepsy, or any other seizure disorder.

Carmustine

▶ Drug Class: Alkylating agent

▶ Available in: Injection

▶ Available OTC? No

▶ As Generic? Yes

Side Effects

SERIOUS
Black or tarry stools; blood-tinged (pink or maroon) urine or stools; cough or shortness of breath; fever and chills; lower back pain or pain in flanks; painful, difficult urination; small, red spots on the skin; bleeding from gums, nose, or other unusual places; easy bruising. These side effects may mean that normal blood cells and special blood-clotting cells have been affected, or that normal immune cells have been affected and an infection is developing somewhere in your body. See your doctor right away if any of these symptoms occur.

COMMON
Nausea and vomiting, weakness, fatigue, loss of appetite, pain or redness at injection site (tell your nurse immediately if this happens while the drug is being administered).

LESS COMMON
Decreased urination, edema (swelling) of the feet and ankles, diarrhea, dizziness, skin discoloration at injection site, skin rash or itching, difficulty swallowing, difficulty walking, hair loss.

PRINCIPAL USES
To treat brain, liver, and gastrointestinal cancers, in addition to lymphomas (cancers of the lymphatic system).

HOW THE DRUG WORKS
Carmustine interferes with the growth of cancer cells by preventing them from reproducing. The drug may also affect the growth and development of normal cells in the body, resulting in unpleasant side effects.

DOSAGE
Adults and children: The dose of carmustine depends on the type of tumor, the patient's body weight, and whether other chemotherapy drugs are being used. Your oncologist (cancer specialist) will determine the proper dose.

ONSET OF EFFECT
Almost immediately following injection.

DURATION OF ACTION
Unknown.

DIETARY ADVICE
Maintain optimal food and fluid intake. Calorie, protein, and vitamin needs increase in patients with cancer. Good nutrition is essential to cope with the demands of chemotherapy.

STORAGE
Refrigerate.

IF YOU MISS A DOSE
Inform your oncologist as soon as possible.

STOPPING THE DRUG
The decision to stop administering carmustine must be made by your doctor.

PROLONGED USE
Use beyond 1 to 2 days is not recommended.

PRECAUTIONS

Over 60: Adverse reactions may be more likely and more severe.

Driving and Hazardous Work: The use of this medication may impair your ability to drive or operate machinery safely, or perform hazardous work.

Alcohol: Avoid alcohol.

Pregnancy: Carmustine may cause birth defects. Persons of childbearing years should take steps to prevent pregnancy during therapy.

Breast Feeding: Not recommended during therapy.

Infants and Children: Consult your pediatrician.

Special Concerns: Patients with cancer are very often weakened by their illness, by poor nutrition, and by the effects of chemotherapy, radiation, and surgery. These patients are more likely to experience undesirable side effects of a medication. In addition, these side effects may be more pronounced. Follow directions very carefully for all medication that you are taking. Read and understand all potential side effects and drug interactions. Infection is the single greatest threat to people receiving chemotherapy. Carmustine may lower your ability to resist infection by lowering the number of white blood cells in the blood. Therefore, do not receive any vaccinations without your doctor's approval. Avoid people with infections. Inform your doctor immediately if you have fever, chills, diarrhea, or a cough. Shortness of breath may develop many years after initial treatment in chil-dren or adolescents who receive higher doses.

OVERDOSE
Symptoms: No cases of overdose have been reported.

What to Do: Although not likely to occur, if you are concerned about the possibility of an overdose of carmustine, contact your doctor.

DRUG INTERACTIONS
Consult your doctor for specific advice if you are taking amphotericin B, thyroid medications, azathioprine, chloramphenicol, colchicine, flucytosine, ganciclovir, interferon, plicamycin, or zidovudine (AZT).

FOOD INTERACTIONS
None are known.

DISEASE INTERACTIONS
Consult your doctor if you have any of the following: chicken pox (or recent exposure to someone with it), shingles, an infection, kidney disease, liver disease, or lung disease.

Carteolol Hydrochloride Ophthalmic

BRAND NAME
Ocupress

▶ Drug Class: Antiglaucoma drug; ophthalmic beta-blocker

▶ Available in: Ophthalmic solution

▶ Available OTC? No

▶ As Generic? No

Side Effects

SERIOUS
Palpitations, breathing difficulty, dizziness and weakness caused by low blood pressure. Call your doctor right away.

COMMON
Temporary eye irritation, tearing, eye inflammation, burning, swelling.

LESS COMMON
Blurred vision, poor night vision, and increased sensitivity to light; headache; insomnia; sinus irritation; odd or bitter taste in the mouth.

PRINCIPAL USES
To treat glaucoma.

HOW THE DRUG WORKS
Glaucoma, a sight-threatening disorder, occurs when aqueous humor (the fluid inside the eye) cannot drain properly, causing an increase in pressure within the eyeball (known as intraocular pressure). Increased intraocular pressure can damage the optic nerve and lead to a gradually progressive loss of vision. Carteolol decreases the production of aqueous humor, thereby reducing intraocular pressure.

DOSAGE
1 drop inside the lower eyelid twice a day.

ONSET OF EFFECT
30 to 60 minutes.

DURATION OF ACTION
From 6 to 8 hours.

DIETARY ADVICE
Can be applied without regard to dietary habits or schedule.

STORAGE
Store in a tightly sealed container away from heat, moisture, and direct light.

IF YOU MISS A DOSE
Apply it as soon as you remember. If it is near the time for the next dose, skip the missed dose and resume your regular dosage schedule. Do not double the next dose.

STOPPING THE DRUG
The decision to stop using the drug should be made by your doctor.

PROLONGED USE
Eye examinations should be done regularly as part of glaucoma follow-up.

PRECAUTIONS
Over 60: Adverse reactions may be more likely and more severe in older patients.

Driving and Hazardous Work: Do not drive or engage in hazardous work until you determine how the medicine affects your vision.

Alcohol: Use with caution.

Pregnancy: Adequate human studies have not been completed. Before taking ophthalmic carteolol, tell your doctor if you are pregnant or plan to become pregnant.

Breast Feeding: Ophthalmic carteolol may pass into breast milk; caution is advised. Consult your doctor for advice.

Infants and Children: Adverse reactions may be more likely and more severe in children.

Special Concerns: To use the eye drops, first wash your hands. Tilt your head back. Gently apply pressure to the inside corner of the eyelid and with the index finger of the same hand, pull downward on the lower eyelid to make a space. Drop the medicine into this space and close your eye. Apply pressure for 1 or 2 minutes while keeping the eye closed without blinking. Then wash your hands again. Make sure the tip of the dropper does not touch your eye, finger, or any other surface. Carteolol may make your eyes more sensitive to sunlight. If this occurs, wear sunglasses or avoid bright light as comfort dictates. Before you have any kind of surgery, emergency treatment, or dental treatment, tell the doctor or dentist that you are taking ophthalmic carteolol.

OVERDOSE
Symptoms: Nervousness, chest pain, confusion, hallucinations, coughing, wheezing, drowsiness, dizziness, irregular or pounding heartbeat, insomnia, fatigue.

What to Do: If a large volume of the drug enters the eyes, flush with water. If the medication is accidentally ingested, seek medical assistance right away.

DRUG INTERACTIONS
It is not recommended to use two ophthalmic beta-blockers at the same time. Special caution is warranted in people taking antidiabetic drugs, since ophthalmic carteolol may mask symptoms of low blood sugar. Other drugs may interact with ophthalmic carteolol. Tell your doctor if you are using any other prescription or over-the-counter medication.

FOOD INTERACTIONS
No known food interactions.

DISEASE INTERACTIONS
Do not use ophthalmic carteolol if you have asthma, chronic obstructive pulmonary disease (COPD), or heart rhythm irregularities. Caution is advised when taking ophthalmic carteolol. Consult your doctor if you have any of the following: hay fever, chronic bronchitis, diabetes, low blood sugar, heart disease, blood vessel disease, myasthenia gravis, or an overactive thyroid. Use of this drug may cause complications in patients with liver or kidney disease, since these organs work together to remove the medication from the body.

Carteolol Hydrochloride Oral

Cartrol 5 mg
(ABBOTT)

▶ Drug Class: Beta-blocker

▶ Available in: Tablets

▶ Available OTC? No

▶ As Generic? No

Side Effects

SERIOUS
Shortness of breath, wheezing; irregular or slow heartbeat (50 beats per minute or less); pain or feelings of tightness or pressure in the chest; swelling of the ankles, feet, and lower legs; mental depression. Call your doctor right away.

COMMON
Dizziness or lightheadedness, especially when rising rapidly to a standing position; rapid heartbeat or palpitations; decreased sexual ability; unusual fatigue, weakness, or drowsiness; muscle cramps; insomnia.

LESS COMMON
Anxiety, irritability, nervousness; constipation; diarrhea; dry, sore eyes; itching; nausea or vomiting; nightmares or intensely vivid dreams; numbness, tingling, or other unusual sensations in the fingers, toes, or scalp.

PRINCIPAL USES
To treat high blood pressure (hypertension).

HOW THE DRUG WORKS
By blocking actions of the sympathetic nervous system, carteolol reduces the rate and force of the heartbeat, thus lowering blood pressure.

DOSAGE
To treat high blood pressure: 2.5 mg once a day, increased to 5 to 10 mg per day if needed. (Dosage schedule for persons with impaired kidney function: 2.5 mg once every 1, 2, or 3 days as needed.)

ONSET OF EFFECT
Three weeks of therapy may be needed for the full effect of the drug to occur.

DURATION OF ACTION
24 hours.

DIETARY ADVICE
Most effective when taken at least 1 hour before or 2 hours after eating.

STORAGE
Store in a tightly sealed container away from heat and direct light.

IF YOU MISS A DOSE
Take it as soon as you remember. If it is within 8 hours of the next dose, skip the missed dose and resume your regular dosage schedule. Do not double the next dose.

STOPPING THE DRUG
The decision to stop taking the drug should be made in consultation with your doctor. Gradual reduction of the dose over 2 to 3 weeks is generally necessary; stopping the drug abruptly may cause potentially serious medical consequences.

PROLONGED USE
Prolonged use may weaken the heart.

PRECAUTIONS
Over 60: Adverse reactions may be more likely and more severe in older patients. Treatment usually begins with small doses that are increased gradually to avoid an excessive reduction in blood pressure.

Driving and Hazardous Work: Do not drive or engage in hazardous work until you determine how the medicine affects you.

Alcohol: Drink in careful moderation if at all. Alcohol may interact with the drug and cause a dangerous drop in blood pressure.

Pregnancy: No birth defects were found in animal studies. Adequate studies in pregnant human patients have not been done. Before taking carteolol, notify your doctor if you are pregnant or plan to become pregnant.

Breast Feeding: Carteolol may pass into breast milk; caution is advised. Consult your doctor for advice.

Infants and Children: The safety and effectiveness of carteolol use in children under 12 have not been determined. It should be used only under close medical supervision.

Special Concerns: Be cautious about exposure to very hot or very cold weather conditions. Heavy exercise or exertion can cause excessive fatigue, muscle cramping, or dangerous increases in your blood pressure.

OVERDOSE
Symptoms: Slow heartbeat, severe dizziness, fainting, fast or irregular heartbeat, difficulty breathing, bluish-colored fingernails or palms, seizures.

What to Do: Call your doctor, emergency medical services (EMS), or the nearest poison control center immediately.

DRUG INTERACTIONS
Consult your doctor for specific advice if you are taking other drugs for high blood pressure, reserpine, theophylline, amiodarone, clonidine, diltiazem, epinephrine, ergot preparations, fluvoxamine, insulin, nifedipine, oral antidiabetic agents, phenothiazines, nonsteroidal anti-inflammatory drugs, or indomethacin.

FOOD INTERACTIONS
No known food interactions.

DISEASE INTERACTIONS
Use of carteolol may cause complications in patients with liver or kidney disease, since these organs work together to remove the medication from the body. Carteolol should be used with caution in people with diabetes, especially insulin-dependent diabetes, since the drug may mask the symptoms of hypoglycemia. Also consult your doctor if you have any of the following disorders: congestive heart failure, coronary artery disease, allergic rhinitis (seasonal allergies), asthma, chronic bronchitis, hyperthyroidism, myasthenia gravis, or blood vessel (vascular) disease.

Carvedilol

BRAND NAME
Coreg

▶ Drug Class: Beta-blocker

▶ Available in: Tablets

▶ Available OTC? No

▶ As Generic? No

Side Effects

SERIOUS
Shortness of breath, wheezing; irregular or slow heartbeat (50 beats per minute or less); pain or feelings of tightness or pressure in the chest; swelling of the ankles, feet, and lower legs; mental depression. If you experience such symptoms, call your doctor immediately.

COMMON
Dizziness or lightheadedness, especially when rising suddenly to a standing position; decreased sexual ability; unusual fatigue, weakness, or drowsiness; insomnia; diarrhea; nausea or vomiting.

LESS COMMON
Anxiety, irritability, nervousness; constipation; dry, sore eyes; itching; nightmares or intensely vivid dreams; numbness, tingling, or other unusual sensations in the fingers, toes, or scalp.

PRINCIPAL USES
To treat mild to moderate congestive heart failure (CHF) in conjunction with digitalis, diuretics, or ACE inhibitors. Also used to treat high blood pressure.

HOW THE DRUG WORKS
It is not known how carvedilol improves CHF and lowers blood pressure.

DOSAGE
Dosages must be tailored individually to each patient, using the following guidelines as starting points. For CHF: Initially, 3.125 mg twice a day for 2 weeks. If the dose is tolerated, it may be increased to 6.25 mg twice a day. Dosing should then be doubled every 2 weeks to the highest level tolerated by the patient. For patients weighing less than 187 lbs, maximum daily dose is 25 mg twice a day. For patients weighing more than 187 lbs, maximum daily dose is 50 mg twice a day. For high blood pressure: Initially, 6.25 mg twice a day for 7 to 14 days. Dose may then be increased to 12.5 mg twice a day for 7 to 14 days, as needed. Dose may be further increased to 25 mg twice a day for 7 to 14 days, if tolerated and needed. Maximum daily dose is 50 mg.

ONSET OF EFFECT
Within 1 to 2 hours.

DURATION OF ACTION
Unknown.

DIETARY ADVICE
Take it with food to reduce the risk of potentially dangerous drop in blood pressure. Follow your doctor's dietary guidelines.

STORAGE
Store in a tightly sealed container away from heat, moisture, and direct light.

IF YOU MISS A DOSE
Take it as soon as you remember. If it is within 4 hours of the next scheduled dose, skip the missed dose and resume your regular dosage schedule. Do not double the next dose.

STOPPING THE DRUG
This drug should not be stopped suddenly, as this may lead to angina and possibly a heart attack in patients with advanced heart disease. Slow reduction of dosage over a period of 1 to 2 weeks is advised.

PROLONGED USE
Regular visits to your doctor are needed to evaluate the drug's ongoing, long-term effectiveness.

PRECAUTIONS
Over 60: Many elderly patients are more sensitive to the drug than younger persons. Smaller doses and frequent blood pressure checks may be warranted.

Driving and Hazardous Work: Use caution in such activities until you determine how the medication affects you.

Alcohol: Drink in careful moderation if at all. Alcohol may interact with the drug and cause a dangerous drop in blood pressure.

Pregnancy: Discuss with your doctor the relative risks and benefits of using this drug while pregnant.

Breast Feeding: Trace amounts of this drug can be found in breast milk; however, adverse effects in infants have not been documented. Consult your doctor for specific advice.

Infants and Children: Not recommended.

Special Concerns: Use of the drug should be considered but one element of a comprehensive therapeutic program that includes weight control, smoking cessation, regular exercise, and a healthy (low-salt, low-fat) diet.

OVERDOSE
Symptoms: Unusually slow heartbeat, severe dizziness or fainting, vomiting, breathing difficulty, seizures.

What to Do: Call your doctor, emergency medical services (EMS), or the nearest poison control center immediately.

DRUG INTERACTIONS
The following drugs may interact with carvedilol. Inform your doctor if you are taking amphetamines, oral antidiabetic agents, insulin, asthma medication (such as aminophylline or theophylline), calcium channel blockers, clonidine, guanabenz, immunotherapy for allergies (allergy shots), MAO inhibitors, reserpine, cyclosporine, other beta-blockers, or any over-the-counter medicine.

FOOD INTERACTIONS
None reported.

DISEASE INTERACTIONS
Carvedilol should be used with caution by people with diabetes, especially insulin-dependent diabetes, since the drug may mask symptoms of hypoglycemia. Consult your doctor for specific advice if you have allergies or asthma; heart or blood vessel disease (including peripheral vascular disease); hyperthyroidism; irregular (slow) heartbeat; a history of mental depression; myasthenia gravis; psoriasis; respiratory problems such as bronchitis or emphysema; or kidney or liver disease.

Castor Oil

BRAND NAMES
Alphamul, Emulsoil, Fleet Flavored Castor Oil, Kellogg's Castor Oil, Neoloid, Purge

▶ Drug Class: Stimulant laxative

▶ Available in: Oral solution

▶ Available OTC? Yes

▶ As Generic? Yes

Side Effects

SERIOUS
Confusion, irregular heartbeat, muscle cramps. Call your doctor immediately.

COMMON
Laxative dependence, skin rashes, stomach cramps, belching, diarrhea, nausea.

LESS COMMON
Fatigue or weakness.

PRINCIPAL USES
For short-term relief of constipation.

HOW THE DRUG WORKS
Castor oil stimulates muscle contractions in the wall of the bowel. These contractions promote the passage of stool.

DOSAGE
The dose will be different for different products. A typical dose is 15 to 60 ml for adults and teenagers. Castor oil should be taken early in the day because the laxative effect is unpredictable and might otherwise interfere with a full night's sleep.

ONSET OF EFFECT
Within 2 to 6 hours.

DURATION OF ACTION
Variable.

DIETARY ADVICE
Laxatives may contain a large amount of sodium or sugar. Regular bowel movements are more likely with a diet that contains an adequate amount of liquid (6 to 8 full 8-oz glasses per day), whole-grain products and bran, fruit, and vegetables.

STORAGE
Store in a tightly sealed container away from heat, moisture, and direct light. Keep the liquid form refrigerated, but do not allow it to freeze.

IF YOU MISS A DOSE
If you are on a prescribed dosage schedule, take a missed dose as soon as you remember, unless the time for your next scheduled dose is within the next 2 hours. If so, do not take the missed dose. Take your next scheduled dose at the proper time, and resume your regular dosage schedule. Do not double the next dose.

STOPPING THE DRUG
Take it as prescribed for the full treatment period. However, you may stop taking the drug if you are feeling better before the scheduled end of the therapy.

PROLONGED USE
Do not use castor oil for more than 3 to 5 days without informing your physician. Prolonged, excessive use of castor oil may be associated with an increased risk of side effects, including laxative dependence.

PRECAUTIONS
Over 60: Adverse reactions may be more likely and more severe in older patients.

Driving and Hazardous Work: Do not drive or engage in hazardous work until you determine how the medicine affects you.

Alcohol: Avoid alcohol when using this medication.

Pregnancy: Castor oil may cause premature contractions and so should be avoided in pregnant women.

Breast Feeding: Castor oil may be used by nursing mothers.

Infants and Children: Do not give laxatives to children under 6 years of age unless prescribed by a physician.

Special Concerns: Occasional missed bowel movements do not constitute constipation; do not use castor oil under such circumstances. Persistent constipation or difficulty in passing stool is serious and requires evaluation.

OVERDOSE
Symptoms: No cases of overdose with castor oil have been reported.

What to Do: An overdose of castor oil is unlikely to be life-threatening. However, if someone takes a much larger dose than prescribed, contact a physician.

DRUG INTERACTIONS
Do not take a prescription medication within 2 hours of taking a laxative (either before or after), since this may diminish the effects of the prescription drug. Consult your doctor for specific advice if you are taking digitalis drugs or a diuretic.

FOOD INTERACTIONS
No known food interactions.

DISEASE INTERACTIONS
Caution is advised when taking castor oil. Do not use any laxative if you have any of the following: stomach or abdominal pain, especially if accompanied by fever; cramping; abdominal swelling or bloating; nausea or vomiting. Consult your doctor if you have any of the following problems: abdominal pain and fever, rectal bleeding, ostomy (an artificial surgical opening in the body to allow the release of urine or feces), diabetes mellitus, heart or kidney disease, or high blood pressure.

Cefaclor

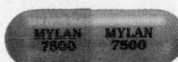

Generic 500 mg
(**MYLAN**)

▶ Drug Class: Cephalosporin antibiotic

▶ Available in: Capsules, oral suspension

▶ Available OTC? No

▶ As Generic? Yes

Side Effects

SERIOUS
Severe allergic reaction (breathing difficulties, confusion, hives, itching, swelling of the face or throat, sweating, and lightheadedness), severe stomach pain and cramps, fever, severe, sometimes bloody diarrhea. Call your doctor immediately.

COMMON
Mild diarrhea or stomach cramps, sore mouth or tongue, nausea and vomiting.

LESS COMMON
Vaginal itching or unusual discharge, anemia, rash, decreased white blood cell count causing increased susceptibility to infection.

PRINCIPAL USES
To treat a variety of bacterial infections, including those of the nose, tonsils, and throat, skin and soft tissues, genitourinary tract, and the respiratory tract. Cefaclor is effective only against infections caused by bacteria; it is ineffective against those caused by viruses, fungi, or other microorganisms.

HOW THE DRUG WORKS
Cefaclor prevents bacteria from forming cell walls.

DOSAGE
Adults and teenagers: 250 to 500 mg every 8 hours. Children 1 month to 12 years: 20 mg per 2.2 lbs (1 kg) of body weight a day in divided doses every 8 hours. It can be given every 12 hours for ear infection or sore throat.

ONSET OF EFFECT
30 to 60 minutes.

DURATION OF ACTION
1 to 2 hours.

DIETARY ADVICE
Cefaclor may be taken on a full or empty stomach, but taking it with food will reduce stomach irritation.

STORAGE
Store in a tightly sealed container away from heat, moisture, and direct light. Keep liquid form refrigerated, but do not allow it to freeze.

IF YOU MISS A DOSE
Take it as soon as you remember. This will help keep a constant level of medication in your system. If it is near the time for the next dose, skip the missed dose and resume your regular dosage schedule. Do not double the next dose.

STOPPING THE DRUG
Take it as prescribed for the full treatment period, even if you begin to feel better before the scheduled end of therapy. Stopping cefaclor prematurely may slow your recovery or lead to a rebound infection, also known as superinfection, in which the heartier strains of bacteria survive and multiply, leading to a more serious and drug-resistant infection. When taking this drug to treat a streptococcal (strep) infection, it is particularly important to take it for the entire treatment period. Serious heart and kidney problems can develop later if the drug is discontinued prematurely.

PROLONGED USE
Cefaclor is generally prescribed for short-term therapy (10 to 14 days). Use of cefaclor beyond this period increases the risk of adverse effects and superinfection.

PRECAUTIONS
Over 60: Adverse reactions may be more likely and more severe in older patients.

Driving and Hazardous Work: Do not drive or engage in hazardous work until you determine how the medicine affects you.

Alcohol: Avoid alcohol.

Pregnancy: Adequate studies of cephalosporin use in pregnant women have not been done. Before taking cefaclor, tell your physician if you are pregnant or are planning to become pregnant.

Breast Feeding: Cefaclor passes into breast milk; caution is advised. Consult your doctor for specific advice.

Infants and Children:
This drug may be used by children 1 month and older. Consult your pediatrician for advice.

Special Concerns: People who are allergic to penicillin may have equally serious allergic reactions to cephalosporin antibiotics such as cefaclor. This drug is useful only against bacteria that are susceptible to its effects, not against colds, flu, or other viral infections. If your condition has not improved within a few days of starting cefaclor, or instead has worsened, tell your doctor.

OVERDOSE
Symptoms: Seizures, severe abdominal pain, bloody diarrhea, vomiting.

What to Do: Call your doctor, emergency medical services (EMS), or the nearest poison control center immediately.

DRUG INTERACTIONS
Consult your doctor for specific advice if you are taking carbenicillin injection, heparin, divalproex, anticoagulants, sulfinpyrazone, dipyridamole, pentoxifylline, plicamycin, ticarcillin, probenecid, or valproic acid.

FOOD INTERACTIONS
No known food interactions.

DISEASE INTERACTIONS
Caution is advised when taking cefaclor. Consult your doctor if you have a history of kidney disease or colitis.

Cefadroxil

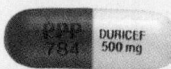

Duricef 500 mg
(BRISTOL-MYERS SQUIBB)

▶ Drug Class: Cephalosporin
antibiotic

▶ Available in: Capsules,
tablets, oral suspension

▶ Available OTC? No

▶ As Generic? Yes

Side Effects

SERIOUS
Severe allergic reaction
(breathing difficulties,
confusion, hives, itching,
swelling of the face or
throat, sweating, and
lightheadedness), severe
stomach pain and
cramps, fever, severe,
sometimes bloody diar-
rhea. Call your doctor
immediately.

COMMON
Mild diarrhea or stomach
cramps, sore mouth or
tongue, nausea and
vomiting.

LESS COMMON
Vaginal itching or dis-
charge, anemia, rash,
decreased white blood
cell count causing
increased susceptibility to
infection, decreased
blood platelets causing
increased risk of bleeding
problems.

PRINCIPAL USES
To treat a variety of bacterial infections, including
those of the throat, skin and
soft tissues, and the genitourinary tract. Cefadroxil is
effective only against infections caused by bacteria; it
is ineffective against those
caused by viruses, fungi, or
other microorganisms.

HOW THE DRUG WORKS
Cefadroxil prevents bacteria
from forming protective cell
walls necessary for survival.

DOSAGE
Adults and teenagers: 500
mg every 12 hours, or 1 to
2 g once a day. Children: 15
mg per 2.2 lbs (1 kg) of
body weight every 12
hours, or 30 mg per 2.2 lbs
once a day.

ONSET OF EFFECT
12 hours.

DURATION OF ACTION
20 to 22 hours.

DIETARY ADVICE
Cefadroxil may be taken on
a full or empty stomach, but
taking it with food will
reduce stomach irritation.

STORAGE
Store in a tightly sealed container away from heat, moisture, and direct light. Keep
liquid form refrigerated, but
do not allow it to freeze.

IF YOU MISS A DOSE
Take it as soon as you
remember. This will help
keep a constant level of
medication in your system.
If it is near the time for the
next dose, skip the missed
dose and resume your regular dosage schedule. Do not
double the next dose.

STOPPING THE DRUG
Take it as prescribed for the
full treatment period, even if
you begin to feel better
before the scheduled end of

therapy. Stopping cefadroxil
prematurely may slow your
recovery or lead to a
rebound infection, also
known as superinfection, in
which the heartier strains of
bacteria survive and multiply, leading to a more serious and drug-resistant
infection. When taking this
drug to treat a streptococcal
(strep) infection, it is particularly important to take it
for the entire treatment
period. Serious heart and
kidney problems can
develop later if the drug is
discontinued prematurely.

PROLONGED USE
Cefadroxil is generally
prescribed for short-term
therapy (10 to 14 days).
Use of cefadroxil beyond
this period increases the
risk of adverse effects and
superinfection.

PRECAUTIONS
Over 60: Adverse reactions
may be more likely and
more severe in older
patients.

**Driving and Hazardous
Work:** Do not drive or
engage in hazardous work
until you determine how the
medicine affects you.

Alcohol: Avoid alcohol.

Pregnancy: Adequate studies of cephalosporin use in
pregnant women have not
been done. Before taking
cefadroxil, tell your doctor if
you are or plan to become
pregnant.

Breast Feeding:
Cefadroxil passes into
breast milk; caution is
advised. Consult your doctor for specific advice.

Infants and Children:
This drug may be used by
children age 1 and older.
Consult your pediatrician
for advice.

Special Concerns: People
who are allergic to penicillin
may have equally serious
allergic reactions to
cephalosporin antibiotics
such as cefadroxil. This
drug is useful only against
bacteria that are susceptible
to its effects, not against
colds, flu, or other viral
infections. If your condition
has not improved within a
few days of starting
cefadroxil, or instead has
worsened, tell your doctor.

OVERDOSE
Symptoms: Seizures,
severe abdominal pain,
bloody diarrhea, vomiting.

What to Do: Call your
doctor, emergency medical
services (EMS), or the
nearest poison control center immediately.

DRUG INTERACTIONS
Consult your doctor for
specific advice if you are
taking carbenicillin injection, heparin, divalproex,
anticoagulants, sulfinpyrazone, dipyridamole,
pentoxifylline, plicamycin,
ticarcillin, probenecid, or
valproic acid.

FOOD INTERACTIONS
No known food interactions.

DISEASE INTERACTIONS
Caution is advised when
taking cefadroxil. Consult
your doctor if you have a
history of kidney disease
or colitis.

Cefamandole Nafate

BRAND NAME
Mandol

▶ Drug Class: Cephalosporin antibiotic

▶ Available in: Injection

▶ Available OTC? No

▶ As Generic? Yes

Side Effects

SERIOUS
Severe allergic reaction (breathing difficulties, confusion, hives, swelling of the face or throat, sweating, and lightheadedness), severe stomach pain and cramps, fever, severe, sometimes bloody diarrhea, unusual bleeding or bruising. Call your doctor immediately.

COMMON
Mild diarrhea or stomach cramps, sore mouth or tongue, nausea and vomiting.

LESS COMMON
Vaginal itching or discharge, pain at site of injection, rash, decreased white blood cell count causing increased susceptibility to infection, decreased blood platelets causing increased risk of bleeding problems.

PRINCIPAL USES
To treat a variety of serious bacterial infections, including those of the lung, genitourinary tract, blood, bones, joints, skin, and other organs. Cefamandole nafate is effective only against infections caused by bacteria; it is ineffective against those caused by viruses, fungi, or other microorganisms. Cephalosporins such as cefamandole nafate are prescribed when other antibiotics are not sufficient to treat the infection.

HOW THE DRUG WORKS
Cefamandole nafate prevents bacteria from forming protective cell walls.

DOSAGE
Adults and teenagers: 500 to 1,000 mg (2,000 mg for life-threatening infections) every 4 to 8 hours, injected into a vein or muscle. Children 1 month to 12 years: 8.3 to 33.3 mg per 2.2 lbs (1 kg) of body weight every 4 to 8 hours into a vein or muscle.

ONSET OF EFFECT
Into a vein: Immediate. Into a muscle: 30 to 120 minutes.

DURATION OF ACTION
Into a vein: 1 hour. Into a muscle: 2 hours.

DIETARY ADVICE
Eat 4 oz of yogurt or drink 4 oz of buttermilk a day to protect against intestinal superinfection. Drink plenty of fluids.

STORAGE
Not applicable; the dose is administered only at a health care facility.

IF YOU MISS A DOSE
Not applicable; the dose is administered by a health care professional.

STOPPING THE DRUG
The decision to stop taking cefamandole nafate should be made by your doctor.

PROLONGED USE
Cefamandole nafate is generally prescribed for short-term therapy (10 to 14 days). Use beyond this period increases the risk of adverse effects and superinfection, a subsequent infection caused by heartier, drug-resistant strains of bacteria.

PRECAUTIONS
Over 60: Adverse reactions may be more likely and more severe in older patients.

Driving and Hazardous Work: Not applicable; the dose is administered only in a health care institution.

Alcohol: Avoid alcohol.

Pregnancy: Adequate studies of cephalosporin use in pregnant women have not been done. Before taking cefamandole nafate, tell your doctor if you are pregnant or plan to become pregnant.

Breast Feeding: Cefamandole nafate passes into breast milk; caution is advised. Consult your doctor for advice.

Infants and Children: This drug may be used by children 1 month and older. Consult your pediatrician for advice.

Special Concerns: People who are allergic to penicillin may have equally serious allergic reactions to cephalosporin antibiotics such as cefamandole nafate. This drug is useful only against bacteria that are susceptible to its effects, not against colds, flu, or other viral infections. If your condition has not improved within a few days of starting cefamandole nafate, or instead has worsened, tell your doctor.

OVERDOSE
Symptoms: An overdose of cefamandole nafate is unlikely to occur.

What to Do: Emergency instructions not applicable.

DRUG INTERACTIONS
Consult your doctor for specific advice if you are taking carbenicillin injection, heparin, divalproex, anticoagulants, sulfinpyrazone, dipyridamole, pentoxifylline, plicamycin, ticarcillin, probenecid, medications containing alcohol, or valproic acid.

FOOD INTERACTIONS
No known food interactions.

DISEASE INTERACTIONS
Caution is advised when taking cefamandole nafate. Consult your doctor if you have a history of kidney disease, bleeding disorders, or colitis.

Cefazolin Sodium

BRAND NAMES
Ancef, Kefzol, Zolicef

▶ Drug Class: Cephalosporin antibiotic

▶ Available in: Injection

▶ Available OTC? No

▶ As Generic? Yes

Side Effects

SERIOUS
Severe allergic reaction (breathing difficulties, confusion, itching, hives, swelling of the face or throat, sweating, and lightheadedness), severe stomach pain and cramps, fever, severe, sometimes bloody diarrhea. Call your doctor immediately.

COMMON
Mild diarrhea or stomach cramps, sore mouth or tongue, nausea and vomiting.

LESS COMMON
Vaginal itching or unusual discharge, pain or itching at the site of injection.

PRINCIPAL USES
To treat a variety of moderately severe bacterial infections, including those of the heart, lung, genitourinary tract, bones, joints, skin and soft tissue, and blood. Cefazolin sodium is effective only against infections caused by bacteria; it is ineffective against those caused by viruses, fungi, or other microorganisms. Cephalosporins such as cefazolin sodium are prescribed when other antibiotics are not sufficient to treat the infection. It is also used prior to some surgeries to prevent infection.

HOW THE DRUG WORKS
Cefazolin sodium prevents bacteria from forming protective cell walls.

DOSAGE
Adults and teenagers: 250 to 1,500 mg every 6 to 8 hours into a vein. Children 1 month to 12 years: 6.25 to 25 mg per 2.2 lbs (1 kg) of body weight every 6 hours, or 8.3 to 33.3 mg per 2.2 lbs every 8 hours into a vein.

ONSET OF EFFECT
Immediate.

DURATION OF ACTION
4 hours.

DIETARY ADVICE
Eat 4 oz of yogurt or drink 4 oz of buttermilk a day to protect against intestinal superinfection. Drink plenty of fluids.

STORAGE
Not applicable; the dose is administered only at a health care facility.

IF YOU MISS A DOSE
Not applicable; the dose is administered by a health care professional.

STOPPING THE DRUG
The decision to stop taking the drug should be made by your doctor.

PROLONGED USE
Cefazolin sodium is generally prescribed for short-term therapy (10 to 14 days). Use beyond this period increases the risk of adverse effects and superinfection, a subsequent infection caused by heartier, drug-resistant strains of bacteria.

PRECAUTIONS
Over 60: Adverse reactions may be more likely and more severe in older patients.

Driving and Hazardous Work: Not applicable; the dose is administered only in a health care institution.

Alcohol: Avoid alcohol.

Pregnancy: Adequate studies of cephalosporin use in pregnant women have not been done. Before taking cefazolin sodium, tell your doctor if you are pregnant or plan to become pregnant.

Breast Feeding: Cefazolin sodium passes into breast milk; caution is advised. Consult your doctor for specific advice.

Infants and Children: This drug may be used by children 1 month and older. Consult your pediatrician for advice.

Special Concerns: People who are allergic to penicillin may have equally serious allergic reactions to cephalosporin antibiotics. Cefazolin sodium is useful only against bacteria that are susceptible to its effects and will not work against colds, flu, or other viral infections. If your condition has not improved within a few days of starting cefazolin sodium, or instead has worsened, tell your doctor.

OVERDOSE
Symptoms: An overdose of cefazolin sodium is unlikely.

What to Do: Emergency instructions not applicable.

DRUG INTERACTIONS
Consult your doctor for specific advice if you are taking carbenicillin injection, heparin, divalproex, anticoagulants, sulfinpyrazone, dipyridamole, pentoxifylline, plicamycin, ticarcillin, probenecid, or valproic acid.

FOOD INTERACTIONS
No known food interactions.

DISEASE INTERACTIONS
Caution is advised when taking cefazolin. Consult your doctor if you have a history of kidney disease or colitis.

Cefepime

BRAND NAME
Maxipime

▶ Drug Class: Cephalosporin antibiotic

▶ Available in: Injection

▶ Available OTC? No

▶ As Generic? No

Side Effects

SERIOUS
Severe allergic reaction (breathing difficulties, confusion, hives, swelling of the face or throat, sweating, and lightheadedness), severe stomach pain and cramps, fever, severe, sometimes bloody diarrhea, unusual bleeding or bruising. Call your doctor immediately.

COMMON
Mild diarrhea or stomach cramps, sore mouth or tongue, nausea and vomiting.

LESS COMMON
Vaginal itching or unusual discharge, pain at the site of injection, itching.

PRINCIPAL USES
To treat a variety of moderate to serious bacterial infections, including those of the ear, nose, tonsils, and throat, skin and soft tissues, genitourinary tract, and the respiratory tract. Cefepime is effective only against infections caused by bacteria; it is ineffective against those caused by viruses, fungi, or other microorganisms. Cephalosporins such as cefepime are prescribed when other antibiotics are not sufficient to treat the infection.

HOW THE DRUG WORKS
Cefepime prevents bacteria from forming cell walls.

DOSAGE
Adults and teenagers—
Mild to moderate urinary tract infections: 500 to 1,000 mg every 12 hours. Severe urinary tract infections: 2,000 mg every 12 hours. Moderate to severe pneumonia: 1,000 to 2,000 mg every 12 hours. Moderate to severe skin infections: 2,000 mg every 12 hours. Injections are usually into a vein. For mild to moderate urinary tract infections, cefepime may be administered into a muscle. Children age 2 months to 16 years and weighing less than 40 kg: 50 mg per 2.2 lbs (1 kg) of body weight every 12 hours. The dose should not exceed the recommended adult dose.

ONSET OF EFFECT
Immediate.

DURATION OF ACTION
Unknown.

DIETARY ADVICE
Eat 4 oz of yogurt or drink 4 oz of buttermilk a day to protect against intestinal superinfection. Drink plenty of fluids.

STORAGE
Not applicable; the dose is administered only at a health care facility.

IF YOU MISS A DOSE
Not applicable; the dose is administered by a health care professional.

STOPPING THE DRUG
The decision to stop taking the drug should be made by your doctor.

PROLONGED USE
Cefepime is generally prescribed for short-term therapy (10 to 14 days). Use of cefepime beyond this period increases the risk of adverse effects and superinfection, a subsequent infection caused by heartier, drug-resistant bacteria.

PRECAUTIONS
Over 60: Adverse reactions may be more likely and more severe in older patients.

Driving and Hazardous Work: Not applicable; the dose is administered only in a health care institution.

Alcohol: Avoid alcohol.

Pregnancy: Adequate studies of cephalosporin use in pregnant women have not been done. Before taking cefepime, tell your doctor if you are pregnant or plan to become pregnant.

Breast Feeding: Cefepime passes into breast milk; caution is advised. Consult your doctor for specific advice.

Infants and Children: This drug is not recommended for use by children under 2 months of age.

Special Concerns: People who are allergic to penicillin may have equally serious allergic reactions to cephalosporin antibiotics such as cefepime. This drug is useful only against bacteria that are susceptible to its effects. Cephalosporins will not work against colds, flu, or other viral infections. If your condition has not improved within a few days of starting cefepime, or instead has worsened, tell your doctor.

OVERDOSE
Symptoms: An overdose of cefepime is unlikely.

What to Do: Emergency instructions not applicable.

DRUG INTERACTIONS
Consult your doctor for specific advice if you are taking carbenicillin injection, heparin, divalproex, anticoagulants, sulfinpyrazone, dipyridamole, pentoxifylline, plicamycin, ticarcillin, probenecid, or valproic acid.

FOOD INTERACTIONS
No known food interactions.

DISEASE INTERACTIONS
Consult your doctor if you have a history of kidney disease, bleeding disorders, or colitis.

Cefixime

Suprax 400 mg
(LEDERLE)

▶ Drug Class: Cephalosporin antibiotic

▶ Available in: Tablets, oral suspension

▶ Available OTC? No

▶ As Generic? No

Side Effects

SERIOUS
Severe allergic reaction (breathing difficulties, confusion, hives, itching, swelling of the face or throat, sweating, and lightheadedness), severe stomach pain and cramps, fever, severe, sometimes bloody diarrhea. Call your doctor immediately.

COMMON
Mild diarrhea or stomach cramps, sore mouth or tongue, nausea and vomiting.

LESS COMMON
Vaginal itching or unusual discharge, decreased white blood cell count causing increased susceptibility to infection, decreased blood platelets causing increased risk of bleeding problems, itching.

PRINCIPAL USES
To treat a variety of bacterial infections, including those of the ear, nose, tonsils, and throat, skin and soft tissues, genitourinary tract, and the respiratory tract. Cefixime is also used to treat gonorrhea. It is effective only against infections caused by bacteria; it is ineffective against those caused by viruses, fungi, or other microorganisms.

HOW THE DRUG WORKS
Cefixime prevents bacteria from forming protective cell walls necessary for survival.

DOSAGE
Adults and teenagers: 200 mg every 12 hours, or 400 mg once a day. Uncomplicated gonorrhea is treated with 400 mg, given in a one-time dose. Children 6 months to 12 years: 4 mg per 2.2 lbs (1 kg) of body weight every 12 hours, or 8 mg per 2.2 lbs once a day.

ONSET OF EFFECT
2 to 4 hours.

DURATION OF ACTION
6 to 18 hours.

DIETARY ADVICE
It may be taken with food to reduce stomach irritation.

STORAGE
Store in a tightly sealed container away from heat, moisture, and direct light. Oral suspension does not need to be refrigerated.

IF YOU MISS A DOSE
Take it as soon as you remember. If it is near the time for the next dose, skip the missed dose and resume your regular dosage schedule. Do not double the next dose.

STOPPING THE DRUG
Take it as prescribed for the full treatment period, even if you begin to feel better before the scheduled end of therapy. Stopping cefixime prematurely may slow your recovery or lead to a rebound infection, also known as superinfection, in which the heartier strains of bacteria survive and multiply, leading to a more serious and drug-resistant infection. When taking this drug to treat a streptococcal (strep) infection, it is particularly important to take it for the entire treatment period. Serious heart and kidney problems can develop later if the drug is discontinued prematurely.

PROLONGED USE
Cefixime, when taken to treat gonorrhea, is prescribed as a one-time dose. For other bacterial infections, cefixime is generally prescribed for short-term therapy (10 to 14 days). Use of cefixime beyond this period increases the risk of adverse effects and superinfection.

PRECAUTIONS

Over 60: Adverse reactions may be more likely and more severe in older patients.

Driving and Hazardous Work: Do not drive or engage in hazardous work until you determine how the medicine affects you.

Alcohol: Avoid alcohol.

Pregnancy: Adequate studies of cephalosporin use in pregnant women have not been done. Before taking cefixime, tell your doctor if you are pregnant or are planning to become pregnant.

Breast Feeding: Cefixime passes into breast milk; caution is advised. Consult your doctor for specific advice.

Infants and Children: May be used by children 6 months and older. Consult your pediatrician for specific advice.

Special Concerns: Those allergic to penicillin may have equally serious allergic reactions to cephalosporin antibiotics such as cefixime. It is useful only against bacteria that are susceptible to its effects, not against colds, flu, or other viral infections. If your condition has not improved within a few days of starting cefixime, or instead has worsened, tell your doctor.

OVERDOSE
Symptoms: Seizures, severe abdominal pain, bloody diarrhea, vomiting.

What to Do: Call your doctor, emergency medical services (EMS), or the nearest poison control center immediately.

DRUG INTERACTIONS
Consult your doctor for specific advice if you are taking carbenicillin injection, heparin, divalproex, anticoagulants, sulfinpyrazone, dipyridamole, pentoxifylline, plicamycin, ticarcillin, probenecid, or valproic acid.

FOOD INTERACTIONS
No known food interactions.

DISEASE INTERACTIONS
Consult your doctor if you have a history of kidney disease or colitis.

Cefotetan Disodium

BRAND NAME
Cefotan

▶ Drug Class: Cephalosporin antibiotic

▶ Available in: Injection

▶ Available OTC? No

▶ As Generic? No

Side Effects

SERIOUS
Severe allergic reaction (breathing difficulties, confusion, hives, swelling of the face or throat, sweating, and lightheadedness), severe stomach pain and cramps, fever, severe, sometimes bloody diarrhea, unusual bleeding or bruising. Call your doctor immediately.

COMMON
Mild diarrhea or stomach cramps, sore mouth or tongue, nausea and vomiting.

LESS COMMON
Vaginal discharge or itching, pain at site of injection, rash, decreased white blood cell count causing increased susceptibility to infection, decreased blood platelets causing increased risk of bleeding problems.

PRINCIPAL USES

To treat a variety of serious bacterial infections, including those of the lung, genitourinary tract, blood, bones, joints, skin and soft tissues, and other organs. Cefotetan disodium is also used to treat gonorrhea. It is effective only against infections caused by certain strains of bacteria; it is ineffective against those caused by viruses, fungi, or other microorganisms. Cephalosporins such as cefotetan disodium are prescribed when other antibiotics are not sufficient to treat the infection. Cefotetan disodium is also used in some cases prior to certain major surgical procedures in order to minimize the risk of infection.

HOW THE DRUG WORKS

Cefotetan disodium prevents bacteria from forming protective cell walls necessary for their survival.

DOSAGE

1 to 3 g into a vein or muscle every 12 hours.

ONSET OF EFFECT

Into a vein: Immediate. Into a muscle: 1 hour.

DURATION OF ACTION

6 to 9 hours.

DIETARY ADVICE

Eat 4 oz of yogurt or drink 4 oz of buttermilk a day to protect against intestinal superinfection. Drink plenty of fluids.

STORAGE

Not applicable; the dose is administered only at a health care facility.

IF YOU MISS A DOSE

Not applicable; the dose is administered by a health care professional.

STOPPING THE DRUG

The decision to stop taking the drug should be made by your doctor.

PROLONGED USE

Cefotetan disodium is generally prescribed for short-term therapy (10 to 14 days). Use beyond this period increases the likelihood of adverse effects and superinfection, a subsequent infection caused by heartier, drug-resistant strains of bacteria.

PRECAUTIONS

Over 60: Adverse reactions may be more likely and more severe in older patients.

Driving and Hazardous Work: Not applicable; the dose is administered only in a health care institution.

Alcohol: Avoid alcohol.

Pregnancy: Adequate studies of cephalosporin use in pregnant women have not been done. Before taking cefotetan disodium, tell your doctor if you are pregnant or plan to become pregnant.

Breast Feeding: Cefotetan disodium passes into breast milk; caution is advised. Consult your doctor for specific advice.

Infants and Children: This drug is not recommended for use by children under the age of 12.

Special Concerns: People who are allergic to penicillin may have equally serious allergic reactions to cephalosporin antibiotics such as cefotetan disodium. This drug is useful only against bacteria that are susceptible to its effects, not against colds, flu, or other viral infections. If your condition has not improved within a few days of starting cefotetan disodium, or instead has worsened, tell your doctor.

OVERDOSE

Symptoms: An overdose of cefotetan disodium is unlikely.

What to Do: Emergency instructions not applicable.

DRUG INTERACTIONS

Consult your doctor for specific advice if you are taking carbenicillin injection, heparin, divalproex, anticoagulants, sulfinpyrazone, dipyridamole, pentoxifylline, plicamycin, ticarcillin, probenecid, medications containing alcohol, or valproic acid.

FOOD INTERACTIONS

No known food interactions.

DISEASE INTERACTIONS

Caution is advised when taking cefotetan disodium. Consult your doctor if you have a history of kidney disease, bleeding disorders, or colitis.

Vantin 100 mg
(UPJOHN)

▶ Drug Class: Cephalosporin antibiotic

▶ Available in: Oral suspension, tablets

▶ Available OTC? No

▶ As Generic? No

Side Effects

SERIOUS
Severe allergic reaction (breathing difficulties, itching, hives, swelling of the face or throat, and sweating), severe stomach pain and cramps, fever, severe, sometimes bloody diarrhea. Call your doctor immediately.

COMMON
Mild diarrhea or stomach cramps, sore mouth or tongue, nausea and vomiting.

LESS COMMON
Vaginal itching or unusual discharge, rash, decreased white blood cell count causing increased susceptibility to infection, decreased blood platelets causing increased risk of bleeding problems.

PRINCIPAL USES
To treat a variety of bacterial infections, including those of the ear, nose, and throat, skin and soft tissues, genitourinary tract, respiratory tract, and other organs. Cefpodoxime is also used to treat gonorrhea. It is effective only against infections caused by bacteria; it is ineffective against those caused by viruses, fungi, or other microorganisms.

HOW THE DRUG WORKS
Cefpodoxime prevents bacteria from forming protective cell walls.

DOSAGE
Adults and teenagers: 100 to 400 mg every 12 hours. Gonorrhea is treated with 200 mg, given in a one-time dose. Children 6 months to 12 years: 5 mg per 2.2 lbs (1 kg) of body weight every 12 hours.

ONSET OF EFFECT
Unknown.

DURATION OF ACTION
Approximately 6 hours.

DIETARY ADVICE
Take it with food to increase the absorption of the drug by the body.

STORAGE
Store in a tightly sealed container away from heat, moisture, and direct light. Keep liquid form refrigerated, but do not allow it to freeze.

IF YOU MISS A DOSE
Take it as soon as you remember. This will help keep a constant level of medication in your system. If it is near the time for the next dose, skip the missed dose and resume your regular schedule. Do not double the next dose.

STOPPING THE DRUG
Take it as prescribed for the full treatment period, even if you begin to feel better before the scheduled end of therapy. Stopping the drug prematurely may slow your recovery or lead to a rebound infection, also known as superinfection, in which the heartier strains of bacteria survive and multiply, leading to a more serious and drug-resistant infection. When taking this drug to treat a streptococcal (strep) infection, it is particularly important to take it for the entire treatment period. Serious heart and kidney problems can develop later if it is discontinued prematurely.

PROLONGED USE
Cefpodoxime is generally prescribed for short-term therapy (10 to 14 days). Use of cefpodoxime beyond this period increases the risk of adverse effects and superinfection.

PRECAUTIONS
Over 60: Adverse reactions may be more likely and more severe.

Driving and Hazardous Work: Avoid such activities until you determine how the medicine affects you.

Alcohol: Avoid alcohol.

Pregnancy: Adequate studies of cephalosporin use in pregnant women have not been done. Before taking cefpodoxime proxetil, tell your doctor if you are pregnant or plan to become pregnant.

Breast Feeding: Cefpodoxime proxetil passes into breast milk and may be hazardous to the nursing infant; caution is advised. Consult your doctor for advice.

Infants and Children: May be used in children 6 months and older. Consult your pediatrician for advice.

Special Concerns: People who are allergic to penicillin may have equally serious allergic reactions to cephalosporin antibiotics. Cefpodoxime is useful only against bacteria that are susceptible to its effects, not against colds, flu, or other viral infections. If your condition has not improved within a few days of starting the drug, or instead has worsened, notify your physician.

OVERDOSE
Symptoms: Seizures, severe abdominal pain, bloody diarrhea, vomiting.

What to Do: Call your doctor, emergency medical services (EMS), or the nearest poison control center immediately.

DRUG INTERACTIONS
Consult your doctor for specific advice if you are taking carbenicillin injection, heparin, divalproex, anticoagulants, sulfinpyrazone, dipyridamole, pentoxifylline, plicamycin, ticarcillin, probenecid, or valproic acid.

FOOD INTERACTIONS
No known food interactions.

DISEASE INTERACTIONS
Caution is advised when taking cefpodoxime proxetil. Consult your doctor if you have a history of kidney disease or colitis.

Cefprozil

BRAND NAME
Cefzil

Cefzil 250 mg
(BRISTOL-MYERS SQUIBB)

▶ Drug Class: Cephalosporin antibiotic

▶ Available in: Oral suspension, tablets

▶ Available OTC? No

▶ As Generic? No

Side Effects

SERIOUS
Severe allergic reaction (breathing difficulties, confusion, lightheadedness, itching, hives, swelling of the face or throat, and unusual sweating), severe stomach pain and cramps, fever, severe, sometimes bloody diarrhea. Call your doctor immediately.

COMMON
Mild diarrhea or stomach cramps, sore mouth or tongue, nausea and vomiting.

LESS COMMON
Vaginal itching or unusual discharge, decreased white blood cell count causing increased susceptibility to infection, decreased blood platelets causing increased risk of bleeding problems.

PRINCIPAL USES
To treat a variety of bacterial infections, including those of the ear, nose, tonsils, and throat, skin and soft tissues, and the respiratory tract. Cefprozil is effective only against infections caused by bacteria; it is ineffective against those caused by viruses, fungi, or other microorganisms.

HOW THE DRUG WORKS
Cefprozil prevents bacteria from forming protective cell walls necessary for survival.

DOSAGE
Adults and teenagers: 250 to 500 mg every 12 to 24 hours. Children ages 2 to 12: 7.5 mg per 2.2 lbs (1 kg) of body weight every 12 hours. Children 6 months to 12 years: 15 mg per 2.2 lbs every 12 hours.

ONSET OF EFFECT
Approximately 90 minutes.

DURATION OF ACTION
Unknown.

DIETARY ADVICE
It may be taken with food to reduce stomach irritation.

STORAGE
Store in a tightly sealed container away from heat, moisture, and direct light. Keep liquid form refrigerated, but do not allow it to freeze.

IF YOU MISS A DOSE
Take it as soon as you remember. This will help keep a constant level of medication in your system. If it is near the time for the next dose, skip the missed dose and resume your regular dosage schedule. Do not double the next dose.

STOPPING THE DRUG
Take it as prescribed for the full treatment period, even if you begin to feel better before the scheduled end of therapy. Stopping cefprozil prematurely may slow your recovery or lead to a rebound infection, also known as superinfection, in which the heartier strains of bacteria survive and multiply, leading to a more serious and drug-resistant infection. When taking this drug to treat a streptococcal (strep) infection, it is particularly important to take it for the entire treatment period. Serious heart and kidney problems can develop later if it is discontinued prematurely.

PROLONGED USE
Cefprozil is generally prescribed for short-term therapy (10 to 14 days). Use of cefprozil beyond this period increases risks of adverse effects and superinfection.

PRECAUTIONS
Over 60: Adverse reactions may be more likely and more severe in older patients.

Driving and Hazardous Work: Do not drive or engage in hazardous work until you determine how the medicine affects you.

Alcohol: Avoid alcohol.

Pregnancy: Adequate studies of cephalosporin use in pregnant women have not been done. Before taking cefprozil, tell your doctor if you are pregnant or are planning to become pregnant.

Breast Feeding: Cefprozil passes into breast milk; caution is advised. Consult your doctor for specific advice.

Infants and Children: Cefprozil may be used by children 6 months and older. Consult your pediatrician for specific advice.

Special Concerns: People who are allergic to penicillin may have equally serious allergic reactions to cephalosporin antibiotics such as cefprozil. This drug is useful only against bacteria that are susceptible to its effects, not against colds, flu, or other viral infections. If your condition has not improved within a few days of starting cefprozil, or instead has worsened, tell your doctor.

OVERDOSE
Symptoms: Seizures, severe abdominal pain, bloody diarrhea, vomiting.

What to Do: Call your doctor, emergency medical services (EMS), or the nearest poison control center immediately.

DRUG INTERACTIONS
Consult your doctor for specific advice if you are taking carbenicillin injection, heparin, divalproex, anticoagulants, sulfinpyrazone, dipyridamole, pentoxifylline, plicamycin, ticarcillin, probenecid, or valproic acid.

FOOD INTERACTIONS
No known food interactions.

DISEASE INTERACTIONS
Caution is advised when taking cefprozil. Consult your doctor if you have a history of kidney disease, phenylketonuria, or colitis.

Cefuroxime

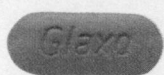
Side Effects

SERIOUS
Severe allergic reaction (breathing difficulties, confusion, hives, swelling of the face or throat, and lightheadedness), severe stomach pain and cramps, fever, severe, sometimes bloody diarrhea. Call your doctor immediately.

COMMON
Mild diarrhea or stomach cramps, sore mouth or tongue, nausea and vomiting.

LESS COMMON
Vaginal itching or discharge, pain at site of injection, rash, decreased white blood cell count causing increased susceptibility to infection, decreased blood platelets causing increased risk of bleeding problems.

PRINCIPAL USES
To treat a variety of bacterial infections, including those of the brain, ear, nose, tonsils, and throat, skin and soft tissues, genitourinary tract, respiratory tract, blood, bones, joints, and other organs. Cefuroxime also is used to treat gonorrhea and is given prior to some surgeries to prevent infection. It is effective only against susceptible infections caused by bacteria; it is ineffective against those caused by viruses, fungi, or other microorganisms.

HOW THE DRUG WORKS
Cefuroxime prevents bacteria from forming cell walls.

DOSAGE
Adults and teenagers— Tablets: 125 to 500 mg every 12 hours for 5 to 10 days. Injection: 750 to 1,500 mg every 6 to 8 hours into a vein or muscle. Children 3 months to 12 years— Tablets: 125 mg every 12 hours for 10 days. Injection: 16.7 to 33.3 mg per 2.2 lbs (1 kg) of body weight every 8 hours into a vein or muscle. Oral suspension: 10 to 15 mg per 2.2 lbs every 12 hours for 10 days. Special note— Gonorrhea is treated with a one-time tablet dose of 1,000 mg or a one-time injected dose of 1,500 mg into a muscle. The injected dose is divided and administered at 2 separate sites on the body, along with a single 1,000 mg oral dose of probenecid.

ONSET OF EFFECT
Into a vein: Immediate. Into a muscle: 15 to 60 minutes. Oral forms: Unknown.

DURATION OF ACTION
5 to 8 hours.

DIETARY ADVICE
Tablets can be taken without regard to meals. Take oral suspension with food to increase the absorption of the drug by the body. Maintain normal fluid intake.

STORAGE
Store in a tightly sealed container away from heat, moisture, and direct light. Keep liquid form refrigerated, but do not allow it to freeze.

IF YOU MISS A DOSE
Take it as soon as you remember. If it is near the time for the next dose, skip the missed dose and resume your regular dosage schedule. Do not double the next dose.

STOPPING THE DRUG
Take it as prescribed for the full treatment period, even if you begin to feel better before the scheduled end of therapy. Stopping prematurely may slow your recovery or lead to a rebound infection, also known as superinfection, in which the heartier strains of bacteria survive and multiply, leading to a more serious and drug-resistant infection. When taking this drug to treat a streptococcal (strep) infection, it is particularly important to take it for the entire treatment period. Serious heart and kidney problems can develop later if the drug is discontinued prematurely.

PROLONGED USE
Cefuroxime is generally prescribed for short-term therapy (5 to 10 days). Use beyond this period increases risks of adverse effects and superinfection.

PRECAUTIONS
Over 60: Adverse reactions may be more likely and more severe in older patients.

Driving and Hazardous Work: Do not drive or engage in hazardous work until you determine how the medicine affects you.

Alcohol: Avoid alcohol.

Pregnancy: Adequate studies of use during pregnancy have not been done. Consult your doctor for advice.

Breast Feeding: Cefuroxime passes into breast milk; caution is advised. Consult your doctor for advice.

Infants and Children: May be used by children 3 months and older. Consult your pediatrician for advice.

Special Concerns: Those who are allergic to penicillin may have equally serious allergic reactions to cephalosporin antibiotics. If your condition has not improved within a few days, or instead has worsened, tell your doctor. The tablets and the oral suspension can not be equally substituted for each other.

OVERDOSE
Symptoms: Seizures, severe abdominal pain, bloody diarrhea, vomiting.

What to Do: Seek medical assistance immediately.

DRUG INTERACTIONS
Consult your doctor for specific advice if you are taking carbenicillin injection, heparin, divalproex, anticoagulants, sulfinpyrazone, dipyridamole, pentoxifylline, plicamycin, ticarcillin, probenecid, or valproic acid.

FOOD INTERACTIONS
No known food interactions.

DISEASE INTERACTIONS
Consult your doctor if you have a history of kidney disease or colitis.

BRAND NAME
Celebrex

▶ Drug Class: Nonsteroidal anti-inflammatory drug (NSAID)/COX-2 inhibitor

▶ Available in: Capsules

▶ Available OTC? No

▶ As Generic? No

Side Effects

SERIOUS
Stomach ulcers. Black, tarry stools may signal stomach bleeding. Symptoms of liver disease (nausea, fatigue, lethargy, itching, yellowish discoloration of the eyes or skin, fluid retention). Call your doctor immediately.

COMMON
Indigestion, diarrhea, and mild abdominal pain.

LESS COMMON
Flatulence, mild swelling, sore throat, and upper respiratory tract infection.

PRINCIPAL USES
To relieve the pain, inflammation, and stiffness of osteoarthritis and rheumatoid arthritis.

HOW THE DRUG WORKS
By inhibiting the activity of the enzyme cyclooxygenase-2 (COX-2), celecoxib reduces the synthesis of prostaglandins that play a role in causing arthritis pain and inflammation. It does not inhibit the activity of COX-1, the enzyme involved in the synthesis of prostaglandins that help protect against stomach ulcers and other health problems.

DOSAGE
For osteoarthritis: 200 mg a day, either as one single dose or 100 mg twice a day. For rheumatoid arthritis: 100 to 200 mg twice a day. To minimize potential gastrointestinal side effects, the lowest effective dose should be used for the shortest possible time.

ONSET OF EFFECT
Within 24 to 48 hours.

DURATION OF ACTION
Unknown.

DIETARY ADVICE
Celecoxib may be taken with or without food.

STORAGE
Store in a tightly sealed container away from heat, moisture, and direct light.

IF YOU MISS A DOSE
Take it as soon as you remember. If it is near the time for the next dose, skip the missed dose and resume your regular dosage schedule. Do not double the next dose.

STOPPING THE DRUG
The decision to stop taking the drug should be made in consultation with your physician.

PROLONGED USE
The risk of gastrointestinal side effects may be increased with extended use.

PRECAUTIONS
Over 60: Adverse reactions may be more likely and more severe in older patients.

Driving and Hazardous Work: No special problems are expected.

Alcohol: Avoid alcohol when using this medication because it increases the risk of stomach irritation.

Pregnancy: Discuss with your doctor the relative risks and benefits of using this drug while pregnant. Do not use celecoxib during the last trimester.

Breast Feeding: Celecoxib may pass into breast milk; caution is advised. Consult your doctor for advice on whether to discontinue nursing or discontinue the drug.

Infants and Children: The safety and effectiveness of this drug have not been established for children under the age of 18.

OVERDOSE
Symptoms: No cases of overdose have been reported. Symptoms may include lethargy, drowsiness, nausea, vomiting, abdominal pain, black, tarry stools, breathing difficulty, and coma.

What to Do: If you suspect an overdose or if someone takes a much larger dose than prescribed, call your doctor, emergency medical services (EMS), or the nearest poison control center immediately.

DRUG INTERACTIONS
Do not take this drug with aspirin or any other NSAIDs without your doctor's approval. In addition, consult your doctor if you are taking furosemide, ACE inhibitors, fluconazole, lithium, or warfarin.

FOOD INTERACTIONS
No known food interactions.

DISEASE INTERACTIONS
Celecoxib should not be taken by people who have experienced asthma, hives, or allergic-type reactions after taking aspirin or other NSAIDs. Consult your doctor if you have any of the following: bleeding problems, inflammation or ulcers of the stomach and intestines, asthma, high blood pressure, or heart failure. Use of celecoxib may cause complications in patients with liver or kidney disease, since these organs work together to remove the medication from the body.

Cephalexin

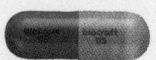

Generic 250 mg
(BIOCRAFT)

799

Additional photographs

▶ Drug Class: Cephalosporin antibiotic

▶ Available in: Capsules, oral suspension, tablets

▶ Available OTC? No

▶ As Generic? Yes

Side Effects

SERIOUS
Severe allergic reaction (breathing difficulties, confusion, hives, itching, swelling of the face or throat, unusual sweating, and lightheadedness), severe stomach pain and cramps, fever, severe, sometimes bloody diarrhea. Call your doctor immediately.

COMMON
Mild diarrhea or stomach cramps, sore mouth or tongue, nausea and vomiting.

LESS COMMON
Vaginal itching or unusual discharge, rash, decreased white blood cell count causing increased susceptibility to infection, decreased blood platelets causing increased risk of bleeding problems.

PRINCIPAL USES
To treat a variety of bacterial infections, including those of the ear, nose, tonsils, and throat, bones, joints, skin and soft tissues, genitourinary tract, and respiratory tract. It is effective only against infections caused by bacteria; it is ineffective against those caused by viruses, fungi, or other microorganisms.

HOW THE DRUG WORKS
Cephalexin prevents bacteria from forming cell walls.

DOSAGE
Adults and teenagers: 250 to 500 mg every 6 to 12 hours. Children: 6.25 to 25 mg per 2.2 lbs (1 kg) of body weight every 6 hours, or 12.5 to 50 mg per 2.2 lbs every 12 hours.

ONSET OF EFFECT
1 hour.

DURATION OF ACTION
Unknown.

DIETARY ADVICE
Cephalexin may be taken on a full or empty stomach, but taking it with food will reduce stomach irritation.

STORAGE
Store in a tightly sealed container away from heat, moisture, and direct light. Keep liquid form refrigerated, but do not allow it to freeze.

IF YOU MISS A DOSE
Take it as soon as you remember. This will help keep a constant level of medication in your system. If it is near the time for the next dose, skip the missed dose and resume your regular dosage schedule. Do not double the next dose.

STOPPING THE DRUG
Take it as prescribed for the full treatment period, even if you begin to feel better before the scheduled end of therapy. Stopping cephalexin prematurely may slow your recovery or lead to a rebound infection, also known as superinfection, in which the heartier strains of bacteria survive and multiply, leading to a more serious and drug-resistant infection. When taking this drug to treat a streptococcal (strep) infection, it is particularly important to take it for the entire treatment period. Serious heart and kidney problems can develop later if it is discontinued prematurely.

PROLONGED USE
Cephalexin is generally prescribed for short-term therapy (10 to 14 days). Further use increases the risk of adverse effects and superinfection.

PRECAUTIONS
Over 60: Adverse reactions may be more likely and more severe in older patients.

Driving and Hazardous Work: Do not drive or engage in hazardous work until you determine how the medicine affects you.

Alcohol: Avoid alcohol.

Pregnancy: Adequate studies of cephalosporin use in pregnant women have not been done. Before taking cephalexin, tell your doctor if you are pregnant or plan to become pregnant.

Breast Feeding: Cephalexin passes into breast milk; caution is advised. Consult your doctor for specific advice.

Infants and Children: Adequate studies of cephalexin use in children have not been done. Consult your pediatrician.

Special Concerns: People who are allergic to penicillin may have equally serious allergic reactions to cephalosporin antibiotics such as cephalexin. This drug is useful only against bacteria that are susceptible to its effects, not against colds, flu, or other viral infections. If your condition has not improved within a few days of starting cephalexin, or instead has worsened, tell your doctor.

OVERDOSE
Symptoms: Seizures, severe abdominal pain, bloody diarrhea, vomiting.

What to Do: Call your doctor, emergency medical services (EMS), or the nearest poison control center immediately.

DRUG INTERACTIONS
Consult your doctor for specific advice if you are taking carbenicillin injection, heparin, divalproex, anticoagulants, sulfinpyrazone, dipyridamole, pentoxifylline, plicamycin, ticarcillin, probenecid, or valproic acid.

FOOD INTERACTIONS
No known food interactions.

DISEASE INTERACTIONS
Caution is advised when taking cephalexin. Consult your doctor if you have a history of kidney disease or colitis.

Cephradine

Generic 250 mg
(BIOCRAFT)

▶ Drug Class: Cephalosporin antibiotic

▶ Available in: Oral suspension, capsules

▶ Available OTC? No

▶ As Generic? Yes

Side Effects

SERIOUS
Severe allergic reaction (breathing difficulties, confusion, hives, itching, swelling of the face or throat, sweating, and lightheadedness), severe stomach pain and cramps, fever, severe, sometimes bloody diarrhea. Call your doctor immediately.

COMMON
Mild diarrhea or stomach cramps, sore mouth or tongue, nausea and vomiting.

LESS COMMON
Vaginal itching or discharge.

PRINCIPAL USES
To treat a variety of bacterial infections, including those of the ear, nose, tonsils, and throat, skin and soft tissues, genitourinary tract, and the respiratory tract. Cephradine is effective only against infections caused by bacteria; it is ineffective against those caused by viruses, fungi, or other microorganisms.

HOW THE DRUG WORKS
Cephradine prevents bacteria from forming cell walls.

DOSAGE
Oral suspension and capsules— Adults and teenagers: 250 to 500 mg every 6 hours, or 500 to 1,000 mg every 12 hours. Children: 6.25 to 25 mg every 6 hours.

ONSET OF EFFECT
1 hour.

DURATION OF ACTION
Unknown.

DIETARY ADVICE
Cephradine may be taken on a full or empty stomach, but taking it with food will reduce stomach irritation.

STORAGE
Store in a tightly sealed container away from heat, moisture, and direct light. Keep liquid form refrigerated, but do not allow it to freeze.

IF YOU MISS A DOSE
Take it as soon as you remember. This will help keep a constant level of medication in your system. If it is near the time for the next dose, skip the missed dose and resume your regular dosage schedule. Do not double the next dose.

STOPPING THE DRUG
Take it as prescribed for the full treatment period, even if you begin to feel better before the scheduled end of therapy. Stopping cephradine prematurely may slow your recovery or lead to a rebound infection, also known as superinfection, in which the heartier strains of bacteria survive and multiply, leading to a more serious and drug-resistant infection. When taking this drug to treat a streptococcal (strep) infection, it is particularly important to take it for the entire treatment period. Serious heart and kidney problems can develop later if it is discontinued prematurely.

PROLONGED USE
Cephradine is generally prescribed for short-term therapy (10 to 14 days). Use of cephradine beyond this period increases the risk of adverse effects and superinfection.

PRECAUTIONS
Over 60: Adverse reactions may be more likely and more severe in older patients.

Driving and Hazardous Work: Do not drive or engage in hazardous work until you determine how the medicine affects you.

Alcohol: Avoid alcohol.

Pregnancy: Adequate studies of cephalosporin use during pregnancy have not been done. Consult your doctor for specific advice.

Breast Feeding: Cephradine passes into breast milk; caution is advised. Consult your doctor for specific advice.

Infants and Children: Cephradine may be used by children age 1 and older. Consult your pediatrician for specific advice.

Special Concerns: People who are allergic to penicillin may have equally serious allergic reactions to cephalosporin antibiotics such as cephradine. This drug is useful only against bacteria that are susceptible to its effects, not against colds, flu, or other viral infections. If your condition has not improved within a few days of starting cephradine, or instead has worsened, tell your doctor.

OVERDOSE
Symptoms: Seizures, severe abdominal pain, bloody diarrhea, vomiting.

What to Do: Call your doctor, emergency medical services (EMS), or the nearest poison control center immediately.

DRUG INTERACTIONS
Consult your doctor for specific advice if you are taking carbenicillin injection, heparin, divalproex, anticoagulants, sulfinpyrazone, dipyridamole, pentoxifylline, plicamycin, ticarcillin, probenecid, or valproic acid.

FOOD INTERACTIONS
No known food interactions.

DISEASE INTERACTIONS
Caution is advised when taking cephradine. Consult your doctor if you have a history of kidney disease or colitis.

Cetirizine

Zyrtec 10 mg
(PFIZER)

▶ Drug Class: Histamine (H1) blocker

▶ Available in: Tablets, syrup

▶ Available OTC? No

▶ As Generic? No

Side Effects

SERIOUS
No serious side effects are associated with the use of cetirizine.

COMMON
Drowsiness, fatigue, headache, dry mouth.

LESS COMMON
Nausea and vomiting.

PRINCIPAL USES
For symptomatic relief of perennial and seasonal allergies (including hay fever), itchy skin, and chronic hives.

HOW THE DRUG WORKS
Cetirizine blocks the effects of histamine, a naturally occurring substance within the body that causes swelling, itching, sneezing, watery eyes, hives, and other symptoms of allergic reaction.

DOSAGE
Adults and children over age 12: 5 to 10 mg once a day. Do not increase the dose to obtain quicker relief of symptoms. A lower dose (no more than 5 mg a day) is recommended for patients with impaired kidney or liver function.

ONSET OF EFFECT
Within 20 to 40 minutes.

DURATION OF ACTION
Approximately 24 hours.

DIETARY ADVICE
Cetirizine can be taken without regard to diet.

STORAGE
Store in a tightly sealed container away from heat, moisture, and direct light. Do not allow the syrup to freeze.

IF YOU MISS A DOSE
This drug is prescribed to be taken once a day. If you miss a day, skip the missed dose and resume your regular dosage schedule. Do not double the next dose.

STOPPING THE DRUG
Take it as prescribed for the full treatment period, even if you feel better before the scheduled end of therapy.

PROLONGED USE
Safety and effectiveness during prolonged use have yet to be established.

PRECAUTIONS
Over 60: The dosage may need to be reduced in elderly patients, especially for those in whom kidney function is impaired.

Driving and Hazardous Work: Do not drive or engage in hazardous work until you determine how the medication affects you.

Alcohol: Avoid alcohol while taking this medication, since it can magnify side effects such as drowsiness and fatigue.

Pregnancy: Adequate human studies of the use of this drug during pregnancy have not been done; caution is advised. Before taking cetirizine, tell your doctor if you are pregnant or plan to become pregnant.

Breast Feeding: Cetirizine passes into breast milk; avoid or discontinue use while nursing.

Infants and Children: The safety and effectiveness of cetirizine use by children under the age of 12 have not been established.

Special Concerns: If cetirizine causes dry mouth as a side effect, use sugarless gum, sugarless sour hard candy, or ice chips for relief.

OVERDOSE
Symptoms: No cases of overdose have been reported.

What to Do: An overdose of cetirizine is unlikely to be life-threatening. However, if someone takes a much larger dose than prescribed, call your doctor, emergency medical services (EMS), or the nearest poison control center immediately.

DRUG INTERACTIONS
No significant drug interactions have been reported. Cetirizine may, however, increase the depressant effects of alcohol, sedatives, tranquilizers, painkillers, barbiturates, or other antihistamines on the central nervous system. Consult your doctor for specific advice.

FOOD INTERACTIONS
No food interactions have been reported.

DISEASE INTERACTIONS
Cetirizine blood levels may increase in patients with liver or kidney disease, since these organs work together to remove the medication from the body. Reduced doses may be required for such persons.

Cevimeline Hydrochloride

BRAND NAME
Evoxac

▶ Drug Class: Cholinergic (muscarinic) agonist

▶ Available in: Capsules

▶ Available OTC? No

▶ As Generic? No

Side Effects

SERIOUS
Serious side effects are rare, but may include: heartbeat irregularities, chest pain, increased bronchial secretions. Some of these side effects may be relevant only to those who have a history of heart problems or respiratory conditions (see Disease Interactions).

COMMON
Excessive sweating, nausea, runny nose.

LESS COMMON
Excessive salivation, weakness, sinusitis, upper respiratory infection, abdominal pain, urinary tract infection, coughing, vomiting, back pain, conjunctivitis, bronchitis, joint pain, fatigue, pain, insomnia, hot flushes.

PRINCIPAL USES
To treat symptoms of dry mouth in patients with Sjogren's syndrome.

HOW THE DRUG WORKS
Cevimeline stimulates the secretion of glands such as salivary and sweat glands and increases the tone of smooth muscle in the gastrointestinal and urinary tracts.

DOSAGE
Adults: 30 mg 3 times a day.

ONSET OF EFFECT
Unknown.

DURATION OF ACTION
Unknown.

DIETARY ADVICE
Cevimeline may be taken with or without food.

STORAGE
Store in a tightly sealed container away from heat, moisture, and direct light.

IF YOU MISS A DOSE
Take it as soon as you remember. If it is near the time for the next dose, skip the missed dose and resume your regular dosage schedule. Do not double the next dose.

STOPPING THE DRUG
The decision to stop taking the drug should be made in consultation with your physician.

PROLONGED USE
See your doctor regularly for tests and examinations if you must take this drug for a prolonged period.

PRECAUTIONS
Over 60: Adverse reactions may be more likely and more severe.

Driving and Hazardous Work: This drug can cause visual blurring, which may affect depth perception, night vision, and general vision. Do not drive or engage in hazardous work until you determine how the medicine affects you.

Alcohol: Avoid alcohol while taking this medication, as the diuretic effect of alcohol may aggravate your condition.

Pregnancy: No human tests have been done. However, discuss with your doctor the relative risks and benefits of using this drug while pregnant.

Breast Feeding: Cevimeline may pass into breast milk; caution is advised. Consult your doctor for advice on whether to discontinue nursing or discontinue the drug.

Infants and Children: The safety and effectiveness of this drug have not been established for children under the age of 18.

Special Concerns: Dehydration may result if you sweat excessively while taking cevimeline. Drink extra water and consult your physician.

OVERDOSE
Symptoms: No cases of overdose have been reported.

What to Do: If you suspect an overdose or if someone takes a much larger dose than prescribed, call your doctor, emergency medical services (EMS), or the nearest poison control center immediately.

DRUG INTERACTIONS
Consult your doctor for specific advice if you are taking a beta-blocker.

FOOD INTERACTIONS
No known interactions.

DISEASE INTERACTIONS
Do not take cevimeline if you have uncontrolled asthma or if you have an eye condition, such as acute iritis or narrow-angle glaucoma, which may be aggravated by the drug's tendency to cause the pupil's to constrict. The drug should be used with caution in people with a history of kidney or gallbladder stones.

Charcoal, Activated

▶ Drug Class: Antidote

▶ Available in: Oral suspension, powder, tablets, capsules

▶ Available OTC? Yes

▶ As Generic? Yes

Side Effects

SERIOUS
Swelling or pain in stomach. If this symptom persists, call your doctor immediately.

COMMON
Black, tarry stools.

LESS COMMON
Nausea, constipation. Notify your doctor if any common or less-common side effects persist.

PRINCIPAL USES
Used as an emergency antidote for treatment of poisonings by most drugs and chemicals; also used to relieve diarrhea or excess gas.

HOW THE DRUG WORKS
Activated charcoal prevents the absorption of certain kinds of drugs and chemicals by the body.

DOSAGE
For treatment of poisoning— Oral suspension and powder: Adults and teenagers: 25 to 100 grams (g). Children: 1 g per 2.2 lbs (1 kg) of body weight, or 25 to 50 g. Mix powder with water. Take 1 time only. For treatment of diarrhea— Capsules: Adults and children age 3 and older: 520 mg every 30 to 60 minutes, as needed. Do not take more than 4.16 g per day. For treatment of excess gas— Tablets and capsules: Adults and teenagers: 975 mg to 3.9 g, 3 times a day.

ONSET OF EFFECT
Immediate.

DURATION OF ACTION
Not applicable. Activated charcoal is not absorbed by the body.

DIETARY ADVICE
As an antidote: No special restrictions. To treat diarrhea: It is important to replace the fluid lost by your body and to eat a proper diet. During the first 24 hours, drink plenty of caffeine-free clear liquids like water, broth, ginger ale, and decaffeinated tea. During the second 24 hours you may eat bland foods such as applesauce, bread, crackers, and oatmeal. Avoid caffeine, fried or spicy foods, bran, candy, fruits, and vegetables. These may worsen your condition.

STORAGE
Store in a tightly sealed container away from heat, moisture, and direct light. Premixed suspension can be stored for up to 1 year. Do not allow the liquid form of activated charcoal to freeze.

IF YOU MISS A DOSE
As an antidote: Not applicable. To treat diarrhea or excess gas: Take it as soon as you rcmcmber. If it is near the time for the next dose, skip the missed dose and resume your regular dosage schedule. Do not double the next dose.

STOPPING THE DRUG
As an antidote: Not applicable. To treat diarrhea or excess gas: Take as prescribed for the full treatment period. However, you may stop taking the drug if you are feeling better before the scheduled end of therapy.

PROLONGED USE
As an antidote: Not applicable. To treat diarrhea: If diarrhea has not improved or if you have developed a fever after 2 days, call your doctor. To treat excess gas: If your condition has not improved after 3 to 4 days, call your doctor.

PRECAUTIONS
Over 60: No special problems are expected.

Driving and Hazardous Work: The use of activated charcoal should not impair your ability to perform such tasks safely.

Alcohol: No special precautions are necessary.

Pregnancy: Activated charcoal has not been reported to cause problems in an unborn child. Consult your doctor for specific advice.

Breast Feeding: No problems have been reported.

Infants and Children: May be used in infants and children only under strict supervision by a doctor.

Special Concerns: Call your doctor, emergency medical services (EMS), or the nearest poison control center before administering activated charcoal. Charcoal will not be effective if you have been poisoned by swallowing alkalies (lye), petroleum products, strong acids, ethyl or methyl alcohol, iron, boric acid, or lithium. Activated charcoal will not prevent these poisons from being absorbed by the body. If inducing vomiting with ipecac syrup, do so 1 to 2 hours before administering activated charcoal.

OVERDOSE
Symptoms: None expected.

What to Do: Emergency procedures not applicable.

DRUG INTERACTIONS
Activated charcoal may decrease the absorption of any medicine taken within 2 hours of administration. Acetylcysteine and ipecac syrup can decrease the effectiveness of activated charcoal.

FOOD INTERACTIONS
Do not eat chocolate syrup, ice cream, or sherbet with activated charcoal. They will decrease the amount of poison the charcoal can absorb.

DISEASE INTERACTIONS
Caution is advised when taking activated charcoal if you also suffer from dysentery or dehydration.

Chloral Hydrate

BRAND NAME
Noctec

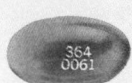

Generic 500 mg
(SCHEIN)

▶ Drug Class: Sedative/hypnotic

▶ Available in: Capsules, syrup

▶ Available OTC? No

▶ As Generic? Yes

Side Effects

SERIOUS
Hallucinations, confusion, excitability, skin rash, hives. Stop taking the drug and call your doctor immediately.

COMMON
Nausea, vomiting, stomach pain or abdominal discomfort, hangover-like symptoms, drowsiness.

LESS COMMON
Diarrhea, loss of coordination, dizziness or light-headedness.

PRINCIPAL USES
For the short-term treatment of insomnia. Chloral hydrate is being replaced by safer, more effective drugs for this purpose.

HOW THE DRUG WORKS
Drugs such as chloral hydrate depress activity in the central nervous system (brain and spinal cord), producing a mild sedative effect.

DOSAGE
Adults: 250 to 1,500 mg, 30 minutes before bedtime.

ONSET OF EFFECT
Within 30 minutes.

DURATION OF ACTION
From 4 to 8 hours.

DIETARY ADVICE
Both oral forms of chloral hydrate should be taken shortly after meals. They may be taken with a full glass of a liquid such as water, fruit juice, or ginger ale to improve flavor and minimize stomach upset.

STORAGE
Store in a tightly sealed container away from heat, moisture, and direct light. Avoid extremes in temperature.

IF YOU MISS A DOSE
If it is near the time for the next dose, skip the missed dose and resume your regular dosage schedule. Do not double the next dose.

STOPPING THE DRUG
The dosage will be gradually reduced to prevent withdrawal effects.

PROLONGED USE
Chloral hydrate may be habit-forming. Prolonged use increases the risk of drug dependency.

PRECAUTIONS
Over 60: Adverse reactions may be more likely and more severe in older patients.

Driving and Hazardous Work: Avoid such activities until you determine how this medication affects you.

Alcohol: Avoid alcohol while taking this drug.

Pregnancy: Adequate studies of the use of chloral hydrate during pregnancy have not been done. Before taking chloral hydrate, tell your doctor if you are pregnant or plan to become pregnant.

Breast Feeding: Chloral hydrate passes into breast milk; caution is advised. Consult your doctor for advice.

Infants and Children: Chloral hydrate should be used by children only under a doctor's supervision.

Special Concerns: Swallow the capsules whole. Do not chew them, since chloral hydrate has an unpleasant taste. Make sure your doctor has specifically indicated to your pharmacist both how many milligrams and how many capsules or teaspoonfuls you or your child should receive in a single dose.

OVERDOSE
Symptoms: Severe nausea, vomiting, or stomach pain; difficulty swallowing; severe drowsiness; continuing confusion; seizures; low body temperature; difficulty breathing or shortness of breath; irregular heartbeat; severe weakness; staggering; slurred speech.

What to Do: Call your doctor, emergency medical services (EMS), or the nearest poison control center immediately.

DRUG INTERACTIONS
The following drugs may interact with chloral hydrate. Consult your doctor for specific advice if you are taking anticoagulants, tricyclic antidepressants, or central nervous system depressants.

FOOD INTERACTIONS
No food interactions have been reported.

DISEASE INTERACTIONS
Caution is advised when taking chloral hydrate. Consult your doctor if you have any of the following: kidney or liver problems, ulcers or other intestinal problems, esophagitis, or sleep apnea.

Chlorambucil

Leukeran 2 mg
(**GLAXO WELLCOME**)

▶ Drug Class: Alkylating agent

▶ Available in: Tablets

▶ Available OTC? No

▶ As Generic? No

Side Effects

SERIOUS
Black or tarry stools; blood-tinged (pink or maroon) urine or stools; cough or hoarseness; fever; chills; lower back pain or pain in flanks; painful, difficult urination; small, red spots on the skin; bleeding from gums, nose, or other unusual places; easy bruising; shortness of breath. These side effects may mean that normal blood cells and special blood-clotting cells have been affected, or that normal immune cells have been affected and an infection is developing somewhere in your body. See your doctor right away if any of these occur.

COMMON
Nausea and vomiting.

LESS COMMON
Painful joints, rash, itching, swelling of feet or lower legs (edema), changes in menstruation.

PRINCIPAL USES
To treat some types of cancer, especially leukemia and lymphoma (cancer of the lymphatic system). More specifically, chlorambucil is used to treat chronic lymphocytic leukemia (a type of leukemia caused by overproduction and abnormal formation of certain white blood cells important in the body's immune system) and Hodgkin's disease (a type of cancer affecting the lymphatic system, characterized by painless swelling of the lymph nodes).

HOW THE DRUG WORKS
Chlorambucil kills cancer cells by interfering with the activity of their genetic material, thus preventing the cells from reproducing. The drug may also affect the growth and development of normal cells in the body, resulting in unpleasant side effects.

DOSAGE
Initial dose: 0.1 to 0.2 mg per 2.2 lbs (1 kg) of body weight daily (approximately 4 to 10 mg per day) for 3 to 6 weeks. Maintenance dose will depend on white blood cell counts.

ONSET OF EFFECT
Within 3 to 4 weeks.

DURATION OF ACTION
Unknown.

DIETARY ADVICE
Swallow with liquid 2 hours after a light meal. Drink plenty of fluids between meals.

STORAGE
Store in a tightly sealed container away from heat and direct light.

IF YOU MISS A DOSE
Take it as soon as you remember. If it is near the time for the next dose, skip the missed dose and resume your regular dosage schedule. Do not double the next dose.

STOPPING THE DRUG
The decision to stop taking chlorambucil should be made by your doctor.

PROLONGED USE
Consult with your doctor about the need for periodic medical exams and blood tests, since adverse reactions are more likely the longer the drug is used.

PRECAUTIONS
Over 60: Adverse reactions may be more likely and severe in elderly patients.

Driving and Hazardous Work: Should not interfere with any activities requiring mental alertness.

Alcohol: Avoid alcohol.

Pregnancy: Chlorambucil may cause birth defects. Persons of childbearing years should take steps to prevent pregnancy when being treated with this medication.

Breast Feeding: Not recommended during therapy.

Infants and Children: No special problems are expected, although children with impaired kidney function may be at greater risk of having seizures while taking chlorambucil.

Special Concerns: Infection is the single greatest threat to people receiving chemotherapy. Chlorambucil may lower your ability to resist infection by lowering the number of white blood cells in the blood. Therefore, do not receive any vaccinations without doctor's approval. Avoid people with infections. Inform your doctor immediately if you have fever, chills, diarrhea, or a cough.

OVERDOSE
Symptoms: Fever, chills, unusual bleeding, seizures, agitation.

What to Do: Call your doctor, emergency medical services (EMS), or the nearest poison control center immediately.

DRUG INTERACTIONS
Consult your doctor for specific advice if you are taking amphotericin B (by injection), other antineoplastic (anticancer) drugs, antithyroid medications, chloramphenicol, colchicine or other antigout drugs, corticosteroid drugs, or immunosuppressant drugs (such as azathioprine, cyclosporine, ganciclovir, and interferon).

FOOD INTERACTIONS
Avoid consuming excess quantities of foods high in fat or sugar.

DISEASE INTERACTIONS
Caution is advised. Consult your doctor if you have any of the following: gout; a history of kidney stones; an active infection; recent exposure to chicken pox or shingles; liver or kidney problems.

Chloramphenicol Ophthalmic and Otic

BRAND NAMES
Ak-Chlor, Chloracol, Chlorofair, Chloromycetin Ophthalmic, Chloromycetin Otic, Chloroptic, Econochlor, I-Chlor, Ocu-Chlor, Ophthoclor, Spectro-Chlor

▶ Drug Class: Antibiotic

▶ Available in: Ophthalmic solution and ointment, otic solution

▶ Available OTC? No

▶ As Generic? Yes

Side Effects

SERIOUS
Bone marrow depression is a rare complication of chloramphenicol use. Other serious side effects include pale skin, sore throat and fever, unusual bleeding or bruising, unusual fatigue, itching, redness, swelling, skin rash, and skin irritation. Stop using the medication and call your doctor immediately.

COMMON
No common side effects are associated with otic chloramphenicol. Ophthalmic chloramphenicol may delay healing of the surface layer of the cornea.

LESS COMMON
Stinging or burning sensation.

PRINCIPAL USES
To treat infections of the eye or of the ear canal.

HOW THE DRUG WORKS
Chloramphenicol inhibits the spread of bacteria by interfering with protein synthesis in bacterial cells, preventing them from multiplying.

DOSAGE
Ophthalmic solution: 1 drop every 1 to 4 hours. Ophthalmic ointment: Apply every 3 hours. Otic solution: 2 or 3 drops every 6 to 8 hours.

ONSET OF EFFECT
Unknown.

DURATION OF ACTION
Unknown.

DIETARY ADVICE
This drug can be used without regard to diet.

STORAGE
Store in a tightly sealed container away from heat, moisture, and direct light. Do not allow the medicine to freeze. You may refrigerate the otic solution.

IF YOU MISS A DOSE
Apply it as soon as you remember. If it is near the time for the next dose, skip the missed dose and resume your regular dosage schedule. Do not double the next dose.

STOPPING THE DRUG
Use this drug as prescribed for the full treatment period, even if you begin to feel better before the scheduled end of therapy.

PROLONGED USE
You should see your doctor regularly for tests and examinations if you take this drug for a prolonged period.

PRECAUTIONS
Over 60: No special problems are expected.

Driving and Hazardous Work: Do not drive or engage in hazardous work until you determine how the drug affects your vision.

Alcohol: Avoid alcohol.

Pregnancy: Caution is advised; consult your doctor about whether the benefits outweigh potential risks to the unborn child.

Breast Feeding: Chloramphenicol may pass into breast milk; caution is advised. Consult your doctor if you are considering breast feeding.

Infants and Children: Do not use this drug on infants or children unless specifically directed by your physician.

Special Concerns: To use the eye drops or the ointment, first wash your hands. Tilt your head back. Gently apply pressure to the inside corner of the eyelid and with the index finger of the same hand, pull downward on the lower eyelid to make a space. Drop the medicine or put a short strip of ointment (about ⅓ inch long) into this space and close your eye. Apply pressure for 1 or 2 minutes while keeping the eye closed without blinking. To use the ear drops, lie down or tilt your head so the infected ear faces up. Gently pull the earlobe up and back for adults (down and back for children) to straighten the ear canal. Drop the medicine into the ear. Keep the ear facing upward for 1 to 2 minutes after inserting the drops to allow the medicine to reach the infection. You may insert a cotton ball to prevent the medicine from leaking out. Make sure the applicator for eye or ear drops does not touch your eye, ear, finger, or any other surface.

OVERDOSE
Symptoms: No specific symptoms have been reported.

What to Do: An overdose of ophthalmic or otic chloramphenicol is unlikely to be life-threatening. If a large volume enters the eye, flush with water. If a large volume enters the ear or someone accidentally ingests the medication, call your physician, emergency medical services (EMS), or the nearest poison control center immediately.

DRUG INTERACTIONS
Other drugs may interact with ophthalmic or otic chloramphenicol. Consult your doctor for specific advice if you are taking any other prescription or over-the-counter medication.

FOOD INTERACTIONS
No known food interactions.

DISEASE INTERACTIONS
Caution is advised when taking ophthalmic or otic chloramphenicol. Consult your doctor if you have a perforated eardrum (for otic solution) or any other medical condition.

Chloramphenicol Oral and Topical

▶ Drug Class: Antibiotic

▶ Available in: Capsules, oral suspension, injection, cream

▶ Available OTC? No

▶ As Generic? Yes

Side Effects

SERIOUS
Pale or sickly appearance, sore throat, fever, unusual bruising or bleeding, unusual fatigue, confusion, delirium, headache, eye pain, blurring or loss of vision, weakness, numbness, tingling, or pain in hands or feet, skin rash, breathing difficulty. Call your doctor immediately.

COMMON
No common side effects are associated with the use of chloramphenicol.

LESS COMMON
Diarrhea, nausea, and vomiting.

PRINCIPAL USES
To treat serious infections caused by bacteria. Because of the risk of dangerous side effects, it is prescribed only when other less toxic antibiotics cannot be used.

HOW THE DRUG WORKS
Chloramphenicol works by killing bacteria or inhibiting their growth.

DOSAGE
Oral forms and injection—Adults and teenagers: 5.7 mg per lb of body weight, 4 times a day. Children: 5.7 mg per lb of body weight, 4 times a day, or 11.4 mg per lb, 2 times a day. Infants under 2 weeks: 2.8 mg per lb, 4 times a day. Cream—Apply to infected area of skin 3 or 4 times a day.

ONSET OF EFFECT
Unknown.

DURATION OF ACTION
Unknown.

DIETARY ADVICE
Oral forms work best when taken on an empty stomach, at least 1 hour before or 2 hours after meals, with a full glass of water.

STORAGE
Store in a tightly sealed container away from heat and direct light. Do not allow liquid forms to freeze.

IF YOU MISS A DOSE
Take it as soon as you remember. If it is near the time for the next dose, skip the missed dose and resume your regular dosage schedule. Do not double the next dose.

STOPPING THE DRUG
Take the medicine as prescribed for the full treatment period, even if you begin to feel better before the scheduled end of therapy.

PROLONGED USE
You should see your doctor regularly for tests and examinations if you must take this medicine for a prolonged period of time.

PRECAUTIONS
Over 60: In older patients it is not known whether chloramphenicol causes side effects different from or more severe than those in younger persons.

Driving and Hazardous Work: Do not drive or engage in hazardous work until you determine how the medicine affects you.

Alcohol: It is advisable to abstain from alcohol when fighting an infection.

Pregnancy: Chloramphenicol has not been shown to cause birth defects in humans. However, its use is not recommended in the weeks immediately before delivery because it can cause temporary adverse side effects in the newborn child. Consult your doctor before using this drug during pregnancy.

Breast Feeding: Chloramphenicol passes into breast milk; avoid or discontinue use while nursing.

Infants and Children: Adverse reactions may be more likely and more severe in newborn babies.

Special Concerns: Chloramphenicol may cause anemia, which may increase the risk of infections and other problems in the gums. Blood must be monitored frequently while using this medicine. Be careful when brushing and flossing. Delay dental work, if possible, until you have stopped taking chloramphenicol. Chloramphenicol may cause false results on blood sugar tests for diabetics. Use of chloramphenicol while you are receiving x-ray treatment can increase the risk of blood problems.

OVERDOSE
Symptoms: Nausea, vomiting, unpleasant taste in the mouth, diarrhea.

What to Do: An overdose of chloramphenicol is unlikely to be life-threatening, Nonetheless, call your doctor, emergency medical services (EMS), or the nearest poison control center immediately.

DRUG INTERACTIONS
Consult your doctor for specific advice if you are taking alfentanil, amphotericin B, antithyroid agents, azathioprine, chemotherapy drugs for cancer, colchicine, clindamycin, cyclophosphamide, ethotoin, erythromycins, oral antidiabetic agents, flucytosine, ganciclovir, interferon, mephenytoin, mercaptopurine, methotrexate, phenytoin, plicamycin, or zidovudine (AZT).

FOOD INTERACTIONS
No known food interactions.

DISEASE INTERACTIONS
Caution is advised when taking chloramphenicol. Consult your doctor if you have anemia or another blood disorder, liver disease, or if you are undergoing radiation therapy.

Chlordiazepoxide

BRAND NAME
Librium

Generic 10 mg
(BARR)

▶ Drug Class: Benzodiazepine tranquilizer; antianxiety agent

▶ Available in: Capsules, tablets, injection

▶ Available OTC? No

▶ As Generic? Yes

Side Effects

SERIOUS
Difficulty concentrating, outbursts of anger, other behavior problems, depression, hallucinations, confusion, memory impairment, faintness, muscle weakness, skin rash or itching, sore throat, fever and chills, sores or ulcers in throat or mouth, unusual bruising or bleeding, extreme fatigue, yellow discoloration of the eyes or skin. Call your doctor immediately.

COMMON
Drowsiness, loss of coordination, unsteady gait, dizziness, lightheadedness, slurred speech.

LESS COMMON
Change in sexual desire or ability, constipation, false sense of well-being, nausea and vomiting, urinary problems, unusual fatigue.

PRINCIPAL USES
To treat anxiety, muscle spasms, and alcohol withdrawal symptoms.

HOW THE DRUG WORKS
In general, chlordiazepoxide produces mild sedation by depressing activity in the central nervous system. In particular, the drug appears to enhance the effect of gamma-aminobutyric acid (GABA), a natural chemical that inhibits the firing of neurons and dampens the transmission of nerve signals, thus decreasing nervous excitation.

DOSAGE
For anxiety— Adults: 5 to 25 mg, 3 or 4 times per day. Patients older than 60 or those who have a chronic illness: Initial dose of 5 to 10 mg, 2 to 4 times per day. Dose may be increased by your doctor to a maximum of 25 mg, 2 to 3 times per day. For alcohol withdrawal— Initial dose is 50 to 100 mg, repeated as recommended by your doctor. Some patients will require up to 300 mg per day in the early stages of alcohol withdrawal. Your doctor will determine a daily maintenance dose once the early stages of withdrawal have passed.

ONSET OF EFFECT
Within 1 to 2 hours.

DURATION OF ACTION
Up to 48 hours.

DIETARY ADVICE
No special restrictions.

STORAGE
Store in a tightly sealed container away from heat, moisture, and direct light.

IF YOU MISS A DOSE
Take it as soon as you remember. If it is near the time for the next dose, skip the missed dose and resume your regular dosage schedule. Do not double the next dose.

STOPPING THE DRUG
Do not stop taking the drug abruptly or without your doctor's approval. Dosage should be reduced gradually to prevent withdrawal symptoms, including seizures.

PROLONGED USE
This medication may slowly lose its effectiveness with prolonged use. You should see your doctor for periodic evaluation if you must take it for an extended time.

PRECAUTIONS
Over 60: Adverse reactions may be more likely and more severe in older patients.

Driving and Hazardous Work: The use of this drug may impair your ability to perform such tasks safely.

Alcohol: Alcohol intake should be extremely moderate or stopped altogether while taking this drug.

Pregnancy: Use during pregnancy should be avoided if possible. Be sure to tell your doctor if you are pregnant or plan to become pregnant.

Breast Feeding: This drug passes into breast milk; do not take it while nursing.

Infants and Children: This drug is not recommended for use by children under the age of 6.

Special Concerns: Chlordiazepoxide use can lead to psychological or physical dependence. Never take more than the prescribed daily dose.

OVERDOSE
Symptoms: Extreme drowsiness, confusion, slurred speech, slow reflexes, poor coordination, staggering gait, tremor, slowed breathing, loss of consciousness.

What to Do: Call your doctor, emergency medical services (EMS), or the nearest poison control center immediately.

DRUG INTERACTIONS
Consult your doctor for specific advice if you are taking any drugs that depress the central nervous system; these include antihistamines, antidepressants or other psychiatric medications, barbiturates, sedatives, cough medicines, decongestants, and painkillers. Be sure your doctor knows about any over-the-counter medication you may take.

FOOD INTERACTIONS
None reported.

DISEASE INTERACTIONS
Consult your doctor if you have a history of alcohol or drug abuse, stroke or other brain disease, any chronic lung disease, hyperactivity, depression or other mental illness, myasthenia gravis, sleep apnea, epilepsy, porphyria, kidney disease, or liver disease.

Chlordiazepoxide/Amitriptyline

Generic 10\25 mg
(**MYLAN**)

▶ Drug Class: Benzodiazepine tranquilizer; antianxiety agent/antidepressant

▶ Available in: Tablets

▶ Available OTC? No

▶ As Generic? Yes

Side Effects

SERIOUS
Blurred vision, confusion, difficulty speaking or swallowing, eye pain, fainting, rapid or uneven heartbeat, hallucinations, poor balance, nervousness or restlessness, problems urinating, shakiness or trembling, shuffling walk, slowed movements, stiffness in the arms and legs.

COMMON
Dizziness, drowsiness, loss of coordination, poor balance, dry mouth, headache, increased appetite, nausea, fatigue or mild weakness, unpleasant taste in mouth or of food, unexpected weight gain.

LESS COMMON
Diarrhea, heartburn, increased sweating, vomiting, increased sensitivity to sunlight.

PRINCIPAL USES
Chlordiazepoxide/amitriptyline is used to treat anxiety occurring simultaneously with depression.

HOW THE DRUG WORKS
Chlordiazepoxide depresses activity in the central nervous system, producing a mild sedative effect. Amitriptyline affects the activity of certain brain chemicals (serotonin and norepinephrine) that are linked to mood, emotions, and mental state.

DOSAGE
Adults: Initial dose is 5 mg of chlordiazepoxide and 12.5 mg of amitriptyline, or 10 mg of chlordiazepoxide and 25 mg of amitriptyline, 3 to 4 times daily. Some patients require higher doses, while some do well with lower doses. Your doctor will determine the correct dose.

ONSET OF EFFECT
The antianxiety and sedation effects occur within the first week of therapy. The antidepressant effect may require several weeks.

DURATION OF ACTION
Unknown.

DIETARY ADVICE
No special restrictions.

STORAGE
Store in a tightly sealed container away from heat, moisture, and direct light.

IF YOU MISS A DOSE
Take it as soon as you remember. If it is near the time for the next dose, skip the missed dose and resume your regular dosage schedule. Do not double the next dose.

STOPPING THE DRUG
Discontinuing the drug abruptly may produce withdrawal symptoms. Dosage should be reduced gradually according to your doctor's instructions.

PROLONGED USE
Short-term therapy (8 weeks or less) is typical; do not take it for a longer period unless so advised by your doctor.

PRECAUTIONS
Over 60: Adverse reactions may be more likely and more severe in older patients.

Driving and Hazardous Work: This drug can impair mental alertness and physical coordination. Adjust your activities accordingly.

Alcohol: Avoid alcohol while using this medication.

Pregnancy: Use during pregnancy should be avoided if possible. Be sure to tell your doctor if you are pregnant or plan to become pregnant.

Breast Feeding: Avoid or discontinue use while breast feeding.

Infants and Children: This drug combination is not recommended for use by infants and children.

Special Concerns: Use of this medication can lead to physical dependence. Never take more than the prescribed daily dose.

OVERDOSE
Symptoms: Confusion; convulsions; poor concentration; severe drowsiness, fatigue, or weakness (some patients will become unusually restless or agitated); dilated pupils; rapid or irregular heartbeat; rapid, shallow breathing, shortness of breath, or other breathing trouble; fever; hallucinations.

What to Do: Call your doctor, emergency medical services (EMS), or the nearest poison control center immediately.

DRUG INTERACTIONS
Consult your doctor for specific advice if you are taking sedatives, tranquilizers, or other medications that cause drowsiness; amphetamines or diet pills; asthma medication; prescription or nonprescription decongestants; prescription or nonprescription medicine for colds, sinus problems, allergies, and hay fever; high blood pressure medication; thyroid medicine; or MAO inhibitors.

FOOD INTERACTIONS
None reported.

DISEASE INTERACTIONS
Consult your doctor if you have a history of alcohol or drug abuse, stroke or other brain disease, any chronic lung disease, glaucoma, hyperactivity, depression or other mental illness, myasthenia gravis, sleep apnea, epilepsy, porphyria, kidney disease, or liver disease.

Chlorhexidine Gluconate

▶ Drug Class: Topical antiseptic; anti-infective

▶ Available in: Skin cleanser, wound cleanser, oral rinse

▶ Available OTC? No

▶ As Generic? No

Side Effects

SERIOUS
Rare severe allergic reaction with swelling, breathing difficulty, and even complete closure of the airways with potentially fatal anaphylactic shock. Seek medical assistance immediately.

COMMON
Staining (sometimes heavy) of the teeth, gums, dental fillings, dentures, and other oral surfaces (staining may be more pronounced in patients with greater pre-existing plaque accumulation); alteration in taste perception (taste perception returns to normal when medicine is discontinued); paradoxical increase in plaque buildup on the teeth.

LESS COMMON
Irritation or allergy of the skin, gums, tongue, or other mouth surfaces with redness, burning, stinging, or rash; swollen glands in the neck or sides of the face.

PRINCIPAL USES
Skin or wound cleanser: To prevent infection. Oral rinse: To treat gingivitis (inflammation of the gums, marked by redness, tenderness, swelling, and bleeding of gum tissue).

HOW THE DRUG WORKS
On the skin, it reduces surface bacteria to prevent infection. In the mouth, chlorhexidine kills the bacteria that cause dental plaque and gingivitis. However, it cannot prevent plaque from forming, nor does it remove plaque that has already formed. Scrupulous brushing and flossing and regular visits to a dentist are still necessary.

DOSAGE
Skin cleanser: 5 ml (1 teaspoon) lathered for 30 seconds to 3 minutes and rinsed. Oral rinse: average adult dose (individual dose may vary): 15 ml (1 capful), used as a mouthwash for 30 seconds, twice a day, after brushing and flossing teeth. Do not dilute the drug with water. Rinse your mouth thoroughly before use and be careful not to swallow any of the product. Do not rinse with water after using the medication.

ONSET OF EFFECT
Within 1 hour.

DURATION OF ACTION
Unknown.

DIETARY ADVICE
Do not eat or drink for 2 to 3 hours following treatment.

STORAGE
Store in a tightly sealed container away from heat and direct light. Do not allow the medication to freeze.

IF YOU MISS A DOSE
Use as soon as you remember. If it is near the time for the next dose, skip the missed dose and resume your regular dosing schedule following the next brushing. Do not double the next dose.

STOPPING THE DRUG
Use for the full treatment period, unless directed otherwise by your doctor or dentist.

PROLONGED USE
See your doctor as recommended; see your dentist every 6 months for professional cleaning and evaluation of the progress of therapy.

PRECAUTIONS
Over 60: No precautions.

Driving and Hazardous Work: No special precautions are necessary.

Alcohol: No special restrictions. Persons with a history of alcoholism, however, should not use chlorhexidine oral rinse since it contains a relatively high percentage of alcohol, which may trigger a relapse of alcohol abuse.

Pregnancy: Adequate human studies have not been done; consult your doctor.

Breast Feeding: No problems have been documented, but be sure your doctor knows if you are breast feeding.

Infants and Children: It is not commonly prescribed for patients under 18 years old; children may be most susceptible to side effects, especially those related to alcohol intoxication (oral rinse contains more than 10% alcohol).

Special Concerns: If the skin or wound being scrubbed with chlorhexidene appears to become infected, notify your doctor immediately. Do not allow the medication to come in contact with eyes or ears, since it may cause permanent injury. Do not use chlorhexidine if you have had a prior allergic reaction to it. Cosmetic dentistry may be needed to treat discoloration of teeth.

OVERDOSE
Symptoms: Slurred speech, staggering, drowsiness or stupor, stomach upset, nausea (overdose is most likely to affect young or underweight patients).

What to Do: Call your doctor or EMS right away if anyone—especially a child—accidentally ingests more than 4 oz of chlorhexidine or exhibits the above symptoms.

DRUG INTERACTIONS
Do not use any other prescription or nonprescription medications for the area of the skin being treated or for the mouth without checking with your doctor or dentist.

FOOD INTERACTIONS
No known food interactions.

DISEASE INTERACTIONS
Do not take chlorhexidine gluconate if you have periodontal disease (various disorders of the bones of the jaw and other tissues surrounding and supporting the teeth).

Chloroquine

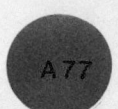

A 77

Aralen Phosphate 500 mg
(Sanofi Winthrop)

▶ Drug Class: Anti-infective/
antimalarial

▶ Available in: Tablets, injection

▶ Available OTC? No

▶ As Generic? Yes

Side Effects

SERIOUS
Blurred or altered vision;
blood problems including
low white blood cell
count (sore throat, fever),
anemia (fatigue, weak-
ness), and low platelet
count (easy bleeding and
bruising). Such side
effects are extremely
rare; call your doctor
immediately if they
occur.

COMMON
No common side effects
are associated with
chloroquine.

LESS COMMON
Diarrhea, loss of appetite,
headache, stomach
cramps or pain, nausea
or vomiting, itching, dizziness, fatigue, confusion,
loss or bleaching of hair,
skin rash. Also blue-black
discoloration of skin,
inside of mouth, or

PRINCIPAL USES
To prevent and treat malaria
caused by specific strains of
plasmodia (the parasite that
causes malaria) that are susceptible to chloroquine.
(The drug is ineffective
against other strains.) It is
also used with another drug
as a second line of therapy
for hard-to-treat amebic
(parasitic) liver abscess.

HOW THE DRUG WORKS
Chloroquine is poisonous to
the malarial parasite.

DOSAGE
Tablets— For malaria pre-
vention: 500 mg (300 mg
base) once a week. For
treatment of malaria: To
start, 1,000 mg (600 mg
base). Then, 500 mg (300
mg base), 6 to 8 hours after
the first dose, and 500 mg
once a day on the second
and third days of treatment.
To treat amebic liver
abscess: To start, 250 mg
(150 mg base), 4 times a
day for 2 days. Then, 250
mg twice a day for at least 2
to 3 weeks. Injection— For
treatment of malaria: 200 to
250 mg (160 to 200 mg
base). If needed, the dose
may be repeated after 6
hours, not to exceed 1,000
mg (800 mg base) in the
first 24 hours. To treat amebic liver abscess: 200 to 250
mg a day for 10 to 12 days.
(Note: All dosages are for
adults and adolescents.
Consult your pediatrician
for children's doses, which
are based on body weight
and should not exceed
adult doses.)

ONSET OF EFFECT
Unknown.

DURATION OF ACTION
Unknown.

DIETARY ADVICE
Take it with food or milk to
reduce stomach upset.

STORAGE
Store in a tightly sealed container away from heat, moisture, and direct light.

IF YOU MISS A DOSE
If taking 1 or more doses a
day, take it as soon as you
remember. If it is near the
time for the next dose, skip
the missed dose and
resume your regular dosage
schedule. Do not double the
next dose. If taking 1
weekly dose, take it as soon
as possible, then resume
regular schedule.

STOPPING THE DRUG
Take it as prescribed for the
full treatment period.

PROLONGED USE
If you are taking this drug
as a preventive, your doctor
may want you to begin 1 to
2 weeks before you travel to
an area where malaria is
prevalent. Keep taking
chloroquine while you are
in the area and for 4 weeks
after you leave.

PRECAUTIONS
Over 60: Adverse reactions
may be more likely and
more severe.

**Driving and Hazardous
Work:** Do not drive or
engage in hazardous work
until you determine how the
medicine affects you.

Alcohol: No special precautions are necessary.

Pregnancy: The use of
chloroquine is discouraged
during pregnancy because
of the risks it poses to the
unborn child. However, in
some cases it may be pre-
scribed to prevent or treat
malaria or amebic liver
abscess, since the risks of
these diseases are poten-
tially more serious than
those posed by the drug.
Consult your doctor for
advice.

Breast Feeding: Chloroquine passes into breast
milk; extreme caution is
advised. Consult your physician for specific advice.

Infants and Children:
Extreme caution is neces-
sary when used by children.

Special Concerns: If you
take chloroquine once a
week, take it on the same
day every week. Malaria is
spread by mosquitoes. Take
appropriate precautions,
such as using mosquito netting, to guard against being
bitten by malaria-carrying
mosquitoes.

OVERDOSE
Symptoms: Increased
excitability, headache,
drowsiness, seizures, vision
changes, heartbeat irregularities, low blood pressure
(causing dizziness or fainting), respiratory and cardiac arrest.

What to Do: Seek medical
assistance immediately.

DRUG INTERACTIONS
Consult your doctor for specific advice if you are taking
magnesium salts, antacids,
cimetidine, or penicillamine.
The intradermal rabies vaccine may not be effective if
chloroquine is being used at
the time of vaccination.

FOOD INTERACTIONS
No known food interactions.

DISEASE INTERACTIONS
Consult your doctor for specific advice if you have a
severe blood disorder, any
eye disorder, liver disease, a
severe nervous system disorder, G6PD deficiency, porphyria, or psoriasis.

Chlorothiazide

BRAND NAMES
Diurigen, Diuril

Generic 250 mg
(WEST POINT)

▶ Drug Class: Thiazide diuretic

▶ Available in: Tablets, oral suspension, injection

▶ Available OTC? No

▶ As Generic? Yes

Side Effects

SERIOUS
Skin rash, hives, intense itching, swelling of the mouth and throat, breathing difficulty, serious heartbeat irregularities or palpitations, lightheadedness or dizziness, unusual bleeding or bruising. Call your doctor immediately.

COMMON
Potassium depletion may lead to heart palpitations and weakness. Fluid depletion may lead to dizziness, especially upon arising from a sitting or lying position.

LESS COMMON
Decreased sexual ability, increased sensitivity to sunlight, loss of appetite, gout, increased blood sugar (a problem for patients with diabetes).

PRINCIPAL USES
To treat high blood pressure and conditions causing edema (swelling of body tissues resulting from excess salt and water retention).

HOW THE DRUG WORKS
Diuretics increase the excretion of salt and water in the urine. By reducing the overall fluid volume in the body, these drugs reduce blood volume and so reduce pressure within the blood vessels.

DOSAGE
Adults— For high blood pressure: 250 mg once a day. To reduce edema: 250 to 500 mg once a day, or 2 or 3 days a week.

ONSET OF EFFECT
2 hours after oral dose; 15 minutes after injection.

DURATION OF ACTION
6 to 12 hours.

DIETARY ADVICE
Tablets should be taken with food.

STORAGE
Store in a tightly sealed container away from heat and direct light. Keep the liquid form from freezing.

IF YOU MISS A DOSE
Take it as soon as you remember. If it is near the time for the next dose, skip the missed dose and resume your regular dosage schedule. Do not double the next dose.

STOPPING THE DRUG
The decision to stop taking the drug should be made by your doctor.

PROLONGED USE
See your doctor regularly for examinations and tests if you must take this medicine for an extended period.

PRECAUTIONS
Over 60: No special problems are expected.

Driving and Hazardous Work: No special precautions are necessary.

Alcohol: No special precautions are necessary.

Pregnancy: Chlorothiazide has caused birth defects in animals. Human studies have not been done. This medicine should not be taken during pregnancy unless recommended by your doctor. Other diuretics are preferred in pregnant women.

Breast Feeding: Chlorothiazide passes into breast milk; avoid or discontinue use during the first month of nursing.

Infants and Children: This drug generally is not prescribed for children.

Special Concerns: Chlorothiazide is usually taken once a day. To prevent it from interfering with sleep, take it in the morning (unless otherwise prescribed by your doctor). If you are taking it for high blood pressure, follow the diet and weight control measures recommended by your doctor. Avoid exposure to sunlight, use a sunblock, or wear protective clothing. This medicine may cause your body to lose potassium. Follow your doctor's instructions about eating potassium-rich foods or taking a potassium supplement.

OVERDOSE
Symptoms: Lethargy, dizziness, drowsiness, muscle weakness, cramps, heartbeat irregularities, fainting.

What to Do: Call your doctor, emergency medical services (EMS), or the nearest poison control center immediately.

DRUG INTERACTIONS
Consult your doctor for specific advice if you are taking anticoagulants, cholestyramine, colestipol, drugs for diabetes, nonsteroidal anti-inflammatory drugs, digitalis drugs, or lithium.

FOOD INTERACTIONS
No known food interactions.

DISEASE INTERACTIONS
Caution is advised when taking chlorothiazide. Consult your doctor if you have any of the following: diabetes, gout, lupus erythematosus, pancreatitis, heart disease, blood vessel disease, liver disease, or kidney disease.

▶ Drug Class: Female sex hormone

▶ Available in: Capsules

▶ Available OTC? No

▶ As Generic? Yes

Side Effects

SERIOUS
Profuse or abnormal vaginal bleeding, blood clots (pain, redness, swelling in arm, leg, or buttock), stroke (slurred speech, loss of sensation, blurry vision), chest pain, shortness of breath. Call your doctor immediately.

COMMON
Nausea, diarrhea, stomach cramps, loss of appetite, breast pain or tenderness. In men: Breast enlargement, reduction in the size of the testicles, diminished sex drive.

LESS COMMON
Rash, joint pain, lumps in breast, depression, dizziness, migraine headaches.

PRINCIPAL USES
To relieve the symptoms of inoperable prostate cancer and ease some of the symptoms of menopause (hot flashes, sweating, chills, faintness). Chlorotrianisene may also be used to prevent breast engorgement following childbirth.

HOW THE DRUG WORKS
In women, chlorotrianisene supplements deficient natural levels of estrogen in the body. In men, the drug inhibits growth of cells in the prostate gland.

DOSAGE
For prostate cancer: 12 to 25 mg a day. For menopausal symptoms: 12 to 25 mg a day for 30 days or a cyclic regimen that requires 3 weeks on and 1 week off.

ONSET OF EFFECT
Unknown.

DURATION OF ACTION
24 hours.

DIETARY ADVICE
Take chlorotrianisene with or immediately following a meal to reduce nausea. If you have difficulty swallowing the capsule whole, open it and take it with liquid or food. Follow a low-sodium diet, since sodium causes your body to retain excess water.

STORAGE
Store in a tightly sealed container away from heat, moisture, and direct light.

IF YOU MISS A DOSE
Take it as soon as you remember, unless the time for your next scheduled dose is within the next 12 hours. If so, skip the missed dose and resume your regular dosage schedule. Do not double the next dose.

STOPPING THE DRUG
Take it as prescribed for the full treatment period, even if you begin to feel better before the scheduled end of therapy. The decision to stop taking the drug should be made in consultation with your doctor.

PROLONGED USE
Prolonged use of chlorotrianisene may lead to an increased risk of uterine or breast cancer and growth of fibroid tumors of the uterus (a common benign tumor). Talk to your doctor about the need for follow-up medical examinations or laboratory tests including Pap smear, mammogram, and liver function tests.

PRECAUTIONS
Over 60: Adverse reactions may be more likely and more severe in elderly patients.

Driving and Hazardous Work: This drug does not interfere with your ability to engage in such activities.

Alcohol: No special precautions are necessary.

Pregnancy: You should not use chlorotrianisene if you are pregnant or plan to become pregnant.

Breast Feeding: Chlorotrianisene is used to prevent breast engorgement and milk production following pregnancy; it should not be used by women wishing to nurse.

Infants and Children: Not prescribed for children.

Special Concerns: If you are on cyclic therapy (3 weeks on, 1 week off) for menopausal symptoms, some minor vaginal bleeding may occur during the week you are not taking the drug. This symptom is common and should diminish at the start of the next treatment cycle.

OVERDOSE
Symptoms: Nausea, vomiting, fluid retention, breast enlargement, abnormal vaginal bleeding.

What to Do: Call your doctor, emergency medical services (EMS), or the nearest poison control center immediately.

DRUG INTERACTIONS
Consult your doctor for specific advice if you are taking antidepressants, aspirin, barbiturates, bromocriptine, calcium supplements, corticosteroids, corticotropin, cyclosporine, dantrolene, nicotine, somatropin, tamoxifen, or warfarin.

FOOD INTERACTIONS
No known food interactions.

DISEASE INTERACTIONS
Caution is advised when taking chlorotrianisene. Consult your doctor if you have any of the following: a history of cancer of the breast or reproductive organs; a family history of breast cancer; breast lumps; heart or blood vessel disease; asthma; bone disease; gallbladder disease; liver or kidney problems; migraines; seizures; or phlebitis.

Chlorpheniramine Maleate Oral

Chlor-Trimeton Allergy 8 Hr. 8 mg
(SCHERING-PLOUGH)

Additional photographs

▶ Drug Class: Antihistamine

▶ Available in: Tablets, sustained-release capsules, syrup

▶ Available OTC? Yes

▶ As Generic? Yes

Side Effects

SERIOUS
Bleeding problems; small red pinpoints on the skin; fever; extreme fatigue; bleeding ulcers in the rectum, mouth, and vagina; reduced count of white blood cells (rare).

COMMON
Drowsiness; unusual excitability; dry mouth, nose, or throat. Symptoms of drowsiness tend to subside after a few days' use as your body adjusts to the drug.

LESS COMMON
Vision changes, loss of appetite, dizziness, painful or difficult urination, less tolerance for contact lenses.

PRINCIPAL USES
To relieve the symptoms of hay fever and other allergies, and for itching skin and hives.

HOW THE DRUG WORKS
Chlorpheniramine maleate works by blocking the effects of histamine, a naturally occurring substance that causes swelling, itching, sneezing, watery eyes, hives, and other symptoms of allergic reaction.

DOSAGE
Tablets— Adults: 4 mg, 3 to 4 times per day as needed, for a maximum dose of 24 mg a day. Sustained-release capsules— 8 mg every 8 hours, or 12 mg every 12 hours, as needed. Syrup— Children ages 6 to 12: 2 mg, 3 to 4 times a day, not exceeding 12 mg a day. Children ages 2 to 6: 1 mg every 6 hours.

ONSET OF EFFECT
15 to 60 minutes.

DURATION OF ACTION
3 to 6 hours for regular form, 8 to 12 hours for sustained-release capsules.

DIETARY ADVICE
Chlorpheniramine maleate may be taken with food or milk to reduce stomach upset. Use sugarless gum, sugarless sour hard candy, or ice chips to ease dry mouth.

STORAGE
Store in a tightly sealed container away from heat and direct light.

IF YOU MISS A DOSE
Take it as soon as you remember, up to 2 hours late. If it is more than 2 hours late, skip the missed dose and resume your regular dosage schedule. Do not double the next dose.

STOPPING THE DRUG
You should take it as prescribed for the full treatment period, but you may stop if you are feeling better before the scheduled end of therapy. Chlorpheniramine may be taken as needed.

PROLONGED USE
No special concerns.

PRECAUTIONS
Over 60: Older persons are more sensitive to antihistamine side effects, particularly confusion, dizziness, drowsiness, restlessness, irritability, nightmares, and dry mouth, nose, and throat.

Driving and Hazardous Work: Do not drive or engage in hazardous work until you determine how the medicine affects you. Use of this drug is a disqualification for piloting aircraft.

Alcohol: Alcohol increases the likelihood and the severity of side effects like drowsiness and confusion.

Pregnancy: In animal studies, no birth defects have been reported. Studies of pregnant women have not been undertaken. Before taking this drug, tell your doctor if you are pregnant or are planning to become pregnant.

Breast Feeding: Chlorpheniramine passes into breast milk; avoid or discontinue use while nursing.

Infants and Children: This drug is not recommended for children under the age of 2.

Special Concerns: Do not break, crush, or chew sustained-release capsules.

OVERDOSE
Symptoms: Marked drowsiness, dilated and sluggish pupils, combativeness, excessive excitability, confusion, loss of coordination, weak pulse, seizures, loss of consciousness.

What to Do: Patient should be made to vomit immediately, using ipecac syrup. If the patient is unconscious, he or she should be taken to the nearest hospital emergency room right away.

DRUG INTERACTIONS
Consult your doctor for specific advice if you are taking anticholinergics, bepridil, medications containing alcohol, or MAO inhibitors.

FOOD INTERACTIONS
No known food interactions.

DISEASE INTERACTIONS
Before taking chlorpheniramine, consult your doctor if you wear contact lenses or if you have glaucoma, prostate enlargement, difficulty with urination, or dry mouth or eyes.

BRAND NAME
Thorazine

Generic 10 mg
(GENEVA)

▶ Drug Class: Neuroleptic; antipsychotic

▶ Available in: Capsules, tablets, liquid concentrate, syrup, suppositories

▶ Available OTC? No

▶ As Generic? Yes

Side Effects

SERIOUS
Extreme and persistent restlessness; uncontrolled movements, including tics, twitching, twisting movements, and muscle spasms in the face, neck, and back; loss of coordination and balance; shuffling gait; trembling, weakness, or stiffness in the extremities; difficulty swallowing or speaking; persistent, uncontrolled chewing, lip-smacking, or tongue movements; staring and absence of facial expression; fainting; difficulty urinating; increased skin sensitivity to the sun; skin rash; yellow discoloration of the eyes or skin (indicating a liver disorder).

COMMON
Constipation, decreased sweating, lightheadedness, dizziness or faintness, drowsiness, dry mouth.

LESS COMMON
Menstrual irregularities; sexual dysfunction; breast pain, swelling, or secretion; weight gain; blurred vision.

PRINCIPAL USES
To treat psychotic conditions such as schizophrenia. It can also be used to ease severe nausea and vomiting, and persistent hiccups.

HOW THE DRUG WORKS
Chlorpromazine inhibits activity of the brain chemical dopamine, thereby helping to prevent the overstimulation of specific nerve centers believed to be responsible for certain psychiatric disorders. The drug also suppresses activity in the trigger zones of the brain and gastrointestinal tract that govern the vomiting reflex and hiccupping.

DOSAGE
Dose, dosage form, and dosing schedule vary based on many factors, including patient's age, medical condition, body weight, tolerance of side effects, and overall response to the drug. Usual adult dose: Initially, 10 to 25 mg, 3 or 4 times a day. Your doctor may increase it as needed and tolerated; maximum dose may reach 200 mg a day for many, or even 800 mg a day for severely psychotic patients. Children: Consult your pediatrician.

ONSET OF EFFECT
For psychotic conditions: 4 to 6 weeks. For nausea and vomiting: 1 hour or less.

DURATION OF ACTION
Unknown.

DIETARY ADVICE
Take it with meals in order to reduce stomach upset.

STORAGE
Store in a tightly sealed container away from heat, moisture, and direct light.

IF YOU MISS A DOSE
Take it as soon as you remember. However, if it is near the time for the next dose, skip the missed dose and resume your regular dosage schedule. Do not double the next dose.

STOPPING THE DRUG
Do not stop taking the drug abruptly or without your doctor's approval. Dosage should be reduced gradually by your doctor to prevent withdrawal symptoms.

PROLONGED USE
Prolonged use may lead to tardive dyskinesia (involuntary movements of the jaw, lips, and tongue). Consult your doctor about the need for follow-up evaluations and tests if you must take this drug for an extended period.

PRECAUTIONS
Over 60: Adverse reactions, especially drowsiness and low blood pressure, are more common in elderly patients. A lower dose may be warranted.

Driving and Hazardous Work: The use of this drug may impair your ability to perform such tasks safely.

Alcohol: Avoid alcohol.

Pregnancy: Avoid using this drug if you are pregnant or plan to become pregnant.

Breast Feeding: Either avoid taking the drug if possible or refrain from breast feeding.

Infants and Children: This drug should not be used by infants and children younger than 2 years old. For older children, use it only under the care of your pediatrician.

OVERDOSE
Symptoms: Extreme drowsiness, heart rhythm irregularities, dry mouth, restlessness or agitation, seizures, unconsciousness.

What to Do: Call your doctor, emergency medical services (EMS), or the nearest poison control center immediately.

DRUG INTERACTIONS
Consult your doctor for specific advice if you are taking amantadine, high blood pressure medication, bromocriptine, deferoxamine, diuretics, levobunolol, heart medication, metoprolol, nabilone, other psychiatric drugs, pentamidine, pimozide, promethazine, trimeprazine, a thyroid agent, central nervous system depressants, epinephrine, lithium, levodopa, methyldopa, metoclopramide, metyrosine, pemoline, a rauwolfia alkaloid, or metrizamide.

FOOD INTERACTIONS
No known food interactions.

DISEASE INTERACTIONS
Consult your doctor if you have a history of alcohol abuse, any blood disorder, breast cancer, benign prostatic hyperplasia (BPH), epilepsy or seizures, glaucoma, heart, lung, or blood vessel disease, liver disease, Parkinson's disease, peptic ulcer, or urinary difficulty.

Chlorpropamide

BRAND NAMES
Chlorabetic, Diabinese,
Glucamide, Insulase

Generic 100 mg
(SIDMAK)

▶ Drug Class: Antidiabetic
agent/sulfonylurea

▶ Available in: Tablets

▶ Available OTC? No

▶ As Generic? Yes

Side Effects

SERIOUS
Low blood sugar; perspiration or a cold sweat; restlessness; rapid pulse; anxious feeling; nausea; difficulty breathing; feelings of dizziness, weakness, or lightheadedness; poor coordination, slurred speech, confusion; sleepiness; seizures or convulsions; weakness of an arm, leg, or an entire side of the body; fainting. Contact your doctor immediately. Administer sugar-containing substances only if the patient is conscious and alert.

COMMON
Mild dizziness, diarrhea, frequent or unusual hunger, nausea, heartburn, itching, changes in taste, constipation, fluid retention, rash.

LESS COMMON
Fatigue, heightened skin sensitivity to light, yellowish tinge to skin and eyes, ringing in the ears.

PRINCIPAL USES
To help control mild to moderate non-insulin-dependent (type 2) diabetes mellitus in patients whose blood sugar cannot be adequately controlled by diet, weight loss, and exercise.

HOW THE DRUG WORKS
Chlorpropamide stimulates the release of additional insulin from the pancreas and makes the tissues of the body more responsive to insulin.

DOSAGE
Initially, 250 mg once a day. After 5 to 7 days, dose can be increased by 50 to 125 mg. It may be increased every 3 to 5 days, if needed, to a maximum dose of 750 mg a day. Adults over age 65: 100 to 125 mg each day, increased as described above.

ONSET OF EFFECT
Within 1 hour.

DURATION OF ACTION
Up to 60 hours.

DIETARY ADVICE
Take 1 dose daily, 30 minutes before breakfast; if stomach upset occurs, divide the daily amount into two equal doses and take them before your morning and evening meals. The tablet may be crushed. Follow the dietary guidelines given to you by your doctor, and restrict intake of sugar-containing snacks.

STORAGE
Store in a tightly sealed container away from heat and direct light.

IF YOU MISS A DOSE
Take it as soon as you remember. If it is near the time for the next dose, skip the missed dose and resume your regular dosage schedule. Do not double the next dose.

STOPPING THE DRUG
Do not stop taking the drug without your doctor's approval. Take it as prescribed for the full treatment period, even if you begin to feel better.

PROLONGED USE
Prolonged use increases the risk of adverse effects. Periodic physical examinations and laboratory tests (blood and urine tests to monitor sugar levels) are needed.

PRECAUTIONS
Over 60: Adverse reactions may be more likely and more severe in elderly patients.

Driving and Hazardous Work: Do not drive or engage in hazardous work until you determine how this medication affects you.

Alcohol: Avoid alcohol. Patients who consume alcohol while taking chlorpropamide are at risk for a severe reaction that may include nausea, vomiting, flushing, lightheadedness, headache, and shortness of breath.

Pregnancy: Avoid using chlorpropamide if you are pregnant or are planning to become pregnant.

Breast Feeding: Chlorpropamide passes into breast milk and may be harmful; avoid or discontinue use while nursing.

Infants and Children: Chlorpropamide is not recommended for infants and children.

OVERDOSE
Symptoms: Excessive hunger, nausea, anxiety, cool skin, cold sweats, drowsiness, rapid heartbeat, tingling of lips and tongue, weakness, unconsciousness, confusion, seizures.

What to Do: Call your doctor, emergency medical services (EMS), or the nearest poison control center immediately.

DRUG INTERACTIONS
Consult your doctor for specific advice if you are taking anabolic steroids or corticosteroids, allopurinol, anticoagulants, aspirin and aspirin-containing cough, cold, and appetite-control drugs, barbiturates, beta-blockers, calcium channel blockers, cimetidine, ranitidine, pentamidine, chloramphenicol, ciprofloxacin, cyclosporine, estrogens, ethanol, thiazide diuretics, fenfluramine, oral miconazole or ketoconazole, lithium, MAO inhibitors, probenecid, rifampin, selegiline or procarbazine, sulfinpyrazone, quinidine.

FOOD INTERACTIONS
No known food interactions.

DISEASE INTERACTIONS
Caution is advised when taking chlorpropamide. Consult your doctor if you have any of the following: malnutrition, heart problems, liver or kidney disease, thyroid disease, a severe infection, fever, or an underactive pituitary or adrenal gland.

Generic 50 mg
(MYLAN)

Additional photographs

▶ Drug Class: Thiazide-like diuretic

▶ Available in: Tablets

▶ Available OTC? No

▶ As Generic? Yes

Side Effects

SERIOUS
Skin rash, hives, intense itching, swelling of the mouth and throat, breathing difficulty, serious heartbeat irregularities or palpitations, lightheadedness or dizziness, unusual bleeding or bruising. Call your doctor immediately.

COMMON
Potassium depletion may lead to heart palpitations and weakness. Fluid depletion may lead to dizziness, especially upon arising from a sitting or lying position.

LESS COMMON
Decreased sexual ability, increased sensitivity to sunlight, loss of appetite, gout, increased blood sugar (a problem for patients with diabetes).

PRINCIPAL USES
To treat high blood pressure (hypertension) and conditions that cause edema (swelling of body tissues resulting from excess salt and water retention).

HOW THE DRUG WORKS
Diuretics increase the excretion of salt and water in the urine. By reducing the overall fluid volume in the body, these drugs reduce blood volume and so reduce pressure within the blood vessels.

DOSAGE
Adults: 25 to 100 mg once a day or every other day.

ONSET OF EFFECT
2 to 3 hours.

DURATION OF ACTION
2 to 3 days.

DIETARY ADVICE
Take it with food to avoid stomach upset.

STORAGE
Store in a tightly sealed container away from heat and direct light.

IF YOU MISS A DOSE
Take it as soon as you remember. However, if it is near the time for the next dose, skip the missed dose and resume your regular dosage schedule. Do not double the next dose.

STOPPING THE DRUG
Unless directed otherwise by your doctor, take this medication as prescribed for the full treatment period, even if you begin to feel better before the scheduled end of therapy.

PROLONGED USE
See your doctor regularly for examinations and tests, if you must take this medicine for an extended period.

PRECAUTIONS
Over 60: Adverse reactions may be more likely and severe in older patients.

Driving and Hazardous Work: No special precautions are warranted.

Alcohol: Avoid alcohol while taking this drug.

Pregnancy: This medicine should not be taken during pregnancy unless recommended by your doctor.

Breast Feeding: Chlorthalidone passes into breast milk; avoid or discontinue use while nursing.

Infants and Children: Although chlorthalidone is rarely prescribed for children, no unusual side effects are expected. The dose must be determined by a pediatrician.

Special Concerns: Chlorthalidone is usually taken once a day. To prevent it from interfering with sleep, take it in the morning. If you are taking it for high blood pressure, follow the diet and weight control measures recommended by your doctor. Avoid exposure to sunlight, use a sunblock, or wear protective clothing. This medicine may cause your body to lose potassium. Follow your doctor's instructions about eating potassium-rich foods or taking a potassium supplement.

OVERDOSE
Symptoms: Fainting, lethargy, dizziness, drowsiness, confusion, gastrointestinal irritation.

What to Do: Call your doctor, emergency medical services (EMS), or the nearest poison control center immediately.

DRUG INTERACTIONS
Consult your doctor for specific advice if you are taking anticoagulants, cholestyramine, colestipol, drugs for diabetes, nonsteroidal anti-inflammatory drugs, digitalis drugs, or lithium.

FOOD INTERACTIONS
No significant food interactions have been reported.

DISEASE INTERACTIONS
Caution is advised when taking chlorthalidone. Consult your doctor if you have any of the following: diabetes, gout, lupus erythematosus, pancreatitis, diabetes, heart disease, blood vessel disease, liver disease, or kidney disease.

Chlorzoxazone

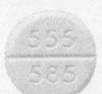

Generic 500 mg
(BARR)

▶ Drug Class: Muscle relaxant

▶ Available in: Caplets, tablets

▶ Available OTC? No

▶ As Generic? Yes

Side Effects

SERIOUS
Fainting; palpitations or
rapid heartbeat; fever;
hives or severe swelling
of face, lips, or tongue
along with shortness of
breath, chest tightness,
or wheezing (indicating a
potentially life-threatening allergic reaction);
mental depression; tem-
porary loss of vision. Call
your doctor right away.

COMMON
Drowsiness, dizziness,
dry mouth.

LESS COMMON
Bruises, feeling of illness,
excitability, stomach
upset, discolored urine,
bloody or black stools,
hiccups.

PRINCIPAL USES
Muscle relaxants are used
to relieve stiffness and discomfort caused by severe
sprains and strains, muscle
spasms, or other muscle
problems. They may be prescribed in conjunction with
other treatment methods,
such as physical therapy.

HOW THE DRUG WORKS
Muscle relaxants such as
chlorzoxazone depress
activity in the central nervous system, which in turn
interferes with the transmission of nerve impulses from
the spinal cord to the skeletal muscles.

DOSAGE
Adults: 250 to 750 mg, 3 or
4 times a day. The dosage
can be reduced as improvement occurs.

ONSET OF EFFECT
15 to 30 minutes.

DURATION OF ACTION
Up to 4 hours.

DIETARY ADVICE
Take it with meals to lessen
stomach upset. Be sure to
eat a well-balanced diet; the
healing of injured tissue
increases the body's protein
and calorie requirements.
To avoid dry mouth, main-
tain adequate fluid intake
and suck on ice chips if
desired.

STORAGE
Store in a tightly sealed container away from heat, moisture, and direct light.

IF YOU MISS A DOSE
Take it as soon as you
remember. If it is near the
time for the next dose, skip
the missed dose and
resume your regular dosage
schedule. Do not double the
next dose.

STOPPING THE DRUG
The decision to stop taking
the drug should be made by
your doctor. Gradual reduction of the dose may be necessary if you have taken the
drug for a long time.

PROLONGED USE
Adult use should generally
be limited to 10 days. Consult your doctor about the
need for follow-up medical
examinations or laboratory
studies. Periodic liver tests
are recommended during
therapy.

PRECAUTIONS
Over 60: Adverse reactions
may be more likely and
more severe in older
patients.

**Driving and Hazardous
Work:** Do not drive or
engage in hazardous work
until you determine how the
medicine affects you.

Alcohol: Avoid alcohol
while taking this drug
because it may compound
the sedative effect and may
cause liver damage.

Pregnancy: Before taking
chlorzoxazone, be sure to
tell your doctor if you are
pregnant or are planning to
become pregnant.

Breast Feeding: Chlorzoxazone passes into breast
milk; avoid or discontinue
use while nursing.

Infants and Children:
Not recommended for use
by children under age 12.

Special Concerns: If your
symptoms do not improve
after 2 days of use, call your
doctor. Use of chlorzoxa-
zone should be accompa-
nied by bed rest, physical
therapy, and other measures
to relieve discomfort. Do
not take this drug if you are
allergic to any skeletal muscle relaxant.

OVERDOSE
Symptoms: Nausea, vomiting, diarrhea, loss of
appetite, headache, severe
weakness, unusual increase
in sweating, fainting, breathing difficulties, irritability,
convulsions, feeling of paralysis, loss of consciousness.

What to Do: An overdose
of chlorzoxazone is unlikely
to be life-threatening, However, if someone takes a
much larger dose than prescribed, seek medical assistance immediately.

DRUG INTERACTIONS
Tell your doctor if you are
taking oral anticoagulants,
antidepressants, antihistamines, clozapine, dronabinol, any mind-altering
medication, MAO inhibitors,
other muscle relaxants, any
narcotic, phenobarbital, sertraline, sleeping pills, or a
tetracycline antibiotic.

FOOD INTERACTIONS
No known food interactions.

DISEASE INTERACTIONS
Use of this drug may cause
complications in patients
with liver or kidney disease,
since these organs work
together to remove the
medication from the body.

Cholestyramine

BRAND NAMES
Questran, Questran Light

▶ Drug Class: Antilipidemic (cholesterol-lowering agent)

▶ Available in: Powder

▶ Available OTC? No

▶ As Generic? Yes

Side Effects

SERIOUS
Severe abdominal pain (a very rare reaction, indicating intestinal obstruction). Stop taking the drug and contact your doctor immediately.

COMMON
Constipation, heartburn, bloating, belching, abdominal discomfort, irritation of the anal area.

LESS COMMON
Hives, rash, gas, diarrhea, nausea, vomiting, gallstones.

PRINCIPAL USES
To reduce cholesterol in people with high blood levels of low-density lipoprotein (LDL), as part of a comprehensive treatment program that includes exercise and special diet. The drug is also used to relieve itching caused by high levels of bile acids in the blood, a problem associated with blockage of the bile ducts. Cholestyramine may also be used to prevent some types of diarrhea or to serve as an antidote to poisoning from or overdose of digitalis drugs.

HOW THE DRUG WORKS
Cholestyramine binds with bile acids in the intestine, forming an insoluble complex that is excreted in the feces. This process reduces the bile acids in the blood. In response to the lower levels of bile acids, the liver converts more cholesterol to bile acids. Consequently, the amount of cholesterol in liver cells declines, and the liver makes more LDL receptors. The resulting increased removal of LDL from the blood lowers LDL cholesterol.

DOSAGE
Initial dose is 4 g, 1 or 2 times a day. Maintenance dose is 8 to 24 g per day in 2 equally divided doses. Always mix the powder thoroughly with appropriate liquid (water or fruit juice; do not use carbonated beverages), and wait 10 to 15 minutes after mixing before drinking. Dosages are increased or decreased according to the individual's response.

ONSET OF EFFECT
Within 1 to 3 weeks.

DURATION OF ACTION
Cholestyramine's effects persist for 2 to 4 weeks after final dose.

DIETARY ADVICE
Follow all special dietary restrictions and guidelines as directed by your doctor.

STORAGE
Store in a tightly sealed container away from heat and direct light. Keep away from moisture.

IF YOU MISS A DOSE
Take it as soon as you remember. However, if it is near the time for the next dose, skip the missed dose and resume your regular dosage schedule. Do not double the next dose.

STOPPING THE DRUG
The drug may be stopped after 1 to 3 months if the therapeutic effect is not adequate. The decision to stop taking the drug should be made by your doctor.

PROLONGED USE
Cholestyramine may be used safely for years; however, periodic evaluation of the drug's effectiveness is necessary.

PRECAUTIONS
Over 60: Adverse reactions (particularly constipation) are more likely and more severe in older patients.

Driving and Hazardous Work: No special precautions are necessary.

Alcohol: No special precautions are necessary.

Pregnancy: The effects on a fetus are unknown. Consult your doctor if you become or plan to become pregnant.

Breast Feeding: At very high doses cholestyramine may interfere with the absorption of vitamins A, D, E, and K, which may affect the nutritional intake of the nursing infant. Consult your doctor for specific advice.

Infants and Children: Prescribed for children only in rare circumstances. Follow doctor's instructions and dosage guidelines carefully in such cases.

Special Concerns: At very high doses cholestyramine may interfere with the absorption of fats and fat-soluble vitamins (vitamins A, D, E, and K); vitamin supplementation may be advised.

OVERDOSE
Symptoms: None reported.

What to Do: Emergency instructions not applicable.

DRUG INTERACTIONS
Cholestyramine may bind with other drugs and hinder their absorption. Therefore, take all other drugs 1 to 2 hours before or 4 hours after taking cholestyramine.

FOOD INTERACTIONS
No known food interactions.

DISEASE INTERACTIONS
Do not take this drug if you have had a prior allergic reaction to it. Do not take Questran Light if you have phenylketonuria. Use of cholestyramine may make the following conditions worse: gallstones, peptic ulcer, intestinal bleeding disorders, hemorrhoids, malabsorption, constipation.

Cidofovir Intravenous

▶ Drug Class: Antiviral

▶ Available in: Intravenous injection

▶ Available OTC? No

▶ As Generic? No

Side Effects

SERIOUS
Kidney damage, causing decreased or increased urination, thirst, and shortness of breath. Impaired vision or other changes in vision may also develop. If such symptoms occur, call your doctor right away.

COMMON
Probenecid, which is given with cidofovir, may cause fever, chills, headache, rash, nausea, or vomiting.

LESS COMMON
Persistent weakness and fatigue or general loss of strength.

PRINCIPAL USES
To treat cytomegalovirus (CMV) retinitis (an eye infection) or other forms of CMV disease in patients with human immunodeficiency virus (HIV) infection. Cidofovir is given in combination with probenecid, a drug that enhances the effectiveness of antimicrobial medications.

HOW THE DRUG WORKS
Cidofovir interferes with the activity of enzymes needed for the replication of DNA in viral cells, thus preventing CMV from reproducing.

DOSAGE
For patients with normal kidney function: Initially, 5 mg per 2.2 lbs (1 kg) of body weight infused intravenously over a period of 60 minutes, once a week, for 2 consecutive weeks. Probenecid is also given at a dose of 2 g, 3 hours before infusion, followed by 1 g, 2 hours later, then again 8 hours later. Maintenance dose of cidofovir: 5 mg per 2.2 lbs of body weight once every 2 weeks. For patients with impaired kidney function: A reduced dose is necessary, as determined by your doctor.

ONSET OF EFFECT
Unknown.

DURATION OF ACTION
Unknown.

DIETARY ADVICE
Cidofovir can be given without regard to diet. Probenecid should be given after food intake. Drink plenty of fluids.

STORAGE
Not applicable; the dose is administered at a health care facility or by a home nurse.

IF YOU MISS A DOSE
If you miss a dose for any reason, contact your doctor and arrange to receive treatment as soon as possible.

STOPPING THE DRUG
The decision to stop taking the drug should be made in consultation with your physician.

PROLONGED USE
See your doctor regularly for tests and examinations if you must take this medication for a prolonged period. See an ophthalmologist regularly for eye examinations.

PRECAUTIONS
Over 60: Older patients are more likely to have impaired kidney function requiring an adjustment in dosage.

Driving and Hazardous Work: Do not drive or engage in hazardous work until you determine how the medicine affects you.

Alcohol: Avoid alcohol if liver function is impaired.

Pregnancy: Cidofovir has been shown to cause birth defects in animals. Human studies have not been done. This medication should be given during pregnancy only if potential benefits outweigh the risks to the unborn child.

Breast Feeding: It is unknown whether cidofovir passes into breast milk; however, women infected with HIV should not nurse, to avoid transmitting the virus to an uninfected child.

Infants and Children: The safety and effectiveness of cidofovir in infants and children have not been established.

Special Concerns: The risk of severe nausea when probenecid is given can be reduced by taking an anti-nausea medication, such as diphenhydramine hydrochloride.

OVERDOSE
Symptoms: No cases of overdose have been reported.

What to Do: An overdose of cidofovir is unlikely to occur. Nonetheless, if you have any reason to suspect an overdose, call your physician, emergency medical services (EMS), or the nearest poison control center immediately.

DRUG INTERACTIONS
Other drugs may interact with cidofovir. Consult your doctor for specific advice if you are taking any other drug that can cause kidney damage, such as aminoglycosides, amphotericin B, foscarnet, nonsteroidal anti-inflammatory drugs, pentamidine, vancomycin, and zidovudine. A seven-day waiting period after use of such drugs is recommended before beginning therapy with cidofovir.

FOOD INTERACTIONS
No known food interactions, but side effects of probenecid are decreased when it is taken with food.

DISEASE INTERACTIONS
Consult your doctor if you have any condition that impairs kidney function.

Cilostazol

▶ Drug Class: Phosphodi-esterase type 3 inhibitor

▶ Available in: Tablets

▶ Available OTC? No

▶ As Generic? No

Side Effects

SERIOUS
No serious side effects have been reported.

COMMON
Headache, heart palpitations, diarrhea, increased risk of infection.

LESS COMMON
Rapid heartbeat, abdominal pain, indigestion, flatulence, nausea, swelling of the extremities, dizziness, sore throat, runny nose.

PRINCIPAL USES
To reduce symptoms of intermittent claudication (leg pain that is induced by walking and which subsides after rest).

HOW THE DRUG WORKS
Intermittent claudication results from impaired blood supply to the legs. Although its precise mechanism of action is not clear, cilostazol appears to improve circulation by dilating blood vessels, especially those supplying the legs. It also appears to inhibit the aggregation (clumping) of platelets and this reduces the formation of blood clots which can block arterial blood flow.

DOSAGE
100 mg 2 times a day.

ONSET OF EFFECT
From 2 to 12 weeks.

DURATION OF ACTION
Unknown.

DIETARY ADVICE
Take on an empty stomach at least 30 minutes before or 2 hours after a meal.

STORAGE
Store in a tightly sealed container away from heat, moisture, and direct light.

IF YOU MISS A DOSE
Take it as soon as you remember. If it is near the time for the next dose, skip the missed dose and resume your regular dosage schedule. Do not double the next dose.

STOPPING THE DRUG
The decision to stop taking the drug should be made in consultation with your physician.

PROLONGED USE
The safety and effectiveness of cilostazol have not been determined beyond 24 weeks of use.

PRECAUTIONS
Over 60: No special problems are expected.

Driving and Hazardous Work: Use caution when driving or engaging in hazardous work until you determine how the medicine affects you.

Alcohol: No special precautions are necessary.

Pregnancy: Adequate human studies have not been done. Before taking cilostazol, tell your doctor if you are pregnant or plan to become pregnant.

Breast Feeding: Cilostazol may pass into breast milk; caution is advised. Consult your doctor for advice on whether to discontinue nursing or discontinue the drug.

Infants and Children: Safety and effectiveness have not been established for children under age 18.

OVERDOSE
Symptoms: Few cases of overdose have been reported. However, if you take a much larger dose than prescribed, you may experience severe headache, diarrhea, dizziness or fainting, and heartbeat irregularities.

What to Do: Call your doctor, emergency medical services (EMS), or the nearest poison control center immediately.

DRUG INTERACTIONS
The following drugs may interact with cilostazol. Consult your doctor for specific advice if you are taking ketoconazole, itraconazole, fluconazole, miconazole, fluvoxamine, fluoxetine, nefazodone, sertraline, erythromycin and other macrolide antibiotics, omeprazole, diltiazem, or clopidogrel.

FOOD INTERACTIONS
Do not take cilostazol with grapefruit juice.

DISEASE INTERACTIONS
Do not take cilostazol if you have congestive heart failure of any severity.

Cimetidine

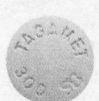

Tagamet 300mg
(SMITHKLINE BEECHAM)

Additional photographs

▶ Drug Class: Histamine (H2) blocker

▶ Available in: Tablets, oral solution, oral suspension

▶ Available OTC? Yes

▶ As Generic? Yes

Side Effects

SERIOUS
Irregular heart rhythm (palpitations), slowed heartbeat, severe blood problems resulting in unusual bleeding, bruising, fever, chills, and increased susceptibility to infection. Call your doctor immediately.

COMMON
Headache, fatigue, drowsiness, dizziness, nausea, vomiting, abdominal pain, diarrhea.

LESS COMMON
Blurred vision, decreased sexual desire or function, swelling of breasts in males or females, temporary hair loss, hallucinations, depression, insomnia, skin rash, hives, or redness.

PRINCIPAL USES
To treat ulcers of the stomach and duodenum, as well as other conditions, such as esophagitis (chronic inflammation of the esophagus), and gastroesophageal reflux (backwash of stomach acid into the esophagus, resulting in heartburn).

HOW THE DRUG WORKS
Cimetidine blocks the action of histamine (a compound produced in the body's cells), which in turn decreases the stomach's secretion of hydrochloric acid. Once stomach acid production is decreased, the body is better able to heal itself.

DOSAGE
For treatment of acute (symptomatic, bothersome) duodenal or gastric ulcers— Adults and teenagers: Various dosage schedules are used, including 300 mg, 4 times a day, with meals and at bedtime; 400 or 600 mg, 2 times a day; or 800 mg taken once daily at bedtime. For prevention of duodenal ulcers— Adults and teenagers: Usual dose is 300 mg, 2 times a day; another common dosage schedule is 400 mg taken once daily at bedtime. For treatment as needed of heartburn and acid indigestion— Adults and teenagers: 200 mg with water when symptoms start; another 200 mg may be taken within the next 24 hours, for a maximum of 400 mg in a 24-hour period. For treatment of gastroesophageal reflux disease— Adults: 800 to 1,600 mg a day, in 2 to 4 divided doses, for approximately 12 weeks.

ONSET OF EFFECT
Within 1 hour.

DURATION OF ACTION
At least 4 to 5 hours.

DIETARY ADVICE
Avoid foods that cause stomach irritation.

STORAGE
Store away from heat and direct light. Keep the liquid form from freezing.

IF YOU MISS A DOSE
Take it as soon as you remember. If it is near the time for the next dose, skip the missed dose and resume your regular dosage schedule. Do not double the next dose.

STOPPING THE DRUG
Prescription-strength: Take it for the full treatment period, even if you begin to feel better before the scheduled end of therapy. Nonprescription-strength: Take as needed.

PROLONGED USE
Do not take nonprescription-strength cimetidine for more than 2 weeks unless instructed to do so by your physician.

PRECAUTIONS
Over 60: Adverse reactions may be more likely and more severe in older patients.

Driving and Hazardous Work: Do not drive or engage in hazardous work until you determine how the medicine affects you.

Alcohol: Avoid alcohol.

Pregnancy: Avoid or discontinue use if you are pregnant or trying to become pregnant.

Breast Feeding: Cimetidine passes into breast milk; avoid or discontinue use while nursing.

Infants and Children: Not recommended for use by children under the age of 16 years old.

Special Concerns: Avoid cigarette smoking because it may increase stomach acid secretion and thus worsen the disease. Do not take cimetidine if you have ever had an allergic reaction to a histamine (H2) blocker. If stomach pain becomes worse while you are using the drug, tell your doctor right away.

OVERDOSE
Symptoms: No symptoms have been reported.

What to Do: An overdose is unlikely to be life-threatening. However, if someone takes a much larger dose than directed, seek medical assistance right away.

DRUG INTERACTIONS
Consult your doctor for specific advice if you are taking aminophylline, anticoagulants, caffeine, metoprolol, oxtriphylline, phenytoin, propranolol, theophylline, tricyclic antidepressants, itraconazole, ketoconazole, metronidazole.

FOOD INTERACTIONS
Carbonated drinks, citrus fruits and juices, caffeine-containing beverages, and other acidic foods or liquids may irritate the stomach or interfere with the therapeutic action of cimetidine.

DISEASE INTERACTIONS
Patients with kidney or liver disease or weakened immune systems should not use cimetidine or should use it in smaller, limited doses under careful medical supervision.

Ciprofloxacin Ophthalmic

▶ Drug Class: Fluoroquinolone antibiotic

▶ Available in: Ophthalmic solution

▶ Available OTC? No

▶ As Generic? No

Side Effects

SERIOUS
Nausea, blurry or decreased vision, skin rash, severe irritation or redness of the eye. Stop using the drug and call your doctor immediately.

COMMON
Burning or crusting in the eye or eyelid.

LESS COMMON
Redness of the edge of the eyelids, bad taste in mouth, tearing or itching of the eye, swelling of the eyelid, sensation of a foreign body in the eye, increased sensitivity of eyes to bright light.

PRINCIPAL USES
To treat or prevent bacterial infections of the eye, such as conjunctivitis or keratitis (infection of the cornea). Often used to prevent infection while a corneal abrasion is healing.

HOW THE DRUG WORKS
Ciprofloxacin interferes with the action of certain enzymes necessary for bacteria to grow and multiply.

DOSAGE
Exact dosing depends on the nature of the infection and its response to treatment. Follow your doctor's instructions precisely. The following is an example of a typical dose for conjunctivitis. Adults and teenagers: 1 drop in eye every 2 hours for 2 days, then 1 drop every 4 hours for the next 5 days (doses administered during waking hours only).

ONSET OF EFFECT
Unknown.

DURATION OF ACTION
Unknown.

DIETARY ADVICE
No special restrictions.

STORAGE
Store in a tightly sealed container away from heat, moisture, and direct light. Do not refrigerate or allow the solution to freeze.

IF YOU MISS A DOSE
Apply it as soon as you remember. If it is near the time for the next dose, skip the missed dose and resume your regular dosage schedule. Do not double the next dose.

STOPPING THE DRUG
Use this drug as prescribed for the full treatment period, even if you begin to feel better before the scheduled end of therapy.

PROLONGED USE
Prolonged use, as directed by your doctor, may be necessary for severe cases of infection. See your doctor regularly for tests and examinations if you take this drug for a prolonged period.

PRECAUTIONS
Over 60: Adverse reactions may be more likely and more severe in older patients.

Driving and Hazardous Work: Do not drive or engage in hazardous work until you determine how the medicine affects your vision.

Alcohol: No special precautions are necessary.

Pregnancy: Adequate human studies have not been done. Before taking ophthalmic ciprofloxacin, tell your doctor if you are pregnant or plan to become pregnant.

Breast Feeding: Ophthalmic ciprofloxacin may pass into breast milk; caution is advised. Ciprofloxacin taken orally has been found in trace amounts in breast milk. Consult your doctor for advice.

Infants and Children: This medication is not recommended for use by children under the age of 12.

Special Concerns: To use the eye drops, first wash your hands. Tilt your head back. Gently apply pressure to the inside corner of the eyelid and with the index finger of the same hand, pull downward on the lower eyelid to make a space. Drop the medicine into this space and close your eye. Apply pressure for 1 or 2 minutes while keeping the

eye closed without blinking. Then wash your hands again. Make sure the tip of the dropper does not touch your eye, finger, or any other surface. If your symptoms do not improve or if they become worse, check with your doctor. You should not share your medication, towels, or washcloths with other people. Call your doctor if anyone else close to you develops similar symptoms.

OVERDOSE
Symptoms: No specific ones have been reported.

What to Do: An overdose of ophthalmic ciprofloxacin is unlikely to be life-threatening. However, if someone takes a much larger dose of the drug than prescribed or accidentally ingests the medicine, seek medical assistance right away.

DRUG INTERACTIONS
Other drugs may interact with ophthalmic ciprofloxacin. Consult your doctor for specific advice if you are taking any other prescription or over-the-counter medication.

FOOD INTERACTIONS
No known food interactions.

DISEASE INTERACTIONS
Caution is advised when taking ophthalmic ciprofloxacin. Consult your doctor if you have ever had an allergic reaction to ciprofloxacin or other fluoroquinolone antibiotics.

Ciprofloxacin Systemic

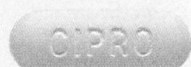

▶ Drug Class: Fluoroquinolone antibiotic

▶ Available in: Tablets, oral suspension

▶ Available OTC? No

▶ As Generic? No

Side Effects

SERIOUS
Serious reactions to ciprofloxacin are rare and include seizures, mental confusion, hallucinations, agitation, nightmares, depression, shortness of breath, unusual swelling in the face or extremities, and loss of consciousness. Also skin burning, redness, blisters, rash, or itching on exposure to sunlight. Call your doctor immediately.

COMMON
Increased sensitivity to sunlight (and increased risk of sunburn) for days following therapy.

LESS COMMON
Diarrhea, nausea and vomiting, stomach pain and upset, gas, headache, dizziness, insomnia, changes in taste perception, drowsiness, itching, dry mouth, unusual body aches or pains.

PRINCIPAL USES
To treat mild to severe bacterial infections, including those of the urinary tract, lower respiratory tract, bones and joints, and the skin. It is also used to treat certain sexually transmitted diseases (such as chancroid and gonorrhea), and diarrhea caused by bacterial infection. Ciprofloxacin is also approved for prophylactic use following known exposure to anthrax bacteria and for treating anthrax infections.

HOW THE DRUG WORKS
Ciprofloxacin inhibits the activity of a bacterial enzyme (gyrase) that is necessary for proper DNA formation and replication. This fights infection by preventing bacteria cells from reproducing.

DOSAGE
250 to 750 mg every 12 hours (2 times a day), for 5 to 14 days, depending on kidney function and the infection being treated. Gonorrhea is usually treated with a one-time dose of 250 mg.

ONSET OF EFFECT
Varies depending on the infection being treated.

DURATION OF ACTION
Unknown.

DIETARY ADVICE
Be sure to drink plenty of fluids, but avoid milk and dairy derivatives.

STORAGE
Store in a tightly sealed container away from heat and direct light.

IF YOU MISS A DOSE
Take it as soon as you remember. If it is near the time for the next dose, skip the missed dose and resume your regular dosage schedule. Do not double the next dose.

STOPPING THE DRUG
Take it as prescribed for the full treatment period, even if you begin to feel better before the scheduled end of therapy.

PROLONGED USE
See your doctor regularly for tests and examinations if you must take this medicine for a prolonged period.

PRECAUTIONS
Over 60: No special problems are expected.

Driving and Hazardous Work: Do not drive or engage in hazardous work until you determine how the medicine affects you.

Alcohol: It is advisable to abstain from alcohol when fighting an infection.

Pregnancy: In some animal tests, ciprofloxacin has caused birth defects. Adequate studies in humans have not been done. It should be used during pregnancy only if potential benefits clearly justify the risks. Before you take ciprofloxacin, tell your doctor if you are pregnant or plan to become pregnant.

Breast Feeding: Ciprofloxacin passes into breast milk and may cause serious side effects in the nursing infant; use of the drug is discouraged when nursing.

Infants and Children: Ciprofloxacin is not recommended for use by persons under the age of 18, as it has been shown to interfere with bone development.

Special Concerns: If ciprofloxacin causes sensitivity to sunlight, stop taking the drug and try to avoid exposure to sunlight for the next 5 days; also wear protective clothing and use a sunblock. Ciprofloxacin should not be taken by patients whose work makes it impossible to avoid exposure to sunlight. It is important to drink plenty of fluids while taking this drug.

OVERDOSE
Symptoms: No specific ones have been reported.

What to Do: If you have any reason to suspect an overdose, call your doctor, emergency medical services (EMS), or the nearest poison control center.

DRUG INTERACTIONS
Consult your doctor for specific advice if you are taking aminophylline, antacids, didanosine, iron supplements, oxtriphylline, sucralfate, theophylline, warfarin, or zinc salts. Also tell your doctor if you are taking any other prescription or over-the-counter medication.

FOOD INTERACTIONS
The effects of caffeine may be magnified by this drug. Milk and dairy products can reduce blood levels of ciprofloxacin by as much as half.

DISEASE INTERACTIONS
Caution is advised when taking ciprofloxacin. Consult your doctor if you have any other medical condition. Use of ciprofloxacin can cause complications in patients with kidney disease, since this organ works to remove the medication from the body.

Citalopram Hydrobromide

BRAND NAME
Celexa

▶ Drug Class: Selective serotonin reuptake inhibitor (SSRI) antidepressant

▶ Available in: Tablet, oral solution

▶ Available OTC? No

▶ As Generic? No

Side Effects

SERIOUS
Chest pain, rapid or irregular heartbeat, lightheadedness or fainting. Call your doctor immediately.

COMMON
Delayed ejaculation (males), dry mouth, increased sweating, nausea, trembling, diarrhea, drowsiness, numbness, tingling, or prickling sensations.

LESS COMMON
Fatigue, fever, loss of appetite, agitation, nasal congestion, sinus infection, erectile dysfunction.

PRINCIPAL USES
To treat symptoms of major depression.

HOW THE DRUG WORKS
Citalopram increases brain levels of serotonin, a chemical that is thought to be linked to mood, emotions, and mental state.

DOSAGE
To start, 20 mg once a day, taken in the morning or evening; dose may be gradually increased by your doctor to 40 mg a day.

ONSET OF EFFECT
Unknown.

DURATION OF ACTION
Unknown.

DIETARY ADVICE
No special restrictions.

STORAGE
Store in a tightly sealed container away from heat, moisture, and direct light.

IF YOU MISS A DOSE
If you miss a dose on one day, do not double the dose the next day.

STOPPING THE DRUG
Take it as prescribed for the full treatment period even if you notice improvement. When it is time to stop therapy, your dosage will be tapered gradually by your doctor.

PROLONGED USE
Usual course of therapy for depression lasts 6 months to 1 year; some patients may benefit from additional therapy.

PRECAUTIONS
Over 60: Adverse reactions may be more likely and more severe in older patients. A lower dose may be warranted.

Driving and Hazardous Work: Use caution when driving or engaging in hazardous work until you determine how the medicine affects you.

Alcohol: Avoid alcohol.

Pregnancy: Citalopram should be used during pregnancy only if the potential benefit justifies the potential risk to the fetus. Before you take this medicine, tell your doctor if you are pregnant or plan to become pregnant.

Breast Feeding: Citalopram passes into breast milk; caution is advised. Consult your doctor for specific advice.

Infants and Children: The safety and effectiveness of the use of citalopram in children have not been established.

OVERDOSE
Symptoms: Dizziness, sweating, nausea, vomiting, trembling, drowsiness, rapid heartbeat.

What to Do: Call your doctor, emergency medical services (EMS), or the nearest poison control center immediately.

DRUG INTERACTIONS
Citalopram and MAO inhibitors should not be used within 14 days of each other. Very serious side effects such as myoclonus (uncontrolled muscle spasms), hyperthermia (excessive rise in body temperature), and extreme stiffness may result. The following drugs may also interact with citalopram; consult your doctor for advice if you are taking cimetidine, warfarin, lithium, carbamazepine, antifungals (such as ketoconazole, itraconazole, and fluconazole), erythromycin antibiotics, omeprazole, tricyclic antidepressants, or any prescription or over-the-counter drugs that depress the central nervous system (including antihistamines, barbiturates, sedatives, cough medicines, and decongestants).

FOOD INTERACTIONS
No known food interactions.

DISEASE INTERACTIONS
Caution is advised when taking citalopram, especially if you have heart disease or a seizure disorder. Use of citalopram may cause complications in patients with liver or kidney disease.

Clarithromycin

BRAND NAME
Biaxin

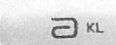

Biaxin 500 mg
(**ABBOTT**)

Additional photographs

▶ Drug Class: Macrolide antibiotic

▶ Available in: Tablets, oral suspension

▶ Available OTC? No

▶ As Generic? No

Side Effects

SERIOUS
Colitis (inflammation of the lower gastrointestinal tract, with symptoms including severe abdominal pain, watery or bloody stools, severe diarrhea, fever); liver toxicity (causing fever, nausea, vomiting, yellowish tinge to eyes or skin); allergic reaction (swelling of the lips, tongue, face, and throat, breathing difficulty, skin rash or hives); blood clotting disorders (causing unusual bleeding and bruising); confusion or change in behavior; heartbeat irregularities in patients with predisposing heart conditions. Such side effects are rare, but if they do occur, stop taking the drug and seek medical assistance immediately.

COMMON
No common side effects.

LESS COMMON
Changes in taste perception; mild abdominal pain or discomfort; mild diarrhea; mild nausea or vomiting; headache; oral thrush (fungal infections of the mouth or throat).

PRINCIPAL USES
To treat various bacterial infections, including those of the sinuses, tonsils, and respiratory tract (such as bronchitis and pneumonia); infections of the ear; and venereal disease due to chlamydial infection. Clarithromycin may also be used to treat certain skin infections, Legionnaires' disease, Lyme disease, and peptic ulcers caused by the bacterium H. pylori. Also used to prevent and, when taken with other drugs, treat a tuberculosis-like disease known as Mycobacterium avium complex (MAC), which is common in people with advanced acquired immunodeficiency syndrome (AIDS).

HOW THE DRUG WORKS
Clarithromycin prevents bacterial cells from manufacturing specific proteins necessary for their survival.

DOSAGE
For bacterial infections— Usual adult dose: 250 to 500 mg every 12 hours, for 7 to 14 days. Children 6 months of age or older: 3.4 mg per lb of body weight, up to 500 mg every 12 hours for 10 days. To prevent MAC— 500 mg, 2 times a day. To treat MAC— 500 mg, 2 times a day in combination with other drugs.

ONSET OF EFFECT
Within 2 hours; full effect may occur in 2 to 5 days.

DURATION OF ACTION
Unknown.

DIETARY ADVICE
Clarithromycin may be taken with or without food. Drink plenty of liquids.

STORAGE
Store in a tightly sealed container away from heat, moisture, and direct light.

IF YOU MISS A DOSE
Take it as soon as you remember. If it is near the time for the next dose, skip the missed dose and resume your regular dosing schedule. Do not double the next dose. If you are taking 2 doses a day, wait 5 to 6 hours before taking the next dose.

STOPPING THE DRUG
For acute infections, take it exactly as prescribed for the full treatment period, even if you feel better before the scheduled end of therapy. Therapy for prevention of MAC should be lifelong.

PROLONGED USE
You may become susceptible to infections caused by germs that are not responsive to clarithromycin. Also, severe drug-induced gastrointestinal problems may result from long-term use.

PRECAUTIONS
Over 60: Older patients, especially those with kidney disease, may require a decrease in dose.

Driving and Hazardous Work: No special precautions are necessary.

Alcohol: No special precautions are necessary.

Pregnancy: Adequate studies of the use of this drug during pregnancy have not been done; discuss potential risks and benefits with your doctor.

Breast Feeding: It is not known if clarithromycin passes into breast milk; consult your doctor for advice.

Infants and Children: No special problems are expected.

OVERDOSE
Symptoms: Severe nausea, vomiting, diarrhea, abdominal discomfort.

What to Do: Call your doctor, emergency medical services (EMS), or the nearest poison control center immediately.

DRUG INTERACTIONS
This drug should not be taken by patients known to have had prior allergic reactions to erythromycins or other macrolide antibiotics. Do not take clarithromycin if you are taking astemizole, or pimozide. Also, alert your doctor if you are taking any of the following drugs: carbamazepine, digoxin, theophylline, warfarin, rifabutin, rifampin, or zidovudine.

FOOD INTERACTIONS
No known food interactions.

DISEASE INTERACTIONS
Consult your doctor if you have a history of a blood disorder, liver disease, or any allergy.

Clemastine Fumarate

Tavist-1 12 Hour 1.34 mg
(**NOVARTIS**)

▶ Drug Class: Antihistamine

▶ Available in: Tablets, syrup, extended-release tablets and caplets

▶ Available OTC? Yes

▶ As Generic? Yes

Side Effects

SERIOUS
Confusion, hallucinations, convulsions, blurred vision, difficulty urinating (urinary obstruction).

COMMON
Drowsiness; nausea; thickening of mucus; dry mouth, nose, and throat; dizziness; disturbed coordination.

LESS COMMON
Chills, headache, fatigue, vomiting, restlessness, irritability, nasal congestion, profuse sweating, diarrhea, constipation.

PRINCIPAL USES
To prevent or relieve symptoms of hay fever and other allergies, and for itching skin and hives.

HOW THE DRUG WORKS
Clemastine blocks the effects of histamine, a naturally occurring substance within the body that causes swelling, itching, sneezing, watery eyes, hives, and other symptoms of allergic reactions.

DOSAGE
Adults and teenagers: 1.34 mg, 2 times a day (for hay fever), or 2.68 mg, 1 to 3 times a day (for hay fever or hives). Children ages 6 to 12: 0.67 mg (syrup) to 1.34 mg, 2 times a day.

ONSET OF EFFECT
15 minutes to 60 minutes.

DURATION OF ACTION
At least 12 hours.

DIETARY ADVICE
Take it with food, water, or milk to avoid stomach irritation. Drinking coffee or tea will help reduce drowsiness. Use sugarless gum, sugarless sour hard candy, or ice chips to ease dry mouth.

STORAGE
Store in a tightly sealed container away from heat and direct light.

IF YOU MISS A DOSE
Take it as soon as you remember. If it is near the time for the next dose, skip the missed dose and resume your regular dosage schedule. Do not double the next dose.

STOPPING THE DRUG
You should take it as prescribed for the full treatment period, but you may stop if you are feeling better before the scheduled end of therapy. It may be taken as needed.

PROLONGED USE
No special problems are expected.

PRECAUTIONS
Over 60: Adverse reactions may be more likely and more severe in older patients.

Driving and Hazardous Work: The use of clemastine may impair your ability to perform such tasks safely. Do not drive or engage in hazardous work until you determine how the medicine affects you.

Alcohol: Alcohol increases the likelihood and the severity of side effects like drowsiness and confusion.

Pregnancy: Animal studies with high doses of clemastine have found no birth defects. Human studies have not been done. Because the studies cannot rule out potential harm, the drug should be used during pregnancy only if it is clearly needed.

Breast Feeding: Clemastine passes into breast milk; do not use it while nursing.

Infants and Children: Children tend to be more sensitive to the effects of antihistamines. Symptoms of excitability, restlessness, and nightmares may occur.

OVERDOSE
Symptoms: Hallucinations, seizures, drowsiness, lethargy, coma.

What to Do: Call your doctor, emergency medical services (EMS), or the nearest poison control center immediately. A conscious patient should be induced to vomit using ipecac syrup.

DRUG INTERACTIONS
Sleeping pills, sedatives, tranquilizers, MAO inhibitors, and antidepressants can increase the sedative effects of clemastine. Anticholinergics may further increase the likelihood that drying of the mucous membranes and urinary obstruction will occur as side effects.

FOOD INTERACTIONS
No known food interactions.

DISEASE INTERACTIONS
Consult your doctor if you have any of the following: asthma, enlarged prostate, difficult urination, glaucoma, sleep apnea, or dry mouth or eyes.

Clindamycin

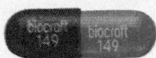

Generic 150 mg
(BIOCRAFT)

▶ Drug Class: Antibiotic

▶ Available in: Capsules, oral solution, injection, gel, topical solution, suspension, cream, vaginal suppositories

▶ Available OTC? No

▶ As Generic? Yes

Side Effects

SERIOUS
For oral forms, injection, gel, solution, and suspension: Severe stomach or abdominal pains and cramps, weight loss, severe diarrhea, fever, sore throat; skin rash, itching, and redness, unusual bleeding or bruising. For vaginal cream and suppositories: Itching of genital area, pain during intercourse, whitish vaginal discharge, diarrhea, dizziness, headache, nausea, vomiting, stomach cramps or pain. Call your doctor right away.

COMMON
For oral forms: Mild diarrhea, nausea, vomiting, stomach pain. For topical forms: Dry, peeling, or scaly skin.

LESS COMMON
For oral forms: Itching of rectal or genital regions. For topical forms: Stomach pain, mild diarrhea, irritated or oily skin, stinging or burning skin, dizziness (cream and suppository), headache (cream and suppository).

PRINCIPAL USES
Orally and by injection, clindamycin is used to treat serious bacterial infections. Topically, it is used to treat acne and vaginal infections.

HOW THE DRUG WORKS
Clindamycin inhibits the synthesis of protein in bacterial organisms.

DOSAGE
For systemic infections, using oral forms— Adults and teenagers: 150 to 300 mg, 4 times a day. For systemic infections, using injection— Adults and teenagers: 300 to 600 mg, 3 or 4 times a day, or 900 mg, 3 times a day. For acne, using gel, solution, or suspension— Adults and teenagers: Apply 2 times a day. Use and dose for children under 12 must be determined by your doctor. For vaginal infections, using vaginal cream— Non-pregnant adults and teenagers: 100 mg inserted in vagina once daily at bedtime for 3 or 7 days (7-day therapy is prescribed for pregnant patients). Dose for children must be determined by your doctor. For bacterial vaginal infections, using vaginal suppositories— Non-pregnant adults and teenagers: 1 suppository (containing 100 mg clindamycin) inserted in vagina once daily at bedtime for 3 days.

ONSET OF EFFECT
Unknown.

DURATION OF ACTION
Unknown.

DIETARY ADVICE
Take the oral forms with food to minimize stomach upset. Take the capsule with a glass of water.

STORAGE
Store in a tightly sealed container away from heat, moisture, and direct light. Do not refrigerate the liquid forms, cream, or suppositories.

IF YOU MISS A DOSE
Take it as soon as you remember. If it is near the time for the next dose, skip the missed dose and resume your regular dosage schedule. Do not double the next dose.

STOPPING THE DRUG
Take it as prescribed for the full treatment period, even if you feel better before the scheduled end of therapy.

PROLONGED USE
See your doctor regularly for tests and examinations if you must take this medicine for a prolonged period.

PRECAUTIONS
Over 60: It is not known whether this drug causes side effects in older patients different from or more severe than those in younger persons.

Driving and Hazardous Work: The use of clindamycin should not impair your ability to perform such tasks safely.

Alcohol: It is advisable to abstain from alcohol when fighting an infection.

Pregnancy: Clindamycin has not been reported to cause birth defects in humans; consult your doctor before taking it during pregnancy.

Breast Feeding: Clindamycin may pass into breast milk; consult your doctor for specific advice.

Infants and Children: Adequate studies of clindamycin use by children have not been done, although no special problems are expected.

Special Concerns: Wash and dry the skin thoroughly before applying the gel, topical solution, or suspension. When using the vaginal cream or suppository, sexual intercourse should be avoided. Clindamycin may weaken latex or rubber products such as condoms and vaginal contraceptive diaphragms; use of such products is not recommended within 72 hours of the application of clindamycin cream or suppositories. Do not use other vaginal products such as tampons or douches when using the vaginal suppositories. Before having surgery with a general anesthetic, tell the doctor or dentist in charge that you are taking clindamycin.

OVERDOSE
Symptoms: No specific ones have been reported.

What to Do: If you have any reason to suspect an overdose, call your doctor, emergency medical services (EMS), or the nearest poison control center.

DRUG INTERACTIONS
Consult your doctor for advice if you are taking chloramphenicol, erythromycin, or any diarrhea medicine containing kaopectate or attapulgite.

FOOD INTERACTIONS
No known food interactions.

DISEASE INTERACTIONS
Consult your doctor if you have a history of kidney disease, liver disease, or intestinal or stomach disease, especially colitis. The vaginal suppositories should not be used if you have a history of enteritis, ulcerative colitis, or "antibiotic-associated" colitis.

Generic 50 mg
(LEMMON)

▶ Drug Class: Antiestrogen

▶ Available in: Tablets

▶ Available OTC? No

▶ As Generic? Yes

Side Effects

SERIOUS
Bloating, stomach or
pelvic pain, changes in
vision or unusual sensi-
tivity to light, yellow discoloration of the eyes or
skin (jaundice). Serious
side effects with
clomiphene are unusual.
If any of these side
effects develop, call your
doctor immediately.

COMMON
Hot flashes, premenstrual
syndrome (PMS). Multi-
ple pregnancies (espe-
cially twin pregnancies)
are more likely in women
who use this drug.

LESS COMMON
Swelling, tenderness, or
discomfort in the breasts;
dizziness; headache;
heavy menstrual periods
or unexpected bleeding
from the vagina; depres-
sion; nausea and vomit-
ing; nervousness;
restlessness; fatigue;
insomnia.

PRINCIPAL USES
To stimulate the release of
eggs by the ovaries (ovulation) in women who wish to
become pregnant.

HOW THE DRUG WORKS
Clomiphene causes an
increase in the level of the
hormones that stimulate the
ovary to release eggs.

DOSAGE
The usual dose is 50 mg
once daily for 5 days, starting on the fifth day of the
menstrual period. Women
who do not have menstrual
cycles can begin taking it
on any convenient day. The
dose may be increased
gradually, up to a maximum
of 250 mg a day.
Clomiphene is usually prescribed for 3 to 4 menstrual
cycles and is stopped if
pregnancy is achieved during that time.

ONSET OF EFFECT
Ovulation occurs 7 to 10
days after the last day of
clomiphene treatment.
There may be considerable
individual variation in this
number, depending on the
patient's sensitivity to
clomiphene.

DURATION OF ACTION
Unknown.

DIETARY ADVICE
No special restrictions.

STORAGE
Store in a tightly sealed container away from heat and
direct light.

IF YOU MISS A DOSE
Take the missed dose as
soon as you remember,
unless the time for your
next scheduled dose is
within the next 2 hours. If
so, take a double dose at
the proper time, and
resume your regular dosage
schedule. Inform your doctor if you miss more than 1
day of treatment.

STOPPING THE DRUG
To be effective, this medication should be taken as prescribed for the full
treatment period. Do not
stop taking clomiphene on
your own.

PROLONGED USE
Do not take clomiphene for
more than 5 days in each
cycle unless otherwise
instructed by your doctor.
Clomiphene is usually prescribed for no more than 3
to 4 cycles; do not take it
for more than 3 to 4 cycles
without your doctor's
approval.

PRECAUTIONS
Over 60: Clomiphene is
usually prescribed only for
women of childbearing age.

**Driving and Hazardous
Work:** Do not drive or
engage in hazardous work
until you determine how the
medicine affects you.

Alcohol: Drink in strict
moderation if at all.

Pregnancy: Clomiphene
must not be used during
pregnancy; discontinue use
immediately if you become
pregnant.

Breast Feeding:
Clomiphene interferes with
the production of breast
milk and should not be
used while nursing.

Infants and Children:
Clomiphene should not be
used by children.

Special Concerns: Use
some means of monitoring
ovulation (for example, by
recording body temperature
changes or by using a home
urine ovulation test kit), as
it is crucial to discontinue
use of this drug when pregnancy occurs. See your doctor with each cycle and be
examined before resuming
clomiphene therapy. There
are many important aspects
to the treatment of infertility; clomiphene is one of
them. Remember to follow
instructions concerning the
frequency and timing of
intercourse with your partner. Try to take clomiphene
at the same time every day.
Maintain a strict dosing
schedule and try not to
miss any doses. Remember
that doses of clomiphene
can be doubled if you miss
one day.

OVERDOSE
Symptoms: No cases of
overdose have been
reported.

What to Do: If you are
concerned about the possibility of an overdose of
clomiphene, call your doctor, emergency medical services (EMS), or the nearest
poison control center.

DRUG INTERACTIONS
None reported.

FOOD INTERACTIONS
No known food interactions.

DISEASE INTERACTIONS
Consult your doctor if you
have any of the following
conditions: large ovary; cyst
on ovary; endometriosis or
excessively painful men-
strual periods; fibroids
(growths on the uterus);
phlebitis (painful inflammation of the veins, usually in
the leg); liver disease;
depression; or unusual
vaginal bleeding.

Clomipramine Hydrochloride

▶ Drug Class: Tricyclic antidepressant

▶ Available in: Capsules

▶ Available OTC? No

▶ As Generic? Yes

Side Effects

SERIOUS
Confusion, sexual dysfunction, heartbeat irregularities, hallucinations, seizures, extreme fatigue or drowsiness, vision problems, breathing difficulty; constipation, staring and absence of facial expression, impaired concentration, difficult urination, fever, extreme and persistent restlessness, loss of coordination and balance, difficulty swallowing or speaking, dilated pupils, eye pain, fainting. Also trembling, weakness, and stiffness in the extremities; shuffling gait. Call your doctor as soon as possible.

COMMON
Drowsiness or dizziness, headache, dry mouth or unpleasant taste, fatigue, heightened sensitivity to light, weight gain, nausea, increased appetite.

LESS COMMON
Heartburn, insomnia, diarrhea, sweating, vomiting.

PRINCIPAL USES
To treat obsessive-compulsive disorder, depression, panic disorder, and chronic pain.

HOW THE DRUG WORKS
Clomipramine affects levels of a specific brain chemical (serotonin) that is thought to be linked to mood, emotions, and mental state.

DOSAGE
Adults: To start, 25 mg once a day; may be increased to 250 mg a day. Children age 10 and older: To start, 25 mg once a day; may be increased to 200 mg a day. Older adults: To start, 25 mg a day; may be increased gradually by your doctor.

ONSET OF EFFECT
1 to 6 weeks.

DURATION OF ACTION
Unknown.

DIETARY ADVICE
To lessen stomach upset, take with food, unless your doctor instructs otherwise. Increase intake of fiber and fluids.

STORAGE
Store in a tightly sealed container away from heat, moisture, and direct light.

IF YOU MISS A DOSE
If you take a one-time daily bedtime dose, do not take a missed dose in the morning because it may cause drowsiness. Call your doctor. If you take more than 1 dose a day, take it as soon as you remember. If it is near the time for the next dose, skip the missed dose and resume your regular dosage schedule. Do not double the next dose.

STOPPING THE DRUG
Take as prescribed for the full treatment period, even if you begin to feel better before the scheduled end of therapy. The decision to stop taking the drug should be made in consultation with your doctor. The dosage should be gradually tapered when stopping.

PROLONGED USE
Usual course of therapy for depression lasts 6 months to 1 year; some patients may benefit from additional therapy. Usual course of therapy for obsessive-compulsive disorder lasts 1 year or more.

PRECAUTIONS
Over 60: Adverse reactions, especially confusion, are more likely and more severe in older patients. A lower dose may be warranted.

Driving and Hazardous Work: Exercise caution until you determine how the medication affects you. Drowsiness, lightheadedness, or confusion can occur.

Alcohol: Avoid alcohol.

Pregnancy: Adequate human studies have not been done. Consult your doctor.

Breast Feeding: Do not use clomipramine while nursing.

Infants and Children: Not prescribed for children under the age of 10.

Special Concerns: This is a potentially dangerous drug, especially if taken in excess. Tricyclic antidepressants should not be within easy reach of suicidal patients. If dry mouth occurs, use sugarless gum or candy.

OVERDOSE
Symptoms: Difficulty breathing, severe fatigue, seizures, confusion, hallucinations, distractibility, dilated pupils, irregular heartbeat, fever.

What to Do: Call your doctor, emergency medical services (EMS), or the nearest poison control center immediately.

DRUG INTERACTIONS
Consult your doctor for specific advice if you are taking antithyroid agents, cimetidine, clonidine, guanadrel, guanethidine, metrizamide, SSRI antidepressants, appetite suppressants, isoproterenol, ephedrine, epinephrine, amphetamines, phenylephrine, antipsychotic drugs, pimozide, methyldopa, metyrosine, metoclopramide, pemoline, promethazine, trimeprazine, rauwolfia alkaloids, MAO inhibitors, or any drugs that depress the central nervous system.

FOOD INTERACTIONS
No known food interactions.

DISEASE INTERACTIONS
Consult your doctor if you have any of the following: a history of alcohol abuse, difficulty urinating, asthma, bipolar disorder, high blood pressure, stomach or intestinal problems, glaucoma, overactive thyroid, enlarged prostate, schizophrenia, seizures, a blood disorder, or kidney, heart, or liver disease.

Clonazepam

Klonopin 0.5 mg
(ROCHE)

▶ Drug Class: Benzodiazepine tranquilizer; antianxiety agent

▶ Available in: Tablets, wafer

▶ Available OTC? No

▶ As Generic? Yes

Side Effects

SERIOUS
Difficulty concentrating, outbursts of anger, other behavior problems, depression, hallucinations, low blood pressure (causing faintness or confusion), memory impairment, muscle weakness, skin rash or itching, sore throat, fever and chills, sores or ulcers in throat or mouth, unusual bruising or bleeding, extreme fatigue, yellowish tinge to eyes or skin. Call your doctor immediately.

COMMON
Drowsiness, loss of coordination, unsteady gait, dizziness, lightheadedness, slurred speech.

LESS COMMON
Change in sexual desire or ability, constipation, false sense of well-being, nausea and vomiting, urinary problems, unusual fatigue.

PRINCIPAL USES
To control seizures; for relief of anxiety and panic attacks.

HOW THE DRUG WORKS
In general, clonazepam produces mild sedation by depressing activity in the central nervous system (the brain and spinal cord). In particular, clonazepam appears to enhance the effect of gamma-aminobutyric acid (GABA), a natural chemical that inhibits the firing of neurons and dampens the transmission of nerve signals, thus decreasing nervous excitation.

DOSAGE
Adults: Initial dose of 0.5 mg, 3 times a day. Patients with seizures may require significantly higher doses. Your doctor will determine the optimal dose. Maximum dose rarely exceeds 20 mg a day. Children: Dose is based on age and body weight.

ONSET OF EFFECT
Within 1 to 2 hours.

DURATION OF ACTION
Less than 24 hours.

DIETARY ADVICE
No special restrictions.

STORAGE
Store in a tightly sealed container away from heat, moisture, and direct light.

IF YOU MISS A DOSE
Take it as soon as you remember, unless your next scheduled dose is within the next 2 hours. If so, do not take the missed dose. Take your next scheduled dose at the proper time and resume your regular dosage schedule. Do not double the next dose.

STOPPING THE DRUG
Discontinuing the drug abruptly may produce withdrawal symptoms (sleep disruption, nervousness, irritability, diarrhea, abdominal cramps, muscle aches, memory impairment). Dosage should be reduced gradually according to your doctor's instructions.

PROLONGED USE
Short-term therapy (8 weeks or less) is typical; do not take it for a longer period unless so advised by your doctor.

PRECAUTIONS

Over 60: Adverse reactions are more likely and more severe in older patients.

Driving and Hazardous Work: Clonazepam can impair mental alertness and physical coordination. Adjust your activities accordingly.

Alcohol: Alcohol must be avoided while taking this medication.

Pregnancy: Taking clonazepam during pregnancy is not recommended.

Breast Feeding: Clonazepam passes into breast milk and may be harmful to the infant; do not take it while nursing.

Infants and Children: This drug is rarely prescribed for young patients.

Special Concerns: Clonazepam use can lead to psychological or physical dependence. Never take more than the prescribed daily dose.

OVERDOSE
Symptoms: Extreme drowsiness, confusion, slurred speech, slow reflexes, poor coordination, staggering gait, tremor, slowed breathing, loss of consciousness.

What to Do: Call your doctor, emergency medical services (EMS), or the nearest poison control center immediately.

DRUG INTERACTIONS
Other drugs may interact with clonazepam. Consult your doctor for specific advice if you are taking any drugs that depress the central nervous system; these include antihistamines, antidepressants or other psychiatric medications, barbiturates, sedatives, cough medicines, decongestants, and painkillers. Be sure your doctor knows about any over-the-counter medication you may take.

FOOD INTERACTIONS
None reported.

DISEASE INTERACTIONS
Caution is advised when taking clonazepam. Consult your doctor if you have a history of alcohol or drug abuse, stroke or other brain disease, any chronic lung disease, hyperactivity, depression or other mental illness, myasthenia gravis, sleep apnea, epilepsy, porphyria, kidney disease, or liver disease.

Clonidine Hydrochloride

BRAND NAMES
Catapres, Catapres-TTS

Generic 0.2 mg
(MYLAN)

Additional photographs

▶ Drug Class: Centrally acting antihypertensive

▶ Available in: Tablets, skin patch

▶ Available OTC? No

▶ As Generic? Yes

Side Effects

SERIOUS
Serious side effects are less likely when clonidine is used as directed.

COMMON
Dry mouth, reduced saliva, drowsiness, dizziness, constipation. Also itching or skin irritation (with skin patch only).

LESS COMMON
Mental depression, swelling of feet and lower legs, pale or cold fingertips and toes, vivid dreams or nightmares. Also darkening of skin (skin patch only).

PRINCIPAL USES
To treat high blood pressure (hypertension).

HOW THE DRUG WORKS
Clonidine acts upon certain areas of the central nervous system (the brain and spinal cord) that regulate the activity of the heart and the smooth muscle tissue surrounding the arteries. It causes the blood vessels to relax and widen, which lowers blood pressure.

DOSAGE
Tablets— Adults: Initial dose is 0.1 mg, 2 times per day. Your doctor may increase this to 0.3 mg, 2 times per day. Most patients achieve adequate blood pressure control with 1 mg or less per day; maximum daily dose is 2.4 mg. Children: Pediatrician will determine proper dosage. Skin patch— The starting dose is one TTS-1 patch per week. Doses above two TTS-3 patches per week are usually not effective. The patch should be applied to a hairless area of skin, ideally on the chest or upper arm. The skin must be free of rashes, blisters, or any form of skin disease.

ONSET OF EFFECT
Tablets: 30 to 60 minutes.
Skin patch: 2 to 3 days.

DURATION OF ACTION
Tablets: Up to 8 hours. Skin patch: 7 days per patch, if patch is left in place as directed; otherwise, up to 8 hours from the time the patch is removed.

DIETARY ADVICE
Follow a healthy diet (low-salt, low-fat, low-cholesterol) as advised by your doctor to help control blood pressure and prevent heart disease.

STORAGE
Store in a tightly sealed container away from heat, moisture, and direct light.

IF YOU MISS A DOSE
Take your missed dose as soon as you remember, unless the time for your next scheduled dose is within the next 2 hours. If so, do not take the missed dose. Take your next dose at the proper time and resume your regular dosage schedule. Do not take a double dose. If you miss more than 1 day of clonidine, inform your doctor.

STOPPING THE DRUG
Stopping clonidine abruptly can lead to a dangerous increase in blood pressure. Do not stop taking clonidine on your own, even if you are feeling better. Your doctor will gradually decrease your dose if necessary.

PROLONGED USE
Long-term use may be necessary and may lead to an increased risk of side effects.

PRECAUTIONS
Over 60: Adverse reactions may be more likely and more severe in older patients.

Driving and Hazardous Work: This medication may cause dizziness and drowsiness; avoid potentially dangerous activities until you know how it affects you.

Alcohol: Avoid alcohol while taking this drug.

Pregnancy: Clonidine use is not recommended during pregnancy.

Breast Feeding: Clonidine passes into breast milk; consult your doctor for advice.

Infants and Children: This drug is not recommended for young patients.

Special Concerns: Blood pressure may rise significantly after missing a few doses. Signs of dangerously high blood pressure are chest pain, dizziness, headache, blurred vision, confusion, restlessness, trembling of hands and fingers, anxiety, stomach pains, nausea, and vomiting. Make sure you have enough clonidine to last through weekends, vacations, or extended trips. Apply each skin patch to a different area of the chest or upper arm.

OVERDOSE
Symptoms: Low blood pressure, slow heartbeat, difficulty breathing, severe dizziness, confusion, weakness or faintness, tiny, constricted pupils.

What to Do: Call your doctor, emergency medical services (EMS), or the nearest poison control center immediately.

DRUG INTERACTIONS
Consult your doctor if you are taking beta-blockers or tricyclic antidepressants.

FOOD INTERACTIONS
No known food interactions.

DISEASE INTERACTIONS
Tell your doctor if you have any of the following problems: heart or blood vessel disease, including strokes and cardiac arrhythmias; skin disease, such as scleroderma (a concern with the skin patch only); kidney disease; mental depression; Raynaud's syndrome; or systemic lupus erythematosus.

Clopidogrel Bisulfate

BRAND NAME
Plavix

▶ Drug Class: Antiplatelet drug

▶ Available in: Tablets

▶ Available OTC? No

▶ As Generic? No

Side Effects

SERIOUS
Gastrointestinal bleeding, fainting, palpitations, extreme fatigue, shortness of breath, chest pain. Call your doctor immediately. In rare instances the drug can block production of white blood cells (a major component of the immune system), leading to potentially severe infections. Seek medical attention promptly at the first signs of infection, especially a high fever.

COMMON
Stomach pain, indigestion, diarrhea, skin rash, itching, flu-like symptoms, body aches or pain, headache, dizziness, joint pain, back pain, increased risk of upper respiratory infection.

LESS COMMON
General weakness, hernia, leg cramps, tingling and numbness in the limbs, vomiting, gout, arthritis, anxiety, insomnia, anemia, dermatitis and skin eruptions, bladder infection, cataract, conjunctivitis.

PRINCIPAL USES
To reduce the risk of recurrence of heart attack or stroke in patients diagnosed with severe arterial disease (atherosclerosis).

HOW THE DRUG WORKS
Heart attacks and strokes occur when a blood clot that forms in a narrowed portion of an artery blocks blood flow and thus cuts off the supply of oxygen and nutrients to the tissue that lies beyond the site of the clot. Clopidogrel can prevent heart attacks and strokes by preventing the aggregation (clumping) of platelets, a type of blood cell that initiates clot formation.

DOSAGE
75 mg once a day.

ONSET OF EFFECT
2 hours or more.

DURATION OF ACTION
Unknown.

DIETARY ADVICE
Clopidogrel can be taken with or without food.

STORAGE
Store in a tightly sealed container away from heat, moisture, and direct light.

IF YOU MISS A DOSE
If you miss a dose on one day, do not double the dose the next day. Resume your regular dosage schedule.

STOPPING THE DRUG
Take it as prescribed for the full treatment period.

PROLONGED USE
Side effects are more likely with prolonged use.

PRECAUTIONS
Over 60: No special problems are expected.

Driving and Hazardous Work: The use of this drug should not impair your ability to perform such tasks safely.

Alcohol: No special precautions are necessary.

Pregnancy: Adequate human studies have not been done. Before taking clopidogrel, tell your doctor if you are pregnant or plan to become pregnant.

Breast Feeding: Clopidogrel passes into breast milk; extreme caution is advised. Consult your doctor for specific advice.

Infants and Children: The safety and effectiveness of clopidogrel use in infants and children have not been established.

Special Concerns: Before you schedule surgery, tell the surgeon or dentist that you are taking this drug.

OVERDOSE
Symptoms: No overdose symptoms have been reported.

What to Do: However, if a greatly excessive dose is taken, call your doctor, emergency medical services (EMS), or the nearest poison control center.

DRUG INTERACTIONS
Consult your doctor for specific advice if you are taking any of the following drugs that may interact with clopidogrel: aspirin or any other nonsteroidal anti-inflammatory drugs (NSAIDs), phenytoin, tamoxifen, tolbutamide, torsemide, fluvastatin, or warfarin.

FOOD INTERACTIONS
No known food interactions.

DISEASE INTERACTIONS
This drug should not be used if you have a peptic ulcer or a history of brain hemorrhage. Caution is advised when taking clopidogrel. Consult your doctor if you have a history of bleeding problems or if you develop bleeding problems while taking this drug. Use of clopidogrel may cause complications in patients with liver disease, since the liver inactivates the drug.

Clorazepate Dipotassium

BRAND NAME
Tranxene

▶ Drug Class: Benzodiazepine tranquilizer; antianxiety agent

▶ Available in: Tablets

▶ Available OTC? No

▶ As Generic? Yes

Side Effects

SERIOUS
Difficulty concentrating, outbursts of anger, other behavior problems, depression, hallucinations, low blood pressure (causing faintness or confusion), memory impairment, muscle weakness, skin rash or itching, sore throat, fever and chills, sores or ulcers in throat or mouth, unusual bruising or bleeding, extreme fatigue, yellowish tinge to eyes or skin. Call your doctor immediately.

COMMON
Drowsiness, loss of coordination, unsteady gait, dizziness, lightheadedness, slurred speech.

LESS COMMON
Change in sexual desire or ability, constipation, false sense of well-being, nausea and vomiting, urinary problems, unusual fatigue.

PRINCIPAL USES
For relief of anxiety and panic attacks.

HOW THE DRUG WORKS
In general, clorazepate produces mild sedation by depressing activity in the central nervous system. In particular, clorazepate appears to enhance the effect of gamma-aminobutyric acid (GABA), a natural chemical that inhibits the firing of neurons and dampens the transmission of nerve signals, thus decreasing nervous excitation.

DOSAGE
For anxiety: Usual dose is 7.5 to 15 mg, 2 to 4 times a day. The dosage may be increased or decreased depending on an individual's response. Older adults are usually started at a total dose of 7.5 to 15 mg a day.

ONSET OF EFFECT
Within 1 to 2 hours.

DURATION OF ACTION
Less than 48 hours.

DIETARY ADVICE
No special restrictions.

STORAGE
Store in a tightly sealed container away from heat, moisture, and direct light.

IF YOU MISS A DOSE
Take it as soon as you remember, unless the time for your next scheduled dose is within 2 hours. If so, skip the missed dose and resume your regular dosage schedule. Do not double the next dose.

STOPPING THE DRUG
Do not stop taking the drug abruptly, as this can cause withdrawal symptoms (seizures, sleep disruption, nervousness, irritability, diarrhea, abdominal cramps, muscle aches, memory impairment). Dosage should be reduced gradually as directed by your doctor.

PROLONGED USE
Clorazepate may slowly lose its effectiveness with prolonged use. See your doctor for periodic evaluation if you must take this drug for an extended time.

PRECAUTIONS
Over 60: Adverse reactions may be more likely and more severe in older patients.

Driving and Hazardous Work: The use of clorazepate may impair your ability to perform such tasks safely.

Alcohol: Avoid alcohol.

Pregnancy: Avoid or discontinue use of this drug during pregnancy.

Breast Feeding: Do not take this drug while breast feeding.

Infants and Children: Not recommended for children under 9 years of age.

Special Concerns: Use of this drug can lead to psychological or physical dependence. Never take more than the prescribed daily dose.

OVERDOSE
Symptoms: Extreme drowsiness, confusion, slurred speech, slow reflexes, poor coordination, staggering gait, tremor, slowed breathing, loss of consciousness.

What to Do: Call your doctor, emergency medical services (EMS), or the nearest poison control center immediately.

DRUG INTERACTIONS
Consult your doctor for specific advice if you are taking any drugs that depress the central nervous system; these include antihistamines, antidepressants or other psychiatric medications, barbiturates, sedatives, cough medicines, decongestants, and painkillers. Be sure your doctor knows about any over-the-counter medication you may take.

FOOD INTERACTIONS
None are known.

DISEASE INTERACTIONS
Consult your doctor if you have a history of alcohol or drug abuse, stroke or other brain disease, any chronic lung disease, hyperactivity, depression or other mental illness, myasthenia gravis, sleep apnea, epilepsy, porphyria, kidney disease, or liver disease.

Clotrimazole

BRAND NAMES
FemCare, Femizole-7, Gyne-Lotrimin, Gyne-Lotrimin 3, Lotrimin, Mycelex, Mycelex Troche, Mycelex Twin Pack, Mycelex-7, Mycelex-G

▶ Drug Class: Antifungal

▶ Available in: Topical cream, lotion, solution, oral lozenges, vaginal cream, tablets

▶ Available OTC? Yes

▶ As Generic? Yes

Side Effects

SERIOUS
Topical: Hives, skin rash, itching, burning, peeling, stinging, redness, or other skin irritation not present prior to treatment. Lozenge and vaginal: None reported.

COMMON
Topical: None reported. Lozenge (when swallowed): Diarrhea, stomach cramping or pain, nausea or vomiting. Vaginal: Vaginal burning, itching, discharge, or other irritation not present prior to treatment.

LESS COMMON
Topical and lozenge: None reported. Vaginal: Headache, stomach cramps or pain, irritation or burning of sexual partner's penis.

PRINCIPAL USES
To treat fungal infections of the mouth and throat (thrush), vaginal area (yeast infection), and the skin, such as tinea corporis (ringworm), tinea cruris (jock itch), tinea pedis (athlete's foot), and pityriasis versicolor ("sun fungus," a fungal skin condition characterized by fine scaly patches of varying shapes, sizes, and colors).

HOW THE DRUG WORKS
Clotrimazole prevents fungal organisms from producing vital substances required for growth and function.

DOSAGE
Topical cream, lotion, solution (for skin infections)—Adults and children: Apply twice a day, in the morning and in the evening. Oral lozenges (to treat thrush)—Adults and children age 5 and older: Dissolve one 10 mg lozenge in mouth 5 times a day for 14 days. To prevent thrush: Adults and children age 5 and older: Dissolve one 10 mg lozenge in mouth 3 times a day. Vaginal cream (for yeast infections)— Adults and teenagers: At bedtime, insert vaginally with an applicator 50 mg of 1% cream for 6 to 14 nights, or 100 mg of 2% cream for 3 nights, or 500 mg of 10% cream for 1 night only. Vaginal tablets (for yeast infections)— Nonpregnant women and teenagers: At bedtime, insert one 100 mg tablet for 6 to 7 nights, or one 200 mg tablet for 3 nights, or one 500 mg tablet for 1 night only. Pregnant women and teenagers: At bedtime, insert one 100 mg tablet for 7 nights.

ONSET OF EFFECT
Unknown.

DURATION OF ACTION
Lozenges: 3 hours. Other forms: Unknown.

DIETARY ADVICE
No special restrictions.

STORAGE
Store in a tightly sealed container away from heat, moisture, and direct light. Do not allow it to freeze.

IF YOU MISS A DOSE
Take it as soon as you remember. If it is near the time for the next dose, skip the missed dose and resume your regular dosage schedule. Do not double the next dose.

STOPPING THE DRUG
If you are using this drug by prescription, take it as prescribed for the full treatment period, even if you begin to feel better before the scheduled end of therapy. Recurrence of the infection is likely if you stop before the full treatment period is complete.

PROLONGED USE
Clotrimazole is generally prescribed for short-term therapy (1 to 14 days). Consult your doctor for further information.

PRECAUTIONS
Over 60: No special problems are expected.

Driving and Hazardous Work: No special precautions are necessary.

Alcohol: No special precautions are necessary.

Pregnancy: Adequate studies on the use of clotrimazole during pregnancy have not been done; however, no problems have been reported. Consult your doctor for specific advice.

Breast Feeding: Clotrimazole may pass into breast milk; caution is advised. Consult your doctor for advice.

Infants and Children: Topical forms: No special warnings. Lozenges are not recommended for children younger than age 5. Vaginal forms: Not commonly prescribed for children under the age of 12.

Special Concerns: Do not chew or swallow lozenges. Clotrimazole lozenges may take 15 to 30 minutes to dissolve completely and are useless if swallowed.

OVERDOSE
Symptoms: An overdose with clotrimazole is unlikely.

What to Do: If someone should swallow a large amount of the medicine, call your doctor, emergency medical services (EMS), or the nearest poison control center immediately.

DRUG INTERACTIONS
No drug interactions have been reported.

FOOD INTERACTIONS
No food interactions have been reported.

DISEASE INTERACTIONS
No disease interactions have been reported.

Clozapine

BRAND NAME
Clozaril

Clozaril 25 mg
(NOVARTIS)

▸ Drug Class: Neuroleptic; antipsychotic

▸ Available in: Tablets

▸ Available OTC? No

▸ As Generic? Yes

Side Effects

SERIOUS
Signs of serious infection including high fever, chills, and sweating, sores or ulcers in the mouth, unusual bruising or bleeding, severe fatigue or weakness. Other serious side effects include seizures, yellow discoloration of the eyes or skin, rapid or irregular heartbeat, severe dizziness, severe low blood pressure (which may cause lightheadedness and fainting, especially when getting up suddenly from sitting or lying positions), and hyperglycemia (elevated blood glucose levels), with symptoms including increased thirst, hunger, and urination. If you experience such symptoms, contact your doctor immediately.

COMMON
Increased salivation, dizziness, drowsiness, mild headache, constipation, nausea or vomiting, weight gain.

LESS COMMON
Abdominal pain, heartburn, sore throat, diarrhea, muscle aches, spasms, or weakness, loss of coordination.

PRINCIPAL USES
Clozapine is used to treat schizophrenia after other standard medications have proved inadequate.

HOW THE DRUG WORKS
Clozapine inhibits activity of the brain chemical dopamine, thereby helping to prevent the overstimulation of specific nerve centers in the brain believed to be responsible for certain psychiatric disorders.

DOSAGE
Adults: 12.5 mg, 1 to 2 times daily; may be increased gradually by your doctor to as much as 900 mg a day. Children: Consult your pediatrician.

ONSET OF EFFECT
Within 2 to 4 weeks. Full effect may not be seen until after 3 months of therapy.

DURATION OF ACTION
Unknown.

DIETARY ADVICE
No special restrictions.

STORAGE
Store in a tightly sealed container away from heat and direct light.

IF YOU MISS A DOSE
Take it as soon as you remember, unless the time for the next scheduled dose is within the next 2 hours. If so, skip the missed dose and resume your regular dosage schedule with the next dose. Do not double the next dose.

STOPPING THE DRUG
Do not stop taking the drug abruptly or without your doctor's approval. Dose must be reduced gradually to prevent withdrawal symptoms from occurring.

PROLONGED USE
The risk of side effects may increase with long-term use of clozapine.

PRECAUTIONS
Over 60: Adverse reactions may be more likely and more severe in older patients.

Driving and Hazardous Work: The use of clozapine may impair your ability to perform such tasks safely.

Alcohol: Avoid alcohol.

Pregnancy: Adequate studies on the use of clozapine during pregnancy have not been done. Consult your doctor for specific advice.

Breast Feeding: Clozapine passes into breast milk; do not use it while nursing.

Infants and Children: Safety and effectiveness of the use of clozapine in children under the age of 16 have not been established.

Special Concerns: Frequent blood tests are required while taking clozapine. This medication can cause a marked decrease in the level of white blood cells in the body. Clozapine prescriptions are sometimes filled only one week at a time, on the condition that the patient be given a blood test to check white cell count before the following week's medication is dispensed. Report symptoms of fever, chills, nausea, vomiting, diarrhea, painful urination, or cough to your doctor when taking this medication.

OVERDOSE
Symptoms: Confusion, restlessness, nervousness, severe drowsiness, hallucinations, fainting, unconsciousness, coma; unusual excitement or agitation; slow, deep breathing or rapid, shallow breathing, or breathing difficulty; increased salivation; rapid or irregular pulse.

What to Do: Call your doctor, emergency medical services (EMS), or the nearest poison control center immediately.

DRUG INTERACTIONS
Other drugs may interact with clozapine. Consult your doctor for specific advice if you are taking sleeping pills or sedatives, antidepressants, amphotericin B, anticancer drugs, thyroid medications, azathioprine, chlorambucil, chloramphenicol, colchicine, cyclophosphamide, flucytosine, haloperidol, interferon, lithium, mercaptopurine, methotrexate, plicamycin, zidovudine (AZT), cimetidine, or erythromycin.

FOOD INTERACTIONS
None reported.

DISEASE INTERACTIONS
Consult your doctor if you have a history of any type of blood disorder, enlarged prostate, difficult urination, stomach or intestinal disorder, heart or blood vessel disease, epilepsy or other seizure disorder, kidney disease, or liver disease.

Coal Tar

▶ Drug Class: Antipsoriasis drug

▶ Available in: Cleansing bar, cream, gel, lotion, ointment, shampoo, liquid

▶ Available OTC? Yes

▶ As Generic? Yes

Side Effects

SERIOUS
Skin irritation or rash not present before use of coal tar. Call your doctor immediately.

COMMON
Mild stinging, increased sensitivity to sunlight.

LESS COMMON
There are no less-common side effects associated with the use of coal tar.

PRINCIPAL USES
To treat skin conditions including dandruff, eczema, seborrheic dermatitis, and psoriasis.

HOW THE DRUG WORKS
Coal tar promotes softening, dissolution, and peeling of hard, scaly, roughened, or irregular surface skin. It also has antiseptic properties and fights fungal, bacterial, and parasitic organisms.

DOSAGE
Cleansing bar: Use 1 or 2 times a day as directed by your doctor. Cream: Apply to affected areas up to 4 times a day. Gel: Apply to affected areas 1 or 2 times a day. Lotion: Apply to affected areas as needed. Ointment: Apply to affected areas 2 or 3 times a day. Shampoo: Use once a day, once a week, or as directed by your doctor. Topical solution: Apply to skin or scalp or use in the bath, depending on product. Topical bath solution: Add appropriate amount to bath water; immerse yourself in the bath for 20 minutes. If you have any questions about its use, consult your doctor.

ONSET OF EFFECT
Unknown.

DURATION OF ACTION
Unknown.

DIETARY ADVICE
Coal tar can be used without regard to diet.

STORAGE
Store in a tightly sealed container away from heat and direct light. Do not allow liquid forms to freeze.

IF YOU MISS A DOSE
Apply it as soon as you remember. If it is near the time for the next dose, skip the missed dose and resume your regular dosage schedule. Do not apply a double dose.

STOPPING THE DRUG
If you are applying coal tar by prescription, the decision to stop using it should be made by your doctor. If you are using the drug without a prescription, you may stop treatment whenever you choose.

PROLONGED USE
Do not use coal tar for longer than your physician prescribes.

PRECAUTIONS
Over 60: Coal tar is not expected to cause different side effects or problems in older patients than it does in younger persons.

Driving and Hazardous Work: The use of coal tar should not impair your ability to perform such tasks safely.

Alcohol: No special restrictions apply.

Pregnancy: Studies of coal tar use during pregnancy have not been done in animals or humans. Before you use coal tar, tell your doctor if you are pregnant or plan to become pregnant.

Breast Feeding: It is not known if coal tar passes into breast milk. Consult your doctor for specific advice.

Infants and Children: Use and dose in infants and children must be determined by your doctor.

Special Concerns: For external use only. Keep coal tar away from the eyes. If you accidentally get some of the medicine in your eyes, flush them thoroughly with water. After applying coal tar, protect the treated area from sunlight for 72 hours, and be sure to remove all coal tar before being exposed to sunlight or using a sunlamp . Do not apply coal tar to infected, blistered, raw, or oozing areas of the skin.

OVERDOSE
Symptoms: None reported.

What to Do: Emergency instructions not applicable.

DRUG INTERACTIONS
Consult your doctor for specific advice if you are using tetracyclines, psoralens, or retinoids. Also tell your doctor if you are using any other prescription or over-the-counter medication.

FOOD INTERACTIONS
No known food interactions.

DISEASE INTERACTIONS
You should not use coal tar if you have had a prior allergic reaction to it.

Codeine

Codeine is available in generic form only.

Generic 15 mg
(ROXANE)

Additional photographs

▶ Drug Class: Opioid (narcotic) analgesic

▶ Available in: Tablets, oral solution

▶ Available OTC? No

▶ As Generic? Yes

Side Effects

SERIOUS
Serious side effects of codeine are indistinguishable from those of overdose: Confusion; sleepiness; slurred speech; unconsciousness; small, pinpoint pupils; cold, clammy skin; slow breathing; seizures; severe drowsiness, weakness, or dizziness.

COMMON
Mild dizziness or lightheadedness, nausea or vomiting, constipation, drowsiness, itching.

LESS COMMON
Headache, sweating, false sense of well-being (euphoria).

PRINCIPAL USES
To treat mild to moderate pain or to control a severe cough.

HOW THE DRUG WORKS
Narcotics such as codeine relieve pain by acting on specific areas of the spinal cord and brain that process pain signals from nerves throughout the body. Codeine dulls the cough reflex, which is why it may be used to treat certain coughs.

DOSAGE
Adults— For pain: 15 to 60 mg every 3 to 6 hours as needed. Usual dose is 30 mg. For cough: 10 to 20 mg every 3 to 6 hours as needed. Children— Oral solution: For pain: 0.5 mg per 2.2 lbs (1 kg) of body weight every 4 to 6 hours as needed. For cough: Age 2: 3 mg every 4 to 6 hours. Take no more than 12 mg a day. Age 3: 3.5 mg every 4 to 6 hours. Take no more than 14 mg a day. Age 4: 4 mg every 4 to 6 hours. Take no more than 16 mg a day. Age 5: 4.5 mg every 4 to 6 hours. Take no more than 18 mg a day. Ages 6 to 12: 5 to 10 mg every 4 to 6 hours. Take no more than 60 mg per day.

ONSET OF EFFECT
30 to 45 minutes.

DURATION OF ACTION
4 to 6 hours.

DIETARY ADVICE
Codeine is constipating; make sure your diet contains adequate amounts of fiber and vegetables.

STORAGE
Store in a tightly sealed container away from heat, moisture, and direct light.

IF YOU MISS A DOSE
Take it as soon as you remember. If it is near the time for the next dose, skip the missed dose and resume your regular dosage schedule. Do not double the next dose.

STOPPING THE DRUG
You should take it as prescribed for the full treatment period, but you may stop taking the drug if you are feeling better before the scheduled end of therapy.

PROLONGED USE
Therapy varies, depending on the cause of the pain. Some patients require long-term narcotic therapy. Side effects may be more likely with prolonged use.

PRECAUTIONS
Over 60: Adverse reactions may be more likely and more severe in older patients.

Driving and Hazardous Work: The use of codeine may impair your ability to perform such tasks safely.

Alcohol: Avoid alcohol.

Pregnancy: Adequate human studies have not been completed. Before taking codeine, tell your physician if you are pregnant or plan to become pregnant.

Breast Feeding: Codeine passes into breast milk; caution is advised. Consult your doctor for specific advice.

Infants and Children: Adverse reactions may be more likely and more severe in children.

Special Concerns: Codeine can cause physical dependence. Some patients may experience withdrawal symptoms when the medication is discontinued. These may include body aches, abdominal pain, stomach cramps, diarrhea, runny nose, gooseflesh, nervousness, agitation, sweating, yawning, loss of appetite, shivering, insomnia, dilated pupils, and weakness. Do not exceed recommended doses or increase the dose on your own.

OVERDOSE
Symptoms: Confusion; sleepiness; slurred speech; unconsciousness; small, pinpoint pupils; cold, clammy skin; slow breathing; seizures; severe drowsiness, weakness, or dizziness.

What to Do: Call your doctor, emergency medical services (EMS), or the nearest poison control center immediately.

DRUG INTERACTIONS
Consult your doctor for specific advice if you are taking carbamazepine or other medicine for seizures, barbiturates, sedatives, cough medicines, decongestants, antidepressants, other prescription pain medications, MAO inhibitors, naltrexone, rifampin, or zidovudine.

FOOD INTERACTIONS
None known.

DISEASE INTERACTIONS
Consult your doctor if you have any of the following: emotional illness; brain disorders or head injury; seizures; lung disease; prostate problems or other problems with urination; gallstones; colitis; heart, kidney, liver, or thyroid disease; or a history of alcohol or drug abuse.

Colchicine

Generic 0.5 mg
(WEST-WARD)

▶ Drug Class: Antigout drug

▶ Available in: Tablets, injection

▶ Available OTC? No

▶ As Generic? Yes

Side Effects

SERIOUS
Allergic reactions, causing rash or hives, swelling of face, lips, tongue, eyelids, and throat; such reactions may interfere with breathing—seek medical help immediately. Unusual or persistent fevers, fatigue, chills, sore throat, bruising, or bleeding; these may be signs of serious anemia or suppression of the immune system.

COMMON
Diarrhea, vomiting, nausea, stomach pain.

LESS COMMON
Muscle weakness; numbness, tingling, or prickling in the hands and feet.

PRINCIPAL USES
To treat painful attacks of gout, as well as to prevent or reduce the frequency of such attacks. Oral colchicine is used for moderate attacks. Injectable colchicine is used for serious attacks or in patients who cannot take the tablets.

HOW THE DRUG WORKS
In gout, crystals of a chemical called monosodium urate are deposited in joints, where they cause inflammation and lead to the sharp, excruciating pain of a gout attack. Colchicine prevents inflammation that may result from the accumulation of monosodium urate crystals.

DOSAGE
For an acute attack: 0.5 to 1.2 mg immediately; then 0.5 or 0.6 mg every 1 or 2 hours, or 1 to 1.2 mg every 2 hours, to a maximum of 6 mg. Stop as soon as you achieve relief. For chronic gout or to prevent attacks: 0.5 or 0.6 mg, usually once a day. Not all patients require daily doses; some may take colchicine periodically. Consult your doctor.

ONSET OF EFFECT
6 to 12 hours.

DURATION OF ACTION
Unknown.

DIETARY ADVICE
No special restrictions.

STORAGE
Store in a tightly sealed container away from heat and direct light. Keep it away from moisture and extremes in temperature.

IF YOU MISS A DOSE
Take it as soon as you remember. If it is near the time for the next dose, skip the missed dose and resume your regular dosage schedule. Do not double the next dose.

STOPPING THE DRUG
You may stop taking the drug if you are feeling better before the scheduled end of therapy. If it was prescribed for long-term use, however, do not stop without first consulting your doctor.

PROLONGED USE
Therapy for a severe attack is usually completed within 1 day. Do not take colchicine for a longer period without your doctor's approval.

PRECAUTIONS
Over 60: Adverse reactions may be more likely and more severe in older patients.

Driving and Hazardous Work: Do not drive or engage in hazardous work until you determine how the medicine affects you.

Alcohol: Avoid alcohol.

Pregnancy: Avoid or discontinue this medication if you are pregnant or trying to become pregnant.

Breast Feeding: Colchicine passes into breast milk; avoid or discontinue use while nursing.

Infants and Children: Not recommended.

Special Concerns: Make sure you understand how to take this drug; colchicine treatments vary. Dosing schedules for an acute attack can be confusing. Read your label carefully; make sure you understand how many tablets constitute the correct dose. Many patients find it helpful to write the dosing plan on an index card and to carry a copy in a wallet or handbag.

Do not continue taking colchicine during an acute gout attack if you begin feeling nauseated, begin vomiting, or develop diarrhea. Call your doctor. Do not continue taking colchicine during an acute attack once you have taken 6 mg; if you still have not achieved relief after reaching this limit, call your doctor.

OVERDOSE
Symptoms: Fever; convulsions; confusion, disorientation, delirium; rapid or irregular breathing; sharp, burning pain in stomach; diarrhea, which may be bloody.

What to Do: Call emergency medical services (EMS), your doctor, or the nearest poison control center immediately.

DRUG INTERACTIONS
Consult your doctor for advice if you are taking phenylbutazone or drugs that may affect your bone marrow including anticonvulsants, certain antibiotics, and chemotherapy drugs for cancer.

FOOD INTERACTIONS
None are likely, but a low-purine diet is recommended to reduce the risk of gout attacks. Foods high in purines include anchovies, sardines, legumes, poultry, sweetbreads, liver, kidneys, and other organ meats.

DISEASE INTERACTIONS
Consult your doctor if you have heart, liver, or kidney disease; blood disorders; or gastrointestinal disorders, such as ulcers, colitis, and intestinal malabsorption.

Colesevelam Hydrochloride

▶ Drug Class: Antilipidemic (cholesterol-lowering agent)

▶ Available in: Tablets

▶ Available OTC? No

▶ As Generic? No

Side Effects

SERIOUS
No serious side effects have been reported in association with the use of colesevelam.

COMMON
Constipation, heartburn.

LESS COMMON
No less common side effects have been reported in association with colesevelam.

PRINCIPAL USES
To reduce cholesterol in people with high blood levels of low-density lipoprotein (LDL), as part of a comprehensive treatment program that includes exercise and special diet. May also be taken in conjunction with another cholesterol drugs called "statins" (such as simvastatin, lovastatin, fluvastatin, pravastatin, or atorvastatin).

HOW THE DRUG WORKS
Colesevelam binds bile acids in the intestine, forming an insoluble complex that is excreted in the feces. This process reduces the amount of bile acids in the blood. In response to the lower levels of bile acids, the liver converts more cholesterol to bile acids. As a consequence, the amount of cholesterol in liver cells declines, and the liver makes more receptors for LDL. The resulting increased removal of LDL from the blood lowers LDL cholesterol.

DOSAGE
3 tablets (625 mg each) twice a day with meals or 6 tablets once a day with a meal, either alone or in combination with a statin. The dose may be increased by your doctor to 7 tablets a day.

ONSET OF EFFECT
Within 2 weeks.

DURATION OF ACTION
For as long as the drug is continued.

DIETARY ADVICE
Follow all special dietary restrictions and guidelines as directed by your doctor. Take colesevelam with a liquid and a meal.

STORAGE
Store in a tightly sealed container away from heat and moisture.

IF YOU MISS A DOSE
Take as soon as you remember. However, if it is near the time for the next dose, skip the missed dose and resume your regular dosage schedule. Do not double the next dose.

STOPPING THE DRUG
The decision to stop taking the drug should be made in consultation with your physician.

PROLONGED USE
Colesevelam may be used safely for years; however, periodic evaluation of the drug's effectiveness and its effects on the liver is necessary.

PRECAUTIONS
Over 60: No special problems are expected.

Driving and Hazardous Work: No special precautions are necessary.

Alcohol: No special precautions are necessary.

Pregnancy: The effects on a fetus are unknown. Consult your doctor if you become or plan to become pregnant.

Breast Feeding: No special precautions are necessary.

Infants and Children: Safety and effectiveness have not been established for patients under 18 years of age. Consult your doctor for specific advice.

Special Concerns: At very high doses, colesevelam may interfere with the absorption of fats and fat-soluble vitamins (vitamins A, D, E, and K); vitamin supplementation may be advised.

OVERDOSE
Symptoms: None reported.

What to Do: Emergency instructions not applicable.

DRUG INTERACTIONS
No known drug interactions.

FOOD INTERACTIONS
No known food interactions.

DISEASE INTERACTIONS
Colesevelam must be used cautiously in patients with blood triglycerides greater than 300 mg/dL and in those with a history of swallowing difficulties, severe abnormalities of gastrointestinal motility, or major gastrointestinal tract surgery.

Colestipol Hydrochloride

▶ Drug Class: Antilipidemic (cholesterol-lowering agent)

▶ Available in: Powder, tablets

▶ Available OTC? No

▶ As Generic? No

Side Effects

SERIOUS
Severe abdominal pain (a very rare reaction, indicating intestinal obstruction). Stop taking the drug and contact your doctor immediately.

COMMON
Constipation, heartburn, bloating, belching, abdominal discomfort, irritation of the anal area.

LESS COMMON
Hives, rash, gas, diarrhea, nausea, vomiting, gallstones.

PRINCIPAL USES
To reduce cholesterol in people with high blood levels of low-density lipoprotein (LDL), as part of a comprehensive treatment program that includes exercise and special diet. The drug is also used to relieve itching caused by high levels of bile acids in the blood, a problem associated with blockage of the bile ducts. It may also be used to prevent some types of diarrhea or serve as an antidote to poisoning from or overdose of digitalis drugs.

HOW THE DRUG WORKS
Colestipol binds with bile acids in the intestine, forming an insoluble complex that is excreted in the feces. This process reduces the amount of bile acids in the blood. In response to the lower levels of bile acids, the liver converts more cholesterol to bile acids. As a consequence, the amount of cholesterol in liver cells declines, and the liver makes more receptors for LDL. The resulting increased removal of LDL from the blood lowers LDL cholesterol.

DOSAGE
Initial dose is 5 g, 1 or 2 times a day. Maintenance dose is 10 to 30 g, given in 2 equally divided doses. Always mix the powder thoroughly with appropriate liquid (water or fruit juice; do not use carbonated beverages) and wait 10 to 15 minutes after mixing before drinking. Doses are increased or decreased according to the individual's response.

ONSET OF EFFECT
Within 1 to 3 weeks.

DURATION OF ACTION
The drug's effects persist for 2 to 4 weeks after the final dose.

DIETARY ADVICE
Follow all special dietary restrictions and guidelines as directed by your doctor.

STORAGE
Store in a tightly sealed container away from heat and direct light. Keep away from moisture.

IF YOU MISS A DOSE
Take as soon as you remember. However, if it is near the time for the next dose, skip the missed dose and resume your regular dosage schedule. Do not double the next dose.

STOPPING THE DRUG
The drug may be stopped after 1 to 3 months if the therapeutic effect is not adequate. The decision to stop taking the drug should be made by your doctor.

PROLONGED USE
Colestipol may be used safely for years; periodic evaluation of the drug's effectiveness is necessary.

PRECAUTIONS
Over 60: Adverse reactions (particularly constipation) are more likely and more severe in older patients.

Driving and Hazardous Work: Colestipol should not impair your ability to perform such tasks safely.

Alcohol: No special precautions are necessary.

Pregnancy: Consult your doctor if you become or plan to become pregnant.

Breast Feeding: At very high doses colestipol may interfere with the absorption of vitamins A, D, E, and K, which may affect the nutritional intake of the nursing infant. Consult your doctor for specific advice.

Infants and Children: Prescribed for children only in rare circumstances. Follow doctor's instructions and dosage guidelines carefully in such cases.

Special Concerns: At very high doses, colestipol may interfere with the absorption of fats and fat-soluble vitamins (vitamins A, D, E, and K); vitamin supplementation may be advised.

OVERDOSE
Symptoms: None reported.

What to Do: Emergency instructions not applicable.

DRUG INTERACTIONS
Colestipol may bind with other drugs and hinder their absorption. Therefore, take all other drugs 1 to 2 hours before or 4 hours after taking colestipol.

FOOD INTERACTIONS
No known food interactions.

DISEASE INTERACTIONS
Do not take this drug if you have had a prior allergic reaction to it. Use of colestipol may make the following conditions worse: gallstones, peptic ulcer, intestinal bleeding disorders, hemorrhoids, malabsorption, constipation.

Colistin/Neomycin/Hydrocortisone

▶ Drug Class: Antibiotic combination drug

▶ Available in: Otic suspension

▶ Available OTC? No

▶ As Generic? No

Side Effects

SERIOUS
Skin rash, itching, redness, swelling, or other signs of irritation that were not present before therapy. Call your doctor immediately.

COMMON
No common side effects are associated with this drug.

LESS COMMON
There are no less-common side effects associated with the use of this drug.

PRINCIPAL USES
To treat infections of the ear canal and other types of ear problems.

HOW THE DRUG WORKS
This drug is a combination of three active ingredients. Colistin and neomycin are both antibiotics that destroy infection-causing bacteria. Hydrocortisone is a steroid hormone that mimics the effects of the body's natural corticosteroids to help reduce redness and pain associated with specific ear problems.

DOSAGE
Adults: 4 drops in the affected ear, 3 or 4 times a day. Children: Up to 3 drops in the affected ear, 3 or 4 times a day.

ONSET OF EFFECT
Unknown.

DURATION OF ACTION
Unknown.

DIETARY ADVICE
No special restrictions.

STORAGE
Store in a tightly sealed container away from heat, moisture, and direct light. Do not allow it to freeze.

IF YOU MISS A DOSE
Apply it as soon as you remember. If it is near the time for the next dose, skip the missed dose and resume your regular dosage schedule. Do not double the next dose.

STOPPING THE DRUG
Use it as prescribed for the full treatment period, even if you feel better before the scheduled end of therapy.

PROLONGED USE
Do not use this medication for more than 10 days unless directed otherwise by your doctor.

PRECAUTIONS
Over 60: No special problems are expected.

Driving and Hazardous Work: The use of this medication should not impair your ability to perform such tasks safely.

Alcohol: No special problems are expected, although it is generally advisable to abstain from alcohol when fighting an infection.

Pregnancy: Problems related to the use of this preparation during pregnancy have not been reported. Consult your doctor before using this medication during pregnancy

Breast Feeding: When used as directed, this medication does not pass into breast milk. Consult your doctor for specific advice.

Infants and Children: No studies on the use of this medication by children have been done. No special problems are expected.

Special Concerns: Before applying this medication, clean the ear canal thoroughly and dry it with a sterile wipe. Tilt the head so that the affected ear is up. Adults should gently pull the earlobe up and back; for children, pull down and back. After the medicine is dropped into the ear canal, keep the ear facing up for 5 minutes (or 1 to 2 minutes for restless children). Your doctor may have further instructions on how to apply the medication.

OVERDOSE
Symptoms: No cases of overdose have been reported.

What to Do: An overdose of this medication is unlikely to be life-threatening. However, if someone takes a much larger dose than prescribed or accidentally ingests the medication, call your doctor, emergency medical services (EMS), or the nearest poison control center immediately.

DRUG INTERACTIONS
It is possible that other drugs may interact with colistin, neomycin, and hydrocortisone. Before you use this medication, tell your doctor if you are taking any other prescription or over-the-counter medication, especially any other kinds of ear drops.

FOOD INTERACTIONS
No known food interactions.

DISEASE INTERACTIONS
Caution is advised when taking this drug. Consult your doctor if you have herpes simplex infection or any other ear problem.

▶ Drug Class: Progestin
(hormone)

▶ Available in: Tablets, injection

▶ Available OTC? No

▶ As Generic? No

Side Effects

SERIOUS
Changes in or cessation of menstrual bleeding, unexpected or increased flow of breast milk, mental depression, skin rash, loss of or change in speech, impaired coordination or vision, severe and sudden shortness of breath. Call your doctor immediately.

COMMON
Stomach pain, swelling of face, ankles, or feet, mild headache, mood changes, unusual fatigue, weight gain, pain or irritation at site of injection.

LESS COMMON
Acne, breast pain or tenderness, hot flashes, insomnia, loss of sexual desire, loss or gain of scalp hair or body hair, brown spots on skin.

PRINCIPAL USES
To prevent pregnancy.

HOW THE DRUG WORKS
Progestin prevents a woman's egg from developing fully; it also causes changes in the uterine lining and the cervical secretions, making it difficult for sperm to reach the egg.

DOSAGE
Tablets: 75 micrograms (mcg) (Ovrette) or 350 mcg (Nor-QD, Miconor) every day beginning on the first day of the menstrual cycle. Injection (Depo-Provera): 150 mg injected into the upper arm or buttock every 13 weeks.

ONSET OF EFFECT
Tablets: Protection begins 3 weeks after first taking the medication. Injection: Immediate if the injection is given within 5 days of the menstrual period.

DURATION OF ACTION
Tablets: 24 hours. Injection: 13 weeks.

DIETARY ADVICE
Tablets can be taken with meals to prevent gastrointestinal upset.

STORAGE
Store in a tightly sealed container away from heat and direct light.

IF YOU MISS A DOSE
Take the missed dose of the tablet as soon as you remember, resume your regular dosage, and use another birth control method for 2 days.

STOPPING THE DRUG
You may stop at any time you choose. This will naturally increase the likelihood of pregnancy unless another birth control method is employed.

PROLONGED USE
You should see your doctor for periodic examinations and laboratory tests if you use these contraceptives for a prolonged period.

PRECAUTIONS
Over 60: Generally not used by older patients.

Driving and Hazardous Work: No special precautions are necessary.

Alcohol: No special precautions are necessary.

Pregnancy: Low-dose progestins for contraception have not been shown to cause problems later if pregnancy occurs.

Breast Feeding: Progestins pass into breast milk but have not been shown to cause problems. They are recommended for nursing mothers who wish to practice contraception.

Infants and Children: Progestin contraceptives have not caused problems in teenagers. Birth control methods that protect against sexually transmitted diseases are also recommended for them.

Special Concerns: No contraceptive method is perfect. If you suspect a pregnancy, call your doctor immediately. If you have any laboratory test, tell the health professional that you are using these contraceptives. Cigarette smoking or alcohol abuse can increase the risk of osteoporosis and may increase the risk of blood clots.

OVERDOSE
Symptoms: No specific ones have been reported.

What to Do: An overdose of these contraceptives is unlikely to be life-threatening. However, if someone takes a much larger dose than prescribed, call your doctor, emergency medical services (EMS), or the nearest poison control center immediately.

DRUG INTERACTIONS
The following drugs may interact with these contraceptives. Consult your doctor for specific advice if you are taking aminoglutethimide, carbamazepine, phenytoin, rifabutin, or rifampin.

FOOD INTERACTIONS
No known food interactions.

DISEASE INTERACTIONS
Caution is advised when taking these contraceptives. Consult your doctor if you have any of the following: asthma, epilepsy, heart problems, circulation problems, kidney disease, liver disease, migraine headaches, breast disease, bleeding problems, diabetes, high blood cholesterol, or central nervous system disorders such as depression.

Contraceptives, Oral (Combination Products)

BRAND NAMES
Brevicon, Demulen, Desogen, Genora, Intercon, Jenest, Levlen, Levora, Lo/Ovral, Loestrin, Mircette, ModiCon, N.E.E., Necon, Nelova, Nordette, Norethin, Norinyl, Ortho Tri-Cyclen, Ortho-Cept, Ortho-Cyclen, Ortho-Novum, Ovcon, Ovral, Tri-Levlen, Tri-Norinyl, Triphasil, Trivora-21, Trivora-28, Zovia

▶ Drug Class: Hormones, estrogen with progestins

▶ Available in: Tablets

▶ Available OTC? No

▶ As Generic? Yes

Side Effects

SERIOUS
Sudden, severe, or continuing stomach pain; sudden or severe headache or migraine; loss of coordination; loss of or change in vision; pains in chest, groin, or leg; sudden slurring of speech; weakness, numbness, or pain in an arm or leg; changes in uterine bleeding pattern; prolonged bleeding at menses; vaginal infection. Call your doctor immediately.

COMMON
Abdominal cramps or bloating; acne; breast pain, tenderness, or swelling; dizziness; nausea; swelling of ankles or feet; unusual fatigue; vomiting; absence of normal menstruation. Call your doctor if you do not have your period at the end of the cycle and before you start a new cycle.

LESS COMMON
Blotchy spots on skin, gain or loss of hair, increased sensitivity to sunlight, changes in sexual interest.

PRINCIPAL USES
To prevent pregnancy.

HOW THE DRUG WORKS
Such products stop a woman's egg from fully developing each month.

DOSAGE
For 21-day cycle: 1 tablet a day for 21 days. Skip 7 days; repeat the cycle. For 28-day cycle: 1 tablet a day for 28 days. Repeat cycle. Each package of pills consists of 21 active tablets only, or 21 active tablets and 7 placebos. During the 7 days of taking placebos or no tablets, menstruation should occur.

ONSET OF EFFECT
At least 7 days.

DURATION OF ACTION
As long as tablets are taken.

DIETARY ADVICE
Take it with food if stomach upset occurs.

STORAGE
Store in a tightly sealed container away from heat and direct light.

IF YOU MISS A DOSE
If you miss the first tablet of a new cycle or 1 tablet during the cycle, take the missed tablet as soon as you remember and take the next tablet at the usual time. If you miss 2 tablets in a row in the first or second week, take 2 tablets the day you remember and 2 the next day, then resume normal dosage schedule and use another birth control method until the next cycle begins. If you miss 2 tablets during the third week or 3 tablets at any time, begin a new cycle on its scheduled starting day, but use another birth control method for 7 days into the new cycle.

STOPPING THE DRUG
You may stop at any time you choose after completing a full 21-day cycle of tablets.

PROLONGED USE
See your doctor at least every 6 months.

PRECAUTIONS
Over 60: Generally not used by older persons.

Driving and Hazardous Work: No special precautions are necessary.

Alcohol: No special precautions are necessary.

Pregnancy: Discontinue use if you become pregnant or suspect that you might be pregnant.

Breast Feeding: Oral contraceptive hormones pass into breast milk; avoid or discontinue use while breast feeding.

Infants and Children: No special problems have been found in teenagers who use oral contraception.

Special Concerns: Limit your exposure to sunlight until you determine how this medication affects you. Smoking can reduce the effectiveness of oral contraceptives and increase the risk of potentially dangerous blood clots.

OVERDOSE
Symptoms: Unexplained vaginal bleeding.

What to Do: An overdose of oral contraceptives is unlikely to be life-threatening. However, if someone takes a much larger dose than prescribed, call your doctor, emergency medical services (EMS), or the nearest poison control center immediately.

DRUG INTERACTIONS
Consult your doctor for specific advice if you are taking: amiodarone, anabolic steroids, androgens, anti-infectives, barbiturates, carbamazepine, carmustine, dantrolene, daunorubicin, disulfiram, divalproex, estrogens, etretinate, gold salts, griseofulvin, hydroxychloroquine, mercaptopurine, methotrexate, naltrexone, phenothiazines, phenylbutazone, phenytoin, plicamycin, primidone, rifabutin, rifampin, troleandomycin, corticosteroids, theophylline, cyclosporine, or ritonavir.

FOOD INTERACTIONS
No known food interactions.

DISEASE INTERACTIONS
Consult your doctor if you have any of the following: endometriosis, fibroid tumors of the uterus, heart or circulation disease, a history of stroke, breast disease, cancer, gallbladder disease, high blood cholesterol, liver disease, mental depression, diabetes, epilepsy, or migraines.

BRAND NAME
Cortone Acetate

Generic 25 mg
(RUGBY)

799

Additional photographs

▶ Drug Class: Corticosteroid

▶ Available in: Tablets

▶ Available OTC? No

▶ As Generic? Yes

Side Effects

SERIOUS
Vision problems, frequent urination, increased thirst, rectal bleeding, blistering skin, confusion, hallucinations, paranoia, euphoria, depression, mood swings, redness and swelling at injection site. Call your doctor immediately.

COMMON
Increased appetite, indigestion, nervousness, insomnia, greater susceptibility to infections, increased blood pressure, slow healing of wounds, weight gain, easy bruising, fluid retention.

LESS COMMON
Change in skin color, dizziness, headache, increased sweating, unusual growth of body or facial hair, increased blood sugar, peptic ulcers, adrenal insufficiency, muscle weakness, cataracts, glaucoma, osteoporosis.

PRINCIPAL USES
To treat numerous conditions that involve inflammation (a response by body tissues, producing redness, warmth, swelling, and pain). Such conditions include arthritis, allergic reactions, asthma, some skin diseases, multiple sclerosis flare-ups, and other autoimmune diseases. Also prescribed to treat deficiency of natural steroid hormones.

HOW THE DRUG WORKS
This hormone mimics the effects of the body's natural corticosteroids. It depresses the synthesis, release, and activity of inflammation-producing body chemicals. It also suppresses the activity of the immune system.

DOSAGE
Adults and teenagers: 25 to 300 mg a day, in 1 or several doses. Doses are individualized, depending on the condition being treated. The dose for children depends on body weight or size and must be determined by your doctor.

ONSET OF EFFECT
Variable.

DURATION OF ACTION
Variable.

DIETARY ADVICE
It can be taken with food or milk to minimize stomach upset. Your doctor may recommend a low-salt, high-potassium, high-protein diet.

STORAGE
Store in a tightly sealed container away from heat, moisture, and direct light.

IF YOU MISS A DOSE
Take it as soon as you remember. If you take several doses a day and it is close to the next dose, double the next dose. If you take 1 dose a day and you do not remember until the next day, skip the missed dose and do not double the next dose.

STOPPING THE DRUG
With long-term therapy, do not stop taking the drug abruptly; the dosage should be decreased gradually.

PROLONGED USE
See your doctor regularly for tests and examinations. Long-term use may lead to cataracts, diabetes, hypertension, or osteoporosis.

PRECAUTIONS
Over 60: Adverse reactions may be more likely and more severe.

Driving and Hazardous Work: Do not drive or engage in hazardous work until you determine how the medicine affects you.

Alcohol: May cause stomach problems; avoid unless your doctor approves occasional moderate drinking.

Pregnancy: Overuse during pregnancy can retard the child's growth and cause other developmental problems. Consult your physician.

Breast Feeding: Do not use while nursing.

Infants and Children: Cortisone may retard the normal growth and development of bone and other tissues. Consult your doctor for advice.

Special Concerns: Avoid immunizations with live vaccines if possible. Remember that this drug can lower your resistance to infection. Patients undergoing long-term therapy should wear a medical-alert bracelet. Call your doctor if you develop a fever.

OVERDOSE
Symptoms: Fever, muscle or joint pain, nausea, dizziness, fainting, breathing difficulty. Prolonged overuse: Moonface, obesity, unusual hair growth, acne, loss of sexual function, muscle wasting.

What to Do: Call your doctor, emergency medical services (EMS), or the nearest poison control center immediately.

DRUG INTERACTIONS
Consult your doctor for specific advice if you are taking aminoglutethimide, antacids, barbiturates, carbamazepine, griseofulvin, mitotane, phenylbutazone, phenytoin, primidone, rifampin, injectable amphotericin B, oral antidiabetes agents, insulin, digitalis drugs, diuretics, or medications containing potassium or sodium.

FOOD INTERACTIONS
Avoid excess sodium.

DISEASE INTERACTIONS
Consult your doctor if you have a history of bone disease, chicken pox, measles, stomach or intestinal disorders, diabetes mellitus, recent serious infection, tuberculosis, glaucoma, heart disease, hypertension, liver or kidney disorders, high blood cholesterol, overactive or underactive thyroid, myasthenia gravis, or lupus.

Cosyntropin

▶ Drug Class: Hormone; diagnostic agent

▶ Available in: Injection

▶ Available OTC? No

▶ As Generic? No

Side Effects

SERIOUS
No serious side effects are associated with cosyntropin.

COMMON
No common side effects are associated with cosyntropin, especially since it is used for diagnostic rather than therapeutic purposes.

LESS COMMON
It has not been established whether cosyntropin produces any minor or rare side effects. In an extremely few number of instances, it has been shown to cause mild allergy-like reactions (mild fever, nausea, vomiting, or skin irritation and redness at the site of injection).

PRINCIPAL USES
The adrenal glands manufacture steroids and other substances that are vital for overall health and well-being. Cosyntropin is used for diagnostic purposes when the adrenal gland is suspected of not working properly. The injection of cosyntropin forms the basis of a very simple, safe, and reliable test, taking 30 to 60 minutes, that measures adrenal gland function.

HOW THE DRUG WORKS
Cosyntropin is a synthetic form of corticotropin, a naturally occurring substance that stimulates the adrenal gland to release the hormone cortisol. After the injection of cosyntropin, blood tests will be performed to measure whether or not your adrenal gland was properly stimulated to produce cortisol.

DOSAGE
Adults: 0.25 mg injected into a vein or into a muscle. Children 2 years of age or less: 0.125 mg injected into a vein or muscle.

ONSET OF EFFECT
Within 30 minutes.

DURATION OF ACTION
Several hours at most.

DIETARY ADVICE
You may be given special dietary instructions for the period prior to diagnostic testing. If not, maintain your usual food and fluid intake. Follow other dietary restrictions, if any, as recommended by your doctor.

STORAGE
Not applicable.

IF YOU MISS A DOSE
Not applicable.

STOPPING THE DRUG
This medication is designed to be administered only once. Your doctor will determine if further injections are needed at a later date.

PROLONGED USE
Cosyntropin is never used for extended periods; it is generally administered on a one-time only basis.

PRECAUTIONS
Over 60: Adverse reactions are not anticipated in older patients.

Driving and Hazardous Work: The use of cosyntropin should not impair your ability to perform such tasks safely.

Alcohol: Alcohol should be avoided during the day or two before diagnostic testing is scheduled.

Pregnancy: Cosyntropin may be used during pregnancy; consult your physician for specific recommendations.

Breast Feeding: It is not known if cosyntropin passes into breast milk. However, no serious problems have been documented.

Infants and Children: Cosyntropin may be used safely in children.

OVERDOSE
Symptoms: No specific ones have been reported.

What to Do: An overdose of cosyntropin is unlikely, since it is administered under the close supervision of your doctor. No cases of overdose have been documented.

DRUG INTERACTIONS
None known.

FOOD INTERACTIONS
None known.

DISEASE INTERACTIONS
None known.

Cromolyn Sodium Inhalant and Nasal

BRAND NAMES
Intal, Nasalcrom

▶ Drug Class: Respiratory inhalant

▶ Available in: Inhalation aerosol, inhalation solution, nasal solution

▶ Available OTC? Yes

▶ As Generic? Yes

Side Effects

SERIOUS
Difficulty swallowing; hives; itching; swelling of face, lips, or eyelids; rash; nosebleeds. Call your doctor immediately.

COMMON
Inhalation: Throat irritation or dryness. Nasal: Increased sneezing; burning, stinging, or irritation in nose.

LESS COMMON
Nasal: Cough, headache, postnasal drip, unpleasant taste.

PRINCIPAL USES
To control, through regular use, chronic bronchial asthma; or it may be used preventively just prior to exposure to certain conditions or substances (allergens such as pollen and dust mites, as well as cold air, chemicals, exercise, or air pollution) that can trigger an acute asthma attack (bronchospasm).

HOW THE DRUG WORKS
Cromolyn sodium inhibits the release of histamine, a naturally occurring substance that causes swelling, itching, sneezing, watery eyes, hives, and other symptoms of allergic reaction, including those that occur in association with an asthma attack.

DOSAGE
Inhalation aerosol— To prevent asthma symptoms: Adults and children age 5 and older: 2 inhalations 4 times a day, 4 to 6 hours apart. To prevent bronchospasm: Adults and children age 5 and older: 2 inhalations at least 10 to 15 minutes before exercise or exposure. Inhalation solution— To prevent asthma symptoms: Adults and children 2 and older: 20 mg, 4 times a day, 4 to 6 hours apart. Nasal solution— For hay fever: Adults and children age 6 and older: 1 spray in each nostril 3 to 6 times a day.

ONSET OF EFFECT
Inhalation: Up to 4 weeks. Nasal: Unknown.

DURATION OF ACTION
Unknown.

DIETARY ADVICE
This medication should be taken 30 minutes before meals.

STORAGE
Store in a tightly sealed container away from heat and direct light.

IF YOU MISS A DOSE
Take it as soon as you remember. If it is near the time for the next dose, skip the missed dose and resume your regular dosage schedule. Do not double the next dose.

STOPPING THE DRUG
The decision to stop taking cromolyn sodium should be made in consultation with your doctor.

PROLONGED USE
If your symptoms do not improve after 4 weeks, consult your doctor.

PRECAUTIONS
Over 60: No studies have been done, but no special problems are expected in older patients.

Driving and Hazardous Work: No special problems are expected.

Alcohol: No special precautions are necessary.

Pregnancy: In animal studies, large doses of cromolyn sodium have caused a decrease in successful pregnancies and a decrease in fetal weight. Human studies have not been done. Before taking cromolyn sodium, tell your doctor if you are currently pregnant or plan to become pregnant.

Breast Feeding: It is not known whether cromolyn sodium passes into breast milk. Mothers who wish to breast feed while taking this drug should discuss the matter with their doctor.

Infants and Children: The inhalation form of cromolyn sodium has not been shown to cause special problems in children. The nasal form has not been studied in children. Consult your pediatrician for advice.

Special Concerns: Clean the inhaler and other devices at least once a week.

OVERDOSE
Symptoms: None reported.

What to Do: An overdose of cromolyn sodium is unlikely to be life-threatening. However, if someone takes a much larger dose than prescribed, call your doctor, emergency medical services (EMS), or the nearest poison control center immediately.

DRUG INTERACTIONS
Before taking cromolyn sodium, check with your doctor if you are using any other prescription or over-the-counter drug.

FOOD INTERACTIONS
No known food interactions.

DISEASE INTERACTIONS
Before taking cromolyn sodium, consult your physician if you are undergoing treatment for any medical condition.

Cromolyn Sodium Ophthalmic

BRAND NAME
Crolom

▶ Drug Class: Antiallergy agent

▶ Available in: Ophthalmic solution

▶ Available OTC? No

▶ As Generic? No

Side Effects

SERIOUS
Rarely, ophthalmic cromolyn sodium causes a rash or redness around the eyes, swelling of the membrane covering the whites of the eyes, red or bloodshot eyes, or other eye irritation. Call your doctor immediately.

COMMON
Mild and temporary burning or stinging of the eyes.

LESS COMMON
Increased watering or itching of the eyes, dryness or puffiness around the eyes.

PRINCIPAL USES
To treat eye disorders associated with seasonal allergies. Such disorders include conjunctivitis (inflammation of the mucous membranes that line the inner surface of the eyelids and whites of the eyes) and keratitis (inflammation of the cornea).

HOW THE DRUG WORKS
Cromolyn inhibits the body's release of certain allergy-related chemicals including histamine, a naturally occurring substance that causes swelling, itching, sneezing, watery eyes, hives, and other symptoms of an allergic reaction.

DOSAGE
Adults and children age 4 and older: 1 drop 4 to 6 times a day in regularly spaced intervals. Children up to 4 years of age: Use and dosage must be determined by your doctor.

ONSET OF EFFECT
The effect might not be felt for several days or possibly several weeks.

DURATION OF ACTION
Unknown.

DIETARY ADVICE
This drug can be used without regard to diet.

STORAGE
Store in a tightly sealed container away from heat, moisture, and direct light. Do not allow it to freeze.

IF YOU MISS A DOSE
Apply it as soon as you remember. If it is near the time for the next dose, skip the missed dose and resume your regular dosage schedule. Do not double the next dose.

STOPPING THE DRUG
Use this drug as prescribed for the full treatment period, even if you begin to feel better before the scheduled end of therapy.

PROLONGED USE
You should see your doctor regularly for tests and examinations if you take this drug for a prolonged period. The therapy may last for as long as 6 weeks.

PRECAUTIONS
Over 60: No special problems are expected.

Driving and Hazardous Work: The use of ophthalmic cromolyn should not impair your ability to perform such tasks safely.

Alcohol: No special precautions are necessary.

Pregnancy: Adequate human studies have not been completed. Before taking ophthalmic cromolyn, tell your doctor if you are pregnant or plan to become pregnant.

Breast Feeding: Ophthalmic cromolyn may pass into breast milk; caution is advised. Consult your doctor for specific advice.

Infants and Children: Use and dosage for infants and children under the age of 4 years must be determined by your doctor.

Special Concerns: To use the eye drops, first wash your hands. Tilt your head back. Gently apply pressure to the inside corner of the eyelid and with the index finger of the same hand, pull downward on the lower eyelid to make a space. Drop the medicine into this space and close your eye. Apply pressure for 1 or 2 minutes while keeping the eye closed without blinking. Then wash your hands again. Make sure the tip of the dropper does not touch your eye, finger, or any other surface. If your symptoms do not improve or if they become worse, check with your doctor.

OVERDOSE
Symptoms: No specific ones have been reported.

What to Do: An overdose of ophthalmic cromolyn is unlikely to be life-threatening. However, if someone takes a much larger dose of the drug than prescribed or accidentally ingests the medicine, call your doctor, emergency medical services (EMS), or the nearest poison control center.

DRUG INTERACTIONS
Other drugs may interact with ophthalmic cromolyn. Consult your doctor for specific advice if you are taking any other prescription or over-the-counter medication.

FOOD INTERACTIONS
No known food interactions.

DISEASE INTERACTIONS
Caution is advised when taking ophthalmic cromolyn. Consult your doctor if you have any other medical condition.

Cyclobenzaprine

BRAND NAME
Flexeril

Generic 10 mg
(**Mylan**)

▶ Drug Class: Muscle relaxant

▶ Available in: Tablets

▶ Available OTC? No

▶ As Generic? Yes

Side Effects

SERIOUS
Unusual heartbeat (racing, pounding, or fluttering), confusion, seizures, hallucinations.

COMMON
Drowsiness, dry mouth, dizziness.

LESS COMMON
Fatigue or excessive tiredness, weakness, nausea, constipation, heartburn, unpleasant bitter or metallic taste in mouth, vision problems, headache, restlessness, nervousness, difficulty urinating, unusual bleeding or bruising.

PRINCIPAL USES
To relieve painful, temporary muscle stiffness and spasms. It is not used for stiffness and spasms due to serious, chronic illnesses of the nervous system and muscles, such as spinal cord injury or cerebral palsy.

HOW THE DRUG WORKS
Cyclobenzaprine appears to work by decreasing nerve impulses from the brain and spinal cord that lead to tensing or tightening of muscle fibers.

DOSAGE
Adults and teenagers 15 years of age and older: Usual dose is 10 mg, 3 times a day, which may be increased by your doctor to a maximum total dose of no more than 60 mg per day. Children and teenagers up to 15 years of age: Consult pediatrician.

ONSET OF EFFECT
Within 1 hour. The maximum effect may require 1 to 2 weeks of therapy.

DURATION OF ACTION
12 to 24 hours following a single dose.

DIETARY ADVICE
Dry mouth is a common complaint with muscle relaxants; maintain adequate fluid intake and suck on ice chips if desired.

STORAGE
Store in a tightly sealed container away from heat and direct light. Keep it away from moisture and extremes in temperature.

IF YOU MISS A DOSE
Take it as soon as you remember. If it is near the time for the next dose, skip the missed dose and resume your regular dosage schedule. Do not double the next dose.

STOPPING THE DRUG
You should take it as prescribed for the full treatment period, but you may stop if you are feeling better before the scheduled end of therapy.

PROLONGED USE
Therapy with cyclobenzaprine is usually completed within 14 to 21 days. Do not take cyclobenzaprine for a longer period without your doctor's approval. Muscle pain and stiffness that does not improve within 14 to 21 days may require a more thorough evaluation.

PRECAUTIONS
Over 60: Adverse reactions may be more likely and more severe in older patients.

Driving and Hazardous Work: The use of cyclobenzaprine may impair your ability to perform such tasks safely; use caution.

Alcohol: Avoid alcohol.

Pregnancy: Adequate studies of cyclobenzaprine use during pregnancy have not been done; discuss the relative risks and benefits with your doctor.

Breast Feeding: Cyclobenzaprine may pass into breast milk; caution is advised. Consult your doctor for advice.

Infants and Children: Cyclobenzaprine is not recommended for use by children under the age of 15.

Special Concerns: Cyclobenzaprine is not meant to be used as the only treatment for sore or stiff muscles. It should be accompanied by bed rest, physical therapy, and other measures to relieve discomfort, such as the application of heat or ice packs (as suggested by your physician).

OVERDOSE
Symptoms: Severe mental confusion, agitation, impaired concentration, difficulty walking or standing, dilated pupils, severe drowsiness, coma.

What to Do: Call emergency medical services (EMS), your doctor, or the nearest poison control center immediately.

DRUG INTERACTIONS
Consult your doctor for specific advice if you are taking sedatives, tranquilizers, or other medications that cause drowsiness (including alcohol); tricyclic antidepressants; or MAO inhibitors.

FOOD INTERACTIONS
No known food interactions.

DISEASE INTERACTIONS
Consult your doctor if you have a history of any of the following: glaucoma, difficult urination, prostate problems, heart disease, or overactive thyroid.

Cyclopentolate

▶ Drug Class: Eye muscle relaxant, pupil enlarger

▶ Available in: Ophthalmic solution

▶ Available OTC? No

▶ As Generic? No

Side Effects

SERIOUS
If absorbed into the bloodstream: Clumsiness or unsteadiness, confusion or changes in behavior, hallucinations, slurred speech, rapid or irregular pulse, flushing, fever, unusual fatigue, dizziness, unusually dry skin, skin rash, dry mouth; in infants, abdominal swelling. Seek medical assistance immediately.

COMMON
Eye irritation and redness not present prior to treatment, swelling of the eyelids, blurred vision, increased sensitivity to bright light.

LESS COMMON
There are no less-common side effects associated with the use of cyclopentolate.

PRINCIPAL USES
To dilate the pupils and temporarily paralyze certain structures within the eye. This is useful in eye examinations to help determine the proper prescription for eyeglasses or for other diagnostic procedures involving the eyes. It may also be needed before or after eye surgery.

HOW THE DRUG WORKS
Cyclopentolate relaxes the ciliary muscle, which controls the shape of the eye's lens as it focuses, and another eye muscle called the sphincter, which controls the narrowing and widening of the pupil. Relaxation of these muscles prevents the lens from focusing and widens the pupil. This allows the doctor to view the interior structures of the eye during an ophthalmologic procedure. And, by immobilizing the tiny structures within the eye, the drug prevents scarring of eye tissue and may alleviate eye pain.

DOSAGE
1 to 2 drops, applied 3 times a day or as needed as determined by your eye doctor.

ONSET OF EFFECT
Maximum effect occurs within 25 to 75 minutes.

DURATION OF ACTION
8 hours, although some effects may persist for up to several days.

DIETARY ADVICE
No special restrictions.

STORAGE
Store in a tightly sealed container away from heat, moisture, and direct light. Do not allow it to freeze.

IF YOU MISS A DOSE
Apply it as soon as you remember. If it is near the time for the next dose, skip the missed dose and resume your regular dosage schedule. Do not double the next dose.

STOPPING THE DRUG
The decision to stop taking the drug should be made by your ophthalmologist.

PROLONGED USE
Not recommended for long-term therapy.

PRECAUTIONS
Over 60: Adverse reactions may be more likely and more severe in older patients.

Driving and Hazardous Work: Do not drive or engage in hazardous work until you determine how the medicine affects your vision. Extreme caution should be observed for activities requiring sharp vision for close objects (less than an arm's length away).

Alcohol: No special precautions are necessary.

Pregnancy: Adequate studies have not been done. Inform your doctor if you are pregnant or are planning to become pregnant.

Breast Feeding: It is not known if cyclopentolate passes into breast milk; caution is advised. Consult your doctor for specific advice.

Infants and Children: Young children with blond hair or blue eyes may be more sensitive to the drug and may have an increased risk of side effects. Use with extreme caution. Infants should not eat for 4 hours following application of drops.

Special Concerns: To use the eye drops, first wash your hands. Tilt your head back. Gently apply pressure to the inside corner of the eyelid and with the index finger of the same hand, pull downward on the lower eyelid to make a space. Drop the medicine into this space and close your eye. Apply pressure for 1 or 2 minutes while keeping the eye closed without blinking. Then wash your hands again. Make sure that the tip of the dropper does not touch your eye, finger, or any other surface.

OVERDOSE
Symptoms: Drowsiness, hallucinations, memory problems, dry mouth, dry skin, restlessness, palpitations, dizziness and disorientation, delirium.

What to Do: Call your doctor, emergency medical services (EMS), or the nearest poison control center immediately.

DRUG INTERACTIONS
Consult your physician if you are taking any other prescription or over-the-counter drugs, especially those designed for use in the eyes.

FOOD INTERACTIONS
No known food interactions.

DISEASE INTERACTIONS
Consult your doctor if you have a history of glaucoma, Down's syndrome, or spastic paralysis.

Cyclophosphamide

Cytoxan 25 mg
(BRISTOL-MYERS SQUIBB)

▶ Drug Class: Antineoplastic (anticancer) agent; immuno-suppressant

▶ Available in: Tablets, liquid for injection

▶ Available OTC? No

▶ As Generic? No

Side Effects

SERIOUS
Shortness of breath, chest tightness, chest or abdominal pain, persistent cough or hoarseness, fever and chills, pain in the lower back or sides, painful or difficult urination, tiny bright red dots on the skin, unusual bleeding or bruising, breathing difficulty, blood in the urine or stool. Call your doctor immediately should any of these occur.

COMMON
Nausea and vomiting, loss of appetite and weight, temporary hair loss, increased susceptibility to infections, loss of hearing or ringing in the ears, sterility in men (usually temporary), unusual fatigue, increased pigmentation in skin and fingernails, dizziness, confusion.

LESS COMMON
Diarrhea, stomach upset, flushing, skin rash, itching, or hives, rapid heartbeat, swelling in the feet or lower legs.

PRINCIPAL USES
To treat a number of cancers, including malignant lymphoma, multiple myeloma, sarcoma, retinoblastoma, leukemia, breast cancer, and ovarian cancer. Cyclophosphamide is sometimes prescribed for other, noncancerous conditions, although this is done with extreme caution in light of the potentially serious side effects associated with this drug.

HOW THE DRUG WORKS
Cyclophosphamide kills cancer cells by interfering with the synthesis of their genetic material, which prevents the malignant cells from multiplying.

DOSAGE
Adults— Oral dose for cancer: 1 to 5 mg for every 2.2 lbs (1 kg) of body weight, once a day, for 5 to 7 days every month. Injection: 40 to 60 mg a day, in divided doses, for 2 to 5 days, depending on the type of cancer treated. This drug should never be administered intravenously without additional intravenous fluids. The dosage may vary considerably, depending on the patient, the disease, and whether any other drugs are being taken. Children— Consult your pediatric oncologist.

ONSET OF EFFECT
2 to 3 hours.

DURATION OF ACTION
Unknown.

DIETARY ADVICE
Take it on an empty stomach; may be taken with small amounts of food or milk if stomach irritation occurs. Be sure to drink plenty of fluids.

STORAGE
Store the tablets in a tightly sealed container away from heat and light.

IF YOU MISS A DOSE
Skip the missed dose and resume your regular dosage schedule. Do not double the next dose.

STOPPING THE DRUG
Continue taking this drug as prescribed, even if you experience side effects such as nausea and vomiting. The decision to stop taking the medication should be made by your doctor.

PROLONGED USE
Prolonged use is associated with an increased risk of adverse effects. Consult your doctor about the need for periodic medical tests and examinations.

PRECAUTIONS
Over 60: Side effects more common in older patients.

Driving and Hazardous Work: Avoid such activities until you determine how the medicine affects you.

Alcohol: Limit alcohol to moderate intake only.

Pregnancy: This drug can cause serious birth defects when taken by the mother or father. Use reliable birth control while taking this drug and for 4 months after therapy.

Breast Feeding: Use is not recommended while nursing.

Infants and Children: Cyclophosphamide can be used in children under close medical supervision.

Special Concerns: Watch for signs of infection, such as fever, sore throat, and fatigue. If your temperature rises above 100°F, call your doctor. To avoid urinary problems, drink a minimum of 3 quarts of water a day. Do not get vaccinated against bacteria or viruses while taking this drug.

OVERDOSE
Symptoms: Shortness of breath, palpitations, chest pain or discomfort, bloody urine, water retention, unusual weight gain, severe infection.

What to Do: Call emergency medical services (EMS) to receive evaluation and treatment in the closest emergency facility.

DRUG INTERACTIONS
Consult your doctor for specific advice if you are taking allopurinol or other gout medications, oral hypoglycemia drugs, clozapine, cyclosporine, digoxin or other antiarrhythmic drugs, other immunosuppressants, insulin, levamisole, lovastatin, phenobarbital, probenecid, sulfinpyrazone, or tiopronin.

FOOD INTERACTIONS
No known food interactions.

DISEASE INTERACTIONS
Consult your doctor if you have a recent history of chicken pox, shingles, gout, kidney stones, or infections. Use of this drug may cause complications in patients with liver or kidney disease, since these organs work together to remove the medication from the body.

Cycloserine

Seromycin 250 mg
(DURA)

▶ Drug Class: Anti-infective
/antitubercular agent

▶ Available in: Capsules

▶ Available OTC? No

▶ As Generic? No

Side Effects

SERIOUS
Dizziness, drowsiness, changes in mental state, depression, anxiety, suicidal thoughts, psychosis, confusion, nightmares, speech difficulties, increased irritability, muscle twitches, increased restlessness, skin rash, seizures. Call your doctor immediately.

COMMON
Headache; numbness, burning pain, prickling, tingling, or weakness in the hands or feet.

LESS COMMON
Abnormal heart rhythm, liver disease (hepatitis).

PRINCIPAL USES
To treat active tuberculosis; used in conjunction with other antitubercular agents after use of the primary antitubercular agents, such as isoniazid, rifampin, ethambutol, pyrazinamide, and streptomycin, have proven ineffective.

HOW THE DRUG WORKS
Cycloserine kills tuberculosis bacteria by interfering with specific enzymes needed for the manufacture of cell walls.

DOSAGE
Adults and teenagers: To start, 250 mg every 12 hours for 2 weeks. If needed, your doctor may increase the dose to 250 mg every 6 to 8 hours; usually not more than 750 to 1,000 mg (6.8 mg per lb of body weight) a day. Children under age 12: 4.5 to 9 mg per lb per day. Cycloserine is taken in conjunction with other antitubercular agents. Vitamin B6 (pyridoxine) should also be taken (at least 100 mg a day) to prevent nerve damage.

ONSET OF EFFECT
Unknown.

DURATION OF ACTION
Unknown.

DIETARY ADVICE
This medication may be taken with liquid or food to minimize stomach irritation.

STORAGE
Store in a tightly sealed container away from heat, moisture, and direct light.

IF YOU MISS A DOSE
Take the drug as soon as you remember. This will help keep a constant level of medication in your system. If it is near the time for the next dose, skip the missed dose and resume your regular dosage schedule. Do not double the next dose.

STOPPING THE DRUG
Take it as prescribed for the full treatment period, even if you begin to feel better before the scheduled end of therapy. Treatment may continue for months or years. The decision to stop taking the drug should be made by your doctor.

PROLONGED USE
Consult your doctor about the need for having periodic medical examinations and laboratory tests.

PRECAUTIONS
Over 60: Adverse reactions may be more likely and more severe in older patients. Smaller doses for shorter treatment periods may be warranted.

Driving and Hazardous Work: Do not drive or engage in hazardous work until you determine how the medicine affects you.

Alcohol: Avoid alcohol.

Pregnancy: No problems have been reported. In any case, tell your doctor if you are pregnant or plan to become pregnant before taking cycloserine.

Breast Feeding: Cycloserine may pass into breast milk; caution is advised. Consult your doctor for specific advice.

Infants and Children: Adequate studies of the use of cycloserine by children have not been done. Consult your pediatrician for specific advice.

Special Concerns: Before taking cycloserine, tell your doctor if you are depressed or have severe anxiety. Persons with a seizure disorder should not take cycloserine.

OVERDOSE
Symptoms: Seizures, drowsiness, confusion, dizziness, headache, extreme irritability, joint pain, psychosis, numbness, tingling, or prickling sensation in the hands or feet.

What to Do: Call your doctor, emergency medical services (EMS), or the nearest poison control center immediately.

DRUG INTERACTIONS
Ethionamide may interact with cycloserine. Consult your doctor for specific advice if you are taking it. Also tell your doctor if you are taking any other prescription or over-the-counter medication.

FOOD INTERACTIONS
No known food interactions.

DISEASE INTERACTIONS
Use of cycloserine may cause complications in patients with kidney disease, since the kidneys play a major role in removing the medication from the body. Caution is advised when taking cycloserine. Consult your doctor if you have any of the following: a seizure disorder such as epilepsy; a history of alcohol abuse; mental depression; psychosis; or severe anxiety.

Cyclosporine

Sandimmune 25 mg
(**NOVARTIS**)

Additional photographs

▶ Drug Class: Immunosuppressant

▶ Available in: Capsules, oral solution, injection

▶ Available OTC? No

▶ As Generic? No

Side Effects

SERIOUS
Frequent urge to urinate; fever or chills; yellow-tinged eyes and skin caused by liver problems; abnormal bleeding; fatigue; high blood pressure. Call your doctor immediately. Psoriasis patients formerly treated with other types of therapy (for example, ultraviolet light or methotrexate) are at increased risk of skin cancer; report any new skin lesion to your doctor immediately.

COMMON
Headache, tremor, unusual hair growth on body and face, swelling or bleeding of gums.

LESS COMMON
Nausea, vomiting, diarrhea, acne or oily skin, sinus inflammation or infection, leg cramps, enlargement and tenderness of the breasts in males (gynecomastia).

PRINCIPAL USES
To slow down or reduce the natural tendency of the immune system to reject organ transplants. Also to treat severe rheumatoid arthritis or severe psoriasis that has not responded to other drug therapy.

HOW THE DRUG WORKS
Cyclosporine suppresses the functioning of the body's immune system. In this way it prevents the normal reaction against foreign substances or tissue that would otherwise cause the body to reject donor organs. Cyclosporine is also used to manage rheumatoid arthritis and psoriasis, as these disorders are classified as autoimmune diseases, that is, those in which the immune system inappropriately attacks healthy tissue.

DOSAGE
Your doctor will determine the correct dose based on a number of individual factors. During therapy, doses may be adjusted according to drug levels in the blood. The various brands of cyclosporine are not interchangeable; any changes in brand or dose should be made only by your doctor.

ONSET OF EFFECT
Unknown.

DURATION OF ACTION
Unknown.

DIETARY ADVICE
Cyclosporine can be taken with food to avoid stomach upset. The oral solution can be taken with orange juice in a glass container, served at room temperature. Do not take cyclosporine with grapefruit juice.

STORAGE
Store in a tightly sealed container away from heat and direct light. Do not store

the oral solution in the refrigerator. Injection: Not applicable; injections are administered only at a health care facility.

IF YOU MISS A DOSE
Take it as soon as you remember, up to 12 hours late. However, if more than 12 hours have elapsed since the time for the missed dose, skip the missed dose and resume your regular dosage schedule. Do not double the next dose.

STOPPING THE DRUG
The decision to stop taking cyclosporine should be made by your doctor.

PROLONGED USE
Prolonged use of cyclosporine may impair kidney function. Periodic examinations and laboratory tests are required.

PRECAUTIONS
Over 60: The dose must be adjusted for a possible decline in kidney function in older patients.

Driving and Hazardous Work: Do not drive or engage in hazardous work until you determine how the medicine affects you.

Alcohol: Avoid alcohol.

Pregnancy: Cyclosporine has been shown to cause serious birth defects in animals. Adequate human studies have not been done. Avoid this drug during pregnancy unless it is clearly needed.

Breast Feeding: Cyclosporine passes into breast milk; avoid or discontinue use while nursing.

Infants and Children: Cyclosporine has not been shown to affect children differently than adults.

Special Concerns: Avoid any immunizations except those approved by your doctor. Do not use plastic or wax-lined cups to take this medicine. Maintain good dental hygiene; this medication can cause gum problems. Cyclosporine can make you more sensitive to sunlight. Limit exposure until you determine how the drug affects you.

OVERDOSE
Symptoms: Yellowish tinge to the skin or eyes (jaundice), lethargy, confusion, swelling of body tissues.

What to Do: Call your doctor, emergency medical services (EMS), or the nearest poison control center immediately.

DRUG INTERACTIONS
Do not take cyclosporine with the herb St. John's wort. Consult your doctor if you are taking androgens, cimetidine, danazol, diltiazem, diuretics, erythromycin, estrogens, other immunosuppressants, ketoconazole, statin (cholesterol-lowering) drugs, or virus vaccines. Many other drugs interact with cyclosporine. Consult your doctor before taking any new medicines, whether by prescription or over the counter.

FOOD INTERACTIONS
Do not take cyclosporine with grapefruit juice.

DISEASE INTERACTIONS
Consult your doctor if you have any of the following: chicken pox, shingles, high blood pressure, infection, a chronic gastrointestinal disorder, or a blood cell disorder. Use of cyclosporine may cause complications in patients with liver or kidney disease, since these organs work together to remove the drug from the body.

Cyproheptadine Hydrochloride

Generic 4 mg
(SIDMAK)

▶ Drug Class: Antihistamine; serotonin blocker

▶ Available in: Syrup, tablets

▶ Available OTC? No

▶ As Generic? Yes

Side Effects

SERIOUS
Confusion, hallucinations, convulsions, restlessness, blurred vision, fainting, unusual or irregular pulse, wheezing.

COMMON
Dry mouth, dry nose, drowsiness (often transient).

LESS COMMON
Difficult urination, dizziness, increased sensitivity to sunlight, rash, weight gain, unusual excitement, irritability, euphoria, or restlessness.

PRINCIPAL USES
To prevent or relieve symptoms of rhinitis (inflammation of the mucous membranes of the nasal passages, often associated with hay fever and other seasonal allergies); skin itching and hives; and tissue swelling (angioedema). Cyproheptadine is also used as an appetite stimulant in patients with anorexia nervosa and to treat vascular headaches.

HOW THE DRUG WORKS
Cyproheptadine blocks the effects of histamine, a naturally occurring substance within the body that causes swelling, itching, sneezing, watery eyes, hives, and other symptoms of allergic reaction. It also blocks the brain chemical serotonin, and so may stimulate appetite and relieve the symptoms of vascular headaches.

DOSAGE
Adults and children over age 14: 4 mg every 8 hours. The dose may gradually be increased by your doctor. Children ages 2 to 6: 2 mg every 8 to 12 hours. Children ages 6 to 14: 4 mg every 8 to 12 hours.

ONSET OF EFFECT
15 to 60 minutes.

DURATION OF ACTION
8 hours.

DIETARY ADVICE
Maintain your usual food and fluid intake. Increase fluid intake during persistent attacks, or if you have a fever or diarrhea.

STORAGE
Store in a tightly sealed container away from heat and direct light. Keep it away from moisture and extremes in temperature. Keep the liquid form of cyproheptadine refrigerated, but do not allow it to freeze.

IF YOU MISS A DOSE
Take it as soon as you remember. However, if it is near the time for the next dose, skip the missed dose and resume your regular dosage schedule. Do not double the next dose.

STOPPING THE DRUG
Take it as prescribed for the full treatment period, but you may stop if you are feeling better before the scheduled end of therapy.

PROLONGED USE
Therapy with cyproheptadine may require days or weeks, depending on the severity of your allergies. Side effects may be more likely with prolonged use.

PRECAUTIONS
Over 60: Adverse reactions may be more likely and more severe in older patients.

Driving and Hazardous Work: Because cyproheptadine may cause drowsiness, its use may impair your ability to perform hazardous tasks safely.

Alcohol: Avoid alcohol.

Pregnancy: Animal studies with high doses of cyproheptadine have found no birth defects. Human studies have not been done. Because the studies cannot rule out harm, the drug should be used during pregnancy only if it is clearly needed.

Breast Feeding: Cyproheptadine may pass into breast milk; caution is advised. Consult your doctor for advice.

Infants and Children: This drug is not recommended for use by children under 2 years of age.

Special Concerns: Children should be observed carefully for signs of side effects; they are more likely to develop serious complications from these medications, and younger children are often unable to describe changes in the way that they are feeling.

OVERDOSE
Symptoms: Hallucinations; convulsions; excitability or severe sedation; blurred vision; flushing or redness of skin; very dry, warm skin; wide, dilated pupils.

What to Do: Call your doctor, emergency medical services (EMS), or the nearest poison control center immediately.

DRUG INTERACTIONS
Consult your doctor for specific advice if you are taking medications containing alcohol or medications that may cause drowsiness such as barbiturates, sedatives, cough medicines, other antihistamines, psychiatric medications (especially MAO inhibitors), and prescription pain medications.

FOOD INTERACTIONS
No known food interactions.

DISEASE INTERACTIONS
Consult your doctor if you have glaucoma or other visual disorders, prostate problems, or other problems urinating.

Cysteamine Bitartrate

▶ Drug Class: Nephropathic cystinosis therapeutic agent

▶ Available in: Capsules

▶ Available OTC? No

▶ As Generic? No

Side Effects

SERIOUS
Loss of appetite, fever, abdominal pain, nausea or vomiting, drowsiness, diarrhea, skin rash, confusion, dizziness, sore throat, mental depression, trembling, headache. Call your doctor as soon as possible. Side effects are most common when cysteamine is first started. Symptoms may improve when the drug is temporarily stopped or the dose is reduced.

COMMON
No common side effects are associated with the use of cysteamine.

LESS COMMON
Constipation, bad breath.

PRINCIPAL USES
To treat the kidney-damaging form of cystinosis. People born without the ability to metabolize the amino acid cystine suffer from cystinosis, a rare inherited disorder characterized by the deposition and accumulation of cystine crystals throughout the body. These crystals cause considerable damage, particularly in the kidney. Kidney failure can occur by the age of 10 in untreated patients. Cysteamine prevents the accumulation of cystine crystals and is prescribed to prevent further kidney damage.

HOW THE DRUG WORKS
Cysteamine helps to convert cystine into less harmful chemical forms that can be removed from cells.

DOSAGE
Adults and teenagers weighing more than 110 pounds: To start, 500 mg a day. Over a period of 4 to 6 weeks, your doctor will gradually increase the dose to a total of 2,000 mg per day, taken in 4 divided doses. Children up to age 12: Dose depends on weight and body surface area. White blood cell counts and cystine levels should be measured every 3 months until the proper dose is determined.

ONSET OF EFFECT
Unknown.

DURATION OF ACTION
As long as it is taken.

DIETARY ADVICE
Children or people who have difficulty swallowing the capsules may open them and sprinkle the contents onto food. Your doctor will recommend dietary and nutritional adjustments should kidney failure develop.

STORAGE
Store in a tightly sealed container away from heat, moisture, and direct light.

IF YOU MISS A DOSE
Take it as soon as you remember, unless the time for your next scheduled dose is within the next 2 hours. If so, skip the missed dose and resume your regular dosage schedule. Do not double the next dose.

STOPPING THE DRUG
Continue to take the medicine as prescribed unless your doctor recommends that the dose be reduced or the drug be discontinued.

PROLONGED USE
Lifelong therapy with cysteamine bitartrate may be necessary.

PRECAUTIONS
Over 60: No studies specifically on older patients have been done.

Driving and Hazardous Work: Do not drive or engage in hazardous work until you determine how the medicine affects you.

Alcohol: Avoid alcohol.

Pregnancy: Adequate human studies have not been done. Before taking cysteamine, tell your physician if you are pregnant or are planning to become pregnant.

Breast Feeding: It is not known whether cysteamine passes into breast milk; caution is advised. Consult your doctor for specific advice.

Infants and Children: Treatment should be started as soon as diagnosis of cystinosis is made. Your pediatrician will determine the size and frequency of the dose.

Special Concerns: If you vomit your dose of cysteamine within 20 minutes of taking it, take the dose again. If you vomit again, do not repeat the dose. Wait until your next scheduled dose. If you vomit 20 minutes after taking the dose, do not repeat the dose.

OVERDOSE
Symptoms: An overdose is unlikely to occur or to be life-threatening.

What to Do: If you have any reason to suspect an overdose, call your doctor, emergency medical services (EMS), or the nearest poison control center.

DRUG INTERACTIONS
No drug interactions have been reported.

FOOD INTERACTIONS
No known food interactions.

DISEASE INTERACTIONS
The dose of cysteamine may need to be adjusted for patients with a medical history of seizures, blood problems, or any form of kidney disease.

Dacarbazine

▶ Drug Class: Antineoplastic (anticancer) agent

▶ Available in: Injection

▶ Available OTC? No

▶ As Generic? Yes

Side Effects

SERIOUS
Black, tarry, or bloody stools; blood-tinged (pink or maroon) urine; cough or hoarseness; fever; chills; lower back pain or pain in flanks; painful, difficult urination; tiny bright red spots on skin; bleeding from gums, nose, or other unusual places; easy bruising; shortness of breath. These side effects may mean that normal blood cells and special blood-clotting cells have been affected, or that normal immune cells have been affected and an infection is developing somewhere in your body. Contact your doctor immediately if any of these occur.

COMMON
Nausea, vomiting, weakness, loss of appetite. If pain or redness occurs at the injection site while dacarbazine is being administered, tell your physician or nurse immediately.

LESS COMMON
Flushing; unusual numbness or tingling of the face; flu-like symptoms (including muscle aches, fever, and joint pain) usually occurring about 7 days after treatment begins.

PRINCIPAL USES
Dacarbazine is used for treatment of malignant melanoma (a type of skin cancer), Hodgkin's disease (a type of lymph node cancer), and occasionally sarcomas (uncommon cancers of the soft tissues).

HOW THE DRUG WORKS
Dacarbazine kills cancer cells by interfering with the synthesis of their genetic material, which prevents the cells from reproducing.

DOSAGE
The dose of dacarbazine depends on the type of tumor, patient weight, and whether other chemotherapy medicines are being used. Your oncologist (cancer specialist) will determine the proper dose.

ONSET OF EFFECT
Immediately after injection.

DURATION OF ACTION
Unknown.

DIETARY ADVICE
Maintain optimal food and fluid intake. Calorie, protein, and vitamin needs increase in patients with cancer. Good nutrition is essential to cope with the demands of chemotherapy.

STORAGE
Refrigerate, but do not allow it to freeze.

IF YOU MISS A DOSE
Inform your oncologist if you miss a dose. Adjustments will be made depending on the other chemotherapy you receive.

STOPPING THE DRUG
The decision to stop dacarbazine must be made in consultation with your physician.

PROLONGED USE
Use beyond 5 to 10 days out of every 28 days in a chemotherapy cycle is not recommended.

PRECAUTIONS
Over 60: Adverse reactions may be more likely and more severe in older patients.

Driving and Hazardous Work: The use of dacarbazine with other chemotherapy agents may impair your ability to perform such tasks safely.

Alcohol: Limit alcohol to moderate intake only.

Pregnancy: The use of chemotherapy during pregnancy could cause birth defects or fetal death. A reliable method of contraception is recommended while using this drug.

Breast Feeding: Dacarbazine passes into breast milk; you should avoid or discontinue use while breast feeding.

Infants and Children: Consult your pediatric oncologist.

Special Concerns: Dacarbazine may lower your ability to resist infection by reducing the number of white blood cells in the blood. Therefore, do not get vaccinated against bacteria or viruses without your doctor's approval. Avoid people with infections. Use care when shaving, trimming nails, or using sharp objects. Inform your doctor immediately if you have fever, chills, unusual bleeding or bruising, diarrhea, or a cough.

OVERDOSE
Symptoms: No specific information is available.

What to Do: If you are concerned about the possibility of an overdose of dacarbazine, call emergency medical services (EMS) to receive evaluation and treatment in the closest emergency facility.

DRUG INTERACTIONS
Consult your doctor if you are taking aspirin, ibuprofen, phenobarbital, phenytoin, amphotericin B, thyroid medications, azathioprine, chloramphenicol, colchicine, flucytosine, ganciclovir, interferon, plicamycin, or zidovudine.

FOOD INTERACTIONS
No known food interactions.

DISEASE INTERACTIONS
Consult your doctor if you have any of the following problems: chicken pox (or possible recent exposure to it), shingles, other infections elsewhere in your body, or kidney, liver, or lung disease.

Dalteparin Sodium

BRAND NAME
Fragmin

▶ Drug Class: Anticoagulant

▶ Available in: Injection

▶ Available OTC? No

▶ As Generic? No

Side Effects

SERIOUS
Easy or unusual bruising or bleeding, especially from the nose and gums, passage of black and tarry stools, vomiting or coughing of bright red blood, unusual weakness, dizziness.

COMMON
Pain or bruising at site of needle injection.

LESS COMMON
Shortness of breath, wheezing, breathing difficulty, confusion, hives, itching, rash, abdominal pain, facial swelling, sweating, weakness, lightheadedness (symptoms of anaphylaxis, a severe allergic reaction).

PRINCIPAL USES
To prevent or inhibit the formation of potentially dangerous blood clots within a blood vessel. Dalteparin is usually prescribed before major surgery, especially for prolonged operations that require general anesthesia. Those most likely to require the drug include patients who are over 40 years old, obese, immobile, suffering from a chronic debilitating disease, or who have had problems in the past with blood clots or who have a history of cancer.

HOW THE DRUG WORKS
Blood clotting (coagulation) is controlled by the interaction of many specialized proteins called coagulation factors. Dalteparin interferes with the normal functioning of several coagulation factors, thereby reducing the risk that a clot will form within a blood vessel. Anticoagulants such as dalteparin are often referred to as blood thinners.

DOSAGE
Adults: 2,500 international units injected under the skin once daily, beginning 1 to 2 hours prior to surgery, and continuing for 5 to 10 days afterward.

ONSET OF EFFECT
Rapid; within minutes.

DURATION OF ACTION
Therapeutic effect will persist for approximately 24 hours.

DIETARY ADVICE
Follow all of your doctor's dietary recommendations and other instructions carefully. Patients recovering from surgery require increased quantities of carbohydrates and proteins.

STORAGE
Not applicable; the dose is administered only at a health care facility.

IF YOU MISS A DOSE
Hospital personnel will ensure that you are administered this medication on schedule, once daily.

STOPPING THE DRUG
The decision to stop taking the drug should be made by your doctor.

PROLONGED USE
Therapy with this medication is usually concluded within 5 to 10 days. Prolonged use may increase the risk of undesirable side effects.

PRECAUTIONS
Over 60: Adverse reactions may be more likely and more severe in older patients.

Driving and Hazardous Work: Consult your doctor regarding the advisability of driving and performing hazardous work while taking an anticoagulant.

Alcohol: No special precautions are necessary.

Pregnancy: Adequate studies of the use of dalteparin during pregnancy have not been done; the drug should be used only if it is determined that benefits clearly outweigh potential risks. One form of dalteparin contains benzyl alcohol; this should not be used in pregnant women.

Breast Feeding: Dalteparin may pass into breast milk; caution is advised. Consult your doctor for specific advice.

Infants and Children: This drug is not recommended for use by children.

Special Concerns: Used properly, dalteparin prevents undesirable blood clots without seriously disrupting your ability to stop bleeding following minor injuries, scrapes, and bruises. Before taking this medication, be sure to inform your doctor if you have had any problem with unusual bleeding in the past. Occasionally, bleeding may occur internally and not be visible; primary symptoms are dizziness or weakness, especially when moving about or changing position. Keep in mind that such symptoms may occur following surgery for many reasons (use of pain medications or other drugs, or prolonged bed rest). It is important to tell your doctor about any changes in the way you are feeling during recovery period.

OVERDOSE
Symptoms: Unusual or uncontrolled bleeding, unusual bruising, weakness, or dizziness.

What to Do: Discontinue use and inform hospital personnel immediately.

DRUG INTERACTIONS
Consult your doctor if you are taking aspirin or other blood thinners.

FOOD INTERACTIONS
No known food interactions.

DISEASE INTERACTIONS
Caution is advised when taking dalteparin. Consult your doctor if you have allergies to pork or pork products, unusual bleeding or bruising, peptic ulcer, or high blood pressure, or if you have had recent surgery.

Danazol

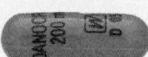

Danocrine 200 mg
(SANOFI WINTHROP)

▶ Drug Class: Gonadotropin inhibitor

▶ Available in: Capsules

▶ Available OTC? No

▶ As Generic? No

Side Effects

SERIOUS
Yellow tinge in the eyes or skin (jaundice); headache, which may be accompanied by nausea, vomiting, and changes in vision; severe abdominal pain; fatigue; skin rashes, which may be extensive and involve the inside of the mouth and nose; unusual nosebleeds, vaginal bleeding, bleeding from gums, or other bruising and bleeding.

COMMON
Cessation of menstruation, irregular or unpredictable vaginal bleeding or spotting, decreased breast size, weight gain, edema (swelling due to fluid retention), flushing, sweating, vaginal dryness, acne.

LESS COMMON
Cataracts; pain or tingling in fingers; increased sensitivity to sunlight; increase in body hair; enlargement of clitoris; hoarseness, sore throat, or deepening of voice.

PRINCIPAL USES
Danazol is used to treat endometriosis, fibrocystic breast disease, and an uncommon condition called hereditary angioedema, which causes abnormal swelling of body tissues.

HOW THE DRUG WORKS
Danazol blocks the production of the hormone estrogen by the ovaries. Without estrogen, endometrial tissue (the uterine lining) shrinks and becomes inactive. Subsequently, menstrual cycles cease, as do the hormone-related flare-ups of endometriosis and fibrocystic breast disease.

DOSAGE
Endometriosis: 100 to 400 mg, 2 times a day, beginning on the first day of menstrual flow. Treatment may take up to 6 months. Fibrocystic breast disease: 50 to 200 mg, 2 times a day, beginning on the first day of menstrual flow. Angioedema: 200 mg, 2 or 3 times a day. Increase in dosage may be necessary depending on results.

ONSET OF EFFECT
The full effect of danazol may take months to occur.

DURATION OF ACTION
Menstrual cycles return within 60 to 90 days after stopping danazol; breast discomfort due to fibrocystic disease may return within one year.

DIETARY ADVICE
Maintain your usual food and fluid intake. Increase fluids if you have a fever or diarrhea.

STORAGE
Store in a tightly sealed container away from heat and direct light. Keep away from moisture and extremes in temperature.

IF YOU MISS A DOSE
Take it as soon as you remember. If it is near the time for the next dose, skip the missed dose and resume your regular dosage schedule. Do not double the next dose.

STOPPING THE DRUG
Take danazol as prescribed for the full treatment period, even if you begin to feel better before the scheduled end of therapy.

PROLONGED USE
Therapy with danazol is usually completed within 3 to 6 months, although it may be extended to 9 months if necessary. Prolonged use may be associated with an increased risk of side effects.

PRECAUTIONS
Over 60: Adverse reactions may be more likely and more severe in older patients.

Driving and Hazardous Work: Do not drive or engage in hazardous work until you determine how the medicine affects you.

Alcohol: Drink alcohol only in moderation.

Pregnancy: Do not use danazol if you are pregnant.

Breast Feeding: Danazol must be avoided by women who are nursing.

Infants and Children: Danazol is not recommended for use by children.

Special Concerns: An effective method of contraception other than birth control pills (such as condoms or other barrier methods) should be used while taking danazol. Exposure of a fetus to danazol may lead to severe deformities. Be sure to report any unusual headache or change in vision to your physician. Some patients are treated successfully with one course of danazol; others require further treatments.

OVERDOSE
Symptoms: No specific ones have been reported.

What to Do: An overdose of danazol is unlikely to be life-threatening. However, if someone takes a much larger dose than prescribed, call your doctor, emergency medical services (EMS), or the nearest poison control center immediately.

DRUG INTERACTIONS
Consult your doctor for advice if you are taking anticoagulants (blood thinners).

FOOD INTERACTIONS
No known food interactions.

DISEASE INTERACTIONS
Consult your doctor if you have any of the following: heart or kidney disease; epilepsy or other seizure disorders; headaches, especially migraines; or any unexplained vaginal bleeding. Such conditions must be evaluated before starting danazol.

Dantrolene Sodium

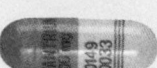

Dantrium 100 mg
(P&GP)

▶ Drug Class: Muscle relaxant

▶ Available in: Capsules, injection

▶ Available OTC? No

▶ As Generic? No

Side Effects

SERIOUS
Seizures, yellowish tinge to eyes and skin (indicating serious liver inflammation), difficulty breathing caused by fluid in the lungs, unusual bleeding, blood in urine or stools, fever, severe diarrhea, weakness, rash, itching, hives. Call your doctor immediately.

COMMON
Muscle weakness, drowsiness, dizziness, headaches.

LESS COMMON
Nervousness, confusion, insomnia, hallucinations, rapid or irregular heartbeat, watery eyes, blood pressure changes, double vision, weight loss, constipation, cramps, difficulty swallowing, frequent urination, sensitivity to sunlight, sweating, unusual hair growth, muscle pain, chills.

PRINCIPAL USES
To control recurrent muscle spasms and cramps, which may occur in association with multiple sclerosis, cerebral palsy, stroke, spinal cord injury, and other conditions. Dantrolene is sometimes used to prevent or control extremely high body temperature (malignant hyperthermia).

HOW THE DRUG WORKS
Calcium is necessary for muscle contraction; dantrolene directly interferes with the release of calcium in skeletal muscle tissue and thereby inhibits muscle cramping and spasms.

DOSAGE
For muscle spasms—Adults: 25 mg once a day to start, increased in 25 mg increments to 100 mg, 2 to 4 times a day, to a maximum of 400 mg a day. Children: 0.5 mg for each 2.2 lbs (1 kg) of body weight, 2 times a day to start; may be increased to a maximum of 100 mg, 4 times a day. For malignant hyperthermia: 4 to 8 mg for each 2.2 lbs of body weight in 3 or 4 doses a day.

ONSET OF EFFECT
1 to 2 weeks.

DURATION OF ACTION
Up to 24 hours.

DIETARY ADVICE
Capsules should be swallowed with milk or meals to prevent stomach upset.

STORAGE
Store in a tightly sealed container in a dry place away from heat and direct light.

IF YOU MISS A DOSE
Take it if you remember within 2 hours. Otherwise, skip the missed dose and resume your regular dosage schedule. Do not double the next dose.

STOPPING THE DRUG
The decision to stop taking the drug should be made by your doctor. Gradual reduction of the dose may be necessary if you have taken the drug for a long time.

PROLONGED USE
Tests that should be conducted periodically during prolonged use include blood counts, liver function studies, and G6PD tests.

PRECAUTIONS
Over 60: Adverse reactions may be more likely and more severe.

Driving and Hazardous Work: Avoid such activites until you determine how the medicine affects you.

Alcohol: Avoid alcohol while taking this drug.

Pregnancy: Dantrolene has not been shown to cause birth defects in humans. Consult your doctor about its use during pregnancy.

Breast Feeding: Dantrolene passes into breast milk; avoid or discontinue use while nursing.

Infants and Children: This drug should be used in children only under close medical supervision.

Special Concerns: You may have trouble swallowing while taking dantrolene; take care to avoid choking. Follow your doctor's advice regarding rest and physical therapy.

OVERDOSE
Symptoms: Bloody urine, chest pains, shortness of breath, convulsions, loss of consciousness.

What to Do: Call your doctor, emergency medical services (EMS), or the nearest poison control center immediately.

DRUG INTERACTIONS
Consult your doctor for specific advice if you are taking acetaminophen, amiodarone, anabolic steroids, androgens, medicines for infections, antithyroid agents, calcium channel blockers (verapamil in particular), carbamazepine, central nervous system depressants, chloroquine, daunorubicin, disulfiram, divalproex, estrogens, etretinate, gold salts, hydroxychloroquine, mercaptopurine, methotrexate, methyldopa, naltrexone, oral contraceptives, phenothiazines, phenytoin, plicamycin, tricyclic antidepressants, or valproic acid.

FOOD INTERACTIONS
No known food interactions.

DISEASE INTERACTIONS
Caution is advised when taking dantrolene. Consult your doctor if you have any of the following: emphysema, asthma, bronchitis, another chronic lung disease, heart disease, or liver disease.

Delavirdine

▶ Drug Class: Antiviral

▶ Available in: Tablets

▶ Available OTC? No

▶ As Generic? No

Side Effects

SERIOUS
Severe skin rash, fever, blistering, mouth sores, muscle or joint aches. Stop taking the medication and call your doctor immediately.

COMMON
Skin rash.

LESS COMMON
Abdominal cramps or pain, back or chest pain, chills, fatigue, lethargy, stiff neck, rapid breathing, migraine headache, fainting, loss of appetite, unusual gain or loss of weight, blood in stools, constipation or diarrhea, loss of appetite, gas, increased thirst, swollen or ulcerated tongue, leg cramps, swollen arms or legs, loss of coordination, amnesia, anxiety, decreased sexual function, depression, disorientation, dizziness, hallucinations, impaired concentration, insomnia, nightmares, restlessness, tremor, cough, breathing difficulty, hair loss, dry eyes, ear pain, ringing in ears, flank pain, blood in urine.

PRINCIPAL USES
To treat HIV infection in combination with other drugs. While not a cure for HIV, it may suppress the replication of the virus and delay the progression of the disease.

HOW THE DRUG WORKS
Delavirdine interferes with the activity of enzymes needed for the replication of DNA in viral cells, thus preventing the human immunodeficiency virus (HIV) from reproducing.

DOSAGE
400 mg, 3 times a day. The tablets can be dissolved in water before being administered. Rinse the glass and drink the rinse water to be sure that the entire dose has been taken.

ONSET OF EFFECT
Unknown. With most antiretroviral drugs, an early response can be seen within the first few days of therapy, but the maximum effect may take 12 to 16 weeks.

DURATION OF ACTION
Unknown. Effects of the drug may be prolonged if delavirdine is used in combination with other effective drugs and the virus is maximally suppressed.

DIETARY ADVICE
No special restrictions.

STORAGE
Store in a tightly sealed container away from heat and direct light.

IF YOU MISS A DOSE
Take it as soon as you remember. If it is near the time for the next dose, skip the missed dose and resume your regular dosage schedule. Do not double the next dose.

STOPPING THE DRUG
Take delavirdine every day, as prescribed. The decision to stop taking the drug should be made in consultation with your doctor.

PROLONGED USE
See your doctor regularly for tests and examinations for the duration of therapy.

PRECAUTIONS
Over 60: A lower dose may be advised for older patients.

Driving and Hazardous Work: Do not drive or engage in hazardous work until you determine how the medicine affects you.

Alcohol: Avoid alcohol if liver function is impaired.

Pregnancy: Delavirdine has been shown to cause birth defects in animals. Nevertheless, it is increasingly being used with other antiretroviral drugs to treat pregnant HIV-infected women.

Breast Feeding: It is not known whether delavirdine passes into breast milk; however, women infected with HIV should not breastfeed, to avoid transmitting the virus to an uninfected child.

Infants and Children: Safety and effectiveness of the use of this drug in children under 16 have not been established.

Special Concerns: Use of delavirdine does not eliminate the risk of passing the AIDS virus to other persons. Be sure to take appropriate preventive measures.

OVERDOSE
Symptoms: No cases of overdose have been reported.

What to Do: An overdose is unlikely to occur. Nonetheless, if you have any reason to suspect an overdose, seek medical assistance right away.

DRUG INTERACTIONS
Some drugs, when combined with delavirdine, may cause severe liver damage and so should not be taken. These drugs include certain nonsedating antihistamines, sedative hypnotic drugs, calcium channel blockers, ergot alkaloid preparations, and amphetamines. Other drugs may interact with delavirdine, requiring changes in your drug regimen; consult your doctor for specific advice if you are taking any other prescription or over-the-counter medication, especially antacids, clarithromycin, fluoxetine, ketoconazole, phenytoin, phenobarbital, carbamazepine, rifabutin, rifampin, cimetidine, famotidine, nizatidine, ranitidine, didanosine, indinavir, ritonavir, nelfinavir, or saquinavir.

FOOD INTERACTIONS
No known food interactions.

DISEASE INTERACTIONS
No disease interactions have been reported.

Desipramine Hydrochloride

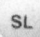

Generic 25 mg
(SIDMAK)

Additional photographs

▶ Drug Class: Tricyclic antidepressant

▶ Available in: Tablets

▶ Available OTC? No

▶ As Generic? Yes

Side Effects

SERIOUS
Confusion, heartbeat irregularities, hallucinations, seizures, extreme fatigue or drowsiness, blurred or altered vision, breathing difficulty, constipation, impaired concentration, difficult urination, fever, extreme and persistent restlessness, loss of coordination and balance, difficulty swallowing or speaking, dilated pupils, eye pain, fainting. Also trembling, shaking, weakness, and stiffness in the extremities; shuffling gait. Call your doctor immediately.

COMMON
Drowsiness or dizziness, headache, dry mouth or unpleasant taste, fatigue, heightened sensitivity to light, weight gain, nausea, increased appetite.

LESS COMMON
Heartburn, difficulty sleeping, diarrhea, sweating, vomiting.

PRINCIPAL USES
To relieve symptoms of major depression.

HOW THE DRUG WORKS
Desipramine affects levels of norepinephrine, a brain chemical that is thought to be linked to mood, emotions, and mental state.

DOSAGE
Adults: 100 to 200 mg once a day; may be increased to 300 mg a day. Older adults: 25 to 50 mg a day; may be increased to 150 mg a day.

ONSET OF EFFECT
1 to 6 weeks.

DURATION OF ACTION
Unknown.

DIETARY ADVICE
To lessen stomach upset, take with food, unless your doctor instructs otherwise. Increase your intake of fiber and fluids.

STORAGE
Store in a tightly sealed container away from heat, moisture, and direct light.

IF YOU MISS A DOSE
If you take a one-time daily bedtime dose, do not take the missed dose in the morning because it may cause drowsiness. Call your doctor. If you take more than 1 dose a day, take it as soon as you remember. If it is near the time for the next dose, skip the missed dose and resume your regular dosage schedule. Do not double the next dose.

STOPPING THE DRUG
Take it as prescribed for the full treatment period, even if you begin to feel better before the scheduled end of therapy. The decision to stop taking desipramine should be made in consultation with your doctor. The dosage should be tapered gradually over a period of 5 to 7 days when stopping treatment.

PROLONGED USE
Usual course of therapy lasts 6 months to 1 year; some patients may benefit from additional therapy.

PRECAUTIONS
Over 60: Adverse reactions may be more likely and more severe in older patients. A lower dose may be warranted.

Driving and Hazardous Work: Use caution when driving or engaging in hazardous work until you determine how the medication affects you. Drowsiness or lightheadedness can occur.

Alcohol: Avoid alcohol.

Pregnancy: Adequate studies have not been done. Consult your doctor for specific advice.

Breast Feeding: Desipramine passes into breast milk; do not use it while nursing.

Infants and Children: Not prescribed for children under age 16. Should not be prescribed for children, as unexplained deaths have occurred.

Special Concerns: This is a potentially dangerous drug, especially if taken in excess. Tricyclic antidepressants should not be within easy reach of suicidal patients.

OVERDOSE
Symptoms: Difficulty breathing, severe fatigue, seizures, confusion, hallucinations, distractibility, dilated pupils, irregular heartbeat, fever.

What to Do: Call your doctor, emergency medical services (EMS), or the nearest poison control center immediately.

DRUG INTERACTIONS
Consult your doctor for specific advice if you are taking antithyroid agents, cimetidine, clonidine, guanadrel, guanethidine, metrizamide, appetite suppressants, isoproterenol, ephedrine, epinephrine, amphetamines, phenylephrine, antipsychotic drugs, pimozide, methyldopa, metyrosine, metoclopramide, pemoline, promethazine, trimeprazine, rauwolfia alkaloids, MAO inhibitors, or any drugs that depress the central nervous system.

FOOD INTERACTIONS
No known food interactions.

DISEASE INTERACTIONS
Consult your doctor if you have any of the following: a history of alcohol abuse, difficulty urinating, asthma, bipolar disorder, high blood pressure, stomach or intestinal problems, glaucoma, overactive thyroid, enlarged prostate, schizophrenia, seizures, a blood disorder, or kidney, heart, or liver disease.

Desmopressin Acetate

BRAND NAMES
DDAVP, Stimate

▶ Drug Class: Antidiuretic; antihemorrhagic

▶ Available in: Injection, nasal solution, tablets

▶ Available OTC? No

▶ As Generic? Yes

Side Effects

SERIOUS
Rare severe allergic reaction (skin rash, itching, wheezing, swelling of lips, tongue, and throat). In some cases water intoxication may occur, causing lethargy, nausea, vomiting, mental impairment, and in severe cases seizures or coma. Seek medical attention immediately.

COMMON
No common side effects are associated with the use of desmopressin.

LESS COMMON
Headache, flushing, nausea, abdominal cramps, and slight rise in blood pressure. Such symptoms are generally associated with excessive doses.

PRINCIPAL USES
To treat diabetes insipidus, a relatively rare disorder characterized by excessive loss of water in the urine. Desmopressin is also used to help manage nighttime bedwetting. It may also be used to increase blood plasma levels of factor VIII, a crucial protein needed for clot formation. A deficiency of factor VIII may result in uncontrolled bleeding, the primary feature of hemophilia and a related disorder known as von Willebrand's disease type 1.

HOW THE DRUG WORKS
Desmopressin simulates the action of the hormone vasopressin, which helps the kidneys reabsorb water from urine, thus maintaining proper fluid balance. It also helps to boost plasma levels of factor VIII.

DOSAGE
For diabetes insipidus— Injection: 2 to 4 mg, 1 or 2 times a day. Nasal solution: 1 to 2 sprays per day. Tablets: 0.1 to 0.8 mg, 2 times a day in divided doses. For bedwetting in patients age 6 and over— Tablets: 0.2 mg at bedtime. May be increased to 0.6 mg. For von Willebrand's type 1— Injection: 0.3 mg per 2.2 lbs (1 kg) of body weight per day, administered over 15 to 30 minutes. Lowest effective dose will be determined by the doctor based on the patient's response to the drug.

ONSET OF EFFECT
Within 1 hour.

DURATION OF ACTION
Injection or nasal spray: 12 to 24 hours. Tablets: Approximately 8 hours.

DIETARY ADVICE
Take it with or between meals.

STORAGE
Keep nasal or injectable forms refrigerated, but do not allow them to freeze. When traveling, these forms remain stable at room temperature for up to 3 weeks. Keep tablets at room temperature, away from heat and direct light.

IF YOU MISS A DOSE
Take it as soon as you remember. If it is near the time for the next dose, skip the missed dose and resume your regular dosage schedule. Do not double the next dose.

STOPPING THE DRUG
The decision to stop taking the drug should be made by your doctor.

PROLONGED USE
No apparent problems with prolonged use of this drug.

PRECAUTIONS
Over 60: Adverse reactions may be more likely and more severe in older patients.

Driving and Hazardous Work: Do not drive or engage in hazardous work until you determine how the medication affects you.

Alcohol: Drink alcohol only in moderation.

Pregnancy: Desmopressin has not been shown to cause birth defects in animals. While no adequate studies have been done in humans, the drug is presumed to be safe.

Breast Feeding: Desmopressin has not been shown to cause problems in nursing babies. Consult your doctor about its use if you are breast feeding.

Infants and Children: Adverse reactions may be more likely and more severe in children under the age of 18.

Special Concerns: Periodic laboratory tests are needed to check your fluid status. Desmopressin tablets used for bedwetting may be taken alone or in conjunction with other kinds of non-medical therapy such as behavioral conditioning.

OVERDOSE
Symptoms: Drowsiness, listlessness, headache, confusion, inability to urinate, unexpected weight gain or fluid retention.

What to Do: An overdose of desmopressin is unlikely to be life-threatening but can cause water intoxication (leading to symptoms above) and spasm of the blood vessels. If someone takes a much larger dose than prescribed, call your doctor, emergency medical services (EMS), or poison control center immediately.

DRUG INTERACTIONS
Large doses of desmopressin should be used with other "pressor" agents only with careful monitoring. Consult your physician for specific advice if you are taking carbamazepine, chlorpropamide, demeclocycline, ethanol, fludrocortisone, heparin, lithium, norepinephrine, or tricyclic antidepressants.

FOOD INTERACTIONS
No known food interactions.

DISEASE INTERACTIONS
Consult your doctor if you have any of the following: seizures, migraine headaches, asthma, heart disease, blood vessel disease, congestive heart failure, or kidney disease.

▶ Drug Class: Respiratory corticosteroid

▶ Available in: Oral inhalation, nasal spray

▶ Available OTC? No

▶ As Generic? No

Side Effects

SERIOUS
No serious side effects are associated with this drug.

COMMON
Nosebleeds or bloody nasal secretions, nasal burning or irritation, sore throat.

LESS COMMON
Eye pain, watering eyes, gradual decrease of vision, stomach pain and digestive disturbances.

PRINCIPAL USES
To treat bronchial asthma; to treat allergic rhinitis (seasonal allergies such as hay fever); to prevent recurrence of nasal polyps after they have been removed surgically.

HOW THE DRUG WORKS
Respiratory corticosteroids such as dexamethasone primarily reduce or prevent inflammation of the lining of the airways, reduce the allergic response to inhaled allergens, and inhibit the secretion of mucus within the airways.

DOSAGE
Oral inhalation— Adults: To start, 3 inhalations 3 or 4 times a day; decreased as needed. Most patients respond to 2 inhalations 2 times a day. Children: 2 inhalations 3 or 4 times a day; decreased as needed. Most patients respond to 2 inhalations 2 times a day. Nasal spray— 2 sprays each nostril 3 times a day; decreased as needed.

ONSET OF EFFECT
Usually within 1 week; it may take 3 weeks for the full effect to occur.

DURATION OF ACTION
Unknown.

DIETARY ADVICE
No special restrictions.

STORAGE
Store in a tightly sealed container away from heat and direct light. Keep from getting cold; the medicine is less effective when cold.

IF YOU MISS A DOSE
Take it as soon as you remember. However, if it is near the time for the next dose, skip the missed dose and resume your regular dosage schedule. Do not double the next dose.

STOPPING THE DRUG
The decision to stop taking the drug should be made by your doctor.

PROLONGED USE
Consult your doctor about the need for regular medical tests and examinations if you must take this drug for a prolonged period of time.

PRECAUTIONS
Over 60: No special problems are expected.

Driving and Hazardous Work: The use of dexamethasone should not impair your ability to perform such tasks safely.

Alcohol: No special precautions are necessary.

Pregnancy: Nasal or inhaled steroids have not been reported to cause birth defects if taken during pregnancy. Before using such drugs, tell your doctor if you are pregnant or plan to become pregnant.

Breast Feeding: Dexamethasone may pass into breast milk; caution is advised. Consult your doctor for advice.

Infants and Children: Inhalation corticosteroids like dexamethasone have not been shown to cause different side effects or problems in children than they do in adults. Consult your doctor for specific advice.

Special Concerns: Inhaled steroids will not help an asthma attack in progress. Inhaled steroids can lower resistance to yeast infections of the mouth, throat, or voice box. To prevent yeast infections, gargle or rinse your mouth with water after each use; do not swallow the water.

Know how to use the spray properly; read and follow the directions that come with the device. Before you have surgery, tell the doctor or dentist that you are using a steroid.

OVERDOSE
Symptoms: No specific ones have been reported.

What to Do: Call your doctor, emergency medical services (EMS), or the nearest poison control center if you have any reason to suspect an overdose.

DRUG INTERACTIONS
Consult your doctor for specific advice if you are taking systemic corticosteroids, other inhaled corticosteroids, or any medications that suppress the immune system.

FOOD INTERACTIONS
No known food interactions.

DISEASE INTERACTIONS
Caution is advised when taking dexamethasone. Consult your doctor if you have osteoporosis or a history of tuberculosis.

Dexamethasone Ophthalmic

BRAND NAMES
AK-Dex, Baldex, Decadron Ophthalmic, Dexair, Dexotic, Maxidex Ophthalmic, Ocu-Dex, Storz-Dexa

▶ Drug Class: Corticosteroid

▶ Available in: Ophthalmic solution, suspension

▶ Available OTC? No

▶ As Generic? Yes

Side Effects

SERIOUS
Decreased vision or blurring of vision (from cataract); eye pain, nausea, vomiting (from increased eye pressure); pain, redness, sensitivity to bright light, discharge (from eye infection). Call your doctor immediately if you experience any of these signs or symptoms. This drug may trigger a recurrence of herpes infection of the eye; mention any previous herpes infection to your doctor.

COMMON
No common side effects are associated with the use of ophthalmic dexamethasone.

LESS COMMON
Burning, stinging, redness, or watering of eyes.

PRINCIPAL USES
To control inflammation and prevent potentially permanent damage that may result from conditions that involve inflammation in the eye tissues.

HOW THE DRUG WORKS
Dexamethasone inhibits the release of natural substances that stimulate an inflammatory reaction.

DOSAGE
Solution or suspension: 1 or 2 drops in each eye up to 16 times a day.

ONSET OF EFFECT
Unknown.

DURATION OF ACTION
Unknown.

DIETARY ADVICE
This drug can be used without regard to diet.

STORAGE
Store in a tightly sealed container away from heat, moisture, and direct light. Do not allow it to freeze.

IF YOU MISS A DOSE
Administer it as soon as you remember. If it is near the time for the next dose, skip the missed dose and resume your regular dosage schedule. Do not double the next dose.

STOPPING THE DRUG
Use this drug as prescribed for the full treatment period, even if symptoms improve before the scheduled end of the therapy.

PROLONGED USE
See your doctor regularly for tests and examinations if you must take this drug for a prolonged period.

PRECAUTIONS
Over 60: No special problems are expected.

Driving and Hazardous Work: Avoid such activities until you determine how the medicine affects your vision.

Alcohol: No special precautions are necessary.

Pregnancy: Ophthalmic dexamethasone has caused birth defects in animals. Reliable human studies have not been done, but no human birth defects have been documented. Before you use this drug, tell your doctor if you are pregnant or plan to become pregnant.

Breast Feeding: This drug has not been reported to cause problems in nursing babies. Consult your doctor for specific advice.

Infants and Children: Children under age 2 may be especially sensitive to the effects of this drug.

Special Concerns: To use the eye drops, first wash your hands. Tilt your head back. Gently apply pressure to the inside corner of the eyelid and with the index finger of the same hand, pull downward on the lower eyelid to make a space. Drop the medicine into this space and close your eye. Apply pressure for 1 or 2 minutes while keeping the eye closed without blinking. Then wash your hands again. Make sure the tip of the dropper does not touch your eye, finger, or any other surface. If your symptoms do not improve in 5 to 7 days or if they become worse, check with your doctor. Wearing contact lenses while using this medication may increase the risk of infection. Your doctor may tell you not to wear contact lenses during and for a day or two after treatment.

OVERDOSE
Symptoms: When applied topically, an overdose of ophthalmic dexamethasone is very unlikely. Inadvertent oral ingestion, however, may cause fever, muscle weakness, nausea, loss of appetite, dizziness, fainting, or difficulty breathing.

What to Do: An overdose of this drug is unlikely to be life-threatening. However, if someone takes a much larger dose than prescribed or accidentally ingests the medicine, call your doctor, emergency medical services (EMS), or the nearest poison control center.

DRUG INTERACTIONS
Other drugs may interact with ophthalmic dexamethasone. Consult your doctor for specific advice if you are taking any other prescription or over-the-counter medication.

FOOD INTERACTIONS
No known food interactions.

DISEASE INTERACTIONS
Caution is advised when taking ophthalmic dexamethasone. Consult your doctor if you have any of the following: diabetes, herpes infection of the eye, glaucoma, cataracts, tuberculosis of the eye, or any other eye infection.

Dexamethasone Systemic

BRAND NAMES
Dalalone, Decaject,
Deronil, Dexacen,
Dexasone, Solurex

Generic 0.75 mg
(ROXANE)

Additional photographs

▶ Drug Class: Corticosteroid

▶ Available in: Elixir, oral
  solution, tablets, injection

▶ Available OTC? No

▶ As Generic? Yes

Side Effects

SERIOUS
Vision problems, frequent urination, increased thirst, rectal bleeding, blistering skin, confusion, hallucinations, paranoia, euphoria, depression, mood swings, redness and swelling at injection site. Call your doctor immediately.

COMMON
Increased appetite, indigestion, nervousness, insomnia, greater susceptibility to infections, increased blood pressure, slow healing of wounds, weight gain, easy bruising, fluid retention.

LESS COMMON
Change in skin color, dizziness, headache, increased sweating, unusual growth of body or facial hair, increased blood sugar, peptic ulcers, adrenal insufficiency, muscle weakness, cataracts, glaucoma, osteoporosis.

PRINCIPAL USES
To treat numerous conditions that involve inflammation (a response by body tissues, producing redness, warmth, swelling, and pain). Such conditions include arthritis, allergic reactions, asthma, some skin diseases, multiple sclerosis flare-ups, and other autoimmune diseases. Also prescribed to treat deficiency of natural steroid hormones.

HOW THE DRUG WORKS
This hormone mimics the effects of the body's natural corticosteroids. It depresses the synthesis, release, and activity of inflammation-producing body chemicals. It also suppresses the activity of the immune system.

DOSAGE
Adults and teenagers— Oral dosage: 25 to 300 mg a day, depending on condition, in 1 or several doses. Injection: 20 to 300 mg once a day, depending on condition. Children— Consult your pediatrician.

ONSET OF EFFECT
Within 2 hours of oral form, 1 hour of injection.

DURATION OF ACTION
More than 2 days for oral form; 6 days after injection.

DIETARY ADVICE
It can be taken with food or milk to minimize stomach upset. Your doctor may recommend a low-salt, high-potassium, high-protein diet.

STORAGE
Store in a tightly sealed container away from heat, moisture, and direct light.

IF YOU MISS A DOSE
Take it as soon as you remember. If you take several doses a day and it is close to the next dose, double the next dose. If you take 1 dose a day and you do not remember until the next day, skip the missed dose and do not double the next dose.

STOPPING THE DRUG
With long-term therapy, do not stop taking the drug abruptly; the dosage should be decreased gradually.

PROLONGED USE
See your doctor regularly for tests and examinations. Long-term use may lead to cataracts, diabetes, hypertension, or osteoporosis.

PRECAUTIONS
Over 60: Adverse reactions may be more likely and more severe in older patients.

Driving and Hazardous Work: Do not drive or engage in hazardous work until you determine how the medicine affects you.

Alcohol: May cause stomach problems; avoid it unless your physician approves occasional moderate drinking.

Pregnancy: Overuse during pregnancy can retard the child's growth and cause other developmental problems. Consult your physician.

Breast Feeding: Do not use while nursing.

Infants and Children: Dexamethasone may retard the normal growth and development of bone and other tissues. Consult your doctor.

Special Concerns: Avoid immunizations with live vaccines if possible. Remember that this drug can lower your resistance to infection. Patients undergoing long-term therapy should wear a medical-alert bracelet. Call your doctor if you develop a fever.

OVERDOSE
Symptoms: Fever, muscle or joint pain, nausea, dizziness, fainting, difficulty breathing. Prolonged overuse: Moonface, obesity, unusual hair growth, acne, loss of sexual function, muscle wasting.

What to Do: Call your doctor, emergency medical services (EMS), or the nearest poison control center immediately.

DRUG INTERACTIONS
Consult your doctor for specific advice if you are taking aminoglutethimide, antacids, barbiturates, carbamazepine, griseofulvin, mitotane, phenylbutazone, phenytoin, primidone, rifampin, injectable amphotericin B, oral antidiabetes agents, insulin, digitalis drugs, diuretics, or medications containing potassium or sodium.

FOOD INTERACTIONS
Avoid excess sodium.

DISEASE INTERACTIONS
Consult your doctor if you have a history of bone disease, chicken pox, measles, gastrointestinal disorders, diabetes, recent serious infection, tuberculosis, glaucoma, heart disease, hypertension, liver or kidney disorders, high blood cholesterol, overactive or underactive thyroid, myasthenia gravis, or lupus.

Dexamethasone Topical

BRAND NAMES
Aeroseb-Dex, Decaderm, Decadron, Decarex, Decaspray, Dexone, DMS, Hexadrol, Maxidex, Mymethasone

▶ Drug Class: Topical corticosteroid

▶ Available in: Gel, aerosol solution, cream

▶ Available OTC? No

▶ As Generic? Yes

Side Effects

SERIOUS
No serious side effects are associated with topical dexamethasone.

COMMON
Burning, itching, irritation, redness, dryness, acne, stinging and cracking of skin, numbness or tingling in the extremities. Such side effects are unlikely to occur except when topical dexamethasone is used with bandages or other occlusive dressings.

LESS COMMON
With prolonged use: Blistering and pus near hair follicles, unusual bleeding or bruising, darkening or prominence of small surface veins, increased susceptibility to infection.

PRINCIPAL USES
To treat skin rash and inflammation. Topical steroids come in many strengths; dexamethasone is a lower-strength steroid, which is safest and most appropriate for certain minor skin conditions.

HOW THE DRUG WORKS
Topical dexamethasone appears to interfere with the formation of natural substances within the body that are directly responsible for the process of inflammation, which produces swelling, redness, and pain.

DOSAGE
Gel (0.1% strength)— Apply 2 or 3 times daily. Aerosol (0.01% and 0.04% strength)— Adults: Apply 2 to 4 times daily. Children: 1 or 2 times daily. Cream (0.1% strength)— Adults: Apply 3 or 4 times daily. Children: once daily.

ONSET OF EFFECT
Soon after application. However, recognizable changes in your condition may take several days or more to develop.

DURATION OF ACTION
Unknown.

DIETARY ADVICE
No special restrictions.

STORAGE
Store in a tightly sealed container away from heat and direct light.

IF YOU MISS A DOSE
Apply it as soon as you remember. If it is near the time for the next dose, skip the missed dose and resume your regular dosage schedule.

STOPPING THE DRUG
Take as prescribed for the full treatment period, even if you begin to feel better before the scheduled end of therapy.

PROLONGED USE
Avoid prolonged use, particularly near the eyes, on the face, genital, or rectal areas, or in the folds of the skin.

PRECAUTIONS
Over 60: Side effects may be more likely and more severe in elderly patients; therapy with topical corticosteroids should therefore be brief and infrequent.

Driving and Hazardous Work: The use of topical dexamethasone should not impair your ability to perform such tasks safely.

Alcohol: No special precautions are necessary.

Pregnancy: This drug should not be used for prolonged periods by pregnant women or women trying to become pregnant.

Breast Feeding: Although problems have not been documented, caution is advised. Do not apply to breasts prior to nursing. Consult your doctor for specific advice.

Infants and Children: It should not be used for more than 2 weeks on children and teenagers, unless otherwise directed by your doctor. Do not use tight-fitting diapers or plastic pants on children when treating skin irritation in the diaper area.

Special Concerns: Take care to avoid use of this medication around the eyes. Take care to apply only to the affected area. Note that dexamethasone is not a treatment for acne, burns, infections, or disorders of pigmentation. Do not bandage or wrap the medicated area of skin with any special dressings or coverings unless specifically told to do so by your doctor. Applying special coverings may increase the chance of an undesirable interaction or side effect.

OVERDOSE
Symptoms: None known.

What to Do: An overdose of a topical corticosteroid is unlikely to be life-threatening. However, in the event of accidental ingestion or an apparent overdose, call your doctor, emergency medical services (EMS), or the nearest poison control center right away.

DRUG INTERACTIONS
Do not mix topical dexamethasone with other products, especially alcohol-containing preparations (which include colognes, aftershave, and many moisturizer lotions), since this may cause dryness and irritation, or increase the risk of an allergic reaction.

FOOD INTERACTIONS
Potassium supplements may decrease this drug's effects. Avoid foods high in sodium.

DISEASE INTERACTIONS
Consult your doctor if you have any of the following: cataracts; diabetes mellitus; glaucoma; infection, sores, or ulcerations of the skin; infection elsewhere in your body; or tuberculosis.

Generic 5 mg
(SMITHKLINE BEECHAM)

▶ Drug Class: Central nervous
system stimulant/amphetamine

▶ Available in: Extended-
release capsules, tablets

▶ Available OTC? No

▶ As Generic? No

Side Effects

SERIOUS
Irregular heartbeat, chest
pain, increased blood
pressure, skin rash,
uncontrollable move-
ments of arms and legs,
mental changes, unusual
weakness, very high
fever. Call your doctor
immediately.

COMMON
Mood changes, insomnia,
drowsiness, restlessness.

LESS COMMON
Blurred vision, constipa-
tion, diarrhea, loss of
appetite, headache,
increased sweating,
stomach cramps or pain,
nausea or vomiting,
changes in sexual
desire or decreased
sexual ability.

PRINCIPAL USES
To treat attention-deficit
hyperactivity disorder,
sometimes referred to as
ADHD or simply hyperactivity. It is also used to treat
narcolepsy (uncontrolled
onset of sleep).

HOW THE DRUG WORKS
Dextroamphetamine acti-
vates nerve cells in the
brain and spinal cord to
increase motor activity and
alertness and lessen drowsiness and fatigue. In hyperactivity disorders and
narcolepsy, amphetamines
improve mental focus and
the ability to stay awake
or concentrate.

DOSAGE
To treat ADHD— Adults: 5
to 60 mg a day. Children
age 6 and older: To start, 5
mg, 1 or 2 times a day. Children ages 3 to 6: To start,
2.5 mg a day. To treat narcolepsy— Adults: 5 to 60
mg a day. Teenagers: To
start, 10 mg once a day.
Children ages 6 to 12: To
start, 5 mg once a day.

ONSET OF EFFECT
Usually within 30 to 45 minutes for tablets, and somewhat later for extended-
release capsules.

DURATION OF ACTION
In adults, 8 to 12 hours; in
children, 6 to 10 hours.
Extended-release capsules
have a somewhat longer
duration of action.

DIETARY ADVICE
Take it with liquid 30 to 45
minutes before meals. Avoid
caffeinated beverages like
tea, coffee, and some colas.
Avoid vitamin C pills and
acidic foods rich in vitamin
C, such as fruit juices and
other citrus products.

STORAGE
Store in a tightly sealed container away from heat, moisture, and direct light.

IF YOU MISS A DOSE
Take it as soon as you
remember. If it is near the
time for the next dose, skip
the missed dose and
resume your regular dosage
schedule. Do not double the
next dose.

STOPPING THE DRUG
Take it as prescribed for the
full treatment period, even
if you begin to feel better
before the scheduled end
of therapy. The decision to
stop taking the drug should
be made by your doctor.
The doctor may decrease
your dosage gradually to
reduce the possibility of
withdrawal symptoms.

PROLONGED USE
Amphetamines can be habit-
forming, and prolonged use
may increase the risk of
dependency.

PRECAUTIONS
Over 60: Adverse reactions
may be more likely and
more severe in older
patients.

**Driving and Hazardous
Work:** Do not drive or
engage in hazardous work
until you determine how the
medicine affects you.

Alcohol: Avoid alcohol.

Pregnancy: Adequate
human studies have not
been completed. Before
taking dextroamphetamine,
tell your doctor if you are
pregnant or plan to become
pregnant.

Breast Feeding: Dex-
troamphetamine passes into
breast milk; caution is
advised. Consult your doctor for advice.

Infants and Children:
Not recommended for use
by children under age 3.

Special Concerns: Take
only as directed and do not
increase the dose on your
own. Remember that
fatigue, excessive drowsiness, sleepiness, or depression while taking stimulants
may mean an emergency
situation is developing.
Difficulty sleeping may be
improved by taking the last
scheduled dose several
hours before bedtime.

OVERDOSE
Symptoms: Extreme restlessness, agitation, or
bizarre behavior; panic;
rapid breathing; confusion;
high fever; hallucinations;
seizures; coma.

What to Do: Call your
doctor, emergency medical
services (EMS), or the
nearest poison control center immediately.

DRUG INTERACTIONS
Consult your doctor for specific advice if you are taking
tricyclic antidepressants,
caffeine, beta-blockers, digitalis drugs, central nervous
system stimulants, meperidine, MAO inhibitors, sympathomimetic agents, or
thyroid hormones.

FOOD INTERACTIONS
Citrus juices and caffeinated
beverages and foods may
interact with this drug.

DISEASE INTERACTIONS
Consult your doctor if you
have any of the following:
advanced blood vessel disease, heart disease, hyperthyroidism, hypertension,
severe anxiety, Tourette's
syndrome, glaucoma, or a
history of drug abuse.

Dextromethorphan

▶ Drug Class: Cough
suppressant

▶ Available in: Capsules,
lozenges, tablets, oral
suspension, syrup

▶ Available OTC? Yes

▶ As Generic? Yes

Side Effects

SERIOUS
Serious side effects occur
only in cases of overdose
(see Overdose).

COMMON
No common side effects
are associated with the
use of this drug.

LESS COMMON
Mild dizziness or seda-
tion, nausea or vomiting,
abdominal pain. Such
symptoms are more
likely to occur at the
beginning of therapy and
tend to diminish as your
body becomes accus-
tomed to taking the drug.
Consult your doctor if
they persist or interfere
with daily activities.

PRINCIPAL USES
To relieve a dry or mini-
mally productive cough
(that is, a mild cough that
rids the lungs of modest
amounts of phlegm or
mucus), commonly associ-
ated with allergies, colds,
influenza, and certain lung
disorders. This medicine is
ideally useful when a mild
or hacking cough would
otherwise interrupt sleep
or interfere with your daily
activities.

HOW THE DRUG WORKS
Dextromethorphan works
by directly reducing the
sensitivity of the cough center—the part of the brain
that responds to stimuli in
the lower respiratory passages that irritate and trigger the cough reflex.

DOSAGE
Adults: 10 to 20 mg every
4 hours or 30 mg every 6 to
8 hours; 30 to 60 mg of
extended-release liquid
twice a day. Children 6 to
12: 5 to 10 mg every 4
hours or 30 mg of extended-
release liquid twice a day.
Children 2 to 6: 2.5 to 5 mg
every 4 hours, or 7.5 mg
every 6 to 8 hours, or 15
mg of the extended-release
liquid twice a day. Children
under 2: Dosage must be
individualized.

ONSET OF EFFECT
15 to 30 minutes.

DURATION OF ACTION
Up to 6 hours.

DIETARY ADVICE
No special restrictions.

STORAGE
Store in a tightly sealed container away from heat, moisture, and direct light.

IF YOU MISS A DOSE
Take it as soon as you
remember. However, if it is
near the time for the next
dose, skip the missed dose
and resume your regular
dosage schedule. Do not
double the next dose.

STOPPING THE DRUG
Take it as prescribed for the
full treatment period. However, you may stop taking
the drug if you are feeling
better before the scheduled
end of therapy. If the cough
does not improve after 7
days, consult your doctor.

PROLONGED USE
No problems are expected.

PRECAUTIONS
Over 60: Side effects
may be more frequent and
severe than in younger persons. Smaller doses for
shorter periods may be
needed. If this drug is used
to control coughing, other
treatment measures may be
needed to liquefy any accumulation of thick mucus
that may form in the
bronchial tubes.

**Driving and Hazardous
Work:** Determine if dex-
tromethorphan causes
drowsiness or dizziness
before you drive or engage
in hazardous work.

Alcohol: Avoid alcohol
while using this drug; it
may increase the risk of
sedation.

Pregnancy: Ask your doctor whether the benefits of
the drug justify the possible
risk to the fetus.

Breast Feeding: Dextromethorphan may pass into
breast milk; caution is
advised. Consult your doctor for specific advice about
taking dextromethorphan
while you are nursing.

Infants and Children:
Doses for children under 2
must be individualized; consult your pediatrician.

Special Concerns: Do not
take dextromethorphan to
relieve a cough caused by
asthma, emphysema, or
smoking.

OVERDOSE
Symptoms: Nausea, vomiting, extreme drowsiness or
dizziness, nervousness and
agitation, extreme irritability or mood changes, hallucinations, blurred vision,
uncontrollable eye move-
ment, inability to urinate,
confusion, loss of consciousness, or coma.

What to Do: Call your
doctor, emergency medical
services (EMS), or the
nearest poison control center immediately.

DRUG INTERACTIONS
Taking a sedative or other
depressant can increase the
sedative effects of both
drugs. Using doxepin
increases the toxic effects
of both drugs. Taking an
MAO inhibitor can cause a
high fever, disorientation, or
loss of consciousness. Using
quinidine increases the risk
of experiencing side effects
with dextromethorphan.

FOOD INTERACTIONS
No known food interactions.

DISEASE INTERACTIONS
Caution is advised when
taking dextromethorphan.
Consult your doctor if you
have a history of asthma or
impaired liver function.

Diazepam

BRAND NAMES
Di-Tran, Diastat, Diazepam Intensol, Diazepm, T-Quil, Valium, Valrelease, Vazepam, X-O'Spaz, Zetran

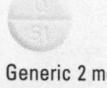

Generic 2 mg
(PUREPAC)

▶ Drug Class: Benzodiazepine tranquilizer; antianxiety agent/muscle relaxant

▶ Available in: Tablets, capsules, injection, rectal gel

▶ Available OTC? No

▶ As Generic? Yes

Side Effects

SERIOUS
Difficulty concentrating, outbursts of anger, other behavior problems, depression, hallucinations, low blood pressure (causing faintness or confusion), memory impairment, muscle weakness, skin rash or itching, sore throat, fever and chills, sores or ulcers in throat or mouth, unusual bruising or bleeding, extreme fatigue, yellowish tinge to eyes or skin. Call your doctor immediately.

COMMON
Drowsiness, loss of coordination, unsteady gait, dizziness, lightheadedness, slurred speech.

LESS COMMON
Change in sexual desire or ability, constipation, false sense of well-being, nausea and vomiting, urinary problems, unusual fatigue.

PRINCIPAL USES
To treat anxiety, panic attacks, and muscle spasms. It is also used in the acute treatment of seizures.

HOW THE DRUG WORKS
In general, diazepam produces mild sedation by depressing activity in the central nervous system. In particular, diazepam appears to enhance the effect of gamma-aminobutyric acid (GABA), a natural chemical that inhibits the firing of neurons and dampens the transmission of nerve signals, thus decreasing nervous excitation.

DOSAGE
For anxiety— Adults: 2 to 10 mg, 4 times a day. Children: 1 to 2.5 mg, 3 or 4 times a day. For muscle spasms— 2 to 10 mg, 2 to 4 times a day. For treatment of seizures— Injection: The dose is determined and administered by your doctor. Rectal gel: The recommended dose is 0.2 to 0.5 mg per 2.2 lbs (1 kg) of body weight depending on age. Your doctor will determine the correct dosage.

ONSET OF EFFECT
30 minutes.

DURATION OF ACTION
Up to 48 hours.

DIETARY ADVICE
No special restrictions.

STORAGE
Store in a tightly sealed container away from heat, moisture, and direct light.

IF YOU MISS A DOSE
Take the missed dose if you remember within 2 hours. If more than 2 hours, skip the missed dose and return to your regular schedule. Do not double the next dose.

STOPPING THE DRUG
Discontinuing the drug abruptly may produce withdrawal symptoms (seizures, sleep disruption, nervousness, irritability, diarrhea, abdominal cramps, muscle aches, memory impairment). Dosage should be reduced gradually according to your physician's instructions.

PROLONGED USE
Diazepam may slowly lose its effectiveness with prolonged use. You should see your doctor for periodic evaluation if you must take it for an extended time.

PRECAUTIONS
Over 60: Dosage is often reduced because adverse reactions are more likely and may be more severe in older patients.

Driving and Hazardous Work: Diazepam can impair mental alertness and physical coordination. Adjust your activities accordingly.

Alcohol: Alcohol intake should be extremely moderate or stopped altogether while taking this drug.

Pregnancy: Use during pregnancy should be avoided if possible. Be sure to tell your doctor if you are pregnant or plan to become pregnant.

Breast Feeding: Diazepam passes into breast milk; do not take it while nursing.

Infants and Children: Diazepam should be used by children only under close medical supervision.

Special Concerns: Diazepam use can lead to psychological or physical dependence. Never take

more than the prescribed daily dose. Your physician will teach you how to determine when it is appropriate and how to properly administer the rectal gel.

OVERDOSE
Symptoms: Extreme drowsiness, confusion, slurred speech, slow reflexes, poor coordination, staggering gait, tremor, slowed breathing, loss of consciousness.

What to Do: Call your doctor, emergency medical services (EMS), or the nearest poison control center immediately.

DRUG INTERACTIONS
Other drugs may interact with diazepam. Consult your doctor for specific advice if you are taking any drugs that depress the central nervous system; these include antihistamines, antidepressants or other psychiatric medications, barbiturates, sedatives, cough medicines, decongestants, and painkillers. Be sure your doctor knows about any over-the-counter medication you may take.

FOOD INTERACTIONS
None reported.

DISEASE INTERACTIONS
Do not take diazepam if you have acute narrow angle glaucoma. Consult your doctor if you have a history of alcohol or drug abuse, stroke or other brain disease, any chronic lung disease, hyperactivity, depression or other mental illness, myasthenia gravis, sleep apnea, epilepsy, porphyria, kidney disease, or liver disease.

Diazoxide

▶ Drug Class: Glucose-elevating agent (capsules); antihypertensive (injection)

▶ Available in: Capsules, injectable solution

▶ Available OTC? No

▶ As Generic? Yes

Side Effects

SERIOUS
Excess sodium and water retention (edema), resulting in decreased urination, rapid weight gain (or bloating), swelling of feet or lower legs. In some cases this condition, if unchecked, may lead to congestive heart failure; call your doctor at once. A diuretic may be prescribed to counteract the edema, but the combination of diazoxide with a thiazide diuretic may further raise blood glucose levels. Attacks of gout may occur since diazoxide can raise uric acid levels.

COMMON
Rapid heartbeat.

LESS COMMON
Fever, rash, stiffness of arms or legs, unusual bleeding or bruising, constipation, loss of appetite, stomach pain, nausea and vomiting. With long-term use: growth of hair on forehead, back, arms, and legs.

PRINCIPAL USES
To correct low blood glucose levels (hypoglycemia) resulting from overproduction of insulin by the pancreas, which may occur when an insulin-producing pancreatic tumor cannot be removed by surgery or when a malignant insulin-producing tumor has spread.

HOW THE DRUG WORKS
Insulin, a hormone produced by the beta cells of the pancreas, lowers blood glucose (sugar) levels by increasing the uptake of glucose by muscles and reducing its release from the liver. Too much insulin causes blood glucose to drop to low levels. Diazoxide inhibits the release of insulin from the pancreas and thus helps to prevent blood glucose from falling to low levels.

DOSAGE
The dose is based on body weight and should be determined by your doctor. Adults, teenagers, and children: Starting at 1 mg per 2.2 lbs (1 kg) of body weight every 8 hours. Can be increased to 3 to 8 mg per 2.2 lbs in 2 or 3 doses a day. Newborn babies and infants: Starting at 3.3 mg per 2.2 lbs of body weight every 8 hours. Can be increased to 8 to 15 mg per 2.2 lbs (3.6 to 6.8 mg per lb) in 2 or 3 doses a day.

ONSET OF EFFECT
1 hour.

DURATION OF ACTION
8 hours.

DIETARY ADVICE
Can be taken with or between meals. A diet rich in carbohydrates may help to raise and maintain blood glucose levels.

STORAGE
Store in a dry place away from heat and light. Keep the solution from freezing.

IF YOU MISS A DOSE
Take it as soon as you remember. If it is near the time for the next dose, skip the missed dose and go back to your regular dosage schedule. Do not double the next dose.

STOPPING THE DRUG
Do not stop taking diazoxide without first consulting your doctor.

PROLONGED USE
Close monitoring of blood sugar levels is necessary. Long-term side effects of diazoxide may include stiffening of limbs; shaking and trembling of hands and fingers; increased hair growth on forehead, back, arms, and legs.

PRECAUTIONS
Over 60: Older persons are more likely to suffer from impaired kidney function and may therefore require a reduced dose.

Driving and Hazardous Work: Do not drive or engage in hazardous work until you determine how diazoxide affects you.

Alcohol: Follow your physician's instructions about alcohol use while taking this drug.

Pregnancy: Use of diazoxide during pregnancy may have adverse effects on the fetus. Consult your doctor if you are pregnant or plan to become pregnant.

Breast Feeding: It is not known whether diazoxide passes into breast milk. Consult your doctor about the drug's relative risks and benefits if you are breast feeding.

Infants and Children: Careful monitoring is required.

Special Concerns: Follow the special diet that your doctor gives you, and be sure to call your doctor if you experience edema (swelling, especially in the lower extremities), excessive rise in your blood glucose levels, or a drop in blood pressure.

OVERDOSE
Symptoms: An excessive rise in blood glucose can cause drowsiness, flushed skin, dry skin, increased urination, or unusual thirst (symptoms of diabetic ketoacidosis or hyperosmolar coma).

What to Do: Call your doctor immediately.

DRUG INTERACTIONS
Drugs that can affect or be affected by diazoxide include alpha- and beta-blockers, anticoagulants, antigout drugs, anticonvulsants, and thiazide diuretics.

FOOD INTERACTIONS
No known food interactions.

DISEASE INTERACTIONS
Your doctor must be aware of any other medical problems, especially angina, gout, heart disease, blood vessel disease, kidney disease, liver disease, or a recent stroke.

Diclofenac Ophthalmic

BRAND NAME
Voltaren Ophthalmic

▶ Drug Class: Nonsteroidal anti-inflammatory drug (NSAID)

▶ Available in: Ophthalmic solution

▶ Available OTC? No

▶ As Generic? No

Side Effects

SERIOUS
Rarely, ophthalmic diclofenac will cause bleeding in the eye, redness or swelling of the eye or eyelid not present before the start of therapy, or tearing or itching of the eye. Call your doctor immediately.

COMMON
Mild and temporary burning or stinging of eyes after application.

LESS COMMON
No less-common side effects are associated with the use of ophthalmic diclofenac.

PRINCIPAL USES
To treat inflammation and eye problems that occur after cataract removal surgery. Also used to control eye pain after corneal refractive surgery (such as the increasingly popular radial keratotomy to correct nearsightedness).

HOW THE DRUG WORKS
Ophthalmic diclofenac inhibits the release of natural substances that stimulate inflammation and can cause pain in eye tissues.

DOSAGE
Adults: 1 drop in each affected eye 4 times a day, beginning 24 hours after surgery and continuing for the next 2 weeks. Children: Use and dosage must be determined by your doctor.

ONSET OF EFFECT
Unknown.

DURATION OF ACTION
Unknown.

DIETARY ADVICE
This medication can be used without regard to diet.

STORAGE
Store in a tightly sealed container away from heat and direct light. Do not refrigerate or allow to freeze.

IF YOU MISS A DOSE
Apply it as soon as you remember. If it is near the time for the next dose, skip the missed dose and resume your regular dosage schedule. Do not double the next dose.

STOPPING THE DRUG
Use this drug as prescribed for the full treatment period, even if you begin to feel better before the scheduled end of therapy.

PROLONGED USE
You should see your doctor regularly for tests and examinations if you take this drug for a prolonged period.

PRECAUTIONS
Over 60: No special problems are expected.

Driving and Hazardous Work: The use of ophthalmic diclofenac should not impair your ability to perform such tasks safely.

Alcohol: No special precautions are necessary.

Pregnancy: Adequate human studies have not been completed. Before taking ophthalmic diclofenac, tell your doctor if you are pregnant or plan to become pregnant.

Breast Feeding: Ophthalmic diclofenac may pass into breast milk; caution is advised. Consult your doctor for specific advice.

Infants and Children: Use and dosage for infants and children must be determined by your doctor.

Special Concerns: To use the eye drops, first wash your hands. Tilt your head back. Gently apply pressure to the inside corner of the eyelid and with the index finger of the same hand, pull downward on the lower eyelid to make a space. Drop the medicine into this space and close your eye. Apply pressure for 1 or 2 minutes while keeping the eye closed without blinking. Then wash your hands again. Make sure the tip of the dropper does not touch your eye, finger, or any other surface. If your symptoms do not improve or if they become worse, check with your doctor. Oph-thalmic diclofenac has caused severe eye irritation in some persons wearing soft contact lenses. Do not wear soft contact lenses while using this medication.

OVERDOSE
Symptoms: No specific ones have been reported.

What to Do: An overdose of ophthalmic diclofenac is unlikely to be life-threatening. However, if someone takes a much larger dose of the drug than prescribed or accidentally ingests the medicine, call your doctor, emergency medical services (EMS), or the nearest poison control center.

DRUG INTERACTIONS
Consult your doctor for advice if you are taking aspirin or another salicylate, diflunisal, etodolac, fenoprofen, floctafenine, flurbiprofen, ibuprofen, indomethacin, ketoprofen, ketorolac, meclofenamate, mefenamic acid, nabumetone, naproxen, oxyphenbutazone, phenylbutazone, piroxicam, sulindac, suprofen, tenoxicam, tiaprofenic acid, tolmetin, or zomepirac.

FOOD INTERACTIONS
No known food interactions.

DISEASE INTERACTIONS
Caution is advised when using ophthalmic diclofenac. Consult your doctor if you have hemophilia or any other bleeding problem.

Diclofenac Systemic

BRAND NAMES
Cataflam, Voltaren

▶ Drug Class: Nonsteroidal anti-inflammatory drug (NSAID)

▶ Available in: Tablets, delayed-release tablets, suppositories

▶ Available OTC? No

▶ As Generic? Yes

Side Effects

SERIOUS
Shortness of breath or wheezing, with or without swelling of legs or other signs of heart failure; chest pain; peptic ulcer disease with vomiting of blood; black, tarry stools; decreasing kidney function. Call your doctor immediately.

COMMON
Nausea, vomiting, heartburn, diarrhea, constipation, headache, dizziness, sleepiness.

LESS COMMON
Ulcers or sores in mouth, depression, rashes or blistering of skin, ringing sound in the ears, unusual tingling or numbness of the hands or feet, seizures, blurred vision. Also elevated potassium levels, decreased blood counts; such problems can be detected by your doctor.

PRINCIPAL USES
To treat mild to moderate pain and inflammation caused by tendinitis, arthritis, bursitis, gout, soft tissue injuries, migraine and other vascular headaches, menstrual cramps, and other conditions. When patients fail to respond to one NSAID, another may be tried. The greatest effectiveness often requires trial and error of several different NSAIDs.

HOW THE DRUG WORKS
NSAIDs work by interfering with the formation of prostaglandins, substances that cause inflammation and make nerves more sensitive to pain impulses. NSAIDs also have other modes of action that are less well understood.

DOSAGE
Adults— For osteoarthritis and rheumatoid arthritis: 50 mg, 2 or 3 times a day. Ankylosing spondylitis: 25 mg, 4 times a day, with another 25 mg at bedtime if needed. Menstrual pain: 50 mg, 3 times a day; an initial dose of 100 mg may be given.

ONSET OF EFFECT
Within 30 minutes.

DURATION OF ACTION
Up to 8 hours.

DIETARY ADVICE
Take it with food.

STORAGE
Store in a tightly sealed container away from heat, moisture, and direct light.

IF YOU MISS A DOSE
Take it as soon as you remember. If it is near the time for the next dose, skip the missed dose and resume your regular dosage schedule. Do not double the next dose.

STOPPING THE DRUG
The decision to stop taking the drug should be made in consultation with your physician.

PROLONGED USE
Prolonged use can cause gastrointestinal problems, including ulceration and bleeding, kidney dysfunction, and liver inflammation. Consult your physician about the need for medical examinations and laboratory studies.

PRECAUTIONS
Over 60: Because of the potentially greater consequences of gastrointestinal side effects, the dose of NSAIDs for older patients, especially those over age 70, is often cut in half.

Driving and Hazardous Work: Do not drive or engage in hazardous work until you determine how the medicine affects you.

Alcohol: Avoid alcohol when using this medication because it increases the risk of stomach irritation.

Pregnancy: Avoid or discontinue this drug if you are pregnant or plan to become pregnant.

Breast Feeding: Diclofenac passes into breast milk; avoid or discontinue use while nursing.

Infants and Children: Diclofenac may be used in exceptional circumstances; consult your pediatrician for specific advice.

Special Concerns: Because NSAIDs can inhibit blood coagulation, this drug should be discontinued at least 3 days prior to any surgery. Do not crush or chew the tablets.

OVERDOSE
Symptoms: Nausea, vomiting, severe headache, confusion, seizures.

What to Do: Call your doctor, emergency medical services (EMS), or the nearest poison control center immediately.

DRUG INTERACTIONS
Do not take this drug with aspirin or any other NSAIDs without your doctor's approval. In addition, consult your doctor if you are taking antihypertensives, steroids, anticoagulants, antibiotics, itraconazole or ketoconazole, plicamycin, penicillamine, valproic acid, phenytoin, cyclosporine, digitalis drugs, lithium, methotrexate, probenecid, triamterene, or zidovudine.

FOOD INTERACTIONS
No known food interactions.

DISEASE INTERACTIONS
Consult your doctor if you have any of the following: bleeding problems, inflammation or ulcers of the stomach and intestines, diabetes mellitus, systemic lupus erythematosus (SLE, lupus), anemia, asthma, epilepsy, Parkinson's disease, kidney stones, or a history of heart disease or alcohol abuse. Use of diclofenac may cause complications in patients with liver or kidney disease, since these organs work together to remove the medication from the body.

Diclofenac/Misoprostol

▶ Drug Class: Antirheumatic

▶ Available in: Tablets

▶ Available OTC? No

▶ As Generic? No

Side Effects

SERIOUS
Irregular heartbeat, fainting, coma, seizures, yellowish tinge to eyes or skin, or pain or tenderness in the upper-right abdomen. Call your doctor immediately.

COMMON
Stomach pain or upset, diarrhea, indigestion, nausea, flatulence.

LESS COMMON
Fatigue, weakness, fever, tremor, dizziness, loss of appetite, dry mouth, gastroesophageal reflux (backwash of stomach acid into the esophagus, resulting in heartburn), breathing difficulty, persistent but unproductive urge to urinate or defecate, hemorrhoids, breast pain, painful menstruation, menstrual irregularities, hives, impotence, unexpected changes in weight, muscle and joint pain, confusion, mental depression, sleeping difficulty, nightmares or unusually vivid dreams, hallucinations, irritability, nervousness, paranoia, bruising, skin rash, blurred or abnormal vision.

PRINCIPAL USES
To relieve the symptoms of osteoarthritis or rheumatoid arthritis in patients at high risk of developing peptic ulcers as a result of therapy with NSAIDs.

HOW THE DRUG WORKS
Diclofenac, a nonsteroidal anti-inflammatory drug (NSAID), works by interfering with the formation of prostaglandins, substances that cause inflammation and make nerves more sensitive to pain impulses. Ongoing therapy with NSAIDs can irritate and damage the stomach lining, increasing the risk of peptic ulcers. Misoprostol, a synthetic prostaglandin, helps prevent ulcers and enhances the stomach's natural healing ability by increasing the production of protective mucus and inhibiting the secretion of stomach acid.

DOSAGE
Osteoarthritis: 1 tablet of Arthrotec 50 (50 mg diclofenac/200 micrograms [mcg] misoprostol), 3 times a day. Rheumatoid arthritis: 1 tablet of Arthrotec 75 (75 mg diclofenac/200 mcg misoprostol), 3 to 4 times a day. Different doses may be warranted in some patients. Consult your doctor.

ONSET OF EFFECT
Unknown.

DURATION OF ACTION
Unknown.

DIETARY ADVICE
The drug should be taken with food to minimize stomach upset and diarrhea.

STORAGE
Store in a tightly sealed container away from heat, moisture, and direct light.

IF YOU MISS A DOSE
Take it as soon as you remember. If it is near the time for the next dose, skip the missed dose and resume your regular dosage schedule. Do not double the next dose.

STOPPING THE DRUG
Take it as prescribed for the full treatment period.

PROLONGED USE
Since side effects are more likely with prolonged use, regular follow-up visits with your doctor are important. To minimize the chance of an adverse effect, the lowest effective dose should be used for the shortest possible duration (misoprostol is generally not prescribed for longer than 4 weeks).

PRECAUTIONS
Over 60: No special problems are expected.

Driving and Hazardous Work: Do not drive or engage in hazardous work until you determine how the medicine affects you.

Alcohol: Avoid alcohol, as it may increase the risk of stomach irritation.

Pregnancy: This drug combination should not be used during pregnancy. The misoprostol component can cause miscarriage and induce abortion. Before it can be prescribed, female patients are required to have had a negative pregnancy test within the previous 2 weeks. Therapy then begins only on the second or third day of the following menstrual period. An effective method of birth control should be used while taking this drug. If you suspect you are pregnant, stop taking the drug immediately and consult your doctor.

Breast Feeding: This drug passes into breast milk and may be harmful; avoid use while nursing.

Infants and Children: Not recommended for use by children under 18.

OVERDOSE
Symptoms: Nausea, vomiting, severe headache, confusion, seizures, tremors, sleepiness, difficulty breathing, stomach pain, severe diarrhea, fever, palpitations, extremely low blood pressure causing dizziness or fainting, slow heartbeat.

What to Do: Call your doctor, emergency medical services (EMS), or the nearest poison control center immediately.

DRUG INTERACTIONS
The following drugs may interact with this drug: aspirin, digoxin, blood pressure medication, warfarin, methotrexate, cyclosporine, oral diabetes drugs, lithium, antacids, diuretics, or any over-the-counter drugs. Consult your doctor. To minimize the risk of diarrhea, avoid the use of magnesium-containing antacids.

FOOD INTERACTIONS
No known food interactions.

DISEASE INTERACTIONS
You should not take this medication if you have ever experienced breathing difficulty, hives, swelling of the face, tongue, or throat, or any other allergic reactions after taking aspirin or other NSAIDs. Caution is advised if you have a history of high blood pressure or asthma. Use of this drug combination may cause complications in patients with liver or kidney disease, since these organs work together to remove the medications from the body.

Dicloxacillin Sodium

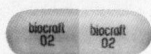

Generic 250 mg
(BIOCRAFT)

Additional photographs

▶ Drug Class: Penicillin antibiotic

▶ Available in: Capsules, liquid

▶ Available OTC? No

▶ As Generic? Yes

Side Effects

SERIOUS
Irregular, rapid, or labored breathing, light-headedness or sudden fainting, joint pain, fever, severe abdominal pain and cramping with watery or bloody stools, severe allergic reaction (marked by sudden swelling of the lips, tongue, face, or throat; breathing difficulty; skin rash, itching, or hives), unusual bleeding or bruising, yellowish tinge to eyes or skin. Call your doctor immediately.

COMMON
Mild rash, mild diarrhea, nausea, vomiting, headache, vaginal discharge and itching, pain or white patches in the mouth or on the tongue.

LESS COMMON
Diminished urine output, chills, weakness, fatigue.

PRINCIPAL USES
To treat bacterial infections, especially those of the skin or bone caused by penicillin-resistant staphylococcus bacteria. Dicloxacillin is ineffective against infections caused by viruses, fungi, or other microorganisms.

HOW THE DRUG WORKS
Dicloxacillin blocks the formation of bacterial cell walls, rendering bacteria unable to multiply and spread. Unlike other penicillin antibiotics, dicloxacillin is resistant to bacterial enzymes that chemically inactivate penicillins.

DOSAGE
Adults and children over 88 lbs: 125 to 250 mg every 6 hours, for a total dosage of 500 to 1,000 mg a day. Children under 88 lbs: Dose is determined by doctor, based on several factors. Usual dose is 1.4 to 2.8 mg per lb of body weight every 6 hours.

ONSET OF EFFECT
Unknown.

DURATION OF ACTION
Up to 6 hours.

DIETARY ADVICE
Take dicloxacillin on an empty stomach, 1 to 2 hours before or 2 to 3 hours after a meal, with a full glass of water.

STORAGE
Store capsules in a dry place away from heat and light. Keep the liquid form refrigerated, but do not allow it to freeze.

IF YOU MISS A DOSE
Take it as soon as you remember. If you take 2 doses a day, take the next dose 5 to 6 hours later and go back to your regular schedule. If you take 3 or more doses a day, take the next dose 2 to 4 hours later, then go back to your regular schedule. Do not double the next dose.

STOPPING THE DRUG
Take it as prescribed for the full treatment period, even if you begin to feel better before the scheduled end of therapy. Stopping the drug prematurely may slow your recovery or lead to a rebound infection, also known as superinfection, in which the heartier strains of bacteria survive and multiply, leading to a more serious and drug-resistant infection.

PROLONGED USE
Prolonged use may make you more susceptible to infections that are resistant to penicillin; caution is advised.

PRECAUTIONS
Over 60: No special problems are expected.

Driving and Hazardous Work: Usually not dangerous, since most hazardous reactions occur a few minutes after the drug is taken.

Alcohol: Alcohol may increase stomach irritation.

Pregnancy: Adequate studies of the use of penicillin antibiotics during pregnancy have not been done; however, no problems have been reported.

Breast Feeding: Dicloxacillin passes into breast milk and may cause diarrhea, fungal infections, and allergic reactions in nursing infants; avoid use while nursing.

Infants and Children: No special problems are expected.

Special Concerns: Dicloxacillin can cause false results on some urine sugar tests for patients with diabetes. Those who are prone to asthma, hay fever, hives, or allergies may be more likely to have an allergic reaction to a penicillin antibiotic. If severe diarrhea occurs as a side effect of this drug, do not take antidiarrheal medications; call your doctor.

OVERDOSE
Symptoms: Severe diarrhea, nausea, vomiting, seizures.

What to Do: Call your doctor, emergency medical services (EMS), or the nearest poison control center immediately.

DRUG INTERACTIONS
Consult your doctor for specific advice if you are taking aminoglycosides, ACE inhibitors, diuretics, potassium supplements or potassium-containing drugs, anticoagulants or other anti-clotting drugs, nonsteroidal anti-inflammatory drugs, sulfinpyrazone, cholestyramine, colestipol, oral contraceptives, methotrexate, probenecid, or rifampin.

FOOD INTERACTIONS
No known food interactions.

DISEASE INTERACTIONS
Consult your doctor if you have a history of allergies, asthma, congestive heart failure, gastrointestinal disorders (especially colitis associated with the use of antibiotics), or impaired kidney function.

Dicyclomine Hydrochloride

BRAND NAMES
A-Spas, Antispas, Bemot, Bentyl, Byclomine, Di-Spaz, Dibent, Or-Tyl, Spasmoject

► Drug Class: Antidiarrheal/antispasmodic

► Available in: Tablets, syrup, capsules, injection

► Available OTC? No

► As Generic? Yes

Side Effects

SERIOUS
No serious side effects are associated with dicyclomine.

COMMON
Headache; dizziness; constipation; dry mouth, nose, throat, or skin; difficulty urinating; heart palpitations.

LESS COMMON
Drowsiness, decreased sweating, confusion, nervousness, rapid pulse, blurred vision, nausea, vomiting.

PRINCIPAL USES
To treat irritable bowel syndrome, and to reduce spasms of the digestive system, bladder, and urethra.

HOW THE DRUG WORKS
Dicyclomine slows bowel action and reduces production of stomach acid.

DOSAGE
Oral forms— Adults and teenagers: 10 to 20 mg, 3 or 4 times a day. Children age 2 and older: 5 to 10 mg, 3 or 4 times a day. Children ages 6 months to 2 years: 5 to 10 mg of the syrup 3 or 4 times a day. Injection— Adults and teenagers: 20 mg into a muscle every 4 to 6 hours. Children: Consult a pediatrician for advice.

ONSET OF EFFECT
Unknown.

DURATION OF ACTION
Unknown.

DIETARY ADVICE
Take this medicine 30 to 60 minutes before meals and bedtime unless your doctor directs otherwise. Bedtime dose should be given at least 2 hours after the last meal of the day.

STORAGE
Store in a tightly sealed container away from heat, moisture, and direct light. Keep liquid forms of the drug refrigerated, but do not allow them to freeze.

IF YOU MISS A DOSE
Take it as soon as you remember, unless the time for your next scheduled dose is within the next 2 hours. If so, skip the missed dose and resume your regular dosage schedule. Do not double the next dose.

STOPPING THE DRUG
Take it as prescribed for the full treatment period. However, you may stop taking the drug if you are feeling better before the scheduled end of therapy. The doctor may want you to reduce the amount you take gradually.

PROLONGED USE
Prolonged use can cause chronic constipation and fecal impaction. Consult your doctor immediately.

PRECAUTIONS
Over 60: Adverse reactions may be more likely and more severe in older patients.

Driving and Hazardous Work: Do not drive or engage in hazardous work until you determine how the drug affects you. The use of dicyclomine disqualifies you from piloting an aircraft.

Alcohol: No special precautions are necessary.

Pregnancy: Consult your doctor about taking dicyclomine if you are pregnant or plan to become pregnant.

Breast Feeding: Dicyclomine passes into breast milk and decreases milk production. Avoid taking this medicine or discontinue breast feeding while you take it. Consult your doctor about maintaining milk flow if you breast feed.

Infants and Children: Give dicyclomine to infants and children only under close medical supervision.

Special Concerns: Tell any other doctor or dentist whom you consult that you take dicyclomine. Strenuous exercise, hot baths, or saunas while you take this medicine can make you dizzy or faint.

OVERDOSE
Symptoms: Blurred vision; dilated pupils; dizziness; rapid pulse; hot, dry skin; slurred speech; confusion; nausea; headache; loss of consciousness.

What to Do: Call your doctor, emergency medical services (EMS), or the nearest poison control center immediately.

DRUG INTERACTIONS
Consult your doctor about any other medicines you are taking, especially antacids, antihistamines, narcotic pain relievers, antiarrhythmic drugs, drugs for Parkinson's disease, antidepressants, or antipsychotic drugs (such as phenothiazines). Large doses of vitamin C can reduce the effect of dicyclomine. Potassium supplements can increase the risk of an intestinal ulcer. Nitrates and nitrites can increase internal pressure of the eye.

FOOD INTERACTIONS
No known food interactions.

DISEASE INTERACTIONS
You may not be able to take dicyclomine if you have intestinal problems, heart disease, bleeding problems, glaucoma, chronic bronchitis, an enlarged prostate, a hernia, liver disease, kidney disease, a fever, brain damage (in children), an overactive thyroid, or urinary problems.

Didanosine (Dideoxyinosine; ddI)

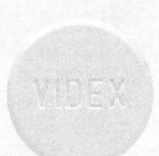

Videx 100 mg
(Bristol-Myers Squibb)

▶ Drug Class: Antiviral

▶ Available in: Tablets, powder for solution

▶ Available OTC? No

▶ As Generic? No

Side Effects

SERIOUS
Nerve damage causing numbness, tingling, prickling, or pain in the hands and feet; pancreatitis (inflammation of the pancreas) causing abdominal pain, nausea, and vomiting. Call your doctor immediately.

COMMON
Temporary toxicity of the central nervous system causing headache, anxiety, irritability, restlessness, or sleep disruption; gastrointestinal disturbances, including stomach pain, gas, nausea, vomiting, and diarrhea; dry mouth.

LESS COMMON
Swollen hands or legs, shortness of breath, yellow discoloration of the eyes or skin, rash, itch, weakness, vision problems, muscle aches or spasms, muscle wasting, pain, pneumonia, cough, hair loss.

PRINCIPAL USES
To treat HIV infection. While not a cure for HIV, this drug may suppress the replication of the virus and delay the progression of the disease.

HOW THE DRUG WORKS
Didanosine (also known as dideoxyinosine or ddI) interferes with the activity of enzymes needed for the replication of DNA in viral cells.

DOSAGE
Tablets— Adults and teenagers weighing 132 lbs or more: 200 mg every 12 hours. Adults and teenagers weighing less than 132 lbs: 125 mg every 12 hours. Children: Dose may range from 25 to 100 mg every 8 to 12 hours. Tablets must be chewed or dissolved in water or apple juice. Always take 2 tablets at the same time; there is not enough medicine in a single tablet to ensure adequate absorption. Powder (dissolved in water)— Adults and teenagers weighing 132 lbs or more: 250 mg every 12 hours. Adults and teenagers weighing less than 132 lbs: 167 mg every 12 hours. Children (a special pediatric formulation is used): Dose may range from 31 to 125 mg every 8 to 12 hours. Didanosine is sometimes given once a day, using the full dose (400 mg in adults).

ONSET OF EFFECT
Unknown.

DURATION OF ACTION
Unknown.

DIETARY ADVICE
Didanosine should be taken on an empty stomach, at least 1 hour before or 2 hours after eating. If you are on a low-salt diet, be aware that this drug contains high quantities of sodium.

STORAGE
Store tablets in a dry place away from heat and direct light. The mixed solution may be refrigerated, but do not allow it to freeze.

IF YOU MISS A DOSE
If it is near the time for the next dose, skip the missed dose and resume your regular dosage schedule. Do not double the next dose.

STOPPING THE DRUG
The decision to stop taking the drug should be made in consultation with your physician.

PROLONGED USE
See your doctor regularly for tests and examinations.

PRECAUTIONS
Over 60: No special problems are expected.

Driving and Hazardous Work: Do not drive or engage in hazardous work until you determine how the medicine affects you.

Alcohol: Avoid alcohol if liver function is impaired. Heavy alcohol use can increase the risk of pancreatitis, an uncommon side effect of didanosine.

Pregnancy: While didanosine has been shown to cause birth defects in animals, it is nonetheless increasingly being used in combination with other anti-retroviral drugs to treat pregnant HIV-infected women.

Breast Feeding: Women infected with HIV should not breast-feed.

Infants and Children: Safety and effectiveness for children under 6 months have not been established.

Special Concerns: Use of didanosine does not eliminate the risk of passing the AIDS virus to other persons. Be sure to take appropriate preventive measures.

OVERDOSE
Symptoms: Seizures, severe nausea and vomiting, extreme fatigue or weakness, unusual bleeding or bruising, clumsiness, involuntary eye movement.

What to Do: Seek medical assistance immediately.

DRUG INTERACTIONS
Consult your doctor for specific advice if you are taking antibiotic or anti-infective drugs, antidepressants, antifungals, antimalarial drugs, antiparkinson's agents, blood pressure medication, cancer drugs, diuretics, estrogens, lithium, nitrous oxide, phenytoin, stavudine, or zalcitabine.

FOOD INTERACTIONS
Food can interfere with the absorption of didanosine.

DISEASE INTERACTIONS
You may not be able to take didanosine if you have had pancreatitis (inflammation of the pancreas), hepatitis (liver inflammation), other liver or kidney problems, high blood pressure, blood disorders, gout, swollen ankles, or numbness and tingling in the hands or feet.

Diethylpropion Hydrochloride

BRAND NAME
Tenuate

▶ Drug Class: Sympatho-mimetic; central nervous system stimulant

▶ Available in: Tablets, extended-release tablets

▶ Available OTC? No

▶ As Generic? Yes

Side Effects

SERIOUS
Chest pain; severe dizziness; headache (especially if associated with nausea or vomiting); convulsions; rash; racing, pounding, or fluttering heartbeat.

COMMON
Lightheadedness; irritability or nervousness, difficulty falling asleep, exaggerated feelings of well-being or confidence (euphoria), increased heartbeat, palpitations, increased blood pressure.

LESS COMMON
Persistent or unusual fever, chills, sore throat, or cough; persistent or unusual bruising or bleeding; gastrointestinal problems.

PRINCIPAL USES
Diethylpropion is used to suppress appetite in obese patients. It is used in conjunction with a strict diet, and should never be prescribed as the sole method of achieving weight loss. Diethylpropion is indicated for patients with an initial body mass index (BMI) of 30 or greater (see Special Concerns for information on BMI calculation).

HOW THE DRUG WORKS
It is believed that the appetite-control center for the body may be found in a part of the brain called the hypothalamus. Diethylpropion probably affects the transmission of nerve impulses in this region.

DOSAGE
Oral tablet: 25 mg, 3 times per day before meals. Oral extended-release tablet: 75 mg, once a day, taken at midmorning.

ONSET OF EFFECT
Within a few hours after ingestion.

DURATION OF ACTION
Regular tablets: 4 hours. Extended-release: 12 hours.

DIETARY ADVICE
Take this medication one hour before meals. Significant weight loss will not occur without carefully adhering to a strict diet as outlined by your physician or nutritionist.

STORAGE
Store in a tightly sealed container away from heat and direct light. Keep away from moisture and extremes in temperature.

IF YOU MISS A DOSE
Take it as soon as you remember. If it is near the time for the next dose, skip the missed dose and resume your regular dosage schedule. Do not double the next dose.

STOPPING THE DRUG
Take as prescribed for the full treatment period. Your dose may need to be reduced gradually to prevent withdrawal effects or a rebound increase in appetite.

PROLONGED USE
This drug is usually prescribed for several weeks. Side effects may become more likely over this period of time. Prolonged use may result in mental or physical dependence.

PRECAUTIONS
Over 60: Adverse reactions may be more likely and more severe in older patients, especially with drugs that act on the central nervous system.

Driving and Hazardous Work: Do not drive or engage in hazardous activities until you determine how the drug affects you.

Alcohol: Avoid alcohol.

Pregnancy: Avoid or discontinue diethylpropion if you are pregnant or trying to become pregnant.

Breast Feeding: Diethylpropion passes into breast milk; avoid or discontinue usage while nursing.

Infants and Children: Not recommended for use by children under age 12.

Special Concerns: The appetite suppressant effect of this medication may diminish after a few weeks. This is known as drug tolerance, and you should inform your physician. Do not increase the dose. The BMI can be calculated by dividing your weight in pounds by your height in inches squared, and then multiplying by 705.

OVERDOSE
Symptoms: Extreme restlessness; tremor or shaking of the hands, muscles of the face, or other areas of the body; confusion; hallucinations; extreme fear or panic; rapid breathing; violent behavior; nausea; vomiting; fainting; coma.

What to Do: Call emergency medical services (EMS), your doctor, or the nearest poison control center immediately.

DRUG INTERACTIONS
Consult your doctor for specific advice if you are taking amantadine; amphetamines; medications for hyperactivity, or other drugs for appetite control; caffeine; chlophedianol; asthma medication; prescription and nonprescription decongestants or medicine for colds, sinus problems, or seasonal allergies such as hay fever (including nose drops or sprays); methylphenidate; nabilone; pemoline; or an MAO inhibitor.

FOOD INTERACTIONS
Avoid food or beverages containing caffeine.

DISEASE INTERACTIONS
Consult your doctor if you have a history of alcohol or drug abuse; diabetes mellitus; glaucoma; heart disease; blood vessel disease, especially of the arteries; strokes or "mini strokes" (transient ischemic attacks); high blood pressure; mental illness; or thyroid or kidney disease. An increased frequency of seizures has been reported in patients with epilepsy.

Diethylstilbestrol (DES)

BRAND NAMES
Stilbestrol, Stilbetin

Generic 5 mg
(LILLY)

Additional photographs

▶ Drug Class: Antineoplastic
(anticancer) agent; hormone
treatment

▶ Available in: Tablets, injection

▶ Available OTC? No

▶ As Generic? Yes

Side Effects

SERIOUS
Breast pain or increased
breast size (in both men
and women), swelling of
feet and lower legs, rapid
weight gain, irregular
vaginal bleeding, painful
menstrual periods, breast
lumps, pain in stomach,
side, or abdomen, jerky
muscle movements, yel-
lowish tinge to eyes or
skin (jaundice), sudden or
severe headache, loss of
coordination, loss of or
change in vision, pain in
chest, groin, or leg, sudden shortness of breath,
slurred speech, weakness
or numbness in arm or
leg. Notify your doctor
promptly.

COMMON
Bloating of or cramps in
stomach, loss of appetite,
nausea, rash, freckles on
the face.

LESS COMMON
Abnormal hair loss or
growth, joint pain,
depression, dizziness,
headache, problems with
contact lenses, change in
level of sexual desire,
vomiting, diarrhea.

PRINCIPAL USES
To slow the progress of
advanced breast and
prostate cancers.

HOW THE DRUG WORKS
Diethylstilbestrol is a form
of the hormone estrogen. It
can block the action of certain other hormones that
promote tumor growth; this
in turn will slow the
progress of the cancer.

DOSAGE
Tablet— For breast cancer:
15 mg once a day. For
prostate cancer: 1 to 3 mg a
day; dose may be decreased
to 1 mg a day. Injection—
500 mg a day. The dose
may be increased to 1 g per
day, then lowered to 250 to
500 mg once a week.

ONSET OF EFFECT
Unknown.

DURATION OF ACTION
Unknown.

DIETARY ADVICE
Drink plenty of fluids.

STORAGE
Store in a tightly sealed container away from heat and
direct light.

IF YOU MISS A DOSE
Take it as soon as you
remember. If it is close to
the time for the next dose,
skip the missed dose and
resume your regular dosage
schedule. Do not double the
next dose.

STOPPING THE DRUG
The decision to stop taking
diethylstilbestrol should be
made in consultation with
your doctor.

PROLONGED USE
You should see your doctor
regularly for tests and
examinations if you take
this drug for a prolonged
period.

PRECAUTIONS
Over 60: No extra problems or side effects are
expected in older patients
as compared with younger
persons.

**Driving and Hazardous
Work:** Do not drive or
engage in hazardous work
until you determine how the
medicine affects you.

Alcohol: Avoid alcohol.

Pregnancy: Diethylstilbestrol can cause birth defects
and should never be taken
during pregnancy.

Breast Feeding: Not
recommended while taking
diethylstilbestrol.

Infants and Children:
Diethylstilbestrol is not
recommended for use in
infants and children.

Special Concerns:
Diethylstilbestrol may
cause tenderness, swelling,
or bleeding of the gums.
Brush and floss your teeth
regularly and see your
dentist regularly. Patients
who take DES may be at
increased risk for cancer.

OVERDOSE
Symptoms: Loss of
appetite, nausea, vomiting,
abdominal cramps, diar-
rhea, vaginal bleeding.

What to Do: Call your
doctor, emergency medical
services (EMS), or the
nearest poison control center immediately.

DRUG INTERACTIONS
Consult your doctor for specific advice if you are taking
acetaminophen, amio-
darone, anabolic steroids,
androgens, anti-infective
medications, antithyroid
agents, carbamazepine,
carmustine, chloroquine,
dantrolene, daunorubicin,
disulfiram, divalproex,
etretinate, gold salts,
hydroxychloroquine, mer-
captopurine, methotrexate,
methyldopa, naltrexone,
oral contraceptives,
phenothiazines, phenytoin,
plicamycin, tamoxifen,
valproic acid, bromocrip-
tine, or cyclosporine.

FOOD INTERACTIONS
No known food interactions.

DISEASE INTERACTIONS
Caution is advised when
taking diethylstilbestrol.
Consult your doctor if you
have a history of blood
clots, changes in vaginal
bleeding, endometriosis,
fibroid tumors of the uterus,
gallbladder disease or gallstones, jaundice, liver disease, porphyria, blood clots,
heart or circulatory disease,
stroke, high blood pressure,
diabetes mellitus, asthma,
kidney disease, liver disease, or depression.

Diflunisal

BRAND NAME
Dolobid

▶ Drug Class: Nonsteroidal anti-inflammatory drug (NSAID)

▶ Available in: Tablets

▶ Available OTC? No

▶ As Generic? Yes

Side Effects

SERIOUS
Shortness of breath or wheezing, with or without swelling of legs or other signs of heart failure; chest pain; peptic ulcer disease with vomiting of blood; black, tarry stools; decreasing kidney function. Call your doctor immediately.

COMMON
Nausea, vomiting, heartburn, diarrhea, constipation, headache, dizziness, sleepiness.

LESS COMMON
Ulcers or sores in mouth, depression, rashes or blistering of skin, ringing sound in the ears, unusual tingling or numbness of the hands or feet, seizures, blurred vision. Also elevated potassium levels, decreased blood counts; such problems can be detected by your doctor.

PRINCIPAL USES
To treat mild to moderate pain and inflammation caused by tendinitis, arthritis, bursitis, gout, soft tissue injuries, migraine and other vascular headaches, menstrual cramps, and other conditions. When patients fail to respond to one NSAID, another may be tried. The greatest effectiveness often requires trial and error of several different NSAIDs.

HOW THE DRUG WORKS
NSAIDs work by interfering with the formation of prostaglandins, naturally occurring substances in the body that cause inflammation and make nerves more sensitive to pain impulses. NSAIDs also have other modes of action that are less well understood.

DOSAGE
Adults and teenagers: 500 to 1,000 mg a day in 2 divided doses. Adults over age 65: 250 to 500 mg a day in 2 divided doses.

ONSET OF EFFECT
Within 1 hour; 3 weeks of regular use may be required for maximum effect.

DURATION OF ACTION
8 to 12 hours.

DIETARY ADVICE
Take with food; maintain your usual food and fluid intake.

STORAGE
Store in a tightly sealed container away from heat, moisture, and direct light.

IF YOU MISS A DOSE
Take it as soon as you remember. If it is near the time for the next dose, skip the missed dose and resume your regular dosage schedule. Do not double the next dose.

STOPPING THE DRUG
The decision to stop taking the drug should be made in consultation with your physician.

PROLONGED USE
Prolonged use can cause gastrointestinal problems, including ulceration and bleeding, kidney dysfunction, and liver inflammation. Consult your physician about the need for medical examinations and laboratory studies.

PRECAUTIONS
Over 60: Because of the potentially greater consequences of gastrointestinal side effects, the dose of NSAIDs for older patients, especially those over age 70, is often cut in half.

Driving and Hazardous Work: Do not drive or engage in hazardous work until you determine how this drug affects you.

Alcohol: Avoid alcohol when using this medication because it increases the risk of stomach irritation.

Pregnancy: Avoid or discontinue this drug if you are pregnant or plan to become pregnant.

Breast Feeding: Diflunisal passes into breast milk; avoid or discontinue use while nursing.

Infants and Children: Diflunisal is not generally prescribed for children under the age of 12, but may be used in exceptional circumstances; consult your pediatrician.

Special Concerns: Because NSAIDs can interfere with blood coagulation, this drug should be stopped at least 3 days prior to any surgery.

OVERDOSE
Symptoms: Nausea, vomiting, severe headache, confusion, seizures.

What to Do: Call your doctor, emergency medical services (EMS), or the nearest poison control center immediately.

DRUG INTERACTIONS
Do not take this drug with aspirin or any other NSAIDs without your doctor's approval. In addition, consult your doctor if you are taking antihypertensives, steroids, anticoagulants, antibiotics, itraconazole or ketoconazole, plicamycin, penicillamine, valproic acid, phenytoin, cyclosporine, digitalis drugs, lithium, methotrexate, probenecid, triamterene, or zidovudine.

FOOD INTERACTIONS
No known food interactions.

DISEASE INTERACTIONS
Caution is advised when taking diflunisal. Consult your doctor if you have any of the following: bleeding problems, inflammation or ulcers of the stomach and intestines, diabetes mellitus, systemic lupus erythematosus (SLE, lupus), anemia, asthma, epilepsy, Parkinson's disease, kidney stones, or a history of heart disease or alcohol abuse. Use of diflunisal may cause complications in patients with liver or kidney disease, since these organs work together to remove the medication from the body.

Digitoxin

BRAND NAME
Crystodigin

Generic 0.1 mg
(Lilly)

▶ Drug Class: Digitalis drug
(cardiac glycoside)

▶ Available in: Tablets

▶ Available OTC? No

▶ As Generic? Yes

Side Effects

SERIOUS
Heartbeat irregularities that may be life-threatening and cause dizziness, palpitations, shortness of breath, sweating, or fainting. Other serious side effects include hallucinations, confusion, and mental changes; extreme drowsiness; and visual disturbances such as double vision or seeing colored halos around objects. Call your doctor right away.

COMMON
Weakness, fatigue, blurred vision, nausea, agitation, erectile dysfunction, male breast enlargement.

LESS COMMON
Headache, vertigo, numbness or tingling sensation, overall feeling of illness, increased sensitivity of eyes to light, diarrhea, vomiting.

PRINCIPAL USES
To treat congestive heart failure and atrial arrhythmias (heart rhythm irregularities). Because this drug carries potentially serious risks, it is seldom prescribed in current medical practice.

HOW THE DRUG WORKS
Digitalis drugs such as digitoxin enhance and strengthen the force of the heart's contractions, and thus help to regulate the rate and the rhythm of the heartbeat.

DOSAGE
Adults: Initial dose is 0.2 mg, 2 times a day for 4 days. Maintenance dosage ranges from 0.05 to 0.3 mg, taken once a day. Children: Dosage must be determined by your pediatrician. Dosages for all patients must be closely regulated by frequently checking drug levels in the blood.

ONSET OF EFFECT
30 minutes to 2 hours.

DURATION OF ACTION
3 to 4 days.

DIETARY ADVICE
Take it on an empty stomach at the same time every day. Taking digitoxin with food can decrease the absorption rate and peak concentration.

STORAGE
Store in a tightly sealed container away from heat, moisture, and direct light.

IF YOU MISS A DOSE
Take it as soon as you remember. However, if it is within 12 hours of the next scheduled dose, skip the missed dose and resume your regular dosage schedule. Do not double the next dose.

STOPPING THE DRUG
Many patients must take digitoxin for extended periods. Do not stop taking digitoxin unless your doctor advises you to do so.

PROLONGED USE
Prolonged use requires your doctor's careful supervision and periodic assessments of the continued need to take the drug. Blood levels of digitoxin must be measured at regular intervals to ensure proper dosing.

PRECAUTIONS
Over 60: Underweight or frail older persons may require a lower maintenance dose.

Driving and Hazardous Work: Digitoxin may cause drowsiness or vision changes. Do not drive or engage in hazardous work until you determine how it affects you.

Alcohol: No interactions are expected.

Pregnancy: Human studies have not been done. In animal studies, no birth defects have been reported. Digitoxin should be used during pregnancy only if your doctor says it is clearly needed.

Breast Feeding: Digitoxin passes into breast milk. The nursing infant should be monitored carefully. Stop using the drug or discontinue breast feeding if adverse effects develop.

Infants and Children: The dosage for infants and children must be determined by your pediatrician.

Special Concerns: You should carry a card that says you are taking digitoxin. Do not take over-the-

counter antacids or cold or allergy remedies without consulting your doctor. Digitoxin causes impotence and enlarged breasts in a third of the men who take it. Mental changes induced by the drug may be mistaken for psychosis or senility.

OVERDOSE
Symptoms: Heart palpitations, abdominal pain, diarrhea, nausea, vomiting, very slow pulse.

What to Do: Call your doctor, emergency medical services (EMS), or the nearest poison control center immediately.

DRUG INTERACTIONS
Numerous drugs interact with digitoxin and may alter blood levels of the drug, leading to toxicity. Consult your doctor for specific advice if you are taking any drug, especially airway-opening drugs (bronchodilators), antacids, antibiotics such as neomycin or tetracycline, anticholinergic drugs such as atropine, cholesterol-lowering drugs, diuretics, steroids, indomethacin, or any other heart drug.

FOOD INTERACTIONS
Ask your doctor about the advisability of eating high-potassium foods.

DISEASE INTERACTIONS
Consult your doctor if you have any other medical condition, especially lung disease, kidney disease, or poor thyroid function.

Lanoxin 0.125 mg
(GLAXO WELLCOME)

Additional photographs

▶ Drug Class: Digitalis drug (cardiac glycoside)

▶ Available in: Tablets, capsules, elixir

▶ Available OTC? No

▶ As Generic? Yes

Side Effects

SERIOUS
Heartbeat irregularities causing dizziness, palpitations, shortness of breath, sweating, or fainting. Other serious side effects include hallucinations, confusion, and mental changes; extreme drowsiness; visual disturbances such as double vision or seeing colored halos around objects; weakness, fatigue, blurred vision; nausea; or agitation. Call your doctor immediately.

COMMON
Erectile dysfunction, male breast enlargement. Notify your doctor if such symptoms occur.

LESS COMMON
Headache, vertigo, numbness or tingling sensation, overall feeling of illness, sensitivity of eyes to light, diarrhea, vomiting. Call your doctor if such symptoms persist.

PRINCIPAL USES
To treat congestive heart failure (CHF) and atrial arrhythmias (heart rhythm irregularities).

HOW THE DRUG WORKS
Digitalis drugs such as digoxin enhance and strengthen the force of the heart's contractions, and help to regulate the rate and the rhythm of the heartbeat.

DOSAGE
Adults: Initial dose is 0.5 mg. Maintenance dosage, starting the next day, ranges from 0.125 to 0.25 mg a day (rarely more) taken once a day. Periodic blood tests are necessary to determine the proper dose. Children: Dosage is determined by your doctor.

ONSET OF EFFECT
30 minutes to 2 hours.

DURATION OF ACTION
3 to 4 days.

DIETARY ADVICE
Take it on an empty stomach, at the same time every day. Taking digoxin with food can decrease the absorption rate and the peak concentration.

STORAGE
Store in a tightly sealed container away from heat, moisture, and direct light.

IF YOU MISS A DOSE
Take it as soon as you remember. If it is within 12 hours of the next scheduled dose, skip the missed dose and resume your regular dosage schedule. Do not double the next dose.

STOPPING THE DRUG
Do not stop taking it unless your doctor advises otherwise. Abrupt discontinuation can cause serious heart problems. Most patients take digoxin for an extended period or for the rest of their lives.

PROLONGED USE
Prolonged use requires your doctor's supervision and periodic assessments of the continued need to take the drug. Blood levels of digoxin must be measured at regular intervals to ensure proper dosing.

PRECAUTIONS
Over 60: Underweight or frail older persons may require a lower maintenance dose.

Driving and Hazardous Work: Digoxin may cause drowsiness or vision changes. Do not drive or engage in hazardous work until you determine how it affects you.

Alcohol: No interactions are expected.

Pregnancy: Human studies have not been done. In animal studies, no birth defects have been reported. Digoxin should be used during pregnancy only if your doctor decides it is clearly needed.

Breast Feeding: Digoxin passes into breast milk. The nursing infant should be monitored carefully. Stop using the drug or discontinue breast feeding if adverse effects develop.

Infants and Children: The dosage for infants and children must be determined by your pediatrician.

Special Concerns: You should carry a card that says you are taking digoxin. Do not take over-the-counter antacids or cold or allergy remedies without consulting your doctor. Digoxin causes impotence and enlarged breasts in a third of the men who take it. Mental changes induced by the drug may be mistaken for psychosis or senility.

OVERDOSE
Symptoms: Heart palpitations, abdominal pain, diarrhea, nausea, vomiting, very slow pulse.

What to Do: Call your doctor, emergency medical services (EMS), or the nearest poison control center immediately.

DRUG INTERACTIONS
Numerous drugs interact with digoxin and may alter blood levels of the drug, leading to toxicity. Consult your doctor for specific advice if you are taking any medications, especially antiarrhythmic drugs, such as quinidine or procainamide, airway-opening drugs (bronchodilators), antacids, antibiotics such as neomycin or tetracycline, anticholinergic drugs such as atropine, cholesterol-lowering drugs, diuretics (water pills), steroids, indomethacin, or any other heart drug.

FOOD INTERACTIONS
Ask your doctor about the advisability of eating high-potassium foods.

DISEASE INTERACTIONS
Tell your doctor if you have any other medical condition, especially lung disease, kidney disease, or poor thyroid function.

Dihydroergotamine Mesylate

BRAND NAMES
D.H.E. 45, Migranal

▶ Drug Class: Antimigraine/antiheadache drug

▶ Available in: Injection, nasal spray

▶ Available OTC? No

▶ As Generic? No

Side Effects

SERIOUS
Blurred vision, headaches, chest pain, pale, cold, bluish-colored hands or feet, numbness or tingling in fingers and toes, gangrene. Such symptoms may indicate inadequate blood circulation owing to excessive blood vessel constriction. Other serious side effects include: rapid or slow heartbeat, itching, weakness in legs, muscle pain, severe anxiety or confusion, and excess water retention. Seek medical attention immediately.

COMMON
Constipation, reduced sweating, dizziness or lightheadedness, drowsiness.

LESS COMMON
Nausea, vomiting.

PRINCIPAL USES
To treat migraine headaches. This drug is ineffective against other kinds of pain or headaches, and because of its potential for serious side effects, it is prescribed only when other treatments prove ineffective.

HOW THE DRUG WORKS
It reduces throbbing pain by constricting the walls of the blood vessels that carry blood in the brain. It may also depress activity in certain areas in the brain, directly suppressing headache pain. Because this drug may cause constriction of blood vessels throughout the body, serious side effects may result from lack of sufficient blood supply to various organ systems.

DOSAGE
Injection: 1 mg per injection, up to 2 mg per attack, with at least 1 or 2 hours between injections. Maximum weekly dosage is 6 mg. Lie down in a quiet, dark room after the injection. Nasal spray: 1 spray (0.5 mg) in each nostril. Fifteen minutes later, an additional 1 spray should be administered in each nostril for a total of 4 sprays (2 mg). Maximum daily dosage is 3 mg; maximum weekly dosage is 4 mg. Do not sniff following administration. The nasal spray should stay in the nose so that it can be absorbed into the bloodstream through the lining of the nose. This drug works best when taken at the first sign of a migraine headache; dihydroergotamine should not be taken preventively.

ONSET OF EFFECT
Injection: Intravenous: Within 5 minutes. Intramuscular: Within 15 to 30 minutes. Nasal spray: Unknown

DURATION OF ACTION
Injection: About 8 hours. Nasal spray: Unknown.

DIETARY ADVICE
Do not fast or skip meals; this may trigger a migraine. Try to eat at least three meals a day, at the same times each day. Avoid foods that contain preservatives (such as nitrates and nitrites), monosodium glutamate (MSG), and large amounts of caffeine or salt.

STORAGE
Store in a tightly sealed container away from moisture, heat, and direct light. Do not refrigerate or freeze the nasal spray.

IF YOU MISS A DOSE
Not applicable. This drug is only taken as needed.

STOPPING THE DRUG
Headaches may get worse if you stop using this drug. Consult your doctor.

PROLONGED USE
Prolonged use can lead to addiction or tolerance to this medicine. Consult your doctor if the usual dose fails to relieve headaches or if the frequency or severity of headaches increases.

PRECAUTIONS
Over 60: Side effects are more likely and may be more severe.

Driving and Hazardous Work: Exercise caution until you determine how this drug affects you.

Alcohol: Limit intake of alcohol, as it may increase the constriction of blood vessels caused by this drug.

Pregnancy: This medicine should not be used during pregnancy because it can cause a miscarriage or serious damage to the fetus.

Breast Feeding: This drug passes into breast milk and can cause vomiting, diarrhea, convulsions, or other untoward effects in nursing infants; avoid use while breast feeding.

Infants and Children: Consult your pediatrician about giving the injection to children age 6 and older. Adequate studies of the use of the nasal spray have not been done.

OVERDOSE
Symptoms: Seizures, nausea, vomiting, stomach pain or bloating, unusually rapid or slow heartbeat, severe headache, dizziness, drowsiness, constipation, shortness of breath, excitability.

What to Do: Call your doctor, emergency medical services (EMS), or the nearest poison control center immediately.

DRUG INTERACTIONS
Do not take dihydroergotamine within 24 hours of taking naratriptan, sumatriptan, or zolmitriptan. Do not take this drug if you are taking an over the counter or prescription allergy or cold remedy. Consult your doctor for specific advice if you are taking any other medicine, especially erythromycin, nicotine, insulin, or beta-blocker heart drugs.

FOOD INTERACTIONS
Caffeine and salt intake should be limited.

DISEASE INTERACTIONS
Tell your doctor if you are overly sensitive to this drug or other ergot derivatives or if you have any other condition, especially high blood pressure, a blood vessel condition, any infection, a liver problem, a heart problem, or a kidney problem.

Diltiazem Hydrochloride

Side Effects

SERIOUS
Irregular or slow heartbeat, shortness of breath, and fatigue caused by heart failure. Call a doctor immediately.

COMMON
Headache, drowsiness, swelling of feet and ankles, constipation, nausea, sudden weight gain, fatigue.

LESS COMMON
Dizziness, weakness, depression, nervousness, insomnia, confusion, slow pulse, vomiting, diarrhea, excessive urination, itch, sensitivity to sunlight, yellowish tinge to eyes or skin due to liver failure, skin rash, overgrowth of the gums.

PRINCIPAL USES
To relieve and control angina (chest pain associated with heart disease), to reduce high blood pressure, and to correct heartbeat irregularities (cardiac arrhythmia).

HOW THE DRUG WORKS
Diltiazem interferes with the movement of calcium into heart muscle cells and the smooth muscle cells in the walls of the arteries. This action relaxes blood vessels (causing them to widen), which lowers blood pressure, increases the blood supply to the heart, and decreases the heart's overall workload.

DOSAGE
Tablets (for chest pain)—30 mg, 3 or 4 times a day to start, increased to 40 to 60 mg, 3 or 4 times a day. Extended-release capsules (for high blood pressure)—120 to 240 mg a day taken in 1 or 2 divided doses. (For heartbeat irregularities, diltiazem is administered by injection by a health care professional.)

ONSET OF EFFECT
Tablets: 30 to 60 minutes. Extended-release capsules: 2 to 3 hours.

DURATION OF ACTION
Tablets: 6 to 8 hours. Extended-release capsules: 10 to 14 hours.

DIETARY ADVICE
Diltiazem is best taken before meals or at bedtime.

STORAGE
Store tablets and capsules in a tightly sealed container away from heat, moisture, and direct light.

IF YOU MISS A DOSE
Take it as soon as you remember. However, if it is near the time for the next dose, skip the missed dose and resume your regular dosage schedule. Do not double the next dose.

STOPPING THE DRUG
Do not stop taking this drug suddenly, as this may cause potentially serious health problems. If therapy is to be discontinued, dosage should be reduced gradually, according to doctor's instructions.

PROLONGED USE
No unusual side effects are expected with prolonged therapy.

PRECAUTIONS
Over 60: Weakness, dizziness, and fainting are more likely in older persons.

Driving and Hazardous Work: Diltiazem can cause dizziness or drowsiness. Do not drive or engage in hazardous work until you determine how the medicine affects you.

Alcohol: Use alcohol with caution because it may increase the effect of the drug and cause an excessive drop in blood pressure.

Pregnancy: Birth defects have occurred in animal studies. Adequate human studies have not been done. Avoid this drug during the first 3 months of pregnancy and take it during the last 6 months only if your doctor says it is clearly needed.

Breast Feeding: Diltiazem passes into breast milk; avoid or discontinue use while breast feeding.

Infants and Children: Usually not prescribed; the safety and effectiveness of diltiazem for children under the age of 12 have not been established.

Special Concerns: It is important to brush and floss your teeth and see your dentist regularly, since using diltiazem may promote dental problems. This drug may make you sensitive to sunlight.

OVERDOSE
Symptoms: Heart block causing unusual shortness of breath; fatigue, excessive dizziness, fainting.

What to Do: Call your doctor, emergency medical services (EMS) or the nearest poison control center immediately.

DRUG INTERACTIONS
Consult your doctor for specific advice if you are taking aspirin, beta-blockers, digitalis preparations, carbamazepine, cyclosporine, digoxin, lithium, oral diabetes agents, phenytoin, rifampin, cimetidine, fluvoxamine, or ranitidine.

FOOD INTERACTIONS
Avoid excessive salt intake.

DISEASE INTERACTIONS
Consult your doctor if you have any of the following: kidney disease, liver disease, high blood pressure, or any kind of heart or blood vessel disease.

Dimenhydrinate

Dramamine 50 mg
(UPJOHN)

Additional photographs

▶ Drug Class: Antihistamine

▶ Available in: Capsules,
tablets, elixir, syrup, injection,
suppositories

▶ Available OTC? Yes

▶ As Generic? Yes

Side Effects

SERIOUS
No serious side effects
are associated with this
drug.

COMMON
Drowsiness.

LESS COMMON
Headache, blurred vision,
palpitations, loss of coordination, dry mouth, low
blood pressure causing
dizziness and weakness,
ringing in ears.

PRINCIPAL USES
To relieve nausea and vomiting and to treat or prevent
motion sickness.

HOW THE DRUG WORKS
Dimenhydrinate directly
inhibits the stimulation of
certain nerves in the brain
and inner ear to suppress
nausea, vomiting, dizziness,
and vertigo.

DOSAGE
Capsules, tablets, liquids—
Adults: 50 to 100 mg every
4 to 6 hours. Children ages
6 to 12: 25 to 50 mg every 6
to 8 hours. Children ages 2
to 6: 12.5 to 25 mg every 6
to 8 hours. Injection—
Adults: 50 mg into a vein
every 4 hours. Children:
1.25 mg per 2.2 lbs (1 kg)
of body weight into a vein
or muscle every 6 hours.
Suppositories— Adults: 50
to 100 mg every 6 to 8
hours. Children over age
12: 50 mg every 8 to 12
hours. Children ages 8 to
12: 25 to 50 mg every 8 to
12 hours. Children ages 6 to
8: 12.5 to 25 mg every 8 to
12 hours. To prevent motion
sickness, take this drug at
least 30 minutes, and preferably 1 to 2 hours, before
traveling.

ONSET OF EFFECT
Oral: Within 20 to 30 minutes. Injection: 2 to 20 minutes. Suppositories: 30 to 45
minutes.

DURATION OF ACTION
3 to 6 hours.

DIETARY ADVICE
This drug can be taken with
food or milk to minimize
gastrointestinal distress.

STORAGE
Store in a tightly sealed container in a dry place away
from heat and direct light.

IF YOU MISS A DOSE
Take it as soon as you
remember. However, if it is
near the time for the next
dose, skip the missed dose
and resume your regular
dosage schedule. Do not
double the next dose.

STOPPING THE DRUG
You should take it as prescribed for the full treatment period, but you may
stop if you are feeling better
before the scheduled end of
therapy.

PROLONGED USE
Take this drug only as long
as it is needed.

PRECAUTIONS
Over 60: Older persons
are more sensitive to the
effects of dimenhydrinate.
Dizziness, drowsiness, confusion, difficult or painful
urination, and other side
effects are more likely to
occur.

**Driving and Hazardous
Work:** Do not drive or
engage in hazardous work
until you determine how the
medicine affects you.

Alcohol: Avoid alcohol.

Pregnancy: Animal studies
with high doses of dimenhydrinate have found no birth
defects. Human studies
have not been done.
Because the studies cannot
rule out harm, the drug
should be used during pregnancy only if it is clearly
needed.

Breast Feeding: Dimenhydrinate may pass into breast
milk; caution is advised;
avoid or discontinue use
while nursing.

Infants and Children:
The safety and efficacy of
this drug in children under
2 years of age (age 6 for the
suppository form) have not

been established. Older
children are especially
sensitive to the drug's
side effects.

Special Concerns: Children should be observed
carefully for signs of side
effects; they are more likely
to develop serious complications from these medica-
tions, and younger children
are often unable to describe
changes in the way that
they are feeling.

OVERDOSE
Symptoms: Seizures, hallucinations, drowsiness, difficulty breathing,
unconsciousness.

What to Do: An overdose
of dimenhydrinate is
unlikely to be life-threatening. However, if someone
takes a much larger dose
than prescribed, call your
doctor, emergency medical
services (EMS), or the
nearest poison control center immediately.

DRUG INTERACTIONS
Consult your doctor for
specific advice if you are
taking any narcotic pain
relievers, sedatives, tranquilizers, antidepressants,
antibiotics, aspirin, barbiturates, cisplatin, diuretics,
or theophylline.

FOOD INTERACTIONS
No known food interactions.

DISEASE INTERACTIONS
Caution is advised when
taking dimenhydrinate.
Consult your doctor if you
have glaucoma or an
enlarged prostate.

Diphenhydramine Hydrochloride

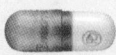

Benadryl Allergy 25 mg
(PARKE-DAVIS)

Additional photographs

▶ Drug Class: Antihistamine

▶ Available in: Capsules, elixir,
  syrup, tablets, injection

▶ Available OTC? Yes

▶ As Generic? Yes

Side Effects

SERIOUS
No serious side effects
are associated with this
drug.

COMMON
Drowsiness, dry mouth,
nausea, thickening of
mucus.

LESS COMMON
Confusion, difficult urination, blurred vision.

PRINCIPAL USES
To relieve hay fever symptoms, itching skin and
hives, motion sickness, non-
productive cough due to
cold or hay fever, and sleeping difficulty; also used to
treat symptoms of Parkin-
son's disease.

HOW THE DRUG WORKS
It blocks the effects of histamine, a naturally occurring
substance that causes
swelling, itching, sneezing,
and watery eyes. In patients
with Parkinson's disease, it
decreases tremors and
muscle stiffness.

DOSAGE
For hay fever symptoms—
Capsules, elixir, syrup,
tablets: Adults and
teenagers: 25 to 50 mg
every 4 to 6 hours. Children
younger than age 6: 6.25 to
12.5 mg every 4 to 6 hours.
Children ages 6 to 12: 12.5
to 25 mg every 4 to 6 hours.
Injection: Adults: 10 to 50
mg into a vein or muscle.
Children: 1.25 mg per 2.2
lbs (1 kg) of body weight
into a muscle 4 times a day.
For nausea, vomiting and
dizziness— Capsules, elixir,
syrup, tablets: Adults: 25 to
50 mg every 4 to 6 hours.
Children: 1 to 1.5 mg per
2.2 lbs every 4 to 6 hours.
Injection: Adults: 10 mg into
a vein or muscle. May be
increased to 25 to 50 mg
every 2 to 3 hours. Chil-
dren: 1 to 1.5 mg per 2.2 lbs
every 6 hours. For Parkinson's disease— Capsules,
elixir, syrup, tablets: Adults:
25 mg, 3 times a day. Doctor may gradually in-crease
dose. Injection: Adults: 10 to
50 mg into a vein or muscle.
Children: 1.25 mg per 2.2
lbs into a muscle, 4 times a
day. As a sedative— Cap-
sules, elixir, syrup, tablets:
Adults: 50 mg 20 to 30 minutes before bedtime. For
cough— Liquid: Adults and
teenagers: 25 mg every 4 to

6 hours. Children ages 2 to
6: 6.25 mg (½ teaspoon)
every 4 to 6 hours. Children
ages 6 to 12: 12.5 mg (1 teaspoon) every 4 to 6 hours.

ONSET OF EFFECT
After capsules, elixir, syrup,
or tablets: 15 minutes. Injection: unknown.

DURATION OF ACTION
6 to 8 hours.

DIETARY ADVICE
Take diphenhydramine with
food or milk to reduce gastrointestinal distress.

STORAGE
Store in a dry place away
from heat and direct light.
Prevent liquid forms from
freezing.

IF YOU MISS A DOSE
Take it as soon as you
remember. If it is near the
time for the next dose, skip
the missed dose and
resume your regular dosage
schedule. Do not double the
next dose.

STOPPING THE DRUG
Stop taking this drug and
call your doctor if it is not
effective after 5 days.

PROLONGED USE
No special problems have
been reported.

PRECAUTIONS
Over 60: Adverse reactions
may be more likely and
more severe.

**Driving and Hazardous
Work:** Do not drive or
engage in hazardous work
until you determine how the
medicine affects you. Use of
this drug is a disqualification for piloting aircraft.

Alcohol: Alcohol may
increase the likelihood and
severity of side effects such
as drowsiness and mental
confusion.

Pregnancy: No birth
defects have been reported
in animals. Studies of pregnant women have found no
significant increase in birth
defects.

Breast Feeding: Diphenhydramine passes into
breast milk; avoid or discontinue use while nursing.

Infants and Children:
This drug is not recom-
mended for children under
the age of 2.

Special Concerns: Children should be observed
carefully for signs of side
effects; they are more likely
to develop serious complications, and younger children
are often unable to describe
changes in the way that
they are feeling.

OVERDOSE
Symptoms: Marked
drowsiness, dilated and
unreactive pupils, fever,
excitability, breathing inter-
ruptions, combativeness,
confusion, loss of coordination, weak pulse, seizures,
loss of consciousness.

What to Do: Call your
doctor, emergency medical
services (EMS), or the
nearest poison control center immediately.

DRUG INTERACTIONS
Consult your doctor for specific advice if you are taking
anticholinergics, alcohol,
disopyramide, central nervous system depressants,
or MAO inhibitors.

FOOD INTERACTIONS
No known food interactions.

DISEASE INTERACTIONS
Consult your doctor if you
have a history of severe respiratory disease, glaucoma,
urinary obstruction, or
prostate enlargement.

Diphenoxylate Hydrochloride/Atropine Sulfate

Lonox 2.5/0.025 mg
(GENEVA)

▶ Drug Class: Antidiarrheal

▶ Available in: Liquid, tablet

▶ Available OTC? No

▶ As Generic? Yes

Side Effects

SERIOUS
Swelling of the hands,
feet, face, lips or throat;
severe stomach pain
accompanied by nausea
and vomiting. Call your
doctor immediately.

COMMON
Dizziness, dry mouth,
sedation.

LESS COMMON
Drowsiness, lethargy,
headache, restlessness,
mental depression, fast
pulse, enlarged pupils,
nausea, vomiting,
abdominal discomfort,
loss of appetite, slowed
breathing, rash, itching,
inability to urinate.

PRINCIPAL USES
To relieve severe diarrhea
and intestinal cramps.

HOW THE DRUG WORKS
This medication blocks
nerve activity in the intestinal tract, which reduces
propulsive contractions
(peristalsis) and diminishes
intestinal secretions.

DOSAGE
Adults and teenagers: 5 mg
(2 tablets or 2 teaspoons), 3
or 4 times a day. Your doctor may reduce the dose
when diarrhea starts to be
controlled. Children: Consult your pediatrician.

ONSET OF EFFECT
Within 45 to 60 minutes.

DURATION OF ACTION
3 to 4 hours.

DIETARY ADVICE
The tablet should be taken
with liquid or food to
reduce stomach irritation. A
mild diet is recommended
when recovering from diarrhea. Bananas, rice, applesauce, and plain toast are
good choices. Be sure to
get plenty of fluids.

STORAGE
Store in a tightly sealed container in a dry place away
from heat, moisture, and
direct light. Keep the liquid
form from freezing.

IF YOU MISS A DOSE
Take it as soon as you
remember. If it is near the
time for the next dose, skip
the missed dose and
resume your regular dosage
schedule. Do not double the
next dose.

STOPPING THE DRUG
Continue taking the medi-
cine until at least 24 to 36
hours after diarrhea has
stopped. Consult with your
doctor if the diarrhea does
not stop after 2 days or if
you develop a fever.

PROLONGED USE
Diphenoxylate and atropine
may be habit-forming if
larger doses are taken for a
long time. Ask your doctor
about the need for follow-up
medical examinations or
laboratory studies to check
liver function if you must
take this medication for a
prolonged period of time.

PRECAUTIONS
Over 60: Adverse reactions
may be more likely and
more severe in older
patients.

**Driving and Hazardous
Work:** Do not drive or
engage in hazardous work
until you determine how the
medicine affects you.

Alcohol: Avoid alcohol
while taking this medicine.

Pregnancy: If you are
pregnant or plan to become
pregnant, consult your doctor; discuss whether the
benefits justify the possible
risks to the unborn child.

Breast Feeding: This
drug passes into breast
milk; caution is advised.
Consult your doctor for specific advice.

Infants and Children:
Not recommended for use
by children under the age
of 2. For children over 2,
use the drug only under a
doctor's supervision.

Special Concerns: During the first 24 hours, drink
plenty of caffeine-free clear
liquids such as broth, ginger ale, and decaffeinated
tea. During the second 24
hours you may eat bland
foods such as applesauce,
bread, toast, crackers, rice,
and oatmeal. Avoid caffeine,
fried or spicy foods, bran,
candy, fruits, and vegetables. They can make your
condition worse.

OVERDOSE
Symptoms: Drowsiness,
dizziness, and weakness
caused by low blood pres-
sure; seizures; slow or
arrested breathing; blurred
vision; reddened face; dryness of the mouth; unusual
behavior.

What to Do: Call your
doctor, emergency medical
services (EMS), or the
nearest poison control center immediately.

DRUG INTERACTIONS
The following drugs may
interact with the combination of diphenoxylate and
atropine. Consult your doctor for specific advice if you
are taking antibiotics; central nervous system depressants; MAO inhibitors;
naltrexone; or anticholinergic medicines to reduce
stomach acid, spasms,
or cramps.

FOOD INTERACTIONS
No known food interactions.

DISEASE INTERACTIONS
Caution is advised when
taking this drug. Before
starting, consult your doctor
if you have liver problems,
Down's syndrome, ulcera-
tive colitis, Crohn's disease,
glaucoma, chronic lung disease (such as emphysema),
heart disease, a history of
alcohol or drug abuse, an
enlarged prostate, gallbladder disease or gallstones,
high blood pressure, an
underactive or overactive
thyroid, kidney disease,
dysentery, myasthenia
gravis, or intestinal or urinary tract blockage.

▶ Drug Class: Vaccine

▶ Available in: Injection

▶ Available OTC? No

▶ As Generic? Yes

Side Effects

SERIOUS
Fever of 105°F or more, seizures, collapse, difficulty breathing or swallowing, hives, unusual irritability, temporary loss of consciousness or awareness. Call your doctor as soon as possible.

COMMON
Fever between 100.4°F and 102.2°F, sometimes accompanied by loss of appetite, drowsiness, vomiting, and fretfulness; redness, swelling, lump, pain, or tenderness at the site of the injection.

LESS COMMON
Fever between 102.2°F and 104°F and skin rash.

Diphtheria, Tetanus Toxoids, and Pertussis Vaccine (DTP)

PRINCIPAL USES
The DTP vaccine is used as a combination immunizing agent to prevent three serious childhood diseases—diphtheria, tetanus, and pertussis. Diphtheria can cause difficulty breathing, pneumonia, nerve damage, heart problems, and possibly death. Tetanus (lockjaw) can cause severe muscle spasms. Pertussis (whooping cough) causes severe bouts of coughing that can interfere with breathing. Pertussis can also cause long-lasting bronchitis, pneumonia, seizures, and brain damage, and can lead to death.

HOW THE DRUG WORKS
The DTP vaccine stimulates the body's immune system to produce protective antibodies against diphtheria, tetanus, and pertussis.

DOSAGE
Children 2 months to 7 years: 0.5 ml injected into muscle 4 to 8 weeks apart for 3 doses, followed by a fourth 0.5 ml dose injected into a muscle 1 year later, usually at 15 to 18 months of age. A fifth dose (booster) may be administered at 4 to 6 years of age. Persons over 7 years of age should not receive the whole-cell pertussis vaccine.

ONSET OF EFFECT
Unknown.

DURATION OF ACTION
Up to 10 years.

DIETARY ADVICE
The vaccine can be administered without regard to diet.

STORAGE
Not applicable; the dose is administered only at a health care facility.

IF YOU MISS A DOSE
If your child misses a scheduled vaccination, contact your pediatrician.

STOPPING THE DRUG
The full schedule of injections should be followed unless a medical problem intervenes.

PROLONGED USE
No special problems are expected.

PRECAUTIONS
Over 60: This vaccine is not intended for use by older persons.

Driving and Hazardous Work: Not applicable.

Alcohol: Not applicable.

Pregnancy: This vaccine is not intended for women of childbearing age.

Breast Feeding: This vaccine is not intended for women of childbearing age.

Infants and Children: Not recommended for use by children over age 7.

Special Concerns: Anyone over the age of 7 should receive a vaccine that contains tetanus and diphtheria toxoids, but not whole-cell pertussis vaccine. Older persons should receive the diphtheria and tetanus booster injections every 10 years for life. Your doctor may want the child to take 1 or more doses of acetaminophen or another medicine that helps prevent fever after receiving the DTP injection. Consult your doctor for specific advice. DTP should not be given to a child who has had a previous serious adverse reaction to a DTP vaccination.

OVERDOSE
Symptoms: Not applicable.

What to Do: No cases of overdose have been reported.

DRUG INTERACTIONS
The following drugs may interact with DTP. Consult your doctor for specific advice if your child is taking an anticoagulant or a drug that suppresses the immune system. DTP can be given with vaccines for other diseases, but should not be given within 3 days of influenza vaccine.

FOOD INTERACTIONS
No known food interactions.

DISEASE INTERACTIONS
Consult your doctor if your child has any of the following: a brain disease, a central nervous system disorder, epilepsy, a fever, muscle spasms, or seizures.

Dipivefrin

▶ Drug Class: Antiglaucoma agent

▶ Available in: Ophthalmic solution

▶ Available OTC? No

▶ As Generic? Yes

Side Effects

SERIOUS
Fast or irregular heartbeat. Call your doctor immediately.

COMMON
In people who have had prior cataract surgery, this drug may cause swelling at the center of the retina that can lead to (in most cases) reversible vision impairment.

LESS COMMON
Increased sensitivity of eyes to light; burning, stinging, or other eye irritation.

PRINCIPAL USES
To treat glaucoma.

HOW THE DRUG WORKS
Glaucoma, a sight-threatening disorder, occurs when the aqueous humor (the fluid inside the eye) cannot drain properly, causing an increase in pressure within the eyeball (intraocular pressure). The increased eye pressure can damage the optic nerve and lead to a gradually progressive loss of vision. Dipivefrin is converted in the eye to epinephrine, which decreases the production of aqueous humor and increases its outflow.

DOSAGE
To start, 1 drop in each eye every 12 hours. The dose may be changed based on patient's response.

ONSET OF EFFECT
Within 30 minutes.

DURATION OF ACTION
12 hours or more.

DIETARY ADVICE
No special restrictions.

STORAGE
Store in a tightly sealed container away from heat, moisture, and direct light. Do not allow the medicine to freeze.

IF YOU MISS A DOSE
Apply it as soon as you remember. If it is near the time for the next dose, skip the missed dose and resume your regular dosage schedule. Do not double the next dose.

STOPPING THE DRUG
The decision to stop using the drug should be made by your doctor.

PROLONGED USE
See your doctor regularly for tests and examinations if you must take this drug for a prolonged period.

PRECAUTIONS
Over 60: No special problems are expected.

Driving and Hazardous Work: The use of dipivefrin should not impair your ability to perform such tasks safely.

Alcohol: No special precautions are necessary.

Pregnancy: Dipivefrin has not caused birth defects in animals. Human studies have not been done. Before you take dipivefrin, tell your doctor if you are pregnant or plan to become pregnant.

Breast Feeding: Dipivefrin may pass into breast milk; caution is advised. Consult your doctor for specific advice.

Infants and Children: No special precautions.

Special Concerns: Dipivefrin should not be used by people with closed-angle glaucoma. To use the eye drops, first wash your hands. Tilt your head back. Gently apply pressure to the inside corner of the eyelid and with the index finger of the same hand, pull downward on the lower eyelid to make a space. Drop the medicine into this space and close your eye. Apply pressure for 1 or 2 minutes while keeping the eye closed without blinking. Then wash your hands again. Make sure the tip of the dropper does not touch your eye, finger, or any other surface. If you are taking the medicine with the compliance cap (C Cap), make sure that the number 1 or the correct day of the week appears in the window of the cap before using the eye drops for the first time. After every dose, rotate the bottle until the cap clicks to the position that tells you the next dose.

OVERDOSE
Symptoms: Rapid or irregular heartbeat.

What to Do: An overdose of dipivefrin is unlikely to be life-threatening. If a large volume enters the eyes, flush with water. If someone accidentally ingests the medicine, call your doctor, emergency medical services (EMS), or the nearest poison control center.

DRUG INTERACTIONS
Other drugs may interact with dipivefrin. Consult your doctor for specific advice if you are taking tricyclic antidepressants, maprotiline, nomifensine, ophthalmic beta-blockers, digitalis drugs, or systemic sympathomimetics.

FOOD INTERACTIONS
No known food interactions.

DISEASE INTERACTIONS
Caution is advised when taking dipivefrin. Consult your doctor if you have closed-angle glaucoma or aphakia (absence of part or all of the lens of the eye).

Dipyridamole

Generic 50 mg
(BARR)

Additional photographs

▶ Drug Class: Antiplatelet drug

▶ Available in: Tablet, injection

▶ Available OTC? No

▶ As Generic? Yes

Side Effects

SERIOUS
Dizziness and weakness caused by low blood pressure (hypotension). Call your doctor.

COMMON
Headache, nausea, rash.

LESS COMMON
Vomiting, diarrhea, flushing, itching, chest pain, liver problems causing nausea, vomiting, yellow-tinged eyes and skin, swelling, bloating.

PRINCIPAL USES
To prevent blood clots during recovery from heart valve replacement surgery; to reduce frequency and intensity of angina attacks (chest pain associated with heart disease).

HOW THE DRUG WORKS
Dipyridamole is believed to increase blood levels of adenosine, a metabolic product that causes blood vessels to expand and prevents platelets, a type of blood cell, from adhering to one another to form a clot.

DOSAGE
Tablets: 75 to 100 mg, 4 times a day, given with an anticoagulant such as warfarin, to prevent blood clots. If at all possible, when dipyridamole is taken with warfarin, the injectable form of dipyridamole should be avoided; injection (when necessary) is administered under doctor's supervision. Aspirin may also be used with dipyridamole, as the two drugs have a synergistic anticoagulant effect.

ONSET OF EFFECT
About 10 minutes; 3 months of continual use is needed for the full effect to occur.

DURATION OF ACTION
About 6 hours.

DIETARY ADVICE
Take this medication 1 hour before or 2 hours after meals. Swallow the tablet with 6 to 8 ounces of water.

STORAGE
Store in a tightly sealed container in a dry place away from heat and direct light.

IF YOU MISS A DOSE
Take it as soon as you remember. However, if it is near the time for the next dose, skip the missed dose and resume your regular dosage schedule as prescribed. Do not double the next dose.

STOPPING THE DRUG
Take as prescribed for the full treatment period.

PROLONGED USE
If you must use dipyridamole for a prolonged period, consult your doctor about the possible need for follow-up medical examinations or laboratory studies.

PRECAUTIONS
Over 60: Older patients should start with smaller doses. Otherwise, no special problems are expected.

Driving and Hazardous Work: Dipyridamole may cause dizziness. Do not drive or engage in hazardous work until you determine how the medicine affects you.

Alcohol: Avoid alcohol while taking this medication because it may lower blood pressure excessively.

Pregnancy: Dipyridamole has not been reported to cause birth defects. Consult your doctor about its use during pregnancy.

Breast Feeding: While dipyridamole passes into breast milk, it has not been reported to cause problems in nursing babies. Consult your doctor for specific advice about its use while nursing.

Infants and Children: Dipyridamole is not recommended for use by children under the age of 12.

Special Concerns: If your doctor tells you to take dipyridamole with aspirin, take only the amount of aspirin that is prescribed. Tell any doctor or dentist whom you consult that you are taking dipyridamole.

OVERDOSE
Symptoms: Dizziness and weakness caused by extremely low blood pressure (hypotension).

What to Do: Discontinue taking the drug. An overdose of dipyridamole is unlikely to be life-threatening; however, if someone takes a much larger dose than prescribed, call your doctor, emergency medical services (EMS), or the nearest poison control center immediately.

DRUG INTERACTIONS
Consult your doctor for specific advice if you are taking anticoagulants (such as warfarin, aspirin, and ticlopidine), valproic acid, or any nonsteroidal anti-inflammatory drug (NSAID) such as indomethacin.

FOOD INTERACTIONS
Taking dipyridamole within 1 hour of eating will decrease the body's absorption of the drug. When possible, take dipyridamole on an empty stomach.

DISEASE INTERACTIONS
Caution is advised when taking dipyridamole. Consult your doctor if you have low blood pressure or liver disease or if you are recovering from a heart attack.

Dirithromycin

DYNABAC
UC5364

Dynabac 250 mg
(BOCK)

▶ Drug Class: Macrolide antibiotic

▶ Available in: Tablets

▶ Available OTC? No

▶ As Generic? No

Side Effects

SERIOUS
Colitis (inflammation of the lower gastrointestinal tract, with symptoms including severe abdominal pain or cramping, watery or bloody stools, severe diarrhea, fever); liver toxicity (causing fever, nausea, vomiting, yellowish tinge to eyes or skin); allergic reaction (swelling of the lips, tongue, face, and throat, breathing difficulty, skin rash or hives); blood clotting disorders (causing unusual bleeding, bruising, and tiny bright red spots on the skin). Such side effects are rare, but if they do occur, stop taking dirithromycin and seek medical assistance immediately.

COMMON
No common side effects are associated with the use of dirithromycin.

LESS COMMON
Dizziness, stomach upset or discomfort, mild diarrhea, mild nausea and vomiting, headache, unusual fatigue.

PRINCIPAL USES
To treat bronchitis, some types of pneumonia such as Legionnaires' disease, skin infections, and tonsillitis or other throat infections such as strep throat. Dirithromycin is effective only against infections caused by bacteria; it is ineffective against those caused by viruses (for example, colds and flu), fungi, or other microorganisms.

HOW THE DRUG WORKS
Dirithromycin prevents bacterial cells from manufacturing specific proteins necessary for their survival.

DOSAGE
Adults and children age 12 and over: 500 mg, once a day for 5 to 14 days (depending on the condition being treated). It is recommended that this medication be taken at the same time every day.

ONSET OF EFFECT
Within 2 hours; full effect may occur in 2 to 5 days.

DURATION OF ACTION
From 30 to 50 hours.

DIETARY ADVICE
Take this medicine with food or within 1 hour of eating. Drink plenty of fluids.

STORAGE
Store in a tightly sealed container away from moisture, heat, and direct light.

IF YOU MISS A DOSE
Take it as soon as you remember, up to 12 hours late. However, if more than 12 hours have passed, skip the missed dose and resume your regular dosage schedule. Do not double the next dose.

STOPPING THE DRUG
Take this drug for the full treatment period, even if you begin to feel better before the scheduled end of therapy.

PROLONGED USE
Prolonged use is not recommended. Your doctor will discontinue the medicine once the infection is cured. Unnecessary or prolonged use of any antibiotic may promote infection by microorganisms that are resistant to the drug's effects. This is known as superinfection.

PRECAUTIONS
Over 60: No special problems are expected.

Driving and Hazardous Work: Do not drive or engage in hazardous work until you determine how dirithromycin affects you.

Alcohol: No special precautions are necessary.

Pregnancy: Adequate studies of the use of dirithromycin during pregnancy have not been done; discuss the potential risks and benefits with your doctor.

Breast Feeding: It is not known if dirithromycin passes into breast milk; consult your doctor for advice.

Infants and Children: Dirithromycin should be given to children under 12 only under close medical supervision.

Special Concerns: Tell any doctor or dentist you consult that you are taking this medicine. Before taking dirithromycin, tell your doctor if you are allergic to any other drug, especially an antibiotic.

OVERDOSE
Symptoms: No cases of dirithromycin overdose have been reported. Symptoms would most likely include diarrhea, nausea, vomiting, and heartburn.

What to Do: An overdose of dirithromycin is unlikely to be life-threatening. However, if someone takes a much larger dose than prescribed, contact a doctor or the nearest poison control center for advice.

DRUG INTERACTIONS
This drug should not be taken by patients known to have had prior allergic reactions to erythromycins or other macrolide antibiotics. Also, consult your doctor for specific advice if you are taking any other drugs, especially allergy drugs, antacids or histamine (H2) blockers, anticoagulants, antiarrhythmics, seizure drugs, cholesterol-lowering drugs, digitalis drugs, ergotamine, bromocriptine, cyclosporine, or valproate.

FOOD INTERACTIONS
No known food interactions.

DISEASE INTERACTIONS
Consult your doctor if you have a blood or liver disorder or any allergy.

Disopyramide

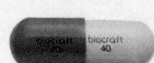

Generic 100 mg
(BIOCRAFT)

▶ Drug Class: Antiarrhythmic

▶ Available in: Capsules, extended-release capsules, tablets

▶ Available OTC? No

▶ As Generic? Yes

Side Effects

SERIOUS
Chest pain, shortness of breath, irregular or rapid heartbeat (palpitations), fainting, sudden weight gain, swelling of fingers or ankles, anxiety. Call your doctor immediately if such symptoms arise.

COMMON
Dizziness, faintness, weakness caused by low blood pressure, blurred vision, constipation, dry eyes, dry nose, dry mouth. Consult your doctor if such symptoms persist.

LESS COMMON
Depression, agitation, fatigue, muscle weakness, decreased urination, nausea, vomiting, severe loss of appetite and weight, abdominal pain, difficulty urinating, yellow-tinged eyes and skin, low blood sugar causing drowsiness, headache, cold sweats, nervousness, confusion, skin rash.

PRINCIPAL USES
To control abnormal or irregular heart rhythms (cardiac arrhythmias).

HOW THE DRUG WORKS
It slows the activity of the heart's natural pacemaker and delays the transmission of electrical impulses through the heart muscle, thus stabilizing heartbeat.

DOSAGE
Adults weighing more than 110 lbs: 150 mg capsules every 6 hours; 300 mg extended-release capsules every 12 hours. Dosage must be individualized for adults weighing less than 110 lbs. Children age 12 to 18: 6 to 15 mg for every 2.2 lbs (1 kg) of body weight daily; ages 4 to 12: 10 to 15 mg per 2.2 lbs daily; ages 1 to 4: 10 to 20 mg per 2.2 lbs of body weight daily; under 1 year: 10 to 30 mg per 2.2 lbs daily. Doses are divided into equal amounts and taken every 6 hours. Initial doses should be smaller in patients suffering from impaired left ventricular function.

ONSET OF EFFECT
30 minutes to 3.5 hours.

DURATION OF ACTION
Up to 8.5 hours (longer in patients with impaired kidney function).

DIETARY ADVICE
Can be taken with or between meals.

STORAGE
Store in a tightly sealed container in a dry place away from heat and direct light.

IF YOU MISS A DOSE
Take it as soon as you remember. However, if it is within 4 hours of the next dose, skip the missed dose and return to your regular dosage schedule as pre-

scribed. Do not double the next dose.

STOPPING THE DRUG
The decision to stop taking the drug should be made by your doctor.

PROLONGED USE
Prolonged use requires supervision and periodic evaluation by your doctor.

PRECAUTIONS
Over 60: Adverse reactions (especially dry mouth and difficulty urinating) may be more likely and more severe in older patients. Dosage reduction may be required.

Driving and Hazardous Work: Avoid such activities until you determine how the medicine affects you.

Alcohol: Avoid alcohol.

Pregnancy: Before taking this medicine, tell your doctor if you are pregnant or plan to become pregnant. Discuss with your doctor whether the benefits of taking disopyramide justify the possible risk to the unborn child.

Breast Feeding: Disopyramide passes into breast milk; avoid or discontinue use while nursing.

Infants and Children: Children using this drug should do so only under close medical supervision.

Special Concerns: Try to take disopyramide exactly at the times prescribed. An alarm clock may be needed for nighttime doses. Tell your doctor if you have had an unfavorable reaction to any other antiarrhythmic medication.

OVERDOSE
Symptoms: Heartbeat irregularities, severe drop in blood pressure, loss of consciousness, breathing difficulty.

What to Do: Call your doctor, emergency medical services (EMS), or the nearest poison control center immediately.

DRUG INTERACTIONS
Consult your doctor if you are taking other antiarrhythmics, anticholinergics, anticoagulants, insulin, drugs for high blood pressure, nimodipine, phenobarbital, phenytoin, pimozide, propafenone, or rifampin.

FOOD INTERACTIONS
No known food interactions.

DISEASE INTERACTIONS
Caution is advised when taking disopyramide. Consult your doctor if you have any of the following: heart disease or heart block, diabetes mellitus, enlarged prostate, glaucoma, myasthenia gravis, kidney or liver disease.

Disulfiram

Generic 250 mg
(SIDMAK)

▶ Drug Class: Alcoholism control drug

▶ Available in: Tablets

▶ Available OTC? No

▶ As Generic? Yes

Side Effects

SERIOUS
Confusion and disorientation, severe skin rash, seizures, neuritis (nerve inflammation causing pain, numbness, or paralysis), low thyroid function, decrease or increase in blood pressure, carpal tunnel syndrome. Call your doctor if such symptoms arise.

COMMON
Drowsiness.

LESS COMMON
Eye pain, vision changes, abdominal discomfort, throbbing headache, mood change, numbness in hands and feet, decreased sexual ability in men, unpleasant taste in mouth, offensive breath and body odor.

PRINCIPAL USES
To help treat chronic alcoholism.

HOW THE DRUG WORKS
Disulfiram interferes with the activity of the liver enzyme that processes and metabolizes alcohol, causing an accumulation of a chemical known as acetaldehyde. A buildup of acetaldehyde in the body leads to a severely unpleasant reaction, including nausea and vomiting. Thus, while not a cure for alcoholism, disulfiram is a deterrent to alcohol consumption.

DOSAGE
Initial dose: 250 to 500 mg a day in a single dose in the morning or evening. Maintenance dose: 125 to 500 mg once a day. Treatment with disulfiram should not start until at least 12 hours after consumption of an alcoholic beverage.

ONSET OF EFFECT
1 to 2 hours.

DURATION OF ACTION
Effects usually last 3 to 4 days but may persist for up to 2 weeks.

DIETARY ADVICE
Take it with or following meals to decrease stomach irritation.

STORAGE
Store in a tightly sealed container in a dry place away from heat and direct light.

IF YOU MISS A DOSE
Take it as soon as you remember. If it is within 12 hours of the next dose, skip the missed dose and return to your normal dosage schedule. Do not double the next dose.

STOPPING THE DRUG
The decision to stop taking the drug should be made in consultation with your physician.

PROLONGED USE
Use of disulfiram on a regular schedule for several months is needed to see if alcohol consumption is deterred. Use should continue until permanent self-control is achieved. Periodic tests of liver function should be done. Gradual reduction of doses may be required when disulfiram has been taken for a prolonged period of time.

PRECAUTIONS
Over 60: Adverse reactions may be more likely and more severe in older patients.

Driving and Hazardous Work: Do not drive or engage in hazardous work until you determine how the medication affects you.

Alcohol: This medication should never be taken by anyone with alcohol in the bloodstream.

Pregnancy: Studies have indicated that disulfiram may lead to birth defects; however, alcohol abuse may lead to births defects as well. Ask your doctor if the possible benefits justify the risk to the unborn baby.

Breast Feeding: It is not known whether disulfiram passes into breast milk. Consult your doctor for advice.

Infants and Children: Not recommended for use by children under age 12.

Special Concerns: Check all liquids that you drink or rub on your skin for the presence of alcohol. Disulfiram may interfere with sexual performance in men. Tell your doctor if you plan to have surgery under general anesthesia while taking disulfiram.

OVERDOSE
Symptoms: Loss of memory, behavior disturbances, confusion, headaches, lethargy, increased blood pressure, nausea, vomiting, stomach pain, diarrhea, unsteady walk, temporary paralysis.

What to Do: Call your doctor, emergency medical services (EMS), or the nearest poison control center immediately.

DRUG INTERACTIONS
Other drugs may interact with disulfiram. Consult your doctor if you are taking anticoagulants, anticonvulsants, antidepressants (especially amitriptyline), barbiturates, cephalosporin antibiotics, clozapine, fluoxetine, guanethidine, guanfacine, isoniazid, leucovorin, methyprion, metronidazole, paraldehyde, sedatives, or sertraline.

FOOD INTERACTIONS
Any food prepared with alcohol, including sauces, fermented vinegar, marinades, or desserts, can produce the unpleasant reaction characteristic of disulfiram.

DISEASE INTERACTIONS
Caution is advised when taking disulfiram. Consult your doctor if you have any of the following: diabetes, epilepsy, kidney disease, liver disease, low thyroid function, lung disease, or a history of psychosis.

Docusate

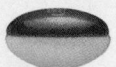

Colace 100 mg
(ROBERTS)

Additional photographs

▶ Drug Class: Stool softener

▶ Available in: Capsules, tablets, liquid, syrup

▶ Available OTC? Yes

▶ As Generic? Yes

Side Effects

SERIOUS
Severe cramping. Stop taking the drug and call your doctor immediately.

COMMON
Diarrhea, mild abdominal cramps.

LESS COMMON
Throat irritation, laxative dependence. Consult your doctor if you cannot maintain normal bowel habits without docusate for more than 2 weeks.

PRINCIPAL USES
To prevent constipation (but not to treat existing constipation). Recommended for persons who should not strain during defecation, such as those recovering from rectal or heart surgery, or women who experience constipation after childbirth.

HOW THE DRUG WORKS
Docusate promotes easier bowel movements by drawing liquid into stools, forming a softer mass.

DOSAGE
Adults and teenagers: 50 to 500 mg once a day until bowel movements return to normal. Children ages 6 to 12: 40 to 140 mg once a day. Liquid forms should be mixed with milk or fruit juice.

ONSET OF EFFECT
Within 24 to 72 hours.

DURATION OF ACTION
Up to 72 hours.

DIETARY ADVICE
Add high-fiber foods like bran and fresh fruits and vegetables to your diet. Drink at least 6 glasses (8 oz each) of water or other liquids a day to help soften stools.

STORAGE
Store in a tightly sealed container away from heat, moisture, and direct light.

IF YOU MISS A DOSE
Take it as soon as you remember. If it is near the time for the next dose, skip the missed dose and resume your regular dosage schedule. Do not double the next dose.

STOPPING THE DRUG
Take it as prescribed for the full treatment period. However, you may stop taking the drug if you are feeling better and normal bowel function has returned before the scheduled end of therapy.

PROLONGED USE
Docusate should not be taken for more than 1 week unless you are under your doctor's supervision. Be aware that overuse can make you dependent on it and may cause damage to the nerves, muscles, and other tissues of the bowel and lead to vitamin and mineral deficiency.

PRECAUTIONS
Over 60: No special problems are expected.

Driving and Hazardous Work: The use of docusate should not impair your ability to perform such tasks safely.

Alcohol: No special precautions are necessary.

Pregnancy: Before taking docusate, tell your doctor if you are pregnant or plan to become pregnant.

Breast Feeding: No special problems are expected if you take docusate while nursing.

Infants and Children: Do not give docusate to children under age 6 unless it is prescribed by your doctor.

Special Concerns: Do not take mineral oil while you are taking docusate.

OVERDOSE
Symptoms: Weakness, sweating, muscle cramps, irregular heartbeat.

What to Do: An overdose of docusate is unlikely to be life-threatening. However, if someone takes a much larger dose than prescribed, call your doctor, emergency medical services (EMS), or the nearest poison control center immediately.

DRUG INTERACTIONS
A number of drugs may interact with docusate if they are ingested at or near the time it is taken. Consult your doctor for specific advice if you are taking any other oral drug within 2 hours before or after taking docusate.

FOOD INTERACTIONS
No known food interactions.

DISEASE INTERACTIONS
This drug cannot be used by people with intestinal obstruction or appendicitis. Symptoms of these conditions include vomiting, abdominal rigidity and tenderness, and fever. Call your doctor or emergency medical services (EMS) immediately if you suspect you may be suffering from intestinal obstruction or appendicitis.

Donepezil

BRAND NAME
Aricept

Aricept 5 mg
(Eisai)

▶ Drug Class: Acetylcholinesterase inhibitor

▶ Available in: Tablets

▶ Available OTC? No

▶ As Generic? No

Side Effects

SERIOUS
No serious side effects
are associated with the
use of donepezil.

COMMON
Nausea, vomiting, diar-
rhea, headache, dizziness,
fatigue, insomnia.

LESS COMMON
Vivid or unusual dreams,
drowsiness, depression,
loss of appetite, unusual
bleeding or bruising,
fainting, muscle cramps,
frequent urination, joint
pain, stiffness, or
swelling.

PRINCIPAL USES
To treat mild to moderate
Alzheimer's disease.

HOW THE DRUG WORKS
Donepezil prevents the
breakdown of acetylcholine,
a brain chemical crucial to
memory. Acetylcholine deficiency is thought to result
in memory loss associated
with Alzheimer's disease.

DOSAGE
To start, 5 mg at bedtime.
The dose may be increased
after 4 to 6 weeks to 10 mg
at bedtime.

ONSET OF EFFECT
Unknown.

DURATION OF ACTION
Unknown.

DIETARY ADVICE
No special restrictions.

STORAGE
Store in a tightly sealed container away from heat, moisture, and direct light.

IF YOU MISS A DOSE
Skip the missed dose and
resume your regular dosage
schedule. Do not double the
next dose.

STOPPING THE DRUG
The decision to stop taking
the drug should be made by
your doctor.

PROLONGED USE
No problems are expected
with long-term use.

PRECAUTIONS
Over 60: No special problems are expected.

**Driving and Hazardous
Work:** Do not drive or
engage in hazardous work
until you determine how the
medicine affects you.

Alcohol: Avoid alcohol
while using this medication.

Pregnancy: In some animal studies, large doses of
donepezil were shown to
cause problems. Before you
take donepezil, tell your
doctor if you are pregnant
or plan to become pregnant.

Breast Feeding: It is not
known whether donepezil
passes into breast milk; caution is advised. Consult your
doctor for specific advice.

Infants and Children:
Donepezil is not intended
for use in children.

Special Concerns: Before
you have any surgery or
dental or emergency treatment, tell the doctor or dentist in charge that you are
taking donepezil. Donepezil
will not cure Alzheimer's
disease and will not stop the
disease from getting worse,
but it will improve cognitive
ability of some patients.

OVERDOSE
Symptoms: Seizures,
severe nausea, slow heartbeat, increased muscle
weakness, vomiting, greatly
increased sweating, greatly
increased watering of the
mouth, weak pulse, irregular breathing, enlargement
of the pupils of the eyes.

What to Do: Call your
doctor, emergency medical
services (EMS), or the
nearest poison control center immediately.

DRUG INTERACTIONS
The following drugs may
interact with donepezil. Consult your doctor for specific
advice if you are taking carbamazepine, dexametha-
sone, ketoconazole,
phenobarbital, phenytoin,
quinidine, or rifampin. Also
tell your doctor if you are
taking any other prescription or over-the-counter
medication.

FOOD INTERACTIONS
No known food interactions.

DISEASE INTERACTIONS
Caution is advised when
taking donepezil. Consult
your doctor if you have any
of the following: asthma,
chronic obstructive pul-
monary disease, urinary difficulties, heart disease, liver
disease, a seizure disorder,
stomach ulcers, or blockage
of the urinary tract.

Dornase Alfa

▶ Drug Class: Cystic fibrosis drug

▶ Available in: Inhalation solution

▶ Available OTC? No

▶ As Generic? No

Side Effects

SERIOUS
Chest pain. Call your doctor immediately.

COMMON
Sore throat, voice changes, such as hoarseness.

LESS COMMON
Skin rash; redness, itching, swelling, pain, or other symptoms of eye irritation.

PRINCIPAL USES
To make breathing easier and help prevent lung infections in patients with cystic fibrosis. It is used in conjunction with other cystic fibrosis drugs such as antibiotics, bronchodilators, and anti-inflammatory agents.

HOW THE DRUG WORKS
The mucus in the lungs of people with cystic fibrosis contains large amounts of DNA; this makes the mucus much thicker than normal. Dornase alfa breaks down the DNA, making the mucus less sticky and easier to cough up.

DOSAGE
Adults and children age 5 and older: 2.5 mg in a nebulizer once a day. Selected patients may require 2 daily doses. Use only the following nebulizers and compressors: Hudson T Up-draft II disposable jet nebulizer with the Pulmo-Aide compressor, Marquest Acorn II disposable jet nebulizer with the Pulmo-Aide compressor, or the PARI LC Jet+ nebulizer with the PARI PRONEB compressor.

ONSET OF EFFECT
Lung function tests improve significantly within 3 days to 1 week. Reduction in respiratory tract infections may occur over the course of weeks to months.

DURATION OF ACTION
The drug is effective only when it is used daily.

DIETARY ADVICE
No special restrictions.

STORAGE
Refrigerate the drug in its protective foil pouch, away from heat, moisture, and direct light. Do not allow it to freeze. Discard the drug if it is cloudy or discolored.

IF YOU MISS A DOSE
Take it as soon as you remember. If it is near the time for the next dose, skip the missed dose and resume your regular dosage schedule. Do not double the next dose.

STOPPING THE DRUG
Take it as prescribed for the full treatment period, even if you begin to feel better before the scheduled end of therapy. The decision to stop taking the drug should be made in conjunction with your doctor.

PROLONGED USE
Prolonged use requires periodic evaluation of response and possible dose adjustment by your doctor. It is expected that dornase alfa will be used for a prolonged period.

PRECAUTIONS
Over 60: No special problems are expected.

Driving and Hazardous Work: The use of this medication should not impair your ability to perform such tasks safely.

Alcohol: No special precautions are necessary.

Pregnancy: Adequate human studies have not been done. Before taking dornase alfa, tell your doctor if you are pregnant or plan to become pregnant.

Breast Feeding: Dornase alfa may pass into breast milk; caution is advised. Consult your doctor for specific advice concerning the relative risks and benefits of using this drug while breast feeding.

Infants and Children: Dornase alfa is not recommended for use by children under the age of 5.

Special Concerns: Breathe only through the mouth while using the nebulizer. A nose clip can help. Use the mouthpiece provided with the nebulizer. Do not use a face mask because less medicine will get into the lungs. If you begin coughing during treatment, turn off the nebulizer taking care not to spill the drug. You can resume treatment when coughing stops. Do not dilute dornase alfa or use other medicines in the nebulizer.

OVERDOSE
Symptoms: An overdose of dornase alfa is unlikely to occur and unlikely to be life-threatening.

What to Do: If you have any reason to suspect an overdose, call your doctor, emergency medical services (EMS), or the nearest poison control center.

DRUG INTERACTIONS
Do not use this medication if you are allergic to Chinese hamster ovary cells. No other drug interactions are known.

FOOD INTERACTIONS
No known food interactions.

DISEASE INTERACTIONS
No disease interactions have been reported.

Dorzolamide Hydrochloride

BRAND NAME
Trusopt

▶ Drug Class: Antiglaucoma agent; carbonic anhydrase inhibitor

▶ Available in: Ophthalmic solution

▶ Available OTC? No

▶ As Generic? No

Side Effects

SERIOUS
Allergic reaction causing redness, itching, and swelling of the eyelid; continued or severe sensitivity to light; feeling that something is in the eye; detachment of the choroid (a thin membrane within the eye) following filtration surgery. Call your doctor immediately.

COMMON
Burning, stinging, or discomfort in the eye when drug is administered; bitter taste in mouth.

LESS COMMON
Eye pain, severe or continued tearing, nausea or vomiting, blood in urine.

PRINCIPAL USES
To treat glaucoma.

HOW THE DRUG WORKS
Glaucoma, a sight-threatening disorder, occurs when aqueous humor (the fluid inside the eye) cannot drain properly, resulting in an increase in pressure within the eyeball (known as intraocular pressure). Increased intraocular pressure can damage the optic nerve and lead to a gradually progressive loss of vision. Dorzolamide inhibits the activity of the enzyme carbonic anhydrase, which is needed in the production of aqueous humor. In this way the drug reduces intraocular pressure.

DOSAGE
Adults and teenagers: 1 drop in each eye 3 times per day.

ONSET OF EFFECT
Unknown.

DURATION OF ACTION
8 hours.

DIETARY ADVICE
No special restrictions.

STORAGE
Store in a tightly sealed container away from heat, moisture, and direct light. Do not refrigerate or allow it to freeze.

IF YOU MISS A DOSE
Apply it as soon as you remember. If it is near the time for the next dose, skip the missed dose and resume your regular dosage schedule. Do not double the next dose.

STOPPING THE DRUG
The decision to stop using the drug should be made by your doctor.

PROLONGED USE
Schedule regular eye examinations with your doctor to be sure the drug is controlling the glaucoma.

PRECAUTIONS
Over 60: No special problems are expected.

Driving and Hazardous Work: Do not drive or engage in hazardous work until you determine how the medicine affects your vision.

Alcohol: No special precautions are necessary.

Pregnancy: One animal study found that very high doses of this drug caused birth defects. Human studies have not been done. Before using this medicine, tell your doctor if you are pregnant or plan to become pregnant.

Breast Feeding: Dorzolamide may pass into breast milk; caution is advised. Consult your doctor for specific advice about whether to use a different medicine or to stop breast feeding.

Infants and Children: Safety and dosage for children have not been established. Dorzolamide should be given to infants and children only under close medical supervision.

Special Concerns: To use the eye drops, first wash your hands. Tilt your head back. Gently apply pressure to the inside corner of the eyelid and with the index finger of the same hand, pull downward on the lower eyelid to make a space. Drop the medicine into this space and close your eye. Apply pressure for 1 or 2 minutes while keeping the eye closed without blinking. Then wash your hands again. Make sure that the tip of the dropper does not touch your eye, finger, or any other surface.

OVERDOSE
Symptoms: No specific ones have been reported.

What to Do: An overdose of dorzolamide is unlikely to be life-threatening. If a large volume enters the eye, flush with water. If someone accidentally ingests the medicine, call your doctor, emergency medical services (EMS), or the nearest poison control center.

DRUG INTERACTIONS
Wait 10 minutes before administering any other eye medicine. Dorzolamide should not be used in conjunction with eye medications containing silver, such as silver nitrate. People allergic to sulfa-type drugs should not use dorzolamide

FOOD INTERACTIONS
No known food interactions.

DISEASE INTERACTIONS
Use of dorzolamide may cause complications in patients with liver disease or kidney disease, since these organs work together to remove the medication from the body.

Doxazosin Mesylate

Cardura 4 mg
(ROERIG)

▶ Drug Class: Antihypertensive;
BPH therapy agent

▶ Available in: Tablets

▶ Available OTC? No

▶ As Generic? No

Side Effects

SERIOUS
Irregular heartbeat. Call
your doctor immediately.
Another serious but rare
side effect is priapism, a
condition characterized
by a prolonged or painful
erection (lasting more
than 4 hours).

COMMON
Dizziness, drowsiness.

LESS COMMON
Headache, weakness, pal-
pitations, rapid pulse,
pain and tingling sensa-
tions in the fingers or
toes, diarrhea or consti-
pation, runny nose, rash
or itchy skin, muscle or
joint pain, headache,
mental depression.

PRINCIPAL USES
To treat mild to moderate
high blood pressure; to ease
urinary tract symptoms due
to benign prostatic hyperplasia (BPH)—that is, noncancerous enlargement of
the prostate gland, which is
extremely common among
men over the age of 50.
Note: Findings from a major
clinical trial indicate that
doxazosin is associated with
an unacceptably high incidence of cardiovascular
complications. The Ameri-
can Academy of Cardiology
has since recommended
that physicians reconsider
the use of doxazosin in the
treatment of their hyperten-
sive patients on a case-by-
case basis.

HOW THE DRUG WORKS
For high blood pressure,
the drug relaxes and
widens blood vessels so
blood passes through them
more easily. For prostate
enlargement, it relaxes muscles in the prostate and the
opening of the bladder.
Note that doxazosin will
not shrink the prostate;
symptoms may worsen
and surgery may eventually
be required.

DOSAGE
For high blood pressure,
initial dose is 1 mg taken
once a day. It can be
increased gradually to a
maximum of 16 mg a day.
For prostate enlargement,
initial dose is 1 mg taken
once a day, which may be
gradually increased to a
maximum of 12 mg a day.

ONSET OF EFFECT
For high blood pressure: 1
to 2 hours. For prostate
enlargement: 1 to 2 weeks.

DURATION OF ACTION
For high blood pressure: 24
hours. For prostate enlargement: Unknown.

DIETARY ADVICE
No special restrictions.

STORAGE
Store in a tightly sealed container in a dry place away
from heat and direct light.

IF YOU MISS A DOSE
Take it as soon as you
remember. If it is near the
time for the next dose, skip
the missed dose and
resume your regular dosage
schedule. Do not double the
next dose.

STOPPING THE DRUG
Take it as prescribed for the
full treatment period, even if
you feel better before the
scheduled end of therapy.

PROLONGED USE
Consult your doctor about
the need for follow-up medical examinations and laboratory studies if you must
take doxazosin for a pro-
longed period.

PRECAUTIONS
Over 60: Adverse reactions
may be more likely and
more severe in older
patients. Dose should be
increased slowly in patients
over 60.

**Driving and Hazardous
Work:** Do not drive or
engage in hazardous work
until you determine how the
medicine affects you.

Alcohol: Alcohol should be
avoided while taking this
medicine because it may
cause an excessive drop in
blood pressure.

Pregnancy: In animal studies, very high doses of doxazosin damaged the fetus.
Before taking this medicine,
tell your doctor if you are
pregnant or plan to become
pregnant.

Breast Feeding: Doxa-
zosin may pass into breast
milk; caution is advised.
Consult your doctor for
specific advice.

Infants and Children:
This drug is not recom-
mended for use by children.

Special Concerns: The
first dose is likely to cause
dizziness or lightheaded-
ness. Take the drug at night
and get out of bed slowly
the next day. Be cautious
while exercising and during
hot weather. Tell your doctor whether you will have
surgery requiring general
anesthesia, including dental
surgery, within the next 2
months.

OVERDOSE
Symptoms: Cold, sweaty
skin, rapid pulse, weakness,
loss of consciousness.

What to Do: Call your
doctor, emergency medical
services (EMS), or the
nearest poison control center immediately.

DRUG INTERACTIONS
Consult your doctor for specific advice if you are taking
amphetamines, other antihypertensive drugs, nons-
teroidal anti-inflammatory
drugs (NSAIDs), estrogen,
or sympathomimetic drugs.

FOOD INTERACTIONS
No known food interactions.

DISEASE INTERACTIONS
Use of doxazosin may cause
complications in patients
with liver or kidney disease,
since these organs work
together to remove the
medication from the body.
Also, consult your doctor if
you have coronary artery
disease, impaired blood
circulation to the brain,
or mental depression.

Doxepin Hydrochloride

BRAND NAMES
Adapin, Sinequan

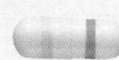

Generic 25 mg
(GENEVA)

Additional photographs

▶ Drug Class: Tricyclic antidepressant

▶ Available in: Capsules, oral solution

▶ Available OTC? No

▶ As Generic? Yes

Side Effects

SERIOUS
Confusion, heartbeat irregularities, hallucinations, seizures, extreme fatigue or drowsiness, blurred or altered vision, breathing difficulty, constipation, impaired concentration, difficult urination, fever, extreme and persistent restlessness, loss of coordination and balance, difficulty swallowing or speaking, dilated pupils, eye pain, fainting. Also trembling, shaking, weakness, and stiffness in the extremities; shuffling gait. Call your doctor immediately.

COMMON
Drowsiness or dizziness, headache, dry mouth or unpleasant taste, fatigue, heightened sensitivity to light, weight gain, nausea, increased appetite.

LESS COMMON
Heartburn, sleeping difficulty, diarrhea, increased sweating, vomiting.

PRINCIPAL USES
To relieve symptoms of major depression.

HOW THE DRUG WORKS
Doxepin affects levels of serotonin, norepinephrine, and acetylcholine, brain chemicals that are thought to be linked to mood, emotions, and mental state.

DOSAGE
Adults: To start, 25 mg, 3 times a day; may be increased to 150 mg a day. Older adults: To start, 25 to 50 mg a day; the dose may be increased gradually by your doctor.

ONSET OF EFFECT
1 to 6 weeks.

DURATION OF ACTION
Unknown.

DIETARY ADVICE
To lessen stomach upset, take it with food, unless your doctor instructs otherwise. Increase intake of fiber and fluids. When taking the oral solution, dilute doxepin in half a glass of water, milk, or fruit juice, but not grapefruit juice. Do not take this drug with a carbonated beverage.

STORAGE
Store in a tightly sealed container away from heat, moisture, and direct light. Do not allow liquid form to freeze.

IF YOU MISS A DOSE
If you take a one-time daily bedtime dose, do not take a missed dose in the morning because it may cause drowsiness. Call your doctor. If you take more than 1 dose a day, take it as soon as you remember. If it is near the time for the next dose, skip the missed dose and resume your regular dosage schedule. Do not double the next dose.

STOPPING THE DRUG
Take as prescribed for the full treatment period, even if you begin to feel better before the scheduled end of therapy. The decision to stop taking the drug should be made in consultation with your doctor.

PROLONGED USE
The usual course of therapy lasts 6 months to 1 year; some patients benefit from additional therapy.

PRECAUTIONS
Over 60: Adverse reactions, especially confusion and urination difficulty, may be more likely and more severe in older patients. Your doctor may prescribe a lower dose.

Driving and Hazardous Work: Use caution when driving or engaging in hazardous work until you determine how the medication affects you. Drowsiness or lightheadedness can occur.

Alcohol: Avoid alcohol.

Pregnancy: Adequate human studies have not been done. Consult your doctor for specific advice.

Breast Feeding: Doxepin passes into breast milk; do not use it while nursing. Doxepin has been found to cause drowsiness in the infant.

Infants and Children: This drug is not prescribed for children under age 6.

Special Concerns: This is a potentially dangerous drug, especially if taken in excess. Tricyclic antidepressants should not be within easy reach of suicidal patients. If dry mouth occurs, use sugarless gum or candy.

OVERDOSE
Symptoms: Difficulty breathing, severe fatigue, seizures, confusion, hallucinations, dilated pupils, irregular heartbeat, fever, impaired concentration.

What to Do: Call your doctor, emergency medical services (EMS), or the nearest poison control center immediately.

DRUG INTERACTIONS
Consult your doctor for specific advice if you are taking antithyroid agents, cimetidine, clonidine, guanadrel, guanethidine, metrizamide, appetite suppressants, isoproterenol, ephedrine, epinephrine, amphetamines, phenylephrine, antipsychotic drugs, pimozide, methyldopa, metyrosine, metoclopramide, pemoline, promethazine, trimeprazine, rauwolfia alkaloids, MAO inhibitors, or any drugs that depress the central nervous system.

FOOD INTERACTIONS
No known food interactions.

DISEASE INTERACTIONS
Consult your doctor if you have any of the following: a history of alcohol abuse, difficulty urinating, asthma, bipolar disorder, high blood pressure, stomach or intestinal problems, glaucoma, overactive thyroid, enlarged prostate, schizophrenia, seizures, a blood disorder, or kidney, heart, or liver disease.

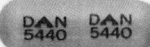

Generic 100 mg
(Schein/Danbury)

Additional photographs

▶ Drug Class: Tetracycline antibiotic

▶ Available in: Capsules, delayed-release capsules, liquid, tablets

▶ Available OTC? No

▶ As Generic? Yes

Side Effects

SERIOUS
Chest pain; increased pressure in the head, causing confusion, sleepiness, and headache; allergic reaction causing severe headache, vision changes, itching, swelling, wheezing, or difficulty breathing; severe rash; severe abdominal pain and diarrhea. Call your doctor immediately.

COMMON
Stomach upset, nausea, mild diarrhea, increased sensitivity to sunlight, increased skin pigmentation, vaginal yeast infection, thrush (oral fungal infection).

LESS COMMON
Sore throat, tongue irritation, loss of appetite, colitis, inflamed anus or genitals, tooth discoloration, pain and swelling of legs.

PRINCIPAL USES
To treat infections caused by bacteria or protozoa (tiny single-celled organisms), including certain sexually transmitted diseases (such as chlamydia, gonorrhea, and syphilis), urinary tract infections, and Lyme disease. Also used to prevent and treat malaria and to treat acne. Doxycycline is also approved for prophylactic use following known exposure to anthrax bacteria and for treating anthrax infections.

HOW THE DRUG WORKS
Doxycycline kills bacteria and protozoa by inhibiting their manufacture of proteins they need for survival.

DOSAGE
For bacterial or protozoal infections— Adults and children over 100 lbs: 100 mg every 12 hours (twice a day) on the first day of therapy, followed by 100 to 200 mg a day. Usual dose for children under 99 lbs: 1 mg per lb of body weight in 2 doses on first day, followed by 1 to 2 mg per lb per day in 1 single or 2 divided doses. For gonorrhea— Adults and children over 100 lbs: 200 mg to start, then 100 mg, 2 times a day for 3 days. For prevention of malaria— Adults and teenagers: 100 mg once a day, starting 1 or 2 days prior to travel, and for 4 weeks after return from a high-risk area. Children ages 8 to 12: 0.9 mg per lb with the same dosage schedule as adults.

ONSET OF EFFECT
Up to 5 days for infection.

DURATION OF ACTION
Several days.

DIETARY ADVICE
Take with a full (8 oz) glass of water.

STORAGE
Store in a tightly sealed container away from heat, moisture, and direct light.

IF YOU MISS A DOSE
Take it as soon as you remember. If it is near the time for the next dose, skip the missed dose and resume your regular dosage schedule. Do not double the next dose.

STOPPING THE DRUG
Take it as prescribed for the full treatment period even if you feel better before the scheduled end of therapy.

PROLONGED USE
Prolonged use may make you more susceptible to infections caused by microorganisms resistant to this antibiotic. Some patients will need periodic monitoring of blood, liver, and kidney function.

PRECAUTIONS
Over 60: Itching in the genital and anal areas may be more common among patients over 60.

Driving and Hazardous Work: No special precautions are necessary.

Alcohol: Avoid alcohol when fighting an infection.

Pregnancy: Studies of pregnant women indicate that this drug can cause discoloration and impaired development of teeth as well as other birth defects. Avoid using doxycycline during pregnancy.

Breast Feeding: Not recommended during therapy.

Infants and Children: Doxycycline should not be used in children younger than 8 years old since it can cause permanent tooth staining.

Special Concerns: To avoid heartburn, do not take capsules or tablets within 1 hour of bedtime. If you take the liquid form, use a specially marked spoon to measure the dose accurately. Do not take outdated capsules or tablets. If this drug causes increased sensitivity to sunlight, use sunscreen when outdoors to prevent sunburn.

OVERDOSE
Symptoms: Nausea and vomiting, diarrhea, difficulty swallowing.

What to Do: An overdose is unlikely to be life-threatening. However, if someone takes a much larger dose than prescribed, call your doctor, emergency medical services (EMS), or the nearest poison control center immediately.

DRUG INTERACTIONS
Consult your doctor for specific advice if you are taking any other antibiotics, antacids, warfarin, antiviral drugs, bismuth salicylate, calcium supplements, cefixime, cholestyramine, oral contraceptives, desmopressin, digitalis drugs, etretinate, lithium, mineral supplements, sodium bicarbonate, or tiopronin.

FOOD INTERACTIONS
Dairy products can decrease absorption of this drug. Take it 2 hours after or 1 hour before consuming milk or another dairy product. Avoid meats and iron-fortified cereals for 2 hours before and after taking doxycycline.

DISEASE INTERACTIONS
Consult your doctor if you have a history of kidney disease, liver disease, lupus, or myasthenia gravis.

Dronabinol

BRAND NAME
Marinol

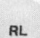

Marinol 2.5 mg
(ROXANE)

▶ Drug Class: Antiemetic; appetite stimulant

▶ Available in: Capsules

▶ Available OTC? No

▶ As Generic? No

Side Effects

SERIOUS
Hallucinations, severe mood changes, irritability, euphoria.

COMMON
Dizziness, drowsiness, poor coordination, trouble thinking.

LESS COMMON
Depression, anxiety, nervousness, headache, hallucinations, blurred vision, rapid heartbeat, frequent or difficult urination, convulsions, dry mouth.

PRINCIPAL USES
To prevent nausea and vomiting caused by cancer drugs, and to stimulate the appetite of AIDS patients.

HOW THE DRUG WORKS
The exact mechanism of action is unknown. Dronabinol may inhibit the centers of the brain that govern the vomiting reflex.

DOSAGE
For nausea and vomiting: 5 mg per square meter of body surface, 1 to 3 hours before chemotherapy is given. The same dose can be taken every 2 to 4 hours after chemotherapy for 4 to 6 doses a day. To stimulate appetite: 2.5 mg twice a day, before lunch and dinner. The dose can be reduced to 2.5 mg taken once in the evening. Maximum dose (if necessary) is up to 20 mg a day, taken in divided doses.

ONSET OF EFFECT
Unknown.

DURATION OF ACTION
From 4 to 6 hours. Appetite stimulation may last 24 hours or longer.

DIETARY ADVICE
For nausea and vomiting control, take it between meals. As an appetite stimulant, take it before lunch and before dinner.

STORAGE
Store in a tightly sealed container away from heat, moisture, and direct light. Keep the medication refrigerated, but do not allow it to freeze.

IF YOU MISS A DOSE
Take it as soon as you remember. If it is near the time for the next dose, skip the missed dose and resume your regular dosage schedule. Do not double the next dose.

STOPPING THE DRUG
The decision to stop taking the drug should be made by your doctor. Withdrawal effects such as insomnia, irritability, sweating, loss of appetite, and hot flashes may follow abrupt termination. These effects will dissipate over the subsequent 24 hours.

PROLONGED USE
Prolonged use increases the risk of side effects and drug dependence.

PRECAUTIONS
Over 60: Adverse reactions may be more likely and more severe in older patients. Older patients should be watched carefully when they take this medicine because of dronabinol's effects on the mind. Changes in mental state due to dronabinol use should not be mistaken for those caused by conditions such as Alzheimer's disease.

Driving and Hazardous Work: Do not drive or engage in hazardous work until you determine how the medicine affects you.

Alcohol: Avoid alcohol.

Pregnancy: Adequate human studies have not been completed. Before taking dronabinol, tell your doctor if you are pregnant or plan to become pregnant.

Breast Feeding: Dronabinol passes into breast milk; avoid or discontinue its use while nursing.

Infants and Children: Dronabinol is not recommended for use by children under age 12 or children with AIDS cachexia.

Special Concerns: Be aware that dronabinol is a derivative of the principal active substance in marijuana and has a high potential for abuse. Prior allergic reaction to marijuana, marijuana by-products, or sesame oil may rule out use of dronabinol.

OVERDOSE
Symptoms: Confusion, slurred speech, red eyes, hallucinations, change in perceptions of taste, sound, touch, smell, or sight, drastic mood changes, rapid, pounding heartbeat, difficulty urinating, nervousness, dry mouth, loss of coordination, fainting, or dizziness.

What to Do: If someone takes a much larger dose of dronabinol than prescribed, call your doctor, emergency medical services (EMS), or the nearest poison control center right away.

DRUG INTERACTIONS
Other drugs may interact with dronabinol. Consult your doctor for specific advice if you are taking anticonvulsants, antidepressants, antihistamines, barbiturates, clozapine, ethinamate, fluoxetine, leucovorin, narcotics, theophylline, muscle relaxants, or any central nervous system depressant.

FOOD INTERACTIONS
No known food interactions.

DISEASE INTERACTIONS
Caution is advised when taking dronabinol. Consult your doctor if you have any of the following: heart disease, high blood pressure, a history of alcohol or drug abuse, schizophrenia, or manic depression (bipolar disorder).

BRAND NAMES
Dilor, Lufyllin, Neothylline

▶ Drug Class: Bronchodilator/ xanthine

▶ Available in: Elixir, tablets

▶ Available OTC? No

▶ As Generic? No

Side Effects

SERIOUS
No serious side effects are associated with dyphylline when used at recommended doses (see Overdose).

COMMON
No common side effects are associated with dyphylline.

LESS COMMON
Heartburn, nausea, vomiting, rapid heartbeat, headache, increased urine output, nervousness, trembling, difficulty.

PRINCIPAL USES
To prevent or treat acute bronchial asthma or episodes of breathing difficulty associated with chronic bronchitis and emphysema.

HOW THE DRUG WORKS
Dyphylline is a mild bronchodilator, similar in effect to drugs like theophylline and aminophylline. It relaxes the smooth muscle tissue surrounding the bronchial passages, helping to widen the airways and aid breathing.

DOSAGE
Adults: Dose is based on individual body weight, usually 15 mg per 2.2 lbs (1 kg), or 6.8 mg per lb, up to 4 times a day. Children: Consult pediatrician for appropriate dose.

ONSET OF EFFECT
Rapid.

DURATION OF ACTION
Unknown.

DIETARY ADVICE
Best when taken on an empty stomach at least 1 hour before or 2 hours after eating. However, it may be taken with meals to minimize the incidence of stomach irritation or upset.

STORAGE
Store in a tightly sealed container away from heat and direct light.

IF YOU MISS A DOSE
Take it as soon as you remember. However, if it is near the time for the next dose, skip the missed dose and resume your regular dosage schedule. Do not double the next dose.

STOPPING THE DRUG
The decision to stop taking the drug should be made in consultation with your physician.

PROLONGED USE
Therapy with this medication may require months or years. See your doctor regularly for tests and examinations if you must take the medication for a prolonged period.

PRECAUTIONS
Over 60: Adverse reactions may be more likely and more severe in older patients.

Driving and Hazardous Work: Do not drive or engage in hazardous work until you determine how the medicine affects you.

Alcohol: No special precautions are necessary.

Pregnancy: Adequate studies of the use of dyphylline during pregnancy have not been done. Discuss the relative risks and benefits with your doctor.

Breast Feeding: Dyphylline passes into breast milk, although no adverse consequences have been reported. Consult your doctor for specific advice.

Infants and Children: The safety and effectiveness of dyphylline use by children have not been established; other medications are generally preferred.

OVERDOSE
Symptoms: Persistent and severe abdominal pain, confusion or changes in mental state, seizures, dark or bloody vomit, rapid or irregular heartbeat, nervousness, restlessness, trembling.

What to Do: Call your doctor, emergency medical services (EMS), or the nearest poison control center immediately.

DRUG INTERACTIONS
Other drugs may interact with dyphylline. Consult your doctor for specific advice if you are taking beta-blockers (including ophthalmic beta-blocker preparations used to treat glaucoma), probenecid, or other xanthine-derivative medications such as theophylline or aminophylline.

FOOD INTERACTIONS
Your doctor may suggest that you restrict your consumption of foods and beverages containing caffeine (including chocolate), since caffeine may heighten dyphylline's stimulating effects to the central nervous system.

DISEASE INTERACTIONS
You should not use dyphylline if you have had a prior allergic reaction to xanthine-derivative drugs such as theophylline or aminophylline. Consult your doctor if you have active gastritis (inflammation of the stomach lining) or a history of peptic ulcer or impaired kidney function.

Econazole Nitrate

BRAND NAME
Spectazole

▶ Drug Class: Antifungal

▶ Available in: Cream

▶ Available OTC? No

▶ As Generic? No

Side Effects

SERIOUS
No serious side effects are associated with econazole.

COMMON
No common side effects are associated with econazole.

LESS COMMON
Itching, burning, stinging, skin redness, or other irritation not present prior to treatment.

PRINCIPAL USES
To treat fungal infections of the skin, such as tinea corporis (ringworm), tinea cruris (jock itch), tinea pedis (athlete's foot), and pityriasis versicolor ("sun fungus," a skin condition characterized by fine scaly patches of varying shapes, sizes, and colors).

HOW THE DRUG WORKS
Econazole prevents fungal organisms from producing vital substances required for growth and function. This drug is effective only for infections caused by fungal organisms. Econazole will not work for bacterial or viral infections.

DOSAGE
Apply to affected area 1 to 2 times a day. When twice a day, apply it in the morning and the evening. Athlete's foot is usually treated for 1 month; jock itch, ringworm, and sun fungus, for 2 weeks.

ONSET OF EFFECT
Unknown.

DURATION OF ACTION
Unknown.

DIETARY ADVICE
Econazole can be applied without regard to diet.

STORAGE
Store in a tightly sealed container away from heat, moisture, and direct light. Do not allow it to freeze.

IF YOU MISS A DOSE
Apply it as soon as you remember. However, if it is near the time for the next application, skip the missed dose and resume your regular dosage schedule.

STOPPING THE DRUG
Use it as prescribed for the full treatment period, even if you begin to feel better before the scheduled end of therapy. Recurrence of the infection is likely if you stop before the full treatment period is complete.

PROLONGED USE
Notify your doctor if no improvement occurs after 2 weeks of treatment for jock itch, ringworm, and sun fungus, or after 4 weeks of treatment for athlete's foot.

PRECAUTIONS
Over 60: No special problems are expected.

Driving and Hazardous Work: The use of econazole should not impair your ability to perform such tasks safely.

Alcohol: No special precautions are necessary.

Pregnancy: Before using econazole, tell your doctor if you are pregnant or plan to become pregnant. Econazole should be used in the first trimester only if the doctor says it is essential to your health, and it should be used in the last two trimesters only if it is clearly needed.

Breast Feeding: Econazole may pass into breast milk; caution is advised. Consult your doctor for specific advice.

Infants and Children: Special problems that would limit the usefulness of this medicine in children are not expected. Consult your pediatrician for specific advice.

Special Concerns: Avoid allowing econazole to come into contact with the eyes. If using the medication for jock itch, do not wear underwear that is tight or made from synthetic materials; wear loose-fitting cotton underwear. If using econazole for athlete's foot, dry your feet carefully after bathing and wear clean cotton socks with sandals or well-ventilated shoes. Before applying the medication, wash the affected area with soap and warm water and dry thoroughly. Econazole may stain your clothing.

OVERDOSE
Symptoms: An overdose of econazole is unlikely.

What to Do: If someone should swallow a large amount of econazole, call your doctor, emergency medical services (EMS), or the nearest poison control center immediately.

DRUG INTERACTIONS
Consult your doctor for specific advice if you are taking topical corticosteroids. They may inhibit the antifungal effect of econazole.

FOOD INTERACTIONS
No food interactions have been reported.

DISEASE INTERACTIONS
No disease interactions have been reported.

Efavirenz

BRAND NAME
Sustiva

▶ Drug Class: Antiviral/reverse transcriptase inhibitor

▶ Available in: Capsules

▶ Available OTC? No

▶ As Generic? No

Side Effects

SERIOUS
Severe depression, mood changes, confusion. Call your doctor immediately.

COMMON
Dizziness, difficulty sleeping, fatigue, impaired concentration, unusual dreams, stomach upset, fever, cough, vomiting, diarrhea. Rash is also common; although the rash usually goes away without a change in treatment, sometimes it may be serious. If you develop a rash, call your doctor immediately.

LESS COMMON
Numerous less common side effects can occur; consult your doctor if you are concerned about any adverse or unusual reactions you experience while taking this drug.

PRINCIPAL USES
To treat human immunodeficiency virus (HIV) infection in combination with other drugs. While not a cure for HIV, such drugs may suppress the replication of the virus and delay the progression of the disease.

HOW THE DRUG WORKS
Efavirenz prevents HIV from reproducing in two ways. A metabolite of the drug inhibits the activity of an enzyme needed for the replication of DNA in viral cells. The metabolite is also incorporated into viral DNA and terminates the formation of the complete DNA.

DOSAGE
Adults: To start, 600 mg once a day. The drug must be taken in combination with other drugs for HIV to delay the development of resistant strains of the virus. For the first two to four weeks of therapy, take the daily dose at bedtime to improve tolerability of certain side effects (such as dizziness, drowsiness, and impaired concentration). Children: The dose may be lower. Consult your doctor.

ONSET OF EFFECT
Unknown. With most antiretroviral drugs, an early response can be seen within the first few days of therapy, but the maximum effect may take 12 to 16 weeks.

DURATION OF ACTION
Unknown. Effects of the drug may be prolonged when efavirenz is used in combination with other effective drugs and the virus is maximally suppressed.

DIETARY ADVICE
Efavirenz should be taken with plenty of water or other liquid. It may also be taken with a meal, but not one high in fat.

STORAGE
Store at room temperature in a tightly sealed container away from heat, moisture, and direct light.

IF YOU MISS A DOSE
Take it as soon as you remember. If it is near the time for the next dose, skip the missed dose and resume your regular dosage schedule. Do not double the next dose. It is especially important to take efavirenz on schedule, to assure constant, proper blood levels of the drug.

STOPPING THE DRUG
The decision to stop taking the drug should be made in consultation with your physician.

PROLONGED USE
See your doctor regularly for tests and examinations.

PRECAUTIONS
Over 60: It is not known whether efavirenz causes different or more severe side effects in older patients.

Driving and Hazardous Work: Do not drive or engage in hazardous work until you determine how the medicine affects you.

Alcohol: Alcohol may raise the blood concentration of the drug.

Pregnancy: Efavirenz has been shown to cause birth defects in animals. Human studies have not been done. This medication should be given during pregnancy only if potential benefits outweigh the risks to the unborn child.

Breast Feeding: Women infected with HIV should not breast feed, to avoid transmitting the virus to an uninfected child.

Infants and Children: Your pediatrician will determine the appropriate dosage based on your child's weight. Call your doctor immediately if you notice rash or any other side effects while your child is taking efavirenz.

Special Concerns: Use of efavirenz does not eliminate the risk of passing the AIDS virus to other persons. You should take appropriate preventive measures.

OVERDOSE
Symptoms: Increased severity of common side effects.

What to Do: Call your doctor, emergency medical services (EMS), or the nearest poison control center immediately.

DRUG INTERACTIONS
Do not take efavirenz with astemizole, midazolam, triazolam, or ergot medications (migraine drugs). Dose adjustments may be necessary if taking indinavir, saquinavir, or clarithromycin. Consult your doctor before taking with warfarin, rifampin, rifabutin, or oral contraceptives.

FOOD INTERACTIONS
Do not take efavirenz with high-fat meals.

DISEASE INTERACTIONS
Caution is advised when taking efavirenz. Consult your doctor if you have a history of mental illness or drug or alcohol abuse. This drug should be used with caution in patients with impaired liver function or risk factors for liver disease.

Emedastine Difumarate

▶ Drug Class: Histamine (H1) blocker

▶ Available in: Ophthalmic solution

▶ Available OTC? No

▶ As Generic? No

Side Effects

SERIOUS
No serious side effects are associated with emedastine.

COMMON
Headache.

LESS COMMON
Bad taste in the mouth, abnormal dreams, eye dryness, blurred vision, burning or stinging of the eye, tearing, runny nose, skin rash, weakness.

PRINCIPAL USES
For short-term therapy of eye itching caused by seasonal allergic conjunctivitis (inflammation of the mucous membranes that line the inner surface of the eyelids and whites of the eyes).

HOW THE DRUG WORKS
Emedastine blocks the effects of histamine, a naturally occurring substance within the body that causes swelling, itching, sneezing, watery eyes, hives, and other symptoms associated with allergic reactions.

DOSAGE
Instill 1 drop in the affected eye(s) up to 4 times a day.

ONSET OF EFFECT
Unknown.

DURATION OF ACTION
Unknown.

DIETARY ADVICE
Emedastine can be used without regard to diet.

STORAGE
Store in a tightly sealed container away from heat, moisture, and direct light. Do not allow it to freeze.

IF YOU MISS A DOSE
Apply it as soon as you remember. If it is near the time for the next dose, skip the missed dose and resume your regular dosage schedule. Do not double the next dose.

STOPPING THE DRUG
You may stop using emedastine whenever you choose.

PROLONGED USE
Emedastine is prescribed for short-term use only.

PRECAUTIONS
Over 60: No special problems are expected.

Driving and Hazardous Work: Do not drive or engage in hazardous work until you determine how the medicine affects you.

Alcohol: No special precautions are necessary.

Pregnancy: No adequate human studies have been done. Before taking emedastine, tell your doctor if you are pregnant or plan to become pregnant.

Breast Feeding: Emedastine may pass into breast milk; caution is advised. Consult your doctor for specific advice.

Infants and Children: Not recommended for use by children under the age of 3 years.

Special Concerns: To use the eye drops, first wash your hands. Tilt your head back. Gently apply pressure to the inside corner of the eyelid and with the index finger of the same hand, pull downward on the lower eyelid to make a space. Drop the medicine into this space and close your eye. Apply pressure for 1 or 2 minutes while keeping the eye closed without blinking. Then wash your hands again. Make sure the tip of the dropper does not touch your eye, finger, or any other surface. You should not wear a contact lens if your eye is red. Emedastine should not be used to treat contact-lens-related irritation. If you wear soft contact lenses and your eyes are not red, wait at least 10 minutes after instilling the drops before inserting your contact lenses.

OVERDOSE
Symptoms: Drowsiness and general feelings of illness have been reported following unintentional oral intake of the drug.

What to Do: An overdose with emedastine is unlikely to be life-threatening. However, if someone accidentally ingests the medicine, seek emergency medical attention immediately.

DRUG INTERACTIONS
None reported.

FOOD INTERACTIONS
None reported.

DISEASE INTERACTIONS
None reported.

Enalapril Maleate

Vasotec 10 mg
(MERCK)

801

Additional photographs

▶ Drug Class: Angiotensin-converting enzyme (ACE) inhibitor

▶ Available in: Tablets

▶ Available OTC? No

▶ As Generic? No

Side Effects

SERIOUS
Fever and chills, sore throat and hoarseness, sudden difficulty breathing or swallowing, swelling of the face, mouth, or extremities, impaired kidney function (ankle swelling, decreased urination), confusion, yellow discoloration of the eyes or skin (indicating liver disorder), intense itching, chest pain or palpitations, abdominal pain. Serious side effects are very rare; contact your doctor immediately.

COMMON
Dry, persistent cough.

LESS COMMON
Dizziness or fainting, skin rash, numbness or tingling in the hands, feet, or lips, unusual fatigue or muscle weakness, nausea, drowsiness, loss of taste, headache, unusual dreams.

PRINCIPAL USES
To control high blood pressure; to treat congestive heart failure; to treat patients with left ventricular dysfunction (damage to the pumping chamber of the heart); and to minimize further kidney damage in diabetic patients with mild kidney disease.

HOW THE DRUG WORKS
Angiotensin-converting enzyme (ACE) inhibitors block an enzyme that produces angiotensin, a naturally occurring substance that causes blood vessels to constrict. As a result, ACE inhibitors relax blood vessels (causing them to widen), which lowers blood pressure and so decreases the workload of the heart.

DOSAGE
Adults: 2.5 to 40 mg a day, taken 1 or 2 times a day. Children ages 1 month to 16 years (for high blood pressure): To start, 0.08 mg per kg (2.2 lbs) once a day, up to 5 mg a day. Your pediatrician may gradually raise the dose up to 40 mg a day, depending upon response to the drug.

ONSET OF EFFECT
Within 1 hour.

DURATION OF ACTION
Up to 24 hours.

DIETARY ADVICE
Take enalapril on an empty stomach, about 1 hour before mealtime. Follow your doctor's dietary advice (such as low-salt or low-cholesterol restrictions) to improve control over high blood pressure and heart disease. Avoid high-potassium foods like bananas and citrus fruits and juices, unless you are also taking medications, such as diuretics, that lower potassium levels.

STORAGE
Keep in a tightly sealed container in a cool, dry place.

IF YOU MISS A DOSE
Take it as soon as you remember. If it is near the time for the next dose, skip the missed dose and resume your regular dosage schedule. Do not double the next dose.

STOPPING THE DRUG
Do not stop taking this drug abruptly, as this may cause potentially serious health problems. Dosage should be reduced gradually, according to your doctor's instructions.

PROLONGED USE
See your doctor regularly for examinations and tests if you must take this medicine for a prolonged period. Remember that enalapril helps control high blood pressure but does not cure it. Lifelong therapy may be necessary.

PRECAUTIONS
Over 60: Some elderly patients may be more sensitive to the effects of this drug; smaller doses may be warranted.

Driving and Hazardous Work: Do not drive or engage in hazardous work until you determine how the medicine affects you.

Alcohol: Consume alcohol only in moderation since it may increase the effect of the drug and cause an excessive drop in blood pressure. Consult your doctor for advice.

Pregnancy: Enalapril use is not recommended, especially during the final 6 months of pregnancy. If you become pregnant, notify your doctor as soon as possible.

Breast Feeding: Trace amounts of enalapril can be found in breast milk; however, adverse effects in infants have not been documented. Consult your doctor for advice.

Infants and Children: Benefits of enalapril use by children must be weighed against risks. Consult your pediatrician for advice.

OVERDOSE
Symptoms: No specific ones have been reported.

What to Do: While overdose is unlikely, call your doctor, emergency medical services (EMS), or the nearest poison control center immediately if you suspect that someone has taken a much larger dose than prescribed.

DRUG INTERACTIONS
Consult your doctor if you are taking diuretics (especially potassium-sparing diuretics), potassium supplements or drugs containing potassium (check ingredient labels), lithium, anticoagulants, anti-inflammatory drugs, or any over-the-counter drugs (especially cold remedies and diet pills).

FOOD INTERACTIONS
Avoid low-salt milk and salt substitutes. Many of these products contain potassium.

DISEASE INTERACTIONS
Consult your doctor if you have systemic lupus erythematosus or if you have had a prior allergic reaction to ACE inhibitors. This medication should be used with caution by patients with severe kidney disease or renal artery stenosis (narrowing of one or both of the arteries that supply blood to the kidneys).

Enalapril Maleate/Diltiazem Malate

BRAND NAME
Teczem

▶ Drug Class: ACE inhibitor/ calcium channel blocker combination

▶ Available in: Extended-release tablets

▶ Available OTC? No

▶ As Generic? No

Side Effects

SERIOUS
Fever and chills; sore throat and hoarseness; sudden difficulty breathing or swallowing; swelling of the face, mouth, or extremities; impaired kidney function (ankle swelling, decreased urination); confusion; yellow discoloration of the eyes or skin (indicating liver disorder); intense itching; chest pain or palpitations; irregular or slow heartbeat, shortness of breath, and fatigue caused by heart failure; abdominal pain. Serious side effects are very rare; contact your doctor immediately.

COMMON
Headache, drowsiness, swelling of feet and ankles, constipation, nausea, sudden weight gain, fatigue, dry, persistent cough.

LESS COMMON
Dizziness or fainting, weakness, depression, nervousness, insomnia, vomiting, diarrhea, excessive urination, skin rash, sensitivity to sunlight, overgrowth of the gums, numbness or tingling in the hands, feet, or lips, unusual muscle weakness, loss of taste.

PRINCIPAL USES
As a secondary treatment for high blood pressure. It is prescribed for people whose blood pressure is not adequately controlled by either enalapril or diltiazem alone and for those taking both drugs separately.

HOW THE DRUG WORKS
Angiotensin-converting enzyme (ACE) inhibitors such as enalapril maleate block an enzyme that produces angiotensin, a naturally occurring substance that causes blood vessels to constrict. Diltiazem, a calcium channel blocker, interferes with the movement of calcium into heart muscle cells and smooth muscle cells in the walls of the arteries. The combined action of enalapril and diltiazem causes blood vessels to relax (causing them to widen), which lowers blood pressure and decreases the workload of the heart.

DOSAGE
Adults: 1 to 4 tablets, each containing 5 mg enalapril and 180 mg diltiazem, in a single dose per day.

ONSET OF EFFECT
Unknown.

DURATION OF ACTION
Unknown.

DIETARY ADVICE
Take enalapril/diltiazem on an empty stomach, about 1 hour before mealtime. Avoid high-potassium foods like bananas and citrus fruits and juices, unless you are also taking medications, such as diuretics, that lower potassium levels.

STORAGE
Store in a tightly sealed container away from heat, moisture, and direct light.

IF YOU MISS A DOSE
If you miss a dose on one day, do not double the dose the next day.

STOPPING THE DRUG
Do not stop taking this drug abruptly, as this may cause potentially serious health problems. Dosage should be reduced gradually.

PROLONGED USE
See your doctor regularly for tests and examinations.

PRECAUTIONS
Over 60: Adverse reactions may be more likely and more severe.

Driving and Hazardous Work: Exercise caution until you determine how the medicine affects you.

Alcohol: Use alcohol with caution because it may increase the effect of the drug and cause an excessive drop in blood pressure.

Pregnancy: This drug can cause injury and even death in the developing fetus. See your doctor and discontinue using the medication as soon as possible when pregnancy is detected.

Breast Feeding: Diltiazem passes into breast milk; avoid use while nursing.

Infants and Children: Safety and effectiveness have not been established for children under 12.

Special Concerns: Brush and floss your teeth and see your dentist regularly, since the diltiazem component may promote dental problems. This drug may make you sensitive to sunlight.

OVERDOSE
Symptoms: None reported. However, heart block (causing shortness of breath), fatigue, excessive dizziness, fainting, and low blood pressure have been attributed to enalapril and diltiazem when taken alone.

What to Do: If someone takes a much larger dose than prescribed, seek medical assistance right away.

DRUG INTERACTIONS
Consult your doctor if you are taking aspirin, beta-blockers, digitalis drugs, carbamazepine, cyclosporine, lithium, oral antidiabetic agents, phenytoin, rifampin, cimetidine, fluvoxamine, ranitidine, diuretics (especially potassium-sparing diuretics), potassium supplements or drugs containing potassium (check ingredient labels), anticoagulants, anti-inflammatory drugs, or any nonprescription drugs (especially cold remedies and diet pills).

FOOD INTERACTIONS
Avoid excessive salt intake. Avoid low-salt milk and salt substitutes. Many of these products contain potassium.

DISEASE INTERACTIONS
Consult your doctor for advice if you have systemic lupus erythematosus or if you have had a prior allergic reaction to ACE inhibitors. This medication should not be used by patients with sick sinus syndrome or heart block (unless a pacemaker is in place), or by those with low blood pressure (hypotension) or history of acute heart attack with lung congestion. This medication should be used with caution by patients with congestive heart failure, liver disease, severe kidney disease, or renal artery stenosis (narrowing of one or both of the arteries that supply blood to the kidneys).

Enalapril Maleate/Felodipine

BRAND NAME
Lexxel

▶ Drug Class: ACE inhibitor/
calcium channel blocker
combination

▶ Available in: Tablets

▶ Available OTC? No

▶ As Generic? No

Side Effects

SERIOUS
Serious side effects are very rare; they include fever and chills, sore throat and hoarseness, sudden difficulty breathing or swallowing, swelling of the face, mouth, or extremities, worsening kidney function (ankle swelling, decreased urination), confusion, jaundice (yellowish tinge to eyes or skin, indicating liver problems), intense itching, chest pain or heart palpitations, abdominal pain, irregular or slow heartbeats, low blood pressure (causing dizziness or faintness). Call your doctor immediately.

COMMON
Mild swelling of arms and legs, fatigue, mild headache, dizziness, cough, flushed skin.

LESS COMMON
Fainting, dry mouth, constipation or diarrhea, gas, nausea, vomiting, rectal pain, gout, neck pain, joint swelling, nervousness, insomnia, sleepiness, skin rash, increased eye pressure, impotence, hot flashes.

PRINCIPAL USES
To control hypertension (high blood pressure).

HOW THE DRUG WORKS
Angiotensin-converting enzyme (ACE) inhibitors such as enalapril maleate block an enzyme that produces angiotensin, a naturally occurring substance that causes blood vessels to constrict and stimulates production of the adrenal hormone, aldosterone, which promotes sodium retention in the body. As a result, ACE inhibitors relax blood vessels (causing them to widen) and reduces sodium retention. Felodipine, a calcium channel blocker, interferes with the movement of calcium into heart muscle cells and the smooth muscle cells in the walls of the arteries. As a result of the combined action of enalapril maleate and felodipine, blood vessels relax (causing them to widen), which lowers blood pressure and thereby decreases the workload of the heart.

DOSAGE
To start, 5 mg once a day. The dose may be increased or decreased gradually by your doctor to 2.5 to 10 mg once a day, as needed. The recommended initial dose for older patients is 2.5 mg a day.

ONSET OF EFFECT
Unknown.

DURATION OF ACTION
Unknown.

DIETARY ADVICE
Enalapril maleate/felodipine is best taken without food. The drug can, however, be taken with grapefruit juice.

STORAGE
Store in a tightly sealed container away from heat, moisture, and direct light.

IF YOU MISS A DOSE
Take it as soon as you remember. If it is near the time for the next dose, skip the missed dose and resume your regular dosage schedule. Do not double the next dose.

STOPPING THE DRUG
The decision to stop taking the drug should be made by your doctor.

PROLONGED USE
See your doctor periodically for tests and examinations.

PRECAUTIONS
Over 60: No special problems are expected.

Driving and Hazardous Work: Avoid such activities until you determine how this medication affects you.

Alcohol: Consume alcohol only in moderation since it may increase the effect of the drug and cause an excessive drop in blood pressure. Consult your doctor for advice.

Pregnancy: Adequate studies have not been done. Before taking enalapril with felodipine, tell your doctor if you are pregnant or plan to become pregnant.

Breast Feeding: This drug passes into breast milk. Discuss with your doctor the relative risks and benefits of using it while nursing.

Infants and Children: The safety and effectiveness of enalapril with felodipine use by infants and children have not been established.

Special Concerns: Enalapril with felodipine is not recommended as the first treatment when high blood pressure is diagnosed. It may be prescribed after other medications have proved unsatisfactory. Before you undergo surgery, tell the doctor or dentist in charge that you are taking this drug.

OVERDOSE
Symptoms: No cases of overdose have been reported.

What to Do: If someone takes a much larger dose than prescribed, call your doctor, emergency medical services (EMS), or the nearest poison control center right away.

DRUG INTERACTIONS
Consult your doctor for specific advice if you are taking diuretics, antihypertensives, lithium, cimetidine, anticonvulsants, or other over-the-counter or prescription medications.

FOOD INTERACTIONS
No known food interactions.

DISEASE INTERACTIONS
Caution is advised when taking enalapril with felodipine. Consult your doctor if you have congestive heart failure (CHF) or any other medical condition. Use of this drug may cause complications in patients with liver or kidney disease, since these organs work together to remove the medication from the body.

Enalapril/Hydrochlorothiazide (HCTZ)

Vaseretic 5/12.5 mg
(MERCK)

▶ Drug Class: Angiotensin-converting enzyme (ACE) inhibitor/diuretic

▶ Available in: Tablets

▶ Available OTC? No

▶ As Generic? No

Side Effects

SERIOUS
Fever and chills, sore throat and hoarseness, sudden difficulty breathing or swallowing, swelling of the face, mouth, or extremities, impaired kidney function (ankle swelling, decreased urination), confusion, yellow discoloration of the eyes or skin (indicating liver disorder), intense itching, chest pain or palpitations, abdominal pain. Serious side effects are very rare; contact your doctor immediately.

COMMON
Dry, persistent cough.

LESS COMMON
Dizziness or fainting, skin rash, numbness or tingling in the hands, feet, or lips, change in color of the hands from white to blue to red (Raynaud's phenomenon) in cold weather, unusual fatigue or muscle weakness, nausea, drowsiness, loss of taste, headache, unusual dreams.

PRINCIPAL USES
To control high blood pressure; to treat congestive heart failure (CHF); to treat patients with left ventricular dysfunction (damage to the pumping chamber of the heart); and to minimize further kidney damage in diabetics with mild kidney disease.

HOW THE DRUG WORKS
Angiotensin-converting enzyme (ACE) inhibitors such as enalapril block an enzyme that produces angiotensin, a naturally occurring substance that causes blood vessels to constrict and stimulates production of the adrenal hormone, aldosterone, which promotes sodium retention in the body. As a result, ACE inhibitors relax blood vessels (causing them to widen) and reduces sodium retention, which lowers blood pressure and so decreases the workload of the heart. Hydrochlorothiazide (HCTZ), a diuretic, increases sodium and water in the urine output. By reducing the overall fluid volume in the body, diuretics reduce blood volume and so reduce blood pressure.

DOSAGE
Adults: 1 to 2 tablets containing 10 mg enalapril and 25 mg hydrochlorothiazide once a day.

ONSET OF EFFECT
Within 1 hour.

DURATION OF ACTION
24 hours.

DIETARY ADVICE
Take on an empty stomach, about 1 hour before mealtime. Follow your doctor's dietary advice (such as low-salt or low-cholesterol restrictions) to improve control over high blood pressure and heart disease.

STORAGE
Store in a tightly sealed container away from heat and direct light.

IF YOU MISS A DOSE
Take it as soon as you remember. If it is near the time for the next dose, skip the missed dose and resume your regular dosage schedule. Do not double the next dose.

STOPPING THE DRUG
Do not stop taking this drug abruptly, as this may cause potentially serious health problems. Dosage should be reduced gradually, according to your doctor's instructions.

PROLONGED USE
See your doctor regularly for examinations and tests if you must take this medication for a prolonged period. Lifelong therapy may be necessary.

PRECAUTIONS
Over 60: Adverse reactions may be more likely and more severe in older patients.

Driving and Hazardous Work: Do not drive or engage in hazardous work until you determine how the medicine affects you.

Alcohol: Consume alcohol only in moderation since it may increase the effect of the drug and cause an excessive drop in blood pressure. Consult your doctor for advice.

Pregnancy: Before taking this medication, tell your doctor if you are pregnant or plan to become pregnant. Use of this drug during the last 6 months of pregnancy may cause severe defects, even death, in the fetus.

Breast Feeding: Enalapril may pass into breast milk; caution is advised. Consult your doctor for specific advice.

Infants and Children: Children may be especially sensitive to the effects of enalapril. Consult your pediatrician about the relative risks and benefits.

OVERDOSE
Symptoms: Overdose has not been reported; symptoms might include dizziness, faintness, or confusion.

What to Do: While overdose is unlikely, call your doctor, emergency medical services (EMS), or the nearest poison control center immediately if you suspect that someone has taken a much larger dose than prescribed.

DRUG INTERACTIONS
Consult your doctor for specific advice if you are taking cholestyramine, colestipol, digitalis drugs, lithium, potassium-containing medicines or supplements, or any over-the-counter drug (especially cold remedies and diet pills).

FOOD INTERACTIONS
Avoid low-salt milk and salt substitutes. Many of these products contain potassium.

DISEASE INTERACTIONS
Consult your doctor if you have systemic lupus erythematosus or if you have had a prior allergic reaction to ACE inhibitors. This medication should be used with caution by patients with severe kidney disease or renal artery stenosis (narrowing of one or both of the arteries that supply blood to the kidneys).

Enoxacin

Generic 400 mg
(RHONE-POULENC RORER)

▸ Drug Class: Fluoroquinolone antibiotic

▸ Available in: Tablets

▸ Available OTC? No

▸ As Generic? No

Side Effects

SERIOUS
Serious reactions are rare and include seizures, confusion, hallucinations, agitation, nightmares, depression, shortness of breath, unusual swelling in the face or extremities, decreased urine output, and loss of consciousness. Also skin burning, redness, blisters, rash, or itching on exposure to sunlight. Call your doctor immediately.

COMMON
Increased sensitivity to sunlight (and increased risk of sunburn) for days following therapy.

LESS COMMON
Diarrhea, nausea and vomiting, stomach pain and upset, gas, headache, dizziness, restlessness, insomnia, changes in taste perception, drowsiness, itching, dry mouth, unusual body aches or pains.

PRINCIPAL USES
To treat bacterial urinary tract infections, including gonorrhea.

HOW THE DRUG WORKS
Enoxacin inhibits the activity of a bacterial enzyme (gyrase) that is necessary for proper DNA formation and replication. This prevents bacteria cells from reproducing.

DOSAGE
For uncomplicated urinary tract infections: 200 mg every 12 hours for 7 days. For severe or complicated urinary tract infections: 400 mg every 12 hours for 14 days. For gonorrhea: 400 mg in a one-time dose. For persons with kidney impairment, doses may be decreased by half.

ONSET OF EFFECT
Varies depending on the infection being treated.

DURATION OF ACTION
Unknown.

DIETARY ADVICE
Take with a full glass of water on an empty stomach, 1 hour before or 2 hours after a meal. Drink plenty of fluids.

STORAGE
Store in a tightly sealed container away from heat, moisture, and direct light.

IF YOU MISS A DOSE
Take it as soon as you remember. If it is near the time for the next dose, skip the missed dose and resume your regular dosage schedule. Do not double the next dose.

STOPPING THE DRUG
Take it as prescribed for the full treatment period, even if you begin to feel better before the scheduled end of therapy.

PROLONGED USE
There are no documented problems with prolonged use, but if you must take this drug for an extended period, see your physician regularly.

PRECAUTIONS
Over 60: No special problems are expected.

Driving and Hazardous Work: Do not drive or engage in hazardous work until you determine how the medicine affects you.

Alcohol: It is advisable to abstain from alcohol when fighting an infection.

Pregnancy: In some animal tests, enoxacin has caused birth defects. Adequate studies in humans have not been done. It should be used during pregnancy only if potential benefits clearly justify the risks. Before you take enoxacin, tell your doctor if you are pregnant or plan to become pregnant.

Breast Feeding: Enoxacin passes into breast milk and may cause serious side effects in the nursing infant; use of the drug is discouraged when nursing.

Infants and Children: Not recommended for use by persons under age 18, as it has been shown to interfere with bone development.

Special Concerns: If enoxacin causes sensitivity to sunlight, stop taking the drug and try to avoid exposure to sunlight for the next 5 days; also wear protective clothing and use a sunblock. Enoxacin should not be taken by patients whose work makes it impossible to stay out of the sun. Avoid smoking. Do not take this medicine if you are allergic

to any quinolone antibiotic. You should avoid people who have an active infection. Refrain from strenuous physical activity while taking this medicine. Be sure to drink at least 8 glasses of water a day while taking enoxacin.

OVERDOSE
Symptoms: No specific ones have been reported.

What to Do: If you have any reason to suspect an overdose, call your doctor, emergency medical services (EMS), or the nearest poison control center.

DRUG INTERACTIONS
Consult your doctor for specific advice if you are taking aminophylline, antacids, didanosine, iron supplements, oxtriphylline, sucralfate, theophylline, warfarin, or zinc salts. Also tell your doctor if you are taking any other prescription or over-the-counter medication.

FOOD INTERACTIONS
The effects of caffeine may be magnified by this drug.

DISEASE INTERACTIONS
Do not use enoxacin if you have a history of hypersensitivity, tendinitis, or tendon rupture associated with the use of enoxacin or any other quinolone antibiotic. Consult your doctor if you have any other medical condition. Use of enoxacin can cause complications in patients with kidney disease, since this organ works to remove the medication from the body.

Enoxaparin Sodium Injection

BRAND NAME
Lovenox

▶ Drug Class: Anticoagulant

▶ Available in: Injection

▶ Available OTC? No

▶ As Generic? No

Side Effects

SERIOUS
Extreme fatigue; abnormal bleeding; bleeding gums; arm or leg bruises; purple or red spots on skin; nosebleeds; black, tarry stools; blood in urine; vomiting of blood. Seek medical assistance immediately.

COMMON
There are no common side effects associated with the enoxaparin use.

LESS COMMON
Nausea, fever, increased menstrual bleeding, confusion, swelling, pain or redness at injection site.

PRINCIPAL USES
To prevent blood clots in the legs after hip or knee replacement surgery, or for other conditions where blood clots could pose a problem.

HOW THE DRUG WORKS
Enoxaparin forms a complex with certain natural body chemicals that prevent clot formation; it also decreases the activity of chemicals that cause clot formation. The combined effect reduces the speed at which blood may coagulate and thus prevents blood clots from developing.

DOSAGE
The appropriate dose will be determined by your doctor and your condition. The usual dosage is 30 mg every 12 hours or 40 mg once a day injected under the skin for 7 to 10 days. It must not be administered intramuscularly or intravenously. Rotate the site of injections from abdomen to thighs to upper arms. After injection, do not massage the site of the injection. Watch for signs of bruising or bleeding at injection sites. Children: Consult your pediatrician for proper dosage.

ONSET OF EFFECT
Within 30 minutes to 3 hours.

DURATION OF ACTION
Up to 24 hours.

DIETARY ADVICE
Injections can be delivered regardless of diet or meal schedule.

STORAGE
Store in a tightly sealed container away from heat and direct light. Do not refrigerate or allow to freeze (for instance, in the trunk of a car during wintertime).

IF YOU MISS A DOSE
Take it as soon as you remember. If it is near the time for the next dose, skip the missed dose and resume your regular dosage schedule. Do not double the next dose.

STOPPING THE DRUG
The decision to stop taking the drug should be made by your doctor.

PROLONGED USE
Enoxaparin should be used only for the period recommended by your doctor.

PRECAUTIONS
Over 60: Older patients may be more susceptible to bleeding during therapy.

Driving and Hazardous Work: Do not drive or engage in hazardous work until you determine how the medicine affects you.

Alcohol: Alcohol should be avoided while taking this medicine.

Pregnancy: Enoxaparin does not appear to cross the placenta. No birth defects have been found in animal studies. Human studies have not been conducted.

Breast Feeding: It is not known if enoxaparin passes into breast milk. Use caution. Consult your doctor for specific advice.

Infants and Children: There is no information about the safety and efficacy of enoxaparin in infants and children. Consult your doctor for specific advice.

Special Concerns: Place used syringes in a disposable, puncture-proof container or follow your doctor's instructions on discarding them. Be sure to tell all doctors and dentists whom you consult that you are using enoxaparin. Before taking enoxaparin, tell your doctor if you have recently given birth, injured your head or body, or had surgery, including dental surgery. Tell your doctor if you are allergic to substances such as pork, preservatives, or dyes.

OVERDOSE
Symptoms: Bleeding complications (such as uncontrolled hemorrhaging).

What to Do: Stop taking enoxaparin, and call your doctor, emergency medical services (EMS), or the nearest poison control center immediately.

DRUG INTERACTIONS
Consult your doctor for specific advice if you are taking aspirin or any other salicylate; inflammation or pain medicine; or drugs that lower blood platelet count, such as famotidine, plicamycin, sulfinpyrazone, ticlopidine, valproic acid, anagrelide, or any other anticoagulant.

FOOD INTERACTIONS
No known food interactions.

DISEASE INTERACTIONS
Caution is advised when taking enoxaparin. Consult your doctor if you have any of the following: blood disease, heart disease, high blood pressure, kidney disease, liver disease, a heart infection, or an ulcer.

Entacapone

BRAND NAME
Comtan

▶ Drug Class: Antiparkinsonism drug/COMT inhibitor

▶ Available in: Tablets

▶ Available OTC? No

▶ As Generic? No

Side Effects

SERIOUS
Dizziness, lightheadedness, or fainting, especially when rising from a sitting or lying position, owing to a sudden drop in blood pressure (orthostatic hypotension). Such symptoms, in addition to nausea, are more common at the beginning of therapy. Hallucinations may also occur and require discontinuation of therapy.

COMMON
Slowed movement, nausea, quirky involuntary muscle movements that may contort the body, discolored urine, abdominal pain, diarrhea.

LESS COMMON
Increased sweating, back pain, anxiety, agitation, drowsiness, vomiting, constipation, dry mouth, indigestion, flatulence, shortness of breath, fatigue, weakness.

PRINCIPAL USES
To treat Parkinson's disease, in conjunction with standard levodopa/carbidopa therapy, in patients who have begun to be less responsive to levodopa and experience worsening symptoms between doses, a phenomenon known as end-of-dose wearing-off.

HOW THE DRUG WORKS
When used with levodopa/carbidopa, entacapone sustains higher levels of levodopa in the blood. Entacapone increases blood levels of levodopa by blocking the action of catechol-O-methyltransferase (COMT), one of the enzymes responsible for breaking down levodopa, before it reaches its receptors in the brain. Levodopa raises the amount of dopamine available in the brain; dopamine plays an essential role in smooth movement of muscles and is deficient in patients with Parkinson's disease.

DOSAGE
Adults: 200 mg in conjunction with each levodopa/carbidopa dose, up to a maximum of 8 times a day (1600 mg a day). Entacapone must be administered with levodopa/carbidopa as entacapone has no antiparkinsonian effect of its own. Patients may require a decrease in their daily dosage of levodopa upon beginning entacapone therapy.

ONSET OF EFFECT
Unknown.

DURATION OF ACTION
Unknown.

DIETARY ADVICE
Entacapone can be taken without regard to meals.

STORAGE
Store in a tightly sealed container away from heat, moisture, and direct light.

IF YOU MISS A DOSE
Take it as soon as you remember. If it is near the time for the next dose, skip the missed dose and resume your regular dosage schedule. Do not double the next dose.

STOPPING THE DRUG
Take it as prescribed for the full treatment period. The decision to stop taking the drug should be made in consultation with your physician. Abrupt discontinuation of entacapone, without a gradual reduction in dose, may increase the risk of adverse effects.

PROLONGED USE
Since Parkinson's disease is a chronic condition, lifelong therapy with entacapone may be required. No special problems are expected.

PRECAUTIONS
Over 60: No specific problems for older people have been reported.

Driving and Hazardous Work: Avoid such activities until you determine how the medicine affects you.

Alcohol: No special precautions are necessary.

Pregnancy: Adequate human studies have not been done. Before taking entacapone, tell your doctor if you are or are planning to become pregnant. Discuss with your doctor the relative risks and benefits of using this drug while pregnant.

Breast Feeding: Entacapone may pass into breast milk; caution is advised. Consult your doctor for specific advice.

Infants and Children: Not applicable. No potential use for entacapone has been identified in children.

Special Concerns: Entacapone may be combined with either the immediate or sustained-release forms of levodopa/carbidopa.

OVERDOSE
Symptoms: An overdose with entacapone is unlikely. However, diarrhea and abdominal pain may occur with an excessive dose.

What to Do: If someone takes a much larger dose than prescribed, call your doctor, emergency medical services (EMS), or the nearest poison control center immediately.

DRUG INTERACTIONS
Consult your doctor for specific advice if you are taking any of the following drugs, which may interact with entacapone: MAO inhibitor antidepressants (such as phenelzine sulfate or tranylcypromine sulfate, but not selegiline), isoproterenol, epinephrine, norepinephrine, dopamine, dobutamine, bitolterol, probenecid, cholestyramine, and some antibiotics (erythromycin, rifampicin, ampicillin, and chloramphenicol).

FOOD INTERACTIONS
No known food interactions.

DISEASE INTERACTIONS
Entacapone should be used with caution in people with liver disease, bile duct obstruction, or low blood pressure.

Ephedrine

▶ Drug Class: Adrenergic
bronchodilator

▶ Available in: Capsules,
injection

▶ Available OTC? Yes

▶ As Generic? Yes

Side Effects

SERIOUS
Irregular heartbeats; hallucinations with high doses; shortness of breath. Call your doctor.

COMMON
Nervousness, rapid heartbeat, paleness, insomnia.

LESS COMMON
Dizziness, loss of appetite, nausea, vomiting, muscle cramps, headache, difficult or painful urination.

PRINCIPAL USES

To relieve bronchial asthma, to decrease nasal and lower respiratory congestion, and to suppress allergic reactions. Ephedrine commonly appears in combination with other drugs in such brand name products as Broncholate, Bronkotuss Expectorant, Quelidrine Cough Formula, and Rynatuss.

HOW THE DRUG WORKS

Ephedrine prevents cells from releasing histamine, a naturally occurring substance that causes swelling, itching, sneezing, watery eyes, hives, and other symptoms of allergic reaction. It also relaxes the smooth muscle surrounding the bronchial tubes, widening the airways, and causes constriction of blood vessels in the nose, which helps to open the nasal passages.

DOSAGE

Capsules— Adults: 25 to 50 mg every 3 or 4 hours, if needed. Children: 3 mg per 2.2 lbs (1 kg) of body weight per day, in 4 to 6 divided doses. Injection— Adults: 1 dose of 12.5 to 25 mg injected into a muscle, a vein, or under the skin. A second dose may be administered if approved by your doctor. Children: 3 mg per 2.2 lbs of body weight a day, in 4 to 6 divided doses.

ONSET OF EFFECT

Capsules: 15 to 60 minutes.
Injection: 10 to 20 minutes.

DURATION OF ACTION

Capsules: 3 to 5 hours.
Injection: 30 minutes to 1 hour after 25 to 50 mg dose.

DIETARY ADVICE

Swallow capsules with water and drink plenty of fluids.

STORAGE

Store in a dry place in a tightly sealed container away from heat and direct light. Keep injection form refrigerated, but do not allow it to freeze. Do not use injection if the liquid is cloudy or unclear.

IF YOU MISS A DOSE

Take it if you remember within 2 hours. If not, skip the missed dose and resume your normal dosage schedule. Do not double the next dose.

STOPPING THE DRUG

You may stop taking this drug at your own discretion. Consult your doctor.

PROLONGED USE

This drug may lose its effectiveness if taken on a continuous basis for 3 to 4 days. Men with an enlarged prostate gland may have difficulty urinating.

PRECAUTIONS

Over 60: Adverse reactions may be more likely and more severe. Small doses are advisable until individual response to the drug has been evaluated.

Driving and Hazardous Work: Ephedrine may cause dizziness. Do not drive or engage in hazardous work until you determine how it affects you.

Alcohol: No special precautions are necessary.

Pregnancy: Consult your doctor; benefits must clearly outweigh risks.

Breast Feeding: Ephedrine passes into breast milk and may be harmful to the child; do not use it while nursing.

Infants and Children: Use caution. Ask your doctor if the benefits of ephedrine justify possible risk to the child.

Special Concerns: Ephedrine can cause insomnia. Take the last dose at least 2 hours before bedtime. Before you take ephedrine, tell your doctor if you will have surgery requiring general anesthesia, including dental surgery, within 2 months.

OVERDOSE

Symptoms: Severe anxiety, convulsions, trouble breathing, coma, confusion, delirium, rapid and irregular pulse, muscle tremors.

What to Do: Call your doctor, emergency medical services (EMS), or the nearest poison control center immediately.

DRUG INTERACTIONS

Consult your doctor for specific advice if you are taking tricyclic antidepressants, high blood pressure medication, beta-blockers, dextrothyroxine, digitalis drugs, ergot-containing preparations, furazolidone, guanadrel, guanethidine, heart medication, methyldopa, MAO inhibitors, nitrates, phenothiazines, pseudoephedrine, rauwolfia alkaloids, sympathomimetic drugs, terazosin, theophylline, or any nonprescription drug for a cough, cold, allergy, or asthma.

FOOD INTERACTIONS

No known food interactions.

DISEASE INTERACTIONS

Caution is advised when taking ephedrine. Consult your doctor if you have any of the following: enlarged prostate, high blood pressure, history of seizures, diabetes, Parkinson's disease, or an overactive thyroid gland.

Epinephrine Hydrochloride

▶ Drug Class: Bronchodilator/sympathomimetic; antiglaucoma agent

▶ Available in: Inhalation aerosols and solutions, injection, eye drops

▶ Available OTC? Yes

▶ As Generic? Yes

Side Effects

SERIOUS
Bluish color of skin, severe dizziness, flushing, and difficulty breathing may indicate an allergic reaction to sulfites in the medication. Contact your doctor immediately.

COMMON
Dry mouth and throat; trembling; headaches. Check with your doctor if these symptoms continue or become bothersome.

LESS COMMON
Eye pain or headache from using eye drops.

PRINCIPAL USES
To treat bronchial asthma, emphysema, and other lung diseases. Epinephrine is also a primary treatment for anaphylaxis; that is, a hypersensitive (allergic) reaction to drugs or other substances. It may also be used to treat nasal congestion, to prolong the action of anesthetics, and to treat cardiac arrest. The ophthalmic form of the drug is used to treat glaucoma.

HOW THE DRUG WORKS
Epinephrine widens constricted airways in the lungs by relaxing smooth muscles that surround bronchial passages. It also raises blood pressure by constricting small blood vessels, increases the heart rate and strength of heart contractions, and decreases fluid pressure in the eye.

DOSAGE
It may be used when needed to relieve breathing difficulty. For adults and children 4 years of age or older with asthma— Inhaled aerosol: 200 micrograms (mcg) to 275 mcg (1 puff), repeated if needed after 1 or 2 minutes, with doses taken at least 3 hours apart. Inhalation solution: 1 puff of 1% solution repeated after 1 or 2 minutes, if needed. Injection: 0.2 to 1 mg, increased if needed. For open-angle glaucoma— 1 or 2 drops of 1% or 2% solution, once or twice daily.

ONSET OF EFFECT
Inhalation: Within 5 minutes. Injection: 1 to 5 minutes.

DURATION OF ACTION
Inhalation: 1 to 3 hours. Injection: 1 to 4 hours.

DIETARY ADVICE
No special concerns.

STORAGE
Store in a tightly sealed container, away from heat, moisture, and direct light.

IF YOU MISS A DOSE
Take your missed dose as soon as you remember, unless the time for your next scheduled dose is within the next 2 hours, in which case skip the missed dose. Take your next scheduled dose at the proper time and resume your regular dosage schedule. Do not take a double dose.

STOPPING THE DRUG
Take the drug exactly as prescribed. Contact your doctor if you do not respond to the strength of the dosage you have been given.

PROLONGED USE
Tolerance to epinephrine may develop with prolonged use.

PRECAUTIONS
Over 60: Adverse reactions may be more likely and more severe in older patients.

Driving and Hazardous Work: Do not drive or engage in hazardous work until you determine how the medicine affects you.

Alcohol: It may increase the excretion of epinephrine in the urine.

Pregnancy: Benefits of taking the drug must outweigh the potential risks; consult your doctor for specific advice.

Breast Feeding: Epinephrine passes into the breast milk. Consult your doctor for specific advice.

Infants and Children: They may be especially sensitive to epinephrine; fainting by children with asthma taking the drug has been reported.

Special Concerns: Do not use without a prescription, unless your problem has been diagnosed as asthma. Take aerosol doses exactly as directed; overuse has caused sudden death. Keep the injectable form ready for use at all times, along with phone numbers of your physician and the local emergency room.

OVERDOSE
Symptoms: Chest discomfort, chills or fever, seizures, dizziness, irregular heartbeat, trouble breathing.

What to Do: Call your doctor, emergency medical services (EMS), or the nearest poison control center immediately.

DRUG INTERACTIONS
Consult your doctor for specific advice if you are taking anesthetics, tricyclic antidepressants, antidiabetic agents, antihypertensives or diuretics, beta-blockers, digitalis drugs, ergoloid mesylates, maprotiline, ergotamine, or MAO inhibitors.

FOOD INTERACTIONS
Avoid any foods that have previously triggered an allergic reaction or asthma attack.

DISEASE INTERACTIONS
The benefits of taking the drug need to be weighed against the potential risks if you have any of the following conditions: organic brain damage, diabetes mellitus, Parkinson's disease, heart or blood vessel disease, or overactive thyroid.

Epoetin Alfa

BRAND NAMES
Epogen, Procrit

▶ Drug Class: Antianemia drug

▶ Available in: Injection

▶ Available OTC? No

▶ As Generic? No

Side Effects

SERIOUS
Chest pain, convulsions, shortness of breath, rapid heartbeat, headache, swelling in the face, hands, and lower extremities, vision problems, unexplained weight gain. Such symptoms are due to an inappropriate elevation of the number of red cells; check with your doctor immediately if such symptoms occur.

COMMON
Influenza-like symptoms, bone pain, burning at the injection site, fatigue. Such symptoms tend to occur at the beginning of therapy but usually diminish as your body adjusts to the medicine. Notify your doctor if such side effects persist or interfere with normal activities.

LESS COMMON
Skin rash, hives.

PRINCIPAL USES
For treating severe anemia due to impaired production of erythropoietin (a hormone that stimulates the bone marrow to produce red blood cells), which may occur with chronic kidney disease, in anemic cancer patients receiving chemotherapy, and anemic HIV-infected patients taking zidovudine.

HOW THE DRUG WORKS
Epoetin alfa stimulates the production of red blood cells in the bone marrow, replacing the hormone erythropoietin, which is depleted in patients suffering from renal (kidney) failure, or who have diseases or take medications that suppress the body's natural erythropoietin production.

DOSAGE
Average dosage range for adults and teenagers: 23 to 68 units per lb of body weight, 3 times a week. May be increased by 11 units per lb every 4 weeks or more, up to 90 units per lb, to produce the desired effect. Once that has been achieved, the dose should be adjusted downward at 4-week intervals to achieve the lowest effective maintenance dose.

ONSET OF EFFECT
Within 2 to 6 weeks.

DURATION OF ACTION
In the presence of impaired erythropoietin production, the drug must be given at least several times per week to maintain its effect.

DIETARY ADVICE
Patients may require iron supplements, but these should be taken only on the advice of a doctor; other vitamins may also be recommended to aid in the manufacture of red blood cells. Patients with kidney problems or high blood pressure are often on restricted diets, which need to be reinforced with vitamin supplementation.

STORAGE
Keep epoetin alfa refrigerated, but do not allow it to freeze.

IF YOU MISS A DOSE
Take it as soon as you remember. If it is near the time for the next dose, skip the missed dose and resume your regular dosage schedule. Do not double the next dose.

STOPPING THE DRUG
Take the drug as prescribed for the full treatment period, in accordance with your doctor's instructions.

PROLONGED USE
Comply with schedules for proper dosage and administration, dialysis, blood tests, and blood pressure tests set by your doctor. If you are performing dialysis at home and self-administering epoetin alfa, follow your doctor's orders carefully and report changes outside of guidelines the doctor has given to you.

PRECAUTIONS
Over 60: Adverse reactions may be more likely and more severe in older patients.

Driving and Hazardous Work: Avoid such activities in the first 90 days of treatment when seizures are most likely to occur.

Alcohol: No special problems are expected.

Pregnancy: Consult your doctor about whether benefits outweigh the potential risk to the unborn child.

Breast Feeding: Epoetin alfa may pass into breast milk; caution is advised. Consult your doctor for specific advice.

Infants and Children: Epoetin alfa is safe for use in children.

Special Concerns: Be sure to follow you doctor's advice, including dietary recommendations and dialysis prescriptions, even if you begin to feel better while taking the drug. Epoetin alfa will correct only anemia, not kidney disease or other medical problems that may be present.

OVERDOSE
Symptoms: Headache, weakness, flushing, dizziness, seizures, chest pain.

What to Do: Call your doctor, emergency medical services (EMS), or the nearest poison control center immediately.

DRUG INTERACTIONS
No known drug interactions.

FOOD INTERACTIONS
No known food interactions.

DISEASE INTERACTIONS
High blood pressure (hypertension) must be controlled before this drug is used. Also, advise your doctor if you have a history of blood clotting disorders, heart or blood vessel disease, blood disorders such as sickle cell anemia, or bone problems.

Ergoloid Mesylates

▶ Drug Class: Psychotherapeutic agent

▶ Available in: Capsules, sublingual tablets, oral solution

▶ Available OTC? No

▶ As Generic? Yes

Side Effects

SERIOUS
No serious side effects
are associated with the
recommended dosage of
ergoloid mesylates.

COMMON
There are no common
side effects.

LESS COMMON
At the recommended
dosage, side effects are
usually rare and remit
when therapy is discon-
tinued. Check with your
doctor if the following
symptoms appear:
drowsiness, slow heart-
beat, dizziness or light-
headedness when getting
up from a sitting or lying
position (orthostatic
hypotension), skin rash,
stomach pain, sensitivity
of eyes to sunlight, soreness under the tongue
(from sublingual tablet)
that does not go away.

PRINCIPAL USES
To treat decline in mental
capacity due to dementia
(progressive breakdown of
mental function).

HOW THE DRUG WORKS
The exact way in which
ergoloid mesylates work
has not been established.

DOSAGE
1 to 2 mg, 3 times a day.
Maximum dose: 12 mg
daily.

ONSET OF EFFECT
Unknown.

DURATION OF ACTION
Unknown.

DIETARY ADVICE
When taking the sublingual
form of the medication, do
not eat, drink, or smoke
while the tablet is dissolving
under your tongue; do not
chew, swallow, or crush it
either.

STORAGE
Store in a tightly sealed container away from heat, moisture, and direct light. Keep
the oral solution form of the
drug refrigerated, but do
not allow it to freeze.

IF YOU MISS A DOSE
Take it as soon as you
remember. However, if it is
near the time for the next
dose, skip the missed dose
and resume your regular
dosage schedule. Do not
double the next dose.

STOPPING THE DRUG
The decision to stop taking
ergoloid mesylates should
be made in consultation
with your doctor.

PROLONGED USE
Regular evaluation by your
doctor is necessary to determine whether or not there
are initial and continuing
therapeutic benefits from
taking ergoloid mesylates;

the medication's effectiveness may not be apparent
for several weeks or even
months.

PRECAUTIONS
Over 60: No special precautions are necessary.

**Driving and Hazardous
Work:** Do not drive or
engage in hazardous work
until you determine how the
medicine affects you.

Alcohol: Avoid alcohol. Be
aware that some over-the-
counter cough, cold, and
allergy medications contain
alcohol; check ingredient
labels carefully.

Pregnancy: Studies of the
use of ergoloid mesylates
during pregnancy have not
been done. Consult your
doctor for specific advice.

Breast Feeding: Studies
of the use of ergoloid mesylates in breast-feeding
women have not been done.
Consult your doctor for
specific advice.

Infants and Children:
Ergoloid mesylates are not
prescribed for children.

Special Concerns: The
therapeutic benefit of
ergoloid mesylates in treating dementia is a matter of
controversy. Some doctors
believe it may be helpful;
others do not.

OVERDOSE
Symptoms: Headache,
blurred vision, dizziness,
fainting, nausea or vomiting,
stomach cramps, flushing,
nasal congestion.

What to Do: Call your
doctor, emergency medical
services (EMS), or the
nearest poison control center immediately.

DRUG INTERACTIONS
Other drugs may interact
with ergoloid mesylates.
Consult your doctor for specific advice if you are taking
any other prescription or
over-the-counter medication.

FOOD INTERACTIONS
No known food interactions.

DISEASE INTERACTIONS
The benefits of the drug
should be weighed against
possible risks for patients
with the following condi-
tions: bradycardia (slow
heartbeat), low blood pressure, or liver disease.
Ergoloid mesylates are not
used to treat acute or
chronic psychosis.

BRAND NAME
Bellergal-S

▶ Drug Class: Antimigraine/antiheadache drug

▶ Available in: Extended-release tablets

▶ Available OTC? No

▶ As Generic? No

Side Effects

SERIOUS
Severe anxiety or confusion; change in vision; chest pain; pale, cold, bluish-colored hands or feet; pain in arms, legs, or lower back; red blisters on hands or feet; gangrene. Seek medical attention immediately.

COMMON
Constipation; swelling of face, fingers, feet, or lower legs; reduced sweating; dizziness or lightheadedness; drowsiness; dry mouth, nose, throat, or skin.

LESS COMMON
Blurred vision; unusual weakness; increased sensitivity of eyes to bright light; diarrhea, nausea, or vomiting; skin rash or itching of skin; sore throat and fever; unusual bruising or bleeding; weakness in legs; yellow discoloration of the eyes or skin; difficulty urinating; difficulty in swallowing; unusual excitability; loss of memory.

PRINCIPAL USES
Used to prevent vascular headaches (those involving the blood vessels to the brain), such as migraines and cluster headaches. Also used to ease symptoms of menopause, such as hot flashes, sweating, restlessness, and insomnia, usually in women for whom estrogen replacement therapy has been ruled out.

HOW THE DRUG WORKS
The above conditions are believed to be caused, in part, by overactivity in the autonomic nervous system, the part that controls involuntary body functions like heart rate, sweating, and digestion. The combination of ergotamine, belladonna alkaloids, and phenobarbital helps to balance and calm this part of the nervous system, thus reducing various kinds of physical distress.

DOSAGE
Adults: 1 tablet in the morning and 1 in the evening. Children: Consult pediatrician. Tablet must be taken whole.

ONSET OF EFFECT
Unknown.

DURATION OF ACTION
Unknown.

DIETARY ADVICE
No special concerns.

STORAGE
Store in a tightly sealed container, away from heat, moisture, and direct light.

IF YOU MISS A DOSE
Skip the missed dose and then resume your regular dosage schedule. Do not double the next dose.

STOPPING THE DRUG
The decision to stop taking the drug should be made by your doctor. Discontinue the drug in gradually diminishing doses, according to your doctor's instructions, to minimize the risk of withdrawal symptoms.

PROLONGED USE
Prolonged use at high doses may produce some degree of physical dependence due to the barbiturate, phenobarbital, and may increase the risk of blood circulation problems.

PRECAUTIONS
Over 60: Adverse reactions may be more likely and more severe in older patients.

Driving and Hazardous Work: Do not drive or engage in hazardous work until you determine how the drug affects you.

Alcohol: Avoid alcohol.

Pregnancy: Do not take the drug combination during pregnancy. Consult your doctor if you become or plan to become pregnant.

Breast Feeding: The drug combination passes into breast milk; avoid or discontinue use while nursing.

Infants and Children: Adverse reactions may be more likely and more severe.

Special Concerns: Avoid smoking, since it may increase the risk of side effects associated with impaired blood circulation. Dress warmly if you have blood circulation problems (most common among elderly patients).

OVERDOSE
Symptoms: Convulsions; severe diarrhea, nausea, vomiting, or stomach pain or bloating; severe dizziness, drowsiness, or weakness; rapid or slow heartbeat; shortness of breath; unusual excitement.

What to Do: Call your doctor, emergency medical services (EMS), or the nearest poison control center immediately.

DRUG INTERACTIONS
Do not take this drug if you are taking naratriptan, sumatriptan, or zolmitriptan. Consult your doctor for specific advice if you are taking antacids, anticoagulants, anticholinergics, carbamazepine, central nervous system depressants, diarrhea medication, digitalis drugs, ketoconazole, MAO inhibitors, other ergot medications, oral contraceptives, potassium chloride, or tricyclic antidepressants.

FOOD INTERACTIONS
No known food interactions.

DISEASE INTERACTIONS
Consult your doctor if you have any of the following: chronic lung disease such as asthma or emphysema, difficult urination, urinary tract blockage, Down's syndrome, enlarged prostate, heart, kidney, or liver disease, blood vessel disease or recent surgery on blood vessels, severe high blood pressure, infection, intestinal conditions, overactive thyroid, porphyria, glaucoma, severe dry mouth, severe itching. In children: brain damage, hyperactivity, spastic paralysis.

▶ Drug Class: Erythromycin antibiotic

▶ Available in: Oral suspension

▶ Available OTC? No

▶ As Generic? Yes

Side Effects

SERIOUS
Skin rash, itching, aching joints and muscles, difficulty swallowing, pale skin or red, blistered, peeling, or loose skin, sore throat and fever, unusual bleeding or bruising, unusual fatigue, yellowish tinge to the eyes or skin, blood in urine, darkened urine, pain in lower back, pain while urinating, pale stools, stomach pain, swollen neck, increased sensitivity to sunlight. Call your doctor immediately.

COMMON
Stomach or abdominal discomfort and cramps, diarrhea, loss of appetite, nausea, vomiting.

LESS COMMON
Sore tongue or mouth.

PRINCIPAL USES
To treat middle ear infections in children.

HOW THE DRUG WORKS
Erythromycin prevents bacterial cells from manufacturing specific proteins necessary for their survival; sulfisoxazole prevents bacteria from utilizing folic acid, a vitamin essential to both cell growth and reproduction.

DOSAGE
Children weighing more than 100 lbs: 2 teaspoons (10 ml) 4 times a day for 10 days. Children weighing 53 to 100 lbs: 1 1/2 tsps (7.5 ml) 4 times a day for 10 days. Children weighing 35 to 53 lbs: 1 tsp (5 ml) 4 times a day for 10 days. Children weighing 18 to 35 lbs: 1/2 tsp (2.5 ml) 4 times a day for 10 days. Children under 18 lbs: The dose must be determined by your pediatrician.

ONSET OF EFFECT
Unknown.

DURATION OF ACTION
Unknown.

DIETARY ADVICE
Give it 1 hour before or 2 hours after meals with a full glass of water. If it causes stomach upset, it can be taken with milk or food. Increase patient's fluid intake.

STORAGE
Store in a tightly sealed container away from heat and direct light. Refrigerate but do not freeze.

IF YOU MISS A DOSE
Give it as soon as you remember. If it is close to the time for the next dose, skip the missed dose and resume the regular dosage schedule. Do not double the next dose.

STOPPING THE DRUG
Give the medicine as prescribed for the full treatment period, even if the child begins to feel better before the scheduled end of therapy.

PROLONGED USE
Your child should see a doctor regularly for tests and examinations if this medicine is prescribed for a prolonged period. Bacteria that are resistant to this medication may develop with long-term use.

PRECAUTIONS
Over 60: This medication is not intended for use by older persons.

Driving and Hazardous Work: This medication should not impair mental alertness or physical coordination.

Alcohol: Not applicable; this drug is for children.

Pregnancy: Adequate studies of the use of this drug during pregnancy have not been done; consult your doctor for specific advice if there is any chance that the patient could become pregnant.

Breast Feeding: Not applicable; the drug is for children.

Infants and Children: This medicine is not recommended for children under 2 months of age.

Special Concerns: If the medicine causes sensitivity to sunlight, take preventive measures: patients should use sunscreens, wear protective clothing, and avoid exposure to sunlight.

OVERDOSE
Symptoms: Severe nausea, vomiting, diarrhea, dizziness, headache, drowsiness, fever, loss of consciousness.

What to Do: Overdose is not likely, but if symptoms occur, call your doctor, emergency medical services (EMS), or the nearest poison control center immediately.

DRUG INTERACTIONS
This drug may interact with acetaminophen, acetohydroxamic acid, alfentanil, amiodarone, aminophylline, oral antidiabetics, carbamazepine, carmustine, chloramphenicol, chloroquine, cholesterol-lowering drugs, dantrolene, dapsone, daunorubicin, divalproex, estrogens, ethotoin, etretinate, gold salts, hydroxychloroquine, lincomycin, methenamine, mephenytoin, methotrexate, mercaptopurine, methyldopa, naltrexone, nitrofurantoin, oral contraceptives, phenytoin, plicamycin, primaquine, procainamide, quinidine, quinine, sulfoxone, or vitamin K. Consult your doctor for specific advice.

FOOD INTERACTIONS
Avoid caffeinated beverages or food.

DISEASE INTERACTIONS
Consult your doctor if the patient has any of the following: anemia or another blood problem, G6PD deficiency, kidney disease, liver disease, hearing loss, or porphyria.

Erythromycin Ophthalmic

BRAND NAME
Ilotycin

▶ Drug Class: Antibiotic

▶ Available in: Ophthalmic ointment

▶ Available OTC? No

▶ As Generic? Yes

Side Effects

SERIOUS
Eye irritation, redness, swelling, or itching that was not present before therapy. Stop using the medication and call your doctor immediately.

COMMON
Blurred vision for up to 30 minutes following application.

LESS COMMON
There are no less-common side effects associated with ophthalmic erythromycin.

PRINCIPAL USES
To treat infections of the eye; to treat inflammation of the edges of the eyelids (blepharitis); to prevent some eye infections in newborn babies (neonatal conjunctivitis and ophthalmia neonatorum).

HOW THE DRUG WORKS
Erythromycin kills bacteria by interfering with the genetic material of bacterial cells, thereby preventing them from multiplying.

DOSAGE
Adults and children— For eye infections: Apply ointment to the affected eye up to 6 times a day, as directed by your doctor. For blepharitis: Apply once a day immediately before bedtime after performing standard eyelid hygiene measures as directed by your doctor. To prevent eye infections in newborns— Ointment is applied once, shortly after birth.

ONSET OF EFFECT
Unknown.

DURATION OF ACTION
Unknown.

DIETARY ADVICE
This medication can be used without regard to diet.

STORAGE
Store in a tightly sealed container away from heat, moisture, and direct light. Do not allow it to freeze.

IF YOU MISS A DOSE
Apply it as soon as you remember. If it is near the time for the next dose, skip the missed dose and resume your regular dosage schedule. Do not double the next dose.

STOPPING THE DRUG
Use it as prescribed for the full treatment period, even if you feel better before the scheduled end of therapy.

PROLONGED USE
You should see your doctor regularly for tests and examinations if you take this drug for a prolonged period.

PRECAUTIONS
Over 60: No special problems are expected.

Driving and Hazardous Work: Do not drive or engage in hazardous work until you determine how the medicine affects your vision.

Alcohol: No special precautions are necessary.

Pregnancy: Erythromycin has not been shown to cause birth defects or other problems during pregnancy. Before using erythromycin, tell your doctor if you are pregnant or are planning to become pregnant.

Breast Feeding: Erythromycin has not been shown to cause problems in nursing babies.

Infants and Children: No special precautions.

Special Concerns: To use the ointment, first wash your hands. Tilt your head back. Gently apply pressure to the inside corner of the eyelid and with the index finger of the same hand, pull downward on the lower eyelid to make a space. Put a short strip of ointment (about ⅓ inch long) into this space and close your eye. Apply pressure for 1 or 2 minutes while keeping the eye closed without blinking. Then wash your hands again. Make sure that the tip of the applicator does not touch your eye, finger, or any other surface. If your symptoms do not improve in a few days or if they become worse, check with your doctor. Do not use this drug if you have a history of allergy to azithromycin, clarithromycin, erythromycin, or lincomycin.

OVERDOSE
Symptoms: No specific ones have been reported.

What to Do: If someone accidentally ingests the medicine, call your doctor, emergency medical services (EMS), or the nearest poison control center.

DRUG INTERACTIONS
Other drugs may interact with ophthalmic erythromycin. Consult your doctor for specific advice if you are taking any other prescription or over-the-counter medication.

FOOD INTERACTIONS
No known food interactions.

DISEASE INTERACTIONS
Caution is advised when taking ophthalmic erythromycin. Consult your doctor if you have any other medical condition.

Erythromycin Systemic

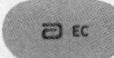

Ery-Tab 250 mg
(ABBOTT)

Additional photographs

▶ Drug Class: Erythromycin antibiotic

▶ Available in: Capsules, tablets, oral suspension, injection

▶ Available OTC? No

▶ As Generic? Yes

Side Effects

SERIOUS

Fever, nausea, skin reddening or itching, severe stomach pain, yellow discoloration of the eyes or skin, fainting, slow or irregular heartbeat in patients with predisposing heart conditions, breathing difficulty, persistent or severe diarrhea, abdominal pain, temporary deafness. Also pain, swelling, or redness at injection site. Although serious side effects are rare, call your doctor immediately.

COMMON

Stomach cramps and abdominal discomfort, diarrhea, nausea, vomiting.

LESS COMMON

Soreness of mouth or tongue, vaginal itching or discharge.

PRINCIPAL USES

To treat bacterial infections, including throat infections, pneumonia, Legionnaires' disease, chlamydia, and diphtheria. It is also prescribed to prevent strep infections that may damage heart valves in susceptible patients (for example, those with a history of rheumatic fever or heart valve replacement) who are allergic to penicillin.

HOW THE DRUG WORKS

Erythromycin prevents bacterial cells from manufacturing specific proteins necessary for their survival.

DOSAGE

To treat infections— Adults and teenagers: 250 to 800 mg, 2 to 4 times a day. Children: 3.4 to 12.5 mg per lb of body weight, 2 to 4 times a day. To prevent strep infections— Adults and teenagers: 1 to 1.6 g before dental appointment or surgery; 500 to 800 mg, 6 hours later. Children: 1.7 to 11.4 mg per lb of body weight before dental appointment or surgery; 4.5 mg per lb of body weight 6 hours later.

ONSET OF EFFECT

Immediate after injection; unknown for oral forms.

DURATION OF ACTION

Unknown.

DIETARY ADVICE

This drug is best taken on an empty stomach, at least 1 hour before or 2 hours after meals, with a full glass of water. If it causes stomach upset, it can be taken with food or milk.

STORAGE

Store in a tightly sealed container away from heat and direct light. Refrigerate liquid form but do not freeze.

IF YOU MISS A DOSE

Take it as soon as you remember. If it is near the time for the next dose, skip the missed dose and resume your regular dosage schedule. Do not double the next dose.

STOPPING THE DRUG

Take it as prescribed for the full treatment period, even if you begin to feel better before the scheduled end of therapy.

PROLONGED USE

You should see your doctor regularly for tests and examinations, including those to evaluate liver function, if this medicine is taken for a prolonged period.

PRECAUTIONS

Over 60: Older patients may be at higher risk of experiencing hearing loss as a side effect.

Driving and Hazardous Work: No special precautions are necessary.

Alcohol: No special precautions are necessary.

Pregnancy: Erythromycin has been shown to cause liver damage in some pregnant women. It has not been shown to cause birth defects or other problems in babies. Before taking erythromycin, tell your doctor if you are pregnant or plan to become pregnant.

Breast Feeding: Erythromycin passes into breast milk; caution is advised. Consult your doctor for specific advice.

Infants and Children: No special problems expected.

Special Concerns: Consult your doctor if your symptoms do not improve, or instead become worse, after a few days of therapy.

OVERDOSE

Symptoms: Severe nausea, vomiting, abdominal pain, diarrhea, dizziness, loss of hearing.

What to Do: Call your doctor, emergency medical services (EMS), or the nearest poison control center immediately.

DRUG INTERACTIONS

Do not use erythromycin if you are taking astemizole. Consult your doctor for specific advice if you are taking acetaminophen, amiodarone, anabolic steroids, androgens, antibiotics, azithromycin, carbamazepine, carmustine, chloramphenicol, chloroquine, clarithromycin, cyclosporine, dantrolene, daunorubicin, disulfiram, divalproex, estrogens, etretinate, gold salts, hydroxychloroquine, lincomycin, methotrexate, mercaptopurine, methyldopa, naltrexone, oral contraceptives, phenothiazines, phenytoin, plicamycin, theophylline, valproic acid, warfarin, tacrolimus, disopyramide, lovastatin, or bromocriptine.

FOOD INTERACTIONS

No known food interactions.

DISEASE INTERACTIONS

Use of this drug is not advised in patients with a history of heart rhythm disorders, kidney disease, liver disease, or hearing problems. Consult your doctor.

Esomeprazole Magnesium

BRAND NAME
Nexium

▶ Drug Class: Antacid/proton pump inhibitor

▶ Available in: Delayed-release capsules

▶ Available OTC? No

▶ As Generic? No

Side Effects

SERIOUS
No serious side effects are associated with this medication.

COMMON
Headache, diarrhea, constipation, nausea, dry mouth, dizziness, stomach pain. Consult your physician if such side effects persist or interfere with daily activities.

LESS COMMON
Many less common side effects can occur; consult your doctor if you are concerned about any adverse or unusual reactions you experience while taking this drug.

PRINCIPAL USES
To treat erosive esophagitis (severe, chronic inflammation of the esophagus) and gastroesophageal reflux (backwash of stomach acid into the esophagus, resulting in heartburn); in combination with amoxicillin and clarithromycin, to reduce the risk of recurrence of duodenal (intestinal) ulcers caused by the bacteria *Helicobacter pylori*.

HOW THE DRUG WORKS
Esomeprazole blocks the action of a specific enzyme in the cells that line the stomach, thereby decreasing the production of stomach acid. Reduction of stomach acid promotes healing of ulcers.

DOSAGE
To treat active erosive esophagitis: 20 or 40 mg a day for 4 to 8 weeks. Maintenance dose for esophagitis: 20 mg a day. To treat gastroesophageal reflux: 20 mg a day for 4 weeks. To reduce risk of duodenal ulcer recurrence: 40 mg esomeprazole a day for 10 days, 1,000 mg amoxicillin twice a day for 10 days, and 500 mg clarithromycin twice a day for 10 days.

ONSET OF EFFECT
Unknown.

DURATION OF ACTION
Unknown.

DIETARY ADVICE
Esomeprazole should be swallowed whole at least one hour before eating. If you have trouble swallowing the pills, mix the contents of the capsules in with food such as applesauce. The applesauce/drug mixture should be swallowed without chewing.

STORAGE
Store in a tightly sealed container away from heat and direct light.

IF YOU MISS A DOSE
Take it as soon as you remember. If it is near the time for the next dose, skip the missed dose and resume your regular dosage schedule. Do not double the next dose.

STOPPING THE DRUG
Take it as prescribed for the full treatment period, even if you begin to feel better before the scheduled end of therapy. The decision to stop taking the drug should be made by your doctor.

PROLONGED USE
Esomeprazole should not be used indefinitely as maintenance therapy for duodenal ulcer or esophagitis; it is generally taken for a limited period of 4 to 8 weeks. Do not take it for a longer period unless instructed to do so by your doctor. See your doctor regularly for tests and examinations if you must take this drug for an extended period of time.

PRECAUTIONS
Over 60: No specific problems for older people have been reported.

Driving and Hazardous Work: Do not drive or engage in hazardous activities until you determine how the drug affects you.

Alcohol: Avoid alcohol while taking this medication, as it may aggravate your condition.

Pregnancy: In animal tests, esomeprazole has not caused problems. Human tests have not been done. Before you take esomeprazole, tell your doctor if you are pregnant or plan to become pregnant.

Breast Feeding: Esomeprazole may pass into breast milk; caution is advised. Consult your doctor for advice.

Infants and Children: Safety and effectiveness have not been established for patients under 18 years of age.

Special Concerns: Tell any doctor or dentist whom you see for treatment that you are taking esomeprazole. If your doctor directs, you may take an antacid along with esomeprazole.

OVERDOSE
Symptoms: No cases of overdose have been reported. However, symptoms may include: blurred vision, confusion, profuse sweating, drowsiness, dry mouth, flushing of the face, headache, nausea, palpitations or unusually rapid heartbeat.

What to Do: Call your doctor, emergency medical services (EMS), or the nearest poison control center immediately.

DRUG INTERACTIONS
Consult your doctor for specific advice if you are taking: ampicillin, sucralfate, iron salts or supplements, cyclosporine, diazepam, disulfiram, ketoconazole, digoxin, or theophylline.

FOOD INTERACTIONS
No significant food interactions have been reported.

DISEASE INTERACTIONS
Caution is advised when taking esomeprazole. Consult your doctor if you have severe liver disease, since it may increase the risk of side effects.

281

Estazolam

ProSom 1 mg
(ABBOTT)

▸ Drug Class: Benzodiazepine tranquilizer

▸ Available in: Tablets

▸ Available OTC? No

▸ As Generic? Yes

Side Effects

SERIOUS
Difficulty concentrating, outbursts of anger, other behavior problems, depression, seizures, hallucinations, low blood pressure (causing faintness or confusion), memory impairment, muscle weakness, skin rash or itching, sore throat, fever and chills, sores or ulcers in throat or mouth, unusual bruising or bleeding, extreme fatigue, yellowish tinge to eyes or skin. Call your doctor immediately.

COMMON
Drowsiness, loss of coordination, unsteady gait, dizziness, lightheadedness, slurred speech.

LESS COMMON
Change in sexual desire or ability, constipation, false sense of well-being, nausea and vomiting, urinary problems, unusual fatigue.

PRINCIPAL USES
To treat insomnia.

HOW THE DRUG WORKS
In general, estazolam produces a mild sedative effect by depressing activity in the central nervous system (the brain and spinal cord). In particular, estazolam appears to enhance the effect of gamma-aminobutyric acid (GABA), a natural chemical that inhibits the firing of neurons and dampens the transmission of nerve signals, thus decreasing nervous excitation.

DOSAGE
Adults: 1 or 2 mg taken at bedtime.

ONSET OF EFFECT
Unknown.

DURATION OF ACTION
Unknown.

DIETARY ADVICE
No special restrictions.

STORAGE
Store in a tightly sealed container away from heat and direct light.

IF YOU MISS A DOSE
Take it as soon as you remember, unless it is late at night. Do not take the medicine unless your schedule permits a full night's sleep.

STOPPING THE DRUG
The decision to stop taking the drug should be made in consultation with your doctor. Stopping it abruptly may cause withdrawal symptoms.

PROLONGED USE
Estazolam can lead to psychological or physical dependence. Short-term therapy (8 weeks or less) is typical; do not take it for a longer period unless so advised by your doctor.

Never take more than the prescribed daily dose.

PRECAUTIONS
Over 60: Adverse reactions are more likely and more severe. A lower dose may be warranted.

Driving and Hazardous Work: Estazolam can impair mental alertness and physical coordination. Adjust your activities accordingly.

Alcohol: Avoid alcohol.

Pregnancy: Estazolam should not be used during the first 3 months (first trimester) of pregnancy and only with great caution and close medical supervision later in pregnancy. Overuse of estazolam during pregnancy may cause drug dependence in the unborn child.

Breast Feeding: Estazolam passes into breast milk; do not take it while nursing.

Infants and Children: Safety and effectiveness have not been determined for children under age 18.

Special Concerns: Estazolam use can lead to psychological or physical dependence.

OVERDOSE
Symptoms: Extreme drowsiness, confusion, slurred speech, slow reflexes, poor coordination, staggering gait, tremor, slowed breathing, loss of consciousness.

What to Do: Call your doctor, emergency medical services (EMS), or the nearest poison control center immediately.

DRUG INTERACTIONS
Other drugs may interact with estazolam. Consult your doctor for specific advice if you are taking any drugs that depress the central nervous system; these include antihistamines, antidepressants or other psychiatric medications, barbiturates, sedatives, cough medicines, decongestants, and painkillers. Be sure your doctor knows about any over-the-counter medication you may take.

FOOD INTERACTIONS
None reported.

DISEASE INTERACTIONS
Caution is advised when taking estazolam. Consult your doctor if you have a history of alcohol or drug abuse, stroke or other brain disease, any chronic lung disease, hyperactivity, depression or other mental illness, myasthenia gravis, sleep apnea, epilepsy, porphyria, kidney disease, or liver disease.

Estradiol

▶ Drug Class: Female sex
   hormone

▶ Available in: Tablets, skin
   patch, vaginal cream,
   injection

▶ Available OTC? No

▶ As Generic? Yes

Side Effects

SERIOUS
For men being treated for
prostate cancer: Sudden
or severe headache, loss
of coordination, sudden
changes in vision, pains
in chest, groin, or leg,
shortness of breath, slurring of speech, weakness
or numbness in arm or
leg. For women: Breast
pain or enlargement,
swelling of legs and feet,
rapid weight gain. Call
your doctor immediately.

COMMON
Abdominal bloating,
stomach cramps, loss of
appetite, skin irritation at
site of patch.

LESS COMMON
Diarrhea, dizziness,
headaches, discomfort
when wearing contact
lenses, decreased sexual
desire in men, increased
sexual desire in women,
vomiting.

PRINCIPAL USES
To provide estrogen when
the body does not produce
enough; to treat carefully
selected cases of advanced
breast cancer; to reduce
risk of osteoporosis after
menopause; to ease
unpleasant symptoms of
menopause, including
vaginal dryness; to prevent
breast engorgement following childbirth; to ease
symptoms of advanced
prostate cancer.

HOW THE DRUG WORKS
In women, estradiol
replaces deficient natural
levels of estrogen in the
body. In men, the hormone
inhibits growth of cells in
the prostate gland.

DOSAGE
To treat breast cancer: 10
mg, 3 times a day. For postmenopausal vaginal dryness
or prevention of osteoporosis: 1 to 2 mg a day of oral
form, or 10 to 20 mg
injected every 4 weeks, or 1
Estraderm, Alora, or Vivelle
patch (0.05 mg) 2 times a
week or 1 Climara patch
weekly. A progestin should
also be taken for 10 to 14
days in each month of use,
except in women who have
had a hysterectomy. To
relieve postmenopausal
vaginal dryness using
intravaginal estrogen
creams: To start, ½ to 1
applicatorful daily and
tapered to 1 applicatorful 1
to 3 times weekly. To treat
menopausal symptoms: 1 to
5 mg injected every 3 to 4
weeks. To prevent breast
engorgement after child-
birth: 10 to 25 mg injected
in a muscle at the time of
delivery. To treat prostate
cancer: 1 to 2 mg, 3 times
daily.

ONSET OF EFFECT
Within 1 hour.

DURATION OF ACTION
Up to 24 hours.

DIETARY ADVICE
No special restrictions.

STORAGE
Keep in a tightly sealed container away from heat and
direct light.

IF YOU MISS A DOSE
Take the missed dose as
soon as you remember. If it
is near time for the next
dose, skip the missed dose
and resume your regular
dosage schedule. Do not
double the next dose.

STOPPING THE DRUG
The decision to stop taking
the drug should be made in
consultation with your
physician.

PROLONGED USE
May increase the risk of
endometrial cancer and perhaps breast cancer. Consult
your doctor about periodic
examinations and other
measures to help prevent
these diseases.

PRECAUTIONS
Over 60: No special problems are expected.

**Driving and Hazardous
Work:** Do not drive or
engage in hazardous work
until you determine how the
medicine affects you.

Alcohol: No special precautions are necessary.

Pregnancy: Not recom-
mended during pregnancy;
estrogens have been shown
to cause birth defects in animals and humans.

Breast Feeding: Do not
use estradiol while nursing.

Infants and Children:
Estradiol is not recom-
mended for use by young

patients in whom bone
growth is not complete.

Special Concerns:
Swelling or bleeding of the
gums may occur; see your
dentist regularly. Do not
apply a patch to the same
site more than once a week.

OVERDOSE
Symptoms: Nausea, unexpected vaginal bleeding.

What to Do: An overdose
of estradiol is unlikely to
occur. However, if someone
takes a much larger dose
than prescribed, seek medical assistance immediately.

DRUG INTERACTIONS
Consult your doctor for
specific advice if you are
taking acetaminophen,
amiodarone, anticonvul-
sants, anti-infective drugs,
antithyroid agents, carmustine, chloroquine, dantrolene, daunorubicin, gold
salts, divalproex, etretinate,
hydroxychloroquine, mer-
captopurine, methotrexate,
oral contraceptives, methyldopa, naltrexone, pheno-
thiazines, plicamycin,
steroids, bromocriptine
or cyclosporine.

FOOD INTERACTIONS
No known food interactions.

DISEASE INTERACTIONS
You should not take estradiol if you have blood clot
disorders, breast cancer,
any hormone-dependent
cancer, or abnormal genital
bleeding.

Estramustine Phosphate Sodium

BRAND NAME
Emcyt

▶ Drug Class: Antineoplastic (anticancer) agent

▶ Available in: Capsules

▶ Available OTC? No

▶ As Generic? No

Side Effects

SERIOUS
Black, tarry stools, blood in urine or stools, cough or hoarseness, fever or chills, severe or sudden headaches, sudden loss of coordination, pain in lower back or side, pain in chest, groin, or leg, painful urination, red spots on skin, sudden shortness of breath, sudden slurred speech, unusual bleeding or bruising, sudden changes in vision, weakness or numbness in arm or leg, skin rash, or fever. Call your doctor or emergency medical services (EMS) immediately.

COMMON
Breast tenderness or enlargement, swelling of feet or lower legs, decreased sexual desire, diarrhea, nausea, general weakness.

LESS COMMON
Insomnia, vomiting.

PRINCIPAL USES
To treat some types of prostate cancer.

HOW THE DRUG WORKS
Estramustine is a combination of two drugs: a form of estrogen (estradiol) and mechlorethamine (nitrogen mustard). It is uncertain precisely how the drug works, but it appears to kill cancer cells by interfering with the synthesis of their genetic material and blocking the activity of hormones and proteins that certain types of prostate tumors need in order to grow.

DOSAGE
10 to 16 mg per 2.2 lbs (1 kg) of body weight daily in 3 or 4 doses.

ONSET OF EFFECT
Unknown.

DURATION OF ACTION
Unknown.

DIETARY ADVICE
Best taken with water 1 hour before or 2 hours after meals. Milk, milk products, or calcium-rich foods should not be taken simultaneously.

STORAGE
Store in a tightly sealed container away from heat and direct light.

IF YOU MISS A DOSE
Take it as soon as you remember. If it is near the time for the next dose, skip the missed dose and resume your regular dosage schedule. Do not double the next dose.

STOPPING THE DRUG
The decision to stop taking the drug should be made in consultation with your physician.

PROLONGED USE
You should see your doctor regularly for tests and examinations if you take this drug for a prolonged period.

PRECAUTIONS
Over 60: Side effects tend to occur more commonly in patients over 60.

Driving and Hazardous Work: Do not drive or engage in hazardous work until you determine how the medicine affects you.

Alcohol: Avoid alcohol while taking this drug.

Pregnancy: Estramustine can cause birth defects if the father is taking it at the time of conception. Before taking estramustine, tell your doctor if you intend to have children; while taking it, a reliable barrier method of birth control is advised.

Breast Feeding: Not applicable for this drug.

Infants and Children: Estramustine is not intended for use in infants and children.

Special Concerns: If you vomit shortly after taking a dose of estramustine, ask your doctor if you should take the dose again or wait for the next scheduled dose. During and after treatment with estramustine, do not get immunized against bacteria or viruses without your doctor's approval. Avoid persons who have recently taken oral polio vaccine. If you must be close to them, consider wearing a protective mask that covers both the nose and mouth.

OVERDOSE
Symptoms: Severe and exaggerated side effects (see Side Effects).

What to Do: Call your doctor, emergency medical services (EMS), or the nearest poison control center immediately.

DRUG INTERACTIONS
Consult your doctor for specific advice if you are taking acetaminophen, amiodarone, anabolic steroids, androgens, antibiotics, antithyroid agents, carbamazepine, carmustine, chloroquine, dantrolene, disulfiram, divalproex, estrogens, etretinate, gold salts, hydrochloroquine, mercaptopurine, methyldopa, naltrexone, phenothiazines, phenytoin, plicamycin, or valproic acid.

FOOD INTERACTIONS
See dietary advice.

DISEASE INTERACTIONS
Caution is advised when taking estramustine. Consult your doctor if you have any of the following: asthma, epilepsy, mental depression, migraine headaches, kidney disease, history of blood clots, history of stroke, a recent heart attack, shingles, diabetes, gallbladder disease, heart or blood vessel disease, liver disease, or a stomach ulcer.

Estrogens, Conjugated

BRAND NAMES
Cenestin, Premarin

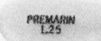

Premarin 1.25 mg
(WYETH-AYERST)

Additional photographs

▶ Drug Class: Female sex hormone

▶ Available in: Tablets, injection, vaginal cream

▶ Available OTC? No

▶ As Generic? Yes

Side Effects

SERIOUS
Women: Breast pain or enlargement; swelling of legs and feet; rapid weight gain. Men being treated for prostate cancer: Sudden or severe headache; loss of coordination; sudden changes in vision; pains in chest, groin, or leg; sudden shortness of breath; slurred speech; weakness or numbness in arm or leg. Call your doctor immediately.

COMMON
Abdominal bloating or cramps, loss of appetite, breast tenderness.

LESS COMMON
Diarrhea, dizziness, headaches, discomfort when wearing contact lenses, decreased sexual desire in men, increased sexual desire in women, vomiting.

PRINCIPAL USES
To provide estrogen after the menopause, when the body produces too little; to treat carefully selected cases of advanced breast cancer; to reduce risk of osteoporosis after menopause; to ease unpleasant symptoms of menopause, including vaginal dryness; to prevent breast engorgement following childbirth; or to ease symptoms of advanced prostate cancer.

HOW THE DRUG WORKS
In women, conjugated estrogens replace deficient natural levels of estrogen in the body. In men, estrogens inhibit growth of cells in the prostate gland.

DOSAGE
Usual adult dose is taken in cycles, with no dosing on certain days of the month. Women must also take a progestin 10 to 14 days in each month of use, except those who have had a hysterectomy (these women may take estrogen daily). To treat breast cancer in men or postmenopausal women: 10 mg, 3 times a day for 3 months or more. To prevent bone loss from osteoporosis: 0.3 to 1.25 mg a day. To ease symptoms of menopause: 0.625 to 1.25 mg a day. To treat prostate cancer: 1.25 to 2.5 mg a day.

ONSET OF EFFECT
Unknown.

DURATION OF ACTION
Unknown.

DIETARY ADVICE
Conjugated estrogens may be taken with food to reduce stomach upset.

STORAGE
Store in a tightly sealed container away from heat, moisture, and direct light. Keep it away from extremes in temperature. Keep the liquid form refrigerated, but do not allow it to freeze.

IF YOU MISS A DOSE
Take it as soon as you remember. If it is near the time for the next dose, skip the missed dose and resume your regular dosage schedule. Do not double the next dose.

STOPPING THE DRUG
The decision to stop taking the drug should be made by your doctor.

PROLONGED USE
Prolonged use of estrogens has been reported to increase the risk of endometrial cancer and perhaps of breast cancer. Consult your doctor about the need for periodic examinations and other measures to screen for these diseases.

PRECAUTIONS
Over 60: No special problems are expected.

Driving and Hazardous Work: Use of this hormone should not impair your ability to perform such tasks safely.

Alcohol: No special precautions are necessary.

Pregnancy: Do not use if you are pregnant. Estrogen use in pregnant women has been associated with birth defects.

Breast Feeding: Talk to your doctor about whether the benefits of the therapy outweigh the potential harm to the nursing infant.

Infants and Children: Should be used with caution by children, as the drug may interfere with bone growth.

OVERDOSE
Symptoms: Nausea, unexpected vaginal bleeding.

What to Do: An overdose of estrogen is unlikely to be life-threatening. However, if someone takes a much larger dose than prescribed, call your doctor, emergency medical services (EMS), or the nearest poison control center immediately.

DRUG INTERACTIONS
Other drugs may interact with estrogens. Consult your doctor if you are taking anticoagulants, anticonvulsants, antidiabetic drugs, thyroid hormones, tricyclic antidepressants, barbiturates, tranquilizers, cyclosporine, corticosteroids, corticotropin, tamoxifen, rifampin, carbamazepine, or bromocriptine.

FOOD INTERACTIONS
Calcium supplements used with estrogen may increase calcium absorption. Vitamin C may increase the effects of estrogen.

DISEASE INTERACTIONS
You should not take conjugated estrogens if you have thrombophlebitis, thromboembolitis, breast cancer, any hormone-dependent cancer, or abnormal genital bleeding. Consult your doctor if you have any of the following: a history of liver disease, heart attack, stroke, a blood clotting disorder, gallbladder disease or gallstones, or if you smoke tobacco heavily.

Estrogens, Conjugated/Medroxyprogesterone Acetate

▶ Drug Class: Female sex hormones

▶ Available in: Tablets

▶ Available OTC? No

▶ As Generic? No

Side Effects

SERIOUS
The most serious side effect is a modest increase in the incidence of breast cancer among women taking estrogen, especially for a long time (10 years or longer). Other side effects requiring your doctor's attention include swelling of legs and feet, rapid weight gain, abnormal menstrual bleeding, mental depression, and skin rash.

COMMON
Nausea, breast tenderness, headache, abdominal pain.

LESS COMMON
Change in appetite, vomiting, stomach cramps or bloating, change in blood pressure, dizziness, nervousness, insomnia, sleepiness, increase or decrease in weight, fatigue, backache.

PRINCIPAL USES
To provide estrogen after the menopause, when the body produces too little; to reduce the risk of osteoporosis; to ease unpleasant symptoms of menopause, including hot flashes and vaginal dryness; and to treat atrophy (wasting) of the vulva or vagina. Estrogen also protects women against coronary artery disease.

HOW THE DRUG WORKS
Estrogen protects against osteoporosis by diminishing the loss of bone that results from estrogen deficiency. Conjugated estrogens replace deficient levels of natural estrogen in women. When given alone to menopausal women, estrogen increases the risk of excessive growth of the uterine lining, which can lead to endometrial cancer. Medroxyprogesterone (a type of progestin) given in conjunction with estrogen nearly eliminates this risk.

DOSAGE
1 tablet, taken once a day. Prempro contains 0.625 mg of estrogen (Premarin) and 2.5 mg of medroxyprogesterone (MPA). Premphase contains 0.625 mg Premarin and 5 mg of MPA.

ONSET OF EFFECT
Unknown.

DURATION OF ACTION
As long as the product is taken.

DIETARY ADVICE
Take it with food to reduce stomach upset.

STORAGE
Store in a tightly sealed container away from heat, moisture, and direct light.

IF YOU MISS A DOSE
If you miss a dose on one day, do not double the dose the next day. Resume your regular dosage schedule.

STOPPING THE DRUG
The decision to stop taking this hormone combination should be made in consultation with your doctor.

PROLONGED USE
You should be reevaluated at 3-month to 6-month intervals to determine whether or not continued treatment is necessary.

PRECAUTIONS
Over 60: No special problems are expected.

Driving and Hazardous Work: Use of this hormone combination should not impair your ability to perform such tasks safely.

Alcohol: No special precautions are necessary.

Pregnancy: Do not use this hormone combination if you are or are planning to become pregnant. Estrogen use in pregnant women has been associated with birth defects.

Breast Feeding: Do not use this hormone combination if you are nursing.

Infants and Children: Not recommended for use by children.

Special Concerns: When this hormone combination is being used in the management or prevention of osteoporosis, regular weight-bearing exercise and good nutrition are important.

OVERDOSE
Symptoms: No serious ill effects have been reported following an overdose. However, nausea, vomiting, and withdrawal bleeding may occur when extremely large doses are ingested.

What to Do: An overdose is unlikely. However, if someone takes a much larger dose than prescribed, seek medical attention.

DRUG INTERACTIONS
Other drugs may interact with this hormone combination. Consult your doctor if you are taking anticoagulants, anticonvulsants, antidiabetic drugs, thyroid hormones, tricyclic antidepressants, barbiturates, tranquilizers, cyclosporine, corticosteroids, corticotropin, tamoxifen, rifampin, carbamazepine, or bromocriptine.

FOOD INTERACTIONS
Estrogen may increase calcium absorption from calcium supplements. Vitamin C may increase the effects of estrogen.

DISEASE INTERACTIONS
You should not take this hormone combination if you have thrombophlebitis, breast cancer, any hormone-dependent cancer, or abnormal vaginal bleeding. Consult your doctor if you have a history of any of the following: liver disease, heart attack, diabetes mellitus, stroke, a blood clotting disorder, thromboembolic disease, gallbladder disease or gallstones, liver disease, or if you smoke cigarettes heavily.

Estropipate

Generic 0.75 mg
(WATSON)

▶ Drug Class: Female sex hormone

▶ Available in: Tablets, vaginal cream

▶ Available OTC? No

▶ As Generic? Yes

Side Effects

SERIOUS
Breast pain or enlargement, swelling of legs and feet, rapid weight gain. Call your doctor immediately.

COMMON
Stomach bloating, lower abdominal cramps, loss of appetite.

LESS COMMON
Diarrhea, dizziness, headaches, discomfort when wearing contact lenses, increased sexual desire in women, vomiting, unusual sensitivity to sunlight.

PRINCIPAL USES
To provide estrogen when the body does not produce enough; to treat selected cases of advanced breast cancer; to reduce risk of osteoporosis after menopause; to ease unpleasant symptoms of menopause, including vaginal dryness; to ease symptoms of advanced prostate cancer.

HOW THE DRUG WORKS
In women, estropipate replaces deficient natural levels of estrogen in the body. In men, it inhibits the growth of cells in the prostate gland.

DOSAGE
For vaginal skin conditions: 0.625 to 5 mg a day of oral form or 2 to 4 grams a day of vaginal cream. For treating menopausal symptoms: 1.25 to 2.5 mg a day of oral form, 3 weeks on, 1 week off. To prevent osteoporosis: 0.625 mg of oral form daily for 25 days of a 31-day cycle. A progestin must also be taken for 10 to 14 days in each month of use, except in women who have had a hysterectomy.

ONSET OF EFFECT
Within 1 hour.

DURATION OF ACTION
Up to 24 hours.

DIETARY ADVICE
This medicine can be taken without regard to meals.

STORAGE
Keep in a tightly sealed container away from heat and direct light.

IF YOU MISS A DOSE
Take the missed dose as soon as you remember. If it is near time for the next dose, skip the missed dose and resume your regular dosage schedule. Do not double the next dose.

STOPPING THE DRUG
The decision to stop taking the drug should be made by your doctor.

PROLONGED USE
Prolonged use of estrogens has been reported to increase the risk of endometrial cancer and perhaps breast cancer. Endometrial cancer is largely prevented by using estropipate in sequence with a progestin. Consult your doctor about the need for periodic examinations and other measures to help detect and prevent these diseases.

PRECAUTIONS

Over 60: No special problems are expected.

Driving and Hazardous Work: Do not drive or engage in hazardous work until you determine how the medicine affects you.

Alcohol: No special precautions are necessary.

Pregnancy: Estrogens have been shown to cause birth defects in animals and humans. Before taking estropipate, be sure to tell your doctor if you are pregnant or plan to become pregnant.

Breast Feeding: Estropipate passes into breast milk; avoid using it while nursing.

Infants and Children: This medicine is not recommended for use by children in whom bone growth is not complete.

Special Concerns: Swelling or bleeding of the gums may occur. See your dentist regularly. You should have a Pap test every 6 to 12 months while taking estropipate. Avoid excessive exposure to sunlight until you determine how the drug affects you.

OVERDOSE
Symptoms: Nausea, unexpected vaginal bleeding.

What to Do: An overdose of estropipate is unlikely to be life-threatening. However, if someone takes a much larger dose than prescribed, call your doctor, emergency medical services (EMS), or the nearest poison control center.

DRUG INTERACTIONS
Consult your doctor for specific advice if you are taking acetaminophen, amiodarone, anabolic steroids, androgens, anti-infective drugs, antithyroid agents, bromocriptine, carbamazepine, carmustine, chloroquine, cyclosporine, dantrolene, daunorubicin, disulfiram, divalproex, etretinate, gold salts, hydroxychloroquine, mercaptopurine, methotrexate, methyldopa, naltrexone, oral contraceptives, phenothiazines, phenytoin, plicamycin, or valproic acid.

FOOD INTERACTIONS
No known food interactions.

DISEASE INTERACTIONS
You should not take estropipate if you have thrombophlebitis, thrombocmbolitis, a history of breast cancer, any hormone-dependent cancer, or abnormal genital bleeding.

Etanercept

BRAND NAME
Enbrel

▶ Drug Class: Biologic response modifier

▶ Available in: Injection

▶ Available OTC? No

▶ As Generic? No

Side Effects

SERIOUS
There are no serious side effects associated with the use of etanercept.

COMMON
Itching, redness, pain, or swelling at the site of injection; upper respiratory infection.

LESS COMMON
Headache, nasal congestion, dizziness, sore throat, cough, general weakness, abdominal discomfort, rash, runny nose.

PRINCIPAL USES
To reduce the signs and symptoms of moderate to severe active rheumatoid arthritis. Etanercept is prescribed for patients who have not responded adequately to one or more antirheumatic medications. It may also be used in combination with methotrexate in patients who have not responded adequately to methotrexate alone.

HOW THE DRUG WORKS
Etanercept works by binding with tumor necrosis factor (TNF), a key protein involved in the inflammatory process. Etanercept reduces inflammation by blocking the interaction of TNF with its receptors on cells.

DOSAGE
Adults: 25 mg, twice a week as a subcutaneous (under the skin) injection. Children: See your pediatrician for the appropriate dosage.

ONSET OF EFFECT
Within 1 to 2 weeks.

DURATION OF ACTION
As long as the drug is taken, but studies have only lasted for 6 months.

DIETARY ADVICE
May be taken without regard to diet.

STORAGE
Keep etanercept refrigerated, but do not allow it to freeze. If not administered immediately after preparing (reconstituting), etanercept may be stored in the vial in the refrigerator for up to 6 hours.

IF YOU MISS A DOSE
Take it as soon as you remember. If it is near the time for the next dose, skip the missed dose and resume your regular dosage schedule. Do not double the next dose.

STOPPING THE DRUG
The decision to stop taking the medication should be made in consultation with your doctor.

PROLONGED USE
No special problems are expected.

PRECAUTIONS
Over 60: No special problems are expected.

Driving and Hazardous Work: The use of etanercept should not impair your ability to perform such tasks safely.

Alcohol: Alcohol may accentuate the side effect of dizziness.

Pregnancy: Adequate human studies have not been done. Before taking etanercept, tell your doctor if you are pregnant or plan to become pregnant.

Breast Feeding: Etanercept may pass into breast milk; caution is advised. Consult your doctor for advice on whether to discontinue nursing or discontinue the drug.

Infants and Children: Not recommended for use by children under age 4.

Special Concerns: Your doctor should instruct you on how to prepare and administer the injection of etanercept before you attempt to do it yourself. Follow your doctor's instructions about selecting and rotating injection sites. Sites for self-injection are the arms, stomach, and thighs. The first injection should be administered under the supervision of your doctor. Other antirheumatic medications may be continued during treatment with etanercept. Consult your doctor for advice.

OVERDOSE
Symptoms: No cases of overdose have been reported.

What to Do: An overdose with etanercept is unlikely. If someone takes a much larger dose than prescribed, call your doctor.

DRUG INTERACTIONS
Avoid live-virus vaccines. No other medications should be added to solutions containing etanercept. Adequate studies involving interactions with other drugs have not been done. Consult your doctor for specific advice.

FOOD INTERACTIONS
No known food interactions.

DISEASE INTERACTIONS
Etanercept should be used with caution in patients with any active infection, including chronic or localized infections, or who are immunosuppressed.

Ethacrynic Acid (Ethacrynate)

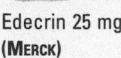

Edecrin 25 mg
(MERCK)

▶ Drug Class: Loop diuretic

▶ Available in: Tablets, injection

▶ Available OTC? No

▶ As Generic? No

Side Effects

SERIOUS
Mood or mental changes, nausea or vomiting, unusual fatigue, black and tarry stools, skin rash. Call your doctor immediately.

COMMON
Muscle cramps or pain. Potassium depletion may lead to heart palpitations and weakness. Fluid depletion may lead to dizziness, especially upon arising from a sitting or lying position, as well as thirst, dry mouth, and constipation.

LESS COMMON
Buzzing or ringing in ears, loss of hearing (particularly after intravenous treatment), diarrhea, loss of appetite, gout, increased blood sugar (a problem for diabetic patients).

PRINCIPAL USES
To reduce fluid (salt and water) accumulation that leads to edema (swelling) and breathlessness in patients who have heart disease, cirrhosis of the liver, and kidney disease.

HOW THE DRUG WORKS
Loop diuretics work on a specific portion of the kidney (the loop of Henle) to increase the excretion of water and salts (including potassium) in urine.

DOSAGE
Adults— Ethacrynic acid (oral dose): 50 to 200 mg a day. Ethacrynate sodium (injection): 50 mg injected into a vein every 2 to 6 hours as needed.

ONSET OF EFFECT
Within 30 minutes after an oral dose; within 5 minutes after intravenous injection.

DURATION OF ACTION
Oral dose lasts 6 to 8 hours; intravenous, 2 hours.

DIETARY ADVICE
Ethacrynic acid may cause depletion of potassium; your doctor may want you to eat high-potassium foods (such as bananas, tomatoes, and citrus fruits) or take potassium supplements. Take the drug with food or milk to minimize stomach upset.

STORAGE
Store in a tightly sealed container away from heat, moisture, and direct light.

IF YOU MISS A DOSE
Take it as soon as you remember. If it is near the time for the next dose, skip the missed dose and resume your regular dosage schedule. Do not double the next dose.

STOPPING THE DRUG
Take it as prescribed for the full treatment period, even if you begin to feel better before the scheduled end of therapy.

PROLONGED USE
Your doctor will schedule regular checkups to determine the medication's effect on your body, and adjust the dosage and dosing frequency. After a maintenance dose is established, diuretic therapy may continue for intermittent periods alternating with periods not using the drug.

PRECAUTIONS
Over 60: No special precautions are warranted.

Driving and Hazardous Work: No special precautions are warranted.

Alcohol: Alcohol should be avoided or used with caution because it may increase the effect of antihypertensive drugs and cause an excessive drop in blood pressure.

Pregnancy: This drug is not usually prescribed during pregnancy. Other diuretics are preferred.

Breast Feeding: It is not known whether the drug is excreted in milk; consult your doctor for specific advice.

Infants and Children: Although ethacrynic acid is rarely prescribed for children, no unusual side effects are expected. The dose must be determined by a pediatrician.

Special Concerns: To prevent sleep disruption, avoid taking this medicine in the evening. You may be advised to in-crease potassium in your diet or take a potassium supplement while taking a diuretic.

OVERDOSE
Symptoms: Weakness, lethargy, dizziness, nausea, vomiting, leg muscle cramps.

What to Do: Call your doctor, emergency medical services (EMS), or the nearest poison control center immediately.

DRUG INTERACTIONS
Consult your doctor if you are taking any of the following: ACE inhibitors, aminoglycosides, cisplatin, digitalis drugs, lithium, nonsteroidal anti-inflammatory drugs, salicylates, or thiazide diuretics.

FOOD INTERACTIONS
No known food interactions.

DISEASE INTERACTIONS
Consult your doctor if you have any of the following conditions: diabetes mellitus, gout, hearing problems, pancreatitis, recent heart attack, kidney or liver disease, or systemic lupus erythematosus.

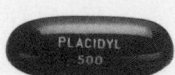

Placidyl 500 mg
(ABBOTT)

Additional photographs

▶ Drug Class: Sedative

▶ Available in: Capsules

▶ Available OTC? No

▶ As Generic? Yes

Side Effects

SERIOUS
Unusual bleeding or bruising; unusual excitement, nervousness, or restlessness; skin rash or hives; yellowish tinge to eyes or skin (jaundice); itching; darkening of urine; pale stools. Call your doctor immediately.

COMMON
Blurred vision, nausea or vomiting, indigestion, bitter or unusual aftertaste, numbness in the face, abdominal pain, dizziness or lightheadedness, unusual fatigue or weakness.

LESS COMMON
Unsteady gait or loss of coordination; confusion; daytime sleepiness. Check with your doctor promptly if such symptoms persist.

PRINCIPAL USES
Used as short-term therapy for insomnia; however, other medications are generally preferred.

HOW THE DRUG WORKS
The exact mechanism of action is unknown; ethchlorvynol appears to depress the central nervous system in a manner similar to that of barbiturates.

DOSAGE
Adults: 500 to 1,000 mg at bedtime.

ONSET OF EFFECT
30 to 60 minutes.

DURATION OF ACTION
5 hours.

DIETARY ADVICE
Take ethchlorvynol with milk or food to minimize temporary dizziness or unsteadiness that may result from the body's rapid absorption of the drug.

STORAGE
Store in a tightly sealed container away from heat, moisture, and direct light.

IF YOU MISS A DOSE
Ethchlorvynol is generally prescribed for once-daily use at bedtime. If you are unable to take it on a particular night, resume your regular scheduled dose the following night.

STOPPING THE DRUG
The decision to stop taking the drug should be made in consultation with your doctor. Generally, therapy lasts no more than 1 week.

PROLONGED USE
Ethchlorvynol should not be prescribed for a period exceeding 1 week, as the body will build up tolerance to the drug, and physical and psychological dependence may develop. Patients abruptly stopping the drug after prolonged use may experience withdrawal symptoms (seizures, delirium, perceptual distortions, agitation, tremors) as late as 9 days after ending therapy. A gradual, progressive reduction of dosage over a period of days or weeks is recommended for patients who have become dependent on ethchlorvynol.

PRECAUTIONS
Over 60: Older patients may be more sensitive to the effects of ethchlorvynol and so should take the smallest effective dose.

Driving and Hazardous Work: The use of this drug may impair your ability to perform such tasks safely.

Alcohol: Avoid alcohol.

Pregnancy: Ethchlorvynol should not be used during the first 2 trimesters (6 months) of pregnancy. Discuss with your doctor the relative risks and benefits of using this drug during the final 3 months (third trimester) of pregnancy.

Breast Feeding: Ethchlorvynol may pass into breast milk. Consult your doctor for specific advice.

Infants and Children: Not recommended for persons under the age of 18.

Special Concerns: Ethchlorvynol may become habit forming. Use only as directed by your doctor. Never take more than the prescribed dose and do not use the drug for a longer period than prescribed.

OVERDOSE
Symptoms: Severe nausea, vomiting, or stomach pain; difficulty swallowing; severe drowsiness; continuing confusion; seizures; low body temperature; difficulty breathing or shortness of breath; irregular heartbeat; severe weakness; staggering; slurred speech.

What to Do: Call your doctor, emergency medical services (EMS), or the nearest poison control center immediately.

DRUG INTERACTIONS
Consult your doctor for specific advice if you are taking barbiturates or other central nervous system depressants, tricyclic antidepressants, MAO inhibitors, or anticoagulants.

FOOD INTERACTIONS
No known food interactions.

DISEASE INTERACTIONS
Your physician should know if you have any of the following conditions: impaired kidney or liver function, a history of alcohol or drug abuse, mental depression, or porphyria.

Ethinyl Estradiol

Estinyl 0.05 mg
(SCHERING-PLOUGH)

▶ Drug Class: Anticancer estrogen

▶ Available in: Tablets

▶ Available OTC? No

▶ As Generic? Yes

Side Effects

SERIOUS
Breast pain or enlargement, swelling of feet and lower legs, rapid weight gain, changes in vaginal bleeding, lumps in or discharge from the breast, visual disturbances, sharp pains in stomach, side, or abdomen, uncontrolled muscle movements, yellowish tinge of eyes or skin (jaundice). Call your doctor immediately.

COMMON
Stomach bloating, lower abdominal cramping and discomfort, loss of appetite.

LESS COMMON
Dizziness, diarrhea, headaches, unusual increase in sexual desire, vomiting, problems with contact lenses.

PRINCIPAL USES
To provide estrogen when the body does not produce enough (hypogonadism); to treat carefully selected cases of advanced breast cancer; to reduce risk of osteoporosis after menopause; to ease unpleasant symptoms of menopause, including vaginal dryness; to ease symptoms of advanced prostate cancer.

HOW THE DRUG WORKS
In women, ethinyl estradiol replaces deficient natural levels of estrogen in the body. In men, it inhibits the growth of cells in the prostate gland.

DOSAGE
For female hypogonadism: 0.05 mg, 1 to 3 times a day for 25 days per month (in conjunction with 10 to 14 days of a progestin, except in women who have had a hysterectomy), for 3 to 6 months. For breast cancer: 1 mg, 3 times a day. For menopausal symptoms: 0.02 to 0.05 mg a day. For prostate cancer: 0.15 to 2 mg a day.

ONSET OF EFFECT
Within 8 hours.

DURATION OF ACTION
Up to 24 hours.

DIETARY ADVICE
This drug can be taken with or immediately after meals to reduce nausea.

STORAGE
Store in a tightly sealed container away from heat and direct light.

IF YOU MISS A DOSE
Take it as soon as you remember. However, if it is near the time for the next dose, skip the missed dose and resume your regular dosage schedule. Do not double the next dose.

STOPPING THE DRUG
The decision to stop taking the drug should be made by your doctor.

PROLONGED USE
Women who take ethinyl estradiol for more than 5 years to treat menopausal symptoms may be at increased risk for endometrial cancer. Consult your physician about the need for discontinuing the drug temporarily. Although the drug may cause menstrual bleeding, it does not restore fertility.

PRECAUTIONS
Over 60: No special problems are expected.

Driving and Hazardous Work: The use of ethinyl estradiol may impair your ability to perform such tasks safely. Do not drive or engage in hazardous work until you determine how the medication affects you.

Alcohol: No special precautions are necessary.

Pregnancy: Drugs of this class have caused serious birth defects in animals and humans. Ethinyl estradiol should not be taken if you are pregnant or are planning to become pregnant.

Breast Feeding: Ethinyl estradiol passes into breast milk; avoid or discontinue use while nursing.

Infants and Children: Not recommended for use by children and adolescents whose bone growth is not complete.

Special Concerns: Ethinyl estradiol may cause dental bleeding and excessive gingival (gum) growth. See your dentist regularly. Nausea may occur in the first weeks after you start taking this drug.

OVERDOSE
Symptoms: Nausea and abnormal vaginal bleeding.

What to Do: An overdose of ethinyl estradiol is unlikely to be life-threatening. However, if someone takes a much larger dose than prescribed, call your doctor, emergency medical services (EMS), or local poison control center.

DRUG INTERACTIONS
Consult your doctor for specific advice if you are taking acetaminophen, amiodarone, anabolic steroids, androgens, anti-infective drugs, antithyroid drugs, carbamazepine, carmustine, chloroquine, dantrolene, daunorubicin, disulfiram, divalproex, etretinate, gold salts, hydroxychloroquine, mercaptopurine, naltrexone, oral contraceptives, phenothiazines, phenytoin, valproic acid, bromocriptine, or cyclosporine.

FOOD INTERACTIONS
No known food interactions.

DISEASE INTERACTIONS
Caution is advised when taking ethinyl estradiol. Consult your doctor if you have any of the following: a history of blood clots while taking estrogens, breast cancer, endometriosis, fibroid tumors of the uterus, gallbladder disease or gallstones, jaundice, liver disease, or porphyria.

Ethosuximide

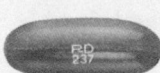

Zarontin 250 mg
(PARKE-DAVIS)

▸ Drug Class: Anticonvulsant/
succinimide

▸ Available in: Capsules, syrup

▸ Available OTC? No

▸ As Generic? Yes

Side Effects

SERIOUS
Sore throat, fever, swollen glands, red or purple point-like rash on the skin or mucous membranes, blistering or peeling skin lesions, mouth sores, easy bruising, paleness, weakness, confusion, lethargy, muscle pain, or seizures may be a sign of a potentially fatal blood reaction or other complication. Call your doctor immediately.

COMMON
Nausea and vomiting, loss of appetite, stomach upset, gastrointestinal cramps, weight loss, diarrhea, sedation, mild sensory nerve impairment.

LESS COMMON
Irritability, headache, dizziness, sleep disturbances. There are numerous additional side effects associated with the use of this drug; consult your physician if you are concerned about any adverse or unusual reactions.

PRINCIPAL USES
To control seizures in patients with certain types of epilepsy.

HOW THE DRUG WORKS
Ethosuximide acts on the central nervous system to control the number and severity of seizures. It is thought to depress the activity of certain parts of the brain and suppress the abnormal transmission of nerve impulses that causes absence seizures.

DOSAGE
Adults: 750 to 1,500 mg a day, in 2 divided doses. A higher dose may be required. Children: 4 to 5 mg a day, in 2 divided doses. A low dose is used to start, and is gradually increased by your doctor.

ONSET OF EFFECT
Several hours.

DURATION OF ACTION
The drug is most effective for 24 hours or longer. After this time, effectiveness gradually decreases.

DIETARY ADVICE
Take it with food to minimize the risk of stomach upset.

STORAGE
Store in a tightly sealed container away from heat and direct light. Do not refrigerate or freeze the syrup.

IF YOU MISS A DOSE
Take it as soon as you remember, unless your next scheduled dose is within the next 4 hours. If so, skip the missed dose. Take your next dose at the proper time, and resume your regular dosage schedule. Do not double the next dose, unless advised to do so by your doctor.

STOPPING THE DRUG
The decision to stop taking the drug should be made by your doctor. Ethosuximide should never be stopped abruptly, since this may cause seizures. The dose is typically tapered over a period of weeks to months.

PROLONGED USE
Ethosuximide can be taken on a long-term basis. Some side effects that are prominent in the first few weeks of therapy usually diminish over time.

PRECAUTIONS
Over 60: Older patients may require lower doses to minimize side effects.

Driving and Hazardous Work: Ethosuximide may cause drowsiness and impair your ability to perform such tasks safely. Do not drive or engage in hazardous work until you determine how the medicine affects you.

Alcohol: May contribute to excessive drowsiness.

Pregnancy: Use of anticonvulsants is associated with an increased risk of birth defects, although studies with ethosuximide are incomplete. However, seizures during pregnancy can also increase risks to the fetus. Discuss with your doctor the potential risks and benefits of using this drug during pregnancy. Folate supplementation is recommended 1 to 2 months prior to conception, and continuing throughout pregnancy.

Breast Feeding: Ethosuximide passes into breast milk, although at low levels. Consult your doctor for specific advice if you are breast feeding.

Infants and Children: No special problems are expected.

Special Concerns: The generic form is not recommended. Your doctor may want you to wear a medical bracelet or carry an identification card saying that you are taking this drug.

OVERDOSE
Symptoms: Severe nausea and vomiting, difficulty breathing, severe drowsiness, coma.

What to Do: Call your doctor, emergency medical services (EMS), or the nearest poison control center immediately.

DRUG INTERACTIONS
Ethosuximide may be affected by other drugs or alter the blood levels of other medications, including other anticonvulsants (carbamazepine, phenacemide, phenobarbital, phenytoin, primidone, valproic acid) and certain psychiatric drugs (tricyclic antidepressants, MAO inhibitors, haloperidol).

FOOD INTERACTIONS
No known food interactions.

DISEASE INTERACTIONS
Special caution is advised if you have liver disease, kidney disease, a blood disorder, or intermittent porphyria.

Etidronate Disodium

Didronel 200 mg
(PROCTER & GAMBLE)

▶ Drug Class: Bisphosphonate inhibitor of bone resorption

▶ Available in: Tablets, injection

▶ Available OTC? No

▶ As Generic? No

Side Effects

SERIOUS
Bone fractures—especially in the long bones of the limbs—may occur, usually in patients on high doses or those taking the drug continuously for longer than 6 months.

COMMON
Bone pain or tenderness, often developing 4 to 6 weeks after treatment begins; it may persist, get worse, or sporadically ease and then return in patients with Paget's disease. Nausea and diarrhea may occur with higher doses. Headache, stomach upset, leg cramps, and joint pain may also occur.

LESS COMMON
Hives, skin rash, itching, swelling of the arms, legs, face, lips, tongue, or throat. The injectable form may cause loss of taste or metallic taste in the mouth.

PRINCIPAL USES
To treat Paget's disease, a disorder characterized by rapid breakdown and reformation of bone, which can lead to fragility and malformation of bones. May also be used to treat elevated blood levels of calcium (hypercalcemia) caused by cancer; to treat and prevent calcium and bone deposits around artificial joint replacements (especially hip replacements) or around an area of spinal cord injury. Etidronate is also commonly used to treat postmenopausal osteoporosis.

HOW THE DRUG WORKS
Etidronate slows bone resorption (the speed at which bone is broken down before it is replaced), promoting the formation of healthy bone. It prevents the bone pain, deformity, and fractures associated with Paget's disease. In cancer-related hypercalcemia, this drug slows bone resorption and thus the flow of calcium from bone into the blood. Etidronate slows the progression of abnormal bone deposition after hip replacement and spinal cord injury. In osteoporosis, it helps to slow the breakdown of bone tissue.

DOSAGE
Usual adult oral dosage for Paget's disease: 2.3 mg per lb of body weight per day, or 2.7 to 4.6 mg per lb, in alternating 6 month courses of treatment and abstention. Or: 5 to 9.1 mg per lb per day for not more than 3 months at a time. For hypercalcemia related to cancer: 9 mg per lb of body weight for 30 to 90 days. For prevention of calcium deposits, with hip replacement: 9 mg per lb for 1 month before and 3 months after surgery; for spinal cord injury: 9 mg per lb for

2 weeks, then 4.5 mg per lb for 10 weeks.

ONSET OF EFFECT
May be observed after 1 month of treatment.

DURATION OF ACTION
Possibly up to a year or more after therapy is stopped.

DIETARY ADVICE
Take the tablets with water on an empty stomach at least 2 hours before or after eating. Eat a well-balanced diet with adequate calcium and vitamin D intake.

STORAGE
Store in a tightly sealed container away from direct light, moisture, and extremes in temperature.

IF YOU MISS A DOSE
Take it as soon as possible. However, if it is near the time for the next dose, skip the missed dose, and resume the normal dosage schedule. Do not double the next dose.

STOPPING THE DRUG
Do not stop taking the drug on your own. Etidronate may take up to 3 months for the full effect to occur.

PROLONGED USE
Regular visits to your doctor are necessary—even between treatments—to evaluate the drug's effect.

PRECAUTIONS
Over 60: Elderly patients may be more prone to excess fluid retention (overhydration) when treated with injected etidronate in conjunction with hydration therapy. Careful monitoring of fluid and electrolyte levels is important.

Driving and Hazardous Work: No special precautions are required.

Alcohol: Alcohol should be restricted in high risk women because it is a risk factor for osteoporosis.

Pregnancy: Consult your doctor about whether the benefits of taking the medicine outweigh the potential risks to the unborn child.

Breast Feeding: It is not known if etidronate passes into breast milk.

Infants and Children: Safety and effectiveness have not been established.

OVERDOSE
Symptoms: Vomiting or diarrhea; palpitations; numbness or tingling in the hands, feet, lips, and tongue; facial pain.

What to Do: Call your doctor, emergency medical services (EMS), or the nearest poison control center immediately.

DRUG INTERACTIONS
Antacids or other medications containing calcium, magnesium, or aluminum may interfere with your body's absorption of oral etidronate. Warfarin may also interact with etidronate; consult your doctor for advice.

FOOD INTERACTIONS
Foods containing large amounts of calcium, such as milk or other dairy products, and mineral supplements containing calcium, iron, magnesium, or aluminum should not be consumed within 2 hours of taking etidronate.

DISEASE INTERACTIONS
Consult your doctor for advice if you have a bone fracture, intestinal or bowel disease, kidney disease, or a heart condition.

Etodolac

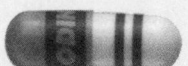

Lodine 200 mg
(WYETH-AYERST)

▶ Drug Class: Nonsteroidal anti-inflammatory drug (NSAID)

▶ Available in: Capsule, tablet, extended-release tablets

▶ Available OTC? No

▶ As Generic? Yes

Side Effects

SERIOUS
Shortness of breath or wheezing, with or without swelling of legs or other signs of heart failure; chest pain; peptic ulcer disease with vomiting of blood; black, tarry stools; decreasing kidney function. Call your doctor immediately.

COMMON
Nausea, vomiting, heartburn, diarrhea, constipation, headache, dizziness, sleepiness.

LESS COMMON
Ulcers or sores in mouth, depression, rashes or blistering of skin, ringing sound in the ears, unusual tingling or numbness of the hands or feet, seizures, blurred vision. Also elevated potassium levels, decreased blood counts; such problems can be detected by your doctor.

PRINCIPAL USES
To treat mild to moderate pain and inflammation caused by tendinitis, arthritis, bursitis, gout, soft tissue injuries, migraine and other vascular headaches, menstrual cramps, and other conditions. When patients fail to respond to one NSAID, another may be tried. The greatest effectiveness often requires trial and error of several different NSAIDs.

HOW THE DRUG WORKS
NSAIDs work by interfering with the formation of prostaglandins, substances in the body that cause inflammation and make nerves more sensitive to pain impulses. NSAIDs have other modes of action that are less well understood.

DOSAGE
For osteoarthritis— Adults: To start, 400 mg, 2 or 3 times a day, or 300 mg, 3 or 4 times a day. For pain— Adults: To start, 400 mg. Then, 200 to 400 mg every 6 to 8 hours as needed. Consult your pediatrician for children's dose.

ONSET OF EFFECT
Within 30 minutes.

DURATION OF ACTION
4 to 6 hours.

DIETARY ADVICE
Take with food; maintain your usual food and fluid intake.

STORAGE
Store in a tightly sealed container away from heat, moisture, and direct light.

IF YOU MISS A DOSE
Take it as soon as you remember. If it is near the time for the next dose, skip the missed dose and resume your regular dosage schedule. Do not double the next dose.

STOPPING THE DRUG
The decision to stop taking the drug should be made in consultation with your physician.

PROLONGED USE
Prolonged use can cause gastrointestinal problems, including ulceration and bleeding, kidney dysfunction, and liver inflammation. See your doctor for regular evaluation.

PRECAUTIONS
Over 60: Because of the potentially greater consequences of gastrointestinal side effects, the dose of NSAIDs for older patients, especially those over age 70, is often cut in half.

Driving and Hazardous Work: Do not drive or engage in hazardous work until you determine how the medicine affects you.

Alcohol: Avoid alcohol when using this medication because it increases the risk of stomach irritation.

Pregnancy: Avoid or discontinue this drug if you are pregnant or are planning to become pregnant.

Breast Feeding: Etodolac passes into breast milk; avoid use while nursing.

Infants and Children: Etodolac may be used in exceptional circumstances; consult your doctor.

Special Concerns: Because NSAIDs can interfere with blood coagulation, this drug should be stopped at least 3 days prior to any surgery.

OVERDOSE
Symptoms: Nausea, vomiting, severe headache, confusion, seizures.

What to Do: Call your doctor, emergency medical services (EMS), or the nearest poison control center immediately.

DRUG INTERACTIONS
Do not take this drug with aspirin or any other NSAIDs without your doctor's approval. In addition, consult your doctor if you are taking antihypertensives, steroids, anticoagulants, antibiotics, itraconazole or ketoconazole, plicamycin, penicillamine, valproic acid, phenytoin, cyclosporine, digitalis drugs, lithium, methotrexate, probenecid, triamterene, or zidovudine.

FOOD INTERACTIONS
No known food interactions.

DISEASE INTERACTIONS
Caution is advised when taking etodolac. Consult your doctor if you have any of the following: bleeding problems, inflammation or ulcers of the stomach and intestines, diabetes mellitus, systemic lupus erythematosus (SLE, lupus), anemia, asthma, epilepsy, Parkinson's disease, kidney stones, or a history of heart disease or alcohol abuse. Use of etodolac may cause complications in patients with liver or kidney disease, since these organs work together to remove the medication from the body.

Etoposide

BRAND NAME
VePesid

▶ Drug Class: Antineoplastic (anticancer) agent

▶ Available in: Capsules, injection

▶ Available OTC? No

▶ As Generic? Yes

Side Effects

SERIOUS
Bone marrow suppression (myelosuppression) causing fatigue, bleeding, bruising, fever, sore throat, chills. Severe gastrointestinal upset. Contact your doctor immediately if such symptoms appear.

COMMON
Loss of appetite, mild to moderate nausea, vomiting. Check with your doctor if these symptoms continue. Hair loss, sometimes progressing to total baldness, is generally temporary; hair will usually begin to grow back when the therapy is discontinued.

LESS COMMON
Allergic reactions, diarrhea, fatigue. Temporary drop in blood pressure (hypotension) causing dizziness and lightheadedness may occur with intravenous infusion.

PRINCIPAL USES
To treat recurrent or persistent testicular cancer or lymphoma (cancer of the lymph nodes). It is also used to treat certain types of lung cancer.

HOW THE DRUG WORKS
Etoposide kills cancer cells by interfering with the activity of their genetic material, which prevents the cells from dividing normally and multiplying. The drug may also affect the growth and development of other kinds of cells in the body, which may cause unpleasant side effects.

DOSAGE
Usual adult dose by intravenous infusion for testicular carcinoma: 50 to 100 mg per square meter of body surface for 5 days to 100 mg per square meter on days 1, 3, and 5. Usual adult oral dose for small-cell lung cancer: 70 mg per square meter of body surface per day for 4 days to 100 mg per square meter per day for 5 days. Both regimens are repeated every 3 to 4 weeks, depending on the severity of any side effects.

ONSET OF EFFECT
Variable.

DURATION OF ACTION
Unknown.

DIETARY ADVICE
No special concerns.

STORAGE
Keep liquid forms of the drug refrigerated, but do not allow them to freeze.

IF YOU MISS A DOSE
Skip the missed dose and continue your normal dosage schedule; do not double the next dose. Notify your doctor about the missed dose right away.

STOPPING THE DRUG
Continue to take the medicine exactly as prescribed by your doctor, even if you begin to feel ill. Certain side effects such as stomach upset and vomiting are common. Notify your doctor if vomiting occurs shortly after dosing.

PROLONGED USE
Follow the treatment schedule determined by your doctor. Periodic evaluation of the drug's effect and blood tests are an important part of treatment; blood cell counts need to be closely monitored.

PRECAUTIONS
Over 60: Adverse reactions may be more likely and more severe in older patients.

Driving and Hazardous Work: Check with your doctor before engaging in activities where you are at risk for bruising or injury.

Alcohol: Limit alcohol to moderate intake.

Pregnancy: Birth defects may result if etoposide is used at the time of conception or during pregnancy. Sterility is another potential side effect. Tell your doctor before taking the drug if you are pregnant; use birth control while taking etoposide, and notify your doctor immediately if you think you have become pregnant while taking the drug.

Breast Feeding: Etoposide is distributed into breast milk and may cause serious side effects; consult your doctor for advice.

Infants and Children: Consult your pediatric oncologist.

Special Concerns: Advise your doctor if you or a family member plans to receive a vaccination; there is a danger you might get the infection the immunization is meant to prevent. Patients with low blood counts should avoid crowds and people with infections, and should be alert for signs of infection and bleeding. Exercise caution when cleaning your teeth, and check with your doctor before having any dental work done.

OVERDOSE
Symptoms: Increased severity of nausea or vomiting, rapid pulse, shortness of breath, fainting.

What to Do: Call your doctor, emergency medical services (EMS), or the nearest poison control center immediately.

DRUG INTERACTIONS
Any or all of the following drugs may cause undesirable effects when taken together with etoposide: bone marrow depressants, antivirals, antifungals, anticoagulants, cyclosporine, or aspirin.

FOOD INTERACTIONS
No known food interactions.

DISEASE INTERACTIONS
Advise your doctor if you have any of the following conditions: chicken pox, shingles, infection, or kidney or liver disease.

Exemestane

▶ Drug Class: Antineoplastic (anticancer) agent

▶ Available in: Tablets

▶ Available OTC? No

▶ As Generic? No

Side Effects

SERIOUS
No serious side effects have been reported.

COMMON
Hot flashes, nausea, fatigue, pain, depression, insomnia, anxiety, shortness of breath.

LESS COMMON
Sweating, flulike symptoms, swelling, dizziness, headache, vomiting, abdominal pain, loss of appetite, constipation, diarrhea, increased appetite, weight gain, cough.

PRINCIPAL USES
To treat advanced breast cancer in postmenopausal women whose tumors stop responding to tamoxifen therapy.

HOW THE DRUG WORKS
The growth of some breast cancers is stimulated by the hormone estrogen. The estrogen in postmenopausal women arises primarily from the conversion by the enzyme aromatase of male hormones (androgens) made in the adrenal and ovaries. Exemestane inactivates aromatase, thus preventing the natural synthesis of estrogen and inhibiting the growth of estrogen-dependent tumors.

DOSAGE
25 mg a day following a meal.

ONSET OF EFFECT
Unknown.

DURATION OF ACTION
Unknown.

DIETARY ADVICE
It is recommended that exemestane be taken after a meal.

STORAGE
Store in a tightly sealed container away from heat, moisture, and direct light.

IF YOU MISS A DOSE
Exemestane is prescribed for once-daily use only. If you are unable to take the medication on a particular day, simply resume your regular dosage schedule the following day. Do not double the next dose.

STOPPING THE DRUG
The decision to stop the drug must be made in consultation with your doctor. Do not stop taking exemestane on your own.

PROLONGED USE
There is no standard duration of therapy with exemestane, although you can expect to remain on it for at least several weeks in order to determine if it is effective. Your doctor will determine whether your response to the drug is satisfactory or not, and will recommend continuation or discontinuation of therapy.

PRECAUTIONS
Over 60: No special problems are expected.

Driving and Hazardous Work: Do not drive or engage in hazardous work until you determine how the medicine affects you.

Alcohol: No special problems are expected, but you should consult your doctor about drinking alcohol while taking exemestane.

Pregnancy: Exemestane must not be used in pregnant women. Although exemestane is only prescribed for postmenopausal women, it is important that patients be sure they are not pregnant before starting treatment with this drug.

Breast Feeding: Not applicable; this drug is prescribed only for postmenopausal women.

Infants and Children: Not applicable.

Special Concerns: Exemestane often lowers blood levels of lymphocytes (a type of infection-fighting white blood cell), but no increase in infections was seen during clinical trials.

OVERDOSE
Symptoms: No cases of overdose have been reported.

What to Do: An overdose is unlikely; however, if you have any reason to suspect that one has occurred, call emergency medical services (EMS) to receive evaluation and treatment at the closest emergency facility.

DRUG INTERACTIONS
None reported.

FOOD INTERACTIONS
None reported.

DISEASE INTERACTIONS
None reported.

Famciclovir

BRAND NAME
Famvir

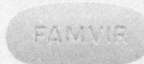

Famvir 500 mg
(SMITHKLINE BEECHAM)

▶ Drug Class: Antiviral

▶ Available in: Tablets

▶ Available OTC? No

▶ As Generic? No

Side Effects

SERIOUS
Extreme drowsiness. Call your doctor immediately.

COMMON
Headache, nausea.

LESS COMMON
Fatigue, vomiting, diarrhea, itchiness, rash, hallucinations, confusion, sore throat, back or joint pain, sinus infection, fever, shivering.

PRINCIPAL USES
To treat shingles (herpes zoster) and recurrent genital herpes.

HOW THE DRUG WORKS
Famciclovir interferes with the activity of specific enzymes needed for the replication of DNA in viral cells, thus preventing the virus from multiplying.

DOSAGE
For shingles (herpes zoster): 500 mg every 8 hours for 7 days. The effectiveness of famciclovir in treating herpes zoster is usually determined after 2 days of regular use. The best effect is achieved if the medicine is prescribed immediately after the diagnosis is made. For recurrent genital herpes: 250 mg twice a day for up to 1 year. It should be taken at the first sign of recurrence.

ONSET OF EFFECT
Within 1 hour.

DURATION OF ACTION
Unknown.

DIETARY ADVICE
No special restrictions.

STORAGE
Store in a tightly sealed container away from heat, moisture, and direct light.

IF YOU MISS A DOSE
Take it as soon as you remember. If it is near the time for the next dose, skip the missed dose and resume your regular dosage schedule. Do not double the next dose.

STOPPING THE DRUG
Take it as prescribed for the full treatment period, even if you feel better before the end of therapy. The decision to stop taking the drug should be made by your doctor.

PROLONGED USE
This drug is not intended for prolonged use, but under some circumstances it may be used for an extended period for the suppression of a chronic herpesvirus infection.

PRECAUTIONS
Over 60: No special problems expected except for older persons with impaired kidney or liver function.

Driving and Hazardous Work: Famciclovir may cause dizziness and fatigue. Do not drive or engage in hazardous work until you determine how the medicine affects you.

Alcohol: No special precautions are necessary.

Pregnancy: Studies of the use of famciclovir in pregnant women have not been done. Consult your doctor about the risk of taking famciclovir during pregnancy.

Breast Feeding: Famciclovir may pass into breast milk; avoid or discontinue use while nursing.

Infants and Children: The safety and effectiveness of famciclovir for anyone under 18 have not been established. It should be used only under close medical supervision.

Special Concerns: This medicine is not recommended for use if you have had a bone marrow transplant or a kidney transplant. Before taking famciclovir, tell the doctor if your immune system is compromised. Do not take famciclovir if you have had an allergic response to it previously. Keep the affected area of skin clean and dry; wear loose-fitting clothing. Your doctor may periodi-

cally wish to take blood tests to evaluate your kidney function.

OVERDOSE
Symptoms: No cases of overdose have been reported.

What to Do: An overdose is unlikely to occur. However, if you have any reason to suspect an overdose, call your doctor, emergency medical services (EMS), or the nearest poison control center immediately.

DRUG INTERACTIONS
Other drugs may interact with famciclovir. Consult your doctor for specific advice if you are taking probenecid or any other prescription or over-the-counter drug.

FOOD INTERACTIONS
No known food interactions.

DISEASE INTERACTIONS
Consult your doctor if you have any disorder or condition associated with a weakened immune system, such as HIV infection or AIDS. Use of famciclovir may cause complications in patients with impaired liver or kidney function, since these organs work together to remove the medication from the body.

Famotidine

Pepcid 20 mg
(MERCK)

Additional photographs

▶ Drug Class: **Histamine (H2) blocker**

▶ Available in: **Tablets, powder for suspension, orally disintegrating tablets, chewable tablets**

▶ Available OTC? **Yes**

▶ As Generic? **No**

Side Effects

SERIOUS
Irregular heart rhythm (palpitations), slowed heartbeat, severe blood problems resulting in unusual bleeding, bruising, fever, chills, and increased susceptibility to infection. Call your doctor immediately.

COMMON
Headache, fatigue, drowsiness, dizziness, nausea, vomiting, abdominal pain, diarrhea, constipation.

LESS COMMON
Blurred vision, decreased sexual desire or function, temporary hair loss, hallucinations, depression, insomnia, skin rash, hives, or redness.

PRINCIPAL USES
To treat heartburn, ulcers of the stomach and duodenum, conditions that cause excess production of stomach acid (such as Zollinger-Ellison syndrome), and gastroesophageal reflux (backwash of stomach acid into the esophagus, resulting in heartburn). Chewable tablets are taken for prevention or treatment of heartburn.

HOW THE DRUG WORKS
Famotidine blocks the action of histamine (a compound produced in the body's cells), which in turn decreases the stomach's secretion of hydrochloric acid. Once the production of stomach acid is decreased, the body is better able to heal itself.

DOSAGE
To prevent heartburn: 10 mg, 1 hour before meals. For excess stomach acid: 20 to 160 mg every 6 hours. For acid reflux disease: 20 mg twice a day for up to 6 weeks. For stomach ulcers: 40 mg once a day for 8 weeks. For duodenal ulcers: To start, 40 mg once a day at bedtime or 20 mg twice a day; later, 20 mg once a day. Chewable tablets— For treatment of heartburn: Chew one tablet (10 mg). For prevention of heartburn: Chew one tablet 15 to 60 minutes before eating.

ONSET OF EFFECT
Prescription form: Within 30 minutes. The lower dosage in the nonprescription form may take 45 minutes to relieve heartburn.

DURATION OF ACTION
Up to 12 hours.

DIETARY ADVICE
Take it after meals or with milk to minimize stomach irritation. Avoid foods that cause stomach irritation. Take chewable tablet with a glass of water.

STORAGE
Store tablets in a tightly sealed container away from heat, moisture, and direct light. After powder vials are reconstituted, store the medicine in the refrigerator, but keep it from freezing. Discard after 30 days.

IF YOU MISS A DOSE
Take it as soon as you remember. If it is near the time for the next dose, skip the missed dose and resume your regular dosage schedule. Do not double the next dose.

STOPPING THE DRUG
The decision to stop taking the prescription drug should be made in consultation with your doctor.

PROLONGED USE
Do not take the prescription drug for more than 8 weeks unless your doctor orders it. Do not take the over-the-counter drug for more than 2 weeks unless otherwise instructed by your doctor.

PRECAUTIONS
Over 60: Adverse reactions may be more likely and more severe in older patients.

Driving and Hazardous Work: Do not drive or engage in hazardous work until you determine how the medicine affects you.

Alcohol: Avoid alcohol while taking this drug; it may slow recovery. Also, this drug increases blood alcohol levels.

Pregnancy: Risks vary, depending on patient and dosage. Consult your physician for advice.

Breast Feeding: Famotidine passes into breast milk; you should avoid or discontinue use while breast feeding.

Infants and Children: Famotidine is not generally prescribed for infants and children.

Special Concerns: If necessary, famotidine may be given with antacids. Avoid cigarette smoking because it may increase secretion of stomach acid and thus worsen the disease.

OVERDOSE
Symptoms: Confusion, slurred speech, rapid heartbeat, difficulty breathing, delirium.

What to Do: Call your doctor, emergency medical services (EMS), or the nearest poison control center immediately.

DRUG INTERACTIONS
None reported.

FOOD INTERACTIONS
Carbonated drinks, citrus fruits and juices, caffeine-containing beverages, and other acidic foods or liquids may irritate the stomach or interfere with the therapeutic action of famotidine.

DISEASE INTERACTIONS
Patients with kidney disease should use famotidine in smaller, limited doses under careful supervision by a physician.

Felbamate

BRAND NAME
Felbatol

Felbatol 400 mg
(WALLACE)

▶ Drug Class: Anticonvulsant

▶ Available in: Oral suspension, tablets

▶ Available OTC? No

▶ As Generic? No

Side Effects

SERIOUS
Fever, weakness, sore throat, swollen glands, purple or red point-like spots on the skin, easy bruising, skin blistering, or yellowing of the eyes or skin may be signs of aplastic anemia, liver failure, or other potentially fatal complications. Call your doctor at once.

COMMON
Headache, nausea and vomiting, loss of appetite, stomach upset, constipation, sleepiness, insomnia, dizziness, anxiety, nervousness, tremor, muscle incoordination, runny nose and upper respiratory tract infection.

LESS COMMON
Blurred or double vision, coughing, diarrhea, abdominal pain, dry mouth. There are numerous additional side effects; consult your doctor if you are concerned about any adverse or unusual reactions.

PRINCIPAL USES
To control certain types of seizures due to epilepsy or other disorders. Because felbamate has a relatively high rate of potentially fatal side effects (including a serious blood disorder called aplastic anemia as well as liver disease), it is used only when other drugs have failed to control seizures. It may be used alone or combined with other anticonvulsants.

HOW THE DRUG WORKS
Felbamate is thought to depress the activity of certain parts of the brain and suppress the abnormal firing of neurons that causes seizures.

DOSAGE
Adults: 1,800 to 3,600 mg a day, in 3 or 4 divided doses. Children: 7 to 20 mg per lb of body weight, in 3 or 4 divided doses. Some patients may require higher doses. Low doses are used to start; the dose is gradually increased by your doctor to achieve the maximum therapeutic benefit. When switching to felbamate from other anticonvulsants, doses of the other drugs should be reduced gradually.

ONSET OF EFFECT
1 to 4 hours.

DURATION OF ACTION
Maximum effect persists for 18 to 24 hours or longer; effectiveness then gradually decreases.

DIETARY ADVICE
Take with food to minimize stomach upset.

STORAGE
Store in a tightly sealed container away from heat, moisture, and direct light.

IF YOU MISS A DOSE
Take it as soon as you remember. If it is near the time for the next dose, skip the missed dose and resume regular dosage schedule. Do not double the next dose, unless so advised by your doctor.

STOPPING THE DRUG
Never stop it abruptly; this may cause seizures. Your doctor will taper the dose over a period of weeks.

PROLONGED USE
Periodic examinations or laboratory tests to check blood counts and liver function may be needed.

PRECAUTIONS
Over 60: Older patients may require lower doses to minimize side effects.

Driving and Hazardous Work: Felbamate may cause drowsiness or dizziness. Do not drive or engage in hazardous work until you determine how the drug affects you.

Alcohol: May contribute to excessive drowsiness.

Pregnancy: Adequate studies of felbamate use during pregnancy have not been done, but many anticonvulsants are associated with an increased rate of birth defects. However, seizures during pregnancy can also increase the risks to the fetus. Discuss with your doctor the potential risks and benefits of using this drug while pregnant. Folate supplementation is recommended beginning 1 to 2 months before conception and throughout pregnancy.

Breast Feeding: Felbamate passes into breast milk, although at low levels. Consult your doctor for advice.

Infants and Children: Close medical supervision is advised for such patients.

Special Concerns: Your doctor may want you to wear a medical bracelet or carry an identification card saying that you are taking this drug.

OVERDOSE
Symptoms: Unknown; reports of felbamate overdose are very rare.

What to Do: If an excessive dose is taken, call your doctor, emergency medical services (EMS), or poison control center immediately.

DRUG INTERACTIONS
Felbamate can increase blood levels of certain anticonvulsants (phenytoin, valproic acid) and decrease blood levels of others (carbamazepine). Phenytoin and carbamazepine can decrease blood levels of felbamate. Patients sensitive to chemically related drugs, such as meprobamate or carisoprodol, may also be sensitive to felbamate.

FOOD INTERACTIONS
No known food interactions.

DISEASE INTERACTIONS
Special caution is advised if you have a history of any blood disorder, bone marrow depression (causing anemia), or liver disease.

Felodipine

Plendil 5 mg
(Astra Merck)

▶ Drug Class: Calcium channel blocker

▶ Available in: Tablets, extended-release tablets

▶ Available OTC? No

▶ As Generic? No

Side Effects

SERIOUS
Irregular or slow heartbeat, low blood pressure (causing dizziness or faintness).

COMMON
Flushing or skin rash; headache; swelling of the lower legs or feet.

LESS COMMON
Dizziness, numbness or tingling sensation, chest pain, palpitations, weakness, runny nose, rapid pulse, sore throat, abdominal discomfort, nausea, constipation or diarrhea, cough, muscle cramps, back pain, overgrowth of the gums.

PRINCIPAL USES
To control high blood pressure (hypertension).

HOW THE DRUG WORKS
Felodipine interferes with the movement of calcium into heart muscle cells and the smooth muscle cells in the walls of the arteries. This action relaxes blood vessels (causing them to widen), which lowers blood pressure, increases the blood supply to the heart, and decreases the heart's overall workload.

DOSAGE
To start, 5 to 10 mg once a day. The dose may be increased if necessary to a maximum of 20 mg once a day. For patients over 65, starting dose is 2.5 mg per day, to a maximum dose of 10 mg per day.

ONSET OF EFFECT
Within 2 to 5 hours.

DURATION OF ACTION
24 hours.

DIETARY ADVICE
Felodipine should be taken either on an empty stomach or with a light meal. Do not crush or chew tablets.

STORAGE
Store in a tightly sealed container away from heat, moisture, and direct light.

IF YOU MISS A DOSE
Take it as soon as you remember. However, if it is near the time for the next dose, skip the missed dose and resume your regular dosage schedule. Do not double the next dose.

STOPPING THE DRUG
Do not stop taking felodipine suddenly, as this may cause potentially serious health problems. If therapy is to be discontinued, the dosage should be reduced gradually, according to your doctor's instructions.

PROLONGED USE
Consult your doctor about the need for medical examinations or laboratory studies to check liver function, kidney function, and heart function.

PRECAUTIONS
Over 60: Older patients are prescribed lower starting doses, which may be gradually increased until the doctor determines the appropriate individual maintenance dose.

Driving and Hazardous Work: Do not drive or engage in hazardous work until you determine how felodipine affects you.

Alcohol: Avoid alcohol while taking this medication as it may cause an excessive drop in blood pressure.

Pregnancy: Consult your physician to determine whether the benefits of felodipine outweigh its possible risks while pregnant.

Breast Feeding: Felodipine may pass into breast milk; caution is advised. Consult your doctor for specific advice.

Infants and Children: Felodipine is generally not prescribed for children.

Special Concerns: Tell all your health care providers that you are taking felodipine and carry a note that says you take this medicine. Felodipine can cause erectile dysfunction in some men. Nicotine can reduce the effectiveness of the medicine. Hot environments can exaggerate the blood-pressure-lowering effect of felodipine.

OVERDOSE
Symptoms: Weakness, light-headedness, rapid pulse, shortness of breath, tremors, flushed skin, fainting, slurred speech.

What to Do: Call your doctor, emergency medical services (EMS), or the nearest poison control center immediately.

DRUG INTERACTIONS
Consult your doctor for advice if you are taking anticonvulsants, beta-blockers, digitalis drugs, carbamazepine, cyclosporine, digoxin, disopyramide, magnesium, phenobarbital, phenytoin, quinidine, rifampin, cimetidine, or erythromycin.

FOOD INTERACTIONS
Grapefruit juice should be avoided because it can amplify the effect of the drug and cause a serious drop in blood pressure. Avoid excessive salt intake.

DISEASE INTERACTIONS
Caution is advised when taking felodipine. Consult your doctor if you have any of the following: congestive heart failure, a history of heart attack or stroke, heart rhythm disturbances, or impaired liver or kidney function.

Fenofibrate

BRAND NAME
Tricor

▶ Drug Class: Antilipidemic (triglyceride-lowering agent)

▶ Available in: Capsules

▶ Available OTC? No

▶ As Generic? No

Side Effects

SERIOUS
Fever, unusual or unexplained muscle aches and tenderness. Call your doctor right away.

COMMON
Skin rash, infection, flu-like symptoms.

LESS COMMON
Fatigue, general feeling of pain, headache, belching, flatulence, nausea, vomiting, constipation, decreased libido, dizziness, nasal congestion, itching, visual disturbances, eye irritation.

PRINCIPAL USES
To treat high levels of blood triglyceride. Usually prescribed after other treatments—including diet, weight loss, exercise, and control of diabetes (when present)—fail to lower triglyceride levels adequately.

HOW THE DRUG WORKS
Fenofibrate speeds the removal of triglycerides from the lipoprotein known as very low density lipoprotein (VLDL), which is converted to low density lipoprotein (LDL). In some people total and LDL cholesterol levels may rise while triglycerides fall.

DOSAGE
Adults: 67 mg (1 capsule) once a day. The dose may be increased by your doctor to no more than 201 mg (3 capsules) a day.

ONSET OF EFFECT
Unknown.

DURATION OF ACTION
Unknown.

DIETARY ADVICE
Follow your doctor's dietary advice to improve control over high blood pressure and help prevent heart disease. The American Heart Association publishes a "Healthy Heart" diet; discuss this with your doctor. Limit intake of alcohol, which can raise triglyceride levels.

STORAGE
Store in a tightly sealed container away from heat, moisture, and direct light.

IF YOU MISS A DOSE
If you miss a dose on one day, do not double the dose the next day.

STOPPING THE DRUG
Do not stop taking fenofibrate on your own; the level of triglycerides in your blood will increase.

PROLONGED USE
During therapy, your doctor will conduct periodic tests to measure triglyceride levels. Therapy should be discontinued if there is an inadequate response to the medication following two months of therapy at the maximum dose of 3 capsules per day.

PRECAUTIONS
Over 60: No special problems are expected.

Driving and Hazardous Work: The use of fenofibrate should not impair your ability to perform such tasks safely.

Alcohol: Alcohol intake should be limited because it can raise triglyceride levels.

Pregnancy: Do not take fenofibrate while pregnant unless your doctor indicates that the risks of stopping the drug are too great. Triglycerides increase substantially during pregnancy and extremely high triglycerides can trigger an attack of acute pancreatitis.

Breast Feeding: Avoid or discontinue use while nursing.

Infants and Children: Safety and effectiveness have not been established for children under age 18.

Special Concerns: The most important treatment for high levels of blood triglycerides is a proper diet, weight loss, regular moderate exercise, the avoidance of certain medications, and control of diabetes. Because fenofibrate has potential side effects, it is important that you maintain a healthy diet and cooperate with other treatment strategies your physician may suggest. Fenofibrate may increase the chances of gallbladder, liver, and pancreas problems; your physician will order periodic blood tests.

OVERDOSE
Symptoms: No specific ones have been reported.

What to Do: If someone takes a much larger dose than prescribed, call your doctor, emergency medical services (EMS), or the nearest poison control center immediately.

DRUG INTERACTIONS
Certain drugs may interact adversely with fenofibrate, particularly anticoagulants such as warfarin, niacin, and any of the group of cholesterol-lowering drugs referred to as "statins." It is usually necessary to reduce the dose of warfarin to prevent bleeding. The combination of fenofibrate with either niacin or a statin drug can cause severe myositis (muscle inflammation), which can release a protein that damages the kidneys. Consult your doctor for specific advice.

FOOD INTERACTIONS
No known food interactions.

DISEASE INTERACTIONS
Inform your doctor if you have any of the following problems: gallstones, stomach or intestinal ulcer, kidney disease, muscle disease, or liver disease. The dose of fenofibrate must be reduced in those with significant kidney damage.

Fenoprofen Calcium

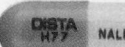

Nalfon 300 mg
(DISTA)

▶ Drug Class: Nonsteroidal anti-inflammatory drug (NSAID)

▶ Available in: Capsules, tablets

▶ Available OTC? No

▶ As Generic? Yes

Side Effects

SERIOUS
Shortness of breath or wheezing, with or without swelling of legs or other signs of heart failure; chest pain; peptic ulcer disease with vomiting of blood; black, tarry stools; decreasing kidney function. Call your doctor immediately.

COMMON
Nausea, vomiting, heartburn, diarrhea, constipation, headache, dizziness, sleepiness.

LESS COMMON
Ulcers or sores in mouth, depression, rashes or blistering of skin, ringing sound in the ears, unusual tingling or numbness of the hands or feet, seizures, blurred vision. Also elevated potassium levels, decreased blood counts; such problems can be detected by your doctor.

PRINCIPAL USES
To treat mild to moderate pain and inflammation caused by tendinitis, arthritis, bursitis, gout, soft tissue injuries, migraine and other vascular headaches, menstrual cramps, and other conditions. When patients fail to respond to one NSAID, another may be tried. The greatest effectiveness often requires trial and error of several different NSAIDs.

HOW THE DRUG WORKS
NSAIDs work by interfering with the formation of prostaglandins, naturally occurring substances in the body that cause inflammation and make nerves more sensitive to pain impulses. NSAIDs also have other modes of action that are less well understood.

DOSAGE
Adults— For arthritis: 300 to 600 mg, 3 or 4 times a day, to a maximum of 3,200 mg a day. Full effect may take 2 to 4 weeks to begin. For mild to moderate pain: 200 mg every 4 to 6 hours.

ONSET OF EFFECT
15 to 30 minutes.

DURATION OF ACTION
4 to 6 hours.

DIETARY ADVICE
Take with food; maintain your usual food and fluid intake.

STORAGE
Store in a tightly sealed container away from heat, moisture, and direct light.

IF YOU MISS A DOSE
Take it as soon as you remember. If it is near the time for the next dose, skip the missed dose and resume your regular dosage schedule. Do not double the next dose.

STOPPING THE DRUG
The decision to stop taking the drug should be made in consultation with your physician.

PROLONGED USE
Prolonged use can cause gastrointestinal problems, including ulceration and bleeding, kidney dysfunction, and liver inflammation. See your doctor for regular evaluation.

PRECAUTIONS
Over 60: Because of the potentially greater consequences of gastrointestinal side effects, the dose of NSAIDs for older patients, especially those over age 70, is often cut in half.

Driving and Hazardous Work: Do not drive or engage in hazardous work until you determine how the medicine affects you.

Alcohol: Avoid alcohol when using this medication because it increases the risk of stomach irritation.

Pregnancy: Avoid or discontinue this drug if you are pregnant or are planning to become pregnant.

Breast Feeding: Fenoprofen passes into breast milk; avoid or discontinue use while nursing.

Infants and Children: May be used in exceptional circumstances; consult your doctor.

Special Concerns: Because NSAIDs can interfere with blood coagulation, this drug should be stopped at least 3 days prior to any surgery.

OVERDOSE
Symptoms: Nausea, vomiting, severe headache, confusion, seizures.

What to Do: Call your doctor, emergency medical services (EMS), or the nearest poison control center immediately.

DRUG INTERACTIONS
Do not take this drug with aspirin or any other NSAIDs without your doctor's approval. In addition, consult your doctor if you are taking antihypertensives, steroids, anticoagulants, antibiotics, itraconazole or ketoconazole, plicamycin, penicillamine, valproic acid, phenytoin, cyclosporine, digitalis drugs, lithium, methotrexate, probenecid, triamterene, or zidovudine.

FOOD INTERACTIONS
No known food interactions.

DISEASE INTERACTIONS
Caution is advised when taking fenoprofen. Consult your doctor if you have any of the following: bleeding problems, inflammation or ulcers of the stomach and intestines, diabetes mellitus, systemic lupus erythematosus (SLE, lupus), anemia, asthma, epilepsy, Parkinson's disease, kidney stones, or a history of heart disease or alcohol abuse. Use of fenoprofen may cause complications in patients with liver or kidney disease, since these organs work together to remove the drug from the body.

Fentanyl Transdermal

BRAND NAME
Duragesic

▶ Drug Class: Opioid (narcotic) analgesic

▶ Available in: Transdermal (skin) patch

▶ Available OTC? No

▶ As Generic? No

Side Effects

SERIOUS
Seizures, severe drowsiness, hallucinations, slow heartbeat, very slow or weak breathing, cold, clammy skin, pinpoint pupils of eyes. Call your doctor immediately.

COMMON
Dizziness, nausea or vomiting, constipation, drowsiness, urine retention, itching.

LESS COMMON
Sweating, skin reaction at patch site, rigid muscles, fainting, jerking body movements (myoclonus).

PRINCIPAL USES
To control severe chronic pain.

HOW THE DRUG WORKS
Fentanyl, a narcotic, relieves pain by acting on specific areas of the spinal cord and brain that process pain signals from nerves throughout the body.

DOSAGE
Attach the patch to the skin using the dose recommended by your doctor. Replace the patch every 72 hours or as your doctor directs. To apply, remove the patch from its protective pouch and remove the liner from the sticky side of the patch. Place the patch on a site that is hairless and dry, and hold it in place for 10 to 30 seconds to ensure adhesion. Wash the area with water if necessary, but do not use soap, lotion, alcohol, or other substances that may irritate the skin. Do not apply it in the same place more than once within a 3-day period. Avoid any area that is burned, irritated, or excessively oily. Wash your hands after applying a new patch. Remove an old patch after 72 hours (3 days), fold it onto itself and dispose of it in the toilet. Fentanyl transdermal patches are available in the following concentrations: 25 micrograms per hour (mcg/hr); 50 mcg/hr; 75 mcg/hr; 100 mcg/hr.

ONSET OF EFFECT
12 to 24 hours.

DURATION OF ACTION
Up to 72 hours.

DIETARY ADVICE
The patch can be applied without regard to diet.

STORAGE
Store the patch in its protective pouch away from heat, moisture, and direct light.

IF YOU MISS A DOSE
Apply a new patch as soon as you remember. Do not apply more than one patch at a time, unless directed to do otherwise by your doctor. Remove the patch 3 days after applying it.

STOPPING THE DRUG
The decision to stop using the drug should be made by your doctor. It may be necessary to reduce the dose gradually if the medication is used for a long time, to decrease the risk of suffering withdrawal symptoms.

PROLONGED USE
Prolonged use may result in physical dependence.

PRECAUTIONS
Over 60: Adverse reactions may be more likely and more severe in older patients. The smallest-dose patch is generally used at the beginning of therapy.

Driving and Hazardous Work: The use of fentanyl may impair your ability to perform such tasks safely.

Alcohol: Avoid alcohol.

Pregnancy: Adequate human studies have not been done. Before taking fentanyl, discuss with your doctor the relative risks and benefits of using this drug while pregnant.

Breast Feeding: This drug passes into breast milk; avoid or discontinue using it while nursing.

Infants and Children: This drug should not be used by patients under age 18 who weigh less than 110 pounds. Safety and effectiveness for children under the age of 12 have not been determined.

Special Concerns: Do not alter your dose or suddenly stop using this drug without consulting your doctor. Abruptly stopping its use may cause withdrawal symptoms. Heat can cause fentanyl to be absorbed more rapidly. Avoid heating pads, sunbathing, or long showers or baths in hot water. Not recommended for postoperative pain.

OVERDOSE
Symptoms: Seizures, severe drowsiness, hallucinations, slow heartbeat, very slow or weak breathing, cold, clammy skin, pinpoint pupils of eyes.

What to Do: Call your doctor, emergency medical services (EMS), or the nearest poison control center immediately.

DRUG INTERACTIONS
Consult your doctor for specific advice if you are taking benzodiazepines; central nervous system depressants such as opiates, barbiturates, and tranquilizers; or antidepressants, amiodarone, clonidine, or MAO inhibitors.

FOOD INTERACTIONS
No known food interactions.

DISEASE INTERACTIONS
Consult your doctor if you have any of the following: liver disease, kidney disease, prostate problems, gallbladder disease, intestinal problems such as colitis, underactive thyroid, brain tumor, any heart disease, anemia, or a history of alcohol or drug abuse. Fever may increase the rate at which the drug is absorbed by the body, thus increasing risk of overdose.

Fentanyl Transmucosal

BRAND NAME
Actiq

▶ Drug Class: Opioid (narcotic) analgesic

▶ Available in: Oral transmucosal (inside the mouth) lozenge

▶ Available OTC? No

▶ As Generic? No

Side Effects

SERIOUS
Seizures, severe drowsiness, hallucinations, slow heartbeat, very slow or weak breathing, cold, clammy skin, pinpoint pupils of eyes. Call your doctor immediately.

COMMON
Dizziness, nausea or vomiting, constipation, drowsiness, urine retention, itching.

LESS COMMON
Sweating, skin reaction at patch site, rigid muscles, fainting, jerking body movements (myoclonus).

PRINCIPAL USES
To manage flare-ups of cancer pain in people who are already receiving and who are tolerant to narcotic (opioid) therapy for underlying cancer pain. People considered opioid tolerant are those taking at least 60 mg of morphine a day, 50 mcg of transdermal fentanyl per hour, or an equivalent dose of another narcotic for a week or longer. Fentanyl lozenges are not for short-term pain, including pain from injuries or surgery.

HOW THE DRUG WORKS
Fentanyl, a narcotic, relieves pain by acting on specific areas of the spinal cord and brain that process pain signals from nerves throughout the body.

DOSAGE
Your oncologist or physician will determine the appropriate dosage. Dosage will be individually adjusted to provide adequate pain relief with minimal side effects. Do not consume more than 4 lozenges per day (no more than 2 per flare-up); if you are not getting adequate pain relief, consult your doctor.

ONSET OF EFFECT
Within 15 to 45 minutes.

DURATION OF ACTION
Unknown.

DIETARY ADVICE
You may drink water before using the drug. Do not eat or drink anything while using it.

STORAGE
Store the lozenge in its protective package away from heat, moisture, and direct light in a child-resistant locked storage space. Do not freeze or refrigerate.

IF YOU MISS A DOSE
Not applicable. This drug is used as needed for breakthrough cancer pain that is not successfully controlled by regularly prescribed pain medication.

STOPPING THE DRUG
The lozenges are used on an as needed basis. However, because fentanyl can be addictive, it may be necessary to reduce the dose gradually if the medication is used for a long time, to decrease the risk of withdrawal symptoms.

PROLONGED USE
Prolonged use may result in physical dependence.

PRECAUTIONS
Over 60: Adverse reactions may be more likely and more severe in older patients. The smallest-dose lozenge is generally used at the beginning of therapy.

Driving and Hazardous Work: The use of fentanyl may impair your ability to perform such tasks safely.

Alcohol: Avoid alcohol.

Pregnancy: Adequate human studies have not been done. Before taking fentanyl, discuss with your doctor the relative risks and benefits of using this drug while pregnant.

Breast Feeding: This drug passes into breast milk; avoid or discontinue using it while nursing.

Infants and Children: Safety and effectiveness for children under the age of 16 have not been determined. The lozenges contain a high concentration of fentanyl which can be fatal to a child.

Special Concerns: You must be opioid tolerant to use this form of fentanyl. The lozenges contain a high concentration of the drug and can cause serious, possibly fatal side effects in those not already taking narcotic pain relievers. If you do not finish the lozenge within 15 minutes, dispose of the remainder appropriately. Your doctor or health care provider will teach you how to do so.

OVERDOSE
Symptoms: Seizures, severe drowsiness, hallucinations, slow heartbeat, very slow or weak breathing, cold, clammy skin, pinpoint pupils of eyes.

What to Do: Call your doctor, emergency medical services (EMS), or the nearest poison control center immediately.

DRUG INTERACTIONS
Consult your doctor for specific advice if you are taking benzodiazepines; central nervous system depressants such as barbiturates, and tranquilizers; or antidepressants, amiodarone, clonidine, or MAO inhibitors.

FOOD INTERACTIONS
No known food interactions.

DISEASE INTERACTIONS
Consult your doctor if you have any of the following: liver disease, kidney disease, prostate problems, gallbladder disease, intestinal problems such as colitis, underactive thyroid, brain tumor, any heart disease, anemia, chronic obstructive pulmonary disease or other respiratory illnesses, or a history of alcohol or drug abuse. Fever may increase the rate at which the drug is absorbed by the body, thus increasing risk of overdose.

Ferrous Salts

BRAND NAMES
Feosol, Fer-In-Sol, Fer-Iron, Fero-Gradumet, Ferospace, Ferra-TD, Ferralyn Lanacaps

Generic 300 mg
(UPSHER-SMITH)

Additional photographs

▶ Drug Class: Dietary supplement

▶ Available in: Capsules, drops, elixir, solution, tablets

▶ Available OTC? Yes

▶ As Generic? Yes

Side Effects

SERIOUS
No serious side effects are associated with ferrous salts, except for iron overload due to prolonged, inappropriate use of the mineral.

COMMON
Nausea, constipation, black stools.

LESS COMMON
Stained teeth (with liquid forms), stomach pain, vomiting, diarrhea.

PRINCIPAL USES
To help increase the body's stores of iron, a mineral essential to the manufacture of red blood cells. An insufficient number of red blood cells results in anemia.

HOW THE DRUG WORKS
Ferrous salts are required for the production of hemoglobin in developing red blood cells. Hemoglobin is a complex iron-based protein in the red cell that carries oxygen to the body's tissues and carries carbon dioxide gas away from the tissues to be exhaled by the lungs.

DOSAGE
For iron deficiency, 325 mg, 3 times a day. Children: 5 to 10 mg for every 2.2 lbs (1 kg) of body weight 3 times a day.

ONSET OF EFFECT
From 5 to 7 days. Depending on the extent of the iron deficiency, more than 3 months of therapy may be needed for maximum benefit to be realized.

DURATION OF ACTION
Depends on the body's ability to utilize it.

DIETARY ADVICE
Take 1 hour before or 2 hours after eating.

STORAGE
Store in a tightly sealed container away from heat and direct light. Keep the liquid form from freezing.

IF YOU MISS A DOSE
Take it as soon as you remember. If it is near the time for the next dose, skip the missed dose and resume your regular dosage schedule. Do not double the next dose.

STOPPING THE DRUG
If the medication was prescribed, the decision to stop taking this supplement should be made by your physician.

PROLONGED USE
Prolonged use may result in the accumulation of iron in the tissues, the effects of which can include liver damage, heart problems, diabetes, erectile dysfunction, and unusually bronzed skin. Do not take iron supplements without consulting your doctor.

PRECAUTIONS
Over 60: Problems in older adults have not been reported with intake of normal daily recommended amounts.

Driving and Hazardous Work: No problems are expected.

Alcohol: Avoid alcohol while taking this medication because it may cause excess absorption of iron.

Pregnancy: This medication should be taken during pregnancy only if your doctor so advises.

Breast Feeding: No problems are expected during breast feeding; however, consult your doctor before taking ferrous salts.

Infants and Children: No unusual problems reported in infants and children. Close medical supervision is nonetheless recommended, and iron tablets should be stored out of reach of small children to avoid accidental ingestion, which can be severely toxic.

Special Concerns: The genetic disorder hemochromatosis, in which iron absorption is excessive, is very common. Iron deficiency may also be the first indication of a gastrointestinal malignancy. Therefore, iron should only be taken on the advice of a physician. Liquid forms of iron can stain the teeth. To prevent stains, mix each dose in water, fruit juice, or tomato juice and drink it through a straw. When using a dropper, place the dose on the back of the tongue and drink a glass of water or juice. Tooth stains can be removed by brushing with baking soda or 3% hydrogen peroxide.

OVERDOSE
Symptoms: Lethargy, nausea, vomiting, weak and rapid pulse, dehydration, loss of consciousness.

What to Do: Call your doctor, emergency medical services (EMS), or the nearest poison control center immediately.

DRUG INTERACTIONS
The following drugs may interact with ferrous salts and prevent their absorption: antacids, antibiotics, fluoroquinalones, levodopa, cholestyramine, or vitamin E. Consult your doctor for specific advice.

FOOD INTERACTIONS
Some foods can reduce the effect of this drug. The following foods should be avoided or taken in small amounts for at least 1 hour before and 2 hours after iron is taken: Eggs, milk, spinach, cheese, yogurt, tea, coffee, whole-grain bread, cereal, and bran.

DISEASE INTERACTIONS
Consult your doctor if you have any of the following: a history of alcoholism; kidney disease; liver disease; porphyria; rheumatoid arthritis; asthma; allergies; heart disease; or a stomach ulcer, colitis, or another intestinal problem.

Fexofenadine

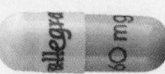

Allegra 60 mg
(HOECHST MARION ROUSSEL)

▶ Drug Class: Antihistamine

▶ Available in: Capsules

▶ Available OTC? No

▶ As Generic? No

Side Effects

SERIOUS
No serious side effects are associated with the use of fexofenadine.

COMMON
No common side effects are associated with the use of fexofenadine.

LESS COMMON
Drowsiness, fatigue, stomach upset, painful menstrual bleeding.

PRINCIPAL USES
To prevent or relieve symptoms of hay fever and other allergies, and to treat itchy skin and hives.

HOW THE DRUG WORKS
Fexofenadine blocks the effects of histamine, a naturally occurring substance within the body that causes swelling, itching, sneezing, watery eyes, hives, and other symptoms of allergic reaction.

DOSAGE
For adults and children age 12 and over: 60 mg, 2 times a day. For patients with decreased kidney function, a starting dose of 60 mg once a day is recommended. Children under age 12: Safety and effectiveness of fexofenadine in this age group have not been established.

ONSET OF EFFECT
Within 1 to 2 hours.

DURATION OF ACTION
12 hours or longer.

DIETARY ADVICE
This drug can be taken without regard to food or drink.

STORAGE
Store in a tightly sealed container in a dry place away from heat and direct light at room temperature.

IF YOU MISS A DOSE
Take it as soon as you remember. If it is near the time for the next dose, skip the missed dose and resume your regular dosage schedule. Do not double the next dose.

STOPPING THE DRUG
You should take it as prescribed for the full treatment period, but you may stop if you are feeling better before the scheduled end of therapy. Fexofenadine can be used as needed to relieve symptoms of hay fever or other allergies.

PROLONGED USE
Tolerance, or decreased responsiveness to the drug, generally does not develop with prolonged use of fexofenadine; if it does, consult your physician. No special problems are expected with long-term use.

PRECAUTIONS
Over 60: No special problems are expected.

Driving and Hazardous Work: In rare cases fexofenadine may cause drowsiness and fatigue. Do not drive or engage in hazardous work until you determine how the medicine affects you.

Alcohol: No special precautions are necessary.

Pregnancy: In animal studies, fexofenadine did not cause birth defects. Adequate, well-controlled studies in humans have not been done. Consult your doctor about taking fexofenadine if you are pregnant or are planning to become pregnant.

Breast Feeding: Fexofenadine may pass into breast milk; caution is advised. Consult your doctor for specific advice about the use of fexofenadine while nursing.

Infants and Children: Side effects are not expected to be any different in children ages 12 to 18 than those in patients 18 and older. The safety and effectiveness of fexofenadine for children up to 12 years of age have not been established.

OVERDOSE
Symptoms: Extreme drowsiness or fatigue.

What to Do: An overdose of fexofenadine is unlikely to be life-threatening. However, if someone takes a much larger dose than prescribed, call your doctor, emergency medical services (EMS), or local poison control center right away.

DRUG INTERACTIONS
There are no known interactions between fexofenadine and other drugs.

FOOD INTERACTIONS
No known food interactions.

DISEASE INTERACTIONS
Consult your physician if you have impaired kidney function.

Fexofenadine/Pseudoephedrine

▶ Drug Class: Antihistamine/ decongestant

▶ Available in: Extended-release tablets

▶ Available OTC? No

▶ As Generic? No

Side Effects

SERIOUS
Palpitations, shortness of breath, breathing difficulty. Stop taking the medication and call your doctor right away.

COMMON
Headache, insomnia, nausea.

LESS COMMON
Dry mouth, indigestion, throat irritation, dizziness, agitation, back pain, anxiety, nervousness, stomach pain, upper respiratory infection.

PRINCIPAL USES
To prevent or relieve symptoms of seasonal allergies such as hay fever.

HOW THE DRUG WORKS
Fexofenadine blocks the effects of histamine, a naturally occurring substance within the body that causes swelling, itching, sneezing, watery eyes, hives, and other symptoms of allergic reaction. Pseudoephedrine narrows and constricts blood vessels to decrease the blood flow to swollen nasal passages and other tissues, which in turn reduces nasal secretions, shrinks swollen nasal mucous membranes, and improves airflow in nasal passages.

DOSAGE
Adults and teenagers: 1 tablet (60 mg fexofenadine/120 mg pseudoephedrine) twice a day.

ONSET OF EFFECT
Within 1 to 2 hours.

DURATION OF ACTION
12 hours or longer.

DIETARY ADVICE
This medication should be taken at least 1 hour before or 2 hours after a meal. Taking it with food delays the onset of the drug's effects. The tablet should be swallowed whole.

STORAGE
Store in a tightly sealed container away from heat, moisture, and direct light.

IF YOU MISS A DOSE
Take it as soon as you remember. If it is near the time for the next dose, skip the missed dose and resume your regular dosage schedule. Do not double the next dose.

STOPPING THE DRUG
You may stop taking the drug before the scheduled end of therapy if you are feeling better.

PROLONGED USE
Consult your doctor about taking this drug for more than 5 to 7 days.

PRECAUTIONS
Over 60: Adverse reactions may be more likely and more severe in older patients.

Driving and Hazardous Work: Do not drive or engage in hazardous work until you determine how the medicine affects you.

Alcohol: No special precautions are necessary.

Pregnancy: Adequate human studies have not been done. Before taking this drug, tell your doctor if you are or are planning to become pregnant. Discuss with your doctor the relative risks and benefits of using this drug while pregnant.

Breast Feeding: The pseudoephedrine component of this drug passes into breast milk; avoid or discontinue taking this drug while breast feeding.

Infants and Children: Not recommended for use by children under age 12.

Special Concerns: If your symptoms do not improve within 7 days, check with your doctor. To help prevent insomnia, take the last dose at least 2 hours before your bedtime.

OVERDOSE
Symptoms: No cases of overdose with this drug have been reported.

What to Do: An overdose is unlikely; however, if you have reason to suspect one has occurred, call emergency medical services (EMS) to receive evaluation and treatment.

DRUG INTERACTIONS
This drug and MAO inhibitors should not be used within 14 days of each other. Consult your doctor for specific advice if you are taking antihypertensives or digitalis drugs.

FOOD INTERACTIONS
No known food interactions.

DISEASE INTERACTIONS
You should not take this drug if you have a history of narrow-angle glaucoma, urinary retention, severe high blood pressure, or severe coronary artery disease. Caution is advised if you have mild to moderate high blood pressure, diabetes mellitus, a history of angina or heart attack, an overactive thyroid gland, impaired kidney function, or an enlarged prostate.

Finasteride

Proscar 5 mg
(MERCK)

▶ Drug Class: 5-alpha reductase inhibitor

▶ Available in: Tablets

▶ Available OTC? No

▶ As Generic? No

Side Effects

SERIOUS
No serious side effects are associated with the use of finasteride.

COMMON
No common side effects are associated with the use of finasteride.

LESS COMMON
Reduced sex drive, erectile dysfunction (impotence), decreased quantity of ejaculate. It should be noted that this decrease is not a sign of reduced fertility.

PRINCIPAL USES
To treat benign prostatic hyperplasia (BPH)—that is, noncancerous enlargement of the prostate gland, which is extremely common among men over 50. Also used to treat male pattern hair loss.

HOW THE DRUG WORKS
Finasteride halts or reverses enlargement of the prostate by blocking the action of the enzyme 5-alpha reductase, which the body needs to produce dihydrotestosterone (DHT), a chemical involved in the mechanism that enlarges the prostate. DHT is also integral to the processs of male pattern hair loss; by decreasing DHT concentrations in the scalp, finasteride may slow or reverse this process.

DOSAGE
For BPH: 5 mg once a day. For male pattern hair loss: 1 mg once a day.

ONSET OF EFFECT
Unknown.

DURATION OF ACTION
For BPH: 24 hours for a single dose; up to 2 weeks after standard therapy is ended. For hair loss: New hair resulting from finasteride treatments will likely regress following discontinuation of the medication.

DIETARY ADVICE
Finasteride can be taken without regard to diet. If you have trouble swallowing the tablet whole, you can crush it and take it with liquid or food.

STORAGE
Store in a tightly sealed container away from heat, moisture, and direct light.

IF YOU MISS A DOSE
If you miss a dose on one day, do not double the dose the next day.

STOPPING THE DRUG
The decision to stop taking the drug should be made by your doctor.

PROLONGED USE
If you take this drug for a prolonged period for BPH, see your doctor regularly so that changes in prostate size can be monitored. For hair loss, continued use is recommended to sustain the drug's benefits.

PRECAUTIONS
Over 60: No special problems are expected.

Driving and Hazardous Work: The use of finasteride should not impair your ability to perform such tasks safely.

Alcohol: No special precautions are necessary.

Pregnancy: Although finasteride is not prescribed for women, those who are pregnant or planning to become pregnant should not handle the medication, especially if it is crushed or broken, because it can have an adverse effect on a male fetus. Men who take finasteride should use a barrier method of birth control (such as a condom), which prevents the female sexual partner from being exposed to small quantities of the drug present in semen.

Breast Feeding: Women who are nursing should avoid contact with finasteride or the sperm of a man who is taking the drug.

Infants and Children: Finasteride is not prescribed for children.

Special Concerns: Before taking this medicine for BPH, you should have a digital rectal examination and other tests for prostate cancer. Note that finasteride may affect the results of the prostate-specific antigen (PSA) test for prostate cancer; be sure any doctor you see for treatment, including your dentist, knows that you are taking this drug.

OVERDOSE
Symptoms: No specific ones have been reported.

What to Do: An overdose of finasteride is unlikely to be life-threatening. However, if someone takes a much larger dose than prescribed, call your doctor, emergency medical services (EMS), or the nearest poison control center.

DRUG INTERACTIONS
Consult your doctor for specific advice if you are taking amantadine, amphetamines, antihistamines, antidepressants, antidyskinetics (medications for Parkinson's disease or similar conditions), antipsychotics, appetite suppressants, anticholinergics (medications for stomach spasms or cramps), bronchodilators, decongestants, ephedrine, or pseudoephedrine.

FOOD INTERACTIONS
No known food interactions.

DISEASE INTERACTIONS
Caution is advised when taking finasteride. Before you start, consult your doctor if you have liver disease, which may magnify the effects of finasteride.

Flavoxate

BRAND NAME
Urispas

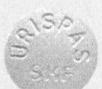

Urispas 100 mg
(SMITHKLINE BEECHAM)

▶ Drug Class: Urinary tract antispasmodic

▶ Available in: Tablets

▶ Available OTC? No

▶ As Generic? No

Side Effects

SERIOUS
Rash, fever, rapid pulse. Call your doctor right away.

COMMON
Confusion, dry mouth and throat, blurred vision, heightened sensitivity of the eyes to light (photophobia), decreased ability to sweat.

LESS COMMON
Dizziness, headache, nervousness, drowsiness, difficulty concentrating, abdominal pain, difficulty focusing the eyes, constipation, nausea, vomiting, hives, fever.

PRINCIPAL USES
To relieve the symptoms of urinary tract spasms, which may include chronic urinary urgency, frequent urination, pain, and incontinence.

HOW THE DRUG WORKS
Flavoxate blocks nerve impulses to the smooth muscles of the urinary tract, preventing muscle contraction in the bladder.

DOSAGE
Adults and children over 12: 100 to 200 mg, 3 or 4 times a day.

ONSET OF EFFECT
45 to 60 minutes.

DURATION OF ACTION
Unknown.

DIETARY ADVICE
Take flavoxate with water 30 minutes before meals unless your physician advises otherwise. If it causes stomach upset, ask your physician if you can take it with food or milk.

STORAGE
Store in a tightly sealed container away from heat, moisture, and direct light.

IF YOU MISS A DOSE
Take it as soon as you remember. If it is near the time for the next dose, skip the missed dose and resume your regular dosage schedule. Do not double the next dose.

STOPPING THE DRUG
Take as prescribed for the full treatment period, even if you begin to feel better before the scheduled end of therapy.

PROLONGED USE
Tell your doctor if symptoms do not improve after prolonged use of this drug.

PRECAUTIONS
Over 60: Adverse reactions, especially confusion, may be more likely and more severe in older patients.

Driving and Hazardous Work: Do not drive or engage in hazardous work until you determine how the medicine affects you.

Alcohol: No special precautions are necessary.

Pregnancy: Flavoxate has not been shown to cause birth defects in animals. Adequate human studies have not been done. Before you take the medicine, tell your doctor if you are pregnant or plan to become pregnant; you must weigh the drug's benefits against the risks.

Breast Feeding: Flavoxate may pass into breast milk; caution is advised. Consult your doctor for advice.

Infants and Children: Not generally recommended for use by children under the age of 12. If flavoxate is prescribed for children, the dose should be determined by your pediatrician, and it should be given under close medical supervision.

Special Concerns: Limit exposure to sunlight and wear sunglasses in bright light. Avoid overexertion, since flavoxate interferes with the ability to sweat, which may lead to heatstroke. Use sugarless gum, candy, or ice chips to relieve dry mouth. Contact your doctor 2 months prior to having any surgery (including dental surgery) that will require general or spinal anesthesia. Tell your doctor if you experience abdominal bloating or difficulty emptying your bladder completely.

OVERDOSE
Symptoms: Rapid pulse and breathing, dilated pupils, dizziness, fever, hallucinations, slurred speech, confusion, agitation, unusual excitability, flushed face, convulsions, loss of consciousness.

What to Do: Call your doctor, emergency medical services (EMS), or the nearest poison control center immediately.

DRUG INTERACTIONS
Certain drugs may interact adversely with flavoxate or interfere with its action. Consult your doctor if you are taking cholinergic drugs. Also, tell your doctor if you are taking any other prescription or over-the-counter medicine before you take flavoxate.

FOOD INTERACTIONS
No known food interactions.

DISEASE INTERACTIONS
Caution is advised when taking flavoxate. Consult your doctor if you have any of the following: severe bleeding, narrow-angle glaucoma, angina, intestinal obstruction, urinary tract blockage, hiatal hernia, an enlarged prostate, myasthenia gravis, or a peptic ulcer.

Flecainide Acetate

Tambocor 100 mg
(3M)

▶ Drug Class: Antiarrhythmic

▶ Available in: Tablets

▶ Available OTC? No

▶ As Generic? No

Side Effects

SERIOUS
Shortness of breath, chest pain, irregular or rapid heartbeat, fainting, swollen feet or lower extremities, shaking or trembling. Call your doctor immediately.

COMMON
Headache; dizziness or lightheadedness; blurred vision or other visual disturbances, such as seeing spots.

LESS COMMON
Nausea, constipation, tremor, fatigue, abdominal pain, swollen hands, skin rash, anxiety, mental depression.

PRINCIPAL USES
To stabilize irregular heartbeats (cardiac arrhythmias).

HOW THE DRUG WORKS
Flecainide slows nerve impulses in the heart and makes heart tissue less sensitive to nerve impulses, thus stabilizing heartbeat.

DOSAGE
For paroxysmal supraventricular tachycardia or paroxysmal atrial fibrillation, or flutter, in persons without structural heart disease: Starting with 50 mg every 12 hours, increased by 50 mg every 4 days if necessary to a maximum of 150 mg every 12 hours. For life-threatening heart arrhythmias: Starting with 100 mg every 12 hours, increased by 50 mg every 4 days if necessary to a maximum of 200 mg every 12 hours. Initial dose should be lower in patients who have impaired heart or kidney function.

ONSET OF EFFECT
1 to 6 hours. May require daily doses for 3 to 5 days for full effect to occur.

DURATION OF ACTION
12 to 27 hours (longer in patients with impaired heart or kidney function).

DIETARY ADVICE
Take tablet with liquid. May be taken with or between meals.

STORAGE
Store in a tightly sealed container in a dry place away from heat and direct light.

IF YOU MISS A DOSE
Take it as soon as you remember, up to 6 hours late. If more than 6 hours, skip the missed dose and resume your regular dosage schedule as prescribed. Do not double the next dose.

STOPPING THE DRUG
Take as prescribed for the full treatment period, even if you begin to feel better before the scheduled end of therapy. The decision to stop taking the drug should be made by your doctor.

PROLONGED USE
Lifelong therapy may be necessary. See your doctor regularly for examinations and diagnostic tests if you must take this medicine for a prolonged period.

PRECAUTIONS
Over 60: Adverse reactions, especially heartbeat irregularities, may be more common and more severe in older patients.

Driving and Hazardous Work: Do not drive or engage in hazardous work until you determine how the medicine affects you.

Alcohol: Alcohol should be avoided while taking this medicine because it may further depress normal heart function.

Pregnancy: In animal studies large doses of flecainide have been shown to cause birth defects. Human studies have not been done. Before taking flecainide, tell your doctor if you are pregnant or plan to become pregnant.

Breast Feeding: Flecainide passes into breast milk and may cause harm to the infant; avoid or discontinue use while nursing.

Infants and Children: Not recommended for use by patients under age 18.

Special Concerns: Before you have any surgery (including dental surgery) or receive emergency medical care, be sure to tell the doctor or dentist that you are using flecainide. If you have a pacemaker, its function should be assessed shortly after starting therapy with flecainide.

OVERDOSE
Symptoms: Dizziness or faintness, rapid or irregular heartbeat, tremor, unusual or profuse sweating, drowsiness, loss of consciousness.

What to Do: Call your doctor, emergency medical services (EMS), or the nearest poison control center immediately.

DRUG INTERACTIONS
The following drugs may interact with flecainide. Consult your doctor if you are taking antacids, amiodarone or other antiarrhythmic drugs, beta-blockers, calcium channel blockers, bone marrow depressants, carbonic anhydrase inhibitors, carbamazepine, cimetidine, digitalis drugs, doxepin, nicotine, phenobarbital, or phenytoin.

FOOD INTERACTIONS
Caffeine-containing beverages can decrease flecainide activity. No other food interactions are expected.

DISEASE INTERACTIONS
Use of flecainide may cause complications in patients with heart disease, heart block, or slow heart rates, and may cause complications in patients with liver or kidney disease, since these organs work together to remove the medication from the body.

Fluconazole

Diflucan 200 mg
(ROERIG)

Additional photographs

▶ Drug Class: Antifungal

▶ Available in: Tablets, oral suspension, injection

▶ Available OTC? No

▶ As Generic? No

Side Effects

SERIOUS
Skin rash or itching, fever or chills. Call your doctor right away.

COMMON
No common side effects have been reported with the use of fluconazole.

LESS COMMON
Diarrhea, nausea, vomiting, constipation, dizziness, headache, redness or flushing of skin.

PRINCIPAL USES
To treat fungal infections of the mouth and throat (thrush), of the vagina (yeast infection), or throughout the body, as well as meningitis (inflammation of the protective membranes surrounding the brain). Often used to treat AIDS-related fungal infections. May also be used to prevent recurring fungal infections in susceptible patients weakened by AIDS or by chemotherapy or radiation treatment.

HOW THE DRUG WORKS
Fluconazole prevents fungal organisms from manufacturing vital substances required for their growth and function. This drug is effective only for infections caused by fungal organisms. It will not work for bacterial or viral infections.

DOSAGE
Adults and teenagers— For fungal infections: 200 to 400 mg on the first day, then 100 to 400 mg once a day, using oral forms or injection. Injections are into a vein. For vaginal yeast infection: 1 dose of 150 mg, tablet or oral suspension.

ONSET OF EFFECT
Oral forms: Unknown. Injection: Immediate.

DURATION OF ACTION
Unknown.

DIETARY ADVICE
Swallow tablets with liquid. Oral suspension should be shaken and carefully measured out before you take it. This drug can be taken without regard to diet.

STORAGE
Store in a tightly sealed container away from heat, moisture, and direct light. Keep any liquid form refrigerated, but do not allow it to freeze.

IF YOU MISS A DOSE
Take it as soon as you remember. This will help keep a constant level of medication in your system. If it is near the time for the next dose, skip the missed dose and resume your regular dosage schedule. Do not double the next dose.

STOPPING THE DRUG
Take it as prescribed for the full treatment period, even if you begin to feel better before the scheduled end of therapy. The decision to stop taking the drug should be made by your doctor. Gradual reduction of the dose may be necessary if you have been taking this medicine for a long time.

PROLONGED USE
Notify your doctor if your condition does not improve, or instead becomes worse, within a few weeks.

PRECAUTIONS
Over 60: Dosage may need to be reduced in older patients with impaired kidney function.

Driving and Hazardous Work: The use of fluconazole should not impair your ability to perform such tasks safely.

Alcohol: No special precautions are necessary.

Pregnancy: Adequate studies of fluconazole use during pregnancy have not been done. Consult your doctor for specific advice if you are currently pregnant or plan to become pregnant.

Breast Feeding: Fluconazole may pass into breast milk; caution is advised. Consult your doctor for specific advice.

Infants and Children: Fluconazole is not generally prescribed for children under 14.

Special Concerns: Your doctor should monitor your kidney function while you take fluconazole. Tell any doctor or dentist whom you consult that you are taking this medicine. Be sure to shake the oral suspension well before taking it.

OVERDOSE
Symptoms: An overdose with fluconazole is unlikely.

What to Do: Emergency instructions not applicable.

DRUG INTERACTIONS
Consult your doctor for specific advice if you are taking oral antidiabetic drugs, cyclosporine, rifampin, phenytoin, rifabutin, tacrolimus, astemizole, or warfarin.

FOOD INTERACTIONS
No food interactions have been reported.

DISEASE INTERACTIONS
Caution is advised when taking fluconazole. Consult your doctor if you have a history of alcohol abuse (and associated liver problems), or any type of liver or kidney disease, since these organs work together to remove the medication from the body.

Flucytosine

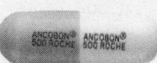

Ancobon 500 mg
(ROCHE)

▶ Drug Class: Antifungal

▶ Available in: Capsules

▶ Available OTC? No

▶ As Generic? No

Side Effects

SERIOUS
Unusual fatigue, yellow eyes or skin, unusual bleeding or bruising, skin rash, redness, or itching, sore throat, fever, increased sensitivity of eyes to sunlight, confusion, hallucinations. Call your doctor immediately.

COMMON
Loss of appetite, abdominal pain, stomach upset, nausea and vomiting, diarrhea.

LESS COMMON
Dizziness or lightheadedness, headache, unusual drowsiness.

PRINCIPAL USES
To treat general fungal infections and severe fungal infections of the bone and bone marrow (osteomyelitis), the protective layers of tissue surrounding the brain (meningitis), the respiratory tract (pneumonia), the blood (septicemia), and the genitourinary tract (particularly those infections associated with AIDS).

HOW THE DRUG WORKS
Flucytosine kills infectious microorganisms by preventing them from synthesizing genetic material (RNA and DNA), thereby preventing the cells from reproducing.

DOSAGE
Adults and children: Usual dose is 12.5 to 37.5 mg per 2.2 lbs (1 kg) of body weight every 6 hours.

ONSET OF EFFECT
Unknown.

DURATION OF ACTION
Unknown.

DIETARY ADVICE
Flucytosine can be taken without regard to diet. You should take a few capsules at a time, over a 15-minute period, with food to reduce stomach distress.

STORAGE
Store in a tightly sealed container away from heat, moisture, and direct light.

IF YOU MISS A DOSE
Take it as soon as you remember. If it is near the time for the next dose, skip the missed dose and resume your regular dosage schedule. Do not double the next dose.

STOPPING THE DRUG
Take it as prescribed for the full treatment period, even if you begin to feel better before the scheduled end of therapy. The decision to stop taking the drug should be made by your doctor.

PROLONGED USE
Prolonged use may cause or aggravate bone marrow depression (reduced bone marrow function), liver damage, or kidney damage. Consult your doctor about the need for periodic blood cell counts and liver and kidney function tests.

PRECAUTIONS
Over 60: Dosage must be reduced in older patients who have impaired kidney function.

Driving and Hazardous Work: Do not drive or engage in hazardous work until you determine how the medicine affects you. Use of this drug may be a disqualification for piloting aircraft.

Alcohol: No special precautions are necessary.

Pregnancy: Adequate studies of flucytosine use during pregnancy have not been done. Consult your doctor for specific advice if you are pregnant or are planning to become pregnant.

Breast Feeding: Flucytosine may pass into breast milk; it is unclear if this poses any risks to the nursing infant. Consult your doctor for specific advice.

Infants and Children: No special problems are expected in young patients.

Special Concerns: Stay out of direct sunlight, especially between 10 am and 3 pm. Wear protective clothing, including a hat, and sunglasses. Apply a sun block with a sun protection factor (SPF) of at least 15. This medicine is generally given in conjunction with amphotericin B to avoid development of drug resistance. Flucytosine may cause infection of the gums. Be careful when using a toothbrush, toothpick, or dental floss. Avoid dental work while taking this drug.

OVERDOSE
Symptoms: Severe nausea, vomiting, abdominal pain, diarrhea, mental confusion.

What to Do: An overdose of flucytosine is unlikely to be life-threatening. However, if someone takes a much larger dose than prescribed, call your doctor, emergency medical services (EMS), or nearest poison control center immediately.

DRUG INTERACTIONS
Other drugs may interact with flucytosine. Consult your doctor for advice if you are taking amphotericin B injection, cytosine, or bone marrow depressants, or if you are undergoing radiation therapy.

FOOD INTERACTIONS
No known food interactions.

DISEASE INTERACTIONS
Caution is advised when taking flucytosine. Consult your doctor if you have bone marrow depression or liver or kidney disease. Use of flucytosine may cause complications in patients with liver or kidney disease, since these organs work together to remove the medication from the body.

Fludrocortisone

BRAND NAME
Florinef

Florinef Acetate 0.1 mg
(Apothecon)

▶ Drug Class: Corticosteroid

▶ Available in: Tablets

▶ Available OTC? No

▶ As Generic? No

Side Effects

SERIOUS
Headache and blurred vision caused by high blood pressure; low body potassium levels, causing cramps, weakness, and heart palpitations. Call your doctor immediately.

COMMON
Mild swelling of hands and feet.

LESS COMMON
Dizziness, difficulty swallowing, headache, hives, itchiness, rash, cough, vomiting, sudden weight gain, retention of sodium and water in the body.

PRINCIPAL USES
To supplement inadequate production of a specific salt-retaining corticosteroid hormone in the body, which leads to conditions known as adrenocortical insufficiency and adrenogenital syndrome. Untreated, these disorders can cause premature puberty in boys, masculinization in females, and even death.

HOW THE DRUG WORKS
Fludrocortisone performs the same functions as one of the body's normal corticosteroid hormones called aldosterone.

DOSAGE
For adrenocortical insufficiency— Adults: 50 to 200 micrograms (mcg) once a day. Children: 50 to 100 mcg once a day. For adrenogenital syndrome— Adults: 100 to 200 mcg once a day.

ONSET OF EFFECT
Variable.

DURATION OF ACTION
1 to 2 days.

DIETARY ADVICE
Can be taken with or between meals. Best taken with a full glass of water. Carefully monitor the amount of sodium in your diet. Excess sodium will increase potassium loss. Eat foods rich in potassium.

STORAGE
Store in a tightly sealed container in a dry place away from heat and direct light.

IF YOU MISS A DOSE
Take it as soon as you remember. If it is near the time for the next dose, skip the missed dose and resume your regular dosage schedule. Do not double the next dose. Notify your physician if more than one dose is missed or a dose cannot be taken due to vomiting or nausea.

STOPPING THE DRUG
The decision to stop taking the drug should be made by your doctor.

PROLONGED USE
Your doctor may need to monitor your blood pressure, blood serum electrolyte (mineral salt) concentration, and other variables if you must take this medicine for a prolonged period.

PRECAUTIONS
Over 60: Adverse reactions may be more likely and more severe in older patients.

Driving and Hazardous Work: Do not drive or engage in hazardous work until you determine how the medicine affects you.

Alcohol: No special precautions are necessary.

Pregnancy: Studies on birth defects in animals and humans have not been done. Before you take fludrocortisone, tell your doctor if you are pregnant or plan to become pregnant, to determine whether benefits outweigh potential risks.

Breast Feeding: Fludrocortisone passes into breast milk; consult your doctor.

Infants and Children: It can be used safely when needed; consult your pediatrician for guidelines.

Special Concerns: Your doctor may ask you to follow a diet that is low in sodium and high in potassium and protein to avoid high blood pressure and excessive accumulation of water in the body. You should drink lots of water every day, unless your doctor directs otherwise.

OVERDOSE
Symptoms: Dizziness, weakness, swelling of the hands and feet, excessive weight gain.

What to Do: Call your doctor, emergency medical services (EMS), or the nearest poison control center immediately.

DRUG INTERACTIONS
Consult your doctor for specific advice if you are taking acetazolamide, amphotericin B, capreomycin, carbenicillin, corticotropin (ACTH), dichlorphenamide, a diuretic, an antiglaucoma drug, insulin or oral antidiabetic agents, laxatives, methazolamide, mezlocillin, piperacillin, a salicylate, aspirin, sodium bicarbonate, ticarcillin, vitamin B, vitamin D, a barbiturate, carbamazepine, griseofulvin, phenylbutazone, phenytoin, primidone, rifampin, digitalis drugs, another steroid, or any medication that contains sodium.

FOOD INTERACTIONS
High-sodium foods should be avoided.

DISEASE INTERACTIONS
Caution is advised if you have any of the following: bone disease, edema (swelling due to fluid retention), heart disease, high blood pressure, kidney disease, liver disease, or thyroid disease. Use of fludrocortisone may cause complications in patients with liver or kidney disease, since these organs work together to remove the medication from the body.

Flunisolide

▶ Drug Class: Respiratory
corticosteroid

▶ Available in: Oral inhalation,
nasal spray

▶ Available OTC? No

▶ As Generic? No

Side Effects

SERIOUS
No serious side effects
are associated with the
use of flunisolide.

COMMON
Oral inhalation: Sore
throat, white patches in
mouth or throat, hoarse-
ness. Nasal spray: Nose-
bleeds or bloody nasal
secretions, nasal burning
or irritation, sore throat.

LESS COMMON
Eye pain, watering eyes,
gradual decrease of
vision, stomach pain and
digestive disturbances.

PRINCIPAL USES
To treat bronchial asthma;
to treat allergic rhinitis (seasonal allergies such as hay
fever); to prevent recur-
rence of nasal polyps after
they have been removed
surgically.

HOW THE DRUG WORKS
Respiratory corticosteroids
such as flunisolide primarily
reduce or prevent inflammation of the lining of the airways (the underlying cause
of asthma), reduce the allergic response to inhaled
allergens, and inhibit the
secretion of mucus within
the airways.

DOSAGE
Oral inhalation— Adults: 2
inhalations of 250 micro-
grams (mcg) each twice a
day, morning and evening.
Maximum dose is 4 inhala-
tions twice a day. Children:
Do not exceed 2 inhalations
twice a day. Nasal spray—
Adults and teenagers 15 and
older: 2 sprays of 25 mcg in
each nostril twice a day.
Maximum dose is 8 sprays
in each nostril a day. Children ages 6 to 14: One
spray of 25 mcg in each
nostril 3 times a day, or 2
sprays in each nostril twice
a day. Maximum dose is 4
sprays in each nostril a day.

ONSET OF EFFECT
Usually within 1 week; it
may take 3 weeks for the
full effect to occur.

DURATION OF ACTION
Unknown.

DIETARY ADVICE
No special restrictions.

STORAGE
Store the inhaler in a dry
place away from heat and
direct light.

IF YOU MISS A DOSE
Take it as soon as you
remember. If it is near the
time for the next dose, skip
the missed dose and
resume your regular dosage
schedule. Do not double the
next dose.

STOPPING THE DRUG
If you have been using flunisolide for a long period,
do not stop taking it suddenly. Consult your doctor
about how to stop.

PROLONGED USE
Consult your doctor about
the need for continuing
medical examinations or
laboratory tests.

PRECAUTIONS
Over 60: No special problems are expected with
older patients.

**Driving and Hazardous
Work:** Do not drive or
engage in hazardous work
until you determine how the
medicine affects you.

Alcohol: No special precautions are necessary.

Pregnancy: Flunisolide
has not been reported to
cause birth defects if taken
during pregnancy. Before
using this drug, tell your
doctor if you are pregnant
or plan to become pregnant.

Breast Feeding: Flu-
nisolide may pass into
breast milk; caution is
advised. Consult your doctor for advice.

Infants and Children:
Not recommended for chil-
dren under the age of 6.
The drug may inhibit
growth and make children
more susceptible to infection. If a younger person
takes this medicine, be
careful to avoid exposure to
chicken pox and measles.

Special Concerns:
Inhaled steroids will not
help an asthma attack in
progress. They can lower
resistance to yeast infections of the mouth, throat,
or voice box. To prevent
yeast infections, gargle or
rinse your mouth with water
after each use; do not swallow the water. Know how to
use the spray; read and follow the directions that come
with the device. Before you
have surgery, tell the doctor
or dentist that you are using
a steroid.

OVERDOSE
Symptoms: No specific
ones have been reported.

What to Do: An overdose
of flunisolide is unlikely to
be life-threatening. How-
ever, if someone takes a
much larger dose than prescribed, or if you have any
reason to suspect an overdose, call your doctor, emergency medical services
(EMS), or the nearest poison control center.

DRUG INTERACTIONS
Consult your doctor for
specific advice if you are
taking systemic cortico-
steroids, other inhaled
corticosteroids, or drugs
that suppress the immune
system.

FOOD INTERACTIONS
No known food interactions.

DISEASE INTERACTIONS
Consult your doctor if you
have a history of tuberculosis, herpes simplex infection
of the eye, chicken pox,
chronic bronchitis or
bronchiectasis, osteoporosis, underactive thyroid,
liver disease, glaucoma,
measles, recent injury to
the nose or nose surgery,
or any active infection.

Fluorometholone

BRAND NAMES
Flarex, Fluor-Op, FML
Forte, FML Liquifilm,
FML S.O.P., FML-S

▶ Drug Class: Corticosteroid

▶ Available in: Ophthalmic
ointment, suspension

▶ Available OTC? No

▶ As Generic? No

Side Effects

SERIOUS
Decreased or blurred
vision (from cataract);
eye pain, nausea, vomit-
ing (from increased eye
pressure); pain, redness,
sensitivity to bright light,
discharge (from eye
infection). Call your doctor immediately if you
experience any of these
signs or symptoms.

COMMON
Increased eye pressure;
this is usually reversed
once the drug is stopped.

LESS COMMON
Burning, stinging, red-
ness, or watering of eyes.

PRINCIPAL USES
To control inflammation and
prevent potentially permanent damage that may
result from various conditions involving inflammation
in the tissues of the eye.

HOW THE DRUG WORKS
Fluorometholone inhibits
the release of substances
that stimulate an inflammatory reaction and pain in
eye tissues.

DOSAGE
Ointment: Apply to eye 1
to 3 times a day, according
to doctor's instructions.
Suspension: 1 or 2 drops,
2 to 4 times a day. For
severe conditions, more
frequent application of
either form may be recom-
mended initially; the dosage
will be decreased as inflammation subsides.

ONSET OF EFFECT
Unknown.

DURATION OF ACTION
Unknown.

DIETARY ADVICE
No special restrictions.

STORAGE
Store in a tightly sealed container away from heat, moisture, and direct light. Do
not allow it to freeze.

IF YOU MISS A DOSE
Apply it as soon as you
remember. If it is near the
time for the next dose, skip
the missed dose and
resume your regular dosage
schedule. Do not double the
next dose.

STOPPING THE DRUG
It is very important to take
this drug as prescribed for
the full treatment period,
even if symptoms improve
before the scheduled end
of therapy.

PROLONGED USE
See your doctor regularly
for tests and examinations if
you must take this drug for
a prolonged period.

PRECAUTIONS
Over 60: No special problems are expected.

**Driving and Hazardous
Work:** Do not drive or
engage in hazardous work
until you determine how
the medicine affects your
vision.

Alcohol: No special precautions are necessary.

Pregnancy: Adequate
human studies have not
been done, although there
have been no reports of
birth defects. Before taking
fluorometholone, tell your
doctor if you are pregnant
or are planning to become
pregnant.

Breast Feeding: This
medicine has not been
reported to cause problems
in nursing babies. Consult
your doctor for specific
advice.

Infants and Children:
Safety and effectiveness
have not been established
for children under 2 years
of age.

Special Concerns: To use
the eye drops or the ointment, first wash your hands.
Tilt your head back. Gently
apply pressure to the inside
corner of the eyelid and
with the index finger of the
same hand, pull downward
on the lower eyelid to make
a space. Drop the medicine
or put a short strip of ointment (about ⅓ inch long)
into this space and close
your eye. Apply pressure for
1 or 2 minutes while keeping the eye closed without
blinking. Then wash your
hands again. Make sure the

tip of the dropper or the
applicator does not touch
your eye, finger, or any
other surface. If your symptoms do not improve in 5 to
7 days or if they become
worse, check with your doctor. Wearing contact lenses
while using this medication
may increase the risk of
infection. Your doctor may
tell you not to wear contact
lenses during treatment and
for a day or two afterward.

OVERDOSE
Symptoms: When used
topically, an overdose of fluorometholone is very
unlikely. Inadvertent oral
ingestion, however, may
cause fever, muscle pain,
loss of appetite, dizziness,
fainting, and difficulty
breathing.

What to Do: In case of
accidental ingestion, call
your doctor, emergency
medical services (EMS), or
the nearest poison control
center right away.

DRUG INTERACTIONS
Other medications may
interact with fluorometh-
olone. Consult your doctor
for specific advice if you are
taking any other prescription or over-the-counter
medication, especially any
preparation designed for
use in the eyes.

FOOD INTERACTIONS
No known food interactions.

DISEASE INTERACTIONS
Consult your doctor if you
have a history of cataracts,
diabetes mellitus, glaucoma,
herpes infection of the eye,
fungal infection of the eye,
or any other eye infection.

Fluorouracil (5-Fluorouracil; 5-FU)

BRAND NAMES
Efudex, Fluoroplex

▶ Drug Class: Antimetabolite

▶ Available in: Cream, topical solution

▶ Available OTC? No

▶ As Generic? No

Side Effects

SERIOUS
Severe redness, swelling, and tenderness of otherwise healthy regions of skin.

COMMON
Burning sensation where medicine is applied, increased sensitivity of skin to sunlight, redness, swelling, itching, rash, tenderness, pain, or oozing and crusting of the skin.

LESS COMMON
Hyperpigmentation (darkening) of skin, scaling, scarring, watery eyes.

PRINCIPAL USES
To treat actinic keratosis (a type of precancerous skin lesion). The drug is prescribed generally for multiple lesions or when limited access to a lesion makes other methods of removal difficult.

HOW THE DRUG WORKS
Topical fluorouracil kills precancerous cells by interfering with the activity of their genetic material, thus preventing the cells from reproducing. The drug selectively destroys cells that multiply rapidly, as many malignant cells do.

DOSAGE
For precancerous skin lesions— Adults: Apply 1% cream or 5% solution to the affected area 1 or 2 times a day. The 5% cream is sometimes prescribed. Children: Use and dose must be determined by your pediatrician.

ONSET OF EFFECT
From 2 to 7 days. The complete effect may require 2 to 6 weeks, or even 12 weeks for some patients. Complete healing may require 1 or 2 months after the drug has been stopped.

DURATION OF ACTION
Up to 24 hours.

DIETARY ADVICE
Fluorouracil may be applied without regard to diet.

STORAGE
Store in a tightly sealed container away from heat and direct light.

IF YOU MISS A DOSE
Apply it as soon as you remember. If it is near the time for the next application, skip the missed dose and resume your regular dosage schedule. Do not double the next dose.

STOPPING THE DRUG
Apply fluorouracil for the entire duration of therapy, as prescribed. The decision to stop the drug should be made by your doctor.

PROLONGED USE
No problems are expected with prolonged use, but check regularly with your physician. Treatment usually lasts 2 to 8 weeks for precancerous lesions. Your physician may order a biopsy if the condition does not clear up.

PRECAUTIONS
Over 60: No special problems are expected.

Driving and Hazardous Work: The use of fluorouracil should not impair your ability to perform such tasks safely.

Alcohol: No special precautions are necessary.

Pregnancy: Some fluorouracil is absorbed through the skin and may affect the unborn child. Before using fluorouracil, tell your doctor if you are pregnant or plan to become pregnant.

Breast Feeding: Fluorouracil passes into breast milk; avoid or discontinue usage while nursing.

Infants and Children: Fluorouracil is generally not prescribed for infants and children, but you should consult your doctor about its use for young patients.

Special Concerns: While you use fluorouracil, and for 1 or 2 months afterward, your skin may become much more sensitive to sunlight, and sunlight may increase the effect of the drug. During this period, stay out of direct sunlight, especially between 10 am and 3 pm. Wear protective clothing, including a hat and sunglasses. Apply a sun block that has a sun protection factor (SPF) of at least 15. When applying fluorouracil, wash the area with soap and water and use a cotton-tipped applicator or your fingertips to apply the drug. Wash your hands immediately to prevent any of the medicine from accidentally getting into your eyes or mouth.

OVERDOSE
Symptoms: No specific ones have been reported.

What to Do: An overdose is unlikely. However, if topical fluorouracil is accidentally swallowed, call your doctor, emergency medical services (EMS), or nearest poison control center.

DRUG INTERACTIONS
None known.

FOOD INTERACTIONS
No known food interactions.

DISEASE INTERACTIONS
Caution is advised when taking fluorouracil. Consult your doctor if you have any other skin problem.

Fluoxetine Hydrochloride

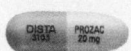

Prozac 20 mg
(DISTA)

▶ Drug Class: Selective serotonin reuptake inhibitor (SSRI) antidepressant

▶ Available in: Capsules, oral solution

▶ Available OTC? No

▶ As Generic? Yes

Side Effects

SERIOUS
Agitation, shaking, difficulty breathing, rash, hives, itching, joint or muscle pain, chills or fever. If such symptoms occur, call your doctor immediately.

COMMON
Nervousness, drowsiness, anxiety, insomnia, headache, diarrhea, excessive sweating, nausea, decreased appetite, decreased initiative.

LESS COMMON
Nasal congestion, unusual or vivid dreams, cough, increased appetite, chest pain, constipation, vision disturbances, abdominal pain, stomach gas, constipation, vomiting, frequent urination, difficulty concentrating, sexual dysfunction, heartbeat irregularities, trembling, fatigue, dizziness, change in taste, flushing of the skin on the face and neck, dry mouth, menstrual pain.

PRINCIPAL USES
To treat major depression, obsessive-compulsive disorder, panic disorder, chronic pain, and premenstrual dysphoric disorder (PMDD).

HOW THE DRUG WORKS
Fluoxetine affects levels of serotonin, a brain chemical that is thought to be linked to mood, emotions, and mental state.

DOSAGE
To start, 20 mg a day, taken in the morning. Your doctor may increase the dose gradually to a maximum of 80 mg a day. Older adults: To start, 10 to 20 mg a day. It may be increased gradually by your doctor to a maximum of 40 to 60 mg a day.

ONSET OF EFFECT
1 to 4 weeks.

DURATION OF ACTION
Unknown.

DIETARY ADVICE
Taking the drug with liquid or food can lessen stomach irritation. Capsules may be opened and mixed with food or juice if the patient has difficulty swallowing them.

STORAGE
Store in a tightly sealed container away from heat, moisture, and direct light. Keep the liquid form refrigerated, but do not allow it to freeze.

IF YOU MISS A DOSE
Take it as soon as you remember. If it is near the time for the next dose, skip the missed dose and resume your regular dosage schedule. Do not double the next dose.

STOPPING THE DRUG
Take it as prescribed for the full treatment period, even if you begin to feel better before the scheduled end of therapy. Discontinuing the drug abruptly may produce unpleasant withdrawal symptoms. Dosage should be reduced gradually according to your doctor's instructions.

PROLONGED USE
The usual course of therapy lasts 6 months to 1 year; some patients benefit from additional therapy. The usual course of therapy for obsessive-compulsive disorder lasts 1 year or more.

PRECAUTIONS
Over 60: Adverse reactions may be more likely and more severe in older patients, since their metabolism is slower. A lower dose may be warranted.

Driving and Hazardous Work: Use caution when driving or engaging in hazardous work until you determine how the medicine affects you.

Alcohol: Avoid alcohol.

Pregnancy: Fluoxetine should be used during pregnancy only if the potential benefit justifies the potential risk to the fetus. Before you take this medicine, tell your doctor if you are pregnant or plan to become pregnant.

Breast Feeding: Fluoxetine may pass into breast milk; caution is advised. Consult your doctor for specific advice.

Infants and Children: Not recommended for use by children under age 12.

Special Concerns: Take it at least 6 hours before bedtime to prevent insomnia, unless the drug causes drowsiness.

OVERDOSE
Symptoms: Agitation, excitement, severe nausea and vomiting, seizures.

What to Do: Call your doctor, emergency medical services (EMS), or the nearest poison control center immediately.

DRUG INTERACTIONS
Fluoxetine should not be used within 5 weeks of taking MAO inhibitors or thioridazine. The following drugs may interact with fluoxetine. Consult your doctor for specific advice if you are taking nortriptyline, caffeine, oral anticoagulants, central nervous system depressants, digitalis preparations, lithium, loratadine, dextromethorphan, ketorolac, buspirone, phenytoin, trazodone, tryptophan, sumatriptan, naratriptan, or zolmitriptan.

FOOD INTERACTIONS
No known food interactions.

DISEASE INTERACTIONS
Use of fluoxetine may cause complications in patients with liver or kidney disease, since these organs work together to remove the medication from the body. Use of the drug may make diabetes or seizures worse.

Fluoxymesterone

BRAND NAMES
Android-F, Halotestin

Halotestin 5 mg
(UPJOHN)

▶ Drug Class: Hormone treatment (androgen); antineoplastic (anticancer) agent

▶ Available in: Tablets

▶ Available OTC? No

▶ As Generic? Yes

Side Effects

SERIOUS
Itching of skin, yellowish tinge to eyes or skin. Call your doctor immediately.

COMMON
Women: Acne or oily skin, decreased breast size, hoarseness or deepening of voice, irregular menstrual periods, male-type baldness, excessive hair growth. Men: Enlarged or sore breasts, frequent or prolonged erections, frequent urination, temporary infertility. Notify your doctor if any of these symptoms occur.

LESS COMMON
Changes in skin coloration, confusion, constipation, dizziness, frequent headaches, increased thirst and urination, depression, nausea, vomiting, swelling of feet or lower legs, unusual bleeding, unusual fatigue, rapid weight gain, diarrhea, increased risk of infection, insomnia, increase or decrease in sexual desire. Men only: Testicular shrinkage, erectile dysfunction, skin irritation of the scrotum. Boys only: Acne, early growth of pubic hair, penis enlargement, increased frequency of erections.

PRINCIPAL USES
For hormone replacement in men; to treat delayed sexual development in boys; to treat certain types of breast cancer in women.

HOW THE DRUG WORKS
Fluoxymesterone replaces natural testosterone in men deficient of the hormone. Fluoxymesterone also blocks the action of certain other hormones that promote the growth of some types of breast tumors.

DOSAGE
For hormone replacement in men: 5 to 20 mg daily, in single or divided doses. For treatment of delayed sexual development in boys: 2.5 to 10 mg a day for 4 to 6 months. For treatment of breast cancer in women: 10 to 40 mg daily, in divided doses.

ONSET OF EFFECT
1 month.

DURATION OF ACTION
Unknown.

DIETARY ADVICE
It can be taken with food to prevent stomach upset.

STORAGE
Store in a tightly sealed container away from heat and direct light.

IF YOU MISS A DOSE
Take it as soon as you remember. If it is near the time for the next dose, skip the missed dose and resume your regular dosage schedule. Do not double the next dose.

STOPPING THE DRUG
The decision to stop taking the drug should be made by your doctor.

PROLONGED USE
You should see your doctor regularly for tests and examinations if you must take this drug for a prolonged period.

PRECAUTIONS
Over 60: An increased risk of prostate enlargement or prostate cancer is found in older men.

Driving and Hazardous Work: Use of this drug should not impair your ability to perform such tasks safely.

Alcohol: No special precautions are necessary.

Pregnancy: Fluoxymesterone can affect both male and female fetuses; it should not be used during pregnancy.

Breast Feeding: Fluoxymesterone passes into breast milk; avoid or discontinue use while nursing.

Infants and Children: Fluoxymesterone can profoundly affect the growth and sexual development of infants and children. Risks must be weighed against benefits; consult your pediatrician for advice.

Special Concerns: This drug contains the dye tartrazine, which may cause allergic reactions in some people. The risk of some cancers is increased with long-term, high-dose use. In some cases this drug can pass to a sexual partner and cause side effects. A non-hormonal (barrier) method of contraception is advised during therapy.

OVERDOSE
Symptoms: No specific ones have been reported.

What to Do: An overdose is unlikely to be life-threatening. However, if someone takes a much larger dose than prescribed, call your doctor, emergency medical services (EMS), or the nearest poison control center immediately.

DRUG INTERACTIONS
Consult your doctor for specific advice if you are taking acetaminophen, amiodarone, anabolic steroids, anticoagulants, anti-infective drugs, antithyroid agents, carbamazepine, carmustine, chloroquine, cyclosporine, dantrolene, daunorubicin, disulfiram, divalproex, estrogens, etretinate, gold salts, hydroxychloroquine, insulin, mercaptopurine, methotrexate, methyldopa, naltrexone, oral contraceptives, phenothiazines, phenytoin, plicamycin, or valproic acid.

FOOD INTERACTIONS
No known food interactions.

DISEASE INTERACTIONS
Consult your doctor if you have a history of prostate cancer, diabetes, edema (swelling owing to excess fluid retention), kidney disease, liver disease, enlarged prostate, heart disease, or blood vessel disease.

Fluphenazine

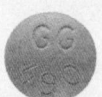

Generic 10 mg
(GENEVA)

Additional photographs

▶ Drug Class: Antipsychotic; phenothiazine

▶ Available in: Tablets, oral concentrate, elixir, injection

▶ Available OTC? No

▶ As Generic? Yes

Side Effects

SERIOUS
Extreme and persistent restlessness; uncontrolled movements, including tics, twitching, twisting movements, and muscle spasms in the face, neck, and back; loss of coordination and balance; trembling, weakness, and stiffness in the extremities; difficulty swallowing or speaking; persistent, uncontrolled chewing, lip-smacking, or tongue movements; staring and absence of facial expression; fainting; increased skin sensitivity to the sun; skin rash; yellowish tinge to eyes or skin.

COMMON
Constipation, decreased sweating, dizziness or faintness, drowsiness, dry mouth, shaking, mild stiffness, shuffling gait, restlessness, blurred vision.

LESS COMMON
Menstrual irregularities, sexual dysfunction, unusual milk secretion, breast pain or swelling, unexpected weight gain, difficulty urinating.

PRINCIPAL USES
To treat psychotic conditions such as schizophrenia.

HOW THE DRUG WORKS
Fluphenazine inhibits the activity of the brain chemical dopamine, thereby helping to prevent the overstimulation of specific nerve centers in the brain that are thought to be responsible for certain psychiatric disorders.

DOSAGE
Oral forms— Adults: To start, 2.5 to 10 mg a day, taken in divided doses every 6 to 8 hours; may be increased to a maximum of 20 mg a day. Maintenance dose is 1 to 20 mg a day. Children: 0.25 to 0.75 mg, 1 to 4 times a day. Older adults: 1 to 2.5 mg a day. Injection— 12.5 to 50 mg every 2 to 4 weeks.

ONSET OF EFFECT
Within 1 hour for oral forms; 24 to 72 hours for injection. Full therapeutic effect may take several weeks.

DURATION OF ACTION
From 6 to 8 hours with oral forms; 1 to 6 weeks with injection.

DIETARY ADVICE
It can be taken with liquid or food to minimize stomach upset. If your medicine comes with a dropper bottle, dilute your dose in half a glass of grapefruit or orange juice or water.

STORAGE
Store in a tightly sealed container in a dry place away from heat and direct light. Do not refrigerate, and keep liquid forms from freezing.

IF YOU MISS A DOSE
Take it as soon as you remember. However, if it is more than 2 hours late, skip the missed dose and resume your regular dosage schedule. Do not double the next dose.

STOPPING THE DRUG
Do not stop taking the drug abruptly or without your doctor's approval. Dosage should be reduced gradually by your doctor to prevent withdrawal symptoms.

PROLONGED USE
Prolonged use may lead to tardive dyskinesia (involuntary movements of the jaw, lips, and tongue). Consult your doctor about the need for follow-up evaluations and tests if you must take this drug for an extended period.

PRECAUTIONS
Over 60: Adverse reactions, especially shuffling gait, shaking, stiffness, and constipation, are more common in older patients.

Driving and Hazardous Work: Do not drive or engage in hazardous work until you determine how the medicine affects you.

Alcohol: Avoid alcohol.

Pregnancy: Discuss with your doctor the relative risks and benefits of taking this drug if you are, or plan to become, pregnant.

Breast Feeding: Either avoid taking the drug if possible or refrain from breast feeding.

Infants and Children: Not for use by children under age 12.

Special Concerns: Avoid getting overheated or chilled. Avoid getting the liquid form of the medicine on the skin, because it can cause irritation or a rash.

OVERDOSE
Symptoms: Extreme drowsiness, heartbeat irregularities, dry mouth, paradoxical restlessness or agitation, seizures, loss of consciousness.

What to Do: Call your doctor, emergency medical services (EMS), or the nearest poison control center immediately.

DRUG INTERACTIONS
The following drugs may interact with fluphenazine. Consult your doctor for specific advice if you are taking anticholinergics, antidepressants, antihistamines, antihypertensives, barbiturates, anesthetics, beta-blockers, diuretics, thyroid drugs, appetite suppressants, epinephrine, bupropion, or calcium supplements.

FOOD INTERACTIONS
Avoid caffeinated beverages, apple juice, and tea.

DISEASE INTERACTIONS
Consult your doctor if you have a history of alcohol abuse, any blood disorder, breast cancer, enlarged prostate, epilepsy or a seizure disorder, glaucoma, lung disease, heart or blood vessel disease, liver disease, Parkinson's disease, peptic ulcer, or urinary difficulty.

Flurazepam Hydrochloride

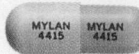

Generic 15 mg
(MYLAN)

▶ Drug Class: Benzodiazepine tranquilizer; sedative/hypnotic

▶ Available in: Capsules

▶ Available OTC? No

▶ As Generic? Yes

Side Effects

SERIOUS
Difficulty concentrating, outbursts of anger, other behavior problems, depression, hallucinations, low blood pressure (causing faintness or confusion), memory impairment, muscle weakness, skin rash or itching, sore throat, fever and chills, sores or ulcers in throat or mouth, unusual bruising or bleeding, extreme fatigue, yellowish tinge to eyes or skin. Call your doctor immediately.

COMMON
Daytime drowsiness, dizziness, lightheadedness, loss of coordination, headaches, slurred speech.

LESS COMMON
Stomach cramps or pain, vision disturbances, change in sexual desire or ability, constipation, false sense of well-being, nausea and vomiting, urinary problems, unusual weakness or fatigue.

PRINCIPAL USES
For the short-term treatment of insomnia.

HOW THE DRUG WORKS
In general, flurazepam produces a mild sedative effect by depressing activity in the central nervous system (the brain and spinal cord). In particular, flurazepam appears to enhance the effect of gamma-aminobutyric acid (GABA), a natural chemical that inhibits the firing of neurons and dampens the transmission of nerve signals, thus decreasing nervous excitation.

DOSAGE
15 or 30 mg, taken in a single dose at bedtime.

ONSET OF EFFECT
From 30 to 60 minutes.

DURATION OF ACTION
Unknown.

DIETARY ADVICE
Limit your intake of caffeine-containing foods and beverages while taking this medication.

STORAGE
Store in a tightly sealed container away from heat, moisture, and direct light.

IF YOU MISS A DOSE
Take it as soon as you remember, unless it is late at night. Do not take the medicine unless your schedule permits a full night's sleep.

STOPPING THE DRUG
Discontinuing the drug abruptly may produce withdrawal symptoms (sleep disruption, nervousness, irritability, diarrhea, abdominal cramps, muscle aches, memory impairment). The dosage should be reduced gradually according to your doctor's instructions.

PROLONGED USE
Do not use flurazepam for more than 8 weeks without consulting your doctor.

PRECAUTIONS
Over 60: Adverse reactions are more likely and more severe. A lower dose may be warranted.

Driving and Hazardous Work: Flurazepam can impair mental alertness and physical coordination. Adjust your activities accordingly.

Alcohol: Avoid alcohol.

Pregnancy: Use during pregnancy should be avoided if possible. Be sure to tell your doctor if you are pregnant or plan to become pregnant.

Breast Feeding: Flurazepam passes into breast milk; do not take it while nursing.

Infants and Children: Flurazepam is not recommended for use by children under the age of 6 months, and it is not generally prescribed for children under age 15. It should be used by older children only under close medical supervision.

Special Concerns: Use of this drug can lead to psychological or physical dependence.

OVERDOSE
Symptoms: Extreme drowsiness, confusion, slurred speech, slow reflexes, poor coordination, staggering gait, tremor, slowed breathing, loss of consciousness.

What to Do: Call your doctor, emergency medical services (EMS), or the nearest poison control center immediately.

DRUG INTERACTIONS
Other drugs may interact with flurazepam. Consult your doctor for specific advice if you are taking any drugs that depress the central nervous system; these include antihistamines, antidepressants or other psychiatric medications, barbiturates, sedatives, cough medicines, decongestants, and painkillers. Be sure your doctor knows about any over-the-counter medication you may take.

FOOD INTERACTIONS
None reported.

DISEASE INTERACTIONS
Caution is advised when taking flurazepam. Consult your doctor if you have a history of alcohol or drug abuse, stroke or other brain disease, any chronic lung disease, hyperactivity, depression or other mental illness, myasthenia gravis, sleep apnea, epilepsy, porphyria, kidney disease, or liver disease.

Flurbiprofen Ophthalmic

BRAND NAME
Ocufen

▶ Drug Class: Nonsteroidal anti-inflammatory drug (NSAID)

▶ Available in: Ophthalmic solution

▶ Available OTC? No

▶ As Generic? No

Side Effects

SERIOUS
Rarely, ophthalmic flurbiprofen will cause bleeding in the eye, redness or swelling of the eye or eyelid not present before the start of therapy, itching of the eye, or excessive tear production. Call your doctor immediately.

COMMON
Mild and temporary burning or stinging of eyes after application.

LESS COMMON
There are no less-common side effects associated with ophthalmic flurbiprofen.

PRINCIPAL USES
To treat some eye conditions and problems that occur during or after eye surgery.

HOW THE DRUG WORKS
Ophthalmic flurbiprofen inhibits the release of substances that stimulate inflammation and cause pain in eye tissues.

DOSAGE
Adults: 1 drop in each eye every 4 hours. Children: Consult your pediatrician.

ONSET OF EFFECT
Unknown.

DURATION OF ACTION
Unknown.

DIETARY ADVICE
No special restrictions.

STORAGE
Store in a tightly sealed container away from heat, moisture, and direct light. Do not allow it to freeze.

IF YOU MISS A DOSE
Apply it as soon as you remember. If it is near the time for the next dose, skip the missed dose and resume your regular dosage schedule. Do not double the next dose.

STOPPING THE DRUG
Use it as prescribed for the full treatment period, even if you feel better before the scheduled end of therapy.

PROLONGED USE
See your doctor regularly for tests and examinations if you must use this drug for a prolonged period.

PRECAUTIONS
Over 60: No special problems are expected.

Driving and Hazardous Work: The use of ophthalmic flurbiprofen should not impair your ability to perform such tasks safely.

Alcohol: No special precautions are necessary.

Pregnancy: Adequate human studies have not been completed. Before taking ophthalmic flurbiprofen, tell your doctor if you are pregnant or plan to become pregnant.

Breast Feeding: Ophthalmic flurbiprofen may pass into breast milk; caution is advised. Consult your doctor for specific advice.

Infants and Children: Use and dosage for infants and children must be determined by your doctor.

Special Concerns: To use the eye drops, first wash your hands. Tilt your head back. Gently apply pressure to the inside corner of the eyelid and with the index finger of the same hand, pull downward on the lower eyelid to make a space. Drop the medicine into this space and close your eye. Apply pressure for 1 or 2 minutes while keeping the eye closed without blinking. Then wash your hands again. Make sure the tip of the dropper does not touch your eye, finger, or any other surface. If your symptoms do not improve or if they become worse, check with your doctor. Ophthalmic flurbiprofen may cause problems in patients who wear soft contact lenses. Your doctor may want you to stop wearing the lenses while you take it.

OVERDOSE
Symptoms: No specific ones have been reported.

What to Do: An overdose of ophthalmic flurbiprofen is unlikely to be life-threatening. However, if someone takes a much larger dose of the drug than prescribed or accidentally ingests the medicine, call your doctor, emergency medical services (EMS), or the nearest poison control center.

DRUG INTERACTIONS
Consult your doctor for specific advice if you are taking aspirin or another salicylate, difunisal, etodolac, fenoprofen, floctafenine, oral flurbiprofen, ibuprofen, indomethacin, ketoprofen, ketorolac, meclofenamate, mefanamic acid, nabumetone, naproxen, oxyphenbutazone, phenylbutazone, piroxicam, sulindac, suprofen, tenoxicam, tiaprofenic acid, tolmetin, or zomepirac. Ophthalmic flurbiprofen reduces the effectivness of acetylcholine or carbachol, two drugs used to treat glaucoma. These drugs are rarely used today, but if you take them, be sure to let your doctor know.

FOOD INTERACTIONS
No known food interactions.

DISEASE INTERACTIONS
Caution is advised when taking ophthalmic flurbiprofen. Consult your doctor if you have hemophilia or any other bleeding problem.

Flurbiprofen Oral

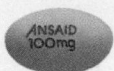

Ansaid 100 mg
(UPJOHN)

▶ Drug Class: Nonsteroidal
anti-inflammatory drug
(NSAID)

▶ Available in: Tablets,
extended-release capsules

▶ Available OTC? No

▶ As Generic? Yes

Side Effects

SERIOUS
Shortness of breath or
wheezing, with or with-
out swelling of legs or
other signs of heart failure; chest pain; peptic
ulcer disease with vomit-
ing of blood; black, tarry
stools; decreasing kidney
function. Call your doctor
immediately.

COMMON
Nausea, vomiting, heart-
burn, diarrhea, constipa-
tion, headache, dizziness,
sleepiness.

LESS COMMON
Ulcers or sores in mouth,
depression, rashes or
blistering of skin, ringing
sound in the ears,
unusual tingling or
numbness of the hands
or feet, seizures, blurred
vision. Also elevated
potassium levels,
decreased blood counts;
such problems can be
detected by your doctor.

PRINCIPAL USES
To treat mild to moderate
pain and inflammation
caused by tendinitis, arthritis, bursitis, gout, soft tissue
injuries, migraine and other
vascular headaches, men-
strual cramps, and other
conditions. When patients
fail to respond to one
NSAID, another may be
tried. The greatest effectiveness often requires trial and
error of several different
NSAIDs.

HOW THE DRUG WORKS
NSAIDs work by interfering
with the formation of
prostaglandins, substances
that cause inflammation and
make nerves more sensitive
to pain impulses. NSAIDs
also have other modes of
action that are less well
understood.

DOSAGE
Adults: Tablets: 50 mg, 4
times daily or 100 mg, 2
times daily. Extended-
release capsules: 200 mg
once a day. Maximum dose
is 300 mg a day. For children's dose, consult your
pediatrician.

ONSET OF EFFECT
Several hours.

DURATION OF ACTION
Varies; some patients
require daily maintenance
doses to control pain.

DIETARY ADVICE
Take flurbiprofen with food.

STORAGE
Store in a tightly sealed container away from heat, moisture, and direct light.

IF YOU MISS A DOSE
Take it as soon as you
remember. If it is near the
time for the next dose, skip
the missed dose and
resume your regular dosage
schedule. Do not double the
next dose.

STOPPING THE DRUG
The decision to stop taking
the drug should be made in
consultation with your
physician.

PROLONGED USE
Prolonged use can cause
gastrointestinal problems,
including ulceration and
bleeding, kidney dysfunc-
tion, and liver inflammation.
Consult your doctor about
the need for medical examinations and laboratory tests.

PRECAUTIONS
Over 60: Because of the
potentially greater consequences of gastrointestinal
side effects, the dose of
NSAIDs for older patients,
especially those over age
70, is often cut in half.

**Driving and Hazardous
Work:** Do not drive or
engage in hazardous work
until you determine how the
medicine affects you.

Alcohol: Avoid alcohol
when using this medication
because it increases the risk
of stomach irritation.

Pregnancy: Do not use
this drug during pregnancy.

Breast Feeding: Flur-
biprofen passes into breast
milk; avoid use while breast
feeding.

Infants and Children:
Flurbiprofen may be used in
exceptional circumstances;
consult your doctor.

Special Concerns:
Because NSAIDs can inter-
fere with blood coagulation,
this drug should be stopped
at least 3 days prior to any
surgery.

OVERDOSE
Symptoms: Severe nausea,
vomiting, headache, confusion, seizures.

What to Do: Call your
doctor, emergency medical
services (EMS), or the
nearest poison control center immediately.

DRUG INTERACTIONS
Do not take this drug with
aspirin or any other NSAIDs
without your doctor's
approval. In addition, consult your doctor if you are
taking antihypertensives,
steroids, anticoagulants,
antibiotics, itraconazole or
ketoconazole, plicamycin,
penicillamine, valproic acid,
phenytoin, cyclosporine,
digitalis drugs, lithium,
methotrexate, probenecid,
triamterene, or zidovudine.

FOOD INTERACTIONS
No known food interactions.

DISEASE INTERACTIONS
Caution is advised when
taking flurbiprofen. Consult
your doctor if you have any
of the following: bleeding
problems, inflammation or
ulcers of the stomach and
intestines, diabetes mellitus,
systemic lupus erythematosus (SLE, lupus), anemia,
asthma, epilepsy, Parkin-
son's disease, kidney
stones, or a history of heart
disease or alcohol abuse.
Use of flurbiprofen may
cause complications in
patients with liver or kidney
disease, since these organs
work together to remove
the drug from the body.

Flutamide

BRAND NAME
Eulexin

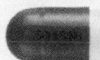

Eulexin 125 mg
(SCHERING-PLOUGH)

▶ Drug Class: Antiandrogen

▶ Available in: Capsules

▶ Available OTC? No

▶ As Generic? No

Side Effects

SERIOUS
Bluish coloring of lips, fingernails, or palms of hands (a sign of inadequate blood and oxygen supply to body tissues), dark urine, extreme dizziness or fainting, feeling of extreme pressure in the head, itching, loss of appetite, nausea or vomiting, pain in the right flank, shortness of breath, weak and rapid heartbeat, yellow discoloration of the skin or eyes (jaundice). Call your doctor immediately.

COMMON
Diarrhea, erectile dysfunction (impotence) or loss of sexual desire, sudden sweating and feeling of warmth.

LESS COMMON
Loss of appetite, tingling or numbness of hands or feet, swollen and tender breasts, swelling of feet or lower legs.

PRINCIPAL USES
To treat cancer of the prostate gland.

HOW THE DRUG WORKS
The growth of some types of prostate tumors is stimulated by the hormone testosterone. Flutamide interferes with the activity of testosterone, thus slowing or halting the growth of such tumors.

DOSAGE
250 mg every 8 hours, in conjunction with leuprolide, a synthetic form of luteinizing hormone-releasing hormone (LHRH), a hormone that also blocks the release of testosterone.

ONSET OF EFFECT
Unknown.

DURATION OF ACTION
Unknown.

DIETARY ADVICE
Take with or without food. Be sure to drink plenty of fluids.

STORAGE
Store in a tightly sealed container away from heat and direct light.

IF YOU MISS A DOSE
Take it as soon as you remember. If it is near the time for the next dose, skip the missed dose and resume your regular dosage schedule. Do not double the next dose.

STOPPING THE DRUG
The decision to stop taking the drug should be made in consultation with your physician.

PROLONGED USE
You should see your doctor regularly for tests and examinations if you take this drug for a prolonged period.

PRECAUTIONS
Over 60: The dosage may be reduced, because the medication takes longer to be eliminated from the body in older patients, but flutamide is not otherwise expected to cause different side effects or problems in older persons than it does in younger people.

Driving and Hazardous Work: Use of flutamide should not impair your ability to perform such tasks safely.

Alcohol: Limit alcohol to moderate intake only.

Pregnancy: Flutamide lowers sperm count, and the medication taken with it causes sterility that may be permanent. If you intend to have children, consult your doctor before you begin to take this medication to discuss utilizing a sperm bank.

Breast Feeding: Not applicable, since flutamide is not given to women.

Infants and Children: Flutamide is not recommended for children.

Special Concerns: If an anticoagulant is taken in combination with flutamide, close monitoring of blood clotting time is necessary, so that the dose of the anticoagulant can be adjusted if needed.

OVERDOSE
Symptoms: Dramatically slowed movement and activity, slow respiration, loss of muscle coordination, excessive tear production (weeping), loss of appetite, breast tenderness, gooseflesh, and vomiting.

What to Do: An overdose of flutamide is unlikely to be life-threatening. However, if someone takes a much larger dose than prescribed, call your doctor, emergency medical services (EMS), or the nearest poison control center immediately.

DRUG INTERACTIONS
The activity of an anticoagulant such as warfarin may be increased by flutamide. Consult your doctor for advice if you are taking an anticoagulant. Also consult your doctor if you are taking cholestyramine, cyclosporine, erythromycin, gemfibrozil, digoxin, cimetidine, ranitidine, omeprazole, or rifampin.

FOOD INTERACTIONS
No known food interactions.

DISEASE INTERACTIONS
You should not take flutamide if you have severe liver impairment. Consult your doctor if you have any other medical condition.

Fluticasone

BRAND NAMES
Flonase, Flovent

▶ Drug Class: Respiratory corticosteroid

▶ Available in: Oral inhalation, nasal spray

▶ Available OTC? No

▶ As Generic? No

Side Effects

SERIOUS
No serious side effects are associated with the use of fluticasone.

COMMON
Oral inhalation: Sore throat, white patches in mouth or throat, hoarseness. Nasal spray: Nosebleeds or bloody nasal secretions, nasal burning or irritation, sore throat.

LESS COMMON
Eye pain, watering eyes, gradual decrease of vision, stomach pain and digestive disturbances.

PRINCIPAL USES
To preventively treat bronchial asthma, and to treat allergic rhinitis (seasonal or perennial allergies such as hay fever).

HOW THE DRUG WORKS
Respiratory corticosteroids such as fluticasone primarily reduce or prevent inflammation of the lining of the airways (the underlying cause of asthma), reduce the allergic response to inhaled allergens, and inhibit the secretion of mucus within the airways.

DOSAGE
For asthma— Oral inhalation: 88 to 220 micrograms (mcg) a day, 2 times per day; not to exceed 440 mcg a day. For patients previously treated with oral corticosteroids: 880 mcg, 2 times a day. Dosage may gradually be reduced after 1 week of therapy. For allergic rhinitis— Nasal spray: Adults: 2 sprays (50 micrograms each) in each nostril once per day, or 1 spray in each nostril twice a day (in the morning and at night). Children ages 4 to 17: One spray in each nostril once a day. Dose, if needed, may be increased to 2 sprays in each nostril once a day. Maximum daily dose should not exceed 200 micrograms. After relief is achieved, the dose may be reduced to 1 spray per day.

ONSET OF EFFECT
Usually within 1 week; it may take 3 weeks for the full effect to occur.

DURATION OF ACTION
Unknown.

DIETARY ADVICE
No special restrictions.

STORAGE
Store the inhaler in a dry place away from heat and direct light.

IF YOU MISS A DOSE
Take it as soon as you remember. If it is near the time for the next dose, skip the missed dose and resume your regular dosage schedule. Do not double the next dose.

STOPPING THE DRUG
If you have been using fluticasone for a long period, do not stop taking it suddenly. Consult your doctor about how to stop.

PROLONGED USE
Consult your doctor about the need for regular medical tests and examinations if you must take this drug for a prolonged period of time.

PRECAUTIONS
Over 60: No special problems are expected.

Driving and Hazardous Work: The use of fluticasone should not impair your ability to perform such tasks safely.

Alcohol: No special precautions are necessary.

Pregnancy: Well-controlled studies of fluticasone use during pregnancy have not been done; it is generally not recommended unless the benefits clearly outweigh the risks. Consult your doctor.

Breast Feeding: Fluticasone may pass into breast milk; caution is advised. Consult your doctor for specific advice.

Infants and Children: Safety and effectiveness have not been established for children under age 4.

Special Concerns:
Inhaled steroids will not help an asthma attack in progress. Inhaled steroids can lower resistance to yeast infections of the mouth, throat, or voice box. To prevent yeast infections, gargle or rinse your mouth with water after each use; do not swallow the water. Know how to use the spray properly; read and follow the directions that come with the device. Before you have surgery, tell the doctor or dentist that you are using a steroid.

OVERDOSE
Symptoms: No cases of overdose have been reported.

What to Do: An overdose of fluticasone is unlikely. If you have any reason to suspect an overdose, contact your doctor or seek medical assistance right away.

DRUG INTERACTIONS
Consult your doctor for specific advice if you are taking systemic corticosteroids, other inhaled corticosteroids, or drugs that suppress the immune system.

FOOD INTERACTIONS
No known food interactions.

DISEASE INTERACTIONS
Caution is advised when taking fluticasone. Consult your doctor if you have any of the following: a lung disease such as tuberculosis; a herpes infection of the eye; nasal ulcers or recent nose surgery or injury; or any bacterial, viral, or fungal infection. If you are exposed to chicken pox or measles, tell your doctor at once.

Fluvastatin

BRAND NAME
Lescol

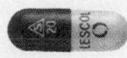

Lescol 20 mg
(NOVARTIS)

▶ Drug Class: Antilipidemic
(cholesterol-lowering agent)

▶ Available in: Capsules

▶ Available OTC? No

▶ As Generic? No

Side Effects

SERIOUS
Fever, unusual or unex-
plained muscle aches and
tenderness. Call your
doctor right away.

COMMON
Side effects occur in only
1% to 2% of patients.
These include constipa-
tion or diarrhea, dizziness
or lightheadedness,
bloating or gas, heart-
burn, nausea, skin rash,
stomach pain, rise in liver
enzymes.

LESS COMMON
Sleeping difficulty.

PRINCIPAL USES
To treat high cholesterol.
Usually prescribed after first
lines of treatment—including diet, weight loss, and
exercise—fail to reduce
total and low-density
lipoprotein (LDL) choles-
terol to acceptable levels.

HOW THE DRUG WORKS
Fluvastatin blocks the action
of an enzyme required for
the manufacture of cholesterol, thereby interfering
with its formation. By lowering the amount of choles-
terol in the liver cells,
fluvastatin increases the
formation of receptors for
LDL, and thereby reduces
blood levels of total and
LDL cholesterol. In addition
to lowering LDL choles-
terol, fluvastatin also modestly reduces triglyceride
levels and raises HDL (the
so-called "good" choles-
terol) levels.

DOSAGE
Initial dose is 20 mg, taken
once a day in the evening.
Dose may be increased by
your doctor to 40 mg, taken
once a day in the evening.

ONSET OF EFFECT
Within 2 to 4 weeks after
starting therapy.

DURATION OF ACTION
The effect persists for the
duration of therapy.

DIETARY ADVICE
Cholesterol-lowering drugs
are only one part of a total
program that should include
regular exercise and a
healthy diet. The American
Heart Association publishes
a "Healthy Heart" diet,
which is recommended.

STORAGE
Store in a tightly sealed container away from heat and
direct light. Keep away from
moisture and extremes in
temperature.

IF YOU MISS A DOSE
Take it as soon as you
remember. Take your next
dose at the proper time and
resume your regular dosage
schedule. Do not double the
next dose.

STOPPING THE DRUG
The decision to stop taking
the drug should be made in
consultation with your doctor. Once the medication is
discontinued, blood cholesterol is likely to return to
original elevated levels.

PROLONGED USE
Side effects are more likely
with prolonged use. As you
continue with fluvastatin,
your doctor will periodically
order blood tests to evaluate
liver function.

PRECAUTIONS
Over 60: No special problems are expected in older
patients.

**Driving and Hazardous
Work:** The use of fluvastatin should not impair your
ability to perform such
tasks safely.

Alcohol: No special precautions are necessary.

Pregnancy: Should not be
used during pregnancy or
by women who plan to
become pregnant in the
near future.

Breast Feeding: Fluvastatin passes into breast milk
and is not recommended
while breast feeding.

Infants and Children:
Rarely used in children.

Special Concerns: Important elements of treatment
for high cholesterol include
proper diet, weight loss,
regular moderate exercise,
and the avoidance of certain
medications that may
increase cholesterol levels.

Because fluvastatin has
potential side effects, it is
important that you maintain
a recommended healthy
diet and cooperate with
other treatments your physician may suggest.

OVERDOSE
Symptoms: An overdose of
fluvastatin is unlikely.

What to Do: Emergency
instructions not applicable.

DRUG INTERACTIONS
Consult your doctor if you
are taking cyclosporine,
gemfibrozil, niacin, antibiotics, especially ery-
thromycin, or medications
for fungus infections. All of
these drugs may increase
the risk of myositis (muscle
inflammation) when taken
with fluvastatin and may
lead to kidney failure.

FOOD INTERACTIONS
No known food interactions.

DISEASE INTERACTIONS
Consult your doctor if you
have any of the following
problems: liver, kidney, or
muscle disease, or a med-
ical history involving organ
transplant or recent
surgery.

Fluvoxamine Maleate

Luvox 100 mg
(SOLVAY)

Additional photographs

▶ Drug Class: Selective serotonin reuptake inhibitor (SSRI) antidepressant/anti-obsessive-compulsive agent

▶ Available in: Tablets

▶ Available OTC? No

▶ As Generic? Yes

Side Effects

SERIOUS
Decreased libido, sexual dysfunction, diarrhea, dizziness, rapid heartbeat, difficulty breathing, seizures, trembling, vomiting, difficulty swallowing, fainting, psychotic reaction. Call your doctor immediately.

COMMON
Insomnia, decreased appetite, constipation, dry mouth, drowsiness, heartburn, runny nose, unexpected weight loss, headache, frequent urination, increased sweating, change in taste, yawning.

LESS COMMON
Swelling of the feet or lower legs, chills, gas, weight gain.

PRINCIPAL USES
To treat obsessive-compulsive disorder.

HOW THE DRUG WORKS
Fluvoxamine affects levels of serotonin, a brain chemical that is thought to be linked to mood, emotions, and mental state.

DOSAGE
Adults: To start, 50 mg taken at bedtime; may be increased gradually by your doctor to 300 mg a day. Doses greater than 100 mg a day may be taken in 2 divided doses. Children ages 8 to 17: To start, 25 mg taken at bedtime; may be increased gradually by your doctor to 200 mg a day. Doses greater than 50 mg a day may be taken in 2 divided doses.

ONSET OF EFFECT
Unknown.

DURATION OF ACTION
Unknown.

DIETARY ADVICE
Fluvoxamine can be taken without regard to diet. Do not chew the tablet.

STORAGE
Store in a tightly sealed container away from heat, moisture, and direct light.

IF YOU MISS A DOSE
Take it as soon as you remember. If it is near the time for the next dose, skip the missed dose and resume your regular dosage schedule. Do not double the next dose.

STOPPING THE DRUG
Take it as prescribed for the full treatment period, even if you begin to feel better before the scheduled end of therapy. Discontinuing the drug abruptly may produce unpleasant withdrawal symptoms. Dosage should be reduced gradually according to your doctor's instructions.

PROLONGED USE
Consult your doctor about the need for follow-up evaluation and tests if you must take this drug for an extended period.

PRECAUTIONS
Over 60: Adverse reactions may be more likely and more severe in older patients. A lower dose may be warranted.

Driving and Hazardous Work: Use caution when driving or engaging in hazardous work until you determine how the medication affects you.

Alcohol: Avoid alcohol.

Pregnancy: Adequate human studies have not been done. Before taking fluvoxamine, tell your doctor if you are pregnant or plan to become pregnant. Discuss with your doctor the relative risks and benefits of using this drug while pregnant.

Breast Feeding: Fluvoxamine passes into breast milk; avoid or discontinue use while nursing.

Infants and Children: Not recommended for use by children under age 8.

OVERDOSE
Symptoms: Severe diarrhea; extreme dizziness, drowsiness, difficulty awakening, or coma; rapid or slow heartbeat; seizures; or severe vomiting.

What to Do: Call your doctor, emergency medical services (EMS), or the nearest poison control center immediately.

DRUG INTERACTIONS
You should not take fluvoxamine if you are taking terfenadine or astemizole. Fluvoxamine and MAO inhibitors should not be used within 14 days of each other. Very serious side effects such as myoclonus (uncontrolled muscle jerking), hyperthermia (excessive rise in body temperature), and extreme stiffness may result. Consult your doctor for specific advice if you are taking or have recently taken alprazolam, diazepam, midazolam, triazolam, beta-blockers, tricyclic antidepressants, carbamazepine, clozapine, theophylline, tryptophan, lithium, warfarin, or methadone. Also consult your doctor if you smoke tobacco.

FOOD INTERACTIONS
No known food interactions.

DISEASE INTERACTIONS
Caution is advised when taking fluvoxamine. Consult your doctor if you have a history of alcohol or drug abuse, mania, or seizures.

Folic Acid (Folacin; Folate)

Side Effects

SERIOUS
Wheezing, breathing difficulty, chest pain, swelling, tightness in throat or chest, dizziness, rash, itching. Such symptoms may indicate a serious allergic reaction, although this is extremely rare.

COMMON
The are no known common side effects associated with the use of folic acid.

LESS COMMON
Mild allergic reactions.

PRINCIPAL USES
The vitamin folic acid (also known as folacin and folate) is prescribed for treatment or prevention of certain types of anemia that result from folic acid deficiency. Such deficiencies may occur due to insufficient intake of folic acid (a result of poor diet or malnutrition), an inability to absorb the vitamin (as occurs in gastrointestinal disease), impaired ability to utilize the vitamin (due to excessive alcohol intake or phenytoin use), or as a result of conditions requiring increased amounts of folic acid (as occurs with pregnancy, breast feeding, hemodialysis, hemolytic anemia, and bone marrow failure).

HOW THE DRUG WORKS
Folic acid enhances chemical reactions that contribute to the production of red blood cells, the manufacture of DNA needed for cell replication, and the metabolism of amino acids (compounds necessary for the manufacture of proteins).

DOSAGE
For severe deficiency— Adults and children, regardless of age: 1 mg daily. For recommended dietary allowances (RDAs)— Adults and adolescents: 400 micrograms (mcg).During pregnancy: 600 mcg, once daily. While breast feeding: 500 mcg, once daily. Children, newborn to 3 years of age: 65 to 250 mcg, once daily; children 4 to 8 years of age: 200 mcg, once daily; children 9 to 13 years of age: 300 mcg, once daily.

ONSET OF EFFECT
Folic acid is used immediately by the body for a number of vital chemical functions.

DURATION OF ACTION
Folic acid is required by your body on a daily basis throughout a lifetime.

DIETARY ADVICE
Maintain your usual food and fluid intake. Increase fluids if you have a fever or diarrhea, in hot weather, or during exercise. Follow your doctor's dietary advice (such as low-fat, low-salt, or low-cholesterol restrictions) to improve control over high blood pressure and heart disease.

STORAGE
Store in a tightly sealed container away from heat and direct light. Keep away from moisture and extremes in temperature.

IF YOU MISS A DOSE
Take it as soon as you remember. If it is near the time for the next dose, skip the missed dose and resume your regular dosage schedule. Do not double the next dose.

STOPPING THE DRUG
The decision to stop taking the drug should be made by your doctor.

PROLONGED USE
Therapy with folacin may require weeks or months.

PRECAUTIONS
Over 60: No special problems are expected in older patients.

Driving and Hazardous Work: The use of folic acid should not impair your ability to perform such tasks safely.

Alcohol: Alcohol impairs the body's utilization of folic acid; avoid it completely if you are taking folic acid.

Pregnancy: Folic acid supplementation is recommended during pregnancy.

Breast Feeding: Folic acid supplementation is recommended while nursing.

Infants and Children: Folic acid may be used regardless of age.

Special Concerns: Folic acid ingestion can mask vitamin B_{12} deficiency and lead to irreversible neurological damage; therefore, folic acid should be taken only upon the recommendation of your doctor. Folic acid deficiency should not occur, and supplementation is not necessary, in healthy individuals who consume a normal balanced diet. However, women who are capable of becoming pregnant are advised to take 400 mcg of supplemental folic acid on a daily basis to prevent certain birth defects.

OVERDOSE
Symptoms: No specific ones have been reported.

What to Do: An overdose of folic acid is not life-threatening. No emergency procedures are warranted.

DRUG INTERACTIONS
Consult your doctor for specific advice if you are taking analgesics (pain relievers), antibiotics, anticonvulsants, epoetin, estrogens, oral contraceptives, methotrexate, pyrimethamine, triamterene, sulfasalazine, or zinc supplements.

FOOD INTERACTIONS
No known food interactions.

DISEASE INTERACTIONS
Consult your doctor if you have pernicious anemia.

Foscarnet Sodium (Phosphonoformic Acid)

BRAND NAME
Foscavir

▶ Drug Class: Antiviral

▶ Available in: Injection

▶ Available OTC? No

▶ As Generic? No

Side Effects

SERIOUS
Kidney damage, causing symptoms such as increased or decreased urine output, increased or decreased urge to urinate, and increased thirst; toxicity of the nervous system, causing twitching or seizures, or numbness, tingling, or prickling in the extremities; fever and chills; pain at injection site; extreme fatigue. Call your doctor right away.

COMMON
Headache, abdominal pain or upset, nausea and vomiting, loss of weight or appetite, nervousness, anxiety, restlessness, mental confusion, lightheadedness, unusual fatigue.

LESS COMMON
Sores on the mouth, throat, penis, or vulva.

PRINCIPAL USES
To treat the eye disorder cytomegalovirus (CMV) retinitis in patients with acquired immunodeficiency syndrome (AIDS). Sometimes prescribed for other viral infections.

HOW THE DRUG WORKS
Foscarnet interferes with the activity of enzymes needed for the replication of viral DNA in cells, thus preventing CMV from multiplying.

DOSAGE
60 mg for every 2.2 lbs (1 kg) of body weight, injected into a vein every 8 hours for 2 to 3 weeks, followed by a maintenance dose of 90 to 120 mg for every 2.2 lbs, injected daily.

ONSET OF EFFECT
Immediate.

DURATION OF ACTION
24 hours.

DIETARY ADVICE
No special restrictions.

STORAGE
Not applicable, since this drug is administered exclusively in a health care facility or by a home intravenous (I.V.) infusion team.

IF YOU MISS A DOSE
Consult your doctor.

STOPPING THE DRUG
The decision to stop taking the drug should be made by your doctor.

PROLONGED USE
Your doctor should check your progress periodically.

PRECAUTIONS
Over 60: Adverse reactions may be more likely and more severe in older patients.

Driving and Hazardous Work: Do not drive or engage in hazardous work until you determine how the medicine affects you.

Alcohol: Avoid alcohol.

Pregnancy: In animal studies, foscarnet has been shown to cause birth defects. Human studies have not been done. Before taking this drug, tell your doctor if you are pregnant or are planning to become pregnant.

Breast Feeding: Foscarnet may pass into breast milk; caution is advised. Consult your doctor for specific advice.

Infants and Children: There is no specific information about the use of foscarnet by infants and children. Consult your doctor about the possible risks and benefits.

Special Concerns: Drink several glasses of water every day unless your doctor advises otherwise. While taking foscarnet, your doctor may conduct periodic tests on the function of your kidneys. Anemia caused by foscarnet may be severe enough to require blood transfusions. If you are receiving the drug as therapy for CMV retinitis, you should periodically receive eye examinations by an ophthalmologist to check for signs of vision loss. Foscarnet may cause sores on the genital organs. Washing the genitals after urinating may decrease the likelihood of this problem.

OVERDOSE
Symptoms: Sudden or severe onset of serious side effects.

What to Do: Call your doctor, emergency medical services (EMS), or the nearest poison control center immediately.

DRUG INTERACTIONS
Other drugs may interact with foscarnet. Consult your doctor for specific advice if you are taking amphotericin B, carmustine, cisplatin, combination pain medicines containing acetaminophen or aspirin, cyclosporine, deferoxamine, gentamicin, gold salts, any pain medicine, lithium, methotrexate, pentamidine, penicillamine, plicamycin, streptozocin, or tiopronin.

FOOD INTERACTIONS
No known food interactions.

DISEASE INTERACTIONS
Caution is advised when taking foscarnet. Consult your doctor if you have anemia, kidney disease, or dehydration.

Fosfomycin Tromethamine

BRAND NAME
Monurol

▶ Drug Class: Antibiotic

▶ Available in: Powder for solution

▶ Available OTC? No

▶ As Generic? No

Side Effects

SERIOUS
No serious side effects are associated with the use of fosfomycin.

COMMON
Diarrhea, headache, vaginal itching, nausea, runny nose, back pain, painful menstruation, throat irritation, dizziness, abdominal pain, generalized pain, weakness, skin rash, indigestion or stomach upset. Call your doctor if such symptoms persist or interfere with daily activities.

LESS COMMON
Abnormal stools, loss of appetite, constipation, dry mouth, failure to urinate, ear disorders, fever, gas, flu-like symptoms, blood in urine, infection, insomnia, swollen lymph glands, nerve pain, nervousness, burning sensation, sleepiness, vomiting.

PRINCIPAL USES
To treat uncomplicated urinary tract infections (acute cystitis) in women.

HOW THE DRUG WORKS
Fosfomycin interferes with the formation of bacterial cell walls, rendering bacteria unable to multiply and spread.

DOSAGE
Adult and teenage females: 3 g in a single dose, given orally.

ONSET OF EFFECT
Within 3 hours.

DURATION OF ACTION
Unknown.

DIETARY ADVICE
No special dietary recommendations. Mix the powder with half a glass of water. (Do not use hot water.)

STORAGE
Store in a tightly sealed container away from heat, moisture, and direct light.

IF YOU MISS A DOSE
Not applicable. Fosfomycin is intended for one-time use.

STOPPING THE DRUG
Not applicable. Fosfomycin is intended for one-time use.

PROLONGED USE
Fosfomycin is intended for one-time use only. Repeated doses increase the likelihood of adverse side effects. Call your doctor if the infection has not improved, or has worsened, within 2 to 3 days.

PRECAUTIONS
Over 60: No special problems are expected.

Driving and Hazardous Work: Do not drive or engage in hazardous work until you determine how the medicine affects you.

Alcohol: No special precautions are necessary.

Pregnancy: Adequate studies of the use of this drug during pregnancy have not been done. Before taking fosfomycin, tell your doctor if you are pregnant or plan to become pregnant; discuss the relative risks and benefits of using the drug, and weigh them carefully.

Breast Feeding: It is not known whether fosfomycin passes into breast milk; caution is advised. Consult your doctor for specific advice.

Infants and Children: Not recommended for use by children under age 12.

Special Concerns: Urine tests to determine the type of bacteria causing the infection and its susceptibility to treatment should be done before and after the completion of therapy with fosfomycin.

OVERDOSE
Symptoms: An overdose with fosfomycin is unlikely to occur; no cases of overdose have been reported.

What to Do: Emergency instructions not applicable.

DRUG INTERACTIONS
Consult your doctor for specific advice if you are concurrently taking metoclopramide. Before taking fosfomycin, tell your doctor if you are taking any other prescription or over-the-counter medication.

FOOD INTERACTIONS
No known food interactions.

DISEASE INTERACTIONS
Caution is advised when taking fosfomycin. Consult your doctor if you have kidney disease or any other medical condition. Use of fosfomycin may cause complications in patients with kidney disease, since this organ works to remove the medication from the body.

Fosinopril Sodium

BRAND NAME
Monopril

Monopril 10 mg
(BRISTOL-MYERS SQUIBB)

Additional photographs

▶ Drug Class: Angiotensin-converting enzyme (ACE) inhibitor

▶ Available in: Tablets

▶ Available OTC? No

▶ As Generic? Yes

Side Effects

SERIOUS
Fever and chills, sore throat and hoarseness, sudden difficulty breathing or swallowing, swelling of the face, mouth, or extremities, impaired kidney function (ankle swelling, decreased urination), confusion, yellow discoloration of the eyes or skin (indicating liver disorder), intense itching, chest pain or palpitations, abdominal pain. Serious side effects are very rare; contact your doctor immediately.

COMMON
Dry, persistent cough.

LESS COMMON
Dizziness or fainting, skin rash, numbness or tingling in the hands, feet, or lips, unusual fatigue or muscle weakness, nausea, drowsiness, loss of taste, headache.

PRINCIPAL USES
To control high blood pressure; to treat congestive heart failure; to treat patients with left ventricular dysfunction (damage to the pumping chamber of the heart); and to minimize further kidney damage in diabetics with mild kidney disease.

HOW THE DRUG WORKS
Angiotensin-converting enzyme (ACE) inhibitors block an enzyme that produces angiotensin, a naturally occurring substance that causes blood vessels to constrict and stimulates production of the adrenal hormone, aldosterone, which promotes sodium retention in the body. As a result, ACE inhibitors relax blood vessels (causing them to widen) and reduces sodium retention, which lowers blood pressure and so decreases the workload of the heart.

DOSAGE
Initial dose: 10 mg once a day. Maintenance dose: 20 to 80 mg a day, in 1 or 2 doses.

ONSET OF EFFECT
Within 1 hour.

DURATION OF ACTION
24 hours.

DIETARY ADVICE
Take fosinopril on an empty stomach, about 1 hour before mealtime. Follow your doctor's dietary advice (such as low-salt or low-cholesterol restrictions) to improve control over high blood pressure and heart disease. Avoid high-potassium foods like bananas and citrus fruits and juices, unless you are also taking medications, such as diuretics, that lower potassium levels.

STORAGE
Store in a tightly sealed container away from heat and direct light. Keep away from moisture and extremes in temperature.

IF YOU MISS A DOSE
Take it as soon as you remember. If it is near the time for the next dose, skip the missed dose and resume your regular dosage schedule. Do not double the next dose.

STOPPING THE DRUG
Do not stop taking this drug abruptly, as this may cause potentially serious health problems. Dosage should be reduced gradually, according to your doctor's instructions.

PROLONGED USE
Therapy with this medication may require months or years. Prolonged use may increase the risk of adverse effects.

PRECAUTIONS
Over 60: Adverse reactions may be more likely and more severe.

Driving and Hazardous Work: Avoid such activities until you determine how this medication affects you.

Alcohol: Consume alcohol only in moderation since it may increase the effect of the drug and cause an excessive drop in blood pressure. Consult your doctor for advice.

Pregnancy: Do not use fosinopril if you are pregnant or trying to become pregnant. Use of this drug during the last 6 months of pregnancy may cause severe defects, even death, in the fetus.

Breast Feeding: Fosinopril passes into breast milk and may be harmful to the infant; avoid using the drug while nursing.

Infants and Children: Fosinopril is generally not recommended for children.

OVERDOSE
Symptoms: No specific ones have been reported.

What to Do: While overdose is unlikely, call your doctor, emergency medical services (EMS), or the nearest poison control center immediately if you suspect that someone has taken a much larger dose than prescribed.

DRUG INTERACTIONS
Consult your doctor if you are taking diuretics (especially potassium-sparing diuretics), potassium supplements or drugs containing potassium (check ingredient labels), lithium, anticoagulants (such as warfarin), indomethacin or other anti-inflammatory drugs, antacids, allopurinol, or any over-the-counter medications (especially cold remedies and diet pills).

FOOD INTERACTIONS
Avoid low-salt milk and salt substitutes. Many brands contain high amounts of potassium. Avoid high-potassium foods like bananas and citrus fruits and juices.

DISEASE INTERACTIONS
Consult your doctor if you have systemic lupus erythematosus or if you have had a prior allergic reaction to ACE inhibitors. This medication should be used with caution by patients with severe kidney disease or renal artery stenosis (narrowing of one or both of the arteries that supply blood to the kidneys).

Furosemide

Generic 20 mg
(ROXANE)

802

Additional photographs

▶ Drug Class: Loop diuretic

▶ Available in: Tablets, oral solution, injection

▶ Available OTC? No

▶ As Generic? Yes

Side Effects

SERIOUS
Skin rash, hives, intense itching, swelling of the mouth and throat, breathing difficulty, mood or mental changes, nausea and vomiting, unusual fatigue, black or tarry stools. Call your doctor immediately.

COMMON
Muscle cramps or pain. Potassium depletion may lead to heart palpitations and weakness. Fluid depletion may lead to dizziness, especially upon arising from a sitting or lying position, as well as thirst, dry mouth, and constipation.

LESS COMMON
Buzzing or ringing in ears, loss of hearing (particularly after intravenous treatment), diarrhea, loss of appetite, gout, increased blood sugar (a problem for diabetic patients).

PRINCIPAL USES
To reduce fluid (salt and water) accumulation that leads to edema (swelling) and breathlessness in patients with heart disease, cirrhosis of the liver, and kidney disease. Furosemide is also sometimes used to help control high blood pressure.

HOW THE DRUG WORKS
Loop diuretics work on a specific portion of the kidney (the loop of Henle) to increase the excretion of water and sodium in urine.

DOSAGE
20 to 600 mg a day. Tablets and solution: dosage is given in 1, 2, or 3 divided doses daily. Injection (given in a hospital setting only): dosage given in divided doses every 2 to 3 hours or as a continuous infusion.

ONSET OF EFFECT
20 to 60 minutes.

DURATION OF ACTION
Tablets and solution: 6 to 8 hours. Injection: 2 hours.

DIETARY ADVICE
Take with food to reduce stomach irritation.

STORAGE
Keep in refrigerator, in a light-resistant container. Do not allow liquid forms to freeze.

IF YOU MISS A DOSE
Take it as soon as you remember. If it is near the time for the next dose, skip the missed dose and resume your regular dosage schedule. Do not double the next dose.

STOPPING THE DRUG
The decision to stop taking the drug should be made by your doctor.

PROLONGED USE
No apparent problems. Regular examinations by your doctor are advised.

PRECAUTIONS
Over 60: No special problems are expected.

Driving and Hazardous Work: No special precautions are required.

Alcohol: No special precautions are required.

Pregnancy: Diuretics are not useful for the normal fluid retention that occurs with pregnancy. In patients who do need diuretic therapy, furosemide is generally preferred, but should be taken only after careful consultation with your primary care doctor or OB/GYN specialist.

Breast Feeding: Furosemide passes into breast milk; avoid or discontinue use while nursing.

Infants and Children: Use furosemide only under careful supervision by a pediatrician.

Special Concerns: To prevent sleep disruption, avoid taking furosemide in the evening. You may have to take a potassium supplement or consume foods or fluids high in potassium while taking this drug. Diabetic patients should monitor their blood sugar levels carefully.

OVERDOSE
Symptoms: Weakness, lethargy, mental confusion, muscle cramps.

What to Do: Call your doctor, emergency medical services (EMS), or the nearest poison control center immediately.

DRUG INTERACTIONS
Consult your doctor about any other drugs you are taking, especially antibiotics, other blood pressure drugs, any ACE inhibitor, any pain reliever, lithium, cortisone-related drugs, digitalis-related drugs, or any nonsteroidal anti-inflammatory drug.

FOOD INTERACTIONS
None reported.

DISEASE INTERACTIONS
Caution is advised when taking this medication. Consult your doctor if you have diabetes, gout, or a hearing problem, or have had a recent heart attack.

Gabapentin

BRAND NAME
Neurontin

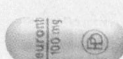

Neurontin 100 mg
(PARKE-DAVIS)

▶ Drug Class: Anticonvulsant

▶ Available in: Capsules, tablets

▶ Available OTC? No

▶ As Generic? No

Side Effects

SERIOUS
Fever, sore throat, swollen glands, red or purple point-like rash on the skin or mucous membranes, blistering or peeling skin lesions, mouth sores, easy bruising, paleness, weakness, confusion, lethargy, or seizures may be a sign of a potentially fatal blood disorder (aplastic anemia) or other complication. Call your physician immediately.

COMMON
Fatigue, dizziness, sedation, clumsiness or unsteadiness, unusual eye movements, blurred or altered vision, nausea, vomiting, tremor.

LESS COMMON
Diarrhea, muscle aches or weakness, dry mouth, headache, sleep disturbances, irritability, slurred speech. There are numerous additional side effects associated with the use of this drug; consult your doctor if you are concerned about any adverse or unusual reactions.

PRINCIPAL USES
To control certain kinds of seizures in the treatment of epilepsy. Gabapentin is often prescribed in combination with another anticonvulsant medication.

HOW THE DRUG WORKS
The mechanism of action is not well understood. It is believed that gabapentin inhibits activity in certain parts of the brain and suppresses the abnormal firing of neurons that causes seizures.

DOSAGE
Adults and teenagers: 900 to 3,600 mg a day, in 3 or 4 divided doses. Some patients require higher doses. The dose is started low and then gradually increased by your doctor to achieve maximum therapeutic benefit with a minimum of side effects. Children ages 3 to 12: To start, 10 to 15 mg per 2.2 lbs (1 kg), in 3 divided doses. The dose is started low and then gradually increased by your doctor to achieve maximum therapeutic benefit with a minimum of side effects.

ONSET OF EFFECT
Several hours.

DURATION OF ACTION
Maximum effectiveness lasts 5 to 8 hours or longer; effectiveness then gradually decreases.

DIETARY ADVICE
No special restrictions.

STORAGE
Store in a tightly sealed container away from heat, moisture, and direct light. Refrigerate the oral solution, but do not allow it to freeze.

IF YOU MISS A DOSE
Take it as soon as you remember. If your next dose is scheduled within the next 2 hours, take the missed dose, and take the next dose 1 to 2 hours later. Resume your regular dosage schedule. Do not double the next dose unless advised to do so by your doctor. Do not wait more than 12 hours between doses.

STOPPING THE DRUG
The decision to stop taking the drug should be made by your doctor. Never stop this drug abruptly because this may cause seizures. The dose is typically tapered over a period of weeks.

PROLONGED USE
Therapy with gabapentin may be required for months or years. Some side effects that are prominent during the first few weeks of therapy may subsequently diminish.

PRECAUTIONS
Over 60: Older persons may require lower doses to minimize side effects.

Driving and Hazardous Work: Avoid such activities until you determine how the medication affects you.

Alcohol: May contribute to excessive drowsiness.

Pregnancy: Adequate human studies of gabapentin during pregnancy have not been done, but the use of other anticonvulsants is associated with an increased risk of birth defects. However, seizures during pregnancy can also increase the risks to the unborn child. Discuss with your doctor the potential risks and benefits of using gabapentin during pregnancy. Folate supplementation is recommended beginning 1 to 2 months before conception and throughout pregnancy.

Breast Feeding:
Gabapentin may pass into breast milk, although at low levels. Consult your doctor for specific advice if you are nursing.

Infants and Children:
There are few published studies regarding the use of gabapentin in children age 12 and younger, but effectiveness should be similar to that seen in older patients. Safety and effectiveness have not been established for children under the age of 3.

Special Concerns: Your doctor may want you to wear a medical bracelet or carry an identification card saying that you are taking this drug.

OVERDOSE
Symptoms: There have been few reports of gabapentin overdose. Symptoms include double vision, slurred speech, drowsiness, lethargy, and diarrhea.

What to Do: Call your doctor, emergency medical services (EMS), or the nearest poison control center immediately.

DRUG INTERACTIONS
Gabapentin has no significant drug interactions.

FOOD INTERACTIONS
No known food interactions.

DISEASE INTERACTIONS
The dose of gabapentin may need to be lower in patients with kidney disease.

Galantamine Hydrobromide

▶ Drug Class: Reversible cholinesterase inhibitor

▶ Available in: Tablets

▶ Available OTC? No

▶ As Generic? No

Side Effects

SERIOUS
No serious side effects are associated with the use of galantamine.

COMMON
Nausea, vomiting, diarrhea, loss of appetite, and weight loss.

LESS COMMON
Fatigue, lightheadedness, dizziness, tremor, headache, abdominal pain, heartburn, depression, insomnia, drowsiness, runny nose, urinary tract infection, blood in the urine.

PRINCIPAL USES
To treat mild to moderate Alzheimer's disease.

HOW THE DRUG WORKS
The exact mechanism of action is unknown. However, galantamine is believed to work by inhibiting acetylcholinesterase enzymes, which reduces the breakdown of acetylcholine, a brain chemical crucial to memory. Acetylcholine deficiency is thought to result in memory loss associated with Alzheimer's disease.

DOSAGE
To start, 4 mg twice a day. After a minimum of four weeks of treatment, your doctor may increase the dose to 8 mg twice a day. The dose may be further increased after no less than a 4-week interval to 12 mg twice a day, if tolerated. People with moderate liver or kidney impairment should not take more than 16 mg a day.

ONSET OF EFFECT
Unknown.

DURATION OF ACTION
Unknown,

DIETARY ADVICE
Rivastigmine should be taken with food in the morning and evening.

STORAGE
Store in a tightly sealed container away from heat, moisture, and direct light.

IF YOU MISS A DOSE
Take it as soon as you remember. If it is near the time for the next dose, skip the missed dose and resume your regular dosage schedule. Do not double the next dose. If therapy has been interrupted for several days or longer, consult your doctor.

STOPPING THE DRUG
The decision to stop taking the drug should be made in consultation with your physician.

PROLONGED USE
No problems are expected with long-term use.

PRECAUTIONS
Over 60: No special problems are expected.

Driving and Hazardous Work: Do not drive or engage in hazardous work until you determine how the medicine affects you.

Alcohol: Avoid alcohol while using this medication.

Pregnancy: Adequate studies on the use of galantamine during pregnancy have not been done. Discuss with your doctor the relative risks and benefits of using this drug while pregnant.

Breast Feeding: It is not known whether galantamine passes into breast milk; caution is advised. Consult your doctor for specific advice.

Infants and Children: Galantamine is not intended for use in children.

Special Concerns: Galantamine will not cure Alzheimer's disease and will not stop the disease from getting worse, but it will improve cognitive ability of some patients.

OVERDOSE
Symptoms: Severe nausea, vomiting, increased salivation, sweating, slow heartbeat, low blood pressure, irregular breathing, unconsciousness, increased muscle weakness, death.

What to Do: Call your doctor, emergency medical services (EMS), or the nearest poison control center immediately.

DRUG INTERACTIONS
The following drugs may interact with galantamine. Consult your doctor for specific advice if you are taking anticholinergic drugs or paroxetine.

FOOD INTERACTIONS
No known food interactions.

DISEASE INTERACTIONS
Do not take galantamine if you have severe liver or kidney impairment. Caution is advised when taking this drug. Consult your doctor if you have any of the following: asthma, obstructive pulmonary disease, epilepsy or a history of seizures, heart problems, intestinal blockage, stomach or duodenal ulcer, liver disease, or urinary problems.

Ganciclovir Sodium

Cytovene 250 mg
(Roche)

▶ Drug Class: Antiviral

▶ Available in: Capsules, injection, intraocular implant

▶ Available OTC? No

▶ As Generic? Yes

Side Effects

SERIOUS
Unusual or persistent fevers, chills, unusual fatigue, sore throat, bruising, or bleeding (these may be signs of serious anemia or problems with the cells of your immune system); skin rash, tremor, eye pain, or sudden change in vision (blurring or partial loss of sight), pain at the injection site. Call your doctor immediately.

COMMON
No common side effects are associated with the use of ganciclovir.

LESS COMMON
Abdominal discomfort, decreased appetite, nausea, vomiting, sweating.

PRINCIPAL USES
To treat or prevent infections caused by cytomegalovirus (CMV). CMV infection of the eyes occurs in patients with weakened immune systems and is prevalent among people with AIDS. A more widespread infection with CMV may occur in patients who have received organ or bone marrow transplants and who are being treated with medications (immunosuppressants) to prevent rejection.

HOW THE DRUG WORKS
Ganciclovir interferes with the activity of enzymes needed for the replication of viral DNA in cells, thus preventing the virus from multiplying.

DOSAGE
Adults: Capsules (for maintenance and prevention therapy only; not for treatment of active infection): 1,000 mg, 3 times a day with food, or 500 mg every 3 hours while awake, for a total of 6 consecutive doses. Patients with kidney problems may require smaller doses. An injection form is available for hospitalized patients and those in special home care situations; the dose is determined by weight. The intraocular insert must be surgically implanted in the eye and replaced every 6 months.

ONSET OF EFFECT
Unknown.

DURATION OF ACTION
About 24 to 48 hours.

DIETARY ADVICE
Take the capsules with food. Increase fluids if you have a fever or diarrhea. Patients with AIDS are often weakened and may be unable to consume adequate amounts of nutritious food. Use special liquid supplements if necessary. Your doctor may refer you to a nutritionist.

STORAGE
Store in a tightly sealed container away from heat and direct light.

IF YOU MISS A DOSE
Take it as soon as you remember. If it is near the time for the next dose, skip the missed dose and resume your regular dosage schedule. Do not double the next dose.

STOPPING THE DRUG
Take it as prescribed for the full treatment period, even if you feel better before the scheduled end of therapy.

PROLONGED USE
Your doctor should check your progress periodically during prolonged use.

PRECAUTIONS
Over 60: Adverse reactions may be more likely and more severe in older patients.

Driving and Hazardous Work: Avoid such activities until you determine how the medicine affects you.

Alcohol: Avoid alcohol.

Pregnancy: Avoid use of this drug if you are pregnant or trying to become pregnant. If you must use the drug, use a reliable birth control method (both men and women) throughout therapy and for at least 3 months afterward.

Breast Feeding: Ganciclovir passes into breast milk and may be harmful to the nursing infant; do not breast feed when taking this drug.

Infants and Children: Not recommended for infants and children.

Special Concerns: Therapy with oral ganciclovir requires many weeks or months. Relapse of eye problems is common, once the drug is stopped. Remember that infection is a great threat to people with weakened immune systems. Do not receive any vaccinations without your doctor's approval, and try to avoid people with infections. Watch for unusual bleeding, bruising, or fevers.

OVERDOSE
Symptoms: Extreme weakness and dizziness, severe diarrhea and stomach upset, shortness of breath.

What to Do: Call your doctor, emergency medical services (EMS), or the nearest poison control center immediately.

DRUG INTERACTIONS
Consult your doctor for specific advice if you are taking amphotericin B, azathioprine, carmustine, chloramphenicol, cisplatin, cyclosporine, dapsone, deferoxamine, didanosine (ddI), flucytosine, gold salts, any pain medicine, lithium, methotrexate, pentamidine, penicillamine, plicamycin, probenecid, streptozocin, tiopronin, trimethoprim/sulfamethoxazole, or zidovudine (AZT).

FOOD INTERACTIONS
No known food interactions.

DISEASE INTERACTIONS
Consult your doctor for advice if you have been diagnosed as having a low white blood cell count, low platelet count, clotting or bleeding problems, or kidney disease.

Gatifloxacin

BRAND NAME
Tequin

▶ Drug Class: Fluoroquinolone antibiotic

▶ Available in: Tablets, injection

▶ Available OTC? No

▶ As Generic? No

Side Effects

SERIOUS
Serious reactions to gatifloxacin are rare and include seizures, rapid heartbeat, mental confusion, hallucinations, agitation, nightmares, depression, shortness of breath, unusual swelling in the face or extremities, and loss of consciousness. Also skin burning, redness, blisters, rash, or itching on exposure to sunlight; increased risk of tendinitis or tendon rupture. Call your doctor immediately.

COMMON
Nausea, vaginitis, diarrhea, headache, dizziness.

LESS COMMON
Chills, fever, back pain, abdominal pain, constipation, heartburn, inflammation of the tongue, mouth sores, vomiting, swelling, insomnia, numbness, shortness of breath, sore throat, sweating, abnormal vision, change in sense of taste, ringing in the ears, painful urination, blood in the urine.

PRINCIPAL USES
To treat mild to severe bacterial infections, including acute sinusitis, community-acquired pneumonia, urinary tract infections, kidney infections, acute bacterial complications due to chronic bronchitis, and gonorrhea.

HOW THE DRUG WORKS
Gatifloxacin inhibits the activity of bacterial enzymes (DNA gyrase and a topoisomerase) that are necessary for proper DNA formation and replication. This fights infection by preventing bacteria from reproducing.

DOSAGE
For most infections: 400 mg once a day for 7 to 10 days (14 days for community-acquired pneumonia). For uncomplicated urinary tract infections: 400 mg as a one-time dose or 200 mg a day for 3 days. For gonorrhea: 400 mg as a one-time dose.

ONSET OF EFFECT
Varies depending on the infection being treated.

DURATION OF ACTION
Unknown.

DIETARY ADVICE
Can be taken without regard to meals.

STORAGE
Store in a tightly sealed container away from heat, moisture, and direct light.

IF YOU MISS A DOSE
Take it as soon as you remember. If it is near the time for the next dose, skip the missed dose and resume your regular dosage schedule. Do not double the next dose.

STOPPING THE DRUG
It is very important to take this drug as prescribed for the full treatment period, even if you begin to feel better before the scheduled end of therapy.

PROLONGED USE
If your symptoms do not improve or instead become worse after a few days, consult your doctor promptly. Gatifloxacin is typically taken for no more than 14 days.

PRECAUTIONS
Over 60: No special advice.

Driving and Hazardous Work: Avoid such activities until you determine how the medicine affects you.

Alcohol: It is advisable to abstain from alcohol when fighting an infection.

Pregnancy: In some animal tests, gatifloxacin has caused birth defects. Adequate human studies have not been done. It should be used during pregnancy only if potential benefits clearly justify the risks. Before you take gatifloxacin, tell your doctor if you are pregnant or plan to become pregnant.

Breast Feeding: Gatifloxacin may pass into breast milk and cause serious side effects in the nursing infant; use of the drug is discouraged when nursing.

Infants and Children: Gatifloxacin is not recommended for use by persons under the age of 18.

Special Concerns: Do not take this medicine if you are allergic to any quinolone antibiotic, such as ciprofloxacin, or lomefloxacin.

OVERDOSE
Symptoms: An overdose is unlikely to occur. Possible symptoms after an excessive dose may include decreased activity and rate of breathing, vomiting, tremors, and seizures.

What to Do: If you have any reason to suspect an overdose, call your doctor, emergency medical services (EMS), or the nearest poison control center.

DRUG INTERACTIONS
Because gatifloxacin can affect the function of the heart, it should not be used if you are taking antiarrhythmic drugs such as amiodarone, quinidine, procainamide, or sotalol. It should be used with caution in patients taking erythromycin, antipsychotics, tricylic antidepressants, warfarin, nonsteroidal anti-inflammatory drugs (NSAIDs; including ibuprofen, aspirin, and naproxen), or digoxin. Gatifloxacin should be taken at least 4 hours before using ferrous sulfate (iron supplement), dietary supplements containing zinc, didanosine, or antacids containing aluminum or magnesium salts.

FOOD INTERACTIONS
No known food interactions.

DISEASE INTERACTIONS
Gatifloxacin should not be taken by people with prolongation of the QT interval on an electrocardiogram, known heart rhythm disturbances, uncorrected hypokalemia (low blood potassium levels), or those taking antiarrhythmic drugs such as amiodarone, quinidine, procainamide, or sotalol. This drug should be used with caution in people with significant bradycardia (slow heart rate), recent myocardial ischemia, known or suspected nervous system disorders, or those predisposed to seizures. People with impaired kidney function may require a reduced dose depending on the severity of kidney dysfunction. Your doctor will determine the appropriate dose.

Gemfibrozil

R

Generic 600 mg
(LEMMON)

▶ Drug Class: Antilipidemic (triglyceride-lowering agent)

▶ Available in: Tablets

▶ Available OTC? No

▶ As Generic? Yes

Side Effects

SERIOUS
Muscle aches and tenderness; crampy abdominal pain, especially in the area under the ribs on the right side, with nausea and vomiting (this is an uncommon, serious side effect that may indicate gallbladder disease); decreased urine output.

COMMON
Diarrhea, nausea, gas.

LESS COMMON
Decreased sexual ability; headache; weight gain; feelings similar to the flu, with muscle aches or cramps, weakness, and unusual tiredness; inflammation of mouth and lips; heartburn.

PRINCIPAL USES
To treat high levels of blood triglyceride. Usually prescribed after other treatments—including diet, weight loss, exercise, and control of diabetes (when present)—fail to lower triglyceride levels adequately.

HOW THE DRUG WORKS
Gemfibrozil speeds the removal of triglycerides from the lipoprotein known as very-low-density lipoprotein (VLDL), which is converted to low-density lipoprotein (LDL). In some people total and LDL cholesterol levels may rise while triglycerides fall.

DOSAGE
Adults: 600 milligrams, 2 times per day. Usually taken 30 to 60 minutes before morning and evening meals.

ONSET OF EFFECT
Improvement begins in about 1 week and becomes most noticeable in about 4 weeks.

DURATION OF ACTION
Blood triglyceride levels increase within a few weeks of stopping gemfibrozil.

DIETARY ADVICE
Follow your doctor's dietary advice to improve control over high blood pressure and help prevent heart disease. The American Heart Association publishes a "Healthy Heart" diet; discuss this with your doctor. Limit intake of alcohol, which can raise triglyceride levels.

STORAGE
Store in a tightly sealed container away from heat and direct light.

IF YOU MISS A DOSE
Take your missed dose as soon as you remember, unless the time for your next scheduled dose is within the next 2 hours. If so, do not take the missed dose. Take your next scheduled dose at the proper time, and resume your regular dosage schedule. Do not double the next dose.

STOPPING THE DRUG
Do not stop taking gemfibrozil on your own; the level of triglycerides in your blood will increase.

PROLONGED USE
Gemfibrozil is often taken for long periods of time. If your blood triglycerides do not diminish, your physician may stop the medication.

PRECAUTIONS
Over 60: Adverse reactions may be more likely and more severe in older patients.

Driving and Hazardous Work: The use of gemfibrozil should not impair your ability to perform such tasks safely.

Alcohol: Alcohol intake should be limited because it can raise triglyceride levels.

Pregnancy: Do not take gemfibrozil while pregnant unless your doctor indicates that the risks of stopping the drug are too great. Triglycerides increase substantially during pregnancy and extremely high triglycerides can trigger an attack of acute pancreatitis.

Breast Feeding: Avoid or discontinue usage while nursing.

Infants and Children: Rarely used in infants and children.

Special Concerns: The most important treatment for high levels of blood triglycerides is a proper diet, weight loss, regular moderate exercise, the avoidance of certain medications, and control of diabetes. Because gemfibrozil has potential side effects, it is important that you maintain a healthy diet and cooperate with other treatment strategies your physician may suggest. Gemfibrozil may increase the chances of gallbladder, liver, and pancreas problems; your physician will order periodic blood tests.

OVERDOSE
Symptoms: No specific ones have been reported.

What to Do: Emergency instructions not applicable.

DRUG INTERACTIONS
Certain drugs may interact adversely with gemfibrozil, particularly anticoagulants (blood thinners, such as warfarin), niacin, and any of the group of cholesterol-lowering drugs referred to as "-statins." It may be necessary to reduce the dose of warfarin to prevent bleeding. The combination of gemfibrozil with either niacin or a statin drug can cause severe myositis (muscle inflammation), which can release a protein that damages the kidneys. Consult your doctor for specific advice.

FOOD INTERACTIONS
No known food interactions.

DISEASE INTERACTIONS
Inform your doctor if you have any of the following problems: gallstones, stomach or intestinal ulcer, kidney disease, muscle disease, or liver disease. The dose of gemfibrozil must be reduced in those with significant kidney damage.

Gentamicin Topical

BRAND NAMES
Ed-Mycin, G-Myticin,
Garamycin, Gentamar

▶ Drug Class: Antibacterial
(topical)

▶ Available in: Cream, ointment

▶ Available OTC? No

▶ As Generic? Yes

Side Effects

SERIOUS
No serious side effects
are associated with topi-
cal gentamicin when
used as directed.

COMMON
No common side effects
are associated with topi-
cal gentamicin when
used as directed.

LESS COMMON
Itching, swelling,
increased redness, or discomfort at the application
site not present prior to
therapy (as a result of
allergic reaction).

PRINCIPAL USES
To treat minor bacterial
infections of the skin,
including infected bites,
burns, abrasions, and other
wounds; infected cysts, hair
follicles, and other skin
structures; and infections
complicating rashes,
eczema, dermatitis, and
other inflammatory skin
conditions. Gentamicin is
not effective against fungal
infections or viruses.

HOW THE DRUG WORKS
Gentamicin works by pre-
venting bacterial organisms
from manufacturing the vital
proteins they require for
growth and function.

DOSAGE
Adults, teenagers, and children over 1 year of age:
Apply it to the affected site
3 or 4 times a day.

ONSET OF EFFECT
Gentamicin begins killing
susceptible bacteria shortly
after contact. The drug's
effects may not be noticeable for several days.

DURATION OF ACTION
The exact duration of action
of gentamicin is not known,
but replenishing the topical
antibiotic 3 or 4 times a day
is sufficient for treatment.

DIETARY ADVICE
No special restrictions.

STORAGE
Store in a tightly sealed container away from heat, moisture, and direct light.

IF YOU MISS A DOSE
Apply it as soon as you
remember. If it is near the
time for the next dose, skip
the missed dose and
resume your regular dosage
schedule. Do not double the
next dose or apply exces-
sive amounts of the drug to
compensate for a missed
application.

STOPPING THE DRUG
Apply the medicine as prescribed by your doctor for
the full treatment period,
even if you begin to feel better before the scheduled
end of therapy.

PROLONGED USE
Therapy with gentamicin is
usually completed within 7
to 14 days. Use of any antibiotic drug for longer than
your doctor recommends
increases your risk of infection by drug-resistant bacteria or other microorganisms
(known as superinfection).

PRECAUTIONS
Over 60: Adverse reactions
may be more likely and
more severe in older
patients.

**Driving and Hazardous
Work:** No special precautions are necessary.

Alcohol: No special precautions are necessary.

Pregnancy: Problems in
pregnant women using gen-
tamicin have not been
reported. Consult your doctor for specific advice.

Breast Feeding: Gentamicin may pass into breast
milk; caution is advised.
Consult your doctor for
specific advice.

Infants and Children:
This drug is not recom-
mended for use by children
under 1 year of age.

Special Concerns: Make
sure you tell your doctor
about allergies that you
might have before taking
any antibiotic. There is
varying opinion as to
whether or not topical
antibiotics are effective to
treat infections. Tell your
doctor if your condition has
not improved within a few
days of starting gentamicin.

As with any other antibiotic,
gentamicin is useful only
against strains of bacteria
that are susceptible to its
effects.

OVERDOSE
Symptoms: No specific
ones have been reported.

What to Do: An overdose
of gentamicin is unlikely to
be life-threatening. How-
ever, if someone takes a
much larger dose than prescribed or accidentally
ingests the cream or ointment, call your doctor,
emergency medical services
(EMS), or the nearest poison control center.

DRUG INTERACTIONS
No drug interactions have
been reported. If you are
concerned about whether a
prescription or nonprescription medication you are taking may interact with topical
gentamicin, consult your
doctor or pharmacist for
current information.

FOOD INTERACTIONS
No known food interactions.

DISEASE INTERACTIONS
Caution is advised when
using gentamicin. Consult
your doctor if you have
hearing problems, kidney
disease, any prior reactions
to a skin cream or ointment,
or any history of allergic
reaction to antibiotics.

Glatiramer Acetate (Copolymer-1)

BRAND NAME
Copaxone

▶ Drug Class: Immunomodulator

▶ Available in: Powder that is used for injection

▶ Available OTC? No

▶ As Generic? No

Side Effects

SERIOUS
Severe pain or rash at injection site immediately after injection. Call your doctor immediately.

COMMON
Flushed skin, dizziness, depression, palpitations, anxiety, difficulty breathing, throat constriction, fast heartbeat, tremor, hives, transient chest pain, enlarged blood vessels, fever, chills, infection, migraine headache, loss of appetite, gastrointestinal disorders, nausea, vomiting, swelling of arms and legs, joint pains, anxiety, muscle tension, bronchitis, nasal inflammation, itching skin, ear pain, urge to urinate frequently.

LESS COMMON
There are no less-common side effects associated with glatiramer acetate.

PRINCIPAL USES
To prevent or reduce the frequency of relapses in patients with relapsing-remitting multiple sclerosis (the most common form of MS, in which periods of active disease alternate with periods of remission or reduced severity of symptoms).

HOW THE DRUG WORKS
Nerves are insulated by a layer of fatty material known as myelin. MS is a frequently progressive, often debilitating, disorder that occurs when the protective myelin is damaged at various (multiple) sites throughout the central nervous system (brain and spinal cord) by the body's own immune system, with the subsequent development of scarlike tissue, a process referred to by doctors as sclerosis. Glatiramer acetate is believed to block the attack on the myelin sheath, slowing the progress of the disease.

DOSAGE
20 mg injected under the skin once a day.

ONSET OF EFFECT
Unknown.

DURATION OF ACTION
Unknown.

DIETARY ADVICE
No special restrictions.

STORAGE
The powder should be kept refrigerated; if refrigeration is not available, it may be stored at room temperature for up to one week. The vials of sterile water with which the powder is mixed should be stored at room temperature. The powder and water should be kept in tightly sealed containers away from direct light.

IF YOU MISS A DOSE
Take it as soon as you remember. However, if it is near the time for the next dose, skip the missed dose and resume your regular dosage schedule. Do not double the next dose.

STOPPING THE DRUG
The decision to stop taking the drug should be made by your doctor.

PROLONGED USE
You should see your doctor regularly for tests and examinations if you must take this medicine for a prolonged period of time.

PRECAUTIONS
Over 60: No special problems are expected.

Driving and Hazardous Work: Do not drive or engage in hazardous activities until you determine how the drug affects you.

Alcohol: No special precautions are necessary.

Pregnancy: Glatiramer acetate has not been shown to cause birth defects in animals. Human studies have not been done. Before you take glatiramer acetate, tell your doctor if you are pregnant or plan to become pregnant.

Breast Feeding: Glatiramer acetate may pass into breast milk; caution is advised. Consult your doctor for specific information.

Infants and Children: The safety and effectiveness of glatiramer acetate in persons under age 18 have not been established.

Special Concerns: Glatiramer acetate should be injected at a different site every day during the week; 7 sites in all. Sites for self-injection are the arms, stomach, thighs, and hips. The injection is best given at the same time every day. To prepare the medication for injection, use a sterile syringe and needle to transfer the sterile water into the glatiramer acetate vial. Swirl the vial gently and let it stand at room temperature until the solid material is completely dissolved. Discard the preparation if it contains visible sediment. Put the preparation into a sterile syringe fitted with a new 27-gauge needle and make the injection under the skin at the selected site of the day. After the injection, a cotton ball should be held against the injection site for a few seconds, but the site should not be rubbed.

OVERDOSE
Symptoms: No specific ones have been reported.

What to Do: If someone receives a much larger dose than prescribed or accidentally ingests glatiramer acetate, call the nearest poison control center immediately.

DRUG INTERACTIONS
Other drugs potentially may interact with glatiramer acetate. Consult your doctor for advice if you are taking any other prescription or over-the-counter drug.

FOOD INTERACTIONS
No known food interactions.

DISEASE INTERACTIONS
Caution is advised when taking glatiramer acetate. Consult your physician if you have any other medical condition.

Glimepiride

BRAND NAME
Amaryl

Amaryl 2 mg
(HOECHST MARION ROUSSEL)

▸ Drug Class: Antidiabetic agent/sulfonylurea

▸ Available in: Tablets

▸ Available OTC? No

▸ As Generic? Yes

Side Effects

SERIOUS
Serious side effects are related to hypoglycemia, or low blood sugar, whose symptoms include perspiration or a cold sweat, restlessness, rapid pulse, anxious feeling, nausea, feelings of dizziness, weakness, or light-headedness, poor coordination, slurred speech, confusion, sleepiness, seizures or convulsions, weakness of an arm, leg, or an entire side of the body, fainting. Seek emergency assistance. Administer sugar-containing substances only if the patient is conscious and alert. Other serious but less common side effects include low white blood cell count and elevation of liver-associated enzymes; these problems can be detected by your doctor.

COMMON
Dizziness, weakness, nausea, headache.

LESS COMMON
Skin reactions, such as itching, peeling, rashes, and hives; blurred vision; edema (swelling due to fluid retention) of face or extremities; severe tiredness; abdominal pain.

PRINCIPAL USES
Glimepiride is used to treat diabetes (high blood sugar) in patients who require little or no injectable insulin. It is used in conjunction with a special diet and exercise. Some patients may fail to respond initially or gradually lose their responsiveness to glimepiride. The antidiabetic agent metformin may be used in conjunction with glimepiride to achieve the desired results.

HOW THE DRUG WORKS
Glimepiride stimulates the release of insulin from the pancreas and makes the tissues of your body more responsive to insulin.

DOSAGE
Adults: 1 to 4 mg once daily, 30 minutes before breakfast. Children: Not recommended for use by children.

ONSET OF EFFECT
2 to 3 hours.

DURATION OF ACTION
12 to 24 hours.

DIETARY ADVICE
Maintain special diets as recommended by your doctor. Restrict excessive intake of sugar-containing snacks. Read food labels carefully.

STORAGE
Keep away from direct light, moisture, and extremes in temperature.

IF YOU MISS A DOSE
Take it as soon as you remember. If it is near the time for the next dose, skip the missed dose and resume your regular dosage schedule. Do not double the next dose.

STOPPING THE DRUG
The decision to stop taking glimepiride should be made by your doctor.

PROLONGED USE
Therapy with glimepiride may require months or years. Its prolonged use may be associated with an increased risk of side effects.

PRECAUTIONS
Over 60: Adverse reactions from this drug may be more likely and more severe.

Driving and Hazardous Work: Do not drive or engage in hazardous work until you determine how the medicine affects you.

Alcohol: Use only in a moderate, responsible fashion. Consult your doctor.

Pregnancy: Glimepiride should not be used during pregnancy.

Breast Feeding: It should not be used by nursing mothers.

Infants and Children: Not recommended for use by children.

Special Concerns: Understand the symptoms of low blood sugar. Always have easy access to sources of simple sugar—juice, candy bars, energy bars, hard candy, honey, sugar cubes, sugar dissolved in water—in the event you experience symptoms of hypoglycemia (low blood sugar). Inform your physician promptly about changes in the way you are feeling, changes in your lifestyle and level of activity, medications that you may have been prescribed by other specialists, medications that you have stopped taking, unusually high or low results for any at-home tests you use to check your urine or blood, episodes of low blood sugar, and pregnancy. Wear a spe-cial medical ID bracelet. Do not miss meals. Use caution when exercising.

OVERDOSE
Symptoms: Symptoms are similar to serious side effects.

What to Do: Call emergency medical services (EMS), your doctor, or the nearest poison control center immediately.

DRUG INTERACTIONS
Consult your doctor for specific advice if you are taking steroids and nonsteroidal anti-inflammatory drugs (such as ibuprofen, aspirin, or aspirin-containing drugs), anticoagulants, certain antibiotics, especially for fungal infections, diuretics, lithium, beta-blockers, ulcer medications, ciprofloxacin, cyclosporine, guanethidine, MAO inhibitors, quinidine, quinine, chloramphenicol, estrogen, isoniazid, thyroid hormones, theophylline, pentamidine phenothiazines, or phenytoin.

FOOD INTERACTIONS
No known food interactions.

DISEASE INTERACTIONS
Consult your doctor if you have diarrhea, persistent vomiting, malabsorption disease, liver, thyroid, kidney, or adrenal gland disease, fever, or infection.

Glipizide

Generic 5 mg
(MYLAN)

▶ Drug Class: Antidiabetic
agent/sulfonylurea

▶ Available in: Tablets,
extended-release tablets

▶ Available OTC? No

▶ As Generic? Yes

Side Effects

SERIOUS
Serious side effects are
related to hypoglycemia,
or low blood sugar, whose
symptoms include perspi-
ration or a cold sweat,
restlessness, rapid pulse,
anxious feeling, nausea,
feelings of dizziness,
weakness, or lightheaded-
ness, poor coordination,
slurred speech, confusion,
drowsiness, seizures,
weakness of an arm, leg,
or an entire side of the
body, and fainting. Seek
emergency assistance.
Administer sugar-contain-
ing substances only if the
patient is conscious and
alert. Other serious but
less common side effects
include low white blood
cell count and elevation of
liver-associated enzymes;
these problems can be
detected by your doctor.

COMMON
Dizziness, constipation,
nausea, heartburn,
unusual or changed taste
of food, or unusual taste
in the mouth.

LESS COMMON
Peeling, red, bruised, or
itching skin, pale skin,
edema (swelling) of face
or extremities, reduced
ability to exercise,
headache, fever.

PRINCIPAL USES
Glipizide is used to treat
diabetes (high blood sugar)
in patients who require little
or no injectable insulin. It is
used in conjunction with a
special diet and exercise.
Some patients may fail to
respond initially or gradually lose their responsiveness to glipizide. Other
antidiabetic agents such as
metformin may be used in
conjunction with glipizide to
achieve the desired results.

HOW THE DRUG WORKS
Glipizide stimulates the
release of insulin from special cells in the pancreas
and therefore helps to lower
blood glucose.

DOSAGE
Usual starting dose: 5 mg
a day, taken 30 minutes
before breakfast. Dosage
should be adjusted by 2.5
to 5 mg per day based on
blood sugar response.
When greater than 15 mg
a day, dosages should be
divided. In the elderly or
patients with liver disease,
the initial dose should be
2.5 mg a day. While the
maximum dose is 40 mg a
day, little additional benefit
is derived from more than
20 mg a day. Extended-
release tablets: 5 to 10 mg,
once daily, usually with
breakfast.

ONSET OF EFFECT
Within 30 minutes.

DURATION OF ACTION
12 to 24 hours.

DIETARY ADVICE
Maintain special diets as
recommended by your doc-
tor, nutritionist, or the
American Diabetes Association. Restrict excessive
intake of sugar-laden
snacks. Read labels care-
fully when buying food.

STORAGE
Store away from direct
light, moisture, and
extremes in temperature.

IF YOU MISS A DOSE
Take it as soon as you
remember. If it is near the
time for the next dose, skip
the missed dose and
resume your regular dosage
schedule. Do not double the
next dose.

STOPPING THE DRUG
The decision to stop taking
it should be made by your
doctor.

PROLONGED USE
Therapy may require
months or years. Prolonged
use may be associated with
an increased risk of side
effects.

PRECAUTIONS
Over 60: Adverse reactions
from this drug may be
more likely and more
severe.

**Driving and Hazardous
Work:** Do not drive or
engage in hazardous work
until you determine how the
medication affects you.

Alcohol: Drink only in
moderation.

Pregnancy: Glipizide
should not be used. Insulin
is the treatment of choice
for pregnant diabetic
women.

Breast Feeding: This
drug passes into breast
milk, although it is uncertain whether this is harmful
to nursing infants. Consult
your doctor.

Infants and Children:
Not recommended for use
by children.

Special Concerns: Keep
simple sugars (juice, candy
bars, hard candy) on hand

in the event of hypogly-
cemia. Inform your doctor
promptly of changes in how
you feel, unusually high or
low results for any at-home
tests, episodes of low blood
sugar, or pregnancy. Wear a
medical ID bracelet. Do not
miss meals. Use caution
when exercising.

OVERDOSE
Symptoms: Symptoms similar to serious side effects.

What to Do: Call emergency medical services
(EMS), your doctor, or the
nearest poison control center immediately.

DRUG INTERACTIONS
Consult your doctor for
specific advice if you are
taking anticoagulants,
antibiotics (especially
sulfa-containing antibiotics
or those used to treat fungal
infections), steroids, diuretics, seizure medications
(such as carbamazepine or
phenytoin), beta-blockers
(which may include eye
drops for glaucoma) or
other blood pressure
medications, lithium,
ulcer drugs, guanethidine,
MAO inhibitors, quinidine,
quinine, salicylates,
chloramphenicol, estrogens,
isoniazid, thyroid
hormones, theophylline,
or pentamidine.

FOOD INTERACTIONS
Food delays the absorption
of immediate-release tablets.

DISEASE INTERACTIONS
Consult your doctor if you
have diarrhea, persistent
vomiting, malabsorption disease, liver, thyroid, kidney,
or adrenal gland disease,
fever, infection, or impend-
ing or recent surgery.

Glucagon

▶ Drug Class: Hormone; antidote; antidiabetic agent

▶ Available in: Injection

▶ Available OTC? No

▶ As Generic? Yes

Side Effects

SERIOUS
No serious side effects
are associated with
glucagon.

COMMON
Nausea may be
associated with higher
dosages.

LESS COMMON
Rare allergic reactions
(wheezing, itching,
weakness); redness and
pain at site of injection.
Consult your doctor if
such side effects persist
or recur.

PRINCIPAL USES
Glucagon is an injectable
drug that is used for the
emergency treatment of low
blood sugar in diabetics
who are unable to take any
sugar-containing foods or
liquids by mouth. These
patients are usually unconscious or very confused
and sleepy.

HOW THE DRUG WORKS
Glucagon stimulates the
liver to release glucose
(sugar) into the blood-
stream.

DOSAGE
Adults and children weighing more than 45 pounds: 1
mg, by injection. Children
less than 45 pounds: 0.5 mg.
Doses may be repeated
twice, at 15 minute intervals. Glucagon emergency
kits usually contain two
vials. One is glucagon. The
other is a fluid that must
be used to dilute glucagon
before it can be drawn up
in a syringe and injected.

ONSET OF EFFECT
Within 15 minutes.

DURATION OF ACTION
The effect persists for 1 to 2
hours.

DIETARY ADVICE
Solutions containing glucose
(sugar) must be adminis-
tered following glucagon
injections for the drug to
work properly.

STORAGE
Store in a tightly sealed container away from heat and
direct light. If you prepared
glucagon for injection but
did not use it, it may be
refrigerated and kept for no
more than 48 hours.

IF YOU MISS A DOSE
Not applicable; glucagon is
used only in emergencies.

STOPPING THE DRUG
If the patient has not
responded within 15 min-
utes of the first injection,
do not stop glucagon treatments. You may administer
2 more injections at 15-
minute intervals.

PROLONGED USE
Not applicable.

PRECAUTIONS
Over 60: No unusual problems are expected.

**Driving and Hazardous
Work:** Not applicable.

Alcohol: Not applicable.

Pregnancy: Glucagon may
be administered.

Breast Feeding: It is
unlikely that glucagon is
hazardous to nursing
infants, since the drug is
used only occasionally,
although no studies have
been done to confirm this.

Infants and Children:
Not applicable.

Special Concerns:
Glucagon is effective only if
given by injection. Therefore, it is very important
that family members or
caregivers know exactly
how to prepare glucagon for
injection. The best time to
read and understand
glucagon instructions is
before an emergency
occurs. Any diabetic patient
who is confused, drowsy,
sleepy, or unconscious
should be assumed to have
low blood sugar. Do not
attempt to feed drowsy, dis-
oriented, or unconscious
individuals. Administer
glucagon promptly. If not
already notified, emergency
personnel should be con-
tacted immediately after the
first glucagon dose has
been injected. Do not wait
for further doses to be
given before calling for
emergency assistance. Do
not wait for additional 15-
minute intervals. Glucagon
is not a cure for low blood
sugar. It is an emergency
treatment that may be life-
saving, but it is only a temporary treatment that buys
time. Even after glucagon
injection, blood sugar may
fall again to dangerously
low levels. Do not assume
that the danger has passed
after successful treatment
with glucagon. Any patient
who was ill enough to
receive glucagon needs to
be evaluated fully by a
physician.

OVERDOSE
Symptoms: Nausea, vomiting, severe weakness, irregular heartbeat, hoarseness,
or cramps.

What to Do: An overdose
of glucagon is unlikely to be
life-threatening. However, if
someone receives a much
larger dose than prescribed,
call your doctor, emergency
medical services (EMS), or
the nearest poison control
center immediately.

DRUG INTERACTIONS
None known.

FOOD INTERACTIONS
No known food interactions.

DISEASE INTERACTIONS
Inform your doctor if you
have insulinoma or
pheochromocytoma. While
these conditions may com-
plicate the use of glucagon,
they do not prohibit a
patient from receiving the
drug in an emergency.

Glyburide

Generic 2.5 mg
(GENEVA)

802

Additional photographs

▶ Drug Class: Antidiabetic
agent/sulfonylurea

▶ Available in: Tablets

▶ Available OTC? No

▶ As Generic? Yes

Side Effects

SERIOUS
Serious side effects are related to hypoglycemia, or low blood sugar, whose symptoms include perspiration or a cold sweat, restlessness, rapid pulse, anxious feeling, nausea, feelings of dizziness, weakness, or lightheadedness, poor coordination, slurred speech, confusion, sleepiness, seizures, weakness of an arm, leg, or an entire side of the body, and fainting. Seek emergency assistance. Administer sugar-containing substances only if the patient is conscious and alert. Other serious but less common side effects include bone marrow suppression, hemolytic anemia, and elevation of liver-associated enzymes; these problems can be detected by your doctor.

COMMON
Bloating, heartburn, nausea, indigestion.

LESS COMMON
Blurred vision, changes in taste, itching, hives, joint or muscle pain.

PRINCIPAL USES
To help control adult-onset (non-insulin-dependent, or type 2) diabetes. Glyburide is sometimes used in conjunction with metformin (another oral antidiabetic).

HOW THE DRUG WORKS
Glyburide stimulates the release of insulin by the pancreas and decreases sugar production in the liver.

DOSAGE
Starting dose is 2.5 to 5 mg daily, 30 minutes before breakfast. It can be increased by your doctor in increments of 2.5 mg to a maximum of 20 mg per day, or decreased if needed. Elderly patients or those with kidney or liver dysfunction should receive an initial dose of 1.25 mg per day. If the daily maintenance dose is increased to 10 mg or more, the total dose should be divided equally between breakfast and dinner.

ONSET OF EFFECT
1 hour.

DURATION OF ACTION
24 hours.

DIETARY ADVICE
It is usually taken 30 minutes before breakfast.

STORAGE
Store in a tightly sealed container away from heat and direct light.

IF YOU MISS A DOSE
Take it as soon as you remember. If it is near the time for the next dose, skip the missed dose and resume your regular dosage schedule. Do not double the next dose.

STOPPING THE DRUG
The decision to stop taking the drug should be made by your doctor. You may need to take glyburide for the rest of your life.

PROLONGED USE
Periodic blood tests should be done to determine how prolonged use affects blood sugar levels.

PRECAUTIONS
Over 60: Treatment should start with lower doses, which should be increased slowly as determined by periodic tests. Adverse reactions may be more likely and more severe in older patients.

Driving and Hazardous Work: Do not drive or engage in hazardous work until you determine how the medication affects you.

Alcohol: Avoid alcohol.

Pregnancy: Uncontrolled blood sugar levels during pregnancy are associated with an increased risk of birth defects, so many experts recommend a switch to insulin during pregnancy.

Breast Feeding: Glyburide may pass into breast milk; caution is advised. Consult your doctor for advice.

Infants and Children: Glyburide does not work in juvenile-onset, insulin-dependent diabetes.

Special Concerns: Carry medical identification that says you have diabetes. If you are under stress due to an infection, fever, an injury, or surgery, you may need insulin therapy in addition to or instead of glyburide.

OVERDOSE
Symptoms: Symptoms are similar to serious side effects.

What to Do: An overdose of glyburide is unlikely to be life-threatening. However, if someone takes a much larger dose than prescribed, call your doctor, emergency medical services (EMS), or the nearest poison control center.

DRUG INTERACTIONS
Consult your doctor for specific advice if you are taking anabolic steroids, aspirin or other salicylates, cimetidine, gemfibrozil, fenfluramine, MAO inhibitors, phenylbutazone, ranitidine, sulfa drugs, beta-blockers, bumetanide, diazoxide, ethacrynic acid, furosemide, phenytoin, rifampin, thiazide diuretics, thyroid hormone, antacids, antifungal agents, enalapril, steroids, or warfarin.

FOOD INTERACTIONS
Glyburide is just part of the treatment for diabetes; be sure to follow the diet recommended by your doctor.

DISEASE INTERACTIONS
Use of this medication may cause complications in patients with liver or kidney disease, since these organs work together to remove the drug from the body.

Glycerin Oral

BRAND NAMES
Glyrol, Osmoglyn

▶ Drug Class: Diuretic, antiglaucoma agent

▶ Available in: Oral solution

▶ Available OTC? No

▶ As Generic? Yes

Side Effects

SERIOUS
Confusion, heart rhythm irregularities. Call your doctor immediately.

COMMON
Headache, nausea, and vomiting.

LESS COMMON
Dizziness, diarrhea, dry mouth, increased thirst.

PRINCIPAL USES
To treat glaucoma.

HOW THE DRUG WORKS
Glaucoma, a sight-threatening disorder, occurs when aqueous humor (the fluid inside the eye) cannot drain properly, causing an increase in pressure within the eyeball (intraocular pressure). This can damage the optic nerve and lead to a gradually progressive loss of vision. Oral glycerin promotes outflow of aqueous humor, thereby reducing intraocular pressure. It is used on a short-term basis to reduce eye pressure until further medical intervention, such as other medications or surgery, can be implemented for more long-term control of glaucoma.

DOSAGE
Adults: To start, 1 dose of 1 to 2 grams (g) per 2.2 lbs (1 kg) of body weight. Additional doses of 500 mg per 2.2 lbs may be given 4 times a day if needed. Children: To start, 1 dose of 1 to 1.5 g per 2.2 lbs. Dose may be repeated in 4 to 8 hours if needed.

ONSET OF EFFECT
Within 10 minutes.

DURATION OF ACTION
About 5 hours.

DIETARY ADVICE
No special restrictions.

STORAGE
Store in a tightly sealed container away from heat and direct light. Do not allow it to freeze.

IF YOU MISS A DOSE
If this drug is prescribed beyond immediate short-term use, take the missed dose as soon as you remember. However, if it is near the time for the next dose, skip the missed dose and resume your regular dosage schedule. Do not double the next dose.

STOPPING THE DRUG
If this drug is prescribed beyond immediate short-term use, take it as prescribed for the full treatment period.

PROLONGED USE
In most cases oral glycerin is used exclusively on a short-term basis, either in a doctor's office or hospital, until other forms of treatment can be implemented.

PRECAUTIONS
Over 60: Excessive dehydration may be more likely to occur in older patients.

Driving and Hazardous Work: Do not drive or engage in hazardous work until you determine how the medicine affects you.

Alcohol: No special precautions are necessary.

Pregnancy: Adequate studies have not been done. Before taking oral glycerin, tell your doctor if you are pregnant or plan to become pregnant.

Breast Feeding: Glycerin may pass into breast milk; caution is advised. Consult your doctor for specific advice.

Infants and Children: No special problems expected.

Special Concerns: To improve the taste of glycerin, it can be mixed with a small amount of unsweetened orange, lemon, or lime juice, poured over ice, and sipped through a straw. If you experience a headache while taking glycerin, you should lie down while you take it and for a short time afterward. If your headaches continue or become severe, consult your doctor. Diabetic patients must be sure their ophthalmologist and other doctors know they have diabetes and that it is under good control. This medication may interfere with blood sugar control.

OVERDOSE
Symptoms: Severe dehydration, heart rhythm abnormalities (cardiac arrhythmias), loss of consciousness, coma.

What to Do: Call your doctor, emergency medical services (EMS), or the nearest poison control center immediately.

DRUG INTERACTIONS
Consult your doctor for specific advice if you are taking a diuretic or any other prescription or over-the-counter medication.

FOOD INTERACTIONS
No known food interactions.

DISEASE INTERACTIONS
Caution is advised when taking glycerin. Consult your doctor if you have any of the following: diabetes mellitus, heart disease, hypovolemia (insufficient fluid volume in the body, due to dehydration or other causes), hypervolemia (excess fluid volume in the body, causing circulatory problems and swelling at various sites, due to fluid retention in the tissues), or a psychological condition associated with persistent confusion. Use of glycerin may cause complications in patients with kidney disease, since this organ works to remove the medication from the body.

Glycerin Rectal

BRAND NAMES
Fleet Babylax, Fleet
Glycerine Laxative,
Sani-Supp

▶ Drug Class: Hyperosmotic laxative

▶ Available in: Rectal solution, rectal suppositories

▶ Available OTC? Yes

▶ As Generic? Yes

Side Effects

SERIOUS
There are no serious side effects associated with the use of glycerin rectal.

COMMON
Cramping.

LESS COMMON
Rectal pain, itching, or burning sensation. This is thought to be more common with dosage forms that require an applicator. If you notice increased pain or bleeding from the rectum after use of glycerin products, call your doctor. Weakness, sweating, and symptoms of dehydration (thirst, dizziness) also may occur.

PRINCIPAL USES
To treat constipation.

HOW THE DRUG WORKS
Glycerin attracts and retains water in the intestine, softening stools and inducing the urge to defecate.

DOSAGE
Adults and children age 6 and older: Insert one suppository or 5 to 15 ml of solution as rectal enema and retain for 15 minutes. Do not lubricate suppositories with anything other than water.

ONSET OF EFFECT
Within 15 to 60 minutes.

DURATION OF ACTION
Only while the solution or suppository is within the rectum.

DIETARY ADVICE
Maintain your usual food and fluid intake. Increase your intake of fluids if you have a fever or diarrhea, during hot weather, or during exercise.

STORAGE
Store solutions and suppositories away from heat, moisture, and direct light. Suppositories may be refrigerated, but do not allow them to freeze.

IF YOU MISS A DOSE
Laxatives are usually prescribed for use only on an as-needed basis and are not meant to be taken regularly or for a prolonged period.

STOPPING THE DRUG
Take rectal glycerin only as needed. However, you may stop using it if you are feeling better before the scheduled end of therapy.

PROLONGED USE
Prolonged, excessive use of glycerin may be associated with an increased risk of side effects, including laxative dependence. Therefore, do not use glycerin for more than 3 to 5 days unless your doctor instructs you to do otherwise.

PRECAUTIONS
Over 60: Adverse reactions may be more likely and more severe in older patients.

Driving and Hazardous Work: Do not drive or engage in hazardous work until you determine how the medicine affects you.

Alcohol: No special precautions are required.

Pregnancy: Adequate human studies have not been done. Before taking glycerin, tell your doctor if you are or are planning to become pregnant.

Breast Feeding: Glycerin suppositories may be used safely by nursing mothers.

Infants and Children: Not recommended for use by children under age 6.

Special Concerns: A single missed bowel movement does not constitute constipation; do not use glycerin under such circumstances. Prolonged constipation or persistent rectal pain and discomfort should be evaluated by your doctor. Remember that chronic use of glycerin or any laxative can lead to laxative dependence. You should be sure to consume adequate amounts of bulk in your diet; good sources include bran or other cereals, fresh fruit, and vegetables.

OVERDOSE
Symptoms: No specific ones have been reported.

What to Do: An overdose of glycerin is unlikely to be life-threatening. However, if someone takes a much larger dose than prescribed, call your doctor.

DRUG INTERACTIONS
No significant drug interactions have been reported.

FOOD INTERACTIONS
No known food interactions.

DISEASE INTERACTIONS
Caution is advised when taking glycerin laxatives. Consult your doctor if you have any of the following: abdominal pain and fever, rectal bleeding, ostomy (an artificial surgical opening in the body to allow the release of urine or feces), diabetes mellitus, heart or kidney disease, or high blood pressure.

Glycopyrrolate

▶ Drug Class: Anticholinergic, antispasmodic

▶ Available in: Tablets

▶ Available OTC? No

▶ As Generic? Yes

Side Effects

SERIOUS
Hives, rash, intense itching, faintness, or swelling soon after a dose. Call your doctor immediately.

COMMON
Enlarged pupils, blurred vision, constipation, dry mouth, difficulty urinating or inability to urinate, breathing difficulty.

LESS COMMON
Disorientation, irritability, incoherence, weakness, rapid or slow pulse, heart palpitations, unusual sensitivity of eyes to light, difficulty swallowing, nausea, vomiting, bloated abdomen, stomach upset, decreased sweating, skin problems, fever, loss of taste, impotence.

PRINCIPAL USES
To treat stomach ulcers and ease cramps and spasms of the stomach and intestines.

HOW THE DRUG WORKS
Glycopyrrolate inhibits gastrointestinal nerve receptor sites that stimulate both the secretion of stomach acid and smooth muscle activity in the digestive tract.

DOSAGE
Usually 1 to 2 mg, 2 to 3 times a day, with a maximum of 8 mg per day.

ONSET OF EFFECT
15 to 30 minutes.

DURATION OF ACTION
Up to 7 hours.

DIETARY ADVICE
Unless your doctor tells you otherwise, take glycopyrrolate 30 minutes to 1 hour before meals.

STORAGE
Store in a tightly sealed container away from heat and direct light.

IF YOU MISS A DOSE
Take it as soon as you remember. If it is near the time for the next dose, skip the missed dose and resume your regular dosage schedule. Do not double the next dose.

STOPPING THE DRUG
Take it as prescribed for the full treatment period, or stop taking it if you are feeling better before the scheduled end of therapy. Do not stop the drug suddenly; consult your doctor about reducing the dose gradually.

PROLONGED USE
Prolonged use may cause chronic constipation and fecal impaction. Consult your doctor immediately.

PRECAUTIONS
Over 60: Adverse reactions may be more likely and more severe in older patients.

Driving and Hazardous Work: Do not drive or engage in hazardous work until you determine how glycopyrrolate affects you. Use of this medicine disqualifies you from piloting aircraft.

Alcohol: No special precautions are necessary.

Pregnancy: Safety of using this drug during pregnancy has not been established. Before taking glycopyrrolate, tell your doctor if you are pregnant or plan to become pregnant and discuss whether the benefits clearly outweigh any potential risks.

Breast Feeding: Glycopyrrolate passes into breast milk; avoid or discontinue use while nursing.

Infants and Children: Smaller doses are recommended for infants and children. Glycopyrrolate should be given to young patients only under close medical supervision.

Special Concerns: Be sure that any doctor or dentist you go to knows that you are taking glycopyrrolate. To prevent heatstroke, avoid becoming overheated during exertion. Take this drug 2 to 3 hours before or after any antacids you are taking.

OVERDOSE
Symptoms: Blurred vision, dry mouth, low blood pressure, decreased breathing rate, rapid heartbeat, drowsiness, inability to urinate, flushed, hot, dry skin.

What to Do: Call your doctor, emergency medical services (EMS), or the nearest poison control center immediately.

DRUG INTERACTIONS
Consult your doctor for specific advice if you are taking antacids, other anticholinergics, tricyclic antidepressants, cyclopropane, cortisone drugs, digitalis drugs, haloperidol, ketoconazole, meperidine, methylphenidate, molindone, narcotic pain relievers, potassium chloride, quinidine, sedatives, or any central nervous system depressants.

FOOD INTERACTIONS
Avoid taking large amounts of vitamin C. No other food interactions are known.

DISEASE INTERACTIONS
Caution is advised while taking glycopyrrolate. Consult your doctor if you have any of the following: open-angle glaucoma, angina, chronic bronchitis, asthma, liver disease, hiatal hernia, enlarged prostate, myasthenia gravis, peptic ulcer, kidney disease, or thyroid disease.

Gold Sodium Thiomalate

BRAND NAME
Myochrysine

▶ Drug Class: Antirheumatic

▶ Available in: Injection

▶ Available OTC? No

▶ As Generic? Yes

Side Effects

SERIOUS
Severe abdominal pain or bloody, black, or tarry stools; confusion; seizures.

COMMON
Temporary joint pain shortly after injection, itching, skin rash, indigestion, heartburn, constipation.

LESS COMMON
Hives, bloody or cloudy urine, sore tongue, bleeding, red, sore, swollen gums; painful sores in the mouth or throat.

PRINCIPAL USES
To treat rheumatoid arthritis. Gold sodium thiomalate is generally prescribed for patients who have not responded adequately to more conservative arthritis treatments, such as aspirin, nonsteroidal anti-inflammatory drugs (NSAIDs), and corticosteroids.

HOW THE DRUG WORKS
Gold sodium thiomalate contains gold. It is not precisely known how gold compounds work, but evidently they reduce some of the painful joint inflammation associated with arthritis. This drug can halt the progress of severe rheumatoid arthritis, preventing further joint damage, and in some cases it may bring about a remission from the disease.

DOSAGE
Adults: 10 mg given once by intramuscular injection during week 1. This is followed by 25 mg given once by injection during week 2, then 25 to 50 mg given once weekly until satisfactory relief is achieved or until 1,000 mg have been administered. If a satisfactory response is achieved, your doctor will begin a maintenance dose of 25 to 50 mg given once by injection every 2 to 4 weeks. Children: 10 mg given once by injection during week 1. This is followed by 1 mg per 2.2 lbs (1 kg) of body weight (but not more than 50 mg) given once by injection during week 2. Further doses are spaced similarly to the adult schedule, with the amount of drug determined by the weight of the child.

ONSET OF EFFECT
Within 6 to 8 weeks at the earliest.

DURATION OF ACTION
Unknown.

DIETARY ADVICE
Maintain your usual food and fluid intake.

STORAGE
Not applicable.

IF YOU MISS A DOSE
Consult your physician.

STOPPING THE DRUG
Your doctor will stop this medication depending on whether you respond satisfactorily, develop side effects that make continuation impossible, or approach the maximum amount of drug that can be taken safely.

PROLONGED USE
Several months of therapy may be necessary to determine whether this medication is helping you. Prolonged use may be associated with an increased risk of side effects.

PRECAUTIONS
Over 60: Adverse reactions may be more likely and severe.

Driving and Hazardous Work: Do not drive or engage in hazardous work until you determine how the medicine affects you.

Alcohol: Avoid alcohol.

Pregnancy: Do not use this drug during pregnancy.

Breast Feeding: This drug may pass into breast milk; caution is advised. Consult your doctor for specific advice.

Infants and Children: Consult your pediatrician.

Special Concerns: Gold compounds may have many adverse effects. Your doctor may order periodic blood tests to determine if you are having any undesirable reactions, such as anemia, low white blood cell count, or protein in the urine. This drug may increase your sensitivity to sunlight. Avoid direct sunlight during peak hours; wear protective clothing and use sunscreens.

OVERDOSE
Symptoms: No specific ones have been reported.

What to Do: Not applicable; an overdose of gold sodium thiomalate is unlikely to be administered by your doctor.

DRUG INTERACTIONS
Consult your doctor for advice if you are taking penicillamine or drugs that may depress bone marrow production, such as seizure medications or chemotherapy agents to treat cancer.

FOOD INTERACTIONS
No known food interactions.

DISEASE INTERACTIONS
Consult your doctor if you have anemia or any other blood disease, skin disease, colitis or any other intestinal disease, ulcers or heartburn, kidney disease, or systemic lupus erythematosus (SLE).

Goserelin Acetate

BRAND NAME
Zoladex

- ▶ Drug Class: Antineoplastic (anticancer) agent

- ▶ Available in: Implant

- ▶ Available OTC? No

- ▶ As Generic? No

Side Effects

SERIOUS
Bone pain; numbness or tingling of hands or feet; difficulty urinating; muscle weakness of the arms or legs. This may occur shortly after therapy begins. Call your doctor.

COMMON
Hot flashes; change in sex drive or decreased interest in sexual activity; erectile dysfunction (impotence); pelvic pain during sex; vaginal dryness and itching.

LESS COMMON
Edema (swelling in the extremities due to fluid retention); dizziness; headache; increased appetite; nausea or vomiting; abdominal pain; pain at application site; sore throat; change in voice; itching; leg cramps; breast pain or swelling; weight gain; chest pain; joint pain; acne or skin rash; increased anxiety or irritability, mood swings, or depression; fatigue; difficulty sleeping; nausea; increase in body or facial hair (in women); decrease in breast size.

PRINCIPAL USES
To treat advanced forms of prostate cancer in men, and to treat advanced forms of breast cancer in women. It may also be used by women to relieve the pain and discomfort of endometriosis.

HOW THE DRUG WORKS
In men, goserelin decreases blood levels of testosterone. This slows the growth of cells in the prostate gland, which may lead to improvement of some of the pain and discomfort of advanced prostate cancer. In women, goserelin decreases blood levels of estrogen and thereby may relieve some of the symptoms of advanced breast cancer. In women with endometriosis, reduced blood levels of estrogen lead to shrinking of endometrial tissue (uterine lining) and thus eases the painful cyclical flare-ups of endometriosis.

DOSAGE
Goserelin implants containing 3.6 mg of medication are placed just under the skin of the upper abdominal wall once every 28 days.

ONSET OF EFFECT
Within 2 to 4 weeks.

DURATION OF ACTION
Blood levels of the hormones testosterone and estrogen remain low for the duration of therapy with goserelin.

DIETARY ADVICE
Maintain your usual food and fluid intake. Increase fluids if you have a fever or diarrhea. Patients with cancer are often weakened by their illness, medications, or other treatments, and may be unable to consume adequate quantities of nutritious food. They should use liquid nutritional supplements if necessary.

STORAGE
Not applicable.

IF YOU MISS A DOSE
Not applicable; the medication is delivered continuously in the form of an implant under the skin.

STOPPING THE DRUG
The decision to stop taking the drug should be made by your doctor.

PROLONGED USE
You should see your doctor regularly for tests and examinations while taking this medicine. Therapy with goserelin for prostate and breast cancer may be required for an indefinite period. Therapy with goserelin for endometriosis is usually completed within 6 months.

PRECAUTIONS
Over 60: Adverse reactions may be more likely and more severe in older patients.

Driving and Hazardous Work: Do not drive or engage in hazardous work until you determine how the medication affects you.

Alcohol: Use alcohol only in moderation.

Pregnancy: Avoid or immediately discontinue taking the drug if you are pregnant or trying to become pregnant.

Breast Feeding: Avoid or discontinue use while breast feeding.

Infants and Children: This drug is not recommended for use by nonmenstruating females under the age of 18.

Special Concerns: Women of childbearing age must use effective non-hormonal contraception (that is, a form other than birth control pills) during treatment with goserelin and for 12 weeks following the end of therapy. In men, goserelin will cause sterility for at least the duration of therapy.

OVERDOSE
Symptoms: No specific ones have been reported.

What to Do: An overdose of goserelin is unlikely to be life-threatening.

DRUG INTERACTIONS
No specific ones known.

FOOD INTERACTIONS
No known food interactions.

DISEASE INTERACTIONS
No specific ones known.

Griseofulvin

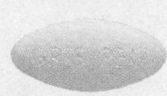

Gris-PEG 125 mg
(WYETH-AYERST)

▶ Drug Class: Antifungal

▶ Available in: Microsize
capsules, oral suspension,
tablets, ultramicrosize tablets

▶ Available OTC? No

▶ As Generic? Yes

Side Effects

SERIOUS
Irritation or soreness of
mouth or tongue; skin
rash, hives, or itching;
confusion; increased
sensitivity of eyes to
sunlight. Call your
doctor immediately.

COMMON
Headache.

LESS COMMON
Insomnia, stomach pain,
nausea or vomiting,
unusual fatigue, dizzi-
ness, diarrhea.

PRINCIPAL USES
To treat various forms of
fungal infection, including
ringworm (tinea barbae,
tinea capitis, tinea corporis),
jock itch (tinea cruris), athlete's foot (tinea pedis), and
nail fungus (tinea unguium).

HOW THE DRUG WORKS
Griseofulvin prevents fungal
organisms from manufacturing vital substances
required for reproduction.

DOSAGE
Microsize capsules, oral
suspension, tablets— Adults
and teenagers: For feet and
nails: 500 mg every 12
hours. For scalp, skin, and
groin: 250 mg every 12
hours or 500 mg once a day.
Children: 5 mg per 2.2 lbs
(1 kg) of body weight every
12 hours, or 10 mg per 2.2
lbs once a day. Ultramicrosize tablets— Adults and
teenagers: For feet and
nails: 250 to 375 mg every
12 hours. For scalp, skin,
and groin: 125 to 187.5 mg
every 12 hours, or 250 to
375 mg once a day. Children
age 2 and older: 2.75 to 3.65
mg per 2.2 lbs every 12
hours, or 5.5 to 7.3 mg per
2.2 lbs once a day.

ONSET OF EFFECT
Unknown.

DURATION OF ACTION
Unknown.

DIETARY ADVICE
Take griseofulvin with or
after meals or milk. Milk,
cheese, and other fatty
foods increase the amount
of medication absorbed
from your stomach. Check
with your physician if you
are on a low-fat diet. Otherwise, maintain your usual
food and fluid intake.

STORAGE
Store in a tightly sealed container away from heat, moisture, and direct light. Keep

the liquid form refrigerated,
but do not allow it to freeze.

IF YOU MISS A DOSE
Take it as soon as you
remember. However, if it is
near the time for the next
dose, skip the missed dose
and resume your regular
dosage schedule. Do not
double the next dose.

STOPPING THE DRUG
Take it as prescribed for the
full treatment period, even if
you begin to feel better
before the scheduled end of
therapy. Recurrence of the
infection is likely if you stop
before the full treatment
period is complete.

PROLONGED USE
Prolonged use may cause or
aggravate bone marrow
depression (reduced bone
marrow function), liver
damage, or kidney damage.
Consult your doctor about
the need for periodic blood
cell counts and liver and
kidney function tests.

PRECAUTIONS
Over 60: Adverse reactions
may be more likely and
more severe in older
patients.

**Driving and Hazardous
Work:** Do not drive or
engage in hazardous work
until you determine how the
medicine affects you.

Alcohol: Avoid alcohol.

Pregnancy: Do not use
griseofulvin if you are pregnant or trying to become
pregnant.

Breast Feeding: The drug
may pass into breast milk;
caution is advised. Consult
your doctor for advice.

Infants and Children:
Griseofulvin is not recommended for use by children
under the age of 2.

Special Concerns: Stay
out of direct sunlight, especially between 10 am and 3
pm. Wear protective clothing, including a hat, and
sunglasses. Apply a sun
block with a sun protection
factor (SPF) of at least 15.
Griseofulvin is usually used
in conjunction with a topical
antifungal to aid in the healing process and to reduce
the likelihood of relapse.

OVERDOSE
Symptoms: An overdose
with griseofulvin is unlikely.

What to Do: Emergency
instructions not applicable.

DRUG INTERACTIONS
Other drugs may interact
with griseofulvin. Consult
your doctor for advice if you
are taking anticoagulants or
oral contraceptives.

FOOD INTERACTIONS
No known food interactions.

DISEASE INTERACTIONS
Caution is advised when
taking griseofulvin. Consult
your doctor if you have
lupus, porphyria, or liver
disease.

Guaifenesin

▶ Drug Class: Expectorant

▶ Available in: Capsules,
tablets, oral solution, syrup,
extended-release forms

▶ Available OTC? Yes

▶ As Generic? Yes

Side Effects

SERIOUS
No serious side effects
are associated with
guaifenesin.

COMMON
No common side effects
are associated with
guaifenesin.

LESS COMMON
Diarrhea; dizziness;
headache; abdominal
pain, nausea, or vomit-
ing; skin rash; itching;
hives.

PRINCIPAL USES
Guaifenesin is classified as
an expectorant; that is, it is
designed to reduce the
thickness of mucus and
phlegm, making it easier to
cough up and out of the
lungs and so improve
breathing. It is used to treat
minor upper respiratory
infections and related conditions, such as bronchitis,
colds, and sinus or throat
infections. Guaifenesin is
not a cough suppressant,
and despite its popularity
and its FDA approval as an
expectorant, there is little
scientific evidence that it is
truly effective at reducing
the thickness of mucus.

HOW THE DRUG WORKS
Guaifenesin supposedly
increases the production of
fluids in the respiratory
tract and helps to liquefy
and thin mucus secretions.

DOSAGE
Adults— Capsules, tablets,
oral solution, syrup: 200 to
400 mg every 4 hours, to a
maximum of 2,400 mg a
day. Extended-release capsules and tablets: 600 to
1,200 mg every 12 hours,
to a maximum of 2,400 mg
a day. Children 2 to 12
years of age— Consult
your pediatrician.

ONSET OF EFFECT
Usually within several
hours.

DURATION OF ACTION
The exact duration of action
is not known.

DIETARY ADVICE
Maintain your usual food
and fluid intake. Increase
fluids if you have a fever or
diarrhea. Coughing also
increases your daily fluid
requirements.

STORAGE
Store in a tightly sealed container away from heat and
direct light. Keep liquid
forms of guaifenesin refrigerated, but do not allow it to
freeze. Keep away from
moisture and extremes in
temperature.

IF YOU MISS A DOSE
Take it as soon as you
remember. If it is near the
time for the next dose, skip
the missed dose and
resume your regular dosage
schedule. Do not double the
next dose.

STOPPING THE DRUG
You may stop taking guaifenesin before the scheduled
end of therapy if you are
feeling better; otherwise,
take as prescribed for the
full treatment period.

PROLONGED USE
Therapy with guaifenesin is
usually completed within 7
to 10 days. Persistent cough
may require special evaluation. Do not take nonpre-
scription guaifenesin for
more than 7 days without
your doctor's approval.

PRECAUTIONS
Over 60: Adverse reactions
may be more likely and
more severe.

**Driving and Hazardous
Work:** Do not drive or
engage in hazardous work
until you determine how the
medicine affects you.

Alcohol: No special precautions are necessary.

Pregnancy: Thorough
studies have not been done,
although no serious prob-
lems have been reported;
consult your doctor for
advice.

Breast Feeding: Guaifenesin may pass into breast
milk, although no problems
have been documented.
Consult your doctor for
advice.

Infants and Children:
Generally, it should not be
given to children under 2
unless directed otherwise
by a pediatrician; children
under 12 who have a persistent cough should be examined by a doctor before they
are given guaifenesin.

Special Concerns: Guaifenesin is present in numerous nonprescription cough
and cold remedies, so ask
your pharmacist if you are
unsure whether a product
you are buying contains it.
Do not treat a persistent
cough on your own for
more than a week or so
without seeking medical
advice. When treating
young children, avoid capsules or tablets, since it is
difficult to rely on children
to swallow these dosage
forms in one piece. Cap-
sules and tablets should
not be chewed.

OVERDOSE
Symptoms: No specific
ones have been reported.

What to Do: An overdose
of guaifenesin is unlikely to
be life-threatening. How-
ever, if someone takes a
much larger dose than prescribed, call your doctor,
emergency medical services
(EMS), or the nearest poison control center.

DRUG INTERACTIONS
None reported.

FOOD INTERACTIONS
None reported.

DISEASE INTERACTIONS
None reported.

Guanabenz Acetate

Generic 4 mg
(COPLEY)

▶ Drug Class: Centrally acting antihypertensive

▶ Available in: Tablets

▶ Available OTC? No

▶ As Generic? Yes

Side Effects

SERIOUS
There are no serious side effects associated with recommended doses of guanabenz. However, serious side effects may occur from missing several doses or upon completion of therapy (see Special Concerns).

COMMON
Dizziness or lightheadedness, faintness, drowsiness, dry mouth, general weakness.

LESS COMMON
Headache, decreased sexual ability, nausea.

PRINCIPAL USES
To treat high blood pressure (hypertension).

HOW THE DRUG WORKS
Guanabenz acts upon certain areas of the central nervous system (the brain and spinal cord) that regulate the activity of the heart and the smooth muscle tissue surrounding the arteries. The drug causes the blood vessels to relax and widen, which in turn lowers blood pressure.

DOSAGE
Adults: Initially, 4 mg, 2 times a day. Your doctor will increase this dose gradually over a period of a few weeks until your blood pressure is acceptable. The usual maximum dose of guanabenz is 32 mg per day, given in divided doses.

ONSET OF EFFECT
Within 1 hour.

DURATION OF ACTION
12 hours.

DIETARY ADVICE
Follow a healthy diet (low-salt, low-fat, low-cholesterol) as advised by your doctor to help control blood pressure and prevent heart disease.

STORAGE
Store in a tightly sealed container away from heat, moisture, and direct light.

IF YOU MISS A DOSE
Take it as soon as you remember. If it is near the time for the next dose, skip the missed dose and resume your regular dosage schedule. Do not double the next dose. Call your doctor if you have missed more than one day of medication.

STOPPING THE DRUG
Do not stop taking this drug suddenly, as this may cause potentially serious health problems. If therapy is to be discontinued, dosage should be reduced gradually, according to doctor's instructions.

PROLONGED USE
Extended therapy with guanabenz may be necessary. Side effects may be more likely with prolonged use.

PRECAUTIONS
Over 60: Adverse reactions may be more likely and more severe.

Driving and Hazardous Work: The use of guanabenz may impair your ability to perform such tasks safely. Do not drive or engage in hazardous work until you determine how the medicine affects you.

Alcohol: Avoid alcohol.

Pregnancy: Avoid or discontinue the drug if you are pregnant or are planning to become pregnant.

Breast Feeding: Guanabenz may pass into breast milk; caution is advised. Consult your doctor for advice.

Infants and Children: Guanabenz is not recommended for use in children.

Special Concerns: If you miss several doses of guanabenz or upon completion of therapy, your blood pressure may return to dangerously high levels (known as rebound effect). Symptoms of rebound hypertension include: severe headache; nausea, vomiting, and abdominal pain; confusion; blurred vision; chest pain; sweating; nervousness, restlessness, anxiety, or trembling; heartbeat irregularities; trouble breathing. Call your doctor immediately. To avoid rebound hypertension, make every effort to follow your dosage schedule. Be sure to have adequate supplies of guanabenz available for vacations, travel, and holidays. Avoid nonprescription decongestants and cough, cold, and flu remedies. Drowsiness is common with guanabenz; take your last dose of the day around bedtime if possible. Remember that control of high blood pressure requires medication, diet, weight loss, and careful supervision by your physician.

OVERDOSE
Symptoms: Very low blood pressure causing faintness, extreme drowsiness, weakness, dizziness, or confusion; unusually slow heartbeat; irritability; tiny, constricted pupils.

What to Do: Call emergency medical services (EMS), your doctor, or the nearest poison control center immediately.

DRUG INTERACTIONS
Consult your doctor for specific advice if you are taking medicines that causes drowsiness, such as barbiturates, sedatives, cough medicines, or decongestants; alcohol; psychiatric medications; pain medications; anti-inflammatory drugs; beta-blockers or other medicines to lower blood pressure.

FOOD INTERACTIONS
No known food interactions.

DISEASE INTERACTIONS
Consult your doctor if you have any of the following: blood vessel disease of the brain, including a history of strokes or transient ischemic attacks (TIAs); angina or other heart disease; liver disease or kidney disease.

Guanadrel Sulfate

BRAND NAME
Hylorel

Hylorel 10 mg
(Fisons)

▶ Drug Class: Peripherally
acting antihypertensive

▶ Available in: Tablets

▶ Available OTC? No

▶ As Generic? Yes

Side Effects

SERIOUS
Excess fluid retention,
which can cause swelling
of lower legs and feet;
chest pain; shortness of
breath; fainting; repeated
episodes of dizziness or
falling, especially when
changing position.

COMMON
Drowsiness; dizziness or
lightheadedness; weight
gain. In men, impotence
and impaired ejaculation.

LESS COMMON
Diarrhea; dry mouth;
headache; muscle aches;
increased urination, especially at night.

PRINCIPAL USES
To treat high blood pres-
sure. Guanadrel is used
in conjunction with other
established treatments,
such as weight loss and
sodium restriction.

HOW THE DRUG WORKS
Guanadrel acts on special
nerve pathways that regu-
late the size of blood vessels by interfering with the
release of a natural sub-
stance called norepineph-
rine, which constricts
muscles surrounding the
vessels. The drug relaxes
these muscles, causing
blood vessels to widen,
which in turn lowers
blood pressure.

DOSAGE
Adults: To start, 5 mg, 2
times a day. Your doctor
will increase this dose as
needed over a period of
weeks until satisfactory
blood pressure is achieved.
This usually requires a dose
of 20 to 75 mg per day,
given in 2 to 4 equally
divided doses.

ONSET OF EFFECT
Within 2 hours.

DURATION OF ACTION
About 9 hours.

DIETARY ADVICE
Follow a healthy diet (low-
salt, low-fat, low-cholesterol)
as advised by your doctor to
help control blood pressure
and prevent heart disease.

STORAGE
Store in a tightly sealed container away from heat and
direct light. Keep it away
from moisture and extremes
in temperature.

IF YOU MISS A DOSE
Take it as soon as you
remember. However, if it is
near the time for the next
dose, skip the missed dose
and resume your regular
dosage schedule. Do not
double the next dose.

STOPPING THE DRUG
Take the drug as prescribed
for the full treatment period,
even if you begin to feel better before the scheduled
end of therapy.

PROLONGED USE
Lifelong therapy may be
necessary. See your doctor
regularly for examinations
and tests if you must take
this medicine for an
extended period of time.

PRECAUTIONS
Over 60: Adverse reactions
may be more likely and
more severe in older
patients.

**Driving and Hazardous
Work:** Do not drive or
engage in hazardous work
until you determine how the
medicine affects you.

Alcohol: Avoid alcohol.

Pregnancy: Before taking
guanadrel, tell your doctor
if you are pregnant or plan
to become pregnant.

Breast Feeding: Gua-
nadrel may pass into breast
milk; caution is advised.
Consult your doctor for
advice.

Infants and Children:
Guanadrel is not recom-
mended for use by children.

Special Concerns: Guanadrel frequently causes
dizziness or lightheaded-
ness, which is most noticeable when you change
position, such as rising from
a seated or lying position, or
when getting out of bed or
bending to pick up some-
thing. This may lead to
fainting, falls, and injury. Sit
or lie down immediately if
you feel dizzy or light-
headed. This side effect
may be worsened by
alcohol, hot weather, dehydration, fever, prolonged
standing, prolonged sitting,
or exercise.

OVERDOSE
Symptoms: Severe dizziness, confusion, weakness,
fainting.

What to Do: Call emergency medical services
(EMS), your doctor, or the
nearest poison control center immediately.

DRUG INTERACTIONS
Consult your doctor for specific advice if you are taking
antidepressants, appetite
suppressants, cyclobenza-
prine, haloperidol, loxapine,
maprotiline, methylpheni-
date, phenothiazines, thioxanthenes, trimeprazine,
MAO inhibitors, metaram-
inol, methoxamine, norepinephrine, or phenylephrine.

FOOD INTERACTIONS
No known food interactions.

DISEASE INTERACTIONS
Consult your doctor if you
have any of the following:
asthma; poor circulation to
the brain, with any history
of stroke, fainting, convulsions, or epilepsy; angina,
recent heart attack, problems with pulse, unusual
heart rhythms, pacemaker,
or heart failure; conditions
that lead to dehydration,
such as fever, diarrhea,
or colitis; diabetes; or
pheochromocytoma.

Guanethidine Monosulfate

BRAND NAME
Ismelin

▶ Drug Class: Peripherally acting antihypertensive

▶ Available in: Tablets

▶ Available OTC? No

▶ As Generic? Yes

Side Effects

SERIOUS
Excess fluid retention, which can cause swelling of lower legs and feet; chest pain; shortness of breath; fainting; dizziness or falling, especially when changing position.

COMMON
Dizziness or lightheadedness, drowsiness, weight gain, slow pulse, stuffy nose. In men, impotence and impaired ejaculation.

LESS COMMON
Diarrhea, dry mouth, headache, muscle aches, increased urination, especially at night, rash, vision problems.

PRINCIPAL USES
To help control moderate to severe high blood pressure, usually after other medications have failed to achieve satisfactory results.

HOW THE DRUG WORKS
Guanethidine interferes with the release of norepinephrine, a natural substance that constricts the muscles surrounding blood vessels. The drug relaxes these muscles, causing blood vessels to widen, thus lowering blood pressure.

DOSAGE
Adults: To start, 10 or 12.5 mg once a day. Your doctor may increase this gradually over weekly intervals until your blood pressure reaches an acceptable level. Your doctor will then prescribe a maintenance dose, usually 25 to 50 mg, taken once a day. Children: Dosage depends on age and weight of the child. Consult your pediatrician.

ONSET OF EFFECT
Blood pressure begins to drop shortly after ingestion; maximum benefits require 1 to 3 weeks.

DURATION OF ACTION
Blood pressure returns to previously high levels within 1 to 3 weeks after stopping.

DIETARY ADVICE
Increase fluids if you have a fever or diarrhea, in hot weather, or during exercise. Follow a healthy diet (low-salt, low-fat, low-cholesterol) as advised by your doctor to help control blood pressure and prevent heart disease.

STORAGE
Store in a tightly sealed container away from heat and direct light.

IF YOU MISS A DOSE
Take it as soon as you remember. However, if it is near the time for the next dose, skip the missed dose and resume your regular dosage schedule. Do not double the next dose. Inform your doctor if you miss more than a full day of medication.

STOPPING THE DRUG
The decision to stop taking the drug should be made by your doctor. Do not stop this medication abruptly.

PROLONGED USE
Lifelong therapy may be necessary. See your doctor regularly for examinations and tests if you must take this drug for an extended period.

PRECAUTIONS
Over 60: Adverse reactions may be more likely and more severe in older patients.

Driving and Hazardous Work: Do not drive or engage in hazardous work until you determine how the medicine affects you.

Alcohol: Avoid alcohol.

Pregnancy: Before taking guanethidine, tell your doctor if you are pregnant or plan to become pregnant.

Breast Feeding: Guanethidine may pass into breast milk; consult your doctor.

Infants and Children: May be used; consult your pediatrician.

Special Concerns: Guanethidine frequently causes dizziness or lightheadedness, especially when you change position. This may lead to fainting, falls, and injury. Sit or lie down immediately if you feel dizzy or lightheaded. This side effect may be worsened by alcohol, hot weather, dehydration, fever, prolonged standing or sitting or exercise.

OVERDOSE
Symptoms: Severe dizziness, confusion, weakness, or fainting; very slow pulse; severe diarrhea; severe nausea; cold, clammy skin; unresponsiveness or loss of consciousness.

What to Do: Call emergency medical services (EMS), your doctor, or the nearest poison control center immediately.

DRUG INTERACTIONS
Consult your doctor for specific advice if you are taking antidepressants, appetite suppressants, cyclobenzaprine, haloperidol, loxapine, maprotiline, methylphenidate, minoxidil, phenothiazines, thioxanthenes, trimeprazine, MAO inhibitors, metaraminol, methoxamine, norepinephrine, phenylephrine, insulin or oral medicines to control blood sugar, or anti-inflammatory drugs, especially NSAIDs.

FOOD INTERACTIONS
No known food interactions.

DISEASE INTERACTIONS
Consult your doctor if you have any of the following: asthma; poor circulation to the brain in association with history of stroke, fainting, epilepsy or other seizure disorders; angina, recent heart attack, heart rhythm irregularities, or heart failure; conditions that lead to dehydration, such as fever, diarrhea, or colitis; diabetes mellitus; pheochromocytoma; or impaired liver or kidney function.

Guanfacine Hydrochloride

Generic 1 mg
(WATSON)

▶ Drug Class: Centrally acting antihypertensive

▶ Available in: Tablets

▶ Available OTC? No

▶ As Generic? Yes

Side Effects

SERIOUS
There are no serious side effects associated with recommended doses of guanfacine. However, serious side effects may occur from missing several doses or upon completion of therapy (see Special Concerns).

COMMON
Dry mouth, dizziness or lightheadedness, fatigue or drowsiness, weakness, constipation.

LESS COMMON
Headache, decreased sexual ability, depression, dry, burning eyes.

PRINCIPAL USES
To treat high blood pressure (hypertension).

HOW THE DRUG WORKS
Guanfacine acts upon certain areas of the central nervous system (the brain and spinal cord) that regulate the activity of the heart and the smooth muscle tissue surrounding the arteries. The drug causes the blood vessels to relax and widen, which in turn lowers blood pressure.

DOSAGE
Adults: To start, 1 mg once daily, at bedtime. Your doctor will increase the dose as needed over a period of 4 to 8 weeks until satisfactory blood pressure is achieved. Maintenance dose is usually 2 to 3 mg per day, taken once daily at bedtime.

ONSET OF EFFECT
Peak effect within 7 days.

DURATION OF ACTION
24 hours.

DIETARY ADVICE
Increase fluid intake in hot weather, during exercise, or if you have a fever or diarrhea. Follow a healthy diet (low-salt, low-fat, low-cholesterol) as advised by your doctor to help control blood pressure and prevent heart disease.

STORAGE
Store in a tightly sealed container away from heat and direct light.

IF YOU MISS A DOSE
Take it as soon as you remember. If it is near the time for the next dose, skip the missed dose and resume your regular dosage schedule. Do not double the next dose. Call your doctor if you have missed more than one day of medication.

STOPPING THE DRUG
Do not stop taking this drug suddenly, as this may cause potentially serious health problems. If therapy is to be discontinued, dosage should be tapered, according to a doctor's instructions.

PROLONGED USE
Extended therapy with this drug may be necessary. Side effects may be more likely with prolonged use.

PRECAUTIONS
Over 60: Adverse reactions may be more likely and more severe.

Driving and Hazardous Work: Do not drive or engage in hazardous work until you determine how the medicine affects you.

Alcohol: Avoid alcohol.

Pregnancy: Avoid or discontinue use if you are pregnant or plan to become pregnant.

Breast Feeding: Guanfacine may pass into breast milk; caution is advised. Consult your doctor.

Infants and Children: Guanfacine is not recommended for use by children.

Special Concerns: If you miss several doses of guanfacine or upon completion of therapy, your blood pressure may return to dangerously high levels (known as rebound effect). Symptoms of rebound hypertension include: severe headache; nausea, vomiting, and abdominal pain; confusion; blurred vision; chest pain; sweating; nervousness, restlessness, anxiety, or trembling; heartbeat irregularities; trouble breathing. Call your doctor immediately. To avoid rebound hypertension, make every effort to follow your dosage schedule. Be sure to have adequate supplies of guanfacine available for vacations, travel, and holidays. Avoid nonprescription decongestants and cough, cold, and flu remedies. Drowsiness is common with guanfacine; take your last dose of the day around bedtime if possible. Remember that control of high blood pressure requires medication, diet, weight loss, and careful supervision by your physician.

OVERDOSE
Symptoms: Extreme drowsiness, weakness, dizziness, or confusion; unusually slow heartbeat; irritability; tiny, constricted pupils.

What to Do: Call emergency medical services (EMS), your doctor, or the nearest poison control center immediately.

DRUG INTERACTIONS
Many patients taking guanfacine also require treatment with a diuretic to control their blood pressure. Consult your doctor for specific advice if you are taking medicines that cause drowsiness, such as barbiturates, sedatives, cough medicines, or decongestants; alcohol; psychiatric medications; pain medications; anti-inflammatory drugs; beta-blockers or other medicines to lower blood pressure.

FOOD INTERACTIONS
No known food interactions.

DISEASE INTERACTIONS
Consult your doctor if you have any of the following: blood vessel disease of the brain, including a history of strokes or transient ischemic attacks (TIAs); angina or other heart disease; liver disease; or kidney disease.

Haloperidol

Generic 5 mg
(GENEVA)

Additional photographs

▶ Drug Class: Neuroleptic; antipsychotic

▶ Available in: Tablets, liquid, injection

▶ Available OTC? No

▶ As Generic? Yes

Side Effects

SERIOUS
Rapid heartbeat, profuse sweating, seizures, difficulty breathing, neck stiffness, swelling of the tongue, difficulty swallowing. Also a rare condition can develop called neuroleptic malignant syndrome, characterized by stiffness or spasms of the muscles, high fever, and confusion or disorientation. Call your doctor immediately.

COMMON
Nausea, reduced sweating, dry mouth, blurred vision, drowsiness, shaking of hands, stiffness, stooped posture.

LESS COMMON
Difficult urination, menstrual irregularities, breast pain or swelling, unexpected weight gain, uncontrolled movements of the tongue, fever, chills, sore throat, unusual bruising or bleeding, heart palpitations, skin rash, itching, increased sensitivity of the skin to sunlight.

PRINCIPAL USES
To treat moderate to severe psychiatric conditions including schizophrenia, manic states, and drug-induced psychosis. It is also used to treat extreme behavior problems in children (including infantile autism), to ease the symptoms of Tourette's syndrome, and to reduce nausea and vomiting associated with chemotherapy for cancer.

HOW THE DRUG WORKS
Haloperidol blocks receptors of dopamine (a chemical that aids in the transmission of nerve impulses) in the central nervous system. Presumably, this produces a tranquilizing or antipsychotic effect.

DOSAGE
For psychotic disorders—Adults: Initial dose is 0.5 to 5 mg, 2 or 3 times a day; maximum dose is 100 mg a day. Children ages 3 to 12: 0.05 to 0.15 mg for every 2.2 lbs (1 kg) of body weight. For Tourette's syndrome— Adults: 0.5 to 5 mg, 2 or 3 times a day. Children ages 3 to 12: 0.075 mg for every 2.2 lbs daily.

ONSET OF EFFECT
Sedation may occur within minutes, but onset of antipsychotic effect may take hours to occur or may not occur until days or weeks after the beginning of therapy.

DURATION OF ACTION
12 to 24 hours, but effects may persist for several days.

DIETARY ADVICE
Take haloperidol with food or a full glass of milk or water. To prevent stomach irritation, the oral solution can be diluted in beverages such as orange, apple, or tomato juice, or cola.

STORAGE
Store in a tightly sealed container away from heat and direct light.

IF YOU MISS A DOSE
Take it as soon as you remember. Do not double the next dose. Space any remaining doses for that day at regular intervals. Return to your regular schedule the next day.

STOPPING THE DRUG
The decision to stop taking the drug should be made in consultation with your doctor. Gradual reduction of doses may be required if you have taken it for an extended period.

PROLONGED USE
Prolonged use may lead to tardive dyskinesia (involuntary movements of the jaw, lips, tongue, and, in rare cases, the arms, legs, hands, or body). Consult your doctor about the need for periodic evaluation and lab tests.

PRECAUTIONS
Over 60: Adverse reactions are more likely and more severe in older patients.

Driving and Hazardous Work: Exercise caution until you determine how the medication affects you.

Alcohol: Avoid alcohol.

Pregnancy: Before taking haloperidol, be sure to tell your doctor if you are, or plan to become, pregnant.

Breast Feeding: Haloperidol passes into breast milk and may be harmful to the child; do not use it while nursing.

Infants and Children: Not recommended for children under age 3 or those weighing less than 33 pounds.

Special Concerns: Avoid prolonged exposure to high temperatures or hot climates. Drink plenty of fluids and stay cool in the summertime. Avoid overexposure to sunlight until you determine if the drug heightens your skin's sensitivity to ultraviolet light.

OVERDOSE
Symptoms: Shallow, slow breathing, weak or rapid pulse, muscle weakness or tremor, dizziness, confusion, seizures, deep sleep, coma.

What to Do: Call your doctor, emergency medical services (EMS), or the nearest poison control center immediately.

DRUG INTERACTIONS
Consult your doctor for specific advice if you are taking anticholinergics, anticonvulsants, antidepressants, antihistamines, antihypertensives, bupropion, central nervous system depressants such as barbiturates, clozapine, dronabinol, ethinamate, fluoxetine, guanethidine, guanfacine, lithium, methyldopa, carbamazepine, rifampin, or trihexyphenidyl.

FOOD INTERACTIONS
No known food interactions.

DISEASE INTERACTIONS
Consult your doctor if you have Parkinson's disease or any movement disorder, glaucoma, epilepsy, or liver or kidney disease.

Haloprogin

BRAND NAME
Halotex

▶ Drug Class: Topical antifungal

▶ Available in: Cream, solution

▶ Available OTC? No

▶ As Generic? No

Side Effects

SERIOUS
No serious side effects have been reported.

COMMON
A mild, temporary stinging when the solution form of haloprogin is applied.

LESS COMMON
Blistering, burning, itching, or other forms of skin irritation that were not present before the start of therapy. Call your doctor immediately.

PRINCIPAL USES
To treat fungal infections of the skin, such as tinea corporis (ringworm), tinea cruris (jock itch), tinea pedis (athlete's foot), tinea manuum ("ringworm of the hand"), pityriasis versicolor ("sun fungus," a skin condition characterized by the formation of fine scaly patches of varying shapes, sizes, and colors).

HOW THE DRUG WORKS
Haloprogin prevents the growth and reproduction of fungus cells.

DOSAGE
For many conditions, rub the medicine gently into the affected area of skin 2 times a day for 2 to 4 weeks. (Note: This is simply the average dose of haloprogin. If the dose recommended by your physician is different, do not change it unless your physician advises you otherwise.)

ONSET OF EFFECT
Unknown.

DURATION OF ACTION
Unknown.

DIETARY ADVICE
Haloprogin can be used without regard to diet.

STORAGE
Store in a tightly sealed container away from heat and direct light. Do not allow the medicine to freeze.

IF YOU MISS A DOSE
Apply it as soon as you remember. If it is near the time for the next dose, skip the missed dose and resume your regular dosage schedule. Do not apply a double dose.

STOPPING THE DRUG
Use the medication as prescribed for the full treatment period, even if you begin to feel better before the scheduled end of therapy. Discontinuing the drug prematurely may lead to an even worse fungal infection later (known as a rebound infection).

PROLONGED USE
If your skin problem does not improve within 4 weeks of starting therapy or if it becomes worse, notify your doctor.

PRECAUTIONS
Over 60: Although there is no specific information comparing use of haloprogin in older patients with use in other age groups, the medicine is not expected to cause different side effects or problems in older people than in younger patients.

Driving and Hazardous Work: The use of haloprogin should not impair your ability to perform such tasks safely.

Alcohol: No special problems are expected with moderate use of alcohol.

Pregnancy: In animal studies, haloprogin has not been shown to cause birth defects or other problems. Human studies have not been done. Before you use haloprogin, be sure to tell your doctor if you are pregnant or plan to become pregnant.

Breast Feeding: It is not known whether haloprogin passes into breast milk; caution is advised. Consult your doctor for specific advice.

Infants and Children: Studies on the relationship of age to the effects of haloprogin have not been done in children. The safety and efficacy of the medicine on children have not been established. Use and dosage should be determined by your doctor.

Special Concerns: Avoid contact of the medicine with the eyes. Do not use haloprogin if you have had a prior allergic reaction to it or to any other topical antifungal medicine.

OVERDOSE
Symptoms: No specific ones have been reported.

What to Do: An overdose of haloprogin is unlikely. However, if someone accidentally ingests the drug, call your doctor, emergency medical services (EMS), or the nearest poison control center right away.

DRUG INTERACTIONS
Consult your doctor for specific advice if you are taking any other antifungal medication for the skin.

FOOD INTERACTIONS
No known food interactions.

DISEASE INTERACTIONS
Caution is advised when taking haloprogin. Consult your doctor if you have any other medical condition.

Hepatitis A Vaccine

BRAND NAMES
Havrix, VAQTA

▶ Drug Class: Vaccine

▶ Available in: Injection

▶ Available OTC? No

▶ As Generic? No

Side Effects

SERIOUS
Serious allergic reaction involving difficulty swallowing or breathing; reddened skin, especially around the ears; itching, particularly of the hands or feet; hives; unusual and severe fatigue; and swollen face, eyes, or nasal passages. Call your doctor immediately.

COMMON
Soreness at the site of injection.

LESS COMMON
Fever, general feeling of illness or discomfort, lack of appetite, headache, nausea, tenderness or warmth at site of injection, aches or pain in joints or muscles, diarrhea or stomach cramps or pain, itching, swelling of the glands in armpits or neck, vomiting, welts.

PRINCIPAL USES
To protect against infection by the hepatitis A virus in people over the age of 2. The vaccine is recommended for people traveling to Africa, Asia (except Japan), parts of the Caribbean, Central and South America, eastern Europe, the Mediterranean basin, the Middle East, and Mexico. The vaccine is also recommended for people who live in or are moving to other areas that have frequent outbreaks of hepatitis A or those who may be at increased risk of infection. These people include military personnel, Alaskan Eskimos, Native Americans, persons engaging in high-risk sexual activity, such as homosexual males; people who use illegal injectable drugs, people working in facilities for the mentally retarded, employees of and children in day-care centers, people who work with hepatitis A virus in the laboratory, people who handle primate animals, food handlers, and people with chronic liver disease.

HOW THE DRUG WORKS
Hepatitis A vaccine stimulates the body's immune system to produce protective antibodies against the disease.

DOSAGE
All doses are administered by a health care professional. Adults: 1 dose injected into a muscle in the upper arm. A booster dose is given 6 months after the first dose. Children ages 2 to 18: 1 pediatric dose injected into a muscle in the upper arm. A similar booster is given 6 to 18 months later.

ONSET OF EFFECT
Within 4 weeks.

DURATION OF ACTION
Unknown.

DIETARY ADVICE
No special restrictions.

STORAGE
Not applicable; the dose is administered only at a health care facility.

IF YOU MISS A DOSE
If you miss a scheduled vaccination, contact your doctor.

STOPPING THE DRUG
The full schedule of injections should be followed unless a medical problem intervenes. A full course of injections must be completed to ensure adequate immunization.

PROLONGED USE
Not applicable.

PRECAUTIONS
Over 60: Hepatitis A vaccine is not expected to cause different or more severe side effects in older patients than it does in younger persons. However, patients over age 50 may not develop as strong an immunity as their younger counterparts.

Driving and Hazardous Work: The vaccine should not impair your ability to perform such tasks safely.

Alcohol: No special precautions are necessary.

Pregnancy: Adequate human studies have not been done. Before taking hepatitis A vaccine, tell your physician if you are pregnant or planning to become pregnant.

Breast Feeding: No problems have been reported in nursing babies, but caution is advised. Consult your doctor.

Infants and Children: Not recommended for use by children under the age of 2. No special problems are expected in children over the age of 2.

OVERDOSE
Symptoms: Not applicable.

What to Do: No cases of overdose have been reported.

DRUG INTERACTIONS
There are no known drug interactions. Tell your doctor if you are taking any prescription or over-the-counter medication.

FOOD INTERACTIONS
No known food interactions.

DISEASE INTERACTIONS
Consult your doctor if you have a bleeding disorder, an immune deficiency condition, or any other medical condition. Vaccine injection may be postponed in persons with a fever or acute illness.

Hepatitis B Vaccine

BRAND NAMES
Engerix-B, Recombivax
HB, Recombivax HB
Dialysis Formulation

▶ Drug Class: Vaccine

▶ Available in: Injection

▶ Available OTC? No

▶ As Generic? No

Side Effects

SERIOUS
Serious allergic reaction involving difficulty swallowing or breathing; reddened skin, especially around the ears; itching, particularly of the hands or feet; hives; unusual and severe fatigue; and swollen face, eyes, or nasal passages. Call your doctor immediately.

COMMON
Soreness at the site of injection.

LESS COMMON
Dizziness, fever, unusual fatigue, headache. Also tenderness, warmth, hard lump, swelling, pain, itching, or purple spot at site of injection.

PRINCIPAL USES
To protect against infection by the hepatitis B virus.

HOW THE DRUG WORKS
Hepatitis B vaccine stimulates the body's immune system to produce protective antibodies against the disease.

DOSAGE
Adults age 20 and older: A first injection of 10 micrograms (mcg) (Recombivax HB) or 20 mcg (Engerix-B) into upper arm, followed by an injection 1 month later and another 6 months after the first dose, for a total of 3 doses. Adults receiving dialysis: A first injection of 40 mcg (Recombivax HD Dialysis Formulation) followed by doses 1 month and 6 months after the first dose; some patients may receive a dose at 2 months. Dialysis patients receiving 4 doses will use Engerix-B. Children ages 11 to 20: A first injection of 5 mcg (Recombivax HB) or 20 mcg (Engerix-B) into upper arm, followed by an injection 1 month later and another 6 months after the first dose, for a total of 3 doses. Infants and children up to age 11: A first dose of 2.5 mcg (Recombivax HB) or 10 mcg (Engerix-B) into the thigh, with doses 1 month and 6 months after the first dose, for a total of 3 doses.

ONSET OF EFFECT
Unknown.

DURATION OF ACTION
Unknown.

DIETARY ADVICE
No special restrictions.

STORAGE
Not applicable; the dose is administered only at a health care facility.

IF YOU MISS A DOSE
If you miss a scheduled vaccination, contact your doctor.

STOPPING THE DRUG
The full schedule of injections should be followed unless a medical problem intervenes. A full course of injections must be completed to ensure adequate immunization.

PROLONGED USE
No special problems are expected.

PRECAUTIONS
Over 60: Hepatitis B vaccine is not expected to cause different or more severe side effects in older patients than it does in younger persons. However, patients over age 50 may not develop as strong an immunity as their younger counterparts.

Driving and Hazardous Work: Hepatitis B vaccine should not impair your ability to perform such tasks safely.

Alcohol: No special precautions are necessary.

Pregnancy: Adequate human studies have not been done. However, problems during pregnancy are not expected. Before you take hepatitis B vaccine, tell your doctor if you are pregnant or plan to become pregnant.

Breast Feeding: Hepatitis B vaccine may pass into breast milk; caution is advised. Consult your doctor for more information.

Infants and Children: Hepatitis B vaccine, with recommended doses, does not cause different or more severe side effects in infants and children than it does in older persons. Studies of the vaccine strength for use by dialysis patients have only been conducted on adult subjects. Consult your pediatrician for specific advice if your child is receiving dialysis.

OVERDOSE
Symptoms: Not applicable.

What to Do: No cases of overdose have been reported.

DRUG INTERACTIONS
Other drugs may interact with hepatitis B vaccine. Tell your doctor if you are taking any prescription or over-the-counter medication.

FOOD INTERACTIONS
No known food interactions.

DISEASE INTERACTIONS
Consult your doctor if you have any of the following: severe heart or lung disease, a moderate or severe illness with or without fever, or an immune deficiency condition.

BRAND NAMES
AK-Homatropine,
I-Homatrine, Isopto
Homatropine, Spectro-
Homatropine

▶ Drug Class: Eye muscle relaxant, pupil enlarger

▶ Available in: Ophthalmic solution

▶ Available OTC? No

▶ As Generic? Yes

Side Effects

SERIOUS

If absorbed into the bloodstream: Loss of coordination or unsteadiness, confusion or changes in behavior, hallucinations, slurred speech, rapid or irregular pulse, flushing, fever, unusual fatigue, dizziness, unusually dry skin, skin rash, dry mouth; in infants, abdominal swelling. Seek medical assistance immediately.

COMMON

Eye irritation and redness not present prior to treatment, swelling of the eyelids, blurred vision, increased sensitivity to bright light.

LESS COMMON

There are no less-common side effects associated with the use of homatropine.

PRINCIPAL USES

To protect the eye before and after surgery, and to treat certain types of eye conditions, including iritis (inflammation of the iris, the colored or pigmented portion of the eye). It may also be used in eye examinations to help determine the proper prescription for eyeglasses.

HOW THE DRUG WORKS

Homatropine relaxes the ciliary muscle, which controls the shape of the eye's lens as it focuses, and another eye muscle called the sphincter, which controls the narrowing and widening of the pupil. Relaxation of these muscles prevents the lens from focusing and widens the pupil. This allows the doctor to view the interior of the eye during an ophthalmologic procedure. And, by immobilizing the tiny structures within the eye, the drug prevents scarring of eye tissue and may also alleviate pain somewhat.

DOSAGE

To aid in ophthalmic surgery or eye examinations: 1 drop (applied by doctor) every 5 to 10 minutes as needed. For treatment of iritis: 1 drop in affected eye(s), 2 or 3 times a day, or up to every 2 or 3 hours in more severe cases.

ONSET OF EFFECT

Within 1 hour.

DURATION OF ACTION

From 24 to 72 hours.

DIETARY ADVICE

It can be taken without regard to diet.

STORAGE

Store in a tightly sealed container away from heat, moisture, and direct light. Do not allow it to freeze.

IF YOU MISS A DOSE

Apply it as soon as you remember. If it is near the time for the next dose, skip the missed dose and resume your regular dosage schedule. Do not double the next dose.

STOPPING THE DRUG

The decision to stop taking the drug should be made by your ophthalmologist.

PROLONGED USE

Not recommended.

PRECAUTIONS

Over 60: Adverse reactions may be more likely and more severe.

Driving and Hazardous Work: Do not drive or engage in hazardous work until you determine how the medicine affects your vision. Extreme caution should be observed for activities requiring sharp vision for close objects (less than an arm's length away).

Alcohol: No special precautions are necessary.

Pregnancy: Adequate studies have not been done. Inform your doctor if you are pregnant or are planning to become pregnant.

Breast Feeding: Small amounts of homatropine pass into breast milk; either discontinue breast feeding or stop taking the drug. Consult your doctor for advice.

Infants and Children: Young children, especially those with blond hair or blue eyes, may be more sensitive to the drug and may have an increased risk of side effects. Use with extreme caution. This medication should not be used at all by infants younger than 3 months old.

Special Concerns: To use the eye drops, first wash your hands. Tilt your head back. Gently apply pressure to the inside corner of the eyelid and with the index finger of the same hand, pull downward on the lower eyelid to make a space. Drop the medicine into this space and close your eye. Apply pressure for 1 or 2 minutes while keeping the eye closed without blinking. Then wash your hands again. Make sure that the tip of the dropper does not touch your eye, finger, or any other surface.

OVERDOSE

Symptoms: Drowsiness, hallucinations, memory problems, dry mouth, dry skin, restlessness, palpitations, dizziness and disorientation, delirium.

What to Do: Call your doctor, emergency medical services (EMS), or the nearest poison control center immediately.

DRUG INTERACTIONS

Consult your doctor if you are taking any other prescription or over-the-counter drugs, especially those preparations designed for use in the eyes.

FOOD INTERACTIONS

No known food interactions.

DISEASE INTERACTIONS

Consult your doctor if you have a history of glaucoma, Down's syndrome, or spastic paralysis.

Hydralazine Hydrochloride

Generic 10 mg
(PAR)

Additional photographs

▶ Drug Class: Antihypertensive vasodilator

▶ Available in: Tablets, injection

▶ Available OTC? No

▶ As Generic? Yes

Side Effects

SERIOUS
Lupus-like syndrome causing fast pulse and palpitations, rapid or irregular heartbeat, hives, itching, or rash, swollen lymph glands, weakness and fainting when standing up, swelling of the feet or legs, and joint pain. Call your doctor immediately.

COMMON
Headache, chest pain, nausea, vomiting, diarrhea, loss of appetite, stomach pain, blood in urine or stools, fatigue.

LESS COMMON
Dizziness; numbness, tingling, and weakness in hands or feet, chills, fever, skin rash.

PRINCIPAL USES
To treat moderate to severe high blood pressure and congestive heart failure.

HOW THE DRUG WORKS
Hydralazine hydrochloride acts upon the smooth muscle tissue surrounding the blood vessels, causing them to relax. The vessels widen and blood pressure decreases.

DOSAGE
To start, 10 mg, 4 times a day for 2 to 4 days. The dose is then increased to 25 mg, 4 times a day. The dose may then be further increased to 50 mg, 4 times a day if needed. The total dose generally should not exceed 200 mg per day, but some patients may require 300 or 400 mg per day.

ONSET OF EFFECT
Within 20 to 30 minutes.

DURATION OF ACTION
3 to 8 hours.

DIETARY ADVICE
This medication should be taken with food. Follow a healthy diet (low-salt, low-fat, low-cholesterol) as advised by your doctor to help control blood pressure and prevent heart disease.

STORAGE
Store in a tightly sealed container away from heat and direct light.

IF YOU MISS A DOSE
Take it as soon as you remember. If it is near the time for the next dose, skip the missed dose and resume your regular dosage schedule. Do not double the next dose.

STOPPING THE DRUG
Take the medicine as prescribed, even if you begin to feel better before the scheduled end of therapy.

PROLONGED USE
Prolonged use may cause an arthritis-like illness similar to lupus, numbness and tingling in hands or feet, and mental effects. Consult your doctor about the need for continuing medical examinations, including blood cell counts and other laboratory studies.

PRECAUTIONS
Over 60: Adverse reactions may be more likely and more severe in older patients.

Driving and Hazardous Work: Do not drive or engage in hazardous work until you determine how the medicine affects you.

Alcohol: Alcohol should be avoided while taking this medication because it may trigger an excessive drop in blood pressure.

Pregnancy: In animal studies, hydralazine has caused birth defects. Human studies have not been done. Before taking hydralazine, tell your doctor if you are pregnant or plan to become pregnant.

Breast Feeding: Hydralazine passes into breast milk; you should avoid or discontinue its use while nursing.

Infants and Children: In children, this medicine is not expected to cause side effects different from those in adults. However, hydralazine should be given to young patients only under close medical supervision.

Special Concerns: It may be necessary to take a diuretic along with hydralazine to reduce its side effects. Several weeks may be needed to determine the effectiveness of hydralazine in reducing blood pressure.

OVERDOSE
Symptoms: Rapid and weak heartbeat, extreme weakness, loss of consciousness, cold and sweaty skin, flushing.

What to Do: Call your doctor, emergency medical services (EMS), or the nearest poison control center immediately.

DRUG INTERACTIONS
Consult your doctor for specific advice if you are taking diazoxide, MAO inhibitors, loop diuretics, beta-blockers, nitrates, or nonsteroidal anti-inflammatory agents such as indomethacin.

FOOD INTERACTIONS
No known food interactions.

DISEASE INTERACTIONS
Caution is advised when taking hydralazine. Consult your doctor if you have any of the following: rheumatic heart disease, mitral valve heart disease, lupus erythematosus, or impaired brain circulation. Use of hydralazine may cause complications in patients with liver or kidney disease, since these organs work together to remove the medication from the body.

Dyazide 25/37.5 mg
(SMITHKLINE BEECHAM)

▶ Drug Class: Thiazide diuretic

▶ Available in: Capsules, tablets

▶ Available OTC? No

▶ As Generic? Yes

Side Effects

SERIOUS
Skin rash, hives, intense itching, swelling of the mouth and throat, breathing difficulty, heart rhythm irregularities or palpitations, lightheadedness or dizziness, unusual bleeding or bruising. Call your doctor immediately.

COMMON
Fluid depletion may lead to dizziness, especially upon arising from a sitting or lying position, as well as thirst, dry mouth, and constipation.

LESS COMMON
Decreased sexual ability, increased sensitivity to sunlight, loss of appetite, gout, increased blood sugar (a problem for diabetic patients).

PRINCIPAL USES
To treat high blood pressure (hypertension); to treat conditions that cause edema (swelling of body tissues resulting from excess salt and water retention).

HOW THE DRUG WORKS
This drug combines a thiazide diuretic (hydrochlorothiazide) and a potassium-sparing diuretic (triamterene) that reduces excess loss of potassium in the body. Diuretics increase the excretion of salt and water in the urine. By reducing the overall fluid volume in the body, these drugs reduce blood volume and so reduce pressure within the blood vessels.

DOSAGE
Adults: 1 or 2 capsules or tablets once a day. Children: The dose must be determined by your doctor.

ONSET OF EFFECT
Within 2 hours.

DURATION OF ACTION
6 to 12 hours.

DIETARY ADVICE
This medication should be taken in the morning after breakfast.

STORAGE
Store in a tightly sealed container away from heat and direct light.

IF YOU MISS A DOSE
Take it as soon as you remember. If it is near the time for the next dose, skip the missed dose and resume your regular dosage schedule. Do not double the next dose.

STOPPING THE DRUG
The decision to stop taking the drug should be made by your doctor.

PROLONGED USE
See your doctor regularly for examinations and tests if you must take this medicine for an extended period.

PRECAUTIONS
Over 60: Adverse reactions may be more likely and more severe.

Driving and Hazardous Work: No special precautions are necessary.

Alcohol: No special precautions are necessary.

Pregnancy: This drug should not be taken during pregnancy unless recommended by your doctor. Other diuretics are generally preferred.

Breast Feeding: This drug passes into breast milk; avoid or discontinue use while nursing.

Infants and Children: No unusual side effects are expected in children. The dose must be determined by a pediatrician.

Special Concerns: To prevent hydrochlorothiazide from interfering with sleep, take it in the morning. If you are taking it for high blood pressure, follow the diet and weight control measures recommended by your doctor. Avoid exposure to sunlight, use a sunblock, or wear protective clothing. This medicine may cause a loss or increase of potassium in your body, so it's important to discuss your diet with your doctor. Follow your doctor's instructions about eating potassium-rich foods or taking a potassium supplement.

OVERDOSE
Symptoms: Dehydration, muscle weakness, cramps, heart arrhythmias.

What to Do: Call your doctor, emergency medical services (EMS), or the nearest poison control center immediately.

DRUG INTERACTIONS
Consult your doctor for specific advice if you are taking ACE inhibitors, cyclosporine, medications or dietary supplements that contain potassium, cholestyramine, colestipol, digitalis drugs, lithium, or any over-the-counter medication.

FOOD INTERACTIONS
Most patients taking this drug should avoid consuming large servings of high-potassium foods, which include bananas, citrus fruits and juices, melons, prunes, (and most fruits in general), avocados, potatoes, nuts, baked beans, brussels sprouts, and skim milk. Check with your doctor if you have questions about your diet.

DISEASE INTERACTIONS
Caution is advised when taking this medicine. Consult your doctor if you have diabetes, gout, kidney stones, lupus erythematosus, pancreatitis, heart disease, blood vessel disease, menstrual problems, liver disease, or kidney disease.

Hydrochlorothiazide (HCTZ)

Generic 25 mg
(GOLDLINE)

▶ Drug Class: Thiazide diuretic

▶ Available in: Tablets, oral suspension

▶ Available OTC? No

▶ As Generic? Yes

Side Effects

SERIOUS
Skin rash, hives, intense itching, swelling of the mouth and throat, breathing difficulty, heart rhythm irregularities, lightheadedness, unusual bleeding or bruising. Call your doctor immediately.

COMMON
Muscle cramps or pain. Potassium depletion may lead to heart palpitations and weakness. Fluid depletion may lead to dizziness, especially upon arising from a sitting or lying position, as well as thirst, dry mouth, and constipation.

LESS COMMON
Decreased sexual ability, increased sensitivity to sunlight, loss of appetite, gout, increased blood sugar (a problem for diabetic patients), pancreatitis (rare).

PRINCIPAL USES
To treat high blood pressure (hypertension); to treat conditions that cause edema (swelling of body tissues resulting from excess salt and water retention).

HOW THE DRUG WORKS
Diuretics increase the excretion of salt and water in the urine. By reducing the overall fluid volume in the body, these drugs reduce pressure within the blood vessels.

DOSAGE
Adults— To reduce excess body water: 25 to 100 mg, 1 or 2 times a day. Your doctor may change the frequency to every other day or 3 to 5 days a week. For high blood pressure: 25 to 100 mg a day. Children, to reduce body water— Ages 2 to 12: 37.5 to 100 mg a day in 2 doses. Ages 6 months to 2 years: 12.5 to 37.5 mg a day in 2 doses. Infants under 6 months: Up to 3.3 mg per 2.2 lbs (1 kg) of body weight in 2 doses.

ONSET OF EFFECT
Within 2 hours.

DURATION OF ACTION
6 to 12 hours.

DIETARY ADVICE
It can be be taken with food to avoid stomach upset.

STORAGE
Store in a tightly sealed container away from heat and direct light. Keep the liquid form from freezing.

IF YOU MISS A DOSE
Take it as soon as you remember. If it is near the time for the next dose, skip the missed dose and resume your regular dosage schedule. Do not double the next dose.

STOPPING THE DRUG
The decision to stop taking the drug should be made by your doctor.

PROLONGED USE
See your doctor regularly for examinations and tests if you must take this medicine for an extended period.

PRECAUTIONS
Over 60: Adverse reactions may be more likely and more severe in older patients.

Driving and Hazardous Work: No special precautions are necessary.

Alcohol: No special precautions are necessary.

Pregnancy: Hydrochlorothiazide has caused birth defects in animals. Human studies have not been done. This medicine should not be taken during pregnancy unless recommended by your doctor; other diuretics are generally preferred for pregnant women.

Breast Feeding: Hydrochlorothiazide passes into breast milk; avoid or discontinue use during the first month of nursing.

Infants and Children: No unusual side effects are expected in children. The dose must be determined by a pediatrician.

Special Concerns: Hydrochlorothiazide is usually prescribed once a day. To prevent it from interfering with sleep, take it in the morning. If you are taking this drug for high blood pressure, follow the diet and weight control measures recommended by your doctor. Avoid exposure to sunlight, use a sunblock, or wear protective clothing. This medicine may cause

your body to lose potassium. Follow your doctor's instructions about eating potassium-rich foods or taking a potassium supplement.

OVERDOSE
Symptoms: Fainting, lethargy, dizziness, drowsiness, confusion, gastrointestinal irritation.

What to Do: Call your doctor, emergency medical services (EMS), or the nearest poison control center immediately.

DRUG INTERACTIONS
Consult your doctor for specific advice if you are taking anticoagulants, cholestyramine, colestipol, drugs for diabetes, nonsteroidal anti-inflammatory drugs, digitalis drugs, or lithium.

FOOD INTERACTIONS
No known food interactions.

DISEASE INTERACTIONS
Caution is advised when taking hydrochlorothiazide. Consult your doctor if you have any of the following: diabetes, gout, lupus erythematosus, pancreatitis, heart disease, blood vessel disease, liver disease, or kidney disease.

Hydrocodone Bitartrate/Acetaminophen

▶ Drug Class: Opioid (narcotic) analgesic

▶ Available in: Capsules, oral solution, tablets

▶ Available OTC? No

▶ As Generic? Yes

Side Effects

SERIOUS
Bloody, dark, or cloudy urine; severe pain in lower back or side; pale or black, tarry stools; yellow-tinged eyes or skin; hallucinations; frequent urge to urinate; painful or difficult urination; sudden decrease in amount of urine; increased sweating; unusual bleeding or bruising; irregular heartbeat; skin rash, hives, or itching; unusual excitement; irregular breathing or wheezing; ringing or buzzing in ears; pinpoint red spots on skin; sore throat and fever; confusion; trembling or uncontrolled muscle movements; flushing or swelling of face. Call your doctor immediately.

COMMON
Dizziness, lightheadedness, nausea or vomiting, drowsiness, constipation, itching.

LESS COMMON
Stomach pain, allergic reaction, false sense of well-being, depression, loss of appetite, blurring or change in vision, feeling of illness, headache, nervousness, insomnia.

PRINCIPAL USES
To relieve moderate to severe pain, when nonprescription pain relievers prove inadequate. Hydrocodone, in combination with acetaminophen, may provide better pain relief at lower doses than either medication used alone at higher doses.

HOW THE DRUG WORKS
Hydrocodone, a narcotic, is believed to relieve pain by acting on specific areas in the spinal cord and brain that process pain signals from nerves throughout the body. Acetaminophen appears to interfere with the action of prostaglandins, substances in the body that cause inflammation and make nerves more sensitive to pain impulses.

DOSAGE
Adults— Capsules: 1 every 4 to 6 hours. Oral solution: 1 to 3 teaspoons every 4 to 6 hours. Tablets: 1 or 2 containing 2.5 mg of hydrocodone, or 1 containing 5, 7.5, or 10 mg of hydrocodone, every 4 to 6 hours.

ONSET OF EFFECT
30 to 60 minutes.

DURATION OF ACTION
4 to 6 hours.

DIETARY ADVICE
This drug can be taken without regard to diet.

STORAGE
Store in a tightly sealed container away from heat, moisture, and direct light.

IF YOU MISS A DOSE
If you are taking this drug on a fixed schedule, take it as soon as you remember. If it is near the time for the next dose, skip the missed dose and resume your regular dosage schedule. Do not double the next dose.

STOPPING THE DRUG
The decision to stop taking the drug should be made by your doctor.

PROLONGED USE
See your doctor regularly for tests and examinations if you take this medication for a prolonged period. Prolonged use can cause mental or physical dependence.

PRECAUTIONS
Over 60: Adverse reactions may be more likely and more severe in older patients.

Driving and Hazardous Work: Do not drive or engage in hazardous work until you determine how the medicine affects you.

Alcohol: Avoid alcohol.

Pregnancy: Overuse during pregnancy can cause drug dependence in the fetus.

Breast Feeding: It is not known whether this drug passes into breast milk; caution is advised. Consult your doctor for specific advice.

Infants and Children: Adverse reactions may be more likely and more severe in children.

Special Concerns: If you feel the drug is not working properly after a few weeks, do not increase the dose.

OVERDOSE
Symptoms: Severe dizziness or drowsiness; cold, clammy skin; difficult or slow breathing or shortness of breath; severe confusion; seizures; stomach cramps or pain; diarrhea; increased sweating; constricted pupils; nausea or vomiting; irregular heartbeat; severe weakness.

What to Do: Call your doctor, emergency medical services (EMS), or the nearest poison control center immediately.

DRUG INTERACTIONS
Consult your doctor for specific advice if you are taking any prescription or over-the-counter medications, especially drugs with acetaminophen or central nervous system depressants such as barbiturates, seizure medicine, muscle relaxants, anesthetics, tranquilizers, or sedatives.

FOOD INTERACTIONS
No known food interactions.

DISEASE INTERACTIONS
Consult your doctor if you have a head injury or brain disease, an underactive thyroid (hypothyroidism), an enlarged prostate, seizures, kidney or liver disease, gall bladder problems, a blood disorder, or a history of alcohol or drug abuse.

Hydrocodone Bitartrate/Ibuprofen

▶ Drug Class: Opioid (narcotic) analgesic

▶ Available in: Tablets

▶ Available OTC? No

▶ As Generic? No

Side Effects

SERIOUS
Shallow or labored breathing; bloody, dark, or cloudy urine; severe pain in lower back or side; frequent urge to urinate; painful or difficult urination; sudden decrease in urine output; unusual bleeding or bruising; irregular heartbeat; skin rash, hives, or itching; confusion; trembling or uncontrolled muscle movements. Call your doctor immediately.

COMMON
Headache, dizziness, lightheadedness, nausea, stomach upset, drowsiness, constipation.

LESS COMMON
Abdominal pain, weakness, insomnia, nervousness, diarrhea, flatulence, dry mouth, swelling of the limbs or other areas, unusual sweating.

PRINCIPAL USES
For short-term (generally less than 10 days) relief of acute pain, when nonprescription pain relievers prove inadequate. Hydrocodone, in combination with ibuprofen, may provide better pain relief at lower doses than either medicine used alone.

HOW THE DRUG WORKS
Hydrocodone, a narcotic, is believed to relieve pain by acting on specific areas in the spinal cord and brain that process pain signals from nerves throughout the body. Ibuprofen, a nonsteroidal anti-inflammatory drug (NSAID), works by interfering with the formation of prostaglandins, substances that cause inflammation and make nerves more sensitive to pain impulses. NSAIDs also have other modes of action that are less well understood.

DOSAGE
Adults and teenagers age 16 and over: 1 tablet every 4 to 6 hours, as needed. Do not take more than 5 tablets in a 24-hour period.

ONSET OF EFFECT
Unknown.

DURATION OF ACTION
Less than 10 hours.

DIETARY ADVICE
Take this drug with food.

STORAGE
Store in a tightly sealed container away from heat, moisture, and direct light.

IF YOU MISS A DOSE
If you are taking this medicine on a fixed schedule, take it as soon as you remember. If it is near the time for the next dose, skip the missed dose and resume your regular dosage schedule. Do not double the next dose.

STOPPING THE DRUG
You may stop taking this drug whenever you choose.

PROLONGED USE
Opioids may be habit-forming, and prolonged use may increase the risk of dependency. Hydrocodone is used only for short-term (10 days or less) treatment of pain.

PRECAUTIONS
Over 60: Adverse reactions may be more likely and more severe in older patients.

Driving and Hazardous Work: The use of this drug may impair your ability to perform such tasks safely.

Alcohol: Avoid alcohol. The combination of alcohol and this drug may increase the depressant effects of the medicine. Drinking alcoholic beverages while taking ibuprofen may increase the risk of stomach irritation.

Pregnancy: Avoid or discontinue this drug if you are pregnant or planning to become pregnant. Overuse during pregnancy can cause drug dependence in the fetus.

Breast Feeding: Ibuprofen passes into breast milk; avoid use while nursing.

Infants and Children: Not recommended for use by children under age 16.

Special Concerns: If you feel the drug is not working properly, do not increase your dose. Call your doctor. Because NSAIDs can interfere with blood coagulation, this drug should be stopped at least 3 days prior to any surgery.

OVERDOSE
Symptoms: Severe nausea, vomiting, difficult or slow breathing or shortness of breath, severe dizziness or drowsiness, cold, clammy or bluish skin, irregular or slow heartbeat, severe weakness, headache, confusion, loss of consciousness.

What to Do: Call your doctor, emergency medical services (EMS), or the nearest poison control center immediately.

DRUG INTERACTIONS
Consult your doctor for specific advice if you are taking any of the following medications that may interact with this drug: ACE inhibitors; anticholinergics; MAO inhibitors; tricyclic antidepressants; aspirin; central nervous system depressants such as barbiturates, seizure medicines, muscle relaxants, anesthetics, tranquilizers, or sedatives; furosemide and other diuretics; lithium; methotrexate; or warfarin.

FOOD INTERACTIONS
No known food interactions.

DISEASE INTERACTIONS
Consult your doctor if you have an underactive thyroid, Addison's disease, an enlarged prostate, urinary difficulty, asthma, any lung disease, bleeding problems, inflammation or ulcers of the stomach and intestine, systemic lupus erythematosus (SLE, lupus), anemia, high blood pressure, or a history of heart disease. Use of this drug may cause complications in patients with severely impaired liver or kidney function.

Hydrocortisone Ophthalmic

▶ Drug Class: Corticosteroid

▶ Available in: Ointment

▶ Available OTC? No

▶ As Generic? No

Side Effects

SERIOUS
Decreased vision or blurring of vision (from cataract); eye pain, nausea, vomiting (from increased eye pressure); pain, redness, sensitivity to bright light, discharge (from eye infection). Call your doctor immediately if you experience any of these signs or symptoms. This drug may trigger a recurrence of herpes infection of the eye; mention any previous herpes infection to your doctor.

COMMON
Mild and temporary blurred vision.

LESS COMMON
Burning, stinging, redness, or watering of eyes.

PRINCIPAL USES
To control inflammation and prevent potentially permanent damage that may result from conditions that involve inflammation in the eye tissues.

HOW THE DRUG WORKS
Hydrocortisone inhibits the release of natural substances that stimulate an inflammatory reaction.

DOSAGE
Adults and children: Ointment is applied to eye 3 or 4 times a day to start; doses are spaced further apart as therapeutic effect is achieved.

ONSET OF EFFECT
Unknown.

DURATION OF ACTION
Unknown.

DIETARY ADVICE
This medication can be used without regard to diet.

STORAGE
Store in a tightly sealed container away from heat and direct light.

IF YOU MISS A DOSE
Apply it as soon as you remember. If it is near the time for the next dose, skip the missed dose and resume your regular dosage schedule. Do not double the next dose.

STOPPING THE DRUG
It is very important to use this drug as prescribed for the full treatment period, even if symptoms improve before the scheduled end of therapy.

PROLONGED USE
You should see your doctor regularly for tests and examinations if you must use this drug for a prolonged period.

PRECAUTIONS
Over 60: While there is no information comparing use of this drug in older patients with use in younger persons, no different side effects or problems are expected.

Driving and Hazardous Work: Do not drive or engage in hazardous work until you determine how the medicine affects you.

Alcohol: No special precautions are necessary.

Pregnancy: This drug has caused birth defects in animals. Reliable human studies have not been done, but no human birth defects have been reported. Before you take ophthalmic hydrocortisone, tell your doctor if you are pregnant or plan to become pregnant.

Breast Feeding: Ophthalmic hydrocortisone has not been reported to cause problems in nursing babies. Consult your doctor for advice.

Infants and Children: Children under 2 years of age may be especially sensitive to the effects of ophthalmic hydrocortisone.

Special Concerns: To use the ointment, first wash your hands. Tilt your head back. Gently apply pressure to the inside corner of the eyelid and with the index finger of the same hand, pull downward on the lower eyelid to make a space. Put a short strip of ointment (about ⅓ inch long) into this space and close your eye. Apply pressure for 1 or 2 minutes while keeping the eye closed without blinking. Then wash your hands again. Make sure the tip of the applicator does not touch your eye, finger, or any other surface. If your symptoms do not improve in a few days or if they become worse, check with your doctor.

OVERDOSE
Symptoms: When used topically, an overdose of ophthalmic hydrocortisone is extremely unlikely. Inadvertent oral ingestion, however, may cause fever, muscle aches, general feeling of weakness and illness, loss of appetite, dizziness, fainting, trouble breathing.

What to Do: An overdose of ophthalmic hydrocortisone is unlikely to be life-threatening. However, if someone applies a much larger dose of the drug than prescribed or accidentally ingests the medicine, call your doctor, emergency medical services (EMS), or the nearest poison control center right away.

DRUG INTERACTIONS
Other drugs may interact with ophthalmic hydrocortisone. Consult your doctor for specific advice if you are taking any other prescription or over-the-counter medication.

FOOD INTERACTIONS
No known food interactions.

DISEASE INTERACTIONS
Caution is advised when taking ophthalmic hydrocortisone. Consult your doctor if you have any of the following: cataracts, diabetes mellitus, glaucoma, herpes infection of the eye, tuberculosis of the eye, or any other eye infection.

Hydrocortisone Systemic

Cortef 5 mg
(UPJOHN)

▶ Drug Class: Corticosteroid

▶ Available in: Oral suspension, tablets, injection, enema, rectal aerosol foam

▶ Available OTC? No

▶ As Generic? No

Side Effects

SERIOUS
Vision problems, frequent urination, increased thirst, rectal bleeding, blistering skin, confusion, hallucinations, paranoia, euphoria, depression, mood swings, redness and swelling at injection site. Call your doctor immediately.

COMMON
Increased appetite, indigestion, nervousness, insomnia, greater susceptibility to infections, increased blood pressure, slowed healing of wounds, rapid weight gain, easy bruising, fluid retention.

LESS COMMON
Change in skin color, dizziness, headache, increased sweating, unusual growth of body or facial hair, increased blood sugar, peptic ulcers, adrenal insufficiency, muscle weakness, cataracts, glaucoma, osteoporosis.

PRINCIPAL USES
To treat numerous conditions that involve inflammation (a response by body tissues, producing redness, warmth, swelling, and pain). Such conditions include arthritis, allergic reactions, asthma, some skin diseases, multiple sclerosis flare-ups, and other autoimmune diseases. Also prescribed to treat deficiency of natural steroid hormones.

HOW THE DRUG WORKS
This hormone mimics the effects of the body's natural corticosteroids. It depresses the synthesis, release, and activity of inflammation-producing body chemicals. It also suppresses the activity of the immune system.

DOSAGE
Oral dose: 20 to 240 mg a day, depending on condition, in 1 or several doses. Injection: 15 to 240 mg a day, injected into a muscle, or 5 to 75 mg every 2 or 3 weeks, injected into a joint or lesion, or 100 to 500 mg every 2 to 6 hours, into muscle or vein or under skin, depending on condition. Enema: 100 mg taken nightly. Rectal aerosol foam: 90 mg, 1 or 2 times a day. Consult pediatrician for children's dosage.

ONSET OF EFFECT
Varies widely depending on the form of the drug used.

DURATION OF ACTION
Variable.

DIETARY ADVICE
Can be taken with food or milk to minimize stomach upset. Your doctor may recommend a special diet.

STORAGE
Store in a tightly sealed container away from heat, moisture, and direct light.

Do not allow liquid form to freeze.

IF YOU MISS A DOSE
If you take several doses a day and it is close to the next dose, double the next dose. If you take 1 dose a day and you do not remember until the next day, skip the missed dose and do not double the next dose.

STOPPING THE DRUG
With long-term therapy, do not stop taking the drug abruptly; the dosage should be decreased gradually.

PROLONGED USE
See your doctor regularly for tests and examinations. Long-term use may lead to cataracts, diabetes, hypertension, or osteoporosis.

PRECAUTIONS
Over 60: Adverse reactions may be more likely and more severe in older patients.

Driving and Hazardous Work: Do not drive or engage in hazardous work until you determine how the medicine affects you.

Alcohol: May cause stomach problems; avoid it unless your physician approves occasional moderate drinking.

Pregnancy: Overuse during pregnancy can retard the child's growth and cause other developmental problems. Consult your doctor for advice.

Breast Feeding: Do not use this drug while nursing.

Infants and Children: Hydrocortisone may retard the normal growth and development of bone and other tissues.

Special Concerns: This drug can lower your resistance to infection. Avoid immunizations with live vaccines. Patients undergoing long-term therapy should wear a medical-alert bracelet. Call your doctor if you develop a fever.

OVERDOSE
Symptoms: Fever, muscle or joint pain, nausea, dizziness, fainting, difficulty breathing. Prolonged overuse: Moonface, obesity, unusual hair growth, acne, loss of sexual function, muscle wasting.

What to Do: Seek medical assistance immediately.

DRUG INTERACTIONS
Consult your doctor for specific advice if you are taking aminoglutethimide, antacids, barbiturates, carbamazepine, griseofulvin, mitotane, phenylbutazone, phenytoin, primidone, rifampin, injectable amphotericin B, oral antidiabetes agents, insulin, digitalis drugs, diuretics, or medications containing potassium or sodium.

FOOD INTERACTIONS
Avoid excess sodium.

DISEASE INTERACTIONS
Consult your doctor if you have a history of bone disease, chicken pox, measles, gastrointestinal disorders, diabetes, recent serious infection, tuberculosis, glaucoma, heart disease, hypertension, liver or kidney disorders, high blood cholesterol, overactive or underactive thyroid, myasthenia gravis, or lupus.

Hydrocortisone Topical

▶ Drug Class: Topical corticosteroid

▶ Available in: Cream, lotion, ointment, topical solution, dental paste

▶ Available OTC? Yes

▶ As Generic? Yes

Side Effects

SERIOUS
Serious side effects from the use of topical hydrocortisone are very rare.

COMMON
Burning, itching, irritation, redness, dryness, acne, stinging and cracking of skin, numbness or tingling in the extremities (in 0.5% to 1% of patients).

LESS COMMON
Blistering and pus near hair follicles, unusual bleeding or easy bruising, darkening or prominence of small surface veins, increased susceptibility to infection.

PRINCIPAL USES
To treat certain skin conditions that are associated with itching, redness, scaling and peeling, pain, and other signs of inflammation. It is also used to treat inflammatory conditions within the mouth.

HOW THE DRUG WORKS
Topical hydrocortisone appears to interfere with the formation of natural substances within the body that are directly responsible for the process of inflammation, which produces swelling, redness, and pain.

DOSAGE
Adults using dental paste: Apply at bedtime to affected areas of the mouth. Adults using cream, lotion, ointment, solution: Apply sparingly to affected areas of the skin 1 to 2 (sometimes 3) times daily. Children: Consult your pediatrician for specific dosage and other advice.

ONSET OF EFFECT
Steroids begin to exert their effect soon after application. However, recognizable changes in your condition may take several days or more to develop.

DURATION OF ACTION
Unknown.

DIETARY ADVICE
Maintain your usual food and fluid intake.

STORAGE
Store in a tightly sealed container away from heat and direct light. Keep away from moisture and extremes in temperature.

IF YOU MISS A DOSE
Apply it as soon as you remember. If it is near the time for the next dose, skip the missed dose and resume your regular dosage schedule. Do not double the next dose.

STOPPING THE DRUG
Take as prescribed for the full treatment period, even if you begin to feel better before the scheduled end of therapy.

PROLONGED USE
Therapy with this medication may require weeks or months; long-term therapy requires monitoring by your physician even with a low-potency product.

PRECAUTIONS
Over 60: Adverse reactions may be more likely and more severe; therapy with topical corticosteroids should therefore be brief and infrequent.

Driving and Hazardous Work: The use of hydrocortisone topical preparation should not impair your ability to perform such tasks safely.

Alcohol: No special precautions are necessary.

Pregnancy: It should not be used for prolonged periods in pregnant women or in those trying to become pregnant.

Breast Feeding: Although problems have not been documented, caution is advised. Do not apply to breasts prior to nursing. Consult your doctor for specific advice.

Infants and Children: Not recommended for prolonged use. Consult your pediatrician.

Special Concerns: Avoid use of this medication around the eye. Hydrocortisone is not a treatment for acne, burns, infections, or disorders of pigmentation. Do not bandage or wrap the medicated area of skin with any special dressings or coverings unless specifically told to do so by your doctor.

OVERDOSE
Symptoms: No specific ones have been reported.

What to Do: An overdose is unlikely to be life-threatening. However, in the event of accidental ingestion or an apparent overdose, call your doctor, emergency medical services (EMS), or the nearest poison control center immediately.

DRUG INTERACTIONS
None reported.

FOOD INTERACTIONS
None reported.

DISEASE INTERACTIONS
Consult your doctor if you have any of the following: diabetes; skin infection, or skin sores and ulcers; infection at another site in your body; tuberculosis; unusual bleeding or bruising; glaucoma; or cataracts.

Hydromorphone Hydrochloride

Generic 2 mg
(ROXANE)

▶ Drug Class: Opioid (narcotic) analgesic

▶ Available in: Oral solution, tablets, injection, rectal suppositories

▶ Available OTC? No

▶ As Generic? Yes

Side Effects

SERIOUS
Serious side effects of hydromorphone are indistinguishable from those of overdose: Confusion; sleepiness; slurred speech; unconsciousness; small, pinpoint pupils; cold, clammy skin; slow breathing; seizures; severe drowsiness, weakness, or dizziness.

COMMON
Dizziness or lightheadedness, nausea or vomiting, constipation, itching.

LESS COMMON
Dry mouth, mood swings or false sense of well-being and euphoria, hallucinations, nightmares.

PRINCIPAL USES
To treat severe pain.

HOW THE DRUG WORKS
Opioids such as hydromorphone relieve pain by acting on specific areas of the spinal cord and brain that process pain signals from nerves throughout the body.

DOSAGE
Adults: Oral solution or tablets: 2 or 2.5 mg every 3 to 6 hours as needed. Injection: 1 to 2 mg into a muscle or under the skin every 3 to 6 hours as needed. Suppositories: 3 mg every 4 to 8 hours as needed. All doses may be increased by your physician, depending on the severity of your pain.

ONSET OF EFFECT
Oral forms and suppositories: Within 30 minutes. Injection: Within 10 to 15 minutes.

DURATION OF ACTION
Oral forms and suppositories: 4 hours. Injection: 2 to 5 hours. These times may decrease as a tolerance to hydromorphone develops.

DIETARY ADVICE
Take hydromorphone with food. Maintain your usual food and fluid intake. Narcotics cause constipation, so make sure your diet contains adequate amounts of fiber and vegetables.

STORAGE
Store in a tightly sealed container away from heat, moisture, and direct light. Keep the liquid form refrigerated, but do not allow it to freeze.

IF YOU MISS A DOSE
If you are taking it on a fixed schedule, take it as soon as you remember. If it is near time for the next dose, skip the missed dose and resume your regular dosage schedule. Do not double the next dose.

STOPPING THE DRUG
You should take it as prescribed for the full treatment period, but you may stop taking the drug if you are feeling better before the scheduled end of therapy.

PROLONGED USE
Therapy with hydromorphone varies, depending on the cause of your pain. Some patients require long-term narcotic therapy. Side effects may be more likely with prolonged use.

PRECAUTIONS
Over 60: Adverse reactions may be more likely and more severe in older patients.

Driving and Hazardous Work: The use of hydromorphone may impair your ability to perform such tasks safely.

Alcohol: Avoid alcohol.

Pregnancy: Adequate human studies have not been done. Before taking hydromorphone, tell your doctor if you are pregnant or are planning to become pregnant.

Breast Feeding: Hydromorphone passes into breast milk; caution is advised. Consult your doctor for advice.

Infants and Children: This drug may be used by young patients. Side effects may be more likely in children under the age of 2. Consult your pediatrician for advice.

Special Concerns: This medication may be habit-forming. Do not exceed recommended doses or increase the dose on your own. This drug is more effective if taken before pain becomes too severe.

OVERDOSE
Symptoms: Confusion; sleepiness; slurred speech; unconsciousness; small, pinpoint pupils; cold, clammy skin; slow breathing; seizures; severe drowsiness, weakness, or dizziness.

What to Do: Call your doctor, emergency medical services (EMS), or the nearest poison control center immediately.

DRUG INTERACTIONS
Consult your doctor for specific advice if you are taking carbamazepine or other medicine for seizures, barbiturates, sedatives, cough medicines, decongestants, antidepressants, other prescription pain medications, MAO inhibitors, naltrexone, rifampin, or zidovudine.

FOOD INTERACTIONS
No known food interactions.

DISEASE INTERACTIONS
Consult your doctor if you have any of the following: history of alcohol or drug abuse; emotional illness; brain disorders or head injury; seizures; lung disease; prostate problems or other problems with urination; gallstones; colitis; or heart, kidney, liver, or thyroid disease.

Hydroxychloroquine Sulfate

Generic 200 mg
(APOTHECON)

▶ Drug Class: Anti-infective/
antimalarial; antirheumatic

▶ Available in: Tablets

▶ Available OTC? No

▶ As Generic? Yes

Side Effects

SERIOUS
Blurred or altered vision;
blood problems including
low white blood cell
count (sore throat, fever),
anemia (fatigue, weak-
ness), and low platelet
count (easy bleeding and
bruising). Such side
effects are extremely
rare; call your doctor
immediately if they
occur.

COMMON
No common side effects
are associated with the
use of this drug.

LESS COMMON
Diarrhea, loss of appetite,
headache, stomach
cramps or pain, nausea
or vomiting, itching, dizziness, fatigue, confusion,
loss or bleaching of hair,
skin rash. Also blue-black
discoloration of the skin,
the inside of the mouth,

PRINCIPAL USES
To prevent and treat malaria
caused by specific strains of
plasmodia (the parasite that
causes malaria) that are
chloroquine-sensitive, but
when chloroquine is not
available. It is also used to
treat rheumatoid arthritis
and systemic lupus erythematosus (SLE, or lupus).

HOW THE DRUG WORKS
Hydroxychloroquine is poisonous to the malarial parasite. For rheumatoid
arthritis and lupus, it may
suppress the release of certain chemicals that cause
inflammation.

DOSAGE
All dosages are for adults
and adolescents. Consult
your pediatrician for children's doses, which are
based on body weight and
should not exceed adult
doses. To prevent malaria:
400 mg (310 mg base) once
a week. To treat malaria:
800 mg (620 mg base)
taken once; or 800 mg, followed by 400 mg (310 mg
base), 6 to 8 hours after the
first dose, then 400 mg once
a day for 2 more days. For
rheumatoid arthritis or
lupus erythematosus: 6.5
mg (5 mg base) per 2.2 lbs
(1 kg) of body weight daily.

ONSET OF EFFECT
Unknown. When taking this
drug for arthritis, it may
take up to 6 months for the
effect to occur. Consult your
physician if your condition
has not improved within
this time.

DURATION OF ACTION
Unknown.

DIETARY ADVICE
Take it with food or milk to
reduce stomach upset.

STORAGE
Store in a tightly sealed container away from heat, moisture, and direct light.

IF YOU MISS A DOSE
Take it as soon as you
remember. However, if it is
near the time for the next
dose, skip the missed dose
and resume your regular
dosage schedule. Do not
double the next dose.

STOPPING THE DRUG
Take it as prescribed for the
full treatment period, even if
you feel better before the
scheduled end of therapy.

PROLONGED USE
You may need to take this
medication for an extended
period of time. If you are
taking it to prevent malaria,
your doctor will want you to
begin 1 to 2 weeks before
you travel to an area where
malaria is prevalent. Keep
taking this medication while
you are in the area and for
4 weeks after you leave.

PRECAUTIONS
Over 60: Adverse reactions
may be more likely and
more severe in older
patients.

**Driving and Hazardous
Work:** The use of this drug
may impair your ability to
perform such tasks safely.
Exercise caution.

Alcohol: No special precautions are necessary.

Pregnancy: The use of
hydroxychloroquine is generally discouraged during
pregnancy because of the
risks it poses to the unborn
child. However, in some
cases it may be prescribed
to prevent or treat malaria,
since the risks of malaria
are potentially more serious
than those posed by the
drug. Discuss with your
doctor the relative risks

and benefits of using this
drug while pregnant.

Breast Feeding: Hydroxychloroquine passes into
breast milk; extreme cau-
tion is advised. Consult your
doctor for specific advice.

Infants and Children:
Children are extremely sensitive to toxic effects of this
drug. Use by children is
considered risky, although it
may be prescribed if benefits outweigh the potential
risks. Consult your pediatrician for advice.

Special Concerns:
Malaria is spread by mos-
quitoes. Take appropriate
precautions to guard against
being bitten by malaria-carrying mosquitoes. Note that
hydroxychloroquine is not
effective against all types of
malaria.

OVERDOSE
Symptoms: Excitability,
headache, drowsiness.

What to Do: Call your
doctor, emergency medical
services (EMS), or the
nearest poison control center immediately.

DRUG INTERACTIONS
Consult your doctor for specific advice if you are taking
magnesium or aluminum
salts, cimetidine, or digoxin.

FOOD INTERACTIONS
No known food interactions.

DISEASE INTERACTIONS
Consult your doctor if you
have any blood disorders,
including anemia, unex-
plained bleeding or bruising, porphyria, or low white
blood cells; liver, neurological, or vision disorders; or
psoriasis.

Hydroxyurea

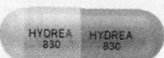

Hydrea 500 mg
(Bristol-Myers Squibb)

▶ Drug Class: Antimetabolite

▶ Available in: Capsules

▶ Available OTC? No

▶ As Generic? Yes

Side Effects

SERIOUS
Cough or hoarseness, fever or chills, pain in lower back or side, painful or difficult urination, black, tarry stools, blood in urine or stools, red spots on skin, unusual bleeding or bruising, sores in mouth or on lips, confusion, seizures, dizziness, hallucinations, headache, joint pain, swelling of feet or lower legs. Call your doctor immediately.

COMMON
Diarrhea, loss of appetite, nausea or vomiting.

LESS COMMON
Constipation, reddening of skin, skin rash and itching, drowsiness.

PRINCIPAL USES
To treat various types of cancer, including malignant melanoma, certain kinds of leukemia, inoperable ovarian tumors, and cancers of the head and neck.

HOW THE DRUG WORKS
Hydroxyurea prevents cancer cell growth by interfering with the synthesis of genetic material. It interferes with the synthesis of DNA in cancer cells and inhibits cell repair, thus decreasing the cell survival rate. The drug may also affect the growth and development of other kinds of cells in the body, resulting in unpleasant side effects.

DOSAGE
For intermittent therapy of solid tumors, with radiation therapy: 60 to 80 mg per 2.2 lbs (1 kg) of body weight every 3 days. For continuous therapy of solid tumors and chronic myelocytic leukemia: 500 to 2,000 mg per day, in 1 or 2 doses.

ONSET OF EFFECT
Unknown.

DURATION OF ACTION
Up to 24 hours.

DIETARY ADVICE
If you cannot swallow the capsule, empty the contents into a glass of water and consume immediately.

STORAGE
Store in a tightly sealed container away from heat and direct light.

IF YOU MISS A DOSE
Take it as soon as you remember. If it is close to the next dose, skip the missed dose and resume your regular dosage schedule. Do not double the next dose.

STOPPING THE DRUG
The decision to stop taking the drug should be made in consultation with your physician.

PROLONGED USE
Hydroxyurea should be discontinued if there is no clinical response as determined by your doctor. If there is a response, the drug may be continued indefinitely.

PRECAUTIONS

Over 60: Adverse reactions may be more likely and more severe in older patients.

Driving and Hazardous Work: Do not drive or engage in hazardous work until you determine how the medicine affects you.

Alcohol: Avoid alcohol.

Pregnancy: Hydroxyurea may cause birth defects if it is taken at the time of conception. Before taking it, tell your doctor if you are pregnant or plan a pregnancy.

Breast Feeding: Not recommended during therapy.

Infants and Children: Adverse reactions may be more likely and more severe in children.

Special Concerns: Be careful when you use a toothbrush, toothpick, or dental floss. Check with your doctor before having any dental work done. Avoid people with infections. Be careful not to cut yourself when you are using sharp objects such as a nail cutter or razor. Wash your hands regularly to decrease the likelihood of spreading bacteria or viruses. Avoid contact sports or other situations where an injury could occur. Watch closely for signs of infection, and take your temperature if you feel ill. Do not receive any immunizations without your doctor's approval. After you stop taking hydroxyurea, check with your doctor if you notice black, tarry stools, blood in urine or stools, cough or hoarseness, fever or chills, pain in lower back or side, painful or difficult urination, red spots on skin, or unusual bleeding or bruising.

OVERDOSE

Symptoms: Excessive side effects.

What to Do: Call your doctor, emergency medical services (EMS), or the nearest poison control center immediately.

DRUG INTERACTIONS
Consult your doctor for specific advice if you are taking amphotericin B, antithyroid agents, azathioprine, chloramphenicol, colchicine, flucytosine, ganciclovir, interferon, plicamycin, zidovudine, probenecid, sulfinpyrazone, didanosine, or stavudine.

FOOD INTERACTIONS
No known food interactions.

DISEASE INTERACTIONS
Caution is advised when taking hydroxyurea. Consult your doctor if you have a history of any of the following: anemia, chicken pox, shingles, gout, kidney stones, any infection, or kidney disease.

Hydroxyzine

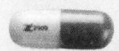

▶ Drug Class: Antihistamine/ mild sedative

▶ Available in: Tablets, syrup, injection

▶ Available OTC? No

▶ As Generic? Yes

Side Effects

SERIOUS
Loss of coordination, seizures, extreme drowsiness, breathing difficulty, inability to urinate.

COMMON
Drowsiness; dryness in the mouth, nasal passages, and other mucous membranes.

LESS COMMON
Difficult urination, dizziness, rash, sore throat, fever, nightmares, restlessness, sleep disruption, irritability, increased skin sensitivity to sunlight, loss of appetite, stomach upset, decreased sexual ability in men.

PRINCIPAL USES
Hydroxyzine is used for several conditions. Its mild sedative effect is useful in treating insomnia and agitation in some patients. It is also used to treat itching, hives, and other allergy symptoms; to control nausea and vomiting; to ease the symptoms of alcohol withdrawal; and to provide mild sedation prior to a dental procedure or to the administration of general anesthesia before surgery.

HOW THE DRUG WORKS
Hydroxyzine is an antihistamine; that is, it blocks the effects of histamine, a naturally occurring substance in the body that causes swelling, itching, sneezing, watery eyes, hives, and other symptoms of allergic reactions. In addition to its antihistamine effect, hydroxyzine also has a sedative effect and appears to suppress activity in some regions of the central nervous system (the brain and spinal cord) associated with nausea and psychological distress.

DOSAGE
For sedation— Adults: 50 to 100 mg a day. For allergy symptoms— Adults: 25 to 100 mg, 3 or 4 times a day, as needed. Children age 6 and older: 12.5 to 25 mg, every 6 hours as needed. Children up to age 6: 12.5 mg every 6 hours as needed. For nausea and vomiting— Adults: 25 to 100 mg, 3 or 4 times a day. Children: 0.6 mg per 2.2 lbs of body weight per day.

ONSET OF EFFECT
15 to 30 minutes.

DURATION OF ACTION
Approximately 6 to 8 hours.

DIETARY ADVICE
Drink plenty of fluids.

STORAGE
Store in a tightly sealed container away from heat and direct light. Keep tablets away from moisture and extremes in temperature. Keep liquid forms refrigerated, but do not allow to freeze.

IF YOU MISS A DOSE
Take it as soon as you remember. If it is near the time for the next dose, skip the missed dose and resume your regular dosage schedule. Do not double the next dose.

STOPPING THE DRUG
The decision to stop taking the drug should be made in consultation with your physician.

PROLONGED USE
Therapy with hydroxyzine may require days or weeks, depending on the condition. Side effects may be more likely with prolonged use.

PRECAUTIONS
Over 60: Adverse reactions may be more likely and more severe in older patients.

Driving and Hazardous Work: Hydroxyzine may impair mental alertness; caution is advised.

Alcohol: Avoid alcohol.

Pregnancy: Adequate studies of hydroxyzine use during pregnancy have not been done; consult your doctor for specific advice.

Breast Feeding: Hydroxyzine may pass into breast milk and cause side effects in the nursing infant; do not use.

Infants and Children: Use this drug only under close supervision by your pediatrician.

Special Concerns: Antihistamines are widely available without prescription; if you are taking a prescription antihistamine, avoid other cough, cold, flu, sinus, or allergy preparations.

OVERDOSE
Symptoms: Severe dryness in mouth, nose, and throat, extreme drowsiness, loss of coordination, faintness, flushing, tremor, hallucinations, breathing difficulty.

What to Do: Call emergency medical services (EMS), your doctor, or the nearest poison control center immediately.

DRUG INTERACTIONS
Consult your doctor for specific advice if you are taking any drugs that depress the central nervous system; these include antidepressants or other psychiatric medications, other antihistamines, barbiturates, sedatives, cough medicines, decongestants, and painkillers. Be sure your doctor knows about any over-the-counter medication you may take.

FOOD INTERACTIONS
None are known.

DISEASE INTERACTIONS
Consult your doctor if you have any of the following: asthma, glaucoma or another eye disorder, thyroid disease, heart or blood vessel disease, high blood pressure, enlarged prostate, or urinary difficulty.

Ibuprofen

Advil 200 mg
(WHITEHALL)

Additional photographs

▶ Drug Class: Nonsteroidal anti-inflammatory drug (NSAID)

▶ Available in: Tablets, oral solution, chewable tablets

▶ Available OTC? Yes

▶ As Generic? Yes

Side Effects

SERIOUS
Shortness of breath or wheezing, with or without swelling of legs or other signs of heart failure; chest pain; peptic ulcer disease with vomiting of blood; black, tarry stools; decreasing kidney function. Call your doctor immediately.

COMMON
Nausea, vomiting, heartburn, diarrhea, constipation, headache, dizziness, sleepiness.

LESS COMMON
Ulcers or sores in mouth, depression, rashes or blistering of skin, ringing sound in the ears, unusual tingling or numbness of the hands or feet, seizures, blurred vision. Also: elevated potassium levels, decreased blood counts; such problems can be detected by your doctor.

PRINCIPAL USES
To treat mild to moderate pain and inflammation caused by tendinitis, arthritis, bursitis, gout, soft tissue injuries, migraine and other vascular headaches, menstrual cramps, and other conditions. It is also used to reduce fever.

HOW THE DRUG WORKS
NSAIDs work by interfering with the formation of prostaglandins, substances that cause inflammation and make nerves more sensitive to pain impulses. NSAIDs also have other modes of action that are less well understood.

DOSAGE
Adults— For mild to moderate pain, arthritis, and menstrual pain: 200 to 400 mg every 4 to 6 hours. For fever: 200 to 400 mg every 4 to 6 hours, but not more than 1,200 mg a day. Children ages 6 months to 12 years— For fevers below 102.5°F, 5 mg for every 2.2 lbs (1 kg) of body weight every 6 to 8 hours. For higher fevers, 10 mg per 2.2 lbs every 6 to 8 hours, but not more than 40 mg per 2.2 lbs a day.

ONSET OF EFFECT
For pain and fever, 30 minutes. For arthritis, up to 3 weeks.

DURATION OF ACTION
4 hours or more.

DIETARY ADVICE
Take ibuprofen with food.

STORAGE
Store in a tightly sealed container away from heat, moisture, and direct light.

IF YOU MISS A DOSE
Take it as soon as you remember. However, if it is near the time for the next dose, skip the missed dose and resume your regular dosage schedule. Do not double the next dose.

STOPPING THE DRUG
If taking this drug by prescription, do not stop without consulting your doctor.

PROLONGED USE
Prolonged use can cause gastrointestinal problems, including ulceration and bleeding, kidney dysfunction, and liver inflammation. See your doctor regularly for laboratory tests and examinations.

PRECAUTIONS
Over 60: Because of the potentially greater consequences of gastrointestinal side effects, the dose of NSAIDs for older patients, especially those over age 70, is often cut in half.

Driving and Hazardous Work: Do not drive or engage in hazardous work until you determine how the medicine affects you.

Alcohol: Avoid alcohol, as it may increase the risk of stomach irritation.

Pregnancy: Avoid or discontinue this drug if you are pregnant or are planning to become pregnant.

Breast Feeding: Ibuprofen passes into breast milk; avoid use while nursing.

Infants and Children: May be used in exceptional circumstances; consult your doctor.

Special Concerns: Because NSAIDs can interfere with blood coagulation, this drug should be stopped at least 3 days prior to any surgery.

OVERDOSE
Symptoms: Severe nausea, vomiting, headache, confusion, seizures.

What to Do: Call your doctor, emergency medical services (EMS), or the nearest poison control center immediately.

DRUG INTERACTIONS
Do not take this drug with aspirin or any other NSAIDs without your doctor's approval. In addition, consult your doctor if you are taking antihypertensives, steroids, anticoagulants, antibiotics, itraconazole or ketoconazole, plicamycin, penicillamine, valproic acid, phenytoin, cyclosporine, digitalis drugs, lithium, methotrexate, probenecid, triamterene, or zidovudine.

FOOD INTERACTIONS
No known food interactions.

DISEASE INTERACTIONS
Consult your doctor if you have any of the following: bleeding problems, inflammation or ulcers of the stomach and intestines, diabetes mellitus, systemic lupus erythematosus (SLE, lupus), anemia, asthma, epilepsy, Parkinson's disease, kidney stones, or a history of heart disease or alcohol abuse. Use of ibuprofen may cause complications in patients with liver or kidney disease, since these organs work together to remove the medication from the body.

Idoxuridine (IDU)

▶ Drug Class: Ophthalmic antiviral drug

▶ Available in: Drops, ointment

▶ Available OTC? No

▶ As Generic? No

Side Effects

SERIOUS
Allergic reaction causing itching, swelling, redness, pain, and constant burning; corneal ulcer causing painful sensation of having something lodged in the eye. In either case, call your doctor or ophthalmologist immediately.

COMMON
Heightened sensitivity of the eyes to bright light, stinging or burning in the eyes.

LESS COMMON
Blurred vision, excessive tear production.

PRINCIPAL USES
To treat viral infections of the eye, especially those caused by the herpes simplex virus.

HOW THE DRUG WORKS
Idoxuridine interferes with the activity of enzymes necessary for the replication of viral DNA in cells, thus preventing the virus from multiplying.

DOSAGE
The dosage may vary considerably from patient to patient, depending on a number of factors. The following guidelines represent typical doses; follow your doctor's specific dosing instruction. Eye drops: Apply 1 drop in the eye every hour during the day and every 2 hours at night. When the condition improves, apply it every 2 hours during the day and every 4 hours at night. Ointment: Apply a ⅜-inch strip of ointment every 4 hours (5 times a day), making the last application at bedtime.

ONSET OF EFFECT
Within 1 hour.

DURATION OF ACTION
Up to 6 hours.

DIETARY ADVICE
No special restrictions.

STORAGE
Keep the liquid form of idoxuridine refrigerated, but do not allow it to freeze.

IF YOU MISS A DOSE
Apply the missed dose as soon as you remember. If it is near time for the next dose, skip the missed dose and resume your regular dosage schedule. Do not double the next dose.

STOPPING THE DRUG
Take the drug as prescribed for the full treatment period, even if you begin to feel better before the scheduled end of therapy.

PROLONGED USE
Idoxuridine is not intended for prolonged use. If your symptoms do not improve in 7 days, consult your physician.

PRECAUTIONS
Over 60: No special problems are expected.

Driving and Hazardous Work: The use of idoxuridine should not impair your ability to perform such tasks safely.

Alcohol: No special precautions are necessary.

Pregnancy: Before taking idoxuridine, tell your doctor if you are pregnant or plan to become pregnant.

Breast Feeding: Idoxuridine may pass into breast milk; caution is advised. Consult your doctor for advice.

Infants and Children: Studies of the use of idoxuridine specifically in children have not been done; this drug should be used by young patients only under close medical supervision.

Special Concerns: Be sure you know how to apply idoxuridine. For the eye drops, first wash your hands. Then apply pressure to the inside corner of the eye with your middle finger. Tilt your head backward and pull the lower lid away from the eye with the index finger of the same hand. Drop the eye drops into the pouch you have created and close your eyes without blinking. Keep your eyes closed for 1 to 2 minutes. Then wash your hands. For the ointment, first wash your hands. Pull the lower lid down from the eye to form a pouch. Squeeze the tube to apply a thin strip of the ointment into the pouch. Close your eyes for 1 to 2 minutes. Then wash your hands. Do not let the applicator touch any surface, including the eye. If you accidentally touch its tip, clean it with warm water and soap. Family members should use separate washcloths and towels to prevent the spread of infection.

OVERDOSE
Symptoms: No specific ones have been reported.

What to Do: An overdose of idoxuridine is unlikely to occur. Emergency instructions are not applicable.

DRUG INTERACTIONS
Consult your doctor if you are using any eye product containing boric acid.

FOOD INTERACTIONS
No known food interactions.

DISEASE INTERACTIONS
Caution is advised when taking idoxuridine; consult your doctor if you have a history of any other eye problems.

Imatinib Mesylate

▶ Drug Class: Antineoplastic (anticancer) agent

▶ Available in: Capsules

▶ Available OTC? No

▶ As Generic? No

Side Effects

SERIOUS
Pleural effusion (excess fluid in the pleural space, which lies between the lungs and the chest wall), ascites (excess fluid in the abdomen), pulmonary edema (fluid in the lungs). Call your doctor immediately.

COMMON
Nausea, vomiting, diarrhea, swelling around the eyes and of the lower limbs, and muscle cramps.

LESS COMMON
Skin rash, headache, fatigue, joint pain, heartburn, fever, abdominal pain, and cough.

PRINCIPAL USES
To treat chronic myeloid leukemia (CML) during blast crisis, accelerated phase, or in chronic phase after failure of interferon-alpha therapy.

HOW THE DRUG WORKS
CML is caused by a genetic abnormality known as the Philadelphia chromosome, which produces a new and abnormal protein that causes the uncontrolled growth of white blood cells. By blocking the action of this protein, imatinib may lower the white blood cell count.

DOSAGE
400 mg once a day during chronic phase. 600 mg once a day during accelerated phase or blast crisis.

ONSET OF EFFECT
Unknown.

DURATION OF ACTION
Unknown.

DIETARY ADVICE
Take with a meal and a large glass of water.

STORAGE
Store in a tightly sealed container away from heat and direct light.

IF YOU MISS A DOSE
If you miss a dose, do not take the missed dose and do not double the next dose. Check with your doctor on what to do.

STOPPING THE DRUG
The decision to stop taking the drug should be made in consultation with your physician.

PROLONGED USE
You should see your doctor regularly for tests and examinations if you must take this drug for a prolonged period.

PRECAUTIONS
Over 60: No special problems are expected.

Driving and Hazardous Work: Do not drive or engage in hazardous work until you determine how the medicine affects you.

Alcohol: Avoid alcohol.

Pregnancy: Use of this drug during pregnancy should be avoided if possible. Be sure to tell your doctor if you are pregnant or plan to become pregnant.

Breast Feeding: It is not known whether this medication passes into breast milk. Breast feeding is not recommended while taking imatinib.

Infants and Children: Safety and effectiveness have not been established for patients under 18 years of age. Consult your pediatric oncologist for advice.

Special Concerns: Consult your doctor if you are taking St. John's wort. It may interact with imatinib.

OVERDOSE
Symptoms: No specific ones have been reported.

What to Do: Call your doctor or emergency medical services (EMS) immediately if you suspect an overdose.

DRUG INTERACTIONS
Consult your doctor if you are taking ketoconazole, itraconazole, erythromycin, clarithromycin, atorvastatin, fluvastatin, lovastatin, pravastatin, simvastatin, phenytoin, dexamethasone, carbamazepine, phenobarbital, cyclosporine, pimozide, benzodiazepine tranquilizers, calcium channel blockers, and warfarin.

FOOD INTERACTIONS
No known food interactions.

DISEASE INTERACTIONS
Use of this drug may cause complications in patients with liver or kidney disease, since these organs work together to remove the medication from the body.

Generic 25 mg
(**BIOCRAFT**)

Additional photographs

▶ Drug Class: Tricyclic
antidepressant

▶ Available in: Tablets,
capsules

▶ Available OTC? No

▶ As Generic? Yes

Side Effects

SERIOUS
Confusion, heartbeat
irregularities, hallucinations, seizures, extreme
fatigue or drowsiness,
blurred or altered vision,
breathing difficulty, constipation, impaired con-
centration, difficult
urination, fever, extreme
and persistent restless-
ness, loss of coordination
and balance, difficulty
swallowing or speaking,
dilated pupils, eye pain,
fainting. Also trembling,
shaking, weakness, and
stiffness in the extremi-
ties; shuffling gait. Call
your doctor immediately.

COMMON
Drowsiness, dizziness, or
lightheadedness, head-
ache, dry mouth or
unpleasant taste, fatigue,
heightened sensitivity of
skin to sunlight, weight
gain, increased appetite,
nausea.

LESS COMMON
Heartburn, insomnia,
diarrhea, increased
sweating, vomiting.

PRINCIPAL USES
To relieve symptoms of
major depression. Also
used to treat bed-wetting
in children age 6 and older
and incontinence in older
women.

HOW THE DRUG WORKS
Imipramine affects levels of
specific brain chemicals
(serotonin and norepinephrine) that are thought to be
linked to mood, emotions,
and mental state.

DOSAGE
For depression— Tablets:
Adults: To start, 25 to 50
mg, 3 to 4 times a day; may
be increased to 200 mg a
day. Teenagers: 25 to 50 mg
a day; may be increased to
100 mg a day. Older adults:
To start, 25 mg a day at
bedtime; may be increased
to 100 mg a day. Children
ages 6 to 12: 10 to 30 mg a
day. Capsules: Adults: To
start, 75 mg a day at bedtime; may be increased to
200 mg a day. For bed-wetting— Tablets: Children age
6 and older: 25 mg a day, 1
hour before bedtime. Dose
may be increased based on
the child's age.

ONSET OF EFFECT
1 to 6 weeks.

DURATION OF ACTION
Unknown.

DIETARY ADVICE
To lessen stomach upset,
take with food, unless your
doctor instructs otherwise.
Increase intake of fiber and
fluids.

STORAGE
Store in a tightly sealed container away from heat, moisture, and direct light.

IF YOU MISS A DOSE
If you take a one-time daily
bedtime dose, do not take a
missed dose in the morning
because it may cause

drowsiness. Call your doctor. If you take more than 1
dose a day, take it as soon
as you remember. If it is
near the time for the next
dose, skip the missed dose
and resume your regular
dosage schedule. Do not
double the next dose.

STOPPING THE DRUG
Take as prescribed for the
full treatment period, even
if you begin to feel better
before the scheduled end
of therapy. The decision to
stop taking the drug should
be made in consultation
with your doctor.

PROLONGED USE
The usual course of therapy
lasts 6 months to 1 year;
some patients benefit from
additional therapy.

PRECAUTIONS
Over 60: Adverse reactions
may be more likely and
more severe in older
patients. A lower dose
may be warranted.

**Driving and Hazardous
Work:** Use caution until
you determine how the
medicine affects you.
Drowsiness and lighthead-
edness can occur.

Alcohol: Avoid alcohol.

Pregnancy: Adequate studies have not been done.
Consult your doctor for
advice.

Breast Feeding: Do not
use this drug while nursing.

Infants and Children:
Not prescribed for children
under age 6.

Special Concerns: This is
a potentially dangerous
drug, especially if taken in
excess. Tricyclic antidepressants should not be within
easy reach of suicidal
patients.

OVERDOSE
Symptoms: Difficulty
breathing, severe fatigue,
seizures, confusion, hallucinations, distractibility,
dilated pupils, irregular
heartbeat, fever.

What to Do: Call your
doctor, emergency medical
services (EMS), or the
nearest poison control
center immediately.

DRUG INTERACTIONS
Consult your doctor for specific advice if you are taking
antithyroid agents, cimetidine, clonidine, guanadrel,
guanethidine, metrizamide,
appetite suppressants, isoproterenol, ephedrine, epinephrine, amphetamines,
phenyl-ephrine, antipsy-
chotic drugs, pimozide,
methyldopa, metyrosine,
metoclopramide, pemoline,
promethazine, trimeprazine,
rauwolfia alkaloids, MAO
inhibitors, or any drugs
that depress the central
nervous system.

FOOD INTERACTIONS
No known food interactions.

DISEASE INTERACTIONS
Consult your physician if
you have any of the following: a history of alcohol
abuse, difficulty urinating,
asthma, bipolar disorder,
high blood pressure, stomach or intestinal problems,
glaucoma, overactive thy-
roid, enlarged prostate,
schizophrenia, seizures a
blood disorder, or kidney,
heart, or liver disease.

Imiquimod

▶ Drug Class: Immunomodulator

▶ Available in: Cream

▶ Available OTC? No

▶ As Generic? No

Side Effects

SERIOUS
Swollen eyelids, face, or lips, wheezing, or rash may be signs of a drug allergy. Call your doctor immediately.

COMMON
Common side effects are limited to the treated area of the skin. The following have been observed: redness, thinning of the skin, flaking, swelling of the treated area.

LESS COMMON
Hardening or stiffening of the treated area, sores, scabbing, blisters.

PRINCIPAL USES
To treat external condylomata acuminata (genital and perianal warts) in adults.

HOW THE DRUG WORKS
Imiquimod's mechanism of action is unknown.

DOSAGE
Apply a thin layer to the affected area 3 times a week at bedtime. Leave it on the skin for 6 to 10 hours. The cream should then be removed by washing with mild soap and water.

ONSET OF EFFECT
Unknown.

DURATION OF ACTION
Unknown.

DIETARY ADVICE
Imiquimod can be used without regard to diet.

STORAGE
Store in a tightly sealed container away from heat, moisture, and direct light. Do not allow it to freeze.

IF YOU MISS A DOSE
If you miss a scheduled dose, skip it and resume your regular dosage schedule on the appointed day; do not apply the cream 2 days in a row.

STOPPING THE DRUG
Treatment should continue until there is total clearance of the warts or for no more than 16 weeks. If the warts do not clear up within this time, do not continue to apply imiquimod to the area; consult your doctor.

PROLONGED USE
Imiquimod is prescribed for no more than 16 weeks.

PRECAUTIONS
Over 60: No special problems are expected.

Driving and Hazardous Work: The use of imiquimod should not impair your ability to perform such tasks safely.

Alcohol: No special precautions are necessary.

Pregnancy: Adequate human studies have not been done. Before taking imiquimod, tell your doctor if you are pregnant or plan to become pregnant.

Breast Feeding: Imiquimod may pass into breast milk; caution is advised. Consult your doctor for specific advice.

Infants and Children: Not recommended for use by children under age 18.

Special Concerns: The treated area should not be covered by tight bandages or clothing. Wash your hands before and after applying imiquimod to the skin. Avoid getting the drug in your eyes. Sexual relations should be avoided while the cream is on the skin. Imiquimod cream may weaken condoms and diaphragms, compromising the protection they provide. If serious irritation of the treated area occurs, discontinue the medication for several days to allow the reaction to subside. You may then resume therapy.

OVERDOSE
Symptoms: No cases of overdose have been reported.

What to Do: An overdose with imiquimod is unlikely. If someone accidentally ingests imiquimod, call your doctor, emergency medical services (EMS), or the nearest poison control center immediately.

DRUG INTERACTIONS
None known.

FOOD INTERACTIONS
No known food interactions.

DISEASE INTERACTIONS
Imiquimod should be used with caution by anyone with a history of inflammatory skin conditions. If you have had any recent medical or surgical treatment in the genital or perianal area, therapy with imiquimod should be delayed until the affected tissue has healed.

Indapamide

Generic 2.5 mg
(Rhone-Poulenc Rorer)

▶ Drug Class: Thiazide diuretic

▶ Available in: Tablets

▶ Available OTC? No

▶ As Generic? Yes

Side Effects

SERIOUS
Skin rash, hives, intense itching, swelling of the mouth and throat, breathing difficulty, heart rhythm irregularities, lightheadedness, unusual bleeding or bruising. Call your doctor immediately.

COMMON
Muscle cramps or pain. Potassium depletion may lead to heart palpitations and weakness. Fluid depletion may lead to dizziness, especially upon arising from a sitting or lying position, as well as thirst, dry mouth, and constipation.

LESS COMMON
Decreased sexual ability, increased sensitivity to sunlight, loss of appetite, gout, increased blood sugar (a problem for diabetic patients).

PRINCIPAL USES
To help control high blood pressure and to treat conditions that cause edema (swelling of body tissues resulting from excess salt and water retention).

HOW THE DRUG WORKS
Diuretics increase the excretion of salt and water in the urine. By reducing the overall fluid volume in the body, these drugs reduce blood volume and so reduce pressure within the blood vessels.

DOSAGE
For high blood pressure: Initial dose is 1.5 mg once a day. It can be increased to 5 mg a day. To reduce edema: 2.5 mg once a day; it can be increased to 5 mg a day.

ONSET OF EFFECT
From 2 to 3 hours.

DURATION OF ACTION
24 hours.

DIETARY ADVICE
A single daily dose should be taken in the morning after breakfast.

STORAGE
Store in a tightly sealed container away from heat and direct light.

IF YOU MISS A DOSE
Take it as soon as you remember. If it is near the time for the next dose, skip the missed dose and resume your regular dosage schedule. Do not double the next dose.

STOPPING THE DRUG
The decision to stop taking the drug should be made by your doctor.

PROLONGED USE
See your doctor regularly for examinations and tests if you must take this medicine for an extended period.

PRECAUTIONS
Over 60: Adverse reactions may be more likely and more severe in older patients.

Driving and Hazardous Work: No special precautions are necessary.

Alcohol: No special precautions are necessary.

Pregnancy: Indapamide should not be used during pregnancy unless recommended by your doctor.

Breast Feeding: Indapamide may pass into breast milk; caution is advised. Consult your doctor for specific advice.

Infants and Children: The safety and effectiveness of indapamide for children under 12 have not been determined. Consult your doctor for specific advice.

Special Concerns: Follow your doctor's instructions about consuming potassium-rich foods or taking a potassium supplement. It may be necessary to discontinue indapamide 5 to 7 days before undergoing major surgery. If you are taking more than 1 dose a day, the last dose should be taken no later than 6 pm unless your doctor advises otherwise.

OVERDOSE
Symptoms: Stomach irritation, thirst, muscle cramps, nausea, vomiting, increased urination, lethargy, loss of consciousness.

What to Do: Call your doctor, emergency medical services (EMS), or the nearest poison control center immediately.

DRUG INTERACTIONS
Consult your doctor for specific advice if you are taking other drugs for high blood pressure, lithium, oral antidiabetic drugs, digitalis preparations, nonsteroidal anti-inflammatory drugs, cholestyramine, or colestipol.

FOOD INTERACTIONS
Follow your doctor's advice about salt use and potassium-rich foods.

DISEASE INTERACTIONS
Caution is advised when taking indapamide. Consult your doctor if you have diabetes, gout, or systemic lupus erythematosus. Use of indapamide may cause complications in patients with liver or kidney disease, since these organs work together to remove the medication from the body.

Indinavir

BRAND NAME
Crixivan

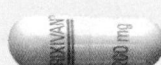

Crixivan 200 mg
(MERCK)

▶ Drug Class: Antiviral/
protease inhibitor

▶ Available in: Capsules

▶ Available OTC? No

▶ As Generic? No

Side Effects

SERIOUS
Blood in urine and sharp back pain caused by kidney stones. High blood sugar (diabetes) has occurred in patients taking drugs of this class, although a cause-and-effect relationship has not been established. Call your doctor if you develop increased thirst or excessive urination.

COMMON
Generalized weakness, abdominal pains, diarrhea, nausea, vomiting, headache, insomnia, changes in taste, dry skin, chapped lips.

LESS COMMON
Dizziness, drowsiness, depression, memory changes, abdominal bloating, muscle wasting.

PRINCIPAL USES
To treat advanced HIV (human immunodeficiency virus) infection and AIDS (acquired immunodeficiency syndrome), usually in combination with other drugs. While not a cure for HIV infection, this drug may suppress the replication of the virus and delay the progression of the disease.

HOW THE DRUG WORKS
Indinavir blocks the activity of a viral protease, an enzyme that is needed by HIV to reproduce. Blocking the protease causes HIV to make copies that cannot infect new cells.

DOSAGE
800 mg every 8 hours, alone or in combination with other antiviral agents. Higher or lower doses are sometimes prescribed when indinavir is being combined with medications such as nevirapine and delavirdine, which alter indinavir blood levels.

ONSET OF EFFECT
Unknown. With most antiretroviral drugs, an early response can be seen within the first few days of therapy, but the maximum effect may take 12 to 16 weeks.

DURATION OF ACTION
Unknown. Effects of the drug may be prolonged if indinavir is used in combination with other effective drugs and the virus is maximally suppressed.

DIETARY ADVICE
Indinavir should be taken with plenty of water or other liquid, preferably at least 1 hour before or 2 hours after a meal. It may also be taken with a light, nonfat snack. Drink at least 48 ounces of water per day.

STORAGE
Store in a tightly sealed container away from heat, moisture, and direct light.

IF YOU MISS A DOSE
Take it as soon as you remember. However, if it is near the time for the next dose, skip the missed dose and resume your regular dosage schedule. Do not double the next dose.

STOPPING THE DRUG
The decision to stop taking the drug should be made by your doctor.

PROLONGED USE
See your doctor regularly for tests and examinations.

PRECAUTIONS

Over 60: No special studies have been done on older patients.

Driving and Hazardous Work: Do not drive or engage in hazardous work until you determine how the medicine affects you.

Alcohol: Avoid alcohol if liver function is impaired.

Pregnancy: Indinavir has been shown to cause birth defects in animals. Human studies have not been done. Nevertheless, indinavir is increasingly being used in combination with other antiretroviral drugs to treat pregnant HIV-infected women.

Breast Feeding: Women infected with HIV should not breast-feed, so as to avoid transmitting the virus to an uninfected child.

Infants and Children: Safety and effectiveness of indinavir for children under the age of 16 have not been established.

Special Concerns: Indinavir should not be taken concurrently with the herb St. John's wort, which can increase blood levels of the drug in the body and lead to possible resistance to indinavir. It is important to drink at least 48 ounces of water or other liquids every 24 hours to help prevent kidney stones. Therapy may be interrupted for patients who develop kidney stones. Be sure to tell any doctor or dentist treating you that you are taking indinavir. Remember that taking indinavir does not eliminate the chance of passing the AIDS virus to other persons. Take appropriate preventive measures.

OVERDOSE

Symptoms: Pain in the lower back, blood in the urine, nausea, vomiting, diarrhea.

What to Do: An overdose of indinavir is unlikely to be life-threatening. However, if someone takes a much larger dose than prescribed, seek medical attention immediately.

DRUG INTERACTIONS
Consult your doctor for specific advice if you are taking any other prescription or over-the-counter drug, especially astemizole, didanosine, delavirdine, efavirenz, itraconazole, ketoconazole, midazolam, triazolam, didanosine, rifabutin, rifampin, phenobarbital, phenytoin, carbamazepine, cholesterol-lowering drugs, or dexamethasone.

FOOD INTERACTIONS
Food, especially fatty foods, will decrease absorption of the drug.

DISEASE INTERACTIONS
Use of indinavir may cause complications in patients with liver disease.

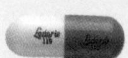

Generic 25 mg
(LEDERLE)

▶ Drug Class: Nonsteroidal
anti-inflammatory drug
(NSAID)

▶ Available in: Capsules, suspension, rectal suppositories

▶ Available OTC? No

▶ As Generic? Yes

Side Effects

SERIOUS
Wheezing or breathing
difficulty, with or without
swelling of the legs or
other signs of heart failure; chest pain; peptic
ulcers with vomiting of
blood; black, tarry stools;
decreased kidney func-
tion causing blood in the
urine, decreased urine
output, and shortness of
breath. NSAIDs may
cause constriction of the
airways or severe allergic
reactions in patients who
are sensitive to aspirin,
especially those with
aspirin-induced nasal
polyps or asthma.

COMMON
Nausea, vomiting, heart-
burn, diarrhea, constipa-
tion, headache, dizziness,
drowsiness.

LESS COMMON
Ulcers or sores in mouth,
rashes or blistering,
unusual tingling or
numbness of the hands
and feet, depression,
ringing in the ears,
seizures, blurred vision.
Also high blood potas-
sium levels and
decreased blood counts;
such problems can be
detected by your doctor.

PRINCIPAL USES
To treat mild to moderate
pain and inflammation
occurring in association
with tendinitis, arthritis,
bursitis, gout, soft tissue
injuries, migraine and other
types of vascular headache,
menstrual cramps, and
other conditions. Because
of its greater risk of toxicity,
indomethacin should be
taken only when other
NSAIDs prove ineffective.

HOW THE DRUG WORKS
NSAIDs such as indometh-
acin work by interfering
with the formation of
prostaglandins. These are
naturally occurring sub-
stances in the body that
cause inflammation and
make nerves more sensitive
to pain impulses. NSAIDs
also have other modes of
action that are less well
understood.

DOSAGE
Adults— Capsules: For
arthritis: 25 to 50 mg, 2 to
4 times daily, up to a usual
maximum of 200 mg a day
at first. For gout: 100 mg
immediately, then 50 mg
taken 3 times a day. This
may be decreased gradually
by your doctor. For bursitis
or tendinitis: 25 mg, 3 to 4
times a day, or 50 mg, 3
times a day. Extended-
release capsules: For arthritis: 75 mg, 1 to 2 times a
day. Rectal suppositories:
For arthritis, gout, bursitis,
and tendinitis: 50 mg suppository, inserted 1 to 4
times a day. Children—
Consult a pediatrician for
dosage for all forms.

ONSET OF EFFECT
30 minutes to several hours.

DURATION OF ACTION
4 hours or more.

DIETARY ADVICE
Take with food; maintain
your usual food and fluid
intake.

STORAGE
Store in a tightly sealed container away from heat, moisture, and direct light.

IF YOU MISS A DOSE
Take it as soon as you
remember. If it is near the
time for the next dose, skip
the missed dose and
resume your regular dosage
schedule. Do not double the
next dose.

STOPPING THE DRUG
Take it as prescribed for the
full treatment period. Ask
your doctor about stopping
the drug if you are feeling
better before the scheduled
end of therapy.

PROLONGED USE
Therapy may require weeks
or months.

PRECAUTIONS
Over 60: Because of the
potentially greater consequences of gastrointestinal
side effects, the dose in
older patients, especially
those over age 70, is often
cut in half.

**Driving and Hazardous
Work:** Avoid such activities
until you determine how the
medicine affects you.

Alcohol: Avoid alcohol.

Pregnancy: Do not use
this drug while pregnant.

Breast Feeding: Do not
use indomethacin while
nursing.

Infants and Children:
May be used in exceptional
circumstances only when
other NSAIDs prove ineffective; consult a pediatrician.

Special Concerns:
Because NSAIDs can inter-
fere with blood coagulation,
this drug should be stopped
at least 3 days prior to any
surgery.

OVERDOSE
Symptoms: Severe nausea,
vomiting, headache, confusion, seizures.

What to Do: Call your
doctor, emergency medical
services (EMS), or the
nearest poison control center immediately.

DRUG INTERACTIONS
Do not take with aspirin or
other NSAIDs. Consult your
doctor if you are taking anticoagulants, antibiotics, itraconazole or ketoconazole,
plicamycin, penicillamine,
valproic acid, phenytoin,
cyclosporine, digitalis
drugs, lithium, medication
for high blood pressure,
methotrexate, probenecid,
steroids, triamterene, or
zidovudine.

FOOD INTERACTIONS
No known food interactions.

DISEASE INTERACTIONS
Consult your doctor if you
have a history of alcohol
abuse, bleeding problems,
inflammation or ulcers of
the stomach and intestines,
diabetes mellitus, heart,
liver, or kidney disease
(including kidney stones),
systemic lupus erythematosus (SLE, lupus), anemia,
asthma, epilepsy, or Parkinson's disease.

Influenza Virus Vaccine

BRAND NAMES
Fluogen, FluShield,
Fluvirin, Fluzone

▶ Drug Class: Vaccine

▶ Available in: Injection

▶ Available OTC? No

▶ As Generic? No

Side Effects

SERIOUS
Serious allergic reaction involving difficulty swallowing or breathing; reddened skin, especially around the ears; itching, particularly of the hands or feet; hives; unusual and severe fatigue; and swollen face, eyes, or nasal passages. Call your doctor immediately.

COMMON
Pain, redness, or hard lump at site of injection.

LESS COMMON
Fever, muscle aches, general feeling of illness.

PRINCIPAL USES
To help prevent infection by the influenza (flu) virus.

HOW THE DRUG WORKS
The influenza vaccine is an injection that works by introducing a dead (inactive) flu virus into the body, which stimulates the immune system to produce protective antibodies against the disease. The virus used for the vaccine at any given time is similar to the one that the World Health Organization and the U.S. Public Health Service believe is likely to appear during the upcoming flu season, since the strains of influenza change from season to season and year to year.

DOSAGE
Adults and children age 9 and older: 1 injection into the upper arm annually, usually in early November. Children ages 6 months to 9 years: 1 or 2 injections into the thigh annually, usually in early November.

ONSET OF EFFECT
Most patients develop immunity within 2 to 4 weeks.

DURATION OF ACTION
Unknown. The antibodies may be available for protection against a particular strain of flu for many years following the injection, but the antibodies will only protect against a flu virus that is identical or very similar to the one that was used in the vaccine. A different strain of the flu may not be affected by the antibodies, leading to infection.

DIETARY ADVICE
No special restrictions.

STORAGE
Not applicable; the dose is administered only at a health care facility.

IF YOU MISS A DOSE
Not applicable.

STOPPING THE DRUG
Not applicable.

PROLONGED USE
Not applicable.

PRECAUTIONS
Over 60: Influenza vaccine is not expected to cause different or more severe side effects in older patients than it does in younger persons. However, older adults may not develop as strong an immunity as younger persons.

Driving and Hazardous Work: The vaccine should not impair your ability to perform such tasks safely.

Alcohol: No special precautions are necessary.

Pregnancy: The vaccine has not been shown to cause problems in pregnant women. Consult your doctor for more information.

Breast Feeding: The vaccine has not been shown to cause any problems in nursing babies. Consult your doctor for advice.

Infants and Children: Not recommended for use by children under the age of 6 months. Only the "split-virus" vaccine should be administered to children under the age of 13.

Special Concerns: If you want to decrease your chances of coming down with the flu, discuss appropriate health care measures with your doctor. Remember that the vaccine is not effective against all strains of the flu. The ability of the vaccine to stimulate your immune system is affected by your age, by the presence of other diseases, and by the use of other medications. Protection from flu infection during the flu season may be less in these circumstances. Make sure to tell your doctor if you or your child are ill on the day the injection is scheduled. Your doctor may decide to reschedule your vaccination.

OVERDOSE
Symptoms: An overdose with the influenza vaccine is unlikely.

What to Do: No cases of overdose have been reported.

DRUG INTERACTIONS
Other drugs may interact with influenza vaccine. Tell your doctor if you are taking any prescription or over-the-counter medication.

FOOD INTERACTIONS
No known food interactions.

DISEASE INTERACTIONS
Consult your doctor if you have any of the following: bronchitis, pneumonia, or other respiratory problems, seizures, allergies to eggs, or allergies to antibiotics, especially gentamicin.

Insulin Glargine (rDNA origin)

BRAND NAME
Lantus

▸ Drug Class: Antidiabetic agent

▸ Available in: Injection

▸ Available OTC? No

▸ As Generic? No

Side Effects

SERIOUS
Symptoms of hypoglycemia can be caused by the release of adrenaline or by an inadequate supply of glucose to the brain. With severe hypoglycemia, lack of sufficient glucose to the brain may cause slurred speech, impaired concentration, confusion, seizures, coma, irreversible brain damage, and death. Mild hypoglycemia may cause restless sleep, nightmares, or a cold sweat that awakens patients at night.

COMMON
Symptoms resulting from release of adrenaline are common manifestations of mild to moderate hypoglycemia. They include cold sweats, anxiety, shakiness, hunger, rapid heartbeat, headache, and nervousness. Weight gain is common when taking insulin.

LESS COMMON
Allergic reactions, lipoatrophy (depressions in the skin due to loss of fat tissue), and lipohypertrophy (excessive accumulation of fat tissue).

PRINCIPAL USES
For long-term treatment of diabetes mellitus. All patients with type 1 diabetes require lifelong insulin treatment. Patients with type 2 diabetes may require insulin if they are unable to control their blood glucose (sugar) levels with diet and oral medications. Insulin glargine is a slightly modified form of human insulin that maintains a relatively constant glucose-lowering effect over a 24-hour period and thus permits dosing once a day.

HOW THE DRUG WORKS
Insulin, a hormone secreted by the beta cells of the pancreas, plays an essential role in controlling the metabolism and storage of carbohydrates, fat, and protein. Insulin is secreted in response to a rise in blood sugar (glucose). Insulin lowers blood glucose by increasing its uptake by body cells, especially muscle, and by reducing the release of glucose from the liver between meals.

DOSAGE
Injected under the skin (stomach, thigh, or upper arm) once a day at bedtime. Doses are determined by your doctor. The solution should be clear and colorless, without any visible particles. Insulin glargine must not be diluted or mixed with any other insulin or solution.

ONSET OF EFFECT
About 1 to 2 hours.

DURATION OF ACTION
At least 24 hours.

DIETARY ADVICE
All patients with diabetes should follow the general dietary recommendations of the American Diabetes Association. Though intake of simple sugars is not forbidden, consuming a large amount of sugary foods at one time may trigger a rapid rise in blood glucose that can increase urination and thirst. In addition, patients who take insulin must remain consistent from day to day in the timing and caloric content of their meals. Depending on the timing, dose, and types of insulin prescribed, snacks may be recommended in the late afternoon, before bedtime, or prior to unusual physical activity. Diabetic patients must always have available a juice, food, or tablets that can raise blood glucose levels rapidly to counter an episode of hypoglycemia.

STORAGE
Refrigerate insulin but do not allow it to freeze. If refrigeration is not possible, the 10 milliliter (mL) vial or 3 mL cartridge in use can be kept unrefrigerated for up to 28 days away from direct heat and light, as long as the temperature is not greater than 86°F. Unrefrigerated 10 mL vials and 3 mL cartridges must be used within the 28-day period or they must be discarded. If refrigeration is not possible, the 5 mL vial in use can be kept unrefrigerated for up to 14 days away from direct heat and light, as long as the temperature is not greater than 86°F. Unrefrigerated 5 mL vials must be used within the 14-day period or they must be discarded. If refrigerated, the 5 mL vial in use can be kept for up to 28 days. Once the 3 mL cartridge is placed into an OptiPen One, it should not be put in the refrigerator.

IF YOU MISS A DOSE
Timing of insulin doses is extremely important. The best approach is to measure blood glucose and add a dose of regular insulin if glucose levels are too high. Otherwise, wait for the next scheduled dose.

STOPPING THE DRUG
Do not stop taking insulin injections unless ordered by your doctor. Patients with diabetes are often given general instructions for modifying their insulin doses based on home blood glucose measurements.

PROLONGED USE
After many years with diabetes, some patients become insensitive to the symptoms of hypoglycemia and are at risk for serious brain complications of prolonged, unrecognized hypoglycemia.

PRECAUTIONS
Over 60: No special warnings. Some older people may, however, have vision problems that may make it difficult to draw up the correct dose of insulin.

Driving and Hazardous Work: Patients taking insulin must be very careful to avoid hypoglycemia when driving or engaging in hazardous work.

Alcohol: Moderate alcohol intake, especially when taken with large meals, does not adversely affect control of diabetes or alter the dose of insulin. However, large amounts of alcohol increase the risk of hypoglycemia.

Pregnancy: Strict metabolic control—using insulin injections in most women—must be maintained during pregnancy to reduce the risk of birth defects, fetal complications, or death at the time of delivery. In women who had diabetes before the onset of pregnancy, the dose of insulin is often smaller during the first third (trimester) of pregnancy and then higher during the final two trimesters. When women first develop diabetes during pregnancy (gestational diabetes), insulin requirements drop rapidly after delivery and most do not need to continue with insulin treatment.

Breast Feeding: Insulin requirements tend to be lower during breast feeding. Home glucose monitoring is important to avoid hypoglycemia. Insulin glargine may pass into breast milk; consult your doctor for advice.

Infants and Children: Treatment with insulin in young patients age 6 and older is the same as that in older people with diabetes. The safety and effectiveness of insulin glargine in children under the age of 6 have not been established.

Special Concerns: Inadequate amounts of insulin in type 1 diabetes may lead to the serious complication of diabetic ketoacidosis, characterized by loss of appetite, excessive thirst and urination, nausea, vomiting, deep breathing, fruity breath odor, drowsiness, confusion, and loss of consciousness. Insulin glargine is not the insulin of choice for treatment of diabetic ketoacidosis. An intravenous short-acting insulin is the preferred treatment.

OVERDOSE

Symptoms: Insulin overdose results in hypoglycemia (see Side Effects for symptoms).

What to Do: For mild to moderate hypoglycemia, ingest drinks or food containing sugar. For more severe hypoglycemia, administer injections of glucagon or call emergency medical services (EMS) immediately.

DRUG INTERACTIONS

A large number of drugs can promote either elevated blood glucose levels or hypoglycemia. Be sure that your doctor knows about all of the medications you take and is informed before you start taking any new drugs, either by prescription or over the counter. Corticosteroids in particular are likely to raise blood glucose levels and insulin requirements. Beta-blockers (commonly prescribed for hypertension) may cause either high blood glucose levels or hypoglycemia; in addition, because these medications may dampen the symptoms of hypoglycemia that are caused by adrenaline release, mild degrees of hypoglycemia may progress unnoticed to more serious hypoglycemia affecting the brain.

FOOD INTERACTIONS

Insulin requirements are increased by the ingestion of large amounts of calories, especially simple sugars and other carbohydrates.

DISEASE INTERACTIONS

Insulin requirements are increased by infections, psychological stress, or an uncontrolled overactive thyroid, and often at a time of surgery. Requirements may diminish with kidney disease or an underactive adrenal or pituitary gland.

Insulin (Intermediate-acting, NPH, Lente)

BRAND NAMES
Humulin L, Humulin N, Insulatard NPH (purified pork), Insulated NPH Human, Lente Iletin I (beef and pork), Lente Iletin II (purified beef), Lente Iletin II (purified pork), Novolin L, Novolin L Pen-Fill Cartridges, Novolin N, NPH Iletin I (beef and pork), NPH Iletin II (purified beef), NPH Iletin II (purified pork)

▶ Drug Class: Antidiabetic agent

▶ Available in: Injection

▶ Available OTC? Yes

▶ As Generic? No

Side Effects

SERIOUS
Symptoms of hypoglycemia can be caused by the release of adrenaline or by an inadequate supply of glucose to the brain. With severe hypoglycemia, lack of sufficient glucose to the brain may cause slurred speech, impaired concentration, confusion, seizures, coma, irreversible brain damage, and death. Mild hypoglycemia may cause restless sleep, nightmares, or a cold sweat that awakens patients at night.

COMMON
Symptoms resulting from the release of adrenaline are common with mild to moderate hypoglycemia. They include cold sweats, anxiety, shakiness, hunger, rapid heartbeat, and headache. Weight gain is also common when taking insulin.

LESS COMMON
Allergic reactions, lipoatrophy (depressions in the skin due to loss of fat tissue), and lipohypertrophy (excessive accumulation of fat tissue).

PRINCIPAL USES
For long-term treatment of diabetes mellitus. All patients with type 1 diabetes require lifelong insulin treatment. Patients with type 2 diabetes may require insulin if they are unable to control their blood glucose (sugar) levels with diet and oral medications.

HOW THE DRUG WORKS
Insulin, a hormone secreted by the beta cells of the pancreas, plays an essential role in controlling the metabolism and storage of carbohydrates, fat, and protein. Insulin is secreted in response to a rise in blood sugar (glucose). Insulin lowers blood glucose by increasing its uptake by body cells, especially muscle, and by reducing the release of glucose from the liver between meals.

DOSAGE
Injected 1 or 2 times a day. Doses and frequency are determined by your doctor. Intermediate-acting (NPH or Lente) insulin can be mixed in the same syringe with rapid-acting insulin; draw up the rapid-acting insulin first. Intermediate-acting insulin solutions are cloudy (insulin settles to the bottom of the bottle) and must be rolled or gently shaken to distribute the insulin evenly in the solution before drawing it up into the syringe.

ONSET OF EFFECT
Within 1 hour; peak effect occurs within 8 to 12 hours.

DURATION OF ACTION
From 12 to 18 hours.

DIETARY ADVICE
All patients with diabetes should follow the general dietary recommendations of the American Diabetes Association. Though intake of simple sugars is not forbidden, consuming a large amount of sugary foods at one time may trigger a rapid rise in blood glucose that can increase urination and thirst. In addition, patients who take insulin must remain consistent from day to day in the timing and caloric content of their meals. Depending on the timing, dose, and types of insulin prescribed, snacks may be recommended in the late afternoon, before bedtime, or prior to unusual physical activity. Diabetic patients must always have available a juice, food, or tablets that can raise blood glucose levels rapidly to counter an episode of hypoglycemia.

STORAGE
Refrigerate insulin but do not allow it to freeze. Insulin does not have to be kept refrigerated when you're traveling for short periods, but exposure to high temperatures must be avoided.

IF YOU MISS A DOSE
Timing of insulin doses is extremely important. The best approach is to measure blood glucose and add a dose of regular insulin if your glucose levels are too high. Otherwise, wait for the next scheduled dose.

STOPPING THE DRUG
Do not stop taking insulin injections unless ordered by your doctor. Patients with diabetes are often given general instructions for modifying their insulin doses based on home blood glucose measurements.

PROLONGED USE
After many years with diabetes, some patients become insensitive to the symptoms of hypoglycemia and are at risk for serious brain complications of prolonged, unrecognized hypoglycemia.

PRECAUTIONS
Over 60: No special warnings. Some older people may, however, have vision problems that may make it difficult to draw up the correct dose of insulin.

Driving and Hazardous Work: Patients taking insulin must be very careful to avoid hypoglycemia when driving or engaging in hazardous work.

Alcohol: Moderate alcohol intake, especially when taken with large meals, does not adversely affect control of diabetes or alter the dose of insulin. However, large amounts of alcohol increase the risk of hypoglycemia.

Pregnancy: Strict metabolic control—using insulin injections in most women—must be maintained during pregnancy to reduce the risk of birth defects, fetal complications, or death at the time of delivery. In women who had diabetes before the onset of pregnancy, the dose of insulin is often smaller during the first third (trimester) of pregnancy and then higher during the final two trimesters. When women first develop diabetes during pregnancy (gestational diabetes), insulin requirements drop rapidly after delivery and most do not need to continue with insulin treatment.

Breast Feeding: Insulin requirements tend to be lower during breast feeding. Home glucose monitoring is important to avoid hypoglycemia. Insulin is not present in breast milk.

Insulin (Intermediate-acting, NPH, Lente)

Infants and Children: Treatment with insulin in children is the same as in older people with diabetes.

Special Concerns: Inadequate amounts of insulin in type 1 diabetes may lead to the serious complication of diabetic ketoacidosis, characterized by loss of appetite, excessive thirst and urination, nausea, vomiting, deep breathing, fruity breath odor, drowsiness, confusion, and loss of consciousness.

OVERDOSE

Symptoms: Insulin overdose results in hypoglycemia (see Side Effects for symptoms).

What to Do: For mild to moderate hypoglycemia, ingest drinks or food containing sugar. For more severe hypoglycemia, administer injections of glucagon or call emergency medical services (EMS) immediately.

DRUG INTERACTIONS

A large number of drugs can promote either elevated blood glucose levels or hypoglycemia. Be sure that your doctor knows about all of the medications you take and is informed before you start taking any new drugs, either by prescription or over the counter. Corticosteroids in particular are likely to raise blood glucose levels and insulin requirements. Beta-blockers (commonly prescribed for hypertension) may cause either high blood glucose levels or hypoglycemia; in addition, because these medications may dampen the symptoms of hypoglycemia that are caused by adrenaline release, mild degrees of hypoglycemia may progress unnoticed to more serious hypoglycemia affecting the brain.

FOOD INTERACTIONS

Insulin requirements are increased when larger amounts of calories are ingested, especially simple sugars and carbohydrates.

DISEASE INTERACTIONS

Insulin requirements are increased by infections, psychological stress, or an uncontrolled overactive thyroid, and often at a time of surgery. Requirements may diminish with kidney disease or an underactive adrenal or pituitary gland.

Insulin Lispro (rDNA origin)

BRAND NAME
Humalog

▶ Drug Class: Antidiabetic agent

▶ Available in: Injection

▶ Available OTC? No

▶ As Generic? No

Side Effects

SERIOUS
Symptoms of hypoglycemia can be caused by the release of adrenaline or by an inadequate supply of glucose to the brain. With severe hypoglycemia, lack of sufficient glucose to the brain may cause slurred speech, impaired concentration, confusion, seizures, coma, irreversible brain damage, and death. Mild hypoglycemia may cause restless sleep, nightmares, or a cold sweat that awakens patients at night.

COMMON
Symptoms resulting from release of adrenaline are common manifestations of mild to moderate hypoglycemia. They include cold sweats, anxiety, shakiness, hunger, rapid heartbeat, headache, and nervousness. Weight gain is common when taking insulin.

LESS COMMON
Allergic reactions, lipoatrophy (depressions in the skin due to loss of fat tissue), and lipohypertrophy (excessive accumulation of fat tissue).

PRINCIPAL USES
For long-term treatment of diabetes mellitus. All patients with type 1 diabetes require lifelong insulin treatment. Patients with type 2 diabetes may require insulin if they are unable to control their blood glucose (sugar) levels with diet and oral medications.

HOW THE DRUG WORKS
Insulin, a hormone secreted by the beta cells of the pancreas, plays an essential role in controlling the metabolism and storage of carbohydrates, fat, and protein. Insulin is secreted in response to a rise in blood sugar (glucose). Insulin lowers blood glucose by increasing its uptake by body cells, especially muscle, and by reducing the release of glucose from the liver between meals.

DOSAGE
It may be taken 1 to 4 times daily, before meals and possibly at bedtime. Doses and frequency are determined by your doctor. Rapid-acting (lispro rDNA origin) insulin should be administered 15 minutes before a meal.

ONSET OF EFFECT
Within 30 to 45 minutes; the peak effect occurs within 1 hour.

DURATION OF ACTION
From 3 to 4 hours.

DIETARY ADVICE
All patients with diabetes should follow the general dietary recommendations of the American Diabetes Association. Though intake of simple sugars is not forbidden, consuming a large amount of sugary foods at one time may trigger a rapid rise in blood glucose that can increase urination and thirst. In addition, patients who take insulin must remain consistent from day to day in the timing and caloric content of their meals. Depending on the timing, dose, and types of insulin prescribed, snacks may be recommended in the late afternoon, before bedtime, or prior to unusual physical activity. Diabetic patients must always have available a juice, food, or tablets that can raise blood glucose levels rapidly to counter an episode of hypoglycemia.

STORAGE
Refrigerate insulin but do not allow it to freeze. Insulin does not have to be kept refrigerated when you're traveling for short periods, but exposure to high temperatures must be avoided.

IF YOU MISS A DOSE
Timing of insulin doses is extremely important. The best approach is to measure blood glucose and add a dose of regular insulin if your glucose levels are too high. Otherwise, wait for the next scheduled dose.

STOPPING THE DRUG
Do not stop taking insulin injections unless ordered by your doctor. Patients with diabetes are often given general instructions for modifying their insulin doses based on home blood glucose measurements.

PROLONGED USE
After many years with diabetes, some patients become insensitive to the symptoms of hypoglycemia and are at risk for serious brain complications of prolonged, unrecognized hypoglycemia.

PRECAUTIONS
Over 60: No special warnings. Some older people may, however, have vision problems that may make it difficult to draw up the correct dose of insulin.

Driving and Hazardous Work: Patients taking insulin must be very careful to avoid hypoglycemia when driving or engaging in hazardous work.

Alcohol: Moderate alcohol intake, especially when taken with large meals, does not adversely affect control of diabetes or alter the dose of insulin. However, large amounts of alcohol increase the risk of hypoglycemia.

Pregnancy: Strict metabolic control—using insulin injections in most women—must be maintained during pregnancy to reduce the risk of birth defects, fetal complications, or death at the time of delivery. In women who had diabetes before the onset of pregnancy, the dose of insulin is often smaller during the first third (trimester) of pregnancy and then higher during the final two trimesters. When women first develop diabetes during pregnancy (gestational diabetes), insulin requirements drop rapidly after delivery and most do not need to continue with insulin treatment.

Breast Feeding: Insulin requirements tend to be lower during breast feeding. Home glucose monitoring is important to avoid hypoglycemia. Insulin is not present in breast milk.

Infants and Children: Treatment with insulin in young patients is the same as that in older people with diabetes.

Special Concerns: Inadequate amounts of insulin in type 1 diabetes may lead to the serious complication of diabetic ketoacidosis, characterized by loss of appetite, excessive thirst and urination, nausea, vomiting, deep breathing, fruity breath odor, drowsiness, confusion, and loss of consciousness.

OVERDOSE

Symptoms: Insulin overdose results in hypoglycemia (see Side Effects for symptoms).

What to Do: For mild to moderate hypoglycemia, ingest drinks or food containing sugar. For more severe hypoglycemia, administer injections of glucagon or call emergency medical services (EMS) immediately.

DRUG INTERACTIONS

A large number of drugs can promote either elevated blood glucose levels or hypoglycemia. Be sure that your doctor knows about all of the medications you take and is informed before you start taking any new drugs, either by prescription or over the counter. Corticosteroids in particular are likely to raise blood glucose levels and insulin requirements. Beta-blockers (commonly prescribed for hypertension) may cause either high blood glucose levels or hypoglycemia; in addition, because these medications may dampen the symptoms of hypoglycemia that are caused by adrenaline release, mild degrees of hypoglycemia may progress unnoticed to more serious hypoglycemia affecting the brain.

FOOD INTERACTIONS

Insulin requirements are increased when larger amounts of calories are ingested, especially simple sugars and carbohydrates.

DISEASE INTERACTIONS

Insulin requirements are increased by infections, psychological stress, or an uncontrolled overactive thyroid, and often at a time of surgery. Requirements may diminish with kidney disease or an underactive adrenal or pituitary gland.

BRAND NAMES
Humulin U Ultralente,
Ultralente Iletin I (beef
and pork)

▶ Drug Class: Antidiabetic
agent

▶ Available in: Injection

▶ Available OTC? Yes

▶ As Generic? No

Side Effects

SERIOUS
Symptoms of hypo-
glycemia can be caused
by the release of adrena-
line or by an inadequate
supply of glucose to the
brain. With severe hypo-
glycemia, lack of suffi-
cient glucose to the
brain may cause slurred
speech, impaired concen-
tration, confusion,
seizures, coma, irre-
versible brain damage,
and death. Mild hypo-
glycemia may cause rest-
less sleep, nightmares, or
a cold sweat that awak-
ens patients at night.

COMMON
Symptoms resulting from
release of adrenaline are
common manifestations
of mild to moderate
hypoglycemia. They
include cold sweats,
anxiety, shakiness,
hunger, rapid heartbeat,
headache, and nervous-
ness. Weight gain is com-
mon when taking insulin.

LESS COMMON
Allergic reactions, lipoatrophy (depressions in the
skin due to loss of fat tissue), and lipohypertrophy
(excessive accumulation
of fat tissue).

PRINCIPAL USES
For long-term treatment
of diabetes mellitus. All
patients with type 1 diabetes
require lifelong insulin treatment. Patients with type 2
diabetes may require insulin
if they are unable to control
their blood glucose (sugar)
levels with diet and oral
medications.

HOW THE DRUG WORKS
Insulin, a hormone secreted
by the beta cells of the
pancreas, plays an essential
role in controlling the
metabolism and storage of
carbohydrates, fat, and protein. Insulin is secreted in
response to a rise in blood
sugar (glucose). Insulin
lowers blood glucose by
increasing its uptake by
body cells, especially muscle, and by reducing the
release of glucose from
the liver between meals.

DOSAGE
Injected 1 or 2 times a day.
Doses and frequency are
determined by your doctor.
Long-acting (Ultralente)
insulin can be mixed in the
same syringe with rapid-
acting insulin; draw up the
rapid-acting insulin first.
Long-acting insulin solu-
tions are cloudy (insulin
settles to the bottom of the
bottle) and must be rolled
or gently shaken to distribute the insulin evenly in the
solution before drawing it
up into the syringe.

ONSET OF EFFECT
Within 6 to 8 hours; the
peak effect occurs within
10 to 20 hours.

DURATION OF ACTION
From 24 to 36 hours.

DIETARY ADVICE
All patients with diabetes
should follow the general
dietary recommendations of
the American Diabetes
Association. Though intake
of simple sugars is not forbidden, consuming a large
amount of sugary foods at
one time may trigger a
rapid rise in blood glucose
that can increase urination
and thirst. In addition,
patients who take insulin
must remain consistent
from day to day in the timing and caloric content of
their meals. Depending on
the timing, dose, and types
of insulin prescribed, snacks
may be recommended in
the late afternoon, before
bedtime, or prior to unusual
physical activity. Diabetic
patients must always have
available a juice, food, or
tablets that can raise blood
glucose levels rapidly to
counter an episode of
hypoglycemia.

STORAGE
Refrigerate insulin but do
not allow it to freeze. Insulin
does not have to be kept
refrigerated when you're
traveling for short periods,
but exposure to high tem-
peratures must be avoided.

IF YOU MISS A DOSE
Timing of insulin doses is
extremely important. The
best approach is to measure
blood glucose and add a
dose of regular insulin if
your glucose levels are too
high. Otherwise, wait for
the next scheduled dose.

STOPPING THE DRUG
Do not stop taking insulin
injections unless ordered by
your doctor. Patients with
diabetes are often given
general instructions for
modifying their insulin
doses based on home blood
glucose measurements.

PROLONGED USE
After many years with
diabetes, some patients
become insensitive to the
symptoms of hypoglycemia
and are at risk for serious
brain complications of
prolonged, unrecognized
hypoglycemia.

PRECAUTIONS
Over 60: No special warnings. Some older people
may, however, have vision
problems that may make it
difficult to draw up the correct dose of insulin.

**Driving and Hazardous
Work:** Patients taking
insulin must be very careful
to avoid hypoglyccmia when
driving or engaging in hazardous work.

Alcohol: Moderate alcohol
intake, especially when
taken with large meals,
does not adversely affect
control of diabetes or alter
the dose of insulin. How-
ever, large amounts of
alcohol increase the risk
of hypoglycemia.

Pregnancy: Strict metabolic control—using insulin
injections in most women—
must be maintained during
pregnancy to reduce the
risk of birth defects, fetal
complications, or death at
the time of delivery. In
women who had diabetes
before the onset of preg-
nancy, the dose of insulin
is often smaller during the
first third (trimester) of
pregnancy and then higher
during the final two
trimesters. When women
first develop diabetes
during pregnancy (gesta-
tional diabetes), insulin
requirements drop rapidly
after delivery and most do
not need to continue with
insulin treatment.

Breast Feeding: Insulin
requirements tend to be
lower during breast feeding.
Home glucose monitoring is
important to avoid hypo-
glycemia. Insulin is not present in breast milk.

Infants and Children: Treatment with insulin in young patients is the same as that in older people with diabetes.

Special Concerns: Inadequate amounts of insulin in type 1 diabetes may lead to the serious complication of diabetic ketoacidosis, characterized by loss of appetite, excessive thirst and urination, nausea, vomiting, deep breathing, fruity breath odor, drowsiness, confusion, and loss of consciousness.

OVERDOSE

Symptoms: Insulin overdose results in hypoglycemia (see Side Effects for symptoms).

What to Do: For mild to moderate hypoglycemia, ingest drinks or food containing sugar. For more severe hypoglycemia, administer injections of glucagon or call emergency medical services (EMS) immediately.

DRUG INTERACTIONS

A large number of drugs can promote either elevated blood glucose levels or hypoglycemia. Be sure that your doctor knows about all of the medications you take and is informed before you start taking any new drugs, either by prescription or over the counter. Corticosteroids in particular are likely to raise blood glucose levels and insulin requirements. Beta-blockers (commonly prescribed for hypertension) may cause either high blood glucose levels or hypoglycemia; in addition, because these medications may dampen the symptoms of hypoglycemia that are caused by adrenaline release, mild degrees of hypoglycemia may progress unnoticed to more serious hypoglycemia affecting the brain.

FOOD INTERACTIONS

Insulin requirements are increased when larger amounts of calories are ingested, especially simple sugars and carbohydrates.

DISEASE INTERACTIONS

Insulin requirements are increased by infections, psychological stress, or an uncontrolled overactive thyroid, and often at a time of surgery. Requirements may diminish with kidney disease or an underactive adrenal or pituitary gland.

▶ Drug Class: Antidiabetic
agent

▶ Available in: Injection

▶ Available OTC? Yes

▶ As Generic? No

Side Effects

SERIOUS
Symptoms of hypo-
glycemia can be caused
by the release of adrena-
line or by an inadequate
supply of glucose to the
brain. With severe hypo-
glycemia, lack of suffi-
cient glucose to the
brain may cause slurred
speech, impaired concen-
tration, confusion,
seizures, coma, irre-
versible brain damage,
and death. Mild hypo-
glycemia may cause rest-
less sleep, nightmares, or
a cold sweat that awak-
ens patients at night.

COMMON
Symptoms resulting from
release of adrenaline are
common manifestations
of mild to moderate
hypoglycemia. They
include cold sweats,
anxiety, shakiness,
hunger, rapid heartbeat,
headache, and nervous-
ness. Weight gain is com-
mon when taking insulin.

LESS COMMON
Allergic reactions, lipoatrophy (depressions in the
skin due to loss of fat tissue), and lipohypertrophy
(excessive accumulation
of fat tissue).

PRINCIPAL USES
For long-term treatment
of diabetes mellitus. All
patients with type 1 diabetes
require lifelong insulin treatment. Patients with type 2
diabetes may require insulin
if they are unable to control
their blood glucose (sugar)
levels with diet and oral
medications.

HOW THE DRUG WORKS
Insulin, a hormone secreted
by the beta cells of the
pancreas, plays an essential
role in controlling the
metabolism and storage of
carbohydrates, fat, and protein. Insulin is secreted in
response to a rise in blood
sugar (glucose). Insulin
lowers blood glucose by
increasing its uptake by
body cells, especially muscle, and by reducing the
release of glucose from
the liver between meals.

DOSAGE
It may be taken 1 to 4 times
daily, before meals and possibly at bedtime. Doses and
frequency are determined
by your doctor. Regular (or
rapid-acting or semilente)
insulin should be administered 30 to 45 minutes
before a meal. It can be
mixed in the same syringe
with intermediate-acting
insulins. Draw up the regular insulin first.

ONSET OF EFFECT
Within 45 minutes; peak
effect occurs within 2 to 4
hours.

DURATION OF ACTION
From 4 to 6 hours.

DIETARY ADVICE
All patients with diabetes
should follow the general
dietary recommendations of
the American Diabetes
Association. Though intake
of simple sugars is not forbidden, consuming a large
amount of sugary foods at

one time may trigger a
rapid rise in blood glucose
that can increase urination
and thirst. In addition,
patients who take insulin
must remain consistent
from day to day in the timing and caloric content of
their meals. Depending on
the timing, dose, and types
of insulin prescribed, snacks
may be recommended in
the late afternoon, before
bedtime, or prior to unusual
physical activity. Diabetic
patients must always have
available a juice, food, or
tablets that can raise blood
glucose levels rapidly to
counter an episode of
hypoglycemia.

STORAGE
Refrigerate insulin but do
not allow it to freeze. Insulin
does not have to be kept
refrigerated when you're
traveling for short periods,
but exposure to high tem-
peratures must be avoided.

IF YOU MISS A DOSE
Timing of insulin doses is
extremely important. The
best approach is to measure
blood glucose and add a
dose of regular insulin if
glucose levels are too high.
Otherwise, wait for the next
scheduled dose.

STOPPING THE DRUG
Do not stop taking insulin
injections unless ordered by
your doctor. Patients with
diabetes are often given
general instructions for
modifying their insulin
doses based on home blood
glucose measurements.

PROLONGED USE
After many years with
diabetes, some patients
become insensitive to the
symptoms of hypoglycemia
and are at risk for serious
brain complications of
prolonged, unrecognized
hypoglycemia.

PRECAUTIONS
Over 60: No special warnings. Some older people
may, however, have vision
problems that may make it
difficult to draw up the correct dose of insulin.

**Driving and Hazardous
Work:** Patients taking
insulin must be very careful
to avoid hypoglycemia when
driving or engaging in hazardous work.

Alcohol: Moderate alcohol
intake, especially when
taken with large meals,
does not adversely affect
control of diabetes or alter
the dose of insulin. How-
ever, large amounts of
alcohol increase the risk
of hypoglycemia.

Pregnancy: Strict metabolic control—using insulin
injections in most women—
must be maintained during
pregnancy to reduce the
risk of birth defects, fetal
complications, or death at
the time of delivery. In
women who had diabetes
before the onset of preg-
nancy, the dose of insulin
is often smaller during the
first third (trimester) of
pregnancy and then higher
during the final two
trimesters. When women
first develop diabetes
during pregnancy (gesta-
tional diabetes), insulin
requirements drop rapidly
after delivery and most do
not need to continue with
insulin treatment.

Breast Feeding: Insulin
requirements tend to be
lower during breast feeding.
Home glucose monitoring is
important to avoid hypo-
glycemia. Insulin is not present in breast milk.

Infants and Children:
Treatment with insulin in
young patients is the same

as that in older people with diabetes.

Special Concerns: Inadequate amounts of insulin in type 1 diabetes may lead to the serious complication of diabetic ketoacidosis, characterized by loss of appetite, excessive thirst and urination, nausea, vomiting, deep breathing, fruity breath odor, drowsiness, confusion, and loss of consciousness.

OVERDOSE

Symptoms: Insulin overdose results in hypoglycemia (see Side Effects for symptoms).

What to Do: For mild to moderate hypoglycemia, ingest drinks or food containing sugar. For more severe hypoglycemia, administer injections of glucagon or call emergency medical services (EMS) immediately.

DRUG INTERACTIONS

A large number of drugs can promote either elevated blood glucose levels or hypoglycemia. Be sure that your doctor knows about all of the medications you take and is informed before you start taking any new drugs, either by prescription or over the counter. Corticosteroids in particular are likely to raise blood glucose levels and insulin requirements. Beta-blockers (commonly prescribed for hypertension) may cause either high blood glucose levels or hypoglycemia; in addition, because these medications may dampen the symptoms of hypoglycemia that are caused by adrenaline release, mild degrees of hypoglycemia may progress unnoticed to more serious hypoglycemia affecting the brain.

FOOD INTERACTIONS

Insulin requirements are increased when larger amounts of calories are ingested, especially simple sugars and carbohydrates.

DISEASE INTERACTIONS

Insulin requirements are increased by infections, psychological stress, or an uncontrolled overactive thyroid, and often at a time of surgery. Requirements may diminish with kidney disease or an underactive adrenal or pituitary gland.

Interferon alfa-2a

BRAND NAME
Roferon-A

▶ Drug Class: Immunomodulator

▶ Available in: Injection

▶ Available OTC? No

▶ As Generic? No

Side Effects

SERIOUS
Confusion, depression, nervousness, distractibility, impaired thinking, or thoughts of suicide; numbness or tingling of fingers, toes, and face; black, tarry, or bloody stools; blood in urine; chest pain; hoarseness; fever or chills after 3 weeks of treatment; irregular heartbeat; pain in lower back or side; difficult or painful urination; red spots on skin; unusual bleeding or bruising; increased incidence of infections. Call your doctor immediately.

COMMON
Flu-like symptoms, fatigue, muscle aches, fever, or chills in first weeks of treatment; general discomfort or ill feeling; headache; loss of appetite; nausea and vomiting; odd, metallic, or altered taste; skin rash; temporary hair loss. Side effects are more common with higher doses. Tolerance to high doses may be improved by gradually increasing the doses over the first weeks of treatment.

LESS COMMON
Back pain, blurred vision, dizziness, dry mouth, dry or itching skin, profuse or unusual sweating, joint pain, leg cramps, lip or mouth sores, weight loss.

PRINCIPAL USES
To treat hairy-cell leukemia, AIDS-associated Kaposi's sarcoma, or chronic myelogenous leukemia.

HOW THE DRUG WORKS
Interferon alfa-2a acts in the same way as the body's natural interferons, which are proteins released by cells of the immune system to fight viruses and cancer cells.

DOSAGE
For hairy-cell leukemia: 3 million units daily by injection for 16 to 24 weeks. Then 3 million units 3 times a week for maintenance. For AIDS-related Kaposi's sarcoma: 36 million units daily for 10 to 12 weeks, then 36 million units 3 times a week. For Philadelphia chromosome-positive (Ph+) chronic myelogenous leukemia: 9 million units daily for the duration of treatment or as determined by your doctor.

ONSET OF EFFECT
Unknown.

DURATION OF ACTION
Unknown.

DIETARY ADVICE
Drink plenty of fluids to reduce the risk of excessively low blood pressure.

STORAGE
Keep interferon alfa-2a refrigerated but do not allow it to freeze.

IF YOU MISS A DOSE
If you miss a dose, do not take the missed dose and do not double the next dose. Check with your doctor on what to do.

STOPPING THE DRUG
The decision to stop taking the drug should be made by your doctor.

PROLONGED USE
See your doctor regularly for tests and examinations if you must take this drug for a prolonged period.

PRECAUTIONS
Over 60: Adverse reactions may be more likely and more severe in older patients.

Driving and Hazardous Work: Avoid such activities until you determine how the medicine affects you. Administering interferon at bedtime may help to minimize daytime sleepiness.

Alcohol: Avoid alcohol.

Pregnancy: Adequate studies have not been done. Consult your doctor for advice.

Breast Feeding: Interferon alfa-2a may pass into breast milk; caution is advised. Consult your doctor for advice.

Infants and Children: Severe adverse effects have been noted in some children treated with high doses of interferon. Consult your pediatrician for advice.

Special Concerns: Do not change to another brand of alfa interferon without consulting your doctor. They have different dosage schedules. Try to avoid people with infections, because this drug can lower white blood cell levels temporarily and increase susceptibility to disease. Be careful when cleaning your teeth, and avoid cutting yourself when using sharp objects such as a razor. Avoid contact sports or other situations where bruising could occur.

OVERDOSE
Symptoms: No specific ones have been reported.

What to Do: Call your doctor or emergency medical services (EMS) immediately if you suspect an overdose.

DRUG INTERACTIONS
Consult your doctor for specific advice if you are taking any prescription or over-the-counter medication, especially theophylline, or central nervous system depressants including antihistamines, alcohol, tranquilizers, or psychiatric medications.

FOOD INTERACTIONS
None are known.

DISEASE INTERACTIONS
Consult your doctor if you have a history of bleeding or clotting disorders, chicken pox, shingles, psychological or neurological disorders, seizures, diabetes, heart attack, heart disease, kidney disease, liver disease, lung disease, autoimmune disorders, or thyroid disease.

Interferon alfa-2b

▶ Drug Class: Immunomodulator

▶ Available in: Injection

▶ Available OTC? No

▶ As Generic? No

Side Effects

SERIOUS
Confusion, depression, nervousness, distractibility, or impaired thinking; numbness or tingling of fingers, toes, and face; sleeping difficulty; black, tarry, or bloody stools; blood in urine; chest pain, cough, or hoarseness; fever or chills after 3 weeks of treatment; irregular heartbeat; pain in lower back or side; difficult or painful urination; red spots on skin; unusual bleeding or bruising; increased incidence of infections. Call your doctor immediately.

COMMON
Flu-like symptoms, fatigue, muscle aches, fever, or chills in first weeks of treatment; general discomfort or ill feeling; headache; loss of appetite; nausea and vomiting; odd, metallic, or altered taste; skin rash; temporary hair loss. Side effects are more common with higher doses. Tolerance to high doses may be improved by gradually increasing the doses over the first weeks of treatment.

LESS COMMON
Back pain, blurred vision, dizziness, dry mouth, dry or itching skin, profuse or unusual sweating, joint pain, leg cramps, lip or mouth sores, weight loss.

PRINCIPAL USES
To treat hairy-cell leukemia, AIDS-associated Kaposi's sarcoma, condylomata acuminata (genital warts), and types of chronic hepatitis; also used as an adjuvant (supplemental) treatment to surgery for malignant melanoma.

HOW THE DRUG WORKS
It acts in the same way as the body's natural interferons, which are proteins released by the cells of the immune system to fight viruses and cancer cells.

DOSAGE
For hairy-cell leukemia: 2 million units per square meter of body surface 3 times a week. For AIDS-related Kaposi's sarcoma: 30 million units 3 times a week. For condylomata acuminata: 1 million units per lesion 3 times a week for 3 weeks. For chronic hepatitis: 3 million units 3 times a week for 6 months (in patients with evidence of response). For malignant melanoma: 20 million units per square meter of body surface for 5 consecutive days per week for 4 weeks, followed by maintenance with 10 million units per square meter 3 times a week for 48 weeks.

ONSET OF EFFECT
Unknown.

DURATION OF ACTION
Unknown.

DIETARY ADVICE
Drink plenty of fluids to reduce the risk of excessively low blood pressure.

STORAGE
Keep interferon alfa-2b refrigerated but do not allow it to freeze.

IF YOU MISS A DOSE
If you miss a dose, do not take the missed dose and do not double the next dose. Check with your doctor on what to do.

STOPPING THE DRUG
The decision to stop taking the drug should be made by your doctor.

PROLONGED USE
See your doctor regularly for tests and examinations if you must take this drug for a prolonged period.

PRECAUTIONS
Over 60: Adverse reactions may be more likely and more severe in older patients.

Driving and Hazardous Work: Do not drive or engage in hazardous work until you determine how the medicine affects you. Administering interferon at bedtime may help to minimize daytime sleepiness.

Alcohol: Avoid alcohol.

Pregnancy: Adequate studies have not been done. Consult your doctor for advice.

Breast Feeding: This drug may pass into breast milk; caution is advised. Consult your doctor for advice.

Infants and Children: May be used to treat chronic hepatitis B in children aged 1 and older; consult your pediatrician for advice and dosage.

Special Concerns: Do not change to another brand without consulting your doctor. They have different dosage schedules. Try to avoid people with infections, because this drug can lower white blood cell levels temporarily and increase susceptibility to disease. Be careful when cleaning your teeth, and avoid cutting yourself when using sharp objects such as a razor. Avoid contact sports or other situations where bruising could occur.

OVERDOSE
Symptoms: No specific ones have been reported.

What to Do: Call your doctor or emergency medical services (EMS) immediately if you suspect an overdose.

DRUG INTERACTIONS
Consult your doctor for specific advice if you are taking any prescription or over-the-counter medication, especially central nervous system depressants including antihistamines, alcohol, tranquilizers, or psychiatric medications.

FOOD INTERACTIONS
None are known.

DISEASE INTERACTIONS
Consult your doctor if you have a history of bleeding or clotting disorders, chicken pox, shingles, psychological or neurological disorders, diabetes, autoimmune disorders, or heart, kidney, liver, lung, or thyroid disease.

Interferon alfa-n1

BRAND NAME
Wellferon

▶ Drug Class: Immunomodulator

▶ Available in: Injection

▶ Available OTC? No

▶ As Generic? No

Side Effects

SERIOUS
Confusion, depression, nervousness, distractibility, impaired thinking, or thoughts of suicide; numbness or tingling of fingers, toes, and face; black, tarry, or bloody stools; blood in urine; chest pain; hoarseness; fever or chills after 3 weeks of treatment; irregular heartbeat; pain in lower back or side; difficult or painful urination; red spots on skin; unusual bleeding or bruising; increased incidence of infections. Call your doctor immediately.

COMMON
Flu-like symptoms, fatigue, muscle aches, fever, or chills in first weeks of treatment; general discomfort or ill feeling; headache; loss of appetite; nausea and vomiting; odd, metallic, or altered taste; skin rash; temporary hair loss. Side effects are more common with higher doses. Tolerance to high doses may be improved by gradually increasing the doses over the first weeks of treatment.

LESS COMMON
Back pain, blurred vision, dizziness, dry mouth, dry or itching skin, profuse or unusual sweating, joint pain, leg cramps, lip or mouth sores, weight loss.

PRINCIPAL USES
To treat hairy-cell leukemia, condylomata acuminata (genital warts), or juvenile laryngeal papillomatosis (abnormal growths in the voice box, occurring in children).

HOW THE DRUG WORKS
It acts in the same way as the body's natural interferons, which are proteins released by the cells of the immune system to fight viruses and cancer cells.

DOSAGE
For hairy-cell leukemia: 3 million units a day by injection for 16 to 24 weeks, then 3 million units 3 times a week. For condylomata acuminata: 1 million units per square meter of body surface 5 times a week, then the same dose 5 times a week for 2 weeks, then 3 times a week for 4 weeks, then 3 times a week for 1 month. For juvenile laryngeal papillomatosis: The dose is based on area of body surface and is given daily for 26 days, followed by maintenance dosage 3 times a week for at least 6 months.

ONSET OF EFFECT
Unknown.

DURATION OF ACTION
Unknown.

DIETARY ADVICE
Drink plenty of fluids to reduce the risk of excessively low blood pressure.

STORAGE
Keep interferon alfa-n1 refrigerated but do not allow it to freeze.

IF YOU MISS A DOSE
If you miss a dose, do not take the missed dose and do not double the next dose. Check with your doctor on what to do.

STOPPING THE DRUG
The decision to stop taking the drug should be made by your doctor.

PROLONGED USE
See your doctor regularly for tests and examinations if you must take this drug for a prolonged period.

PRECAUTIONS
Over 60: Adverse reactions may be more likely and more severe in older patients.

Driving and Hazardous Work: Do not drive or engage in hazardous work until you determine how the medicine affects you. Administering interferon at bedtime may help to minimize daytime sleepiness.

Alcohol: Avoid alcohol.

Pregnancy: Adequate studies have not been done. Consult your doctor for advice.

Breast Feeding: Interferon alfa-n1 may pass into breast milk; caution is advised. Consult your doctor for advice.

Infants and Children: No special studies have been done; consult your pediatrician.

Special Concerns: Do not change to another brand of alfa interferon without consulting your doctor. They have different dosage schedules. Try to avoid people with infections, because this drug can lower white blood cell levels temporarily and increase susceptibility to disease. Be careful when cleaning your teeth, and avoid cutting yourself when using sharp objects such as a razor. Avoid contact sports or other situations where bruising could occur.

OVERDOSE
Symptoms: No specific ones have been reported.

What to Do: Call your doctor or emergency medical services (EMS) immediately if you suspect an overdose.

DRUG INTERACTIONS
Consult your doctor for specific advice if you are taking any prescription or over-the-counter medication, especially central nervous system depressants including antihistamines, alcohol, tranquilizers, or psychiatric medications.

FOOD INTERACTIONS
None are known.

DISEASE INTERACTIONS
Consult your doctor if you have a history of bleeding or clotting disorders, chicken pox, shingles, psychological or neurological disorders, diabetes, autoimmune disorders, heart disease, kidney disease, liver disease, lung disease, or thyroid disease.

Interferon alfa-n3

▶ Drug Class: Immunomodulator

▶ Available in: Injection

▶ Available OTC? No

▶ As Generic? No

Side Effects

SERIOUS
Confusion, depression, nervousness, distractibility, impaired thinking, or thoughts of suicide; numbness or tingling of fingers, toes, and face; black, tarry, or bloody stools; blood in urine; chest pain; hoarseness; fever or chills after 3 weeks of treatment; irregular heartbeat; pain in lower back or side; difficult or painful urination; red spots on skin; unusual bleeding or bruising; increased incidence of infections. Call your doctor immediately.

COMMON
Flu-like symptoms, fatigue, muscle aches, fever, or chills in first weeks of treatment; general discomfort or ill feeling; headache; loss of appetite; nausea and vomiting; odd, metallic, or altered taste; skin rash; temporary hair loss. Side effects are more common with higher doses. Tolerance to high doses may be improved by gradually increasing the doses over the first weeks of treatment.

LESS COMMON
Back pain, blurred vision, dizziness, dry mouth, dry or itching skin, profuse or unusual sweating, joint pain, leg cramps, lip or mouth sores, weight loss.

PRINCIPAL USES
To treat condylomata acuminata (genital or venereal warts) in patients 18 years of age or older.

HOW THE DRUG WORKS
It acts in the same way as the body's natural interferons, which are proteins released by the immune system to fight viruses, cancer cells, and other types of disease. Interferon alfa-n3 is derived from human white blood cells and has an antiviral effect.

DOSAGE
0.05 ml injected into each wart 2 times a week for up to 8 weeks. Total dose for each session should not exceed 0.5 ml (2.5 million units).

ONSET OF EFFECT
Unknown.

DURATION OF ACTION
Unknown; however, warts will continue to disappear after completion of 8 weeks of therapy and discontinuation of the drug.

DIETARY ADVICE
Drink plenty of fluids to reduce risk of excessively low blood pressure.

STORAGE
Keep interferon alfa-n3 refrigerated but do not allow it to freeze.

IF YOU MISS A DOSE
If you miss a dose, do not take the missed dose and do not double the next dose. Check with your doctor on what to do.

STOPPING THE DRUG
The decision to stop taking the drug should be made by your doctor.

PROLONGED USE
See your doctor regularly for tests and examinations if you must take this drug for a prolonged period.

PRECAUTIONS
Over 60: Adverse reactions may be more likely and more severe in older patients.

Driving and Hazardous Work: Do not drive or engage in hazardous work until you determine how the medicine affects you. Administering interferon at bedtime may help to minimize daytime sleepiness.

Alcohol: Avoid alcohol.

Pregnancy: Adequate studies have not been done. Consult your doctor for advice.

Breast Feeding: Interferon alfa-n3 may pass into breast milk; caution is advised. Consult your doctor for advice.

Infants and Children: No special studies have been done; consult your pediatrician.

Special Concerns: Do not change to another brand of alfa interferon without consulting your doctor. They have different dosage schedules. Try to avoid people with infections, because this drug can lower white blood cell levels temporarily and increase susceptibility to disease. Be careful when cleaning your teeth, and avoid cutting yourself when using sharp objects such as a razor. Avoid contact sports or other situations where bruising could occur.

OVERDOSE
Symptoms: No specific ones have been reported.

What to Do: Call your doctor or emergency medical services (EMS) immediately if you suspect an overdose.

DRUG INTERACTIONS
Consult your doctor for specific advice if you are taking any prescription or over-the-counter medication, especially central nervous system depressants including antihistamines, alcohol, tranquilizers, or psychiatric medications.

FOOD INTERACTIONS
None are known.

DISEASE INTERACTIONS
Caution is advised when taking interferon alfa-n3. Consult your doctor if you have a history of bleeding or clotting disorders, chicken pox, shingles, psychological or neurological disorders, diabetes, autoimmune disorders, heart disease, kidney disease, liver disease, lung disease, or thyroid disease.

Interferon alfacon-1

Side Effects

SERIOUS
Confusion, depression, nervousness, distractibility, or impaired thinking; numbness or tingling of fingers, toes, and face; sleeping difficulty; black, tarry, or bloody stools; blood in urine; chest pain, cough, or hoarseness; fever or chills after 3 weeks of treatment; irregular heartbeat; pain in lower back or side; difficult or painful urination; red spots on skin; unusual bleeding or bruising; increased incidence of infections. Call your doctor immediately.

COMMON
Flu-like symptoms, fatigue, muscle aches, fever, or chills in first weeks of treatment; general discomfort or ill feeling; headache; loss of appetite; nausea and vomiting; odd, metallic, or altered taste; skin rash; temporary hair loss. Side effects are more common with higher doses. Tolerance to high doses may be improved by gradually increasing the doses over the first weeks of treatment.

LESS COMMON
Back pain, blurred vision, dizziness, dry mouth, dry or itching skin, profuse or unusual sweating, joint pain, leg cramps, lip or mouth sores, weight loss.

PRINCIPAL USES
To treat chronic hepatitis C infection in people age 18 and older who have developed liver disease.

HOW THE DRUG WORKS
It acts in the same way as the body's natural interferons, which are proteins released by the cells of the immune system to fight viruses.

DOSAGE
For people who have never been treated with interferons: 9 micrograms (mcg) injected under the skin 3 times a week for 24 weeks, with at least 48 hours between doses. For people who have undergone previous interferon therapy and either did not respond to it or relapsed following discontinuation of therapy: 15 mcg under the skin 3 times a week for 6 months.

ONSET OF EFFECT
Unknown.

DURATION OF ACTION
Unknown.

DIETARY ADVICE
Drink plenty of fluids to reduce the risk of excessively low blood pressure.

STORAGE
Refrigerate the drug but do not allow it to freeze. Do not expose it to high temperatures or direct sunlight. Store it on a separate shelf or in a drawer, away from food. Just prior to administration, interferon alfacon-1 may be allowed to reach room temperature.

IF YOU MISS A DOSE
If you miss a dose, do not take the missed dose and do not double the next dose. Check with your doctor on what to do.

STOPPING THE DRUG
The decision to stop taking the drug should be made by your doctor.

PROLONGED USE
See your doctor regularly for tests and examinations if you take this drug for a prolonged period.

PRECAUTIONS
Over 60: Adverse reactions may be more likely and more severe in older patients.

Driving and Hazardous Work: Do not drive or engage in hazardous work until you determine how the medicine affects you.

Alcohol: No special precautions are necessary.

Pregnancy: Adequate human studies have not been done. Interferon alfacon-1 should not be used during pregnancy.

Breast Feeding: Interferon alfacon-1 may pass into breast milk; caution is advised. Consult your doctor for specific advice.

Infants and Children: Not recommended for patients under age 18.

Special Concerns: Do not shake the vial prior to administration. If the liquid in the vial is cloudy or discolored, do not use it. Discard any unused portion. Do not change to another brand of interferon without consulting your doctor. They have different dosage schedules. To help prevent the spread of hepatitis C, do not share razors or toothbrushes; cover any cuts or wounds; dispose of wound dressings in a sealed bag in the trash; keep used syringes for injecting interferon, insulin, or other medications capped and in a needle disposal container; use a condom if you have multiple sexual partners or if you have a genital herpes infection; and do not donate blood. It is safe to have close contact with others, to dispose of facial tissues normally, to share dinnerware, and to breast-feed.

OVERDOSE
Symptoms: An overdose with interferon alfacon-1 is unlikely. However, with a very high dose, you may experience some side effects more acutely, particularly loss of appetite, chills, fever, and muscle pain.

What to Do: If you take a much larger dose than prescribed, call your doctor or get emergency medical attention immediately.

DRUG INTERACTIONS
Consult your doctor for specific advice if you are taking any prescription or over-the-counter medication, especially central nervous system depressants including antihistamines, alcohol, tranquilizers, or psychiatric medications.

FOOD INTERACTIONS
No known food interactions.

DISEASE INTERACTIONS
Interferon alfacon-1 should not be taken by patients with severe depression, suicidal feelings, or a history of other severe psychiatric disorders. Those with pre-existing heart disease must use this drug with special caution. Consult your doctor for specific advice if you have a history of bleeding or clotting disorders, chicken pox, shingles, psychological or neurological disorders, diabetes, autoimmune disorders, kidney disease, liver disease, lung disease, or thyroid disease.

Interferon beta-1a

Avonex

▶ Drug Class: Immunomodulator

▶ Available in: Powder for injection

▶ Available OTC? No

▶ As Generic? No

Side Effects

SERIOUS
Seizures, swelling and fluid retention, pelvic pain, pounding in the chest, breast pain, frequent urination, sweating, anxiety, confusion, joint pain, breathing difficulty, mental depression, suicidal thoughts or impulses. Call your physician right away.

COMMON
Pain, inflammation, or allergic reaction at injection site (most common side effect); flu-like symptoms, including headache, fever, muscle aches, general weakness, and fatigue (these symptoms tend to diminish as the body adjusts to therapy); insomnia; increased susceptibility to infection; nausea and vomiting; diarrhea; abdominal pain; temporary hair loss.

LESS COMMON
Dizziness, dry mouth, dry or itching skin, increased sweating, joint pain, changes in vision, hearing problems.

PRINCIPAL USES
To treat relapsing-remitting multiple sclerosis (the most common form of MS, in which periods of active disease alternate with periods of remission or reduced severity of symptoms).

HOW THE DRUG WORKS
It acts in the same way as the body's natural interferons, which are proteins released by the immune system to fight viruses, cancer cells, and other types of disease. The exact way in which the drug fights MS is unknown, but it appears to interfere with the immune system's attack on healthy tissue (the apparent cause of MS).

DOSAGE
6 million units once a week by injection.

ONSET OF EFFECT
Unknown.

DURATION OF ACTION
Unknown.

DIETARY ADVICE
Drink plenty of fluids to reduce the risk of excessively low blood pressure.

STORAGE
Keep liquid form of interferon beta-1a refrigerated but do not allow it to freeze.

IF YOU MISS A DOSE
If you miss a dose, do not take the missed dose and do not double the next dose. Check with your doctor on what to do.

STOPPING THE DRUG
The decision to stop taking the drug should be made by your doctor.

PROLONGED USE
See your doctor regularly for tests and examinations if you must take this drug for a prolonged period.

PRECAUTIONS
Over 60: Adverse reactions may be more likely and more severe in older patients.

Driving and Hazardous Work: Do not drive or engage in hazardous work until you determine how the medicine affects you.

Alcohol: Avoid alcohol.

Pregnancy: Adequate studies have not been done. Consult your doctor for advice.

Breast Feeding: Interferon beta-1a may pass into breast milk; caution is advised. Consult your doctor for advice.

Infants and Children: No special studies have been done on the effects of beta interferon in children.

Special Concerns: Interferon beta-1a should be used with caution in patients with a history of depression, since it has been linked to an increase in suicidal impulses. Try to avoid people with infections, because this drug can lower white blood cell levels temporarily and increase susceptibility to disease. Be careful when using a toothbrush, dental floss, or toothpick. Your doctor or dentist may recommend other ways to clean your teeth. Check with your doctor before having any dental work done. Be careful not to cut yourself when using sharp objects such as a razor. Avoid contact sports or other situations where bruising could occur. Do not touch your eyes or the inside of your mouth unless you have just washed your hands.

OVERDOSE
Symptoms: No specific ones have been reported.

What to Do: Call your doctor or emergency medical services (EMS) immediately if you suspect an overdose.

DRUG INTERACTIONS
Consult your doctor for specific advice if you are taking any prescription or over-the-counter medication.

FOOD INTERACTIONS
None are known.

DISEASE INTERACTIONS
Caution is advised when taking interferon beta-1a. Consult your doctor if you have a history of bleeding or clotting disorders, chicken pox, shingles, psychological or neurological disorders, diabetes, autoimmune disorders, heart disease, kidney disease, liver disease, lung disease, or thyroid disease.

BRAND NAME
Betaseron

▶ Drug Class: Immunomodulator

▶ Available in: Powder for injection

▶ Available OTC? No

▶ As Generic? No

Side Effects

SERIOUS
Seizures, swelling and fluid retention, pelvic pain, pounding in the chest, breast pain, frequent urination, sweating, anxiety, confusion, joint pain, breathing difficulty, mental depression, suicidal thoughts or impulses. Call your doctor right away.

COMMON
Pain, inflammation, or allergic reaction at injection site (most common side effect); flu-like symptoms, including headache, fever, muscle aches, general weakness, and fatigue (these symptoms tend to diminish as the body adjusts to therapy); insomnia; increased susceptibility to infection; nausea and vomiting; diarrhea; abdominal pain; temporary hair loss.

LESS COMMON
Dizziness, dry mouth, dry or itching skin, increased sweating, joint pain, vision or hearing problems. Tissue death at the site of injection has occurred in a few patients.

PRINCIPAL USES
To treat relapsing-remitting multiple sclerosis (the most common form of MS, in which periods of active disease alternate with periods of remission or reduced severity of symptoms).

HOW THE DRUG WORKS
It acts in the same way as the body's natural interferons, which are proteins released by the immune system to fight viruses, cancer cells, and other types of disease. The exact way in which this drug fights MS is unknown, but it appears to interfere with the immune system's attack on healthy tissue.

DOSAGE
8 million units (0.25 mg) by injection every other day.

ONSET OF EFFECT
Unknown.

DURATION OF ACTION
Unknown.

DIETARY ADVICE
Drink plenty of fluids to reduce the risk of excessively low blood pressure.

STORAGE
Keep the liquid form refrigerated but do not allow it to freeze.

IF YOU MISS A DOSE
If you miss a dose, do not take the missed dose and do not double the next dose. Notify your doctor.

STOPPING THE DRUG
The decision to stop taking the drug should be made by your doctor.

PROLONGED USE
See your doctor regularly for tests and examinations if you must take this drug for a prolonged period.

PRECAUTIONS
Over 60: Adverse reactions may be more likely and more severe in older patients.

Driving and Hazardous Work: Do not drive or engage in hazardous work until you determine how the medicine affects you.

Alcohol: Avoid alcohol.

Pregnancy: Adequate studies have not been done. Consult your doctor for advice.

Breast Feeding: Interferon beta-1b may pass into breast milk; caution is advised. Consult your doctor for specific advice.

Infants and Children: No special studies have been done on the effects of beta interferon in children.

Special Concerns: Interferon beta-1b should be used with caution in patients with a history of depression, since it has been linked to an increase in suicidal impulses. Try to avoid people with infections, because this drug can lower white blood cell levels temporarily and increase susceptibility to disease. Be careful when using a toothbrush, dental floss, or toothpick. Your doctor or dentist may recommend other ways to clean your teeth. Check with your doctor before having any dental work done. Be careful not to cut yourself when using sharp objects such as a razor. Avoid contact sports or other situations where bruising could occur. Do not touch your eyes or the inside of your mouth unless you have just washed your hands.

OVERDOSE
Symptoms: No specific ones have been reported.

What to Do: Call your doctor or emergency medical services (EMS) immediately if you suspect an overdose.

DRUG INTERACTIONS
Consult your doctor for specific advice if you are taking any prescription or over-the-counter medication.

FOOD INTERACTIONS
None are known.

DISEASE INTERACTIONS
Caution is advised when taking interferon beta-1b. Consult your doctor if you have a history of bleeding or clotting disorders, chicken pox, shingles, psychological or neurological disorders, diabetes, autoimmune disorders, heart disease, kidney disease, liver disease, lung disease, or thyroid disease.

Interferon gamma-1b

BRAND NAME
Actimmune

▶ Drug Class: Immunomodulator

▶ Available in: Injection

▶ Available OTC? No

▶ As Generic? No

Side Effects

SERIOUS
Black, tarry, or bloody stools; blood in the urine; painful or difficult urination; pain in the lower back or side; loss of balance or coordination; mental confusion and impaired thinking; mask-like facial expression; trouble walking or shuffling gait; red spots on the skin; stiffness of arms or legs; trembling and shaking of hands and fingers; trouble speaking or swallowing. Call your doctor right away.

COMMON
Muscle aches, diarrhea, fever and chills, general discomfort or feelings of illness, headache, nausea or vomiting, skin rash, unusual fatigue, increased incidence of infections, unusual bleeding or bruising.

LESS COMMON
Dizziness, joint pain, loss of appetite, weight loss, cough or hoarseness.

PRINCIPAL USES
To treat chronic granulomatous disease (an inherited disorder characterized by recurring infections and the widespread growth of lesions or tumors in the skin, lungs, and lymphatic system).

HOW THE DRUG WORKS
It acts in the same way as the body's natural interferons, which are proteins released by the immune system to fight viruses, cancer cells, and other types of disease. Of all the interferons, interferon gamma has the greatest immunomodulator properties (ability to alter the efficacy of the immune system).

DOSAGE
For adults with body surface area greater than 0.5 square meters: 1.5 million units (50 micrograms) per square meter by injection 3 times a week. For adults with body surface area less than 0.5 square meters: 1.5 micrograms per 2.2 lbs (1 kg) of body weight 3 times a week. The preferred injection sites are the deltoid (shoulder) muscle or the front thigh muscle.

ONSET OF EFFECT
Unknown.

DURATION OF ACTION
Unknown.

DIETARY ADVICE
Drink plenty of fluids to reduce the risk of excessively low blood pressure.

STORAGE
Keep interferon gamma-1b refrigerated but do not allow it to freeze.

IF YOU MISS A DOSE
If you miss a dose, do not take the missed dose and do not double the next dose. Check with your doctor on what to do.

STOPPING THE DRUG
The decision to stop taking the drug should be made by your doctor.

PROLONGED USE
See your doctor regularly for tests and examinations if you must take this drug for a prolonged period.

PRECAUTIONS
Over 60: No special problems are expected.

Driving and Hazardous Work: Do not drive or engage in hazardous work until you determine how the medicine affects you.

Alcohol: Avoid alcohol.

Pregnancy: Very large doses of interferon gamma-1b have increased fetal deaths and uterine bleeding in animals. Before you take interferon gamma-1b, tell your doctor if you are pregnant or plan to become pregnant.

Breast Feeding: Interferon gamma-1b may pass into breast milk; caution is advised. Consult your doctor for specific advice.

Infants and Children: Interferon gamma-1b is not expected to cause different side effects or problems in infants and children than it does in other age groups.

Special Concerns: Taking interferon gamma-1b at bedtime can help to minimize its flu-like side effects. Your doctor may want you to take acetaminophen before each injection to avoid such side effects. Your doctor may tell you to drink extra fluids to prevent low blood pressure caused by loss of too much water. Interferon gamma-1b may make you more sensitive to sunlight. Use sunscreen or wear protective clothing.

OVERDOSE
Symptoms: No specific ones have been reported.

What to Do: Call your doctor or emergency medical services (EMS) immediately if you have any reason to suspect an overdose.

DRUG INTERACTIONS
Consult your doctor for specific advice if you are taking any prescription or over-the-counter medication.

FOOD INTERACTIONS
No known food interactions.

DISEASE INTERACTIONS
Caution is advised when taking interferon gamma-1b. Consult your doctor if you have a history of seizures, mental or psychiatric illness, heart disease, multiple sclerosis, or systemic lupus erythematosus (which may be worsened by gamma interferon).

BRAND NAMES
Lugol's Solution, Strong
Iodine (generic)

▶ Drug Class: Thyroid agent

▶ Available in: Oral solution

▶ Available OTC? No

▶ As Generic? Yes

Side Effects

SERIOUS
Fever, swollen glands,
rash, joint pain. Call your
doctor immediately.

COMMON
Nausea, metallic taste.

LESS COMMON
Fever, headache,
inflamed salivary glands,
runny nose, stained
teeth, swelling around
eyes, warm and red-
dened skin, pinkeye,
stomach upset, vomiting,
diarrhea, sores on
mucous membranes.

PRINCIPAL USES
To treat an overactive
thyroid gland (hyperthy-
roidism); to treat iodine
deficiency; to prepare for
thyroid surgery.

HOW THE DRUG WORKS
Strong iodine blocks
production and release of
thyroid hormone by the
thyroid gland.

DOSAGE
For overactive thyroid
gland, adults and children
over age 10: 1 ml, 3 times a
day. To prepare for thyroid
surgery: 0.1 ml, 3 times a
day for 10 to 14 days.

ONSET OF EFFECT
Unknown.

DURATION OF ACTION
Unknown.

DIETARY ADVICE
Take with a glass of fruit
juice, milk, or broth to minimize stomach upset. Drink
all of the liquid to get the
full dose of the medicine.

STORAGE
Keep the solution refrigerated, but do not allow it to
freeze.

IF YOU MISS A DOSE
Take it as soon as you
remember. If it is near the
time for the next dose, skip
the missed dose and
resume your regular dosage
schedule. Do not double the
next dose.

STOPPING THE DRUG
The decision to stop taking
the drug should be made by
your doctor.

PROLONGED USE
It is necessary to see your
physician regularly to check
the progress of treatment
when taking strong iodine
for a prolonged period.

PRECAUTIONS
Over 60: While no specific
studies of the use of strong
iodine in older persons have
been done, no special problems or side effects are
expected in older patients.

**Driving and Hazardous
Work:** Use of strong iodine
should not impair your ability to perform such tasks
safely.

Alcohol: No special precautions are necessary.

Pregnancy: Iodine can
cross the placenta and
cause thyroid problems or
goiter in the fetus. Before
you take strong iodine, tell
your doctor if you are pregnant or plan to become
pregnant.

Breast Feeding: Strong
iodine passes into breast
milk; avoid or discontinue
use while nursing.

Infants and Children:
The use and dose of strong
iodine in an infant or a child
must be determined by
your doctor.

Special Concerns: Take
the oral solution by mouth
even if it comes in a dropper bottle. Do not use the
medicine if the solution
turns reddish brown. If
crystals form in the solution, they can be dissolved
by warming the closed container in warm water and
then shaking the container
gently. Take the liquid
through a straw to lessen
tooth discoloration. If stomach upset continues, consult
your doctor.

OVERDOSE
Symptoms: Gastrointestinal pain and diarrhea, sometimes bloody; loss of
consciousness.

What to Do: Call your
doctor, emergency medical
services (EMS), or the
nearest poison control center immediately.

DRUG INTERACTIONS
Other drugs may interact
with strong iodine. Consult
your doctor for specific
advice if you are taking
amiloride, spironolactone,
triamterene, other thyroid
agents, or lithium.

FOOD INTERACTIONS
This medicine contains
potassium. Consult your
doctor if you are on a low-
potassium diet.

DISEASE INTERACTIONS
Caution is advised when
taking strong iodine. Consult your doctor if you have
any of the following: bronchitis or another lung condition, kidney disease, or
hyperkalemia (excess
potassium in the blood).

Iodine Topical

BRAND NAMES
Iodine Tincture, Iodopen

- Drug Class: Antibacterial (topical); antiseptic
- Available in: Topical solution
- Available OTC? Yes
- As Generic? Yes

Side Effects

SERIOUS
Used as directed, topical iodine is not expected to produce any serious side effects.

COMMON
Momentary burning or tingling at the site of application.

LESS COMMON
Irritation or skin allergy, with blistering, crusting, itching, or reddening of skin at site of application.

PRINCIPAL USES
Iodine is a very effective disinfectant used for prevention and treatment of minor skin infections caused by bacteria. It is also used to disinfect the skin prior to needle procedures and minor surgeries (such as blood drawing, dialysis, and injections).

HOW THE DRUG WORKS
Iodine poisons bacteria on contact, by causing the proteins comprising the organism to congeal.

DOSAGE
Adults: Apply to affected site as directed by a physician or according to manufacturer's instructions on the label. Children 1 month of age and over: Consult a pediatrician.

ONSET OF EFFECT
Immediate.

DURATION OF ACTION
Unknown.

DIETARY ADVICE
Maintain your usual food and fluid intake. Increase fluids if you have a fever or diarrhea, in hot weather, or during exercise.

STORAGE
Store in a tightly sealed container away from heat and direct light. Keep away from moisture and extremes in temperature.

IF YOU MISS A DOSE
Apply as soon as you remember. If it is near the time for the next dose, skip the missed dose and resume your regular dosage schedule.

STOPPING THE DRUG
Use as prescribed for the full treatment period, even if you begin to feel better before the scheduled end of therapy.

PROLONGED USE
Therapy with this medication should be concluded within 7 to 10 days. Consult your physician if your condition has not improved—or especially if it has worsened—anytime after starting therapy with iodine.

PRECAUTIONS
Over 60: No special problems are expected.

Driving and Hazardous Work: The use of iodine should not impair your ability to perform such tasks safely.

Alcohol: No special precautions are necessary.

Pregnancy: Avoid or discontinue using iodine if you are pregnant or trying to become pregnant.

Breast Feeding: Iodine passes into breast milk; avoid or discontinue usage while nursing.

Infants and Children: Iodine is not recommended for use on children under 1 month of age.

Special Concerns: Iodine has serious side effects if it is absorbed in large amounts into your blood. Therefore, do not apply excessive amounts to affected skin. Do not swallow iodine solutions. Above all, never apply this medication to open wounds, to deep cuts, or to bleeding or ulcerated skin. Do not use this medication near your eyes; therefore, use caution when applying iodine to the skin of your forehead or cheeks, and be sure to use small quantities applied carefully, rather than large volumes of liquid. If iodine gets into your eyes, wash with water immediately.

OVERDOSE
Symptoms: Overdose with topical iodine is unlikely when used as directed. If this medication is swallowed, symptoms include abdominal pain, diarrhea, nausea, vomiting, fever, excessive thirst, decreased passage of urine.

What to Do: Call your doctor, emergency medical services (EMS), or the nearest poison control center immediately.

DRUG INTERACTIONS
No specific drug interactions have yet been documented. If you are concerned about whether a prescription or nonprescription medication you are taking may interact with topical iodine, consult your doctor or pharmacist for current information.

FOOD INTERACTIONS
No known food interactions.

DISEASE INTERACTIONS
Consult your doctor if you have any of the following: animal bites; large sores, blisters, ulcerations, or broken skin at the application site; severe injury at the application site; puncture wounds or other deep wounds; serious burns; or allergies to shellfish.

399

Ipecac Syrup

▶ Drug Class: Emetic

▶ Available in: Syrup

▶ Available OTC? Yes

▶ As Generic? Yes

Side Effects

SERIOUS
Heartbeat irregularities;
nausea or vomiting last-
ing for more than 30
minutes; excessive diar-
rhea; weakness or stiff-
ness of the muscles in
the neck, arms, and legs;
stomach pain or cramps;
unusual fatigue; difficulty
breathing. Call your doc-
tor right away.

COMMON
Drowsiness and mild
diarrhea.

LESS COMMON
There are no less-
common side effects
associated with the
use of ipecac syrup.

PRINCIPAL USES
To cause vomiting in per-
sons who have ingested
certain toxic substances or
have taken an overdose of
a drug.

HOW THE DRUG WORKS
Ipecac induces vomiting by
chemically irritating the
stomach lining, triggering
the vomiting reflex.

DOSAGE
Adults and teenagers: 15
to 30 ml, followed by 1 full
glass of water. Children
ages 1 to 12: 15 ml followed
by ½ to 1 full glass of water.
Children ages 6 months to 1
year: 5 to 10 ml, followed by
½ to 1 full glass of water. If
vomiting does not occur, the
first dose may be repeated
one time after 20 minutes.

ONSET OF EFFECT
Within 20 to 30 minutes.

DURATION OF ACTION
From 20 to 25 minutes.

DIETARY ADVICE
Drink water immediately
after taking ipecac syrup.

STORAGE
Store in a tightly sealed container away from heat, moisture, and direct light.

IF YOU MISS A DOSE
Not applicable. It should be
used more than 1 time only
if clearly necessary.

STOPPING THE DRUG
Do not give more than 2
doses. If not effective, consult your doctor, emergency
medical services (EMS), or
local poison control center.

PROLONGED USE
Ipecac is not intended for
prolonged use.

PRECAUTIONS
Over 60: No special problems are expected.

**Driving and Hazardous
Work:** Do not drive or
engage in hazardous work
until you determine how the
drug affects you.

Alcohol: Avoid alcohol.

Pregnancy: No studies of
the use of ipecac syrup during pregnancy have been
done. Discuss with your
doctor the relative risks and
benefits of using it while
pregnant.

Breast Feeding: Ipecac
syrup may pass into breast
milk; caution is advised.
Consult your doctor for
advice.

Infants and Children:
Use by children should be
under strict supervision.
There is an increased risk
of swallowing the vomited
substance in children under
1 year of age. Consult your
doctor before using ipecac
syrup.

Special Concerns: Before
giving ipecac syrup, consult
your doctor, emergency
medical services (EMS), or
the nearest poison control
center. Ipecac syrup should
not be given to anyone who
has ingested gasoline, paint
thinner, kerosene, or a caus-
tic substance such as lye.
Do not give ipecac syrup to
anyone who is unconscious
or very drowsy, because of
an increased risk that the
vomited substance can
enter the lung. If you have
a child over 1 year of age
in the house, keep 30 ml (1
oz) of ipecac syrup on hand
for emergencies. Ipecac
syrup should not be used to
induce vomiting as a means
of losing weight. It can be
toxic to the heart.

OVERDOSE
Symptoms: Breathing difficulty, muscle stiffness,
diarrhea.

What to Do: Call your
doctor, emergency medical
services (EMS), or the
nearest poison control center immediately.

DRUG INTERACTIONS
Do not give any other medicines, including over-the-
counter drugs, with ipecac
unless you first consult your
doctor. Antiemetics can
decrease the syrup's effect
and increase its toxicity. If
using activated charcoal,
wait until vomiting (induced
by ipecac) has stopped
before administering it.

FOOD INTERACTIONS
Ipecac syrup should not
be taken with milk, milk
products, or carbonated
beverages. Milk and milk
products prevent ipecac
syrup from working prop-
erly. Carbonated beverages
can cause the stomach to
swell.

DISEASE INTERACTIONS
You should not take ipecac
syrup if you suffer from
or have heart disease, a
history of seizures, shock,
reduced gag reflex, drowsiness, or unconsciousness.

Ipratropium Bromide

BRAND NAME
Atrovent

▶ Drug Class: Respiratory inhalant

▶ Available in: Inhalation aerosol, inhalation solution

▶ Available OTC? No

▶ As Generic? Yes

Side Effects

SERIOUS
Persistent constipation; lower abdominal pain or bloating; wheezing or difficulty breathing; tightness in chest; severe eye pain; skin rash or hives; swelling of face, lips, or eyelids. Call your doctor immediately.

COMMON
Dry mouth, cough, unpleasant taste.

LESS COMMON
Blurred vision, other changes in vision, burning eyes, difficult urination, dizziness, headache, nausea, pounding heartbeat, nervousness, sweating, trembling.

PRINCIPAL USES
To control the symptoms of lung diseases, such as asthma, chronic bronchitis, and emphysema.

HOW THE DRUG WORKS
It inhibits the cough reflex by blocking the activity of acetylcholine, a chemical that, in the lungs, causes the smooth muscles surrounding the airways to constrict. Therefore, when inhaled, ipratropium bromide causes the airways to widen (bronchodilation).

DOSAGE
The drug may be used as needed to relieve respiratory symptoms. For chronic obstructive lung disease such as bronchitis or emphysema— Inhalation aerosol: Adults and children 6 and over: 2 to 4 inhalations 3 or 4 times a day at regularly spaced intervals. Some patients may need 6 to 8 inhalations a day. Inhalation solution, adults and children 12 and over: 250 to 500 micrograms in a nebulizer 3 or 4 times a day, every 6 to 8 hours.

ONSET OF EFFECT
5 to 15 minutes.

DURATION OF ACTION
3 to 4 hours.

DIETARY ADVICE
Sugarless hard candy or gum can be taken to relieve dry mouth.

STORAGE
Store in a tightly sealed container away from heat and direct light. Open bottles of the solution should be refrigerated, but do not allow the solution to freeze.

IF YOU MISS A DOSE
Take it as soon as you remember. If it is near the time for the next dose, skip the missed dose and resume your regular dosage schedule. Do not double the next dose.

STOPPING THE DRUG
It may not be necessary to continue using the medication for as long as originally prescribed; consult your doctor.

PROLONGED USE
You should see your doctor regularly if you must take this drug for a prolonged period.

PRECAUTIONS
Over 60: Ipratropium is not expected to cause different problems in older patients than in younger persons.

Driving and Hazardous Work: Do not drive or engage in hazardous work until you determine how the medicine affects you.

Alcohol: No special precautions are necessary.

Pregnancy: Ipratropium has not caused birth defects in animals. Human studies have not been done. Before you take ipratropium, tell your doctor if you are pregnant or plan to become pregnant.

Breast Feeding: It is not known whether ipratropium passes into breast milk; caution is advised. Consult your doctor for specific advice.

Infants and Children: Ipratropium has been tested in children and has not been shown to cause different effects than in adults.

Special Concerns: To test the inhaler, insert the canister into the mouthpiece, take the cap off the mouthpiece, shake the inhaler 3 or 4 times, and spray once into the air. To use the inhaler, hold it upright, with the mouthpiece end down, shake it 3 or 4 times, then breathe out. Spray into open mouth or with mouth closed over inhaler, as recommended by your doctor. Clean the inhaler, mouthpiece, and spacer at least twice a week. To take the inhalation solution, use a power-operated nebulizer with a face mask or mouthpiece. Get instructions for using the nebulizer from your doctor.

OVERDOSE
Symptoms: No specific ones have been reported.

What to Do: An overdose of ipratropium is unlikely to be life-threatening. However, if someone takes a much larger dose than prescribed, call your doctor, emergency medical services (EMS), or the nearest poison control center.

DRUG INTERACTIONS
Before you use ipratropium, tell your doctor if you are using any other prescription or over-the-counter drug.

FOOD INTERACTIONS
No known food interactions.

DISEASE INTERACTIONS
Consult your doctor if you have glaucoma or difficulty urinating.

Irbesartan

▶ Drug Class: Antihypertensive/
angiotensin II antagonist

▶ Available in: Tablets

▶ Available OTC? No

▶ As Generic? No

Side Effects

SERIOUS
No serious side effects are associated with the use of irbesartan. (In clinical trials, the incidence of adverse effects was not significantly greater with the medication than with a placebo.)

COMMON
No common side effects are associated with the use of irbesartan.

LESS COMMON
Diarrhea, indigestion, heartburn, fatigue, muscle pain, edema, sexual dysfunction, low blood pressure.

PRINCIPAL USES
To control high blood pressure. This drug appears to have the same benefits as the class of antihypertensive drugs known as ACE inhibitors, without producing the common side effect (experienced by as many as 30% of patients) of a dry cough. Irbesartan may be used by itself or in conjunction with other antihypertensive medications.

HOW THE DRUG WORKS
Irbesartan blocks the effects of angiotensin II, a naturally occurring substance that causes blood vessels to narrow. Irbesartan causes the blood vessels to dilate, thereby lowering blood pressure and decreasing the workload of the heart.

DOSAGE
To start, 150 mg once a day. It may be increased by your doctor to a maximum dose of 300 mg per day.

ONSET OF EFFECT
Within 2 to 4 hours.

DURATION OF ACTION
More than 24 hours.

DIETARY ADVICE
No special restrictions, unless your doctor has advised a low-sodium diet or other dietary modifications to help you control your blood pressure.

STORAGE
Store in a tightly sealed container away from heat, moisture, and direct light.

IF YOU MISS A DOSE
If you miss a dose on one day, do not double the dose the next day. Resume your regular dosage schedule.

STOPPING THE DRUG
Take it as prescribed for the full treatment period. The decision to stop taking the drug should be made in consultation with your physician.

PROLONGED USE
Lifelong therapy may be necessary. However, if you do change certain health habits (for example, increasing exercise or losing weight), a reduced dose may be possible under a doctor's supervision.

PRECAUTIONS
Over 60: Adverse reactions may be more likely and more severe in older patients.

Driving and Hazardous Work: Do not drive or engage in hazardous work until you determine how the medicine affects you.

Alcohol: No special precautions are necessary.

Pregnancy: Irbesartan should not be used by pregnant women. Discontinue taking the drug as soon as possible when pregnancy is detected and discuss treatment alternatives with your doctor.

Breast Feeding: Irbesartan may pass into breast milk; caution is advised. Consult your doctor for specific advice.

Infants and Children: The safety and effectiveness of use in children have not been established.

Special Concerns: Irbesartan may cause excessively low blood pressure with dizziness or lightheadedness, which is most noticeable when you change position. This may lead to fainting, falls, and injury. Sit or lie down immediately if you feel dizzy or lightheaded. This side effect may be worsened by alcohol, hot weather, dehydration, salt depletion from diuretic use, fever, prolonged standing, prolonged sitting, or exercise.

OVERDOSE
Symptoms: No cases of overdose have been reported. However, if you take a much larger dose than prescribed, you may experience extremely low blood pressure or heartbeat irregularities.

What to Do: If you take a much larger dose than prescribed, contact your doctor.

DRUG INTERACTIONS
No drug interactions have yet been observed with irbesartan. Consult your doctor for specific advice if you are taking any other medication, including other drugs for high blood pressure. Irbesartan can be taken together with diuretics or other medications for high blood pressure, if your doctor approves.

FOOD INTERACTIONS
No known food interactions.

DISEASE INTERACTIONS
Patients with liver or kidney disease are advised to exercise caution when taking irbesartan.

Isoetharine

BRAND NAMES
Arm-a-Med Isoetharine,
Bronkometer, Bronkosol,
Dey-Lute Isoetharine S/F

▶ Drug Class: Bronchodilator/
sympathomimetic

▶ Available in: Inhalation
solution, inhalation aerosol

▶ Available OTC? No

▶ As Generic? Yes

Side Effects

SERIOUS
Isoetharine may become
ineffective if used too
often, resulting in more-
severe breathing diffi-
culty that does not
improve. Signs include
persistent wheezing,
coughing, or shortness of
breath; confusion; bluish
color to lips or finger-
nails; inability to speak.
Other side effects include
chest pain or heaviness;
irregular, racing, fluttering, or pounding heart-
beat; lightheadedness;
fainting; severe weak-
ness; severe headache.

COMMON
Trouble sleeping, dry
mouth, sore throat, ner-
vousness, restlessness.

LESS COMMON
Trembling, sweating,
headache, nausea or
vomiting, flushing or redness to cheeks or other
skin, muscle aches,
unpleasant or unusual
taste in mouth.

PRINCIPAL USES
Isoetharine is used to dilate
air passages in the lungs
that have become narrowed
as a result of disease or
inflammation. It is used in
the treatment of asthma and
chronic obstructive pul-
monary disease (COPD).

HOW THE DRUG WORKS
Isoetharine widens con-
stricted airways in the lungs
by relaxing the smooth
muscles that surround the
bronchial passages.

DOSAGE
May be used when needed
to relieve breathing difficulty. Adults, using inhalation solution for nebulizers:
Usual dose is 4 inhalations,
not to be taken more fre-
quently than every 4 hours,
for a usual maximum of 3
to 4 times a day. Note that
isoetharine for nebulizers
may or may not require
dilution with saline. Check
with your physician to
determine whether your
medication requires dilu-
tion; if so, follow directions
accordingly. Children: Consult your pediatrician.
Adults using inhalation
aerosol: A treatment con-
sists of 340 micrograms (1
puff), repeated after 1 to 2
minutes if necessary. Treatments may be repeated
every 4 hours if necessary.
Children: Not recom-
mended in children younger
than 12 years of age.

ONSET OF EFFECT
Within 5 minutes.

DURATION OF ACTION
1 to 4 hours.

DIETARY ADVICE
Maintain your usual food
and fluid intake.

STORAGE
Store in a tightly sealed container away from heat and

direct light. Do not refrigerate inhalation solutions.

IF YOU MISS A DOSE
Skip the missed dose and
resume your regular dosage
schedule. Do not double the
next dose.

STOPPING THE DRUG
It may not be necessary to
finish the recommended
course of therapy. Consult
your doctor.

PROLONGED USE
Therapy may require
months or years. Excessive
use may result in temporary
loss of effectiveness.

PRECAUTIONS
Over 60: Adverse reactions
may be more likely and
more severe in older
patients.

**Driving and Hazardous
Work:** Do not drive or
engage in hazardous work
until you determine how the
medicine affects you.

Alcohol: No special precautions are necessary.

Pregnancy: Adequate studies have not been done;
benefits must be weighed
against potential risks. Consult your doctor for specific
advice.

Breast Feeding: It is not
known if isoetharine passes
into breast milk. Mothers
who wish to breast-feed
while taking this drug
should discuss the matter
with their doctor.

Infants and Children:
Nebulized solutions may be
used to treat breathing difficulties in infants and children. Consult your
pediatrician. Use of the
inhalation aerosol is not recommended in children
younger than 12 years old.

Special Concerns: Pay
heed to any asthma attack
or other breathing problem
that does not improve after
your usual nebulizer treatment or usual number of
puffs. Seek help immedi-
ately if you feel your lungs
are persistently constricted,
if you are using more than
the recommended number
of treatments or puffs per
day, or if you feel a recent
attack is somehow different
from others.

OVERDOSE
Symptoms: See Serious
Side Effects.

What to Do: Call your
doctor, emergency medical
services (EMS), or the
nearest poison control
center immediately.

DRUG INTERACTIONS
Consult your doctor for specific advice if you are taking
a beta-blocker, ergotamine
or ergotamine-like medications, antidepressants, digitalis drugs, or an MAO
inhibitor.

FOOD INTERACTIONS
No known food interactions.

DISEASE INTERACTIONS
Consult your doctor if you
have a history of substance
abuse (especially cocaine),
seizures, brain damage,
heart disease, heartbeat
irregularities, high blood
pressure, anxiety disorders,
or a thyroid condition.

Isoniazid

Generic 100 mg
(BARR)

Additional photographs

▶ Drug Class: Anti-infective/
antitubercular agent

▶ Available in: Syrup, tablets,
injection

▶ Available OTC? No

▶ As Generic? Yes

Side Effects

SERIOUS
Numbness, pain, burning,
or tingling in hands and
feet, loss of appetite,
stomach pain, clumsi-
ness, yellowish tinge to
the eyes or skin, nausea,
vomiting, darkened urine,
unusual fatigue. Call your
doctor immediately.

COMMON
Diarrhea, rash, fever.

LESS COMMON
Irritability, seizures.

PRINCIPAL USES
To prevent and treat tuberculosis (TB). It may be
taken alone to prevent TB,
but must be used with other
antitubercular agents to
treat an active case of TB.

HOW THE DRUG WORKS
Isoniazid interferes with
the formation of DNA and
lipids, needed to manufacture the TB bacteria's cell
walls.

DOSAGE
For prevention— Adults and
teenagers: 300 mg once a
day. Children: 4.5 to 9 mg
per lb of body weight once
a day (not more than 300
mg a day). For treatment—
Adults and teenagers: 300
mg once a day, or 6.8 mg
per lb twice a week (not
more than 900 mg per
dose). Children: 4.5 to 9.1
mg per lb (not more than
300 mg a day) once a day,
or 9.1 to 18.2 mg per lb
twice a week (not more
than 900 mg per dose). Vitamin B6 may be given in a
dosage of 10 to 25 mg a day
to prevent nerve damage.

ONSET OF EFFECT
Unknown.

DURATION OF ACTION
Unknown.

DIETARY ADVICE
Take this medicine 1 hour
before or 2 hours after
meals. Taking it with food
or an antacid will prevent
stomach irritation but
decrease the absorption
of the drug. Do not take
an antacid containing
aluminum within 1 hour
of taking isoniazid.

STORAGE
Store in a tightly sealed container away from heat, moisture, and direct light. Do
not freeze the liquid forms.

IF YOU MISS A DOSE
Take it as soon as you
remember, to help keep a
constant level of medication
in your system. If it is near
the time for the next dose,
skip the missed dose and
resume your regular dosage
schedule. Do not double the
next dose.

STOPPING THE DRUG
Take it as prescribed for the
full treatment period, even if
you feel better before the
scheduled end of therapy.
Treatment may continue for
months or years. The decision to stop the drug should
be made by your doctor.

PROLONGED USE
See your doctor regularly
for tests and examinations if
you must take this medicine
for a prolonged period.
If your symptoms do not
improve or instead become
worse after 3 weeks, consult
your doctor.

PRECAUTIONS
Over 60: Adverse reactions
may be more likely and
more severe in older
patients.

**Driving and Hazardous
Work:** Do not drive or
engage in hazardous work
until you determine how the
medicine affects you.

Alcohol: Avoid alcohol; it
may diminish isoniazid's
effectiveness and may interact with the drug, increasing the risk of hepatitis
(liver inflammation).

Pregnancy: In human
studies, isoniazid has not
caused birth defects. Tell
your doctor if you are pregnant or are planning to
become pregnant and dis-
cuss the relative risks and
benefits of using this drug.

Breast Feeding: Isoniazid
passes into breast milk; cau-

tion is advised. Consult your
doctor for specific advice.

Infants and Children:
No special problems are
expected. Discuss with your
pediatrician the relative
risks and benefits of your
child's using this drug.

Special Concerns: Isoniazid can cause false results
on urine sugar tests for
diabetics.

OVERDOSE
Symptoms: Severe
seizures, nausea, vomiting,
difficulty breathing, slurred
speech, blurred vision, hallucinations, dizziness, loss
of consciousness, stupor.

What to Do: Call your
doctor, emergency medical
services (EMS), or the
nearest poison control center immediately.

DRUG INTERACTIONS
Consult your doctor for specific advice if you are taking
narcotic pain relievers,
antacids, acetaminophen,
carbamazepine, disulfiram,
phenytoin, rifampin, ketoconazole, itraconazole, warfarin, or diazepam. Ask your
doctor if any of the medications you take are toxic to
the liver; such drugs should
be avoided.

FOOD INTERACTIONS
Swiss cheese, fish, chocolate, and beer can react with
this medication. Consult
your doctor for advice.

DISEASE INTERACTIONS
Consult your doctor if you
have epilepsy or another
seizure disorder, or a history of alcohol abuse. Use
of isoniazid may cause complications in patients with
liver or kidney disease,
since these organs work
together to remove the
medication from the body.

Isoproterenol

BRAND NAMES
Isuprel, Isuprel
Mistometer, Medihaler-Iso

▶ Drug Class: Bronchodilator/
sympathomimetic

▶ Available in: Inhalation
solution or aerosol

▶ Available OTC? No

▶ As Generic? Yes

Side Effects

SERIOUS
Isoproterenol may
become ineffective if
used too often, resulting
in more-severe breathing
difficulty that does not
improve. Signs include
persistent wheezing,
coughing, or shortness of
breath; confusion; bluish
color to lips or finger-
nails; inability to speak.
Other side effects include
chest pain or heaviness;
irregular, racing, fluttering, or pounding heart-
beat; lightheadedness;
fainting; severe weak-
ness; severe headache.

COMMON
Trouble sleeping, dry
mouth, sore throat, pink-
ish color to saliva, ner-
vousness, restlessness.

LESS COMMON
Trembling, sweating,
headache, nausea or
vomiting, flushing or redness to cheeks or other
skin surfaces.

PRINCIPAL USES
To dilate air passages in the
lungs that have become narrowed as a result of disease
or inflammation. It is used
in the treatment of asthma
and chronic obstructive pulmonary disease (COPD).

HOW THE DRUG WORKS
Isoproterenol widens con-
stricted airways in the lungs
by relaxing smooth muscles
that surround the bronchial
passages.

DOSAGE
For use when needed to
relieve wheezing or difficulty breathing— By nebu-
lizer: Adults: 6 to 12
inhalations of 0.25% solution. May be repeated if
necessary every 15 minutes
for a maximum of 3 doses.
Take no more than 8 treatments every 24 hours. Or:
5 to 10 inhalations of 0.5%
solution, or 3 to 7 inhalations of 1.0% solution,
repeated once after 5 to 10
minutes if necessary. Take
no more than 5 treatments
per day. If you are on a program of scheduled, daily
isoproterenol treatments,
do not take a treatment
more often than every 3 to
4 hours. Children: Follow
directions above for 0.25%
and 0.5% solutions. A 1.0%
solution is not used in children. By inhalation aerosol,
adults and children: 1 puff.
Wait 1 minute to assess
effect. May be repeated
after 1 to 5 minutes if
needed. This treatment
may be repeated 4 to 6
times per day. For sched-
uled, daily use— 1 puff
every 3 to 4 hours.

ONSET OF EFFECT
Within 5 minutes.

DURATION OF ACTION
From 30 to 120 minutes.

DIETARY ADVICE
Maintain your usual food
and fluid intake.

STORAGE
Store at room temperature
in a tightly sealed container
away from heat and direct
light.

IF YOU MISS A DOSE
Skip the missed dose and
resume your regular dosage
schedule. Do not double the
next dose.

STOPPING THE DRUG
It may not be necessary to
finish the recommended
course of therapy. Consult
your doctor.

PROLONGED USE
Therapy may require
months or years. Excessive
use may result in temporary
loss of effectiveness.

PRECAUTIONS
Over 60: Adverse reactions
may be more likely and
more severe in older
patients.

**Driving and Hazardous
Work:** Do not drive or
engage in hazardous work
until you determine how the
medicine affects you.

Alcohol: No special precautions are necessary.

Pregnancy: Benefits must
be weighed against potential
risks; consult your doctor.

Breast Feeding: Mothers
who wish to breast feed
while taking this drug
should discuss the matter
with their doctor.

Infants and Children:
May be used to treat
breathing difficulties in
infants and children.

Special Concerns: Pay
heed to any breathing problem that does not improve
after your usual nebulizer
treatment or usual number
of puffs. Seek help immediately if you feel your lungs
are persistently constricted,
if you are using more than
the recommended number
of treatments per day, or if
you feel a recent attack is
somehow different from
others.

OVERDOSE
Symptoms: Chest pain or
heaviness; irregular, racing,
fluttering, or pounding
heartbeat; dizziness; lightheadedness; fainting; severe
weakness; severe headache.

What to Do: Call your
doctor, emergency medical
services (EMS), or the
nearest poison control
center immediately.

DRUG INTERACTIONS
Consult your doctor for
specific advice if you are
taking a beta-blocker, ergotamine or ergotamine-like
medications, antidepres-
sants, digitalis drugs, or
an MAO inhibitor.

FOOD INTERACTIONS
No known food interactions.

DISEASE INTERACTIONS
Consult your doctor if you
have a history of substance
abuse (especially cocaine),
seizures, brain damage,
heart disease, heartbeat
irregularities, high blood
pressure, anxiety disorders,
or a thyroid condition.

BRAND NAMES
Dilatrate-SR, Iso-Bid,
Isonate, Isorbid, Isordil,
Isotrate, Sorbitrate

Generic 20 mg
(GENEVA)

Additional photographs

▶ Drug Class: Nitrate

▶ Available in: Capsules,
tablets, chewable tablets,
sublingual and buccal forms

▶ Available OTC? No

▶ As Generic? Yes

Side Effects

SERIOUS
Blurred vision, dry
mouth, severe or pro-
longed headache. Call
your doctor immediately.

COMMON
Dizziness or lightheaded-
ness, especially when
getting up from a seated
or lying position, flushing
of the face and neck,
unusually rapid pulse or
heartbeat, nausea and
vomiting, restlessness.

LESS COMMON
Skin rash.

PRINCIPAL USES
To prevent or relieve
attacks of angina (chest
pain associated with heart
disease).

HOW THE DRUG WORKS
Isosorbide dinitrate relaxes
the smooth muscle of the
blood vessels and increases
the supply of blood and
oxygen to the heart. It also
reduces the heart's work-
load and demand for
oxygen.

DOSAGE
To prevent angina attacks:
Extended-release capsules
or tablets, 20 to 80 mg
every 8 to 12 hours. For
short-acting capsules or
tablets, 5 to 40 mg, 4 times
a day. To treat angina
attack: When you feel an
attack of angina starting,
place a sublingual (under
tongue) or buccal (inside
the cheek) tablet in your
mouth or chew a chewable
tablet. If pain is not relieved
in 5 minutes with a sublingual tablet, take a second
tablet. A third tablet may
be used after another 5
minutes. If pain continues
to persist, call your doctor
or go to the nearest hospital
emergency room.

ONSET OF EFFECT
Chewable and sublingual
(under the tongue) tablets:
2 to 5 minutes; tablets: 15
to 40 minutes; extended-
release capsules and tablets:
30 minutes.

DURATION OF ACTION
1 to 2 hours for chewable
tablets, 4 to 6 hours for
tablets and capsules, 12
hours for extended-release
forms.

DIETARY ADVICE
Take capsules or tablets 30
minutes before or 1 to 2
hours after meals.

STORAGE
Store in a tightly sealed container away from heat and
direct light.

IF YOU MISS A DOSE
Take it as soon as you
remember. If it is near the
time for the next dose, skip
the missed dose and
resume your regular dosage
schedule as prescribed. Do
not double the next dose.

STOPPING THE DRUG
The decision to stop taking
the drug should be made by
your doctor. Do not stop
taking this medicine sud-
denly. Consult your doctor
about reducing the dose
gradually.

PROLONGED USE
You should see your doctor
regularly if you must take
this medicine for an
extended period.

PRECAUTIONS
Over 60: Adverse reactions
may be more likely and
more severe in older
patients.

**Driving and Hazardous
Work:** Do not drive or
engage in hazardous work
until you determine how the
medicine affects you.

Alcohol: Alcohol should be
avoided.

Pregnancy: Animal tests
have shown adverse effects
on the fetus. Human tests
have not been done. Before
taking isosorbide dinitrate,
tell your doctor if you are
pregnant or plan to become
pregnant.

Breast Feeding: Isosorbide dinitrate may pass
into breast milk; caution
is advised. Consult your
doctor for advice.

Infants and Children:
No studies on the use of
this medicine in children
have been done. Use and
dose should be determined
by your doctor.

Special Concerns: Use
extra care in hot weather or
during exercise, or when
standing for long periods
of time.

OVERDOSE
Symptoms: Bluish fingernails, lips, or palms;
extreme dizziness or fainting; unusual weakness,
fever, weak and rapid heartbeat, seizures.

What to Do: Call your
doctor, emergency medical
services (EMS), or the
nearest poison control center immediately.

DRUG INTERACTIONS
Do not take isosorbide
dinitrate within 24 hours
of taking sildenafil citrate.
Sildenafil can enhance the
action of nitrates (such as
isosorbide), causing potentially dangerous decreases
in blood pressure. Consult
your doctor for specific
advice if you are taking
other heart medicines,
or antihypertensives.

FOOD INTERACTIONS
No known food interactions.

DISEASE INTERACTIONS
Caution is advised when
taking isosorbide dinitrate.
Consult your doctor if you
have any of the following:
anemia, glaucoma, a recent
head injury or stroke,
hyperthyroidism, or a
recent heart attack. Use
of isosorbide dinitrate may
cause complications in
patients with severe liver or
kidney disease, since these
organs work together to
remove the medication
from the body.

Isosorbide Mononitrate

IMDUR 30 mg
(KEY)

▶ Drug Class: Nitrate

▶ Available in: Tablets, extended-release tablets

▶ Available OTC? No

▶ As Generic? Yes

Side Effects

SERIOUS
Blurred vision, dry mouth, severe or prolonged headache. Call your doctor immediately.

COMMON
Dizziness or lightheadedness, especially when rising suddenly to a standing position, flushing of the face and neck, rapid pulse or heartbeat, nausea or vomiting, restlessness.

LESS COMMON
Skin rash.

PRINCIPAL USES
To prevent or relieve attacks of angina (chest pain associated with heart disease).

HOW THE DRUG WORKS
Isosorbide relaxes the smooth muscle of the blood vessels and increases the supply of blood and oxygen to the heart. It also reduces the heart's workload and demand for oxygen.

DOSAGE
To prevent angina attacks—Tablets: 20 mg, 2 times a day, with doses 7 hours apart. Extended-release tablets: 30 to 240 mg once a day.

ONSET OF EFFECT
60 minutes.

DURATION OF ACTION
Unknown.

DIETARY ADVICE
Take tablets on an empty stomach, at least 30 minutes before or 1 to 2 hours after mealtime.

STORAGE
Store in a tightly sealed container away from heat and direct light.

IF YOU MISS A DOSE
Take it as soon as you remember. If it is near the time for the next dose, skip the missed dose and resume your regular dosage schedule as prescribed. Do not double the next dose.

STOPPING THE DRUG
The decision to stop taking the drug should be made by your doctor.

PROLONGED USE
You should see your doctor regularly if you take this medicine for an extended period.

PRECAUTIONS
Over 60: Adverse reactions may be more likely and more severe in older patients.

Driving and Hazardous Work: Avoid such activities until you determine how the medicine affects you.

Alcohol: Avoid alcohol.

Pregnancy: Animal tests have shown adverse effects on the fetus. Human tests have not been done. Before taking this drug, tell your doctor if you are pregnant or plan to become pregnant.

Breast Feeding: Isosorbide mononitrate may pass into breast milk; caution is advised. Consult your doctor for specific advice.

Infants and Children: No studies on the use of this medicine in children have been done. Use and dose should be determined by your doctor.

Special Concerns: Do not stop taking this medicine suddenly because it can cause a spasm of the blood vessels in the heart. Consult your doctor about reducing the dose gradually. Use extra care in hot weather or during exercise, or when you must stand for long periods of time. This medicine may cause headaches at the beginning of therapy. Headaches can be treated with aspirin or acetaminophen and usually stop after your body becomes accustomed to the medication. The dose may be reduced temporarily because of headaches. The effectiveness of the medicine may decrease over time; notify your doctor if this occurs.

OVERDOSE
Symptoms: Bluish fingernails, lips or palms; extreme dizziness or fainting; unusual weakness, fever, weak and fast heartbeat, seizures.

What to Do: Call your doctor, emergency medical services (EMS), or the nearest poison control c enter immediately.

DRUG INTERACTIONS
Do not take isosorbide mononitrate within 24 hours of taking sildenafil citrate. Sildenafil can enhance the action of nitrates (such as isosorbide), causing potentially dangerous decreases in blood pressure. Consult your doctor for specific advice if you are taking other heart medicines, or antihypertensives.

FOOD INTERACTIONS
No known food interactions.

DISEASE INTERACTIONS
Consult your doctor if you have any of the following: anemia, glaucoma, a recent head injury or stroke, an overactive thyroid, or a recent heart attack. Use of isosorbide mononitrate may cause complications in patients with severe liver or kidney disease, since these organs work together to remove the medication from the body.

Isotretinoin

Side Effects

SERIOUS

Severe headache that may occur in conjunction with blurred vision, nausea, and vomiting. Discontinue isotretinoin and contact your doctor immediately as this may be an indication of a very serious condition known as pseudotumor cerebri, marked by increased pressure within the skull, which may damage the brain. Severe central abdominal pain, penetrating through to the back, may indicate acute pancreatitis (inflammation of the pancreas); call your doctor or get to an emergency room immediately.

COMMON

Dry, itching, or cracked skin or lips; easy bruising; nosebleeds; dry, red, or inflamed eyes, difficulty wearing contact lenses; increased susceptibility to sunburn; muscle or joint pain. Consult your doctor if such symptoms persist or interfere with daily activities.

LESS COMMON

Rashes, peeling of skin on palms and soles, nausea, dizziness, poor night vision (night blindness), cataracts, appearance of small spots or shadows passing slowly across the line of vision ("floaters"), thinning hair, weight loss, swelling in the feet and ankles (known as edema) due to excess fluid retention in the body tissues, mental depression.

PRINCIPAL USES

Isotretinoin is used to treat severe acne that has not responded adequately to other treatments, such as oral antibiotics. Because of the risk for potentially serious side effects, isotretinoin is prescribed only as a last resort.

HOW THE DRUG WORKS

Isotretinoin decreases the size of and interferes with the functioning of structures in the skin called sebaceous glands. These tiny glands, located along hair shafts all over the body's surface, produce sebum—a thick, oily substance that serves as the skin's natural lubricant. Hormonal activity (during pregnancy, puberty, or menstruation, for example) can stimulate overproduction of sebum by the sebaceous glands so that it is secreted faster than it can exit the pores. This may lead to blockage of the hair follicle and result in the sort of skin lesion that characterizes acne. By thinning the composition of sebum and reducing sebum production (as well as causing other, only partly-understood changes), isotretinoin improves acne.

DOSAGE

Adults and teenagers: 0.5 to 1 mg per 2.2 lbs (1 kg) of body weight, in 1 or 2 doses per day, taken for a total period of 20 weeks (average) for complete treatment. Children: Not recommended. Capsules should be swallowed whole; do not open, crush, or chew them.

ONSET OF EFFECT

Variable, usually within several weeks after starting therapy.

DURATION OF ACTION

Most patients have complete and prolonged improvement of acne following therapy with isotretinoin, while others do not. Good results are usually achieved only with the appropriate dose and length of treatment.

DIETARY ADVICE

Isotretinoin should be taken with food. Maintain your usual food and fluid intake. Do not take vitamin supplements containing vitamin A while taking isotretinoin.

STORAGE

Store in a tightly sealed container away from heat and direct light. Keep away from moisture and extremes in temperature.

IF YOU MISS A DOSE

Take it as soon as you remember. If it is near the time for the next dose, skip the missed dose and resume your regular dosage schedule. Do not double the next dose.

STOPPING THE DRUG

Take it as prescribed for the full treatment period, even if your acne clears before the scheduled end of therapy. Special exception: Stop taking the medication immediately if you become pregnant or believe that there is a possibility that you are pregnant.

PROLONGED USE

Therapy with isotretinoin usually lasts 15 to 20 weeks. A second course of therapy may be initiated if the first yields less-than-satisfactory results; a period of two months without using the drug is required between the first and second course of therapy.

PRECAUTIONS

Over 60: It is possible that adverse reactions may be more likely or more severe in older patients.

Driving and Hazardous Work: The use of isotretinoin should not impair your ability to perform such tasks safely during daytime. Exercise caution at night, since the drug may impair night vision.

Alcohol: Simultaneous use of alcohol and isotretinoin may cause an unhealthy rise in triglyceride levels.

Pregnancy: Do not use this medication under any circumstances during pregnancy or within one month of intended pregnancy.

Breast Feeding: Do not use this medication while nursing.

Infants and Children: Not recommended for use by children under age 13.

Special Concerns: Isotretinoin can lead to a severely deformed infant if used during pregnancy, even if only for a very short time. Therefore, this medication should not be used by any woman of childbearing age who is not using established methods of contraception. If you are a woman starting on isotretinoin, you should first be using two reliable forms of contraception and have a pregnancy test done to exclude the possibility of pregnancy. Then, begin isotretinoin on the third day of the subsequent menstrual cycle to further ensure that you are not pregnant. You must also avoid pregnancy for 1 full month after discontinuing therapy. Your doctor may require you to sign a consent form before prescribing this medication.

Once you have started isotretinoin, expect some drying, cracking, peeling, or itching of your skin, as well as dry nasal passages and mouth. About 9 out of every 10 people taking isotretinoin experience these problems. Avoid prolonged exposure to the sun and be sure to use sunblock when spending time outdoors, since isotretinoin may increase your skin's sensitivity to ultraviolet light and thus your risk of sunburn.

OVERDOSE

Symptoms: Headache, vomiting, facial flushing, dry or cracked lips, abdominal pain, dizziness. Such symptoms usually resolve on their own in a short period of time.

What to Do: An overdose is unlikely to be life-threatening. However, if overdose symptoms occur and persist, or if someone accidentally ingests isotretinoin, call your doctor, emergency medical services (EMS), or the nearest poison control center immediately.

DRUG INTERACTIONS

Consult your doctor for specific advice if you are taking etretinate, tretinoin, vitamin A supplements, multivitamins, tetracycline, topical sulfur, or topical benzoyl peroxide.

FOOD INTERACTIONS

No known food interactions. (Isotretinoin should be taken with food.)

DISEASE INTERACTIONS

Consult your doctor if you have any of the following: a history of alcohol abuse, diabetes mellitus, pancreatitis, high blood levels of cholesterol or triglycerides, severe weight problems, vision problems, or severe headaches.

Isoxsuprine Hydrochloride

Generic 20 mg
(GENEVA)

▶ Drug Class: Vasodilator

▶ Available in: Tablets

▶ Available OTC? No

▶ As Generic? No

Side Effects

SERIOUS
Chest pain, dizziness, or faintness; rapid heartbeat; skin rash; shortness of breath; continuing nausea and repeated vomiting. Such side effects are rare but potentially serious; if they do occur, call your doctor immediately.

COMMON
There are no common side effects associated with the use of isoxsuprine.

LESS COMMON
Nausea, vomiting.

PRINCIPAL USES
To treat problems resulting from poor blood circulation to the brain (cerebrovascular insufficiency) or the body (arteriosclerosis obliterans, thromboangiitis obliterans, and Raynaud's disease).

HOW THE DRUG WORKS
Isoxsuprine acts upon the smooth muscle tissue surrounding the arteries, causing it to relax, which widens the blood vessels and lowers blood pressure, as well as increasing heart output and improving blood circulation.

DOSAGE
10 to 20 mg, 3 or 4 times a day.

ONSET OF EFFECT
1 hour.

DURATION OF ACTION
Unknown.

DIETARY ADVICE
Isoxsuprine can be taken with meals or milk.

STORAGE
Store in a tightly sealed container in a dry place away from heat and direct light.

IF YOU MISS A DOSE
Take a missed dose as soon as you remember. If it is near the time for the next dose, skip the missed dose and resume your regular dosage schedule. Do not double the next dose.

STOPPING THE DRUG
Take as prescribed for the full treatment period, even if you begin to feel better before the scheduled end of therapy. The decision to stop taking the drug should be made by your doctor.

PROLONGED USE
You should see your doctor regularly for tests and examinations if you take this drug for a prolonged period.

PRECAUTIONS
Over 60: There is no specific information comparing use of isoxsuprine in older patients with use in other age groups. However, older patients may be more likely to experience an increased sensitivity to cold temperatures.

Driving and Hazardous Work: Do not drive or engage in hazardous work until you determine how the medicine affects you.

Alcohol: Alcohol should be avoided while taking this medication.

Pregnancy: Isoxsuprine has not been shown to cause birth defects. Given prior to delivery, it may cause low blood sugar, bowel problems, low blood pressure, and other problems in a newborn baby.

Breast Feeding: Isoxsuprine has not been shown to cause problems in nursing babies.

Infants and Children: Isoxsuprine is generally not prescribed for infants and children.

Special Concerns: You should avoid sudden changes in position to reduce the possibility of dizziness, lightheadedness, and falling. You should not smoke cigarettes if you take isoxsuprine. Taking blood pressure measurements in sitting, lying, and standing positions is recommended to detect the likelihood of episodes of low blood pressure in patients receiving isoxsuprine. Be sure to tell your doctor if you have had any unusual or allergic reaction to isoxsuprine in the past. Also tell your doctor if you are allergic to any other substances, such as foods, dyes, and preservatives.

OVERDOSE
Symptoms: Headache, vomiting, flushed face, abdominal pain, dizziness, loss of muscle coordination.

What to Do: Call your doctor, emergency medical services (EMS), or the nearest poison control center immediately.

DRUG INTERACTIONS
Consult your doctor for specific advice if you are taking any prescription or over-the-counter medicine. In some cases your doctor may want to change the dose or have you take other precautions.

FOOD INTERACTIONS
No known food interactions.

DISEASE INTERACTIONS
Caution is advised when taking isoxsuprine. Consult your doctor if you have any of the following: angina, bleeding problems, glaucoma, hardening of the arteries, pulmonary hypertension, low blood pressure, a recent heart attack, or a recent stroke.

Isradipine

BRAND NAME
DynaCirc

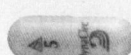

DynaCirc 5 mg
(**Novartis**)

▸ Drug Class: Calcium channel blocker

▸ Available in: Capsules

▸ Available OTC? No

▸ As Generic? No

Side Effects

SERIOUS
Breathing difficulty, coughing, or wheezing; irregular or pounding heartbeat; chest pain; fainting. Call your doctor immediately.

COMMON
Headache, dizziness, skin flushing and feeling of warmth, swelling in the feet, ankles, or calves, palpitations.

LESS COMMON
Constipation or diarrhea, nausea, unusual fatigue and weakness, skin rash, increased urination.

PRINCIPAL USES
To treat high blood pressure (hypertension).

HOW THE DRUG WORKS
Isradipine interferes with the movement of calcium into heart muscle cells and the smooth muscle cells in the walls of the arteries. This action relaxes blood vessels (causing them to widen), which lowers blood pressure, increases the blood supply to the heart, and decreases the heart's overall workload.

DOSAGE
2.5 mg twice a day to start. The dose may be increased.

ONSET OF EFFECT
Within 20 minutes.

DURATION OF ACTION
More than 12 hours.

DIETARY ADVICE
No special restrictions.

STORAGE
Store in a tightly sealed container away from heat and direct light. Keep away from moisture and extremes in temperature.

IF YOU MISS A DOSE
Take it as soon as you remember. If it is near the time for the next dose, skip the missed dose and resume your regular dosage schedule. Do not double the next dose.

STOPPING THE DRUG
Do not stop taking this drug suddenly, as this may cause potentially serious health problems. If therapy is to be discontinued, dosage should be reduced gradually, according to doctor's instructions.

PROLONGED USE
See your doctor regularly for examinations and tests if you take this medicine for a prolonged period. Remember that isradipine controls high blood pressure but does not cure it. Lifelong therapy may be necessary.

PRECAUTIONS
Over 60: Adverse reactions may be more likely and more severe in older patients.

Driving and Hazardous Work: Do not drive or engage in hazardous work until you determine how the medicine affects you.

Alcohol: Avoid alcohol.

Pregnancy: In animal studies, large doses of isradipine have caused birth defects. Human studies have not been done. Before you take isradipine, tell your doctor if you are currently pregnant or plan to become pregnant.

Breast Feeding: Isradipine may pass into breast milk; caution is advised. Consult your doctor for specific advice.

Infants and Children: Safety and effectiveness of isradipine have not been determined for young patients.

Special Concerns: In addition to taking isradipine, be sure to follow all special instructions on weight control and diet. Your doctor will tell you which specific factors are most important for you. Check with your doctor before changing your diet.

OVERDOSE
Symptoms: Dizziness, slurred speech, nausea, weakness, drowsiness, and confusion.

What to Do: Call your doctor, emergency medical services (EMS), or the nearest poison control center immediately.

DRUG INTERACTIONS
Consult your physician for specific advice if you are taking acetazolamide, amphotericin B, corticosteroids, dichlorphenamide, diuretics, methazolamide, beta-blockers, carbamazepine, cyclosporine, procainamide, quinidine, digitalis, disopyramide or the following eye medicines: betaxolol, levobunolol, metipranolol, or timolol.

FOOD INTERACTIONS
Avoid foods high in sodium.

DISEASE INTERACTIONS
Caution is advised when taking isradipine. Consult your doctor if you have any of the following: abnormal heart rhythm (cardiac arrhythmia), or other disorders of the heart and blood vessels, mental depression, or Parkinson's disease. Use of isradipine may cause complications in patients with liver or kidney disease, since these organs work together to remove the medication from the body.

Itraconazole

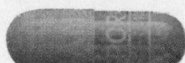

Sporanox 100 mg
(JANSSEN)

▶ Drug Class: Antifungal

▶ Available in: Capsules, oral solution

▶ Available OTC? No

▶ As Generic? Yes

Side Effects

SERIOUS
Skin rash or itching, fever or chills. Call your doctor right away.

COMMON
No common side effects have been reported with the use of itraconazole.

LESS COMMON
Diarrhea, nausea, vomiting, constipation, dizziness, headache, redness or flushing of skin.

PRINCIPAL USES
To treat serious fungal infections in the lungs and other parts of the body. These infections may occur in patients who do not have other illnesses, although they frequently occur in patients with weakened immune systems. Itraconazole is sometimes prescribed for fungal infections that are limited only to the nails.

HOW THE DRUG WORKS
Itraconazole prevents fungal organisms from producing vital substances required for growth and function. This drug is effective only for fungal infections. It will not work against bacterial or viral infections.

DOSAGE
Capsules— Adults and teenagers 16 and older: 200 to 400 mg, taken once daily. Children under age 16: Consult your pediatrician for proper dosage. Oral solution— Adults and teenagers: 100 to 200 mg once a day for days or weeks, depending on the condition being treated. Children: Consult your pediatrician. Swish the solution vigorously in your mouth for several seconds before swallowing.

ONSET OF EFFECT
Unknown.

DURATION OF ACTION
Unknown.

DIETARY ADVICE
Take capsules with food, but do not take the oral solution with food. Maintain your usual food and fluid intake. Patients with compromised immune systems are often weakened by their illness, by medications, or by other treatments, and may be unable to consume adequate amounts of nutritious food. Use liquid supplements if necessary.

STORAGE
Store in a tightly sealed container away from heat, moisture, and direct light.

IF YOU MISS A DOSE
Take it as soon as you remember. This will help keep a constant level of medication in your system. If it is near the time for the next dose, skip the missed dose and resume your regular dosage schedule. Do not double the next dose.

STOPPING THE DRUG
Take it as prescribed for the full treatment period, even if you begin to feel better before the scheduled end of therapy. The decision to stop taking the drug should be made by your doctor. Gradual reduction of the dose may be necessary if you have been taking this medicine for a long time.

PROLONGED USE
Therapy with this medication may require months. Prolonged use may increase the risk of adverse effects.

PRECAUTIONS
Over 60: Adverse reactions may be more likely and more severe.

Driving and Hazardous Work: Avoid such activites until you determine how the medicine affects you.

Alcohol: Avoid alcohol throughout therapy and for two days afterwards.

Pregnancy: Adequate studies of itraconazole use during pregnancy have not been done. Consult your doctor for specific advice if you are or are planning to become pregnant.

Breast Feeding: Itraconazole passes into breast milk; avoid or discontinue use while nursing.

Infants and Children: Itraconazole is not recommended for use by children under the age of 16.

Special Concerns: Women should use effective contraception to prevent pregnancy while taking this medication. Continue these measures for at least 2 months following the end of therapy. The capsules and the oral solution should not be used interchangeably.

OVERDOSE
Symptoms: An overdose with itraconazole is unlikely.

What to Do: Emergency instructions not applicable.

DRUG INTERACTIONS
While taking itraconazole, do not take astemizole, oral midazolam, pimozide, quinidine, dofetilide, triazolam, statin (anti-cholesterol) drugs. You should not take medications containing alcohol, such as cough syrups, elixirs, and tonics. Consult your doctor if you are taking antacids, anticholinergics, histamine H2-blockers, omeprazole, oral antidiabetics, erythromycin, sucralfate, carbamazepine, cyclosporine, isoniazid, didanosine, digoxin, phenytoin, rifampin, or warfarin. If you are taking an antacid, take it at least 2 hours after taking itraconazole.

FOOD INTERACTIONS
No known food interactions.

DISEASE INTERACTIONS
Do not take itraconazole for onychomycosis (a fungal nail infection) if you have congestive heart failure (CHF). Consult your doctor if you have any of the following conditions: liver or kidney disease, low levels or absence of stomach acid, or a history of alcohol abuse.

Kaolin with Pectin

BRAND NAMES
K-P, Kao-Spen, Kapectolin

▶ Drug Class: Antidiarrheal

▶ Available in: Oral suspension

▶ Available OTC? Yes

▶ As Generic? Yes

Side Effects

SERIOUS
No serious side effects have been reported.

COMMON
No common side effects have been reported.

LESS COMMON
Constipation.

PRINCIPAL USES
To treat diarrhea.

HOW THE DRUG WORKS
Kaolin with pectin absorbs fluids and binds to and removes bacteria and toxins from the digestive tract.

DOSAGE
Adults: 4 to 8 tablespoons (60 to 120 ml) after each loose bowel movement. Children age 12 and older: 3 to 4 tbsp (45 to 60 ml) after each loose bowel movement. Children ages 6 to 12: 2 to 4 tbsp (30 to 60 ml) after each loose bowel movement. Children ages 3 to 6: 1 to 2 tbsp (15 to 30 ml) after each loose bowel movement.

ONSET OF EFFECT
Unknown.

DURATION OF ACTION
Unknown.

DIETARY ADVICE
A mild diet is recommended when recovering from diarrhea. Bananas, rice, applesauce, and plain toast are good choices. Be sure to get plenty of fluids.

STORAGE
Store in a tightly sealed container away from heat, moisture, and direct light.

IF YOU MISS A DOSE
Take it as soon as you remember. If it is nearly time for another dose, skip the missed dose. Do not double the next dose.

STOPPING THE DRUG
Do not use this drug for more than 2 days without consulting your doctor.

PROLONGED USE
This drug is not intended for prolonged use. Consult your doctor if diarrhea continues for more than 2 days.

PRECAUTIONS
Over 60: Adverse reactions associated with diarrhea may be more severe in older patients. They should be sure to consume enough liquids to replace body fluids lost because of diarrhea.

Driving and Hazardous Work: The use of kaolin with pectin should not impair your ability to perform such tasks safely.

Alcohol: Avoid alcohol.

Pregnancy: It is not absorbed into the body and is not expected to cause problems during pregnancy.

Breast Feeding: It is not absorbed into the body and is not expected to cause problems during breast feeding.

Infants and Children: Kaolin with pectin should be used in children under the age of 3 only under the supervision of a doctor.

Special Concerns: In addition to taking medicine for diarrhea, it is important to replace the fluid lost by your body and to eat a proper diet. During the first 24 hours, drink plenty of caffeine-free clear liquids like water, broth, ginger ale, and decaffeinated tea. During the second 24 hours you may eat bland foods such as applesauce, bread, crackers, and oatmeal. Avoid caffeine, fried or spicy foods, bran, candy, fruits, and vegetables. They can make your condition worse.

OVERDOSE
Symptoms: Constipation.

What to Do: An overdose of kaolin with pectin is unlikely to be life-threatening. However, if someone takes a much larger dose than prescribed, call your doctor, emergency medical services (EMS), or the nearest poison control center immediately.

DRUG INTERACTIONS
Consult your doctor for specific advice if you are taking anticholinergics, antidyskinetics, digitalis drugs, lincomycins, loxapine, phenothiazines, thioxanthenes, or any other oral medication. Do not take any medication within 2 to 3 hours of taking kaolin with pectin.

FOOD INTERACTIONS
Fruits, fried or spicy foods, bran, candy, and caffeine-containing beverages can make diarrhea worse.

DISEASE INTERACTIONS
Caution is advised when taking kaolin with pectin. Consult your doctor if the diarrhea is suspected to be caused by parasites or dysentery.

Ketoconazole Oral

Nizoral 200 mg
(JANSSEN)

▶ Drug Class: Antifungal

▶ Available in: Tablets

▶ Available OTC? No

▶ As Generic? No

Side Effects

SERIOUS
Skin rash, itching, fever, chills. Call your doctor right away.

COMMON
No common side effects have been reported.

LESS COMMON
Diarrhea, nausea, vomiting, constipation, dizziness, headache, redness or flushing of skin.

PRINCIPAL USES
To treat serious fungal infections occurring in the lungs and other parts of the body. Ketoconazole is used to treat fungal infections of the skin, such as tinea corporis (ringworm), tinea cruris (jock itch), tinea pedis (athlete's foot), and pityriasis versicolor ("sun fungus," a condition characterized by fine scaly patches of varying shapes, sizes, and colors), that are severe or are unresponsive to griseofulvin.

HOW THE DRUG WORKS
Ketoconazole prevents fungal organisms from producing vital substances required for growth and function. This drug is effective only for infections caused by fungal organisms. It will not work for bacterial or viral infections.

DOSAGE
Adults and teenagers: 200 to 400 mg once a day. Children over age 2: 3.3 to 6.6 mg per 2.2 lbs of body weight once a day. Treatment may last from 1 week to 6 months, depending on the type of infection being treated.

ONSET OF EFFECT
Unknown.

DURATION OF ACTION
Unknown.

DIETARY ADVICE
Take it with food to reduce stomach upset. Tablets may be crushed and mixed with a beverage or food to reduce the bitter taste.

STORAGE
Store in a tightly sealed container away from heat, moisture, and direct light.

IF YOU MISS A DOSE
Take it as soon as you remember. This will help keep a constant level of medication in your system. If it is near the time for the next dose, skip the missed dose and resume your regular dosage schedule. Do not double the next dose.

STOPPING THE DRUG
Take it as prescribed for the full treatment period, even if you begin to feel better before the scheduled end of therapy. The decision to stop taking the drug should be made by your doctor. Dose should be reduced gradually if you have used the drug for a long time.

PROLONGED USE
Months of therapy may be necessary. Prolonged use increases the risk of adverse effects and may interfere with the body's synthesis of steroid hormones, which may cause erectile dysfunction in men and cessation of menstrual periods in women.

PRECAUTIONS
Over 60: Adverse reactions may be more likely and more severe.

Driving and Hazardous Work: Avoid such activities until you determine how the medication affects you.

Alcohol: Avoid alcohol.

Pregnancy: Adequate studies of ketoconazole use during pregnancy have not been done. Consult your doctor for advice if you are pregnant or planning to become pregnant.

Breast Feeding: Ketoconazole passes into breast milk; caution is advised. Consult your doctor for specific advice.

Infants and Children: Not recommended for use by children under 2 years.

Special Concerns: Ketoconazole may make your eyes more sensitive to sunlight. If this occurs, avoid exposure to bright light and wear sunglasses. For full effectiveness, ketoconazole should be taken at the same time every day.

OVERDOSE
Symptoms: An overdose is unlikely to occur.

What to Do: Emergency instructions not applicable.

DRUG INTERACTIONS
While taking ketoconazole, do not take astemizole or terfenadine. Serious side effects involving the heart may result. Do not take medications containing alcohol, such as cough syrups, elixirs, and tonics. Consult your doctor for advice if you are taking cyclosporine, isoniazid, didanosine, phenytoin, rifampin, or warfarin. If you are taking antacids, anticholinergics, histamine H2-blockers, omeprazole, or sucralfate, take them at least 2 hours after taking ketoconazole.

FOOD INTERACTIONS
No known food interactions.

DISEASE INTERACTIONS
Caution is advised when taking ketoconazole. Consult your doctor if you have any of the following: history of alcohol abuse, decreased amount of stomach acid, liver disease, or kidney disease. Use of ketoconazole can cause complications in patients with liver or kidney disease, since these organs work together to remove the medication from the body. If you have no stomach acid or a decreased amount of stomach acid, your doctor may prescribe a special solution.

Ketoconazole Topical

Nizoral A-D, Nizoral Cream

▶ Drug Class: Topical antifungal

▶ Available in: Cream, shampoo

▶ Available OTC? Yes

▶ As Generic? Yes

Side Effects

SERIOUS
Blistering or ulceration of the skin; blistering of the lips, nose, and mouth.

COMMON
Brief burning, itching, or irritation after application of cream; peeling.

LESS COMMON
Severe burning, itching, swelling, increased redness, or any discomfort at the application site not present prior to therapy (as a result of allergic reaction).

PRINCIPAL USES
Ketoconazole is used to treat fungal infections of the skin. These infections include tinea pedis (athlete's foot), tinea corporis (ringworm), tinea cruris (jock itch), yeast infections of the skin, seborrheic dermatitis, and others.

HOW THE DRUG WORKS
Ketoconazole prevents fungal organisms from manufacturing vital substances required for growth and function.

DOSAGE
Adults, for tinea and yeast: Apply once daily to affected skin. Treatment generally requires 2 to 6 weeks. Adults, for seborrheic dermatitis: Apply two times a day to affected skin. Treatment generally requires 4 weeks. Children: Consult your pediatrician.

ONSET OF EFFECT
Ketoconazole begins killing susceptible fungi shortly after contact. The effects may not be noticeable for several days or weeks.

DURATION OF ACTION
Unknown.

DIETARY ADVICE
Maintain your usual food and fluid intake. Increase fluid intake in hot weather, during exercise, or if you have a fever or diarrhea.

STORAGE
Store in a tightly sealed container away from heat and direct light.

IF YOU MISS A DOSE
Apply it as soon as you remember. If it is near the time for the next dose, skip the missed dose and resume your regular dosage schedule. Do not double the next dose or apply an excessively thick film of topical medication to compensate for a missed application.

STOPPING THE DRUG
Apply ketoconazole as prescribed for the full treatment period, even if you notice marked improvement before the scheduled end of therapy.

PROLONGED USE
Therapy with this medication should not exceed 4 weeks.

PRECAUTIONS
Over 60: Adverse reactions may be more likely and more severe in older patients.

Driving and Hazardous Work: The use of ketoconazole cream should not impair your ability to perform such tasks safely.

Alcohol: No special precautions are necessary.

Pregnancy: Avoid or discontinue use of ketoconazole if you are pregnant or trying to become pregnant.

Breast Feeding: Ketoconazole may pass into breast milk; avoid or discontinue usage while nursing. Consult your doctor for specific advice.

Infants and Children: Not recommended for use by young children.

Special Concerns: Avoid contact with eyes. Wash hands thoroughly after application. Tell your doctor if your condition has not improved within a few days of starting ketoconazole. As with any other antifungal, ketoconazole is useful only against organisms that are vulnerable to its effects. Therefore, it is important to tell your doctor if your condition has not improved—or has worsened—within a few days of starting ketoconazole. The particular organism causing your illness may be resistant to this medication.

OVERDOSE
Symptoms: No specific ones have been reported.

What to Do: An overdose of ketoconazole is unlikely to be life-threatening. However, if someone applies a much larger dose than prescribed or ingests the medication, call your doctor, emergency medical services (EMS), or the nearest poison control center.

DRUG INTERACTIONS
No specific drug interactions are known as of this writing. If you are concerned whether a prescription or over-the-counter medication you are taking may interact with ketoconazole, consult your physician or pharmacist for current information.

FOOD INTERACTIONS
No known food interactions.

DISEASE INTERACTIONS
Consult your physician if you have had previous allergies or an undesirable reaction to any other topical medication.

Ketoprofen

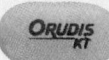

Orudis KT Caplets 12.5 mg
(WHITEHALL-ROBINS)

Additional photographs

▶ Drug Class: Nonsteroidal anti-inflammatory drug (NSAID)

▶ Available in: Tablets and capsules (also extended-release forms), rectal suppositories

▶ Available OTC? Yes

▶ As Generic? Yes

Side Effects

SERIOUS
Shortness of breath or wheezing, with or without swelling of legs or other signs of heart failure; chest pain; peptic ulcer disease with vomiting of blood; black, tarry stools; decreasing kidney function. Call your doctor immediately.

COMMON
Nausea, vomiting, heartburn, diarrhea, constipation, headache, dizziness, sleepiness.

LESS COMMON
Ulcers or sores in mouth, depression, rashes or blistering of skin, ringing sound in the ears, unusual tingling or numbness of the hands or feet, seizures, blurred vision. Also elevated potassium levels, decreased blood counts; such problems can be detected by your doctor.

PRINCIPAL USES
To treat mild to moderate pain and inflammation caused by tendinitis, arthritis, bursitis, gout, soft tissue injuries, migraine and other vascular headaches, menstrual cramps, and other conditions. When patients fail to respond to one NSAID, another may be tried. The greatest effectiveness often requires trial and error of several different NSAIDs.

HOW THE DRUG WORKS
NSAIDs work by interfering with the formation of prostaglandins, naturally occurring substances in the body that cause inflammation and make nerves more sensitive to pain impulses. NSAIDs also have other modes of action that are less well understood.

DOSAGE
Adults— Tablets or capsules: 50 mg, 4 times a day, or 75 mg, 3 times a day. Extended-release tablets or capsules: 200 mg once a day. Suppositories: 50 to 100 mg inserted twice a day (morning and evening). Sometimes, suppositories may be used only at night by people who take an oral dose during the day. Maximum dosage for all forms is 300 mg per day.

ONSET OF EFFECT
1 to 2 hours.

DURATION OF ACTION
3 to 4 hours.

DIETARY ADVICE
Take oral forms with food.

STORAGE
Store in a tightly sealed container away from heat, moisture, and direct light.

IF YOU MISS A DOSE
Take it as soon as you remember. If it is near the time for the next dose, skip the missed dose and resume your regular dosage schedule. Do not double the next dose.

STOPPING THE DRUG
If taking this drug by prescription, do not stop without consulting your doctor.

PROLONGED USE
Prolonged use can cause gastrointestinal problems, including ulceration and bleeding, kidney dysfunction, and liver inflammation. Consult your doctor about the need for medical examinations and lab tests.

PRECAUTIONS
Over 60: Because of the potentially greater consequences of gastrointestinal side effects, the dose of NSAIDs for older patients, especially those over age 70, is often cut in half.

Driving and Hazardous Work: Do not drive or engage in hazardous work until you determine how the medicine affects you.

Alcohol: Avoid alcohol when using this medication because it increases the risk of stomach irritation.

Pregnancy: Do not use ketoprofen while pregnant.

Breast Feeding: Ketoprofen passes into breast milk; avoid use while nursing.

Infants and Children: Ketoprofen may be used in exceptional circumstances; consult your doctor.

Special Concerns: Because NSAIDs can interfere with blood coagulation, this drug should be stopped at least 3 days prior to any surgery.

OVERDOSE
Symptoms: Severe nausea, vomiting, headache, confusion, seizures.

What to Do: Call your doctor, emergency medical services (EMS), or the nearest poison control center immediately.

DRUG INTERACTIONS
Do not take this drug with aspirin or any other NSAIDs without your doctor's approval. In addition, consult your doctor if you are taking antihypertensives, steroids, anticoagulants, antibiotics, itraconazole or ketoconazole, plicamycin, penicillamine, valproic acid, phenytoin, cyclosporine, digitalis drugs, lithium, methotrexate, probenecid, triamterene, or zidovudine.

FOOD INTERACTIONS
No known food interactions.

DISEASE INTERACTIONS
Consult your doctor if you have any of the following: bleeding problems, inflammation or ulcers of the stomach and intestines, diabetes mellitus, systemic lupus erythematosus (SLE, lupus), anemia, asthma, epilepsy, Parkinson's disease, kidney stones, or a history of heart disease or alcohol abuse. Use of ketoprofen may cause complications in patients with liver or kidney disease, since these organs work together to remove the medication from the body.

Ketorolac Tromethamine Ophthalmic

BRAND NAMES
Acular, Acular PF

▶ Drug Class: Nonsteroidal anti-inflammatory drug (NSAID)

▶ Available in: Ophthalmic solution

▶ Available OTC? No

▶ As Generic? No

Side Effects

SERIOUS
Rarely, ophthalmic ketorolac tromethamine will cause bleeding in the eye, redness or swelling of the eye or eyelid not present before the start of therapy, or tearing or itching of the eye. Call your doctor immediately.

COMMON
Mild and temporary burning or stinging of eyes after application; eye infection.

LESS COMMON
There are no less-common side effects associated with ophthalmic ketorolac.

PRINCIPAL USES
For short-term therapy of eye itching caused by seasonal allergic conjunctivitis. It is also used to treat inflammation and eye problems that may occur after cataract surgery.

HOW THE DRUG WORKS
Ophthalmic ketorolac inhibits the release of substances that stimulate inflammation and cause pain in eye tissues.

DOSAGE
Adults: 1 drop in each eye 4 times a day. Children: Consult your pediatrician.

ONSET OF EFFECT
Unknown.

DURATION OF ACTION
Unknown.

DIETARY ADVICE
No special restrictions.

STORAGE
Store this medication in a tightly sealed container away from heat, moisture, and direct light. Do not refrigerate or allow it to freeze.

IF YOU MISS A DOSE
Apply it as soon as you remember. If it is near the time for the next dose, skip the missed dose and resume your regular dosage schedule. Do not double the next dose.

STOPPING THE DRUG
Use it as prescribed for the full treatment period, even if you feel better before the scheduled end of therapy.

PROLONGED USE
See your doctor regularly for tests and examinations if you must use this drug for a prolonged period.

PRECAUTIONS
Over 60: Adverse reactions may be more likely and more severe.

Driving and Hazardous Work: Avoid such activities until you determine how the medicine affects your vision.

Alcohol: Avoid alcohol.

Pregnancy: Adequate human studies have not been completed. Before taking ophthalmic ketorolac, tell your doctor if you are pregnant or plan to become pregnant.

Breast Feeding: Ophthalmic ketorolac may pass into breast milk; caution is advised. Consult your doctor for specific advice.

Infants and Children: Use and dosage for infants and children must be determined by your doctor.

Special Concerns: To use the eye drops, first wash your hands. Tilt your head back. Gently apply pressure to the inside corner of the eyelid and with the index finger of the same hand, pull downward on the lower eyelid to make a space. Drop the medicine into this space and close your eye. Apply pressure for 1 or 2 minutes while keeping the eye closed without blinking. Then wash your hands again. Make sure the tip of the dropper does not touch your eye, finger, or any other surface. If your symptoms do not improve or if they become worse, check with your doctor. Ophthalmic ketorolac may cause problems in patients who wear soft contact lenses. Your physician may want you to stop wearing the lenses while you take the medicine.

OVERDOSE
Symptoms: No specific ones have been reported.

What to Do: An overdose of ophthalmic ketorolac is unlikely to be life-threatening. However, if someone applies a much larger dose of the drug than prescribed or accidentally ingests the medicine, call your doctor, emergency medical services (EMS), or the nearest poison control center.

DRUG INTERACTIONS
Consult your doctor for specific advice if you are taking aspirin or another salicylate, diflunisal, etodolac, fenoprofen, floctafenine, flurbiprofen, ibuprofen, indomethacin, ketoprofen, oral ketorolac, meclofenamate, mefenamic acid, nabumetone, naproxen, oxyphenbutazone, phenylbutazone, piroxicam, sulindac, suprofen, tenoxicam, tiaprofenic acid, tolmetin, or zomepirac.

FOOD INTERACTIONS
No known food interactions.

DISEASE INTERACTIONS
Caution is advised when taking ophthalmic ketorolac. Consult your doctor if you have hemophilia or any other bleeding problem.

Ketorolac Tromethamine Systemic

▶ Drug Class: Nonsteroidal anti-inflammatory drug (NSAID)

▶ Available in: Tablets, injection

▶ Available OTC? No

▶ As Generic? Yes

Side Effects

SERIOUS
Gastrointestinal bleeding causing dark or bloody stools or vomiting; severe high blood pressure causing headache and blurred vision; prolonged bleeding from a cut; burnlike rash. Call your doctor immediately. This drug may cause breathing difficulty or a severe allergic reaction in persons who are sensitive to aspirin, especially those with aspirin-induced nasal polyps or asthma.

COMMON
Stomach distress.

LESS COMMON
Drowsiness, diarrhea, confusion, ringing in ears, sensitivity to sunlight, water retention, hives, headache.

PRINCIPAL USES
To treat moderate to severe pain and inflammation, usually following surgery.

HOW THE DRUG WORKS
NSAIDs work by interfering with the action of prostaglandins, naturally occurring substances that cause inflammation and make nerves more sensitive to pain impulses. NSAIDs also have other modes of action that are less well understood.

DOSAGE
For acute pain— Initial adult dose is usually by injection, which may be followed (if necessary) by injections or tablets. Injection: 30 mg into a vein every 6 hours. Some people may receive one 60 mg dose into a muscle. The dose should not exceed 120 mg per 24-hour period. Tablets: 10 mg, 4 times a day, taken every 4 to 6 hours. Your doctor may recommend a different dose, though it should not exceed 40 mg per day. For pain in children— Consult your pediatrician.

ONSET OF EFFECT
Into a vein: Immediate. Into a muscle: Within 10 minutes. Tablets: 30 to 60 minutes.

DURATION OF ACTION
6 to 8 hours.

DIETARY ADVICE
Tablets should be taken with food; maintain your usual food and fluid intake.

STORAGE
Not applicable for injection form; it is administered only at a health care facility. Store tablets in a tightly sealed container away from heat and direct light.

IF YOU MISS A DOSE
Take tablets as soon as you remember. If it is near the time for the next dose, skip the missed dose and resume your regular dosage schedule. Do not double the next dose.

STOPPING THE DRUG
Take it as prescribed for the full treatment period. Ask your doctor about stopping the drug if you are feeling better before the scheduled end of therapy.

PROLONGED USE
Therapy generally does not last more than 5 days. Use beyond that period may cause serious side effects.

PRECAUTIONS
Over 60: Because of the potentially greater consequences of gastrointestinal side effects, the dose of NSAIDs for older patients, especially those over age 70, is often cut in half.

Driving and Hazardous Work: Avoid such activities until you determine how the medicine affects you.

Alcohol: Avoid alcohol.

Pregnancy: Avoid or discontinue ketorolac if you are pregnant or are planning to become pregnant.

Breast Feeding: Ketorolac passes into breast milk; avoid use while nursing.

Infants and Children: May be used in exceptional circumstances; consult your doctor.

OVERDOSE
Symptoms: Nausea, vomiting, severe headache, confusion, seizures.

What to Do: Call your doctor, emergency medical services (EMS), or the nearest poison control center immediately.

DRUG INTERACTIONS
Do not take this drug with aspirin or any other NSAIDs. In addition, consult your doctor if you are taking acetaminophen, anticoagulants, enoxaparin, lithium, methotrexate, diuretics, beta-blockers, sulfinpyrazone, valproic acid, or warfarin.

FOOD INTERACTIONS
No known food interactions.

DISEASE INTERACTIONS
Caution is advised when taking ketorolac. Consult your doctor if you have any of the following: nasal polyps, severe hives, any stomach or intestinal disorder, high blood pressure, a blood coagulation defect, or a history of heart disease. Use of ketorolac may cause complications in patients with liver or kidney disease, since these organs work together to remove the medication from the body.

Ketotifen Fumarate

▶ Drug Class: Histamine (H1) blocker

▶ Available in: Ophthalmic solution

▶ Available OTC? No

▶ As Generic? No

Side Effects

SERIOUS
No serious side effects are associated with ketotifen.

COMMON
Headache, runny nose.

LESS COMMON
Allergic reaction, burning or stinging of the eye, tearing, eye dryness, eye pain, itching, corneal inflammation, pupil dilation, light sensitivity, rash, flu-like symptoms, sore throat.

PRINCIPAL USES
For short-term therapy of eye itching caused by seasonal allergic conjunctivitis (inflammation of the mucous membranes that line the inner surface of the eyelids and whites of the eyes).

HOW THE DRUG WORKS
Ketotifen blocks the effects of histamine, a naturally occurring substance within the body that causes swelling, itching, sneezing, watery eyes, hives, and other symptoms associated with allergic reactions.

DOSAGE
Instill 1 drop in the affected eye(s) every 8 to 12 hours.

ONSET OF EFFECT
Unknown.

DURATION OF ACTION
Unknown.

DIETARY ADVICE
Ketotifen can be used without regard to diet.

STORAGE
Store in a tightly sealed container away from heat, moisture, and direct light. Do not allow it to freeze.

IF YOU MISS A DOSE
Apply it as soon as you remember. If it is near the time for the next dose, skip the missed dose and resume your regular dosage schedule. Do not double the next dose.

STOPPING THE DRUG
You may stop using ketotifen whenever you choose.

PROLONGED USE
Ketotifen is prescribed for short-term use only.

PRECAUTIONS
Over 60: No special problems are expected.

Driving and Hazardous Work: Do not drive or engage in hazardous work until you determine how the medicine affects you.

Alcohol: No special precautions are necessary.

Pregnancy: No adequate human studies have been done. Before taking ketotifen, tell your doctor if you are pregnant or plan to become pregnant.

Breast Feeding: Ketotifen may pass into breast milk; caution is advised. Consult your doctor for specific advice.

Infants and Children: Not recommended for use by children under the age of 3 years.

Special Concerns: To use the eye drops, first wash your hands. Tilt your head back. Gently apply pressure to the inside corner of the eyelid and with the index finger of the same hand, pull downward on the lower eyelid to make a space. Drop the medicine into this space and close your eye. Apply pressure for 1 or 2 minutes while keeping the eye closed without blinking. Then wash your hands again. Make sure the tip of the dropper does not touch your eye, finger, or any other surface. You should not wear a contact lens if your eye is red. Ketotifen should not be used to treat contact-lens-related irritation. If you wear soft contact lenses and your eyes are not red, wait at least 10 minutes after instilling the drops before inserting your contact lenses.

OVERDOSE
Symptoms: No specific ones have been reported.

What to Do: An overdose with ketotifen is unlikely to be life-threatening. However, if someone accidentally ingests the medicine, seek emergency medical attention immediately.

DRUG INTERACTIONS
None reported.

FOOD INTERACTIONS
None reported.

DISEASE INTERACTIONS
None reported.

Labetalol Hydrochloride

Trandate 200 mg
(GLAXO WELLCOME)

Additional photographs

▶ Drug Class: Beta-blocker

▶ Available in: Tablets (Injection is for hospital use only.)

▶ Available OTC? No

▶ As Generic? Yes

Side Effects

SERIOUS
Shortness of breath, wheezing; chest pain or tightness; swelling of the ankles, feet, and lower legs; mental depression. If you experience such symptoms, stop taking the drug and call your doctor immediately.

COMMON
Dizziness or lightheadedness, especially when rising suddenly to a standing position; decreased sexual ability; unusual fatigue, weakness, or drowsiness; insomnia; scalp tingling, especially at the beginning of treatment.

LESS COMMON
Changes in taste; itching, numbness, or tingling; vivid dreams or nightmares; nausea or vomiting; irregular or slow heartbeat (50 beats per minute or less).

PRINCIPAL USES
To treat severe high blood pressure (hypertension).

HOW THE DRUG WORKS
Labetalol hydrochloride is a beta-blocker with alpha-blocker activity. Such drugs work by preventing—or blocking—nerve impulses from exerting an accelerating or intensifying effect on specific parts of the body, especially the blood vessels and heart. Unlike other beta-blockers, this drug does not significantly slow the heart rate.

DOSAGE
Usual adult dose: 100 mg twice daily, 6 to 12 hours apart, increased to a maintenance dose of 200 to 400 mg twice daily. Maximum dose: 800 mg, 3 times daily.

ONSET OF EFFECT
Within 20 minutes.

DURATION OF ACTION
12 to 24 hours.

DIETARY ADVICE
Follow your doctor's dietary restrictions, such as a low-salt or low-fat diet, to improve control over high blood pressure and heart disease. Take the tablets with food.

STORAGE
Store in a tightly sealed container away from heat and direct light.

IF YOU MISS A DOSE
Take it as soon as you remember. If it is within 8 hours of your next dose, skip the missed dose, and go back to your regular schedule. Do not double the next dose.

STOPPING THE DRUG
Do not stop this drug suddenly, as this may lead to angina or a heart attack in patients with advanced heart disease. Slow reduction of the dose over a period of 2 to 3 weeks is advised. Do not stop taking the drug or make any changes in dosage without consulting your doctor.

PROLONGED USE
Lifelong therapy may be necessary. See your doctor regularly for examinations and tests if you must take this medication for a prolonged period.

PRECAUTIONS
Over 60: Adverse reactions may be more likely and more severe in older patients.

Driving and Hazardous Work: Do not drive or engage in hazardous work until you determine how the medicine affects you.

Alcohol: Drink in careful moderation if at all. Alcohol may interact with the drug and cause a dangerous drop in blood pressure.

Pregnancy: Discuss with your doctor the relative risks and benefits of using this drug while pregnant.

Breast Feeding: Adverse effects in infants have not been reported. Consult your doctor for specific advice.

Infants and Children: No special problems.

Special Concerns: Get up slowly from a sitting or lying position to avoid dizziness or lightheadedness, especially when you first start taking the drug or if the dosage has been increased.

OVERDOSE
Symptoms: Unusually slow or rapid heartbeat, severe dizziness or fainting, poor circulation in the hands (bluish skin), breathing difficulty, seizures.

What to Do: Call your doctor, emergency medical services (EMS), or the nearest poison control center immediately.

DRUG INTERACTIONS
Consult your physician for specific advice if you are taking amphetamines, oral antidiabetic agents, asthma medication (such as aminophylline or theophylline), calcium channel blockers, clonidine, guanabenz, halothane, allergy shots, insulin, MAO inhibitors, reserpine, other beta-blockers, any over-the-counter medicine, sodium bicarbonate injection.

FOOD INTERACTIONS
None reported.

DISEASE INTERACTIONS
Labetalol hydrochloride should be used with caution in people with diabetes, especially insulin dependent diabetes, since the drug may mask symptoms of hypoglycemia. Consult your doctor if you have allergies or asthma, heart or blood vessel disease (including congestive heart failure and peripheral vascular disease), hyperthyroidism, irregular (slow) heartbeat, myasthenia gravis, psoriasis, respiratory problems such as bronchitis or emphysema, kidney or liver disease, or a history of depression.

Lactulose

BRAND NAMES
Cholac, Chronulac,
Constilac, Constulose,
Duphalac, Enulose,
Evalose, Heptalac,
Portalac

▶ Drug Class: Hyperosmotic laxative

▶ Available in: Syrup

▶ Available OTC? No

▶ As Generic? Yes

Side Effects

SERIOUS
Unusual weakness, confusion, muscle cramps, dizziness or lightheadedness, irregular heartbeat.

COMMON
Diarrhea, gas, intestinal cramps, increased thirst.

LESS COMMON
No less-common side effects are associated with lactulose.

PRINCIPAL USES
For long-term treatment of chronic constipation. It is also sometimes used for treatment of severe liver disease.

HOW THE DRUG WORKS
Lactulose draws water into the bowel to help loosen and soften the stool and stimulate bowel activity.

DOSAGE
For constipation: 15 to 30 ml once a day. The dose may be increased to 60 ml once a day, if needed. For severe liver disease: 30 to 45 ml, 3 or 4 times a day until 2 or 3 soft stools are produced daily.

ONSET OF EFFECT
24 to 48 hours.

DURATION OF ACTION
Up to 24 hours.

DIETARY ADVICE
Take it with a full glass (8 oz) of water or fruit juice, or 2 glasses of water if your doctor directs. You should not use lactulose if you are on a low-galactose diet.

STORAGE
Store in a tightly sealed container away from heat, moisture, and direct light. Do not allow to freeze.

IF YOU MISS A DOSE
Take it as soon as you remember. If it is near the time for the next dose, skip the missed dose and resume your regular dosage schedule. Do not double the next dose.

STOPPING THE DRUG
Take it as prescribed for the full treatment period. However, you may stop taking the drug if you are feeling better before the scheduled end of therapy.

PROLONGED USE
Do not take lactulose for more than 1 week unless you are under a doctor's supervision. Prolonged use may cause laxative dependence.

PRECAUTIONS
Over 60: No special problems are expected in older patients.

Driving and Hazardous Work: The use of lactulose should not impair your ability to perform such tasks safely.

Alcohol: No special precautions are necessary.

Pregnancy: Caution is advised. Discuss with your doctor the relative risks and benefits of using this drug while pregnant.

Breast Feeding: Lactulose may pass into breast milk; caution is advised. Consult your doctor for advice.

Infants and Children: Lactulose is not recommended for use by children under the age of 6 unless prescribed by your doctor.

Special Concerns: Excessive use of lactulose or any laxative in teenagers may indicate an eating disorder such as anorexia nervosa or bulimia nervosa. Consult your doctor if you observe such behavior. If you have a sudden change in bowel function or habits that lasts more than 2 weeks, consult your doctor.

OVERDOSE
Symptoms: Diarrhea, severe abdominal cramps.

What to Do: An overdose of lactulose is unlikely to be life-threatening. However, if someone takes a much larger dose than prescribed, call your doctor, emergency medical services (EMS), or the nearest poison control center.

DRUG INTERACTIONS
Consult your doctor for specific advice if you are taking other laxatives, antacids, antibiotics, anticoagulants, digitalis drugs, oral tetracyclines, sodium polystyrene sulfonate, ciprofloxacin, or potassium supplements.

FOOD INTERACTIONS
If you are on a low-calorie, low-salt, or low-sugar diet, check with your doctor before taking lactulose.

DISEASE INTERACTIONS
Caution is advised when taking lactulose. Consult your doctor if you have symptoms of appendicitis or an inflamed bowel (abdominal pain, cramps, soreness, bloating, nausea, and vomiting), diabetes mellitus, difficulty swallowing, heart disease or blood pressure disorder, intestinal problems, or kidney disease.

Lamivudine (3TC)

Epivir 150 mg
(GLAXO WELLCOME)

▶ Drug Class: Antiviral

▶ Available in: Solution, tablets

▶ Available OTC? No

▶ As Generic? No

Side Effects

SERIOUS
Severe stomach or abdominal pain, nausea, vomiting, unusual fatigue, fever, chills, sore throat, numbness, burning, tingling, or pain in hands, arms, legs or feet, breathing difficulty, itching, hives, skin rash, swelling of face, mouth, lips, throat, or tongue. Call your doctor immediately if any of these side effects arise.

COMMON
No common side effects are associated with lamivudine.

LESS COMMON
Mild to moderate abdominal pain, diarrhea, dizziness, cough, headache, mild nausea or vomiting, insomnia, loss of hair.

PRINCIPAL USES
To treat HIV (human immunodeficiency virus) infection in combination with zidovudine (AZT) or other antiretroviral agents. While not a cure for HIV infection, these drugs may suppress the replication of the virus and delay the progression of the disease. Also used to treat chronic hepatitis B.

HOW THE DRUG WORKS
Lamivudine interferes with the activity of enzymes needed for the replication of DNA in viral cells, thus preventing HIV and hepatitis B from reproducing. HIV that has become resistant to lamivudine may be less likely to become resistant to zidovudine.

DOSAGE
To treat HIV (Epivir)— Adults and teenagers weighing 110 lbs or more: 150 mg, 2 times a day. Adults weighing less than 110 lbs: 2 mg per 2.2 lbs (1 kg) of body weight 2 times a day. Children 3 months to 12 years: 4 mg per 2.2 lbs of body weight 2 times a day, up to 150 mg per dose. In all cases lamivudine should be taken with other antiretroviral agents. To treat hepatitis B (Epivir-HBV)— Adults: 100 mg once a day. Epivir and Epivir-HBV are not interchangeable; Epivir tablets and oral solution contain a higher dose of the same active ingredient then Epivir-HBV preparations.

ONSET OF EFFECT
Unknown. Maximum effect may take 12 to 16 weeks.

DURATION OF ACTION
Unknown. Effects of the drug may be prolonged if lamivudine is used in combination with other effective drugs and the virus is maximally suppressed.

DIETARY ADVICE
Can be taken with or without food. Be sure to drink plenty of fluids.

STORAGE
Store in a tightly sealed container away from heat and direct light.

IF YOU MISS A DOSE
Take it as soon as you remember. If it is near the time for the next dose, skip the missed dose and resume your regular dosage schedule. Do not double the next dose. It is especially important to take lamivudine on schedule, to assure constant, proper blood levels of the drug.

STOPPING THE DRUG
Take it as prescribed for the full treatment period, even if you begin to feel better.

PROLONGED USE
See your doctor regularly for tests and examinations if you must take this medicine for a prolonged period.

PRECAUTIONS
Over 60: No special studies have been done on older patients. A lower dose may be warranted, especially if liver or kidney function is impaired.

Driving and Hazardous Work: Do not drive or engage in hazardous work until you determine how the medicine affects you.

Alcohol: Avoid alcohol if liver function is impaired.

Pregnancy: In animal studies, lamivudine has been shown to cause birth defects. Nevertheless, lamivudine is increasingly being used in combination with other antiretroviral drugs to treat pregnant HIV-infected women.

Breast Feeding: Women infected with HIV should not breast feed, so as to avoid transmitting the virus to an uninfected child.

Infants and Children: Adverse reactions may be more likely and more severe in young patients.

Special Concerns: If you are taking the solution, use a special measuring spoon or other precisely marked scoop to dispense the proper dose. The risk of transmitting the HIV or hepatitis B to other persons is not reduced by lamivudine. Be sure to take precautionary measures.

OVERDOSE
Symptoms: No cases of overdose have been reported. The symptoms would likely include diarrhea or abdominal cramps.

What to Do: An overdose of lamivudine is unlikely to occur. Nonetheless, if you have any reason to suspect an overdose, call your doctor, emergency medical services (EMS), or the nearest poison control center as soon as possible.

DRUG INTERACTIONS
Consult your doctor for specific advice if you are taking any other prescription or over-the-counter medication.

FOOD INTERACTIONS
No known food interactions.

DISEASE INTERACTIONS
Consult your doctor if you have any other medical condition. Use of lamivudine may cause complications in patients with impaired liver or kidney function, since these organs work together to remove the medication from the body.

Lamivudine/Zidovudine

▶ Drug Class: Antiviral

▶ Available in: Tablets

▶ Available OTC? No

▶ As Generic? No

Side Effects

SERIOUS
Severe stomach or abdominal pain; anemia (low red blood cell count) causing paleness, fatigue, or shortness of breath; fever; chills; sore throat. Also numbness, burning, tingling, or pain in the hands, arms, legs or feet, breathing difficulty, itching, hives, skin rash, swelling of the face, mouth, lips, throat, or tongue. Call your doctor immediately.

COMMON
Headaches, nausea and vomiting, insomnia, stomach upset, loss of appetite, diarrhea, dizziness, cough.

LESS COMMON
Mild to moderate abdominal pain or cramping, muscle aches and pain, hepatitis (liver inflammation, which may cause yellowish discoloration of skin and eyes), joint pain, loss of hair.

PRINCIPAL USES
To treat HIV (human immunodeficiency virus) infection. While not a cure for HIV, this combination of lamivudine (3TC) and zidovudine (AZT) may suppress the replication of the virus and delay the progression of the disease.

HOW THE DRUG WORKS
This drug combination interferes with the activity of enzymes needed for the replication of DNA in viral cells, thus preventing HIV from reproducing.

DOSAGE
Adults and teenagers: 1 tablet (containing 150 mg of lamivudine and 300 mg of zidovudine) twice a day. Children: Should not be taken by children because it is a fixed-dose combination that cannot be adjusted.

ONSET OF EFFECT
Unknown. With most antiretroviral drugs, an early response can be seen within the first few days of therapy, but the maximum effect may take 12 to 16 weeks.

DURATION OF ACTION
Unknown. Effects of the drug combination may be prolonged if the virus is maximally suppressed.

DIETARY ADVICE
Can be taken with or without food. Be sure to drink plenty of fluids.

STORAGE
Store in a tightly sealed container away from heat, moisture, and direct light.

IF YOU MISS A DOSE
Take it as soon as you remember. If it is near the time for the next dose, skip the missed dose and resume your regular dosage schedule. Do not double the next dose. It is especially important to take this medication on schedule, to assure constant, proper blood levels of the drug.

STOPPING THE DRUG
The decision to stop taking the drug should be made in consultation with your physician.

PROLONGED USE
See your doctor regularly for tests and examinations as long as you take this medication.

PRECAUTIONS
Over 60: No special studies have been done on older patients. A lower dose may be warranted, especially if liver or kidney function is impaired.

Driving and Hazardous Work: Use of this drug combination should not diminish your ability to perform such tasks safely.

Alcohol: Avoid alcohol if liver function is impaired.

Pregnancy: Adequate human studies have not been done. Discuss with your doctor the relative risks and benefits of using this drug while pregnant.

Breast Feeding: Women infected with HIV should not breast-feed, so as to avoid transmitting the virus to an uninfected child.

Infants and Children: Not recommended for children under the age of 12.

Special Concerns: Use of this drug combination does not eliminate the risk of passing the AIDS virus (HIV) to other persons. Be sure to take all appropriate preventive measures. This medication should not be used in patients with low body weight.

OVERDOSE
Symptoms: No cases of overdose with this combination have been reported. However, cases of overdose have been reported for zidovudine taken alone (see Zidovudine).

What to Do: If you suspect an overdose or if someone takes a much larger dose than prescribed, call your doctor, emergency medical services (EMS), or the nearest poison control center immediately.

DRUG INTERACTIONS
Consult your doctor for specific advice if you are taking amphotericin B (by injection), anticancer agents, thyroid drugs, azathioprine, chloramphenicol, colchicine, cyclophosphamide, flucytosine, ganciclovir, interferon, mercaptopurine, methotrexate, plicamycin, clarithromycin, or probenecid. Also consult your doctor for specific advice if you are taking any other prescription or over-the-counter medication.

FOOD INTERACTIONS
No known food interactions.

DISEASE INTERACTIONS
Caution is advised when taking this drug combination. Consult your doctor if you have anemia or another blood problem. Use of this drug is not recommended in patients with impaired kidney function or risk factors for liver disease.

Lamotrigine

Lamictal 100 mg
(GLAXO WELLCOME)

Additional photographs

▶ Drug Class: Anticonvulsant

▶ Available in: Tablets, chewable tablets

▶ Available OTC? No

▶ As Generic? No

Side Effects

SERIOUS
Fever, sore throat, swollen glands, red or purple point-like rash on the skin or mucous membranes, blistering or peeling skin lesion, weakness, confusion, lethargy, or seizures may be a sign of a potentially fatal blood reaction or other complication. Call your doctor immediately.

COMMON
Dizziness, blurred or double vision, clumsiness or incoordination, drowsiness, nausea, vomiting, headache.

LESS COMMON
Indigestion, runny nose, loss of strength, insomnia, depression, mood changes, trembling or shaking, slurred speech. Numerous additional side effects are associated with the use of this drug; consult your doctor if you are concerned about any adverse or unusual reactions.

PRINCIPAL USES
To control certain kinds of seizures in the treatment of epilepsy. Lamotrigine is generally taken in conjunction with other anticonvulsants.

HOW THE DRUG WORKS
Lamotrigine acts on the central nervous system to control the number and severity of seizures. It is thought to depress the activity of certain parts of the brain and suppress the abnormal firing of ncurons that causes seizures.

DOSAGE
Adults: 200 to 900 mg a day, in 2 divided doses. Some patients may require higher doses. A low dose is used to start; the dose is gradually increased by your doctor. The increase in dose is very slow if you are also taking valproic acid (Depakene, Depakote). Lamotrigine is generally not recommended for use in children younger than age 16.

ONSET OF EFFECT
Several hours.

DURATION OF ACTION
Maximum effectiveness lasts 24 hours or longer; effectiveness then gradually decreases.

DIETARY ADVICE
Take it with food to minimize the likelihood of stomach upset. Chewable tablets can be taken with a small amount of water or diluted fruit juice.

STORAGE
Store in a tightly sealed container away from heat, moisture, and direct light.

IF YOU MISS A DOSE
Take it as soon as you remember. If it is near the time for the next dose, skip the missed dose and resume your regular dosage schedule. Do not double the next dose, unless advised to do so by your doctor.

STOPPING THE DRUG
Never stop taking this drug abruptly because seizures may ensue. The dose is typically tapered over a period of weeks under your doctor's supervision.

PROLONGED USE
See your doctor regularly for tests if you must take this drug for an extended period.

PRECAUTIONS
Over 60: Adverse reactions may be more likely in older patients. Lower dosages may be warranted.

Driving and Hazardous Work: This drug may cause drowsiness or dizziness. Do not drive or engage in hazardous work until you determine how it affects you.

Alcohol: May contribute to excessive drowsiness.

Pregnancy: Anticonvulsants have been associated with an increased risk of birth defects, though adequate studies of lamotrigine have not been done. However, seizures during pregnancy can also increase the risks to the fetus. Discuss with your doctor the potential risks and benefits of using this drug during pregnancy. Folate supplementation is advised beginning 1 to 2 months before conception, continuing throughout pregnancy.

Breast Feeding: Lamotrigine passes into breast milk, although at low levels. Caution is advised; consult your doctor for specific advice.

Infants and Children: Because side effects are more common and may be more severe in young patients, lamotrigine is generally not recommended.

Special Concerns: Your doctor may want you to wear a medical bracelet or carry an identification card saying that you are taking this drug.

OVERDOSE
Symptoms: Severe clumsiness and unsteadiness, severe dizziness or drowsiness, extremely slurred speech, severe, unusual, rapid, side-to-side, or rolling eye movements, rapid heartbeat, loss of consciousness, dry mouth.

What to Do: Call your doctor, emergency medical services (EMS), or the nearest poison control center immediately.

DRUG INTERACTIONS
Lamotrigine can interact with many other drugs, including other anticonvulsants (carbamazepine, phenobarbital, phenytoin, primidone, valproic acid), as well as acetaminophen, methotrexate, pyrimethamine, and trimethoprim.

FOOD INTERACTIONS
No known food interactions.

DISEASE INTERACTIONS
Special caution is advised in those with kidney or liver disease or folate deficiency.

Lansoprazole

BRAND NAMES
Prevacid, Prevpac

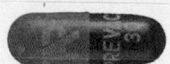

Prevacid 30 mg
(TAP)

Additional photographs

▶ Drug Class: Antacid/proton pump inhibitor

▶ Available in: Delayed-release capsules

▶ Available OTC? No

▶ As Generic? No

Side Effects

SERIOUS
No serious side effects are associated with the use of this medication.

COMMON
Diarrhea, itching or rash, headache, dizziness.

LESS COMMON
Abdominal or stomach pain, nausea, increase or decrease in appetite, anxiety, flu-like symptoms, constipation, coughing, mental depression, muscle pain.

PRINCIPAL USES

To treat stomach and duodenal (intestinal) ulcers, gastroesophageal reflux disease (chronic heartburn caused by the backwash of stomach acid into the esophagus), and conditions that cause increased stomach acid secretion, such as Zollinger-Ellison syndrome. To treat and prevent nonsteroidal anti-inflammatory drug (NSAID)-associated stomach ulcers. Lansoprazole is also prescribed in conjunction with the antibiotics amoxicillin and clarithromycin to eradicate the bacterium *H. pylori* and thus prevent the recurrence of duodenal ulcers caused by this bacterium.

HOW THE DRUG WORKS

Lansoprazole blocks the action of a specific enzyme in the cells that line the stomach, thus decreasing the production of stomach acid. Reduction of stomach acid creates a more favorable environment for the eradication of *H. pylori* and promotes the healing of ulcers.

DOSAGE

Prevacid— To treat duodenal ulcers: Initial dose is 15 mg once a day; it may later be increased. To treat gastroesophageal reflux disease: 15 mg once a day for up to 8 weeks. To treat NSAID-associated stomach ulcers: 30 mg once a day for 8 weeks. To reduce the risk of NSAID-associated stomach ulcer: 15 mg once a day for up to 12 weeks. To treat other conditions: Initial dose is 60 mg once a day; it may be increased. Treatment usually runs 4 to 8 weeks. A second course of treatment may be necessary. For Zollinger-Ellison syndrome: Initial dose is 60 mg once a day; it may be increased. Prevpac— To prevent duo-

denal ulcers: 30 mg lansoprazole, 1 gram amoxicillin, and 500 mg clarithromycin every 12 hours for 14 days.

ONSET OF EFFECT

1 to 3 hours.

DURATION OF ACTION

More than 24 hours.

DIETARY ADVICE

The drug is best taken 30 minutes or more before a meal, preferably breakfast.

STORAGE

Store in a tightly sealed container away from heat, moisture, and direct light.

IF YOU MISS A DOSE

Take it as soon as you remember. However, if it is near the time for the next dose, skip the missed dose and resume your regular dosage schedule. Do not double the next dose.

STOPPING THE DRUG

Take as prescribed for the full treatment period, even if your symptoms improve before the scheduled end of therapy.

PROLONGED USE

Lansoprazole should not be used indefinitely as maintenance therapy for duodenal ulcer or esophagitis; other treatments are advised.

PRECAUTIONS

Over 60: No special problems are expected.

Driving and Hazardous Work: Avoid such activities until you determine how the drug affects you.

Alcohol: Avoid alcohol throughout the duration of therapy with this drug.

Pregnancy: Adequate human studies have not been done. Before taking lansoprazole, tell your doc-

tor if you are pregnant or plan to become pregnant.

Breast Feeding: Lansoprazole may pass into breast milk; consult your doctor for advice.

Infants and Children: Use and dose for anyone under 18 should be determined by your doctor or pediatrician.

Special Concerns: Tell any doctor or dentist whom you see for treatment that you are taking lansoprazole. Do not chew the capsules. If you have trouble swallowing them, you may open them and sprinkle the contents on one tablespoon of applesauce, cottage cheese, yogurt, or similar food. If your doctor directs, you may take an antacid along with lansoprazole.

OVERDOSE

Symptoms: No cases of overdose have been reported.

What to Do: An overdose is unlikely to be life-threatening. However, if someone takes a much larger dose than prescribed, seek medical attention immediately.

DRUG INTERACTIONS

Consult your doctor for specific advice if you are taking ampicillin, sucralfate, iron salts or supplements, cyclosporine, diazepam, disulfiram, ketoconazole, phenytoin, or theophylline.

FOOD INTERACTIONS

No significant food interactions have been reported.

DISEASE INTERACTIONS

Caution is advised when taking lansoprazole. Consult your doctor if you have liver disease, since it may increase the risk of side effects.

Latanoprost

▶ Drug Class: Antiglaucoma agent

▶ Available in: Ophthalmic solution

▶ Available OTC? No

▶ As Generic? No

Side Effects

SERIOUS
Chest pain, difficulty breathing. Call your doctor right away.

COMMON
Blurred vision, burning and stinging of the eye, sensation of something in the eye, increased brown pigmentation of the iris, eye redness.

LESS COMMON
Dry eye, excessive tearing, eye pain, lid crusting, swollen eyelid, eyelid pain or discomfort, sensitivity to light, upper respiratory tract infection, double vision, pain in the chest and back.

PRINCIPAL USES
To treat glaucoma.

HOW THE DRUG WORKS
Glaucoma, a sight-threatening disorder, occurs when the aqueous humor (fluid inside the eye) cannot drain properly, causing increased pressure within the eyeball (intraocular pressure). Increased eye pressure can damage the optic nerve and lead to a gradually progressive loss of vision. Latanoprost promotes outflow of aqueous humor, thereby reducing intraocular pressure.

DOSAGE
1 drop of latanoprost in each eye once daily in the evening.

ONSET OF EFFECT
3 to 4 hours.

DURATION OF ACTION
24 hours or more.

DIETARY ADVICE
This medication can be used without regard to diet.

STORAGE
Store in a tightly sealed container away from heat, moisture, and direct light. Do not allow the medicine to freeze.

IF YOU MISS A DOSE
Apply it as soon as you remember. If it is near the time for the next dose, skip the missed dose and resume your regular dosage schedule. Do not double the next dose.

STOPPING THE DRUG
The decision to stop using the drug should be made by your doctor.

PROLONGED USE
See your doctor regularly for tests and examinations if you must take this drug for a prolonged period.

PRECAUTIONS
Over 60: No special problems are expected.

Driving and Hazardous Work: Do not drive or engage in hazardous work until you determine how the medicine affects your vision.

Alcohol: No special precautions are necessary.

Pregnancy: Latanoprost has not caused birth defects in animals. Human studies have not been done. Before you take latanoprost, tell your doctor if you are pregnant or plan to become pregnant.

Breast Feeding: Latanoprost may pass into breast milk; caution is advised. Consult your doctor for advice.

Infants and Children: The safety and effectiveness of latanoprost in infants and children have not been established.

Special Concerns: To use the eye drops, first wash your hands. Tilt your head back. Gently apply pressure to the inside corner of the eyelid and with the index finger of the same hand, pull downward on the lower eyelid to make a space. Drop the medicine into this space and close your eye. Apply pressure for 1 or 2 minutes while keeping the eye closed without blinking. Then wash your hands again. Make sure the tip of the dropper does not touch your eye, finger, or any other surface. Latanoprost may make your eyes more sensitive to sunlight. If this occurs, wear sunglasses or avoid exposure to bright light as necessary. Latanoprost may change eye color, increasing the brown pigment in the iris over a period of months or years. The color change may be permanent. Latanoprost contains ingredients that may damage contact lenses. Contact lenses should be removed 15 minutes before applying the medication and reinserted 15 minutes or more afterward.

OVERDOSE
Symptoms: No specific ones have been reported.

What to Do: An overdose of latanoprost is unlikely to be life-threatening. If a large volume enters the eyes, flush with water. If someone accidentally ingests the medicine, call your doctor, emergency medical services (EMS), or the nearest poison control center.

DRUG INTERACTIONS
Other drugs may interact with latanoprost. Consult your doctor for specific advice if you are taking any other prescription or over-the-counter medication. If you are using other ophthalmic medications to reduce fluid pressure in the eye, administer them at least 5 minutes apart.

FOOD INTERACTIONS
No known food interactions.

DISEASE INTERACTIONS
Use of latanoprost may cause complications in patients with liver or kidney disease, since these organs work together to remove the drug from the body.

Leflunomide

BRAND NAME
Arava

▶ Drug Class: Antirheumatic

▶ Available in: Tablets

▶ Available OTC? No

▶ As Generic? No

Side Effects

SERIOUS
Liver toxicity may occur; it can be detected by your doctor with blood tests; it may be discerned by the patient if it causes jaundice, characterized by yellowish discoloration of the skin and eyes. Call your doctor immediately.

COMMON
Diarrhea, hair loss, rash.

LESS COMMON
Allergic reaction, back pain, bronchitis, pneumonia, nasal congestion, itching.

PRINCIPAL USES
To reduce the signs and symptoms of moderate to severe active rheumatoid arthritis. Leflunomide is prescribed for patients who have not responded adequately to one or more antirheumatic medications.

HOW THE DRUG WORKS
Leflunomide appears to suppress overactivity of the immune system, which is believed to cause rheumatoid arthritis. It also appears to reduce inflammation.

DOSAGE
Adults: To start, 100 mg a day for 3 days. Maintenance dose: 20 mg a day. Dose may be lowered by your doctor to 10 mg a day, if necessary.

ONSET OF EFFECT
Unknown.

DURATION OF ACTION
Unknown.

DIETARY ADVICE
Maintain your usual food and fluid intake.

STORAGE
Store in a tightly sealed container away from heat, moisture, and direct light.

IF YOU MISS A DOSE
If you miss a dose on one day, do not double the dose the next day.

STOPPING THE DRUG
Take it as prescribed for the full treatment period, even if you begin to feel better.

PROLONGED USE
See your doctor regularly for liver function tests while taking this medication.

PRECAUTIONS
Over 60: No special problems are expected.

Driving and Hazardous Work: The use of leflunomide should not impair your ability to perform such tasks safely.

Alcohol: Drink only in moderation.

Pregnancy: Leflunomide can cause serious birth defects. Do not take the drug if you are pregnant. Before you start taking leflunomide, you must have had a negative pregnancy test within the previous 2 weeks. An effective method of birth control should be used while you are taking leflunomide. If you suspect you are pregnant, stop taking the drug immediately and consult your doctor.

Breast Feeding: It is unknown whether leflunomide passes into breast milk. However, do not take the drug while nursing. Consult your doctor for advice.

Infants and Children: Safety and effectiveness have not been established for children under age 18.

Special Concerns: Upon completion of treatment, it is recommended that you follow a specific procedure to lower the levels of leflunomide in the blood. Take 8 grams cholestyramine 3 times a day for 11 days (does not have to be 11 consecutive days, unless there is a need to reduce levels rapidly). Your doctor will conduct two tests (each at least 2 weeks apart) to monitor blood levels of the medication. Without following this procedure, it may take up to 2 years to reach undetectable blood levels of the drug.

OVERDOSE
Symptoms: No cases of overdose have been reported.

What to Do: If someone takes a much larger dose than prescribed, call your doctor, emergency medical services (EMS), or the nearest poison control center immediately.

DRUG INTERACTIONS
The following drugs may interact with leflunomide. Consult your doctor for specific advice if you are taking: methotrexate, rifampin, cholestyramine, charcoal, or tolbutamide.

FOOD INTERACTIONS
No known food interactions.

DISEASE INTERACTIONS
Do not take leflunomide if you have liver disease. Caution is advised in patients with kidney disease. Consult your doctor for advice.

Letrozole

▶ Drug Class: Antiestrogen; antineoplastic (anticancer) agent

▶ Available in: Tablets

▶ Available OTC? No

▶ As Generic? No

Side Effects

SERIOUS
No serious side effects have been reported.

COMMON
Fatigue, nausea and vomiting, muscle and joint pain, headache, shortness of breath.

LESS COMMON
Chest pain, edema (swelling around the feet and ankles), weakness, increase in weight, high blood pressure, constipation, diarrhea, abdominal pain, loss of appetite, indigestion, viral infection, drowsiness or dizziness, cough, hot flashes, rash, itching.

PRINCIPAL USES
Letrozole is used for the treatment of advanced breast cancer in postmenopausal women. It is also prescribed for women whose breast cancer has progressed following treatment with other antiestrogens, such as tamoxifen.

HOW THE DRUG WORKS
The growth of some breast tumors is stimulated by estrogens. After the menopause, women's ovaries produce little estrogen, but androgens formed in the adrenals can be converted to estrogen. Letrozole blocks the enzyme that carries out this conversion. Thus, letrozole is not directly toxic to cancer cells but rather inhibits the growth of some breast tumors by reducing blood levels of estrogen.

DOSAGE
2.5 mg once a day.

ONSET OF EFFECT
Unknown.

DURATION OF ACTION
Unknown.

DIETARY ADVICE
Letrozole can be taken without regard to meals. Maintain adequate food and fluid intake, since calorie, protein, and vitamin needs increase in patients with cancer.

STORAGE
Store in a tightly sealed container away from heat, moisture, and direct light.

IF YOU MISS A DOSE
Letrozole is prescribed for once-daily use only. If you are unable to take this medication on a particular day, resume your regularly scheduled dose the following day. Do not double the next dose.

STOPPING THE DRUG
This medication is used to treat a chronic condition. You may need to remain on this drug for an extended period, and you should take letrozole exactly as prescribed throughout the course of treatment. The decision to stop the drug must be made in consultation with your doctor. Do not stop taking letrozole on your own.

PROLONGED USE
There is no standard duration of therapy with letrozole, although you can expect to remain on it for several weeks in order to determine if it is effective. Your doctor will decide whether your response to the drug is satisfactory or not, and will recommend continuation or discontinuation of therapy.

PRECAUTIONS
Over 60: No special problems are expected.

Driving and Hazardous Work: Use of this medication should not impair your ability to engage in such tasks safely.

Alcohol: No special precautions are necessary.

Pregnancy: Letrozole must not be used in pregnant women. Although letrozole is not generally prescribed for premenopausal women, it is important that patients be sure they are not pregnant before starting treatment with this drug.

Breast Feeding: Use of this drug is not recommended while nursing; the benefits must clearly outweigh potential risks. Consult your doctor for advice.

Infants and Children: Use of letrozole is not approved for infants and children.

Special Concerns: Patients with cancer are very often weakened by their illness, by poor nutrition, and by the effects of chemotherapy, radiation, and surgery. Such patients are more likely to experience undesirable side effects of a medication. In addition, these side effects may be more pronounced. Follow all medication directions carefully.

OVERDOSE
Symptoms: No cases of overdose have been reported.

What to Do: An overdose is unlikely; however, if you have any reason to suspect that one has occurred, call emergency medical services (EMS) to receive evaluation and treatment in the closest emergency facility.

DRUG INTERACTIONS
No significant drug interactions are associated with the use of letrozole.

FOOD INTERACTIONS
No known food interactions.

DISEASE INTERACTIONS
No significant interactions.

Leucovorin Calcium

Generic 25 mg
(BARR)

Additional photographs

▶ Drug Class: Folic acid derivative

▶ Available in: Tablets, injection

▶ Available OTC? No

▶ As Generic? Yes

Side Effects

SERIOUS
Skin rash, hives, itching, seizures. These may be signs of a serious allergic reaction; call your doctor right away.

COMMON
No common side effects have been reported.

LESS COMMON
There are no less-common side effects associated with leucovorin.

PRINCIPAL USES
To serve as an antidote to the toxic effects of high doses of methotrexate (a cancer drug) and other drugs that antagonize (block the action of) the essential nutrient folic acid. Leucovorin is also used in conjunction with another drug, fluorouracil, to treat some kinds of colon cancer. It may also be used to treat some forms of anemia.

HOW THE DRUG WORKS
Folic acid is needed by healthy cells in the body to grow, survive, and multiply. Leucovorin is a derivative of folic acid and thus prevents some of the damage done to healthy cells by therapy with methotrexate and other drugs that deplete folic acid in the body. Because leucovorin acts in the body the same way as folic acid, it is useful against anemia due to folic acid deficiency.

DOSAGE
To prevent drug side effects: 10 mg per square meter of body surface every 6 hours for 10 doses. For colon cancer, there are 3 accepted regimens: (a) 200 mg per square meter of body surface daily for 5 days; (b) 20 mg per square meter of body surface daily for 5 days; or (c) 500 mg per square meter of body surface in a single dose. In each regimen leucovorin is followed by appropriate doses of fluorouracil. The drug combination is cycled depending on the regimen. To treat megaloblastic anemia caused by congenital enzyme deficiency: 3 to 6 mg to start, then 1 mg per day. To treat folate-deficient megaloblastic anemia: Up to 1 mg of leucovorin daily; duration of treatment depends upon the response of the individual.

ONSET OF EFFECT
From 5 to 20 minutes after injection; 20 to 30 minutes after oral ingestion.

DURATION OF ACTION
From 3 to 6 hours.

DIETARY ADVICE
Leucovorin can be given between meals. The doses must be evenly spaced, day and night.

STORAGE
Store in a tightly sealed container away from heat and direct light.

IF YOU MISS A DOSE
As soon as you remember, check with your doctor to learn if you should take an extra dose. Do not take more medicine without consulting your doctor. Resume your regular dosage schedule as soon as possible.

STOPPING THE DRUG
The decision to stop taking the drug should be made by your doctor.

PROLONGED USE
See your doctor regularly for tests and examinations if you take this medication for a prolonged period.

PRECAUTIONS
Over 60: There is no specific information comparing use of leucovorin in older patients with use in younger persons.

Driving and Hazardous Work: The use of leucovorin should not impair your ability to perform such tasks safely.

Alcohol: Avoid alcohol while taking this medication, since alcohol only further depletes folic acid.

Pregnancy: Neither animal nor human studies on the effects of using leucovorin during pregnancy have been done. Before taking leucovorin, tell your doctor if you are pregnant or plan to become pregnant. It should be used during pregnancy only under the close supervision of a doctor who is experienced in antimetabolite cancer therapy.

Breast Feeding: It is not known whether leucovorin passes into breast milk. It has not been reported to cause problems in nursing infants. Consult your doctor for specific advice.

Infants and Children: In children who suffer from seizure disorders, treatment with leucovorin may increase the frequency of seizures.

Special Concerns: Inform your doctor if you cannot tolerate the oral dose and it causes vomiting. Injection therapy may be warranted.

OVERDOSE
Symptoms: No specific ones have been reported.

What to Do: An overdose of leucovorin is unlikely to be life-threatening. However, if someone takes a much larger dose than prescribed, seek medical assistance right away.

DRUG INTERACTIONS
Consult your doctor for specific advice if you are taking any other prescription or over-the-counter drugs.

FOOD INTERACTIONS
No known food interactions.

DISEASE INTERACTIONS
Caution is advised when taking leucovorin. Consult your doctor if you have kidney disease or vitamin B12 deficiency.

Leuprolide Acetate

▸ Drug Class: Synthetic hormone

▸ Available in: Injection, implanted capsule

▸ Available OTC? No

▸ As Generic? No

Side Effects

SERIOUS
In men: Pain in groin or leg, chest pain. In women: Increased hair growth, deepening of voice. In men and women: Rapid or irregular heartbeat. Call your doctor immediately. Implanted capsule— If reactions such as itching and redness around the insertion site do not heal within 2 weeks contact your doctor.

COMMON
Injection— In women: Light, irregular vaginal bleeding, cessation of menstrual periods (amenorrhea), vaginal dryness. In both men and women: Sudden sweating and feelings of warmth (hot flashes). Implanted capsule— Hot flashes, lack of energy, depression, sweating, headache, bruising, and breast enlargement.

LESS COMMON
In men: Bone pain, constipation, decreased testicle size, impotence, loss of appetite, swollen and tender breasts. In women: Burning, itching, or dryness of vagina, decreased interest in sex, breast tenderness, pelvic pain, mood changes. In men and women: Blurred vision, burning or itching at injection or implant site, headache, nausea or vomiting, swollen feet or lower legs, insomnia, weight gain, numbness or tingling of the hands or feet.

PRINCIPAL USES
To ease symptoms of advanced forms of prostate cancer in men (this is the only FDA-approved use for the implanted capsule), and to relieve the pain and discomfort of endometriosis in women. It is also used by children with precocious (early onset) puberty and in certain patients with anemia owing to bleeding from fibroids.

HOW THE DRUG WORKS
In men, leuprolide decreases blood levels of testosterone. This slows the growth of cells in the prostate gland, which may lead to improvement of some of the pain and discomfort of advanced prostate cancer. In women, leuprolide decreases blood levels of estrogen. Reduced blood estrogen leads to shrinking of endometrial tissue (uterine lining) and thus eases the painful cyclical flare-ups of endometriosis. It will suppress menstrual periods and thus help to correct the anemia associated with bleeding from fibroids.

DOSAGE
Injection— Men: 1 mg injected under the skin once a day or 7.5 mg of the Depot form injected into muscle once a month. Women: 3.75 mg injected into muscle once a month for up to 6 months. Children: Consult your pediatrician. Implanted capsule— Men: 1 capsule is implanted under the skin of the upper arm. The implant contains 65 mg of leuprolide that is continuously released for 12 months. After 12 months the implant must be removed. Another implant may be inserted to continue therapy.

ONSET OF EFFECT
Injection— Men: 2 to 4 weeks. Women: 1 to 2 months. Implanted capsule— Unknown.

DURATION OF ACTION
Injection— Men: 4 to 12 weeks. Women: 60 to 90 days. Implanted capsule— 12 months.

DIETARY ADVICE
This drug can be taken without regard to diet.

STORAGE
Keep the liquid form of this medicine refrigerated until the first dose, but do not allow it to freeze. Then store it in a tightly sealed container at room temperature away from heat and direct light. Implanted capsule: Not applicable.

IF YOU MISS A DOSE
If you are taking this medicine every day, take the missed dose as soon as you remember. If you do not remember until the next day, skip the missed dose and resume your regular dosage schedule. Do not double the next dose. Implanted capsule: Not applicable.

STOPPING THE DRUG
The decision to stop taking the drug should be made by your doctor.

PROLONGED USE
Consult your doctor about the need for periodic examinations and laboratory tests if you use leuprolide for a prolonged period.

PRECAUTIONS
Over 60: No special problems are expected.

Driving and Hazardous Work: Do not drive or engage in hazardous work until you determine how the medicine affects you.

Alcohol: No special precautions are necessary.

Pregnancy: Leuprolide may cause birth defects if taken during pregnancy. Notify your doctor immediately if you think you are pregnant.

Breast Feeding: Leuprolide may pass into breast milk; caution is advised. Consult your doctor for specific advice.

Infants and Children: Leuprolide (injection only) should be given to children only under close medical supervision to treat precocious puberty.

Special Concerns: Use only the syringes provided in the kit. Other types may not deliver the same dose. When taking leuprolide, women should use nonhormonal contraception (that is, methods other than birth control pills).

OVERDOSE
Symptoms: No specific ones have been reported.

What to Do: An overdose of leuprolide is unlikely to be life-threatening. However, if someone takes a much larger dose than prescribed, seek medical attention immediately.

DRUG INTERACTIONS
Other drugs may interact with leuprolide. Consult your doctor if you are taking any prescription or nonprescription drugs or herbal remedies.

FOOD INTERACTIONS
No known food interactions.

DISEASE INTERACTIONS
Consult your doctor if you experience vaginal bleeding of unknown cause or, in men, difficulty urinating.

Levamisole Hydrochloride

Ergamisol 50 mg
(JANSSEN)

▶ Drug Class: Immunomodulator; antineoplastic (anticancer) agent

▶ Available in: Tablets

▶ Available OTC? No

▶ As Generic? No

Side Effects

SERIOUS
Flu-like symptoms (such as fever or chills, body aches, general feeling of discomfort, weakness, and cough), unusual bleeding or bruising, blurred vision, trouble walking, uncontrolled movements of the arms or legs. Although such side effects are rare, they are serious; call your physician immediately if you experience such symptoms.

COMMON
Nausea, vomiting, and diarrhea.

LESS COMMON
Anxiety or nervousness, dizziness, headache, depression, nightmares, pain in joints or muscles, skin rash or itching, insomnia, unusual sleepiness or tiredness, metallic taste, sores in the mouth or on the lips.

PRINCIPAL USES
Levamisole enhances the effectiveness of fluorouracil, a drug used to treat cancer of the colon.

HOW THE DRUG WORKS
It is unknown precisely how levamisole works. It appears that it improves the responsiveness of the immune system, which is suppressed by other chemotherapy agents such as fluorouracil. Therefore it improves the patient's overall ability to fight disease. Unlike many other cancer drugs, levamisole does not directly attack malignant cells.

DOSAGE
50 mg every 8 hours for 3 days, beginning no later than 30 days after surgery. Usual maintenance dose is 50 mg for 3 days every 2 weeks for 1 year.

ONSET OF EFFECT
Unknown.

DURATION OF ACTION
Unknown.

DIETARY ADVICE
Maintain adequate food and fluid intake. Calorie, protein, and vitamin needs increase in patients with cancer. Good nutrition is essential to cope with the demands of chemotherapy.

STORAGE
Store in a tightly sealed container away from heat and direct light.

IF YOU MISS A DOSE
Take it as soon as you remember. If it is near the time for the next dose, skip the missed dose and resume your regular dosage schedule. Do not double the next dose.

STOPPING THE DRUG
The decision to stop taking the drug should be made by your doctor.

PROLONGED USE
You should see your doctor regularly for tests and examinations if you take levamisole for a prolonged period.

PRECAUTIONS
Over 60: Levamisole is not expected to cause different side effects or problems in older persons than it does in younger patients.

Driving and Hazardous Work: Do not drive or engage in hazardous work until you determine how the medicine affects you.

Alcohol: Avoid alcohol completely while taking this medication. When alcohol is consumed with the combination of levamisole and fluorouracil, severe nausea and vomiting may result.

Pregnancy: Levamisole has not been shown to cause birth defects in animals. Human studies have not been done. Consult your doctor for advice if you are pregnant or plan to become pregnant.

Breast Feeding: It is not known whether levamisole passes into breast milk; caution is advised. Consult your doctor for specific advice.

Infants and Children: There is no information comparing the use of levamisole in infants and children with use in older persons.

Special Concerns: If you vomit after taking a dose of levamisole, ask your doctor whether you should take the dose again or wait for the next dose. Avoid contact with persons who have infections. Do not receive any immunizations while you take this medication. Before you have dental work done, tell the dentist that you are taking levamisole. Rinse your mouth after eating and drinking and use a soft toothbrush and an electric razor.

OVERDOSE
Symptoms: Nausea, vomiting, infection, inflammation of the mouth.

What to Do: Call your doctor, emergency medical services (EMS), or the nearest poison control center immediately.

DRUG INTERACTIONS
Consult your doctor for specific advice if you are taking phenytoin or the anticoagulant warfarin. Side effects of levamisole may be more frequent when taken with fluorouracil.

FOOD INTERACTIONS
No known food interactions.

DISEASE INTERACTIONS
Caution is advised when taking levamisole. Consult your doctor if you have any other medical condition.

Levetiracetam

▶ Drug Class: Anticonvulsant

▶ Available in: Tablets

▶ Available OTC? No

▶ As Generic? No

Side Effects

SERIOUS
Extreme drowsiness, psychotic symptoms. Call your doctor immediately.

COMMON
Drowsiness, fatigue, increased susceptibility to infection, dizziness.

LESS COMMON
Coordination difficulties, agitation, hostility, anxiety, nervousness, depression, hallucinations, attempted suicide, loss of appetite, amnesia, emotional instability, numbness, prickling or tingling sensations, cough, sore throat, runny nose, sinusitis, double vision.

PRINCIPAL USES
Used in combination with one or more other anticonvulsant drugs to control partial seizures (those which begin with an abnormal burst of electrical activity in a small portion of the brain, often resulting in twitching or numbness in a localized part of the body).

HOW THE DRUG WORKS
The precise mechanism of action is unknown.

DOSAGE
To start, 500 mg twice a day. Dosage may be gradually increased by your doctor (1,000 mg a day every 2 weeks) to a maximum of 3,000 mg a day. People with impaired kidney function may require an adjustment in dose.

ONSET OF EFFECT
Within 48 hours.

DURATION OF ACTION
Unknown.

DIETARY ADVICE
Can be taken without regard to meals.

STORAGE
Store in a tightly sealed container away from heat, moisture, and direct light.

IF YOU MISS A DOSE
Take it as soon as you remember. If it is near the time for the next dose, skip the missed dose and resume your regular dosage schedule. Do not double the next dose.

STOPPING THE DRUG
The decision to stop taking the drug should be made by your doctor. Never stop this drug abruptly because this may cause seizures. The dose is typically tapered over a period of weeks.

PROLONGED USE
This drug is often taken for prolonged periods. See your physician for periodic checkups.

PRECAUTIONS
Over 60: Decreased kidney function is more common in older persons. Because levetiracetam is eliminated from the body through the kidney, the risk of side effects is increased. Kidney function should be carefully monitored. A dosage adjustment may be warranted.

Driving and Hazardous Work: This drug may cause drowsiness or dizziness, particularly in the first few weeks it is used. Do not drive or engage in hazardous work until you determine how the medicine affects you.

Alcohol: Avoid alcohol; it may contribute to excessive drowsiness.

Pregnancy: Levetiracetam has caused birth defects in animal studies. Human studies with this drug have not been done, but other anticonvulsants are known to increase the risk of birth defects. However, seizures during pregnancy can also increase the risks to the fetus. Discuss with your doctor the potential risks and benefits of using this drug during pregnancy.

Breast Feeding: Levetiracetam may pass into breast milk; caution is advised. Consult your doctor for specific advice.

Infants and Children: Not recommended for use by children under age 16.

Special Concerns: See your doctor for regular check-ups to detect the onset of any serious side effects. Your doctor may advise you to carry an ID card or bracelet that says you are taking this drug.

OVERDOSE
Symptoms: Few cases of overdose have been reported. In clinical trials, the most common symptom following overdose was drowsiness.

What to Do: If an excessive dose is taken, call your doctor, emergency medical services (EMS), or poison control center immediately.

DRUG INTERACTIONS
No known drug interactions.

FOOD INTERACTIONS
No known food interactions.

DISEASE INTERACTIONS
A lower dose of levetiracetam may be needed in patients with decreased kidney function.

Levobunolol

BRAND NAME
Betagan

▶ Drug Class: Antiglaucoma drug; ophthalmic beta-blocker

▶ Available in: Ophthalmic solution

▶ Available OTC? No

▶ As Generic? No

Side Effects

SERIOUS
Palpitations, trouble breathing, dizziness, and weakness caused by low blood pressure. Call your doctor right away.

COMMON
Burning, stinging, tearing, and irritation of the eye when medication is taken.

LESS COMMON
Eyebrow pain, itching, decreased night vision, crusted eyelashes, increased sensitivity of eye to light, dry eye.

PRINCIPAL USES
To treat glaucoma.

HOW THE DRUG WORKS
Glaucoma, a sight-threatening disorder, occurs when aqueous humor (fluid inside the eye) cannot drain properly, causing an increase in pressure within the eyeball (intraocular pressure). The increased eye pressure can damage the optic nerve and lead to a gradually progressive loss of vision. Levobunolol decreases the production of aqueous humor and promotes its outflow, thereby reducing intraocular pressure.

DOSAGE
Adults and older children: 1 drop in each affected eye, 1 or 2 times a day. Children: The dose must be determined by your doctor.

ONSET OF EFFECT
Within 60 minutes.

DURATION OF ACTION
Up to 24 hours.

DIETARY ADVICE
No special restrictions.

STORAGE
Store in a tightly sealed container away from heat, moisture, and direct light. Do not allow it to freeze.

IF YOU MISS A DOSE
Apply it as soon as you remember. If it is near the time for the next dose, skip the missed dose and resume your regular dosage schedule.

STOPPING THE DRUG
The decision to stop using the drug should be made by your doctor.

PROLONGED USE
See your doctor regularly for tests and examinations if you take this drug for a prolonged period.

PRECAUTIONS
Over 60: Adverse reactions may be more likely and more severe.

Driving and Hazardous Work: Avoid such activities until you determine how the medication affects your vision.

Alcohol: Consume alcohol in moderation only.

Pregnancy: Levobunolol has not been shown to cause birth defects in animals. Human studies have not been done. Before you take levobunolol, tell your doctor if you are pregnant or plan to become pregnant.

Breast Feeding: Levobunolol may pass into breast milk; caution is advised. Consult your doctor for advice.

Infants and Children: Adverse reactions may be more likely and more severe in young patients.

Special Concerns: To use the eye drops, first wash your hands. Tilt your head back. Gently apply pressure to the inside corner of the eyelid and with the index finger of the same hand, pull downward on the lower eyelid to make a space. Drop the medicine into this space and close your eye. Apply pressure for 1 or 2 minutes while keeping the eye closed without blinking. Then wash your hands again. Make sure the tip of the dropper does not touch your eye, finger, or any other surface. If you are taking the medicine with the compliance cap (C Cap), make sure the number 1 or the correct day of the week appears in the window of the cap before using the eye drops for the first time. After every dose, rotate the bottle until the cap clicks to the position that tells you the next dose. Before you have any kind of surgery, dental treatment, or emergency treatment, tell the person in charge that you are taking levobunolol. This medication may make you more sensitive to sunlight. If this occurs, wear sunglasses or avoid bright light as comfort dictates.

OVERDOSE
Symptoms: Nervousness, chest pain, confusion, hallucinations, coughing, wheezing, drowsiness, dizziness, nausea or vomiting, irregular or pounding heartbeat, insomnia, unusual fatigue.

What to Do: If a large volume enters the eye, flush with water. If someone accidentally ingests the drug, call your doctor, emergency medical services (EMS), or the nearest poison control center immediately.

DRUG INTERACTIONS
It is not recommended to use two ophthalmic beta-blockers at the same time. Special caution is warranted in people taking antidiabetic drugs, since levobunolol may mask symptoms of low blood sugar. Other drugs may interact with levobunolol. Tell your doctor about any other prescription or over-the-counter medication that you take.

FOOD INTERACTIONS
No known food interactions.

DISEASE INTERACTIONS
Consult your doctor if you have asthma, emphysema or other lung disease, heart disease, hyperthyroidism, or diabetes mellitus.

Levocabastine

▶ Drug Class: Histamine (H1) blocker

▶ Available in: Ophthalmic suspension

▶ Available OTC? No

▶ As Generic? No

Side Effects

SERIOUS
Cough, breathing difficulty, swelling around the eyes, eye pain or discharge, excessive tear production, unusual fatigue, nausea, sore throat, redness or irritation not present prior to treatment, visual disturbances. Such side effects are very rare, but if they occur, stop using the drug and call your doctor immediately.

COMMON
Temporary burning or stinging in the eyes upon application of the drops.

LESS COMMON
Headache, dry eyes, dry mouth, and drowsiness. Call your doctor if such symptoms persist or begin to interfere with daily activities.

PRINCIPAL USES
For temporary symptomatic relief of itching and irritation of the eyes associated with seasonal allergies.

HOW THE DRUG WORKS
Levocabastine blocks the effects of histamine, a naturally occurring substance within the body that causes swelling, itching, sneezing, watery eyes, hives, and other symptoms associated with allergic reactions.

DOSAGE
Instill 1 drop in affected eye(s), 4 times a day, for up to 2 weeks. Shake well before using the drug.

ONSET OF EFFECT
Within 10 to 15 minutes.

DURATION OF ACTION
From 2 to 4 hours.

DIETARY ADVICE
This drug can be used without regard to diet.

STORAGE
Store in a tightly sealed container away from heat, moisture, and direct light. Do not allow it to freeze.

IF YOU MISS A DOSE
Apply it as soon as you remember. If it is near the time for the next dose, skip the missed dose and resume your regular dosage schedule. Do not double the next dose.

STOPPING THE DRUG
Take it as prescribed for the full treatment period, even if you feel better before the scheduled end of therapy.

PROLONGED USE
This medicine is for short-term symptomatic relief only; treatment should not exceed 2 weeks. Check with your doctor if symptoms do not improve, or if your condition becomes worse, after 3 days.

PRECAUTIONS
Over 60: No special problems are expected.

Driving and Hazardous Work: No problems are expected, but it is advisable not to engage in such activities until you determine how this drug affects your vision.

Alcohol: No special precautions are necessary.

Pregnancy: Adequate studies have not been done, although no problems have been reported. Before taking levocabastine, tell your doctor if you are pregnant or plan to become pregnant.

Breast Feeding: Levocabastine passes into breast milk; do not use it when nursing.

Infants and Children: The safety and effectiveness of levocabastine have not been established in children under the age of 12. This drug should not be used by patients in this age group.

Special Concerns: To use the eye drops, first wash your hands. Tilt your head back. Gently apply pressure to the inside corner of the eyelid and with the index finger of the same hand, pull downward on the lower eyelid to make a space. Drop the medicine into this space and close your eye. Apply pressure for 1 or 2 minutes while keeping the eye closed without blinking. Then wash your hands again. Make sure the tip of the dropper does not touch your eye, finger, or any other surface. The manufacturer of this drug recommends that soft contact lenses not be worn while undergoing treatment with levocabastine.

OVERDOSE
Symptoms: No cases of overdose have been reported.

What to Do: An overdose of levocabastine is unlikely to occur. In case of accidental ingestion, call your doctor, emergency medical services (EMS), or the nearest poison control center immediately.

DRUG INTERACTIONS
No drug interactions have been reported. Nonetheless, it is wise to consult your doctor before taking any other prescription or over-the-counter eye medication.

FOOD INTERACTIONS
No food interactions have been reported.

DISEASE INTERACTIONS
No disease interactions have been reported.

Levodopa

BRAND NAMES
Dopar, Larodopa

Larodopa 100 mg
(ROCHE)

▶ Drug Class: Antiparkinsonism drug

▶ Available in: Tablets, capsules

▶ Available OTC? No

▶ As Generic? Yes

Side Effects

SERIOUS
Irregular heartbeat, heart rhythm abnormalities, low blood pressure, fainting or near fainting, hallucinations.

COMMON
Nausea, confusion.

LESS COMMON
Breathing difficulty.

PRINCIPAL USES
To treat Parkinson's disease and Parkinson-like syndromes. Such syndromes can occur following injury to or infection of the central nervous system, damage to the blood vessels in the brain (for example, after a stroke), or exposure to certain toxins.

HOW THE DRUG WORKS
Levodopa replenishes the supply of dopamine in the brain. Dopamine is a chemical in the central nervous system that plays an essential role in the initiation and smooth control of voluntary muscle movement.

DOSAGE
Adults: To start, 0.5 g per day in 2 or more divided doses. The dose is increased gradually (by 0.5 to 0.75 g per day) over the course of 4 to 7 days, until the desired therapeutic response is achieved. The onset of adverse side effects may preclude the use of higher doses. The maximum beneficial dose is usually 5 to 6 g per day. Children: Smaller doses are used; consult your pediatrician for specific information.

ONSET OF EFFECT
Within 1 to 2 hours.

DURATION OF ACTION
From 4 to 5 hours.

DIETARY ADVICE
Eating food shortly after taking this medication may minimize the chance of stomach upset. Eating food before taking the medicine or at the same time may blunt levodopa's effects.

STORAGE
Store in a tightly sealed container away from heat, moisture, and direct light.

IF YOU MISS A DOSE
Take it as soon as you remember. However, if it is near the time for the next dose, skip the missed dose and resume your regular dosage schedule. Do not double the next dose.

STOPPING THE DRUG
Consult your doctor for the best approach to stopping the drug. The dose should be decreased very gradually. Abruptly stopping the drug can cause an acute (sudden-onset) adverse reaction.

PROLONGED USE
Prolonged use of levodopa can result in a less predictable therapeutic response and bothersome involuntary muscle movements.

PRECAUTIONS
Over 60: Adverse reactions to levodopa may be more likely and more severe in older patients. The dose should be increased very gradually in this age group.

Driving and Hazardous Work: Do not drive or engage in hazardous work until the full dose has been attained and you determine how the drug affects you.

Alcohol: Do not consume alcohol. Alcohol can cause pronounced confusion or delirium in patients taking this medication.

Pregnancy: Adequate human studies have not been done, and the effects of levodopa during pregnancy have not been determined. Pregnant women should therefore avoid taking levodopa.

Breast Feeding: Levodopa passes into breast milk; levodopa should not be used by nursing mothers.

Infants and Children: Levodopa should be used with caution by infants and children. The dose should be smaller than that for adults and should be determined by your pediatrician.

Special Concerns: Patients taking levodopa should not eat a high-protein diet, because it can reduce the medication's effectiveness.

OVERDOSE
Symptoms: The symptoms of levodopa overdose are unknown.

What to Do: If you have any reason to suspect an overdose, call your doctor, emergency medical services (EMS), or the nearest poison control center.

DRUG INTERACTIONS
Consult your doctor for specific advice if you are taking any of the following drugs that may interact with levodopa: MAO inhibitor antidepressants (such as phenelzine sulfate or tranylcypromine sulfate) or antihypertensives.

FOOD INTERACTIONS
A high-protein diet can reduce the effectiveness of levodopa. Persons taking levodopa should therefore decrease their protein intake if it is high.

DISEASE INTERACTIONS
Caution is advised when taking levodopa. Consult your doctor if you have any of the following: heart disease or heart rhythm abnormalities, bronchial asthma, glaucoma, malignant melanoma, or changes in mental state.

Sinemet 200/50 mg
(DUPONT)

Additional photographs

▶ Drug Class: Antiparkinsonism
drug

▶ Available in: Tablets,
sustained-release tablets

▶ Available OTC? No

▶ As Generic? Yes

Side Effects

SERIOUS
Nausea, fatigue, depression, dizziness or lightheadedness when
standing or sitting up
suddenly (orthostatic
hypotension), fainting or
near fainting.

COMMON
With long-term use,
quirky involuntary muscle
movements, an unpredictable therapeutic
response.

LESS COMMON
Confusion, delirium; dark
saliva, urine, or sweat.

PRINCIPAL USES
To treat Parkinson's disease
and Parkinson-like syndromes, which can occur
following injury to or infection of the central nervous
system, damage to the
blood vessels in the brain,
or exposure to certain toxins. Levodopa/carbidopa
improves or alleviates such
symptoms as rigidity, slowness, loss of smoothness of
movement, and tremor.

HOW THE DRUG WORKS
Levodopa/carbidopa
increases brain levels of
dopamine, a chemical that
plays an essential role in
the smooth movement
of muscles.

DOSAGE
Adults: To start, 1 tablet of
100/10 levodopa/carbidopa
(containing 100 mg of
levodopa and 10 mg of carbidopa), 3 or 4 times a day;
or 1 tablet of 100/25 levodopa/carbidopa (containing
100 mg of levodopa and 25
mg of carbidopa), 3 times a
day. The dose is gradually
increased every 5 to 7 days
until the maximum therapeutic benefit is achieved
without the onset of serious
side effects. The maximum
dose is variable, ranging
from the equivalent of 4 to
10 tablets (either 100/10 or
100/25 levodopa/carbidopa)
per day. Children: Smaller
doses can be used; consult
your pediatrician.

ONSET OF EFFECT
Within 90 to 120 minutes.

DURATION OF ACTION
From 3 to 4 hours.

DIETARY ADVICE
Eating food shortly after
taking the medication may
minimize the chance of
stomach upset. Eating food
before taking the medicine
or at the same time may
blunt levodopa's effects.

STORAGE
Store in a tightly sealed container away from heat, moisture, and direct light.

IF YOU MISS A DOSE
Take it as soon as you
remember, unless the time
for your next scheduled
dose is within the next 2
hours. If so, skip the missed
dose and resume your regular dosage schedule. Do not
double the next dose.

STOPPING THE DRUG
Consult your doctor before
stopping the drug. The
dosage should be decreased
very gradually. Abruptly
stopping the medication can
result in an acute (sudden-onset) adverse reaction.

PROLONGED USE
Prolonged use may result in
a less predictable therapeutic response as well as the
onset of involuntary muscle
movements.

PRECAUTIONS
Over 60: Adverse reactions
may be more likely and
more severe.

**Driving and Hazardous
Work:** Avoid such activities
until you determine how the
medicine affects you.

Alcohol: Avoid alcohol
while using this medication.

Pregnancy: This combination drug should not be
used by pregnant women.

Breast Feeding: Levodopa
passes into breast milk.
This combination drug
should not be used by
nursing mothers.

Infants and Children:
Levodopa/carbidopa can be
used by children, with caution. The appropriate
dosage will be determined
by your pediatrician. Use of
the sustained-release tablets

in children under the age of
18 is not recommended.

Special Concerns: Levodopa/carbidopa should be
used with special caution if
you are also taking other
antiparkinsonism drugs. Do
not crush or chew the sustained-release tablets. Swallow them whole.

OVERDOSE
Symptoms: Sudden or
severe confusion, delirium,
hallucinations.

What to Do: Seek emergency medical attention
immediately.

DRUG INTERACTIONS
Do not take levodopa/carbidopa if you are taking, or
took within the past 14
days, an MAO inhibitor
(such as phenelzine sulfate
or tranylcypromine sulfate).
Consult your doctor for specific advice if you are taking
selegiline, tricyclic antidepressants, risperidone,
fluphenazine, phenytoin,
papaverine, iron salts, metoclopramide, or any antihypertensive drugs.

FOOD INTERACTIONS
The effectiveness of levodopa/carbidopa may be
impaired by a high-protein
diet. Persons taking the
drug should take care to
limit their protein intake.

DISEASE INTERACTIONS
You should not take levodopa/carbidopa if you
have malignant melanoma,
ischemic heart disease,
heart rhythm abnormalities,
bronchial asthma, narrow-angle glaucoma, or any
changes in mental state.
Levodopa/carbidopa should
be used with caution in people who have kidney, liver,
or endocrine disease, a history of heart attack, peptic
ulcer, or chronic wide-angle
glaucoma.

Levofloxacin

Levaquin 250 mg
(**McNeil**)

▶ Drug Class: Fluoroquinolone antibiotic

▶ Available in: Tablets, injection

▶ Available OTC? No

▶ As Generic? No

Side Effects

SERIOUS
Serious reactions to levofloxacin are rare and include seizures, mental confusion, hallucinations, agitation, nightmares, depression, shortness of breath, unusual swelling in the face or extremities, and loss of consciousness. Also skin burning, redness, blisters, rash, or itching on exposure to sunlight; increased risk of tendinitis or tendon rupture. Call your doctor immediately.

COMMON
Increased sensitivity to sunlight (and increased risk of sunburn) for days following therapy.

LESS COMMON
Diarrhea, nausea and vomiting, stomach pain and upset, gas, headache, dizziness, restlessness, insomnia, changes in taste perception, drowsiness, itching, dry mouth, unusual body aches or pains.

PRINCIPAL USES
To treat pneumonia, chronic bronchitis, and other infections caused by bacteria.

HOW THE DRUG WORKS
Levofloxacin inhibits the activity of a bacterial enzyme (gyrase) that is necessary for proper DNA formation and replication. This fights infection by preventing bacteria cells from reproducing.

DOSAGE
Adults: 250 to 500 mg once a day for 7 to 14 days. After an initial dose of 250 to 500 mg, patients with kidney problems receive 250 mg every day for 7 to 14 days.

ONSET OF EFFECT
Varies depending on the infection being treated.

DURATION OF ACTION
Unknown.

DIETARY ADVICE
Drink plenty of fluids.

STORAGE
Store in a tightly sealed container away from heat and direct light. Do not allow the injection form to freeze.

IF YOU MISS A DOSE
Take it as soon as you remember. If it is near the time for the next dose, skip the missed dose and resume your regular dosage schedule. Do not double the next dose.

STOPPING THE DRUG
It is very important to take this drug as prescribed for the full treatment period, even if you begin to feel better before the scheduled end of therapy (unless you experience intolerable side effects, including increased sensitivity to sunlight).

PROLONGED USE
See your doctor regularly for tests and examinations if you must take this medicine for a prolonged period.

PRECAUTIONS
Over 60: No special problems are expected.

Driving and Hazardous Work: Do not drive or engage in hazardous work until you determine how the medicine affects you.

Alcohol: It is advisable to abstain from alcohol when fighting an infection.

Pregnancy: In some animal tests, levofloxacin has caused birth defects. Adequate studies in humans have not been done. It should be used during pregnancy only if potential benefits clearly justify the risks. Before you take levofloxacin, tell your doctor if you are pregnant or plan to become pregnant.

Breast Feeding: Levofloxacin passes into breast milk and may cause serious side effects in the nursing infant; use of the drug is discouraged when nursing.

Infants and Children: Levofloxacin is not recommended for use by persons under the age of 18, as it has been shown to interfere with bone development.

Special Concerns: If levofloxacin causes sensitivity to sunlight, stop taking the drug and try to avoid exposure to sunlight for the next 5 days; also wear protective clothing and use a sunblock. Levofloxacin should not be taken by patients whose work makes it impossible to avoid exposure to sunlight. It is important to drink plenty of fluids while taking this drug.

OVERDOSE
Symptoms: No specific ones have been reported.

What to Do: If you have any reason to suspect an overdose, call your doctor, emergency medical services (EMS), or the nearest poison control center.

DRUG INTERACTIONS
Consult your doctor for specific advice if you are taking aminophylline, antacids, didanosine, iron supplements, sucralfate, or zinc salts. Also tell your doctor if you are taking any other prescription or over-the-counter drug.

FOOD INTERACTIONS
No known food interactions.

DISEASE INTERACTIONS
Caution is advised when taking levofloxacin. Consult your doctor if you have any other medical condition. Use of levofloxacin can cause complications in patients with kidney disease, since this organ works to remove the medication from the body.

Levomethadyl Acetate Hydrochloride

Side Effects

SERIOUS
Some serious side effects of levomethadyl are indistinguishable from those of overdose: Confusion; slurred speech; severe drowsiness; small, pinpoint pupils; cold, clammy skin; slow breathing; seizures; unconsciousness. Other serious side effects are depression; enlarged pupils; swelling of fingers, feet, face, and lower legs; skin rash; diarrhea; insomnia; rapid heartbeat; nervousness; runny nose; trembling; stomach cramps; fever. Call your doctor immediately.

COMMON
Abdominal or stomach pains, nausea, and constipation.

LESS COMMON
Back pain, watering eyes, anxiety, blurred vision, flu symptoms, chills, decreased sexual desire, dizziness when getting up, headache, cough, hot flashes, muscle pain, unusual dreams.

PRINCIPAL USES
To prevent or ease withdrawal symptoms during detoxification from illegal narcotics, and to serve as maintenance therapy during narcotic addiction treatment programs.

HOW THE DRUG WORKS
Levomethadyl serves as a substitute for other narcotics that tend to produce more-pronounced effects.

DOSAGE
Addicts who have not begun treatment with methadone: To start, between 20 and 40 mg per day, 3 times a week. Addicts who have been receiving methadone: To start, the dose will be a little higher than the amount of methadone per day, but not more than 120 mg, 3 times a week. The dose will be reduced in detoxification programs, continued as long as needed in maintenance programs. Levomethadyl should not be taken daily because of the risk of overdose.

ONSET OF EFFECT
Levomethadyl may not be fully effective for several days. For this reason methadone may be the first drug used in a detoxification program, since its effect is more immediate; levomethadyl may then be used since, unlike methadone, it does not need to be taken every day.

DURATION OF ACTION
48 to 72 hours.

DIETARY ADVICE
No special restrictions.

STORAGE
Not applicable; dose may be taken only at approved treatment facilities.

IF YOU MISS A DOSE
Not applicable; the dose is administered by a health care professional specializing in addiction treatment.

STOPPING THE DRUG
The decision to stop taking levomethadyl should be made by the addiction treatment specialist.

PROLONGED USE
See your health care professional regularly for tests and examinations.

PRECAUTIONS
Over 60: Studies on older patients have not been conducted.

Driving and Hazardous Work: Do not drive or engage in hazardous work until you determine how the medicine affects you.

Alcohol: Avoid alcohol.

Pregnancy: Using this drug during pregnancy may cause withdrawal symptoms in the newborn baby. Federal law requires pregnancy tests before starting treatment and once-a-month exams during treatment.

Breast Feeding: Levomethadyl may pass into breast milk; caution is advised. Consult your doctor for advice.

Infants and Children: Federal law prohibits use of levomethadyl by persons under 18 years of age.

Special Concerns: Tell any doctor or dentist you see for treatment that you are taking levomethadyl. To prevent constipation, you may be advised to increase the fiber in your diet, drink a lot of fluids, or take laxatives.

OVERDOSE
Symptoms: See Serious Side Effects.

What to Do: Call your doctor, emergency medical services (EMS), or the nearest poison control center immediately.

DRUG INTERACTIONS
Consult your doctor for specific advice if you are taking barbiturates, buprenorphine, butorphanol, carbamazepine, central nervous system depressants, chloramphenicol, cimetidine, corticosteroids, dezocine, diltiazem, disulfiram, divalproex, erythromycin, griseofulvin, isoniazid, oral contraceptives, nalbuphine, naltrexone, pentazocine, phenylbutazone, phenytoin, primidone, quinine, rifampin, ranitidine, tricyclic antidepressants, valproic acid, or verapamil.

FOOD INTERACTIONS
No known food interactions.

DISEASE INTERACTIONS
Consult your doctor if you have any of the following: chronic lung disease, brain disease, head injury, colitis, Crohn's disease, enlarged prostate, gallbladder disease, heart disease, high blood pressure, kidney or liver disease, or an underactive thyroid.

Levonorgestrel Implants

▶ Drug Class: Progestin (hormone)

▶ Available in: Implanted capsule

▶ Available OTC? No

▶ As Generic? No

Side Effects

SERIOUS
Changes in or cessation of menstrual bleeding, unexpected or increased flow of breast milk, mental depression, skin rash, loss of or change in speech, impaired coordination or vision, severe and sudden shortness of breath. Call your doctor immediately.

COMMON
Stomach pain, swelling of face, ankles, or feet, mild headache, mood changes, unusual fatigue, weight gain, pain or irritation at site of implant.

LESS COMMON
Acne, breast pain or tenderness, hot flashes, insomnia, loss of sexual desire, loss or gain of scalp hair or body hair, brown spots on skin.

PRINCIPAL USES
As a birth control method.

HOW THE DRUG WORKS
The implant slowly releases levonorgestrel, a synthetic hormone, into the bloodstream. It prevents a woman's egg from developing fully and causes changes in the uterine lining that make it difficult for sperm to reach the egg. It may prevent ovulation in some patients.

DOSAGE
6 capsules are implanted under the skin of the upper arm. The capsules are placed in a fanlike position, 15 degrees apart. They are removed after 5 years.

ONSET OF EFFECT
Within 24 hours if implanted within 7 days of the menstrual period.

DURATION OF ACTION
Up to 5 years.

DIETARY ADVICE
No special restrictions.

STORAGE
Not applicable.

IF YOU MISS A DOSE
Not applicable; the drug is delivered continuously from the implant under the skin.

STOPPING THE DRUG
The decision to stop using the implant can be made whenever you choose, but the implants should be removed by your doctor.

PROLONGED USE
See your doctor at least once a year for periodic examinations and lab tests.

PRECAUTIONS
Over 60: Not normally prescribed for postmenopausal women.

Driving and Hazardous Work: No special precautions are necessary.

Alcohol: No special precautions are necessary.

Pregnancy: Extensive studies have shown that no special risks to mother or child are associated with pregnancies occurring prior to or shortly after implantation of levonorgestrel capsules. Nonetheless, it is advisable to have the implants removed if pregnancy occurs.

Breast Feeding: Levonorgestrel passes into breast milk but has not been shown to cause problems. It can be used by nursing mothers who desire contraception.

Infants and Children: Levonorgestrel implants have not been shown to cause problems in teenagers. However, birth control methods that protect against sexually transmitted diseases (for example, condoms) are preferred for those in this age group.

Special Concerns: Do not have this implant inserted until you are sure you are not pregnant. Call your doctor immediately if one of the capsules falls out before the skin heals over the implant. No contraceptive method is perfect: If you suspect a pregnancy, you should call your doctor immediately. If you have any laboratory test, tell the health professional that you are using these contraceptives. Cigarette smoking or alcohol abuse can increase the risk of osteoporosis and blood clot formation. Implants should be removed if you develop active thrombophlebitis (pain caused by a blot clot lodged in a blood vessel), thromboembolic disease, or jaundice (yellowish tinge to the eyes or skin), or if you will be immobilized for a significant period of time because of illness or some other factor. If you have sudden unexplained vision problems, including changes in tolerance for contact lenses, you should be evaluated by an ophthalmologist.

OVERDOSE
Symptoms: Not applicable.

What to Do: Emergency instructions not applicable.

DRUG INTERACTIONS
Consult your doctor for specific advice if you are taking aminoglutethimide, carbamazepine, phenytoin, rifabutin, or rifampin.

FOOD INTERACTIONS
No known food interactions.

DISEASE INTERACTIONS
Caution is advised when using this contraceptive. Consult your doctor if you have any of the following: asthma, epilepsy, heart or circulation problems, kidney disease, liver disease, migraine headaches, breast disease, bleeding disorders, central nervous system disorders (including depression), diabetes, or high blood cholesterol.

Levothyroxine Sodium

Levoxyl 0.1 mg
(DANIELS)

804

Additional photographs

▶ Drug Class: Hypothyroid
agent

▶ Available in: Tablets, injection

▶ Available OTC? No

▶ As Generic? Yes

Side Effects

SERIOUS
In rare instances levothyroxine may cause severe
headaches, skin rash,
hives, rapid or irregular
heartbeat, chest pain, or
shortness of breath.
These symptoms may
signal an overdose or an
allergic reaction. Seek
emergency medical assis-
tance immediately.

COMMON
No common side effects
are associated with the
use of levothyroxine.

LESS COMMON
Leg cramps, diarrhea,
changes in menstrual
cycle, changes in
appetite, sweating,
sensitivity to heat, shaking of the hands, fever,
headache, insomnia, irri-
tability, weight loss, vomiting, nervousness. These
symptoms may indicate
your dose needs adjust-
ment by your doctor.

PRINCIPAL USES
To treat patients with an
underactive thyroid gland,
goiter (enlarged thyroid
gland), and benign and
malignant (noncancerous
and cancerous) thyroid
nodules.

HOW THE DRUG WORKS
Levothyroxine acts in the
body as a substitute for
natural thyroid hormone.

DOSAGE
Tablets— Adults and
teenagers: 0.0016 mg per
2.2 lbs (1 kg) a day. Children less than 6 months
old: 0.025 to 0.05 mg once a
day. Children 6 to 12
months old: 0.05 to 0.075
mg once a day. Children
ages 1 to 5: 0.075 to 0.1 mg
once a day. Children ages 6
to 12: 0.1 to 0.15 mg a day.
Injection— Adults and
teenagers: 0.05 to 0.1 mg
into a vein or muscle once a
day. Children less than 6
months old: 0.019 to 0.038
mg once a day. Children 6
to 12 months old: 0.038 to
0.056 mg once a day. Children ages 1 to 5: 0.056 to
0.075 mg once a day. Children ages 6 to 10: 0.075 to
0.113 mg once a day. Children ages 10 to 12: 0.113
to 0.15 mg once a day.

ONSET OF EFFECT
24 hours.

DURATION OF ACTION
1 to 3 weeks.

DIETARY ADVICE
Take it before breakfast on
an empty stomach.

STORAGE
Store in a tightly sealed container away from heat, moisture, and direct light.

IF YOU MISS A DOSE
If you miss your dose on
one day, you may double
the dose on the next day. If

you miss two or more doses
in a row, call your doctor.

STOPPING THE DRUG
The decision to stop taking
the drug should be made in
consultation with your
physician.

PROLONGED USE
If you must take this drug,
it is very likely that lifelong
therapy will be necessary.
See your doctor regularly
for routine tests and examinations to evaluate your
condition.

PRECAUTIONS
Over 60: Older patients
may require modification
of dosage size.

**Driving and Hazardous
Work:** Do not drive or
engage in hazardous work
until you determine how the
medicine affects you.

Alcohol: Avoid alcohol.

Pregnancy: Using the recommended dose of levothy-
roxine has not been shown
to cause birth defects.
The dose may need to be
changed during pregnancy.
Consult your doctor for
specific advice.

Breast Feeding: Using the
recommended dose of
levothyroxine has not been
shown to cause problems
while nursing. Consult your
doctor for specific advice.

Infants and Children:
No special problems are
expected.

Special Concerns: You
should wear a medical
bracelet or carry an identification card saying that you
are taking this medication.

OVERDOSE
Symptoms: Rapid heartbeat, chest pain, shortness
of breath.

What to Do: Call your
doctor, emergency medical
services (EMS), or the
nearest poison control center immediately.

DRUG INTERACTIONS
Consult your doctor for
advice if you are taking anticoagulants, cholestyramine,
colestipol, amphetamines,
appetite suppressants,
asthma medication, or
cold, sinus, or allergy
medications.

FOOD INTERACTIONS
No known food interactions.

DISEASE INTERACTIONS
Caution is advised when
taking levothyroxine. Consult your doctor if you have
any of the following: diabetes mellitus, diabetes
insipidus, myxedema, an
overactive thyroid gland,
atherosclerosis (so-called
hardening of the arteries),
heart disease, high blood
pressure, an underactive
adrenal gland, or an underactive pituitary gland.

Lidocaine Hydrochloride Topical

▶ Drug Class: Topical analgesic

▶ Available in: Gel, ointment, aerosol spray, transdermal patch

▶ Available OTC? No

▶ As Generic? Yes

Side Effects

SERIOUS
Hives, itching, rash, swelling of face, mouth, lips, throat, or tongue; burning, swelling, worsening redness, or pain at site of application. These may be signs of a potentially serious allergic reaction, which is rare.

COMMON
There are no significant common side effects of topical lidocaine when used in recommended amounts.

LESS COMMON
Mild redness, blanching (whitening), or swelling of skin at application sites. If irritation or a burning sensation occurs during application of the transdermal patch, remove the patch and do not reapply until the irritation recedes.

PRINCIPAL USES
For topical therapy of certain skin conditions associated with itching or pain. Some such conditions are minor burns, including sunburn; insect stings and bites; inflammatory skin rashes associated with intense itching, like those caused by poison ivy, poison oak, or poison sumac; and minor cuts and scratches. The transdermal patch is used to relieve pain associated with post-herpetic neuralgia. Topical lidocaine is not meant to be used to relieve the pain of severe injuries, nor should it be prescribed for large or actively bleeding wounds.

HOW THE DRUG WORKS
Lidocaine interferes with the ability of certain nerves to conduct electrical signals, which blocks the transmission of nerve impulses that carry pain messages.

DOSAGE
Gel, ointment, and spray— Adults: Apply to affected area 3 to 4 times a day as needed. Children: Consult a pediatrician for advice. Transdermal patch— Adults: Apply a patch to intact skin to cover the most painful area. Up to 3 patches may be applied simultaneously, for no more than 12 hours at a time per 24-hour period.

ONSET OF EFFECT
Within minutes.

DURATION OF ACTION
Gel, ointment, and spray: About 45 minutes. Transdermal patch: Up to 12 hours.

DIETARY ADVICE
Maintain your usual food and fluid intake. Increase fluids if you have a fever or diarrhea, in hot weather, or during exercise.

STORAGE
Store in a tightly sealed container away from heat and direct light. Keep away from moisture and extremes in temperature.

IF YOU MISS A DOSE
Apply it as soon as you remember. If it is near the time for the next dose, skip the missed dose and resume your regular dosage schedule. Do not double the next dose or apply an excessively thick film of topical lidocaine to compensate for a missed application.

STOPPING THE DRUG
Apply it as prescribed for the full treatment period. However, you may stop using the drug if you are feeling better before the scheduled end of the therapy.

PROLONGED USE
Therapy with this medication is generally finished within several days. Prolonged use may increase the risk of side effects.

PRECAUTIONS
Over 60: Adverse reactions may be more likely and more severe.

Driving and Hazardous Work: No special warnings.

Alcohol: No special precautions are necessary.

Pregnancy: Lidocaine may be used during pregnancy, but first consult your physician for advice.

Breast Feeding: Lidocaine may pass into breast milk; caution is advised. Consult your doctor for advice.

Infants and Children: Not recommended for use by children under age 2. The transdermal patch is not recommended for children under the age of 18.

Special Concerns: Lidocaine has serious side effects if it is absorbed in large amounts into the blood. Therefore, do not apply excessive amounts of gel or ointment to the affected skin or wear a patch longer than 12 hours. Use only enough medication to make a thin film. Above all, never apply this medication to open wounds, deep cuts, or bleeding or ulcerated skin. Dispose of the patch to prevent access by children or pets because a significant amount of lidocaine remains in the patch following use.

OVERDOSE
Symptoms: Dizziness, slow or irregular heartbeat, confusion, seizures, shivering, unusual restlessness or agitation, hallucinations, difficulty breathing, bluish color to skin, lips, or fingertips.

What to Do: Call your doctor, emergency medical services (EMS), or the nearest poison control center immediately.

DRUG INTERACTIONS
The following drugs may interact with topical lidocaine, especially if excessive amounts of lidocaine are applied to the skin: medications to control heart rhythms, such as mexiletine or tocainide; beta-blockers; and cimetidine.

FOOD INTERACTIONS
No known food interactions.

DISEASE INTERACTIONS
Caution is advised when taking lidocaine. Consult your doctor if you have any of the following: skin infection at or close to the application site; large sores, blisters, ulcerations, or broken skin at the application site; or severe injury at the application site.

BRAND NAMES
Bio-Well, G-Well, GBH, Kildane, Kwell, Kwildane, Scabene, Thionex

▶ Drug Class: Insecticide

▶ Available in: Cream, lotion, shampoo

▶ Available OTC? No

▶ As Generic? Yes

Side Effects

SERIOUS
Seizures; dizziness, clumsiness, or unsteady gait; rapid heartbeat; muscle cramps; nervousness, restlessness, or irritability; vomiting. Call your doctor immediately.

COMMON
There are no common side effects associated with lindane. However, when you stop using lindane, itching may occur and persist for 1 or more weeks; notify your doctor if this continues for more than a few weeks or interferes with daily activity.

LESS COMMON
Skin rash; redness or skin irritation that was not present prior to therapy.

PRINCIPAL USES
Lindane cream and lotion are used to treat scabies infestation. The shampoo form is used to treat lice infestation.

HOW THE DRUG WORKS
Lindane is absorbed directly into the bodies of scabies and lice, where it overstimulates nerve activity, ultimately causing convulsions and death of the insect.

DOSAGE
Cream and lotion: Wash, rinse, and dry your skin thoroughly before applying. Apply enough lindane to cover the entire surface of your body from the neck down, including the soles of the feet. Rub in well. Leave it on for no more than 8 hours, then remove it by washing thoroughly. Shampoo: Rinse and dry your hair and scalp. Apply enough lindane to thoroughly wet the scalp and affected areas. Allow it to remain in place for 4 minutes, then lather. Rinse thoroughly and dry with a clean towel. Then use a fine-tooth comb to remove nits. Treatment may be repeated after 7 days if necessary.

ONSET OF EFFECT
Unknown.

DURATION OF ACTION
Unknown.

DIETARY ADVICE
Lindane can be used without regard to diet. After applying the medication, be sure to wash your hands thoroughly before eating.

STORAGE
Store in a tightly sealed container away from heat and direct light.

IF YOU MISS A DOSE
If you require a second dose of the shampoo (usually applied 7 days after the first dose) and forget it, administer it as soon as you remember.

STOPPING THE DRUG
In most cases lindane is needed only once; a second application may be necessary if living nits are found after initial treatment.

PROLONGED USE
Not applicable, since lindane is generally used only once or twice.

PRECAUTIONS
Over 60: Adverse reactions may be more likely in older patients.

Driving and Hazardous Work: Do not drive or engage in hazardous work until you determine how the medicine affects you.

Alcohol: No special precautions are necessary.

Pregnancy: Lindane is absorbed through the skin and could reach the fetus. Before you use lindane, tell your doctor if you are currently pregnant or plan to become pregnant. Do not use lindane more than twice during pregnancy.

Breast Feeding: Lindane passes into breast milk; caution is advised. You should not breast feed for 2 days after using lindane. Consult your doctor for advice.

Infants and Children: Adverse reactions may be more likely and more severe in infants and children. Do not use lindane on premature infants.

Special Concerns: Lindane is a poison that can depress the activity of the central nervous system (brain and spinal cord). Keep it away from the eyes and mouth. It may be fatal if swallowed. If you accidentally get some lindane in your eyes, wash them thoroughly with water and call your doctor. Do not use lindane on open wounds, such as cuts and sores. When applying lindane to another person, wear disposable plastic or rubber gloves, especially if you are breast feeding or pregnant. Do not keep lindane in your home any longer than needed. Be sure that any discarded lindane is out of the reach of children and pets.

OVERDOSE
Symptoms: Seizures, dizziness, vomiting.

What to Do: Call your doctor, emergency medical services (EMS), or the nearest poison control center immediately.

DRUG INTERACTIONS
Consult your doctor for specific advice if you are taking any prescription or over-the-counter medication.

FOOD INTERACTIONS
No known food interactions.

DISEASE INTERACTIONS
Caution is advised when using lindane. Consult your doctor if you have a seizure disorder, a skin rash, or any raw and broken skin.

Linezolid

▶ Drug Class: Oxazolidinone antibiotic

▶ Available in: Injection, tablets, oral suspension

▶ Available OTC? No

▶ As Generic? No

Side Effects

SERIOUS
Serious side effects are rare, but may include: thrombocytopenia (reduced blood platelet numbers, resulting in uncontrolled bleeding) and pseudomembranous colitis. Consult your doctor immediately.

COMMON
Diarrhea, headache, nausea.

LESS COMMON
Insomnia, vomiting, constipation, dizziness.

PRINCIPAL USES
To treat certain hospital- or community-acquired pneumonias and some bacterial infections of the skin and bloodstream, including vancomycin-resistant *Enterococcus faecium* infections and *Staphylococcus aureus*.

HOW THE DRUG WORKS
Linezolid inhibits the growth of bacteria by interfering with the process of translating DNA messages into proteins. Because this drug works differently from other antibiotics, the development of cross-resistance between linezolid and other classes of antibiotics is unlikely.

DOSAGE
For vancomycin-resistant *E. faecium* infections: 600 mg every 12 hours for 14 to 28 days. For pneumonia and complicated skin infections: 600 mg every 12 hours for 10 to 14 days. For uncomplicated skin infections: 400 mg every 12 hours for 10 to 14 days.

ONSET OF EFFECT
Unknown.

DURATION OF ACTION
Unknown.

DIETARY ADVICE
Linezolid may be taken with or without food.

STORAGE
Injection: Not applicable; injections are administered only at a health care facility. Tablets and oral solution: Store in a tightly sealed container away from heat, moisture, and direct light.

IF YOU MISS A DOSE
Take it as soon as you remember. If it is near the time for the next dose, skip the missed dose and resume your regular dosage schedule. Do not double the next dose.

STOPPING THE DRUG
Take it as prescribed for the full treatment period, even if your symptoms improve before the scheduled end of therapy.

PROLONGED USE
Prolonged use of any antibiotic increases the risk of superinfection (a more severe and drug-resistant infection); caution is advised. Use is generally limited to 10 to 28 days. People who are at increased risk for bleeding disorders or have low platelets should have their blood platelet counts monitored by their doctor while taking linezolid.

PRECAUTIONS
Over 60: No special problems are expected.

Driving and Hazardous Work: Avoid such activities until you determine how the medicine affects you.

Alcohol: It is advisable to abstain from alcohol when treating a serious infection.

Pregnancy: Adequate human studies have not been done. Before taking linezolid, discuss with your doctor the relative risks and benefits of using this drug while pregnant.

Breast Feeding: Linezolid may pass into breast milk; caution is advised.

Infants and Children: Safety and effectiveness have not been established for children under age 18.

Special Concerns: The oral suspension is supplied in powder form. Tap the bottle gently to loosen the powder. Add a total of 123 milliliters (mL) distilled water in two portions. After adding the first half, shake the bottle well to wet all of the powder. Add the second portion of water and shake vigorously to mix the suspension. After constitution, each 5 mL of suspension contains 100 mg linezolid. Before using, gently mix by inverting the bottle 3 to 5 times. Do not shake. Store at room temperature and use the suspension within 21 days of reconstitution.

OVERDOSE
Symptoms: No overdoses have been reported. Symptoms may include lethargy, impaired coordination, vomiting, and tremor.

What to Do: If you suspect an overdose or if someone takes a much larger dose than prescribed, seek emergency medical attention (EMS) immediately.

DRUG INTERACTIONS
Consult your doctor for specific advice if you are taking an MAO inhibitor (such as phenelzine or tranylcypromine), pseudoephedrine, dopamine, epinephrine, or SSRI antidepressants.

FOOD INTERACTIONS
Avoid tyramine-rich foods, which include aged cheeses, avocados, banana skins, bean curd, bologna and other processed lunch meats, chicken livers, chocolate, figs, canned or dried fish, pickled herring, meat extracts, pepperoni, raisins, raspberries, soy sauce, unpasteurized beer, Chianti, sherry, vermouth, and red wines in general.

DISEASE INTERACTIONS
Consult your doctor if you have a history of high blood pressure, hyperthyroidism, pheochromocytoma, carcinoid syndrome, thrombocytopenia or other bleeding disorders, diarrhea, or decreased kidney function.

Liothyronine Sodium

Cytomel 25 mcg
(SMITHKLINE BEECHAM)

▶ Drug Class: Thyroid hormone

▶ Available in: Tablets

▶ Available OTC? No

▶ As Generic? Yes

Side Effects

SERIOUS
Severe headache in children; skin rash or hives. Call your physician immediately.

COMMON
Changes in appetite, changes in menstrual period, headache, hand tremors, increased sensitivity to heat, irritability, leg cramps, nervousness, sweating, insomnia, vomiting, weight loss, clumsiness, coldness, constipation, dry skin, muscle aches, weakness, weight gain.

LESS COMMON
Diarrhea or other forms of gastrointestinal upset.

PRINCIPAL USES
Liothyronine is prescribed when the thyroid gland does not naturally produce enough thyroid hormone.

HOW THE DRUG WORKS
Liothyronine is a synthetic form of thyroid hormone. It functions in the same manner as (and so serves as a substitute for) the natural hormone when the body does not produce enough on its own.

DOSAGE
25 micrograms (mcg) per day to start. It can be increased to 50 mcg per day, taken in 2 or more daily doses.

ONSET OF EFFECT
Within 48 to 72 hours.

DURATION OF ACTION
Up to 72 hours after the drug is discontinued.

DIETARY ADVICE
Best if taken before breakfast, to minimize risk of insomnia.

STORAGE
Store in a tightly sealed container away from heat and direct light.

IF YOU MISS A DOSE
Take it as soon as you remember. If it is near the time for the next dose, skip the missed dose and resume your regular dosage schedule. Do not double the next dose.

STOPPING THE DRUG
The decision to stop taking the drug should be made by your doctor.

PROLONGED USE
No special problems are expected.

PRECAUTIONS
Over 60: A different dose may be needed for older patients. Consult your doctor about the proper dose.

Driving and Hazardous Work: The use of liothyronine should not impair your ability to perform such tasks safely.

Alcohol: Avoid alcohol.

Pregnancy: Use of proper amounts of liothyronine during pregnancy has not been shown to cause problems. Your doctor may want you to change the dose while you are pregnant. Regular visits to the doctor during pregnancy are advised.

Breast Feeding: Use of proper amounts of liothyronine in nursing women has not been shown to cause problems in their babies.

Infants and Children: The dose for infants and children must be carefully adjusted by the doctor.

Special Concerns: Before undergoing any kind of medical or dental procedure, be sure to tell the doctor or dentist in charge that you are taking liothyronine.

OVERDOSE
Symptoms: Headache, irritability, nervousness, sweating, rapid heartbeat, fever, palpitations or other heartbeat irregularities, increased bowel movements, menstrual irregularities, vomiting, seizures.

What to Do: An overdose of liothyronine is unlikely to be life-threatening. However, if someone takes a much larger dose than prescribed, call your doctor, emergency medical services (EMS), or nearest poison control center immediately.

DRUG INTERACTIONS
Consult your doctor for specific advice if you are taking amphetamines, anticoagulants, appetite suppressants, cholestyramine, colestipol, medicine for asthma or other breathing problems, or medicine for colds, sinus problems or hay fever.

FOOD INTERACTIONS
No known food interactions.

DISEASE INTERACTIONS
Caution is advised when taking liothyronine. Consult your doctor if you have any of the following: diabetes mellitus, hardening of the arteries, heart disease, high blood pressure, history of overactive thyroid, or underactive adrenal gland, underactive pituitary gland. If you have certain kinds of heart disease, this medicine may cause chest pains or shortness of breath during exertion. If these symptoms occur, consult your doctor.

Lisinopril

Prinivil 5 mg
(MERCK)

Additional photographs

▶ Drug Class: Angiotensin-converting enzyme (ACE) inhibitor

▶ Available in: Tablets

▶ Available OTC? No

▶ As Generic? No

Side Effects

SERIOUS
Fever and chills, sore throat and hoarseness, sudden difficulty breathing or swallowing, swelling of the face, mouth, or extremities, impaired kidney function (ankle swelling, decreased urination), confusion, yellow discoloration of the eyes or skin (indicating liver disorder), intense itching, chest pain or palpitations, abdominal pain. Serious side effects are very rare; contact your doctor immediately.

COMMON
Dry, persistent cough.

LESS COMMON
Dizziness or fainting, skin rash, numbness or tingling in the hands, feet, or lips, unusual fatigue or muscle weakness, nausea, drowsiness, loss of taste, headache.

PRINCIPAL USES
To control high blood pressure (hypertension). Also used to treat congestive heart failure (CHF) and left ventricular dysfunction (damage to the primary pumping chamber of the heart), and to minimize further kidney damage in diabetic patients with mild kidney disease.

HOW THE DRUG WORKS
Angiotensin-converting enzyme (ACE) inhibitors block an enzyme that produces angiotensin, a naturally occurring substance that causes blood vessels to constrict and stimulates production of the adrenal hormone, aldosterone, which promotes sodium retention in the body. As a result, ACE inhibitors relax blood vessels (causing them to widen) and reduces sodium retention, which lowers blood pressure and so decreases the workload of the heart.

DOSAGE
For high blood pressure: 5 to 40 mg once a day. For congestive heart failure: 2.5 to 20 mg once a day.

ONSET OF EFFECT
Within 1 hour.

DURATION OF ACTION
24 hours.

DIETARY ADVICE
Take lisinopril on an empty stomach, about 1 hour before mealtime. Follow your doctor's dietary advice (such as low-salt or low-cholesterol restrictions) to improve control over high blood pressure and heart disease. Avoid high-potassium foods like bananas and citrus fruits and juices, unless you are also taking medications, such as diuretics, that lower potassium levels.

STORAGE
Store in a tightly sealed container away from heat and direct light.

IF YOU MISS A DOSE
Take it as soon as you remember. If it is near the time for the next dose, skip the missed dose and resume your regular dosage schedule. Do not double the next dose.

STOPPING THE DRUG
Do not stop taking this drug abruptly, as this may cause potentially serious health problems. Dosage should be reduced gradually, according to your doctor's instructions.

PROLONGED USE
Lifelong therapy with lisinopril may be necessary. See your doctor regularly for examinations and tests if you must take this medicine for a prolonged period.

PRECAUTIONS
Over 60: No unusual problems are expected in older patients.

Driving and Hazardous Work: Do not drive or engage in hazardous work until you determine how the medicine affects you.

Alcohol: Consume alcohol only in moderation since it may increase the effect of the drug and cause an excessive drop in blood pressure. Consult your doctor for advice.

Pregnancy: Use of lisinopril during the last 6 months of pregnancy may cause severe defects, even death, in the fetus. The drug should be discontinued if you are pregnant or plan to become pregnant.

Breast Feeding: Lisinopril may pass into breast milk;

caution is advised. Consult your doctor for advice.

Infants and Children: Children may be especially sensitive to the effects of lisinopril. Benefits must be weighed against potential risks; consult your pediatrician for advice.

OVERDOSE
Symptoms: Dizziness, confusion, faintness.

What to Do: Call your doctor, emergency medical services (EMS), or the nearest poison control center immediately.

DRUG INTERACTIONS
Consult your doctor if you are taking diuretics (especially potassium-sparing diuretics), potassium supplements or drugs containing potassium (check ingredient labels), lithium, anticoagulants (such as warfarin), indomethacin or other anti-inflammatory drugs, or any over-the-counter medications (especially cold remedies and diet pills).

FOOD INTERACTIONS
Avoid low-salt milk and salt substitutes. Many of these products contain potassium.

DISEASE INTERACTIONS
Consult your doctor if you have systemic lupus erythematosus (SLE) or if you have had a prior allergic reaction to ACE inhibitors. Lisinopril should be used with caution by patients with severe kidney disease or renal artery stenosis (narrowing of one or both of the arteries that supply blood to the kidneys).

Lisinopril/Hydrochlorothiazide

BRAND NAMES
Prinzide, Zestoretic

▶ Drug Class: Angiotensin-converting enzyme (ACE) inhibitor/diuretic

▶ Available in: Tablets

▶ Available OTC? No

▶ As Generic? No

Side Effects

SERIOUS
Fever and chills, sore throat and hoarseness, sudden difficulty breathing or swallowing, swelling of the face, mouth, or extremities, impaired kidney function (ankle swelling, decreased urination), confusion, yellow discoloration of the eyes or skin (indicating liver disorder), intense itching, chest pain or heartbeat irregularities, abdominal pain. Serious side effects are very rare; contact your doctor immediately.

COMMON
Dry, persistent cough.

LESS COMMON
Dizziness or fainting, skin rash, numbness or tingling in the hands, feet, or lips, change in color of the hands from white to blue to red (Raynaud's phenomenon) in cold weather, unusual fatigue or muscle weakness, nausea, drowsiness, loss of taste, headache, unusual dreams.

PRINCIPAL USES
To treat high blood pressure (hypertension). Used in patients for whom both lisinopril and hydrochlorothiazide have been prescribed.

HOW THE DRUG WORKS
Angiotensin-converting enzyme (ACE) inhibitors such as lisinopril block an enzyme that produces angiotensin, a naturally occurring substance that causes blood vessels to constrict and stimulates production of the adrenal hormone, aldosterone, which promotes sodium retention in the body. As a result, ACE inhibitors relax blood vessels (causing them to widen) and reduces sodium retention, which lowers blood pressure and so decreases the workload of the heart. Hydrochlorothiazide (HCTZ), a diuretic, increases sodium and water in the urine output. By reducing the overall fluid volume in the body, diuretics reduce blood volume and so reduce blood pressure.

DOSAGE
This combination medication comes in three strengths: lisinopril/hydrochlorothiazide 10/12.5, 20/12.5, and 20/25. The dose ranges from 10 to 40 mg of lisinopril and 12.5 to 50 mg of hydrochlorothiazide per day. 1 or 2 tablets are taken once a day in the morning after breakfast.

ONSET OF EFFECT
Within 1 hour.

DURATION OF ACTION
Unknown.

DIETARY ADVICE
Follow your doctor's dietary advice (such as low-salt or low-cholesterol restrictions) to improve control over high blood pressure and heart disease.

STORAGE
Store in a tightly sealed container away from heat, moisture, and direct light.

IF YOU MISS A DOSE
Take it as soon as you remember. If it is near the time for the next dose, skip the missed dose and resume your regular dosage schedule. Do not double the next dose.

STOPPING THE DRUG
Discontinuing this drug abruptly may cause potentially serious problems. The dosage should be reduced gradually, according to your doctor's instructions.

PROLONGED USE
See your doctor regularly for evaluation if you must take this medicine for a prolonged period. Lifelong therapy may be necessary.

PRECAUTIONS
Over 60: Adverse reactions may be more likely and more severe.

Driving and Hazardous Work: Do not drive or engage in hazardous work until you determine how the medicine affects you.

Alcohol: Consume alcohol only in moderation since it may increase the effect of the drug and cause an excessive drop in blood pressure. Consult your doctor for advice.

Pregnancy: Before taking this medication, tell your doctor if you are pregnant or plan to become pregnant. Use of this drug during the last 6 months of pregnancy may cause severe defects, even death, in the fetus.

Breast Feeding: Lisinopril may pass into breast milk; caution is advised. Consult your doctor for advice.

Infants and Children: Children may be especially sensitive to the effects of lisinopril. Consult your pediatrician about the relative risks and benefits.

OVERDOSE
Symptoms: Overdose has not been reported; symptoms might include dizziness, faintness, or confusion.

What to Do: While overdose is unlikely, call your doctor, emergency medical services (EMS), or the nearest poison control center immediately if you suspect that someone has taken a much larger dose than prescribed.

DRUG INTERACTIONS
Consult your doctor for specific advice if you are taking cholestyramine, colestipol, digitalis drugs, lithium, potassium-containing medicines or supplements, or any over-the-counter drug (especially cold remedies and diet pills).

FOOD INTERACTIONS
Avoid low-salt milk and salt substitutes. Many of these products contain potassium.

DISEASE INTERACTIONS
Consult your doctor if you have systemic lupus erythematosus or if you have had a prior allergic reaction to ACE inhibitors. This medication should be used with caution by patients with severe kidney disease or renal artery stenosis (narrowing of one or both of the arteries that supply blood to the kidneys).

Lithium

BRAND NAMES
Cibalith-S, Eskalith,
Eskalith CR, Lithane,
Lithobid, Lithonate,
Lithotabs

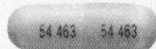

Generic 300 mg
(ROXANE)

▶ Drug Class: Antimanic agent

▶ Available in: Capsules, syrup,
tablets, extended-release
tablets

▶ Available OTC? No

▶ As Generic? Yes

Side Effects

SERIOUS
Sedation, pronounced
muscle weakness, confu-
sion or disorientation,
muscle twitching, vomit-
ing, increased urination,
slow heartbeat, fatigue,
weight gain, dizziness,
cold arms and legs, dry
and rough skin, hoarse-
ness, sensitivity to cold,
swollen feet or legs,
swollen neck. Call your
physician immediately.

COMMON
Increased thirst,
increased urination, nau-
sea, loss of appetite, diarrhea, a slight tremor in
the hands, fatigue, unex-
pected weight gain,
metallic taste in mouth.

LESS COMMON
Skin rash, acne, hair loss.

PRINCIPAL USES
To treat the manic phase
of bipolar disorder (also
known as manic-depression)
and to enhance the effect
of other antidepressant
medications in patients
with recurrent depression.

HOW THE DRUG WORKS
The exact mechanism of
action of lithium is
unknown.

DOSAGE
The dose is determined by
measuring blood levels of
lithium 12 hours after the
drug is administered. The
average adult dose is 900 to
1,800 mg a day. For older
adults, the average dose is
150 to 900 mg a day.

ONSET OF EFFECT
1 to 2 weeks for mania.
When used in conjunction
with an antidepressant,
symptoms may improve
within a few days.

DURATION OF ACTION
24 hours.

DIETARY ADVICE
Can be taken with meals to
lessen stomach upset. You
should drink 8 to 10 glasses
of water or caffeine-free
beverages every day.

STORAGE
Store in a tightly sealed container away from heat and
direct light.

IF YOU MISS A DOSE
Take it as soon as you
remember. If it is near the
time for the next dose, skip
the missed dose and
resume your regular dosage
schedule. Do not double the
next dose.

STOPPING THE DRUG
The decision to stop taking
the drug should be made in
consultation with your
physician.

PROLONGED USE
You should see your doctor
regularly for tests and
examinations if you take
this medicine. Blood levels
of lithium must be mea-
sured carefully to prevent
lithium toxicity.

PRECAUTIONS
Over 60: Adverse reactions
may be more likely and
more severe in older
patients. A lower dose may
be warranted.

**Driving and Hazardous
Work:** Avoid such activities
until you determine how the
medicine affects you.

Alcohol: No special precautions are necessary.

Pregnancy: Lithium can
cause problems in the
unborn child, especially
during the first 3 months of
pregnancy. Before you take
lithium, tell your doctor if
you are pregnant or plan to
become pregnant.

Breast Feeding: Lithium
passes into breast milk; caution is advised. Consult your
doctor for specific advice.

Infants and Children:
Lithium can weaken the
bones of infants and children. Use and dosage for
children under the age of
12 must be determined by
your pediatrician.

Special Concerns: Take
care to avoid dehydration
in hot weather and while
engaging in vigorous
activities. Be sure to drink
plenty of fluids when using
lithium. If you cannot consume enough fluids or you
develop severe diarrhea
while taking lithium, stop
taking the drug and con-
tact your doctor. Nons-
teroidal anti-inflammatory
drugs (NSAIDs) such as
ibuprofen increase blood
levels of lithium.

OVERDOSE
Symptoms: Twitching,
tremor, slurred speech,
extreme drowsiness,
disorientation, confusion,
seizures, muscle weakness,
loss of consciousness,
diarrhea, vomiting.

What to Do: Call your
doctor, emergency medical
services (EMS), or the
nearest poison control
center immediately.

DRUG INTERACTIONS
Other drugs may increase
blood levels of lithium; consult your doctor for specific
advice if you are taking
another medicine for mental
illness, a diuretic, medicine
for pain or inflammation
(especially NSAIDs),
tetracycline, metronidazole,
or ACE inhibitors. Some
drugs lower blood levels of
lithium; consult your doctor
for advice if you are taking
theophylline, caffeine, or
acetazolamide.

FOOD INTERACTIONS
Avoid drinks and foods that
contain caffeine.

DISEASE INTERACTIONS
You should not take lithium
if you have seriously
impaired kidney function,
cardiovascular disease, or a
history of leukemia. Before
taking lithium, consult your
doctor for specific advice if
you have a history of brain
disease, schizophrenia, diabetes, difficulty urinating,
any infection, epilepsy,
thyroid disease, Parkinson's
disease, psoriasis, or
leukemia.

Lomefloxacin Hydrochloride

Maxaquin

Maxaquin 400 mg
(SEARLE)

▶ Drug Class: Fluoroquinolone antibiotic

▶ Available in: Tablets

▶ Available OTC? No

▶ As Generic? No

Side Effects

SERIOUS
Serious reactions to lomefloxacin are rare and include seizures, mental confusion, hallucinations, agitation, nightmares, depression, shortness of breath, unusual swelling in the face or extremities, and loss of consciousness. Also severe skin burning, redness, blisters, rash, or itching on exposure to sunlight. Call your doctor immediately.

COMMON
Increased sensitivity to sunlight (and increased risk of sunburn) for days following therapy.

LESS COMMON
Diarrhea, nausea and vomiting, stomach pain and upset, gas, headache, dizziness, restlessness, insomnia, changes in taste perception, drowsiness, itching, dry mouth, unusual body aches or pains.

PRINCIPAL USES
To treat bacterial infections of the lower respiratory tract and urinary tract; to prevent urinary tract infections in patients preparing to undergo transurethral surgery (such as that performed to treat an enlarged prostate).

HOW THE DRUG WORKS
Lomefloxacin inhibits the activity of a bacterial enzyme (gyrase) that is necessary for proper DNA formation and replication. This prevents bacteria cells from reproducing.

DOSAGE
To treat infection— Adults age 18 and over: 400 mg, once a day for 10 to 14 days, depending on the type of infection being treated. To prevent infections presurgically— 400 mg, 2 to 6 hours before surgery.

ONSET OF EFFECT
Varies depending on the infection being treated.

DURATION OF ACTION
Unknown.

DIETARY ADVICE
Take it without regard to meals, although the drug is absorbed faster when taken on an empty stomach. Take it with a full glass of water, and drink lots of fluids, particularly citrus or cranberry juices.

STORAGE
Store in a tightly sealed container away from heat and direct light.

IF YOU MISS A DOSE
Take it as soon as you remember. If it is near the time for the next dose, skip the missed dose and resume your regular dosage schedule. Do not double the next dose.

STOPPING THE DRUG
Take lomefloxacin as prescribed for the full treatment period, even if you begin to feel better before the scheduled end of therapy.

PROLONGED USE
See your doctor regularly for tests and examinations if you must take this medicine for a prolonged period.

PRECAUTIONS
Over 60: No special problems are expected.

Driving and Hazardous Work: Avoid such activities until you determine how the medicine affects you.

Alcohol: It is advisable to abstain from alcohol when fighting an infection.

Pregnancy: In some animal tests, lomefloxacin has caused birth defects. Adequate studies in humans have not been done. It should be used during pregnancy only if potential benefits clearly justify the risks. Before you take lomefloxacin, tell your doctor if you are pregnant or plan to become pregnant.

Breast Feeding: Lomefloxacin passes into breast milk and may cause serious side effects in the nursing infant; use of the drug is discouraged when nursing.

Infants and Children: Lomefloxacin is not recommended for use by persons under the age of 18, as it has been shown to interfere with bone development.

Special Concerns: If lomefloxacin makes you unusually sensitive to sunlight, wear protective clothing, apply a sunblock, and try to stay out of direct sunlight, particularly between 10 am and 3 pm. Do not take any antacid or vitamin 4 hours before or 2 hours after taking this drug.

OVERDOSE
Symptoms: Severely reduced urination, weight gain, confusion, dryness and flakiness of skin, trembling, seizures.

What to Do: Call your doctor, emergency medical services (EMS), or the nearest poison control center immediately.

DRUG INTERACTIONS
Other drugs may interact with lomefloxacin. Consult your doctor for specific advice if you are taking aminophylline, antacids, didanosine, iron supplements, oxtriphylline, sucralfate, theophylline, warfarin, or zinc salts.

FOOD INTERACTIONS
No known food interactions.

DISEASE INTERACTIONS
Consult your doctor if you have a brain or spinal cord condition, epilepsy, or any other condition causing seizures. Use of lomefloxacin may cause complications in patients with liver or kidney disease, since these organs work together to remove the medication from the body.

Lomustine

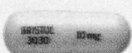

CeeNU 10 mg
(**BRISTOL-MYERS SQUIBB**)

▶ Drug Class: Alkylating agent

▶ Available in: Capsules

▶ Available OTC? No

▶ As Generic? No

Side Effects

SERIOUS
Black, tarry, or bloody stools; blood in urine; fever and chills, cough or hoarseness; pain in lower back or side; difficult, decreased, or painful urination; red spots on skin; unusual bleeding or bruising; confusion; loss of coordination; slurred speech; sores on lips or in mouth; swollen feet or lower legs; unusual fatigue; cough; shortness of breath. Call your doctor immediately.

COMMON
Loss of appetite; nausea and vomiting (for periods of less than 24 hours); temporary hair loss.

LESS COMMON
Darkened skin, diarrhea, itching or skin rash.

PRINCIPAL USES
To treat brain tumors and Hodgkin's disease (a type of cancer affecting the lymph nodes and spleen).

HOW THE DRUG WORKS
Lomustine kills cancer cells by interfering with the activity of their genetic material, thus preventing the cells from reproducing. The drug may also affect the growth and development of normal cells in the body, resulting in unpleasant side effects.

DOSAGE
130 mg per square meter of body surface once every 6 weeks. The dose may need to be lowered, based on red blood cell counts.

ONSET OF EFFECT
Unknown.

DURATION OF ACTION
Unknown.

DIETARY ADVICE
Lomustine is best taken on an empty stomach at bedtime to minimize stomach upset.

STORAGE
Store in a tightly sealed container away from heat and direct light.

IF YOU MISS A DOSE
Take it as soon as you remember. Do not double the next dose.

STOPPING THE DRUG
The decision to stop taking the drug should be made by your doctor.

PROLONGED USE
See your doctor regularly for tests and examinations if you take this medication for a prolonged period.

PRECAUTIONS
Over 60: No special precautions are necessary.

Driving and Hazardous Work: Do not drive or engage in hazardous work until you determine how the medicine affects you.

Alcohol: Avoid alcohol.

Pregnancy: Lomustine can cause birth defects if taken by either the father or the mother. Persons of childbearing years should take steps to prevent pregnancy while being treated with this drug.

Breast Feeding: Not recommended while undergoing therapy with this drug.

Infants and Children: Lomustine is expected to have the same therapeutic effect and cause the same side effects in infants and children as it does in adults.

Special Concerns: Do not receive any immunizations without your doctor's approval. Avoid persons who have recently had oral polio vaccine and those with any infection. Consult your doctor or dentist about appropriate ways to clean your teeth to avoid injury. Be careful not to cut yourself when using sharp objects such as a safety razor or nail cutters. Avoid activities and contact sports where bruising or injury could occur. If you vomit shortly after taking a dose of lomustine, check with your doctor. You may be told to take the dose again. Lomustine may have cumulative effects on bone marrow, causing low blood counts. This drug has been reported to have an effect on the lungs, causing shortness of breath up to 15 years after taking it.

OVERDOSE
Symptoms: Swelling of the abdomen or glands, weakness, nosebleed.

What to Do: Call your doctor, emergency medical services (EMS), or the nearest poison control center immediately.

DRUG INTERACTIONS
Consult your doctor for specific advice if you are taking amphotericin B, anti-thyroid agents, aspirin, azathioprine, chloramphenicol, colchicine, coumadin, flucytosine, ganciclovir, interferon, plicamycin, or zidovudine (AZT). Also consult your doctor if you are taking any over-the-counter medications.

FOOD INTERACTIONS
No known food interactions.

DISEASE INTERACTIONS
Consult your doctor if you have any of the following: shingles, chicken pox, any infection, kidney disease, or lung disease.

Loperamide Hydrochloride

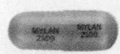

Generic 2 mg
(MYLAN)

Additional photographs

▸ Drug Class: Antidiarrheal

▸ Available in: Capsules, oral solution, tablets

▸ Available OTC? Yes

▸ As Generic? Yes

Side Effects

SERIOUS
Bloating, skin rash, constipation, loss of appetite, stomach pains, nausea, vomiting. Call your doctor immediately.

COMMON
No common side effects are associated with loperamide.

LESS COMMON
Dizziness or drowsiness, dry mouth.

PRINCIPAL USES
To treat diarrhea.

HOW THE DRUG WORKS
Loperamide eases diarrhea by slowing the activity of the intestines.

DOSAGE
Capsules— Adults and teenagers: 4 mg after the first loose bowel movement, 2 mg after each subsequent loose bowel movement. Take no more than 16 mg every 24 hours. Children ages 8 to 12: 2 mg, 3 times a day. Children ages 6 to 8: 2 mg, 2 times a day. Oral solution— Adults and teenagers: 4 mg (4 teaspoons) after the first loose bowel movement, 2 mg after each subsequent loose bowel movement. No more than 8 mg every 24 hours. Children ages 9 to 11: 2 mg after the first loose bowel movement, 1 mg after each subsequent loose bowel movement. No more than 6 mg every 24 hours. Children ages 6 to 8: 2 mg after the first loose bowel movement, 1 mg after each subsequent loose bowel movement. No more than 4 mg every 24 hours. Tablets— Adults and teenagers: 4 mg after the first loose bowel movement, 1 mg after each subsequent loose bowel movement. No more than 8 mg every 24 hours. Children ages 9 to 11: 2 mg after the first loose bowel movement, 1 mg after each subsequent loose bowel movement. No more than 6 mg every 24 hours. Children ages 6 to 8: 2 mg after the first loose bowel movement, 1 mg after each subsequent loose bowel movement. No more than 4 mg every 24 hours.

ONSET OF EFFECT
Unknown.

DURATION OF ACTION
Up to 24 hours.

DIETARY ADVICE
Take it on an empty stomach (1 hour before or 2 hours after eating). A mild diet is recommended when recovering from diarrhea. Bananas, rice, applesauce, and plain toast are good choices. Be sure to drink plenty of fluids.

STORAGE
Store in a tightly sealed container away from heat, moisture, and direct light.

IF YOU MISS A DOSE
Skip the missed dose and resume your regular dosage schedule. Do not double the next dose.

STOPPING THE DRUG
You may stop taking the drug whenever you choose.

PROLONGED USE
Loperamide should not be used for more than 2 days unless directed otherwise by your doctor.

PRECAUTIONS

Over 60: Diarrhea may easily lead to dehydration, especially in older patients, and loperamide may mask the effects of dehydration. When using loperamide, older persons should be sure to get plenty of fluids.

Driving and Hazardous Work: Avoid such activities until you determine how the medicine affects you.

Alcohol: Avoid alcohol.

Pregnancy: Discuss with your doctor the relative risks and benefits of using loperamide while pregnant.

Breast Feeding: It is not known whether loperamide passes into breast milk; cau-

tion is advised. Consult your doctor for specific advice.

Infants and Children: Do not give to children under 6 years of age unless otherwise directed by your doctor.

Special Concerns: During the first 24 hours, drink plenty of caffeine-free clear liquids like water, broth, ginger ale, and decaffeinated tea. During the second 24 hours you may eat bland foods such as applesauce, bread, crackers, and oatmeal.

OVERDOSE
Symptoms: Constipation, central nervous system depression, gastrointestinal irritation.

What to Do: An overdose of loperamide is unlikely to be life-threatening. However, if someone takes a much larger dose than prescribed, call your doctor, emergency medical services (EMS), or the nearest poison control center.

DRUG INTERACTIONS
Consult your doctor for specific advice if you are taking antibiotics such as cephalosporin, erythromycin, and tetracycline; or any narcotic pain medication.

FOOD INTERACTIONS
Fruits, fried or spicy foods, bran, candy, and caffeine-containing beverages can make diarrhea worse.

DISEASE INTERACTIONS
Consult your doctor if you have any of the following: dysentery, severe colitis, or liver disease.

Loperamide/Simethicone

▶ Drug Class: Antidiarrheal/ antigas combination

▶ Available in: Chewable tablet

▶ Available OTC? Yes

▶ As Generic? No

Side Effects

SERIOUS
Skin rash, bloating, constipation, loss of appetite, stomach pain, nausea, vomiting. Call your doctor immediately.

COMMON
Expulsion of excess gas, causing belching and flatulence.

LESS COMMON
Dizziness or drowsiness, dry mouth.

PRINCIPAL USES
To treat diarrhea and to relieve bloating, pain, pressure, and cramps caused by excess gas in the stomach and intestines.

HOW THE DRUG WORKS
Loperamide eases diarrhea by slowing the activity of the intestines. Simethicone disperses and prevents the formation of gas bubbles in the gastrointestinal tract.

DOSAGE
Adults and teenagers: Chew 2 tablets and drink a full glass of water after the first loose stool. If needed, chew 1 tablet and drink more water after the next loose stool. Take no more than 4 tablets per day. Children ages 6 to 11: Chew 1 tablet after the first loose stool. If needed, chew half a tablet after the next loose stool. Children ages 9 to 11 (or weighing 60 to 95 lbs) should take no more than 3 tablets per day. Children ages 6 to 8 (or weighing 48 to 59 lbs) should take no more than 2 tablets per day. Follow each dose with plenty of clear liquids.

ONSET OF EFFECT
Unknown.

DURATION OF ACTION
Unknown.

DIETARY ADVICE
A mild diet is recommended when recovering from diarrhea. Bananas, rice, applesauce, and plain toast are good choices. Be sure to drink plenty of fluids.

STORAGE
Store in a tightly sealed container away from heat, moisture, and direct light.

IF YOU MISS A DOSE
Not applicable, since the drug is taken only when necessary.

STOPPING THE DRUG
You may stop taking the drug whenever you choose.

PROLONGED USE
This drug should not be used for more than 2 days unless directed otherwise by your doctor.

PRECAUTIONS
Over 60: Diarrhea may easily lead to dehydration, especially in older patients, and this drug may mask the symptoms of dehydration. When using this drug, older persons should be sure to get plenty of fluids.

Driving and Hazardous Work: No special precautions are necessary.

Alcohol: Avoid alcohol, as it may irritate the lining of the gastrointestinal tract and promote dehydration.

Pregnancy: Discuss with your doctor the relative risks and benefits of using this drug while pregnant.

Breast Feeding: This drug may pass into breast milk; caution is advised. Consult your doctor for specific advice.

Infants and Children: Not recommended for use by children younger than age 6 or who weigh less than 48 lbs.

Special Concerns: Chew the tablets thoroughly before swallowing for quicker and more complete relief. You should change position frequently and walk about to help eliminate gas. During the first 24 hours, drink plenty of caffeine-free clear liquids like water, broth, ginger ale, and decaffeinated tea. During the second 24 hours you may eat bland foods such as applesauce, bread, crackers, and oatmeal. Tell your doctor if you are on a low-sodium, low-sugar or other special diet. Do not smoke before meals.

OVERDOSE
Symptoms: Constipation, gastrointestinal irritation, drowsiness, confusion.

What to Do: An overdose of this drug is unlikely to be life-threatening. However, if someone takes a much larger dose than prescribed, call your doctor.

DRUG INTERACTIONS
Consult your doctor for specific advice if you are taking antibiotics such as cephalosporin, erythromycin, and tetracycline; or any narcotic pain medication.

FOOD INTERACTIONS
Fruits, fried or spicy foods, bran, candy, and caffeine-containing beverages can make diarrhea worse. Avoid any foods that increase gas formation. Chew your food slowly and thoroughly.

DISEASE INTERACTIONS
Do not use this drug if you have a high fever (over 101°F) or stools containing blood or mucus. Consult your physician if you have dysentery, severe colitis, or liver disease.

Loracarbef

BRAND NAME
Lorabid

Lorabid 200 mg
(LILLY)

▶ Drug Class: Antibiotic

▶ Available in: Capsules, oral suspension

▶ Available OTC? No

▶ As Generic? No

Side Effects

SERIOUS
Severe diarrhea, skin rash, hives, intense itching. Call your doctor right away.

COMMON
Loss of appetite, mild diarrhea, stomach pain, nausea, vomiting. Consult your doctor.

LESS COMMON
Dizziness, drowsiness, headache, discharge from or itching of the vagina, insomnia, general nervousness. Consult your doctor if such symptoms persist.

PRINCIPAL USES
To treat bacterial infections including urinary tract infections, bronchitis, pneumonia, and strep throat (streptococcal pharyngitis).

HOW THE DRUG WORKS
Loracarbef, an antibiotic similar to those in the cephalosporin family, kills bacteria or inhibits their growth and multiplication.

DOSAGE
For infections of the urinary tract— Adults and teenagers: 200 to 400 mg, 1 or 2 times a day for 7 to 14 days. For bronchitis— Adults and teenagers: 200 to 400 mg, 2 times a day for 7 days. For pneumonia— Adults and teenagers: 400 mg, 2 times a day for 14 days. For infections of skin and soft tissue— Adults and teenagers: 200 mg, 2 times a day for 7 days. For strep throat— Adults and teenagers: 200 mg, 2 times a day for 10 days. For all conditions, use and dosage of loracarbef for children ages 6 months to 12 years must be determined by your doctor.

ONSET OF EFFECT
Unknown.

DURATION OF ACTION
Unknown.

DIETARY ADVICE
Loracarbef should be taken on an empty stomach at least 1 hour before or 2 hours after meals. Drink plenty of fluids.

STORAGE
Store in a tightly sealed container away from heat and direct light.

IF YOU MISS A DOSE
Take it as soon as you remember. If it is near the time for the next dose, skip the missed dose and resume your regular dosage schedule. Do not double the next dose.

STOPPING THE DRUG
It is very important to take antibiotics as prescribed for the full treatment period, even if you begin to feel better before the scheduled end of therapy. This is especially important when being treated for streptococcal infections.

PROLONGED USE
You should see your doctor regularly for tests and examinations if you must take this medicine for a prolonged period.

PRECAUTIONS
Over 60: In older patients, loracarbef is not expected to cause side effects different from or more severe than those in younger persons.

Driving and Hazardous Work: Do not drive or engage in hazardous work until you determine how the medicine affects you.

Alcohol: No special problems are expected, although it is generally advisable to abstain from alcohol when fighting an infection.

Pregnancy: Loracarbef has not been shown to cause birth defects in animals. Human studies have not been done. Before you take loracarbef, tell your doctor if you are pregnant or plan to become pregnant.

Breast Feeding: Loracarbef may pass into breast milk; caution is advised. Consult your doctor for advice.

Infants and Children: Consult your doctor about use of loracarbef by children 12 years or younger.

Special Concerns: It is important to maintain consistent blood levels of loracarbef. You should be very careful not to miss a dose. If you have difficulty maintaining a proper dosage schedule, consult your physician.

OVERDOSE
Symptoms: Unusually rapid or slow heartbeat, unusual drop in blood pressure (causing dizziness, lightheadedness, confusion, or fainting).

What to Do: An overdose of loracarbef is unlikely to be life-threatening. However, if someone takes a larger dose than prescribed, call your doctor, emergency medical services (EMS), or the nearest poison control center right away.

DRUG INTERACTIONS
Other drugs may interact with loracarbef. Consult your doctor for specific advice if you are taking diuretics (water pills) or probenecid. Also tell your doctor if you are taking any other prescription or over-the-counter medication.

FOOD INTERACTIONS
No known food interactions.

DISEASE INTERACTIONS
Use of loracarbef may cause complications in patients with liver or kidney disease, since these organs work together to remove the medication from the body.

Loratadine

BRAND NAME
Claritin

Claritin 10 mg
(SCHERING-PLOUGH)

▶ Drug Class: Antihistamine

▶ Available in: Tablets, syrup

▶ Available OTC? No

▶ As Generic? No

Side Effects

SERIOUS
No serious side effects are associated with the use of loratadine.

COMMON
No common side effects are associated with the use of loratadine.

LESS COMMON
In rare cases adverse reactions have been reported in persons taking loratadine, but none of these reactions is clearly linked to use of the drug.

PRINCIPAL USES
To prevent or relieve symptoms of hay fever and other allergies, such as watery or itchy eyes, runny nose, sneezing, or itchy skin. Loratadine is also used sometimes to treat chronic (persistent) hives.

HOW THE DRUG WORKS
Loratadine blocks the effects of histamine, a naturally occurring substance that causes swelling, itching, sneezing, watery eyes, hives, and other symptoms of allergic reaction.

DOSAGE
Tablets and syrup— Adults and children age 10 and older: 10 mg once a day. Children ages 2 to 9: 5 mg once a day. Do not increase the dose in an attempt to achieve quicker relief of symptoms.

ONSET OF EFFECT
Within 1 hour.

DURATION OF ACTION
24 hours or more.

DIETARY ADVICE
Loratadine can be taken without regard to diet, but taking this medicine with food may be beneficial because it may increase absorption of the drug from the gastrointestinal tract by up to 40%.

STORAGE
Store in a tightly sealed container at room temperature, away from heat, moisture, and direct light.

IF YOU MISS A DOSE
Take it as soon as you remember. However, if it is near the time for the next dose, skip the missed dose and resume your regular dosage schedule. Do not double the next dose.

STOPPING THE DRUG
The decision to stop taking the drug should be made in consultation with your physician.

PROLONGED USE
Loratadine can be taken safely for prolonged periods. Long-term use is not associated with decreased effectiveness of the drug (a problem with certain allergy medications and other drugs).

PRECAUTIONS
Over 60: Adverse reactions may be more likely and more severe in older patients.

Driving and Hazardous Work: The use of loratadine, at recommended doses, should not impair your ability to perform such tasks safely.

Alcohol: No special precautions are necessary.

Pregnancy: Before you take loratadine, tell your doctor if you are pregnant or plan to become pregnant.

Breast Feeding: Loratadine passes into breast milk; avoid or discontinue use while nursing.

Infants and Children: Adverse reactions may be more likely and more severe in children.

Special Concerns: Stop taking loratadine 4 to 7 days before you have an allergy skin test.

OVERDOSE
Symptoms: Rapid heartbeat, headache, drowsiness.

What to Do: An overdose of loratadine is unlikely to be life-threatening. However, if someone takes a much larger dose than pre-scribed, call your doctor, emergency medical services (EMS), or the nearest poison control center.

DRUG INTERACTIONS
Consult your doctor for advice if you are taking clarithromycin, erythromycin, troleandomycin, itraconazole, or ketoconazole.

FOOD INTERACTIONS
There are no known interactions between loratadine and specific foods.

DISEASE INTERACTIONS
There are no known disease interactions.

BRAND NAME
Claritin-D

▶ Drug Class: Antihistamine/decongestant

▶ Available in: Extended-release tablets

▶ Available OTC? No

▶ As Generic? No

Side Effects

SERIOUS
No serious side effects are associated with the use of this drug.

COMMON
Insomnia, dry mouth, drowsiness.

LESS COMMON
Nervousness, dizziness, indigestion.

PRINCIPAL USES
To relieve the symptoms of seasonal allergic rhinitis (hay fever), which include runny nose, nasal congestion, and sneezing.

HOW THE DRUG WORKS
Loratadine blocks the effects of histamine, a naturally occurring substance that causes swelling, itching, sneezing, nasal discharge and congestion, and other symptoms of an allergic reaction. Pseudoephedrine narrows and constricts blood vessels to reduce the blood flow to swollen nasal passages, which reduces nasal secretions, shrinks swollen nasal mucous membranes, and improves airflow through the nasal passages.

DOSAGE
The 12-hour formulation may be taken twice a day (every 12 hours). The 24-hour formulation should only be taken once a day. Tablets should be taken with a full glass of water.

ONSET OF EFFECT
Within 1 to 3 hours.

DURATION OF ACTION
12 to 24 hours or more.

DIETARY ADVICE
This drug can be taken without regard to meals. Take it with a full glass of water.

STORAGE
Store in a tightly sealed container away from heat, moisture, and direct light.

IF YOU MISS A DOSE
Not applicable. This drug is taken as needed.

STOPPING THE DRUG
Not applicable. This drug is taken as needed.

PROLONGED USE
This drug is prescribed for short-term (seasonal) use only.

PRECAUTIONS
Over 60: Adequate studies have not been done. However, older patients are more susceptible to the effects of the pseudoephedrine component (see Pseudoephedrine).

Driving and Hazardous Work: The use of this drug should not impair your ability to perform such tasks safely. However, exercise caution if the medication makes you drowsy.

Alcohol: No special precautions are necessary.

Pregnancy: Adequate human studies have not been done. Discuss with your doctor the relative risks and benefits of using this drug while pregnant.

Breast Feeding: Both drugs pass into breast milk. Discuss with your doctor the relative risks and benefits of using this drug while nursing.

Infants and Children: Not recommended for use by children under age 12.

Special Concerns: Do not break or chew the tablet. Patients with a history of esophageal narrowing or swallowing difficulty should not take this drug.

OVERDOSE
Symptoms: Drowsiness, heartbeat irregularities, headache, giddiness, nausea, vomiting, sweating, increased thirst, chest pain, urination difficulties, muscle weakness and tenseness, anxiety, restlessness, insomnia, hallucinations, delusions, seizures, difficulty breathing.

What to Do: Call your doctor, emergency medical services (EMS), or the nearest poison control center immediately.

DRUG INTERACTIONS
This drug and MAO inhibitors should not be used within 14 days of each other. Consult your doctor for specific advice if you are taking beta-blockers, digitalis drugs, or over-the-counter antihistamines or decongestants.

FOOD INTERACTIONS
No known food interactions.

DISEASE INTERACTIONS
You should not take this drug if you have narrow-angle glaucoma, severe hypertension, urinary retention, or severe coronary artery disease. Caution is advised when taking this drug if you have any of the following: high blood pressure, diabetes mellitus, heart disease, increased eye pressure, hyperthyroidism, or enlarged prostate. Use of this drug may cause complications in patients with liver or kidney disease, since these organs work together to remove the medication from the body.

Lorazepam

Generic 0.5 mg
(SCHEIN/DANBURY)

▶ Drug Class: Benzodiazepine tranquilizer; antianxiety agent

▶ Available in: Oral solution, tablets, injection

▶ Available OTC? No

▶ As Generic? Yes

Side Effects

SERIOUS
Difficulty concentrating, outbursts of anger, other behavior problems, depression, hallucinations, low blood pressure (causing faintness or confusion), memory impairment, muscle weakness, skin rash or itching, sore throat, fever and chills, sores or ulcers in throat or mouth, unusual bruising or bleeding, extreme fatigue, yellowish tinge to eyes or skin. Call your doctor immediately.

COMMON
Drowsiness, loss of coordination, unsteady gait, dizziness, lightheadedness, slurred speech.

LESS COMMON
Change in sexual desire or ability, constipation, false sense of well-being, nausea and vomiting, urinary problems, unusual fatigue.

PRINCIPAL USES
To treat anxiety and insomnia. The injection form of lorazepam, administered in a hospital setting, is used to treat a type of seizure disorder (status epilepticus) and is used before surgery to sedate patients prior to the administration of anesthesia.

HOW THE DRUG WORKS
In general, lorazepam produces mild sedation by depressing activity in the central nervous system. In particular, lorazepam appears to enhance the effect of gamma-aminobutyric acid (GABA), a natural chemical that inhibits the firing of neurons and dampens the transmission of nerve signals, thus decreasing nervous excitation.

DOSAGE
For anxiety— Adults and teenagers: 1 to 2 mg every 8 or 12 hours, up to 6 mg a day. Older adults: 0.5 mg, 2 times a day to start; the dose may be increased. For insomnia— Adults and teenagers: 1 to 2 mg taken at bedtime. Note: In all cases, use and dosage for children under 12 years of age must be determined by your doctor.

ONSET OF EFFECT
30 minutes to 2 hours for oral forms.

DURATION OF ACTION
12 to 24 hours.

DIETARY ADVICE
Can be taken with food to prevent gastrointestinal upset.

STORAGE
Store in a tightly sealed container away from heat, moisture, and direct light.

IF YOU MISS A DOSE
Take it as soon as you remember. However, if it is near the time for the next dose, skip the missed dose and resume your regular dosage schedule. Do not double the next dose. For insomnia, do not take it unless your schedule allows a full night's sleep.

STOPPING THE DRUG
Never stop taking the drug abruptly, as this can cause withdrawal symptoms (seizures, sleep disruption, nervousness, irritability, diarrhea, abdominal cramps, muscle aches, memory impairment). Dosage should be reduced gradually as directed by your doctor.

PROLONGED USE
Lorazepam may slowly lose its effectiveness with prolonged use. See your doctor for periodic evaluation if you must take this drug for an extended length of time.

PRECAUTIONS
Over 60: Adverse reactions may be more likely and more severe in older patients. A lower dose may be warranted.

Driving and Hazardous Work: Lorazepam can impair mental alertness and physical coordination. Adjust your activities accordingly.

Alcohol: Avoid alcohol.

Pregnancy: Use during pregnancy should be avoided if possible. Tell your doctor if you are pregnant or plan to become pregnant.

Breast Feeding: Lorazepam passes into breast milk; do not take it while nursing.

Infants and Children: Lorazepam should be used by children only under close medical supervision.

Special Concerns: Lorazepam use can lead to psychological or physical dependence. Short-term therapy (8 weeks or less) is typical; do not take the drug for a longer period unless so advised by your doctor. Never take more than the prescribed daily dose.

OVERDOSE
Symptoms: Extreme drowsiness, confusion, slurred speech, slow reflexes, poor coordination, staggering gait, tremor, slowed breathing, loss of consciousness.

What to Do: Call your doctor, emergency medical services (EMS), or the nearest poison control center immediately.

DRUG INTERACTIONS
Consult your doctor for specific advice if you are taking any drugs that depress the central nervous system (such as antihistamines, antidepressants or other psychiatric medications, barbiturates, sedatives, cough medicines, decongestants, and painkillers). Be sure your doctor knows about any over-the-counter drug you may take.

FOOD INTERACTIONS
None reported.

DISEASE INTERACTIONS
Consult your doctor if you have a history of alcohol or drug abuse, stroke or other brain disease, any chronic lung disease, hyperactivity, depression or other mental illness, myasthenia gravis, sleep apnea, epilepsy, porphyria, kidney disease, or liver disease.

Losartan Potassium

Cozaar 25 mg
(MERCK)

▶ Drug Class: Antihypertensive/
angiotensin II antagonist

▶ Available in: Tablets

▶ Available OTC? No

▶ As Generic? No

Side Effects

SERIOUS
Sudden difficulty breathing or swallowing, hoarseness, swelling of the face, mouth, hands, or throat, dizziness, cough, fever or sore throat. Call your doctor immediately.

COMMON
Headache.

LESS COMMON
Back pain, fatigue, diarrhea, nasal congestion.

PRINCIPAL USES
To control high blood pressure. This drug appears to have the same benefits as the class of antihypertensive drugs known as ACE inhibitors, without producing the common side effect (experienced by as many as 30% of patients) of a dry cough. Losartan may be used alone or in conjunction with other antihypertensive medications.

HOW THE DRUG WORKS
Losartan blocks the effects of angiotensin II, a naturally occurring substance that causes blood vessels to narrow. Losartan causes the blood vessels to dilate, thereby lowering blood pressure and decreasing the workload of the heart.

DOSAGE
Adults: To start, 25 to 50 mg once a day. Usual maintenance dose is 25 to 100 mg, taken once a day or divided into 2 doses. Children: Not recommended.

ONSET OF EFFECT
Within 1 hour.

DURATION OF ACTION
24 hours.

DIETARY ADVICE
Follow a healthy diet (low-salt, low-fat, low-cholesterol) as advised by your doctor to help control blood pressure and prevent heart disease.

STORAGE
Store in a tightly sealed container away from heat, moisture, and direct light.

IF YOU MISS A DOSE
Take it as soon as you remember. If it is near the time for the next dose, skip the missed dose and resume your regular dosage schedule. Do not double the next dose.

STOPPING THE DRUG
Take it as prescribed for the full treatment period. The decision to stop taking the drug should be made in consultation with your physician.

PROLONGED USE
Lifelong therapy may be necessary. However, if you do change certain health habits (for example, increasing exercise or losing weight), it may be possible, under your doctor's supervision, to reduce the dose.

PRECAUTIONS
Over 60: Adverse reactions may be more likely and more severe in older patients.

Driving and Hazardous Work: Do not drive or engage in hazardous work until you determine how the medicine affects you.

Alcohol: Drink only in careful moderation. (See Special Concerns.)

Pregnancy: In certain ways losartan is similar to a class of drugs that have caused damage to the unborn child when taken in the second or third trimester of pregnancy. Because safer, more effective medications can lower blood pressure during pregnancy, and because adequate studies on the use of losartan during pregnancy have not been done, women who are pregnant or planning to become pregnant should not take this drug.

Breast Feeding: Losartan passes into breast milk; avoid use while nursing.

Infants and Children: The safety and effectiveness of this drug have not been established for children.

Special Concerns: Losartan may cause dizziness or lightheadedness, which is most noticeable when you change position. This may lead to fainting, falls, and injury. Sit or lie down immediately if you feel dizzy or lightheaded. This side effect may be worsened by alcohol, hot weather, dehydration, fever, prolonged standing, prolonged sitting, or exercise.

OVERDOSE
Symptoms: Fainting, dizziness, weak pulse that might be very slow or very fast, nausea and vomiting, chest pain.

What to Do: Call your doctor, emergency medical services (EMS), or the nearest poison control center immediately.

DRUG INTERACTIONS
Consult your doctor for specific advice if you are taking diuretics, potassium-containing medicines or supplements, salt substitutes, low-salt milk, NSAIDs, allopurinol, over-the-counter medications for colds, coughs, hay fever, asthma, sinus problems, or appetite control, or other prescription drugs.

FOOD INTERACTIONS
No known food interactions.

DISEASE INTERACTIONS
Use of losartan may cause complications in patients with liver or kidney disease, since these organs work together to remove the medication from the body.

Loteprednol Etabonate

BRAND NAMES
Alrex, Lotemax

▶ Drug Class: Corticosteroid

▶ Available in: Ophthalmic suspension

▶ Available OTC? No

▶ As Generic? No

Side Effects

SERIOUS
Decreased vision or blurring of vision (from cataract); eye pain, nausea, vomiting (from increased intraocular pressure); pain, redness, sensitivity to bright light, discharge (from eye infection). Call your doctor immediately if you experience any of these signs or symptoms. The drug may trigger a recurrence of herpes infection of the eye; mention any previous herpes infection to your doctor.

COMMON
Burning, stinging, redness, or watering of eyes.

LESS COMMON
Headache, runny nose, sore throat.

PRINCIPAL USES
Alrex is prescribed for temporary relief of eye symptoms due to seasonal allergic inflammation of the conjunctiva. Lotemax is used to control inflammation and prevent potentially permanent damage that may result from eye problems such as conjunctivitis, herpes of the eye, and corneal injuries. It is also used to help relieve redness, irritation, and discomfort in the eye, and may be used after eye surgery to control any inflammatory response. Loteprednol is less potent than prednisolone but also less likely to cause adverse effects.

HOW THE DRUG WORKS
Ophthalmic loteprednol inhibits the release of natural substances that cause inflammation and pain in eye tissues.

DOSAGE
Alrex (0.2%)— To treat seasonal allergic conjunctivitis: 1 drop into the affected eye 4 times a day. Lotemax (0.5%)— 1 to 2 drops into the affected eye 4 times a day. Within the first week of treatment, dose may be increased, up to 1 drop per hour, if needed. For postoperative inflammation: 1 to 2 drops into the operated eye 4 times a day beginning 24 hours following surgery and for the next 2 weeks.

ONSET OF EFFECT
Unknown.

DURATION OF ACTION
Unknown.

DIETARY ADVICE
No special restrictions.

STORAGE
Store in a tightly sealed container away from heat, moisture, and direct light. Do not allow it to freeze.

IF YOU MISS A DOSE
Apply it as soon as you remember. If it is near the time for the next dose, skip the missed dose and resume your regular dosage schedule. Do not double the next dose.

STOPPING THE DRUG
It is very important to use this drug as prescribed for the full treatment period, even if symptoms improve before the scheduled end of therapy.

PROLONGED USE
You should see your ophthalmologist to have your eye pressure monitored if you use this drug for 10 days or longer.

PRECAUTIONS

Over 60: No special problems are expected.

Driving and Hazardous Work: Do not drive or engage in hazardous work until you determine how the medicine affects your vision.

Alcohol: No special precautions are necessary.

Pregnancy: Adequate human studies have not been done, though no birth defects have been reported. Before taking ophthalmic loteprednol, tell your doctor if you are pregnant or plan to become pregnant.

Breast Feeding: Ophthalmic loteprednol has not been reported to cause problems in nursing babies. Consult your doctor.

Infants and Children: Safety and effectiveness have not been established.

Special Concerns: Shake the bottle vigorously before administering. Wash your hands and tilt your head back. Gently apply pressure to the inside corner of the eyelid and with the index finger of the same hand, pull downward on the lower eyelid to make a space. Drop the medicine into this space and close your eye. Apply pressure for 1 or 2 minutes while keeping the eye closed without blinking. Then wash your hands again. Make sure the tip of the dropper does not touch your eye, finger, or any other surface. If your symptoms do not improve in 2 days or if they become worse, check with your doctor. Wearing contact lenses while using this medication may increase the risk of infection. Your doctor may tell you not to wear contact lenses during and for a day or two after treatment.

OVERDOSE

Symptoms: When used topically, an overdose is very unlikely. Inadvertent oral ingestion, however, may cause fever, muscle pain, loss of appetite, dizziness, fainting, and trouble breathing.

What to Do: An overdose is unlikely to be life-threatening. However, if someone accidentally ingests the medicine, call your doctor, emergency medical services (EMS), or the nearest poison control center.

DRUG INTERACTIONS
Consult your doctor for specific advice if you are taking any other medication.

FOOD INTERACTIONS
No known food interactions.

DISEASE INTERACTIONS
Consult your doctor if you have any of the following: cataracts, diabetes, glaucoma, herpes infection or tuberculosis of the eye, or any other eye infection.

Lovastatin

BRAND NAME
Mevacor

Mevacor 20 mg
(MERCK)

▶ Drug Class: Antilipidemic
(cholesterol-lowering agent)

▶ Available in: Tablets

▶ Available OTC? No

▶ As Generic? No

Side Effects

SERIOUS
Fever, unusual or unexplained muscle aches and tenderness. Call your doctor right away.

COMMON
Side effects occur in only 1% to 2% of patients. These include constipation or diarrhea, dizziness or lightheadedness, bloating or gas, heartburn, nausea, skin rash, stomach pain, rise in liver enzymes.

LESS COMMON
Sleeping difficulty.

PRINCIPAL USES
To treat high cholesterol. Usually prescribed after first lines of treatment—including diet, weight loss, and exercise—fail to reduce total and low-density lipoprotein (LDL) cholesterol to acceptable levels. Lovastatin has also been approved for the primary prevention of coronary artery disease (CAD) in persons with no symptoms of CAD, but who have average to modestly elevated levels of total and LDL cholesterol and below average HDL.

HOW THE DRUG WORKS
Lovastatin blocks the action of an enzyme required for the manufacture of cholesterol, thereby interfering with its formation. By lowering the amount of cholesterol in the liver cells, lovastatin increases the formation of receptors for LDL, and thereby reduces blood levels of total and LDL cholesterol. In addition to lowering LDL cholesterol, lovastatin also modestly reduces triglyceride levels and raises HDL (the so-called "good") cholesterol.

DOSAGE
20 to 80 mg per day, taken with meals. The 20 mg dose is taken with the evening meal; doses greater than 20 mg per day are taken in the morning and evening.

ONSET OF EFFECT
2 to 4 weeks.

DURATION OF ACTION
The effect persists for the duration of therapy.

DIETARY ADVICE
Cholesterol-lowering drugs are only one part of a total program that should include regular exercise and a healthy diet. The American Heart Association publishes a "Healthy Heart" diet, which is recommended.

STORAGE
Store in a tightly sealed container away from heat, moisture, and direct light.

IF YOU MISS A DOSE
Take your missed dose as soon as you remember. Take your next scheduled dose at the proper time, and resume your regular dosage schedule. Do not take a double dose.

STOPPING THE DRUG
The decision to stop taking the drug should be made in consultation with your doctor. Once the medication is discontinued, blood cholesterol is likely to return to original elevated levels.

PROLONGED USE
Side effects are more likely with prolonged use. As you continue with lovastatin, your doctor will periodically order blood tests to evaluate liver function.

PRECAUTIONS
Over 60: No special problems are expected in older patients.

Driving and Hazardous Work: The use of lovastatin should not impair your ability to perform such tasks safely.

Alcohol: No special precautions are necessary.

Pregnancy: Lovastatin should not be used during pregnancy nor by women who are trying to become pregnant.

Breast Feeding: This drug is not recommended for women who are nursing.

Infants and Children: The drug can be effective, but safety is not known; rarely used in children. Consult your pediatrician.

Special Concerns: Important elements of treatment for high cholesterol include proper diet, weight loss, regular moderate exercise, and the avoidance of certain medications that may increase cholesterol levels. Because lovastatin has potential side effects, it is important that you maintain a recommended healthy diet and cooperate with other treatments your physician may suggest.

OVERDOSE
Symptoms: An overdose of lovastatin is unlikely.

What to Do: Emergency instructions not applicable.

DRUG INTERACTIONS
Consult your doctor if you are taking cyclosporine, gemfibrozil, niacin, antibiotics, especially erythromycin, or medications for fungus infections. All of these drugs may increase the risk of myositis (muscle inflammation) when taken with lovastatin and may lead to kidney failure.

FOOD INTERACTIONS
None reported.

DISEASE INTERACTIONS
Consult your doctor if you have any of the following problems: liver, kidney, or muscle disease, or a medical history involving organ transplant or recent surgery.

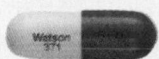

Generic 25 mg
(WATSON)

Additional photographs

▶ Drug Class: Neuroleptic;
antipsychotic

▶ Available in: Tablets, oral
solution, capsules, injection

▶ Available OTC? No

▶ As Generic? Yes

Side Effects

SERIOUS
Seizures, breathing difficulty, heartbeat irregularities, high fever, unusual
sweating, loss of bladder
control, lip puckering or
smacking, uncontrolled
chewing and tongue
movements, uncontrolled
limb or body movements,
difficulty speaking or
swallowing, loss of bal-
ance, trembling, muscle
spasms, severe constipa-
tion, difficulty urinating,
rash, sore throat and
fever, unusual bleeding
or bruising, jaundice. Call
your doctor immediately.

COMMON
Blurred vision, dizziness,
confusion, fainting,
drowsiness, shuffling
gait, slow movements,
staring and absence of
facial expression, dry
mouth.

LESS COMMON
Mild constipation, sexual
dysfunction, headache,
increased sensitivity of
skin to sun, nausea or
vomiting, insomnia,
menstrual irregularities,
breast swelling, unusual
milk secretion, unex-
pected weight gain.

PRINCIPAL USES
To treat moderate to severe
psychiatric conditions such
as schizophrenia.

HOW THE DRUG WORKS
Loxapine appears to block
receptors of dopamine (a
chemical that aids in the
transmission of nerve
impulses) in the central nervous system. Presumably,
this produces a tranquilizing
or antipsychotic effect.

DOSAGE
Oral forms: To start, 10 mg,
2 times a day. The dose may
be gradually increased by
your physician to a maxi-
mum of 250 mg a day. Injection: 12.5 to 50 mg, 4 to 6
times per day, injected into
a muscle.

ONSET OF EFFECT
Sedation may occur within
minutes, but onset of
antipsychotic effect may
take hours to occur or may
not occur until days or
weeks after the beginning
of therapy.

DURATION OF ACTION
12 to 24 hours.

DIETARY ADVICE
Oral solution should be
mixed with orange juice or
grapefruit juice.

STORAGE
Store in a tightly sealed container away from heat, moisture, and direct light. Do
not allow the solution or
injection forms to freeze.

IF YOU MISS A DOSE
Take it as soon as you
remember. However, if it is
near the time for the next
dose, skip the missed dose
and resume your regular
dosage schedule. Do not
double the next dose.

STOPPING THE DRUG
The decision to stop taking
the drug should be made in
consultation with your
physician.

PROLONGED USE
Prolonged use may lead to
tardive dyskinesia (involuntary movements of the jaw,
lips, tongue, and, in rare
cases, the arms, legs,
hands, or body). Consult
your doctor about the need
for follow-up evaluations and
tests if you must take this
drug for an extended
period.

PRECAUTIONS

Over 60: Adverse reactions
may be more likely and
more severe in older
patients.

**Driving and Hazardous
Work:** Do not drive or
engage in hazardous work
until you determine how the
medicine affects you.

Alcohol: Avoid alcohol.

Pregnancy: Adequate
studies have not been completed; consult your doctor
for more information.

Breast Feeding: It is not
known whether loxapine
passes into breast milk,
although no problems have
been reported.

Infants and Children:
The safety and effectiveness
of loxapine in children have
not been established. Use
and dose for children up
to age 16 should be determined by your doctor.

Special Concerns: Avoid
prolonged exposure to
high temperatures in hot
climates. Drink plenty of
fluids and stay cool in the
summer time. Avoid overexposure to sunlight until
you determine if the drug
heightens your skin's sensitivity to ultraviolet light.

OVERDOSE

Symptoms: Severe drowsiness, severe dizziness, muscle jerking, trembling, or
stiffness, trouble breathing,
unusual fatigue.

What to Do: Call your
doctor, emergency medical
services (EMS), or the
nearest poison control
center immediately.

DRUG INTERACTIONS
Do not take loxapine within
2 hours of taking an antacid
or an antidiarrheal medication. Consult your doctor for
specific advice if you are
taking amoxapine, methyl-
dopa, metoclopramide,
metyrosine, other drugs for
mental illness, pemoline,
pimozide, promethazine,
rauwolfia alkaloids,
trimeprazine, any medica-
tion that depresses the
central nervous system, tricyclic antidepressants, guanadrel, or guanethidine.

FOOD INTERACTIONS
None are known.

DISEASE INTERACTIONS
Consult your doctor if you
have a history of alcohol or
drug abuse, difficulty urinating, benign prostatic hyperplasia (BPH), glaucoma,
Parkinson's disease, heart
or blood vessel disease,
liver disease, or a seizure
disorder.

Lyme Disease Vaccine (Recombinant OspA)

▶ Drug Class: Vaccine

▶ Available in: Injection

▶ Available OTC? No

▶ As Generic? No

Side Effects

SERIOUS
No serious side effects have been reported.

COMMON
Soreness or redness at the site of injection.

LESS COMMON
Muscle pain, chills, fever, flu-like symptoms.

PRINCIPAL USES
To protect against, but not treat, Lyme disease in people ages 15 to 70. The vaccine is recommended for people who live or work in grassy or wooded areas infested with ticks infected with *Borrelia burgdorferi* (the bacteria that causes Lyme disease) as well as for people planning to travel to those areas.

HOW THE DRUG WORKS
Lyme disease vaccine stimulates the body's immune system to produce antibodies against a protein on the outer surface of the tick. When infected ticks bite vaccinated humans, the vaccine-induced antibodies enter the tick and attack the B. burgdorferi inside the gut of the tick, thereby preventing transmission of the disease.

DOSAGE
All doses are administered by a health care professional. Adults and teenagers: 1 dose injected into a muscle in the upper arm. Booster doses are given 1 month and 12 months after the first dose. All three doses are required to confer optimal protection.

ONSET OF EFFECT
Unknown.

DURATION OF ACTION
Unknown.

DIETARY ADVICE
No special restrictions.

STORAGE
Not applicable; the dose is administered only at a health care facility.

IF YOU MISS A DOSE
If you miss a scheduled vaccination, contact your doctor. According to the Centers for Disease Control and Prevention (CDC), if you miss the one-month booster, you may take it as soon as possible within the first year. All 3 injections should be completed within 1 year.

STOPPING THE DRUG
The full schedule of injections should be followed unless a medical problem intervenes. A full course of injections must be completed to ensure adequate immunization.

PROLONGED USE
Periodic booster shots may be recommended.

PRECAUTIONS
Over 60: Lyme disease vaccine is not expected to cause different or more severe side effects in older patients than in younger persons.

Driving and Hazardous Work: The vaccine should not impair your ability to perform such tasks safely.

Alcohol: No special precautions are necessary.

Pregnancy: Adequate human studies have not been done. Before taking Lyme disease vaccine, tell your physician if you are pregnant or planning to become pregnant.

Breast Feeding: Lyme disease vaccine may pass into breast milk; caution is advised. Consult your doctor for specific advice.

Infants and Children: Not recommended for use by children under the age of 15. No special problems are expected in persons over the age of 15.

Special Concerns: Previous infection with *B. burgdorferi* does not mean that you are immune to future infections of Lyme disease. As with any vaccine, Lyme disease vaccine may not protect all individuals. In clinical studies, the vaccine was effective in approximately 78% of cases after receiving all three doses. In addition to vaccination, people can decrease their chances of acquiring tick-borne infections by wearing pants and long-sleeved shirts, tucking pants into socks, spraying tick repellent on clothing, checking for ticks in a tick-infested area, and removing attached ticks.

OVERDOSE
Symptoms: Not applicable.

What to Do: No cases of overdose have been reported.

DRUG INTERACTIONS
No drug interactions have been reported. However, as with other intramuscular injections, Lyme disease vaccine should not be administered to people taking anticoagulant drugs such as warfarin unless the potential benefit outweighs the risks.

FOOD INTERACTIONS
No known food interactions.

DISEASE INTERACTIONS
No known disease interactions. However, as with other intramuscular injections, Lyme disease vaccine should not be administered to people with blood clotting disorders. The safety of the vaccine has not been tested in people with joint or neurological complications of Lyme disease, disorders associated with chronic joint swelling, and in those with a pacemaker.

Magaldrate

BRAND NAMES
Losopan, Riopan

▶ Drug Class: Antacid

▶ Available in: Oral suspension

▶ Available OTC? Yes

▶ As Generic? Yes

Side Effects

SERIOUS
Severe and continuing constipation, dizziness, lightheadedness, and heartbeat irregularities. Bone loss (osteomalacia) may occur, especially with prolonged use in dialysis patients. Hypophosphatemia (too little phosphate in the blood) may occur with prolonged use and a low-phosphate diet; symptoms include bone pain, fractures (due to bone loss), muscle weakness, loss of appetite, mood changes, a general feeling of discomfort, swelling of the wrists and ankles, unusual weight loss, and anemia (decreased number of red blood cells; symptoms include weakness and fatigue). Call your doctor immediately.

COMMON
Chalky taste.

LESS COMMON
Increased thirst, speckling or whitish color of stools, stomach cramps, diarrhea, mild constipation.

PRINCIPAL USES
To relieve symptoms of heartburn, acid indigestion, sour stomach, and gastro-esophageal reflux. Also prescribed to treat hyperacidity associated with peptic ulcers, gastritis, and esophagitis.

HOW THE DRUG WORKS
Magaldrate neutralizes stomach acid and reduces the action of pepsin, a digestive enzyme. This provides symptomatic relief from excess stomach acid.

DOSAGE
Adults: 540 to 1,080 mg (5 to 10 ml). Children: 5 to 10 mg. Take it between meals and at bedtime.

ONSET OF EFFECT
Within 20 minutes.

DURATION OF ACTION
20 to 60 minutes in fasting patients; 3 hours when taken after meals.

DIETARY ADVICE
Eat a balanced diet.

STORAGE
Store in a tightly sealed container away from heat, moisture, and direct light.

IF YOU MISS A DOSE
Take it as soon as you remember. If it is near the time for the next dose, skip the missed dose and resume your regular dosage schedule. Do not double the next dose.

STOPPING THE DRUG
Take as directed for the full treatment period.

PROLONGED USE
Do not take magaldrate for more than 2 weeks unless your doctor advises you to do otherwise.

PRECAUTIONS
Over 60: Constipation and intestinal trouble are more common in older persons. Older patients who have or who are at high risk for osteoporosis or other bone disorders should avoid frequent use of magaldrate.

Driving and Hazardous Work: No special precautions are necessary.

Alcohol: Avoid alcohol.

Pregnancy: Adequate studies have not been done. Before taking magaldrate, tell your doctor if you are pregnant or plan to become pregnant.

Breast Feeding: Magaldrate may pass into breast milk but has not been reported to cause problems in nursing babies. Consult your doctor for advice.

Infants and Children: Do not give antacids and other magnesium-containing medicines to young children unless prescribed by a physician.

Special Concerns: Use over-the-counter antacids only occasionally unless otherwise directed by your doctor. Persistent heartburn not readily relieved by antacids may be signaling a heart attack or other serious disorder. Seek medical help promptly.

OVERDOSE
Symptoms: Diarrhea, nausea, vomiting, constipation, confusion, palpitations, weakness, fatigue, bone pain, stupor.

What to Do: An overdose of magaldrate is unlikely to be life-threatening. However, if someone takes a much larger dose than prescribed, call your doctor, emergency medical services (EMS), or the nearest poison control center.

DRUG INTERACTIONS
Magaldrate and other magnesium-containing antacids may interact with vitamin D (including calcitediol and calcitriol), and may decrease the effectiveness of pancrelipase. Note that other medications may lose their effectiveness when taken within 1 hour of antacids. Consult your doctor for specific advice if you are taking amphetamines, bisacodyl, cellulose sodium phosphate, citrates, chenodiol, digoxin, enteric-coated medications, fluoroquinolones, isoniazid, ketoconazole, mecamylamine, methenamine, nitrofurantoin, penicillamine, phosphates, sodium polystyrene sulfonate resin, quinidine, or tetracyclines.

FOOD INTERACTIONS
No known food interactions.

DISEASE INTERACTIONS
Do not take magaldrate if you have any symptoms of appendicitis or an inflamed bowel (abdominal pain, cramps, soreness, bloating, nausea, and vomiting). Magaldrate is not recommended for Alzheimer's patients. Consult your doctor if you have any of the following: broken bones, colitis, diarrhea, intestinal blockage or bleeding, colostomy or ileostomy, edema, hypophosphatemia, heart disease, liver disease, toxemia of pregnancy, or kidney disease.

Magnesium Citrate

BRAND NAMES
Citrate of Magnesia,
Citro-Nesia, Citroma

▶ Drug Class: Hyperosmotic laxative

▶ Available in: Oral solution

▶ Available OTC? Yes

▶ As Generic? Yes

Side Effects

SERIOUS
Confusion, dizziness or lightheadedness, intestinal blockage, skin rash or itching, difficulty swallowing. Call your doctor immediately.

COMMON
Cramping, diarrhea, gas, increased thirst.

LESS COMMON
Sweating, weakness.

PRINCIPAL USES
To treat short-term constipation and for rapid emptying of the colon for rectal and bowel examinations.

HOW THE DRUG WORKS
Magnesium citrate attracts and retains water in the intestine, softening stools and inducing the urge to defecate.

DOSAGE
Adults and teenagers: 11 to 25 g daily in 1 or more doses. Children ages 6 to 12: 5.5 to 12.5 g daily in 1 or more doses.

ONSET OF EFFECT
30 minutes to 3 hours.

DURATION OF ACTION
Variable.

DIETARY ADVICE
Take it on an empty stomach with a full glass of cold water or juice.

STORAGE
Store in a tightly sealed container away from heat, moisture, and direct light.

IF YOU MISS A DOSE
If you are taking this drug on a fixed schedule, take the missed dose as soon as you remember. If it is near the time for the next dose, skip the missed dose and resume your regular dosage schedule. Do not double the next dose.

STOPPING THE DRUG
Take it as prescribed for the full treatment period. However, you may stop taking the drug if you are feeling better before the scheduled end of the therapy.

PROLONGED USE
Magnesium citrate is intended for short-term therapy only.

PRECAUTIONS
Over 60: No special problems are expected in older patients.

Driving and Hazardous Work: The use of magnesium citrate should not impair your ability to perform such tasks safely.

Alcohol: Avoid alcohol.

Pregnancy: Pregnant women with impaired kidney function should avoid taking magnesium citrate.

Breast Feeding: Magnesium citrate may pass into breast milk; caution is advised. Consult your doctor for advice.

Infants and Children: Do not give magnesium citrate and other laxatives to children under 6 years of age unless prescribed by a doctor.

Special Concerns: Chilling the medication or taking it with ice or following it with citrus fruit juice or citrus-flavored carbonated beverages may make it more palatable. Remember that chronic use of magnesium citrate or any laxative can lead to laxative dependence. You should consume adequate amounts of fiber in your diet, like bran, whole-grain cereals, fruit, and vegetables. Magnesium citrate should be taken on a schedule that doesn't interfere with activities or sleep, as it produces watery stools in 3 to 6 hours. It should not be taken within 2 hours of taking other medications.

OVERDOSE
Symptoms: Severe or protracted diarrhea.

What to Do: An overdose of magnesium citrate is unlikely to be life-threatening. However, if someone takes a much larger dose than prescribed, call your doctor, emergency medical services (EMS), or the nearest poison control center right away.

DRUG INTERACTIONS
Consult your doctor for specific advice if you are taking cellulose sodium phosphate; other magnesium-containing medications such as antacids; other laxatives; sodium polystyrene sulfonate; and oral tetracycline antibiotics.

FOOD INTERACTIONS
No known food interactions.

DISEASE INTERACTIONS
Caution is advised when taking magnesium citrate. Consult your doctor if you have kidney problems, symptoms of appendicitis (abdominal pain, nausea, vomiting), heart damage, intestinal obstruction or perforation, heart block, or rectal fissures.

Magnesium Oxide

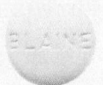

Generic 400 mg
(BLAINE)

▶ Drug Class: Antacid

▶ Available in: Capsules, tablets

▶ Available OTC? Yes

▶ As Generic? Yes

Side Effects

SERIOUS
Dizziness, lightheadedness, continuing feeling of discomfort, irregular heartbeat, loss of appetite, mental or mood changes, muscle weakness, unusual fatigue or weakness, unusual weight loss. Call your doctor immediately.

COMMON
Chalky taste, laxative effect.

LESS COMMON
Diarrhea, increased thirst, speckling or discoloration of stools, stomach cramps, nausea or vomiting, elevated magnesium in the blood (detectable by your doctor).

PRINCIPAL USES
To treat low magnesium in the blood (hypomagnesemia). Also used to replace or prevent magnesium loss resulting from other medications or conditions. It is used as an antacid to relieve heartburn, sour stomach, and acid indigestion.

HOW THE DRUG WORKS
Magnesium oxide neutralizes stomach acid and reduces the action of pepsin, a digestive enzyme. This provides symptomatic relief from excess stomach acid and heartburn.

DOSAGE
Capsules: 140 mg, 3 to 4 times a day. Tablets: 400 to 800 mg a day in evenly divided doses.

ONSET OF EFFECT
Within 20 minutes.

DURATION OF ACTION
For 20 minutes in fasting patients; 3 hours when taken after meals.

DIETARY ADVICE
Take this medication at least 1 hour after meals.

STORAGE
Store in a tightly sealed container away from heat, moisture, and direct light.

IF YOU MISS A DOSE
Take it as soon as you remember. If it is near the time for the next dose, skip the missed dose and resume your regular dosage schedule. Do not double the next dose.

STOPPING THE DRUG
Take it as prescribed for the full treatment period. However, when magnesium oxide is used as an antacid, it may be taken as needed.

PROLONGED USE
You should see your doctor regularly for tests and examinations if you must take this drug for a prolonged period.

PRECAUTIONS
Over 60: Adverse reactions may be more likely and more severe.

Driving and Hazardous Work: Do not drive or engage in hazardous work until you determine how the medicine affects you.

Alcohol: Avoid alcohol.

Pregnancy: Adequate studies have not been done. Before taking magnesium oxide, tell your doctor if you are pregnant or planning to become pregnant.

Breast Feeding: Magnesium oxide may pass into breast milk; consult your doctor for advice.

Infants and Children: Not recommended for use by children under 6 unless prescribed by a doctor.

Special Concerns: Using magnesium oxide in large amounts or for prolonged periods may have a laxative effect; the drug should not be used regularly for this purpose. In general, do not take other medicines within 2 hours of taking magnesium-containing antacids. Heartburn or upper abdominal pain not readily relieved by antacids may be signaling a heart attack or other serious disorder. In such cases, seek medical help promptly.

OVERDOSE
Symptoms: Diarrhea, bloating, change in mental state, muscle pain or twitching, slowed or shallow breathing, coma.

What to Do: An overdose of magnesium oxide is unlikely to be life-threatening. However, if someone takes a much larger dose than prescribed, call your doctor, emergency medical services (EMS), or the nearest poison control center immediately.

DRUG INTERACTIONS
Consult your doctor if you are taking fluoroquinolones, ketoconazole, methenamine, mecamylamine, sodium polystyrene sulfonate, tetracyclines, urinary acidifiers, digitalis drugs, misoprostol, pancrelipase, iron salts, phosphates, salicylates, or vitamin D (including calcifediol and calcitriol). Also, certain medications may lose their effectiveness or cause unexpected side effects when taken within 2 hours of magnesium oxide. These include enteric-coated medicines, folic acid, penicillamine, phenothiazines, and phenytoin. Take at least 2 hours apart (3 hours with phenytoin).

FOOD INTERACTIONS
No known food interactions.

DISEASE INTERACTIONS
Do not take magnesium oxide if you have any symptoms of appendicitis or an inflamed bowel (abdominal pain, cramps, soreness, bloating, nausea, and vomiting). Magnesium-containing antacids should not be taken by patients with kidney disease. Consult your doctor if you have any of the following: bone fractures, colitis, severe and continuing constipation, hemorrhoids, intestinal or rectal bleeding, a colostomy or ileostomy, persistent diarrhea, edema, heart disease, liver disease, toxemia of pregnancy, sarcoidosis, or underactive parathyroid glands.

Magnesium Sulfate

▶ Drug Class: Laxative/dietary supplement

▶ Available in: Crystals, tablets

▶ Available OTC? Yes

▶ As Generic? Yes

Side Effects

SERIOUS
Abdominal cramps, nausea, diarrhea. Call your doctor immediately.

COMMON
There are no common side effects associated with the use of magnesium sulfate.

LESS COMMON
There are no less-common side effects associated with the use of magnesium sulfate.

PRINCIPAL USES
Magnesium sulfate is used to evacuate the bowel before surgery, and as a dietary supplement for people with a magnesium deficiency due to illness or as a result of the use of certain medications.

HOW THE DRUG WORKS
As a laxative, magnesium sulfate attracts and retains water in the intestine, softening stools and inducing the urge to defecate.

DOSAGE
As a laxative— Adults and teenagers: 10 to 30 g daily in 1 or more doses. Children ages 6 to 12: 5 to 10 g daily in 1 or more doses. To treat magnesium deficiency— The dose is determined by your doctor according to the severity of the deficiency.

ONSET OF EFFECT
Within 30 minutes to 3 hours.

DURATION OF ACTION
Variable.

DIETARY ADVICE
Take it on an empty stomach with a full glass of cold water or juice.

STORAGE
Store in a tightly sealed container away from heat, moisture, and direct light.

IF YOU MISS A DOSE
If you are taking this drug on a fixed schedule, take the missed dose as soon as you remember. If it is near the time for the next dose, skip the missed dose and resume your regular dosage schedule. Do not double the next dose.

STOPPING THE DRUG
You should not take magnesium sulfate for more than one week unless your physician prescribes its continued use.

PROLONGED USE
You should see your doctor regularly for tests and examinations if you must take this drug for a prolonged period.

PRECAUTIONS
Over 60: No special problems are expected.

Driving and Hazardous Work: The use of magnesium sulfate should not impair your ability to perform such tasks safely.

Alcohol: Avoid alcohol.

Pregnancy: Magnesium sulfate is used as a treatment, in the hospital only, for certain symptoms of toxemia of pregnancy. In proper amounts it can be used if necessary as a dietary supplement during pregnancy.

Breast Feeding: Magnesium sulfate passes into breast milk; caution is advised. Consult your doctor for advice.

Infants and Children: Magnesium sulfate and other laxatives should not be given to children under 6 years of age unless prescribed by your pediatrician.

Special Concerns: Taking it with ice or following it with citrus fruit juice or citrus-flavored carbonated beverages may make it more palatable. Remember that chronic use of magnesium sulfate or any laxative can lead to laxative dependence. Consume adequate amounts of fiber in your diet, such as bran, whole-grain cereals, fruit, and vegetables. Magnesium sulfate should be taken on a schedule that does not interfere with activities or sleep, as it produces watery stools within 3 to 6 hours. It should not be taken within 2 hours of taking other medications.

OVERDOSE
Symptoms: Blurred or double vision, dizziness or fainting, severe drowsiness, increased or decreased urination, slow heartbeat, trouble breathing.

What to Do: Call your doctor, emergency medical services (EMS), or the nearest poison control center immediately.

DRUG INTERACTIONS
Consult your doctor for specific advice if you are taking oral tetracycline, other magnesium-containing preparations, cellulose sodium phosphate, sodium polystyrene sulfonate, or digitalis drugs.

FOOD INTERACTIONS
No known food interactions.

DISEASE INTERACTIONS
Caution is advised when taking magnesium sulfate. Consult your doctor if you have any of the following: myasthenia gravis, severe kidney disease, heart blockage, intestinal obstruction or perforation, or any respiratory disease.

Maprotiline Hydrochloride

Generic 50 mg
(MYLAN)

▶ Drug Class: Tetracyclic antidepressant

▶ Available in: Tablets

▶ Available OTC? No

▶ As Generic? Yes

Side Effects

SERIOUS
Severe constipation, trembling, weight loss, unusual excitability, severe dizziness or drowsiness, seizures, nausea or vomiting, palpitations or heartbeat irregularities, difficulty breathing, fever, restlessness, severe muscle stiffness or fatigue. Also skin redness, swelling, itching, or rash. Call your doctor right away.

COMMON
Dizziness, lightheadedness, drowsiness, visual disturbances, dry mouth, headache, sexual dysfunction, fatigue.

LESS COMMON
Diarrhea, constipation, heartburn, increased sensitivity to sunlight, increased sweating, weight loss, insomnia, increased appetite with weight gain.

PRINCIPAL USES
To relieve symptoms of major depression.

HOW THE DRUG WORKS
Maprotiline affects levels of norepinephrine, a brain chemical that is thought to be linked to mood, emotions, and mental state.

DOSAGE
Adults: To start, 25 mg, 1 to 3 times a day. The dose may be increased gradually by your doctor to 150 mg a day. Children: Dosage is determined by your doctor.

ONSET OF EFFECT
1 to 3 weeks.

DURATION OF ACTION
Unknown.

DIETARY ADVICE
No special restrictions.

STORAGE
Store in a tightly sealed container away from heat, moisture, and direct light.

IF YOU MISS A DOSE
If you take a one-time daily bedtime dose, do not take a missed dose in the morning because it may cause drowsiness. Call your doctor. If you take more than 1 dose a day, take it as soon as you remember. If it is near the time for the next dose, skip the missed dose and resume your regular dosage schedule. Do not double the next dose.

STOPPING THE DRUG
Take it as prescribed for the full treatment period, even if you feel better before the scheduled end of therapy. The decision to stop taking the drug should be made by your doctor.

PROLONGED USE
See your doctor regularly for tests and examinations if you must take maprotiline for a prolonged period.

PRECAUTIONS
Over 60: Adverse reactions may be more likely and more severe in older patients.

Driving and Hazardous Work: Use caution while driving or engaging in hazardous work until you determine how the medicine affects you. Drowsiness or lightheadedness can occur.

Alcohol: Avoid alcohol.

Pregnancy: In animal studies, maprotiline has not caused problems. Human studies have not been done. Before you take maprotiline, tell your doctor if you are pregnant or plan to become pregnant.

Breast Feeding: Maprotiline passes into breast milk; caution is advised. Consult your doctor for specific advice.

Infants and Children: Use and dosage for infants and children must be determined by your doctor. It is not known whether maprotiline causes different or more severe side effects in infants and children than it does in older persons.

Special Concerns: Risk of seizures is increased if more than 150 mg is taken within a 24-hour period. If maprotiline causes dry mouth, use sugarless candy, gum, or ice chips for relief.

OVERDOSE
Symptoms: Severe dizziness or drowsiness, seizures, nausea or vomiting, heartbeat irregularities, difficulty breathing, fever, restlessness, muscle stiffness or fatigue.

What to Do: Call your doctor, emergency medical services (EMS), or the nearest poison control center immediately.

DRUG INTERACTIONS
Maprotiline and MAO inhibitors should not be used within 14 days of each other. Consult your doctor for specific advice if you are taking asthma medicine, amphetamines, cold medicine, medicines that depress the central nervous system, or appetite suppressants.

FOOD INTERACTIONS
No known food interactions.

DISEASE INTERACTIONS
Caution is advised when taking maprotiline. Consult your doctor if you have any of the following: epilepsy or another seizure disorder, gastrointestinal problems, asthma, urinary problems, glaucoma, a history of alcohol abuse, an enlarged prostate, heart disease, blood vessel disease, liver disease, or an overactive thyroid.

Masoprocol

▶ Drug Class: Topical antineoplastic (anticancer) agent

▶ Available in: Cream

▶ Available OTC? No

▶ As Generic? No

Side Effects

SERIOUS
Shortness of breath,
wheezing, difficulty
breathing, confusion,
hives, itching, rash,
abdominal pain, facial
swelling, sweating, weak-
ness, and lightheaded-
ness (allergic reaction to
sulfites or other compo-
nents of the preparation).

COMMON
Redness, pain, swelling,
and dry, flaking skin at
the site of application.

LESS COMMON
Blistering or wet dis-
charge at the site of
application; burning or
other discomfort follow-
ing application; rough,
wrinkled skin.

PRINCIPAL USES
Masoprocol is used for therapy of actinic keratoses
(precancerous skin growths
that can become malignant
if left untreated).

HOW THE DRUG WORKS
It is not known exactly how
masoprocol works. Labora-
tory experiments have
shown that masoprocol prevents cells similar to the
ones found in actinic keratoses from multiplying.

DOSAGE
Adults: Apply cream to
lesions 2 times a day. Use
sufficient cream to cover
lesions entirely. Do not
apply a covering bandage or
dressing to the site. Children: Consult a pediatrician.

ONSET OF EFFECT
The anticancer effect of
masoprocol begins as soon
as the medication comes in
contact with diseased skin.
Significant improvement,
however, may not be visible
to the patient or physician
until after therapy has continued for a period of time.

DURATION OF ACTION
Unknown.

DIETARY ADVICE
Maintain your usual food
and fluid intake. Increase
intake of fluids if you have a
fever or diarrhea, in hot
weather, or during exercise.

STORAGE
Store in a tightly sealed container away from heat and
direct light. Keep away from
moisture and extremes in
temperature.

IF YOU MISS A DOSE
Apply it as soon as you
remember. If it is near the
time for the next dose, skip
the missed dose and
resume your regular dosage
schedule. Do not double the
next dose.

STOPPING THE DRUG
Take it as prescribed for the
full treatment period, even
if you begin to feel better
before the scheduled end
of the therapy.

PROLONGED USE
Therapy with this medica-
tion may require many
weeks. The risk of an undesirable side effect increases
with prolonged use.

PRECAUTIONS
Over 60: Adverse reactions
may be more likely and
more severe in older
patients.

**Driving and Hazardous
Work:** Masoprocol may
cause dizziness and allergic
reactions. Therefore, do not
drive or engage in haz-
ardous work until you determine how the medicine
affects you.

Alcohol: No special precautions are necessary.

Pregnancy: The effects
are unknown. Consult your
physician if you are pregnant or trying to become
pregnant.

Breast Feeding: Masoprocol may pass into breast
milk; caution is advised.
Consult your doctor for
advice.

Infants and Children:
Safety and effectiveness of
masoprocol are unknown in
young patients. Your pediatrician will weigh the risks
of using it.

Special Concerns: Masoprocol contains sulfites; be
sure to inform your physician if you are allergic to
sulfites or sulfur-containing
compounds. This medica-
tion should be kept away
from your eyes and mouth.
Wash your hands thor-
oughly immediately after

applying masoprocol to prevent accidental contact with
these sensitive areas. Your
skin may appear reddened
and blotchy wherever masoprocol has been in contact
with it. These reactions usually disappear completely
within 2 weeks of stopping
the medication.

OVERDOSE
Symptoms: No specific
ones have been reported.

What to Do: An overdose
of masoprocol is unlikely to
be life-threatening. How-
ever, if someone applies a
much larger dose than prescribed, call your doctor,
emergency medical services
(EMS), or the nearest poison control center.

DRUG INTERACTIONS
No specific interactions are
known at this time. Consult
your doctor or pharmacist if
you are concerned whether
a prescription or nonpre-
scription medication you
are using may interact
with masoprocol.

FOOD INTERACTIONS
No known food interactions.

DISEASE INTERACTIONS
Caution is advised when
taking masoprocol. Consult
your doctor if you have
allergies to sulfites or had
previous allergic reactions
to masoprocol.

Measles, Mumps, and Rubella Vaccine, Live

BRAND NAME
M-M-R II

▶ Drug Class: Vaccine

▶ Available in: Injection

▶ Available OTC? No

▶ As Generic? No

Side Effects

SERIOUS
Serious allergic reaction involving difficulty swallowing or breathing; reddened skin, especially around the ears; itching, particularly of the hands or feet; hives; severe fatigue; swelling of face, eyes, or nasal passages; eye pain or tenderness; or high fever. Call your doctor immediately.

COMMON
Burning or stinging at site of injection, fever, skin rash.

LESS COMMON
Mild headache, sore throat, nausea, vomiting, diarrhea. Also redness, itching, swelling, or hard lump at site of injection; general feeling of illness; aches or pain in joints.

PRINCIPAL USES
To prevent infection by the measles, mumps, and rubella (German measles) viruses.

HOW THE DRUG WORKS
The measles, mumps, and rubella vaccine is an injection that works by introducing small amounts of live strains of the viruses into the body, which stimulate the immune system to produce its own protective antibodies against these viruses.

DOSAGE
The first dose, injected under the skin, should be given at 12 to 15 months of age. A second dose should be given between either ages 4 and 6 or ages 11 and 12. Adults born before 1957 are generally considered to be immune to measles and mumps.

ONSET OF EFFECT
Most patients develop immunity within 2 to 6 weeks.

DURATION OF ACTION
Up to 11 years or more.

DIETARY ADVICE
No special restrictions.

STORAGE
Not applicable; the dose is administered only at a health care facility.

IF YOU MISS A DOSE
If your child misses a scheduled vaccination, contact your pediatrician.

STOPPING THE DRUG
The full schedule of injections should be followed unless a medical problem intervenes.

PROLONGED USE
No special problems are expected.

PRECAUTIONS
Over 60: Measles, mumps, and rubella vaccine is not expected to cause different or more severe side effects in older patients than it does in younger persons.

Driving and Hazardous Work: The use of measles, mumps, and rubella vaccine should not impair your ability to perform such tasks safely.

Alcohol: No special precautions are necessary.

Pregnancy: Generally, its use during pregnancy should be avoided. Before you have a measles, mumps, and rubella vaccination, tell your doctor if you are pregnant or plan to become pregnant. A pregnancy test should be done before the vaccine is given. Women should avoid pregnancy for 3 months following vaccination.

Breast Feeding: Components of the vaccine may pass into breast milk; caution is advised. Consult your doctor for specific advice.

Infants and Children: Measles, mumps, and rubella vaccine is not recommended for children younger than 12 months. The presence of the mother's antibodies in children under 12 months may prevent the vaccine from working. If a child is vaccinated before 12 months, another dose is recommended at 12 to 15 months of age.

Special Concerns: Applying a warm compress to the injection site can reduce redness and swelling. Do not use the vaccine within 3 months of an infusion of immunoglobulin. Immunosuppressive drugs and corticosteroids may decrease the vaccine's effect.

OVERDOSE
Symptoms: An overdose with measles, mumps, and rubella vaccine is unlikely.

What to Do: No cases of overdose have been reported.

DRUG INTERACTIONS
Other drugs may interact with measles, mumps, and rubella vaccine. Consult your doctor for specific advice if you are taking any prescription or over-the-counter medication.

FOOD INTERACTIONS
No known food interactions.

DISEASE INTERACTIONS
Consult your doctor if you have any of the following: a history of immune system deficiency, cancer, a blood disease, active tuberculosis, an allergic reaction to eggs or egg products, or an allergic reaction to neomycin.

Mebendazole

BRAND NAME
Vermox

Generic 100 mg
(COPLEY)

▶ Drug Class: Anthelmintic

▶ Available in: Chewable tablets

▶ Available OTC? No

▶ As Generic? Yes

Side Effects

SERIOUS
Fever, sore throat, skin rash or itching, unusual fatigue. Call your doctor immediately.

COMMON
There are no common side effects associated with the use of this drug.

LESS COMMON
Nausea, vomiting, stomach pain or upset, diarrhea. Such symptoms tend to be short-lived and resolve on their own.

PRINCIPAL USES
To treat various intestinal roundworm infections, including ascariasis (common roundworm), hookworm infection, trichuriasis (whipworm), and enterobiasis or oxyuriasis (pinworm). It may be used to treat nonintestinal roundworm infections or more than one worm infection at a time.

HOW THE DRUG WORKS
Mebendazole interferes with the worm's energy-producing processes, including preventing the worm from absorbing glucose (sugar).

DOSAGE
For roundworms, hookworms, and whipworms—Adults and children age 2 and over: 100 mg, 2 times a day, in the morning and evening, for 3 days. Treatment may be repeated in 2 to 3 weeks. For pinworms—Adults and children age 2 and over: 100 mg for 1 day, repeated in 2 to 3 weeks. For multiple worm infections— Adults and children age 2 and over: 100 mg, 2 times a day, in the morning and evening, for 3 days. Treatment may be repeated in 2 to 3 weeks.

ONSET OF EFFECT
Unknown.

DURATION OF ACTION
Unknown.

DIETARY ADVICE
Take it with meals high in fat content to help the body better absorb the medication. If you are on a low-fat diet, consult your doctor for specific advice.

STORAGE
Store in a tightly sealed container away from heat, moisture, and direct light.

IF YOU MISS A DOSE
Take it as soon as you remember. If it is near the time for the next dose, skip the missed dose and resume your regular dosage schedule. Do not double the next dose.

STOPPING THE DRUG
Take as prescribed for the full treatment period, even if you begin to feel better before the scheduled end of therapy.

PROLONGED USE
You should see your doctor regularly for tests and examinations if you take this medicine for a prolonged period.

PRECAUTIONS

Over 60: No studies have been done specifically on older patients; adverse reactions may be more likely or more severe.

Driving and Hazardous Work: The use of mebendazole should not impair your ability to perform such tasks safely.

Alcohol: No special precautions are necessary.

Pregnancy: The use of mebendazole while pregnant is not recommended. Consult your doctor for advice.

Breast Feeding: Mebendazole may pass into breast milk; caution is advised. Consult your doctor for advice.

Infants and Children: Use and dose for children up to 2 years of age must be determined by your doctor.

Special Concerns: For pinworm infection, clothing, bedding, and towels should be washed daily. All members of the family may have

to be treated to eradicate the infestation. A second treatment for all household members may be necessary after 2 or 3 weeks. All bedding and nightclothes should be washed after treatment. To prevent reinfection, you should wash the anal region daily, change your underwear and bedding every day, and wash your hands and fingernails before each meal and after bowel movements. Hookworm infection can cause anemia, and your doctor may tell you to take iron supplements during and after treatment.

OVERDOSE
Symptoms: Gastrointestinal upset lasting several hours; possible respiratory arrest or seizures.

What to Do: Call your doctor, emergency medical services (EMS), or the nearest poison control center immediately.

DRUG INTERACTIONS
Other drugs may interact with mebendazole. Consult your doctor for specific advice if you are taking carbamazepine or any other prescription or over-the-counter medication.

FOOD INTERACTIONS
No known food interactions.

DISEASE INTERACTIONS
Consult your doctor if you have liver disease, Crohn's disease, or ulcerative colitis.

Meclizine

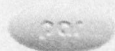

Generic 25 mg
(PAR)

Additional photographs

▶ Drug Class: Antiemetic; antivertigo agent

▶ Available in: Capsules, tablets, chewable tablets

▶ Available OTC? Yes

▶ As Generic? Yes

Side Effects

SERIOUS
No serious side effects are associated with the use of meclizine.

COMMON
Drowsiness.

LESS COMMON
Blurred or double vision; upset stomach; constipation or diarrhea; insomnia; painful or difficult urination; dizziness; dry mouth, nose, and throat; headache; loss of appetite; fast heartbeat; nervousness; restlessness; skin rash.

PRINCIPAL USES
To treat and prevent nausea, vomiting, and dizziness caused by motion sickness and vertigo (dizziness) associated with other medical problems.

HOW THE DRUG WORKS
Meclizine acts on brain centers that control nausea, vomiting, and dizziness.

DOSAGE
To prevent and treat motion sickness— Adults and teenagers: 25 to 50 mg, 1 hour before travel; the dose may be repeated every 24 hours. To prevent and treat vertigo— Adults and teenagers: 25 to 100 mg a day as needed, in divided doses.

ONSET OF EFFECT
Within 1 hour.

DURATION OF ACTION
Up to 24 hours.

DIETARY ADVICE
Can be taken with food.

STORAGE
Store in a tightly sealed container away from heat, moisture, and direct light.

IF YOU MISS A DOSE
Take it as soon as you remember. If it is near the time for the next dose, skip the missed dose and resume your regular dosage schedule. Do not double the next dose.

STOPPING THE DRUG
Take it as prescribed for the full treatment period. However, you may stop taking the medication if you are feeling better before the scheduled end of therapy.

PROLONGED USE
See your doctor regularly for tests and examinations if you must use this drug for a prolonged period.

PRECAUTIONS
Over 60: Adverse reactions may be more likely and more severe in older patients.

Driving and Hazardous Work: Do not drive or engage in hazardous work until you determine how the medicine affects you.

Alcohol: Avoid alcohol when using this medication.

Pregnancy: Adequate human studies have not been completed. Before taking meclizine, tell your doctor if you are pregnant or plan to become pregnant.

Breast Feeding: Meclizine may pass into breast milk but has not been reported to cause problems in nursing babies. It may reduce the flow of breast milk. Consult your doctor for advice.

Infants and Children: Meclizine is not recommended for use by children under the age of 12.

Special Concerns: If dry mouth occurs, use sugarless candy or gum or bits of ice for temporary relief. If constipation occurs, a high-fiber diet and drinking plenty of fluids can help relieve the problem. Meclizine can cause false-negative results in allergy skin testing.

OVERDOSE
Symptoms: Extreme excitability, seizures, drowsiness, hallucinations.

What to Do: Call your doctor, emergency medical services (EMS), or the nearest poison control center immediately.

DRUG INTERACTIONS
Consult your doctor for specific advice if you are taking medications that can depress the central nervous system, such as antihistamines, medicines for hay fever, tranquilizers, sleep medications, prescription pain medicines, or muscle relaxants, or if you are taking any over-the-counter medication.

FOOD INTERACTIONS
No known food interactions.

DISEASE INTERACTIONS
Caution is advised when taking meclizine. Consult your doctor if you have any of the following: urinary tract blockage, glaucoma, asthma, bronchitis, emphysema, any other chronic lung disease, enlarged prostate, heart failure, or intestinal blockage.

Meclofenamate Sodium

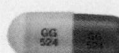

Generic 50 mg
(GENEVA)

▶ Drug Class: Nonsteroidal anti-inflammatory drug (NSAID)

▶ Available in: Capsules

▶ Available OTC? No

▶ As Generic? Yes

Side Effects

SERIOUS
Shortness of breath or wheezing, with or without swelling of legs or other signs of heart failure; chest pain; peptic ulcer disease with vomiting of blood; black, tarry stools; decreasing kidney function. Call your doctor immediately.

COMMON
Nausea, vomiting, heartburn, diarrhea, constipation, headache, dizziness, sleepiness.

LESS COMMON
Ulcers or sores in mouth, depression, rashes or blistering of skin, ringing sound in the ears, unusual tingling or numbness of the hands or feet, seizures, blurred vision. Also elevated potassium levels, decreased blood counts; such problems can be detected by your doctor.

PRINCIPAL USES
To treat mild to moderate pain and inflammation caused by tendinitis, arthritis, bursitis, gout, soft tissue injuries, migraine and other vascular headaches, menstrual cramps, and other conditions. When patients fail to respond to one NSAID, another may be tried. The greatest effectiveness often requires trial and error of several different NSAIDs.

HOW THE DRUG WORKS
NSAIDs work by interfering with the formation of prostaglandins, naturally occurring substances in the body that cause inflammation and make nerves more sensitive to pain impulses. NSAIDs also have other modes of action that are less well understood.

DOSAGE
Adults: 50 mg, 4 to 6 times a day. Maximum dose is 400 mg a day. Children: Consult your pediatrician.

ONSET OF EFFECT
From 30 minutes to several hours or longer.

DURATION OF ACTION
4 hours or more.

DIETARY ADVICE
Take with food; maintain your usual food and fluid intake.

STORAGE
Store in a tightly sealed container away from heat, moisture, and direct light. Keep away from extremes in temperature.

IF YOU MISS A DOSE
Take it as soon as you remember. If it is near the time for the next dose, skip the missed dose and resume your regular dosage schedule. Do not double the next dose.

STOPPING THE DRUG
The decision to stop taking the drug should be made in consultation with your physician.

PROLONGED USE
Prolonged use can cause gastrointestinal problems, including ulceration and bleeding, kidney dysfunction, and liver inflammation. See your doctor regularly for evaluation.

PRECAUTIONS
Over 60: Because of the potentially greater consequences of gastrointestinal side effects, the dose of NSAIDs for older patients, especially those over age 70, is often cut in half.

Driving and Hazardous Work: Do not drive or engage in hazardous work until you determine how the medicine affects you.

Alcohol: Avoid alcohol when using this medication because it increases the risk of stomach irritation.

Pregnancy: Avoid or discontinue this drug if you are pregnant or plan to become pregnant.

Breast Feeding: Meclofenamate passes into breast milk; avoid or discontinue use while nursing.

Infants and Children: May be used in exceptional circumstances; consult your doctor.

Special Concerns: Because NSAIDs can interfere with blood coagulation, this drug should be stopped at least 3 days prior to any surgery.

OVERDOSE
Symptoms: Severe nausea, vomiting, headache, confusion, seizures.

What to Do: Call your doctor, emergency medical services (EMS), or the nearest poison control center immediately.

DRUG INTERACTIONS
Do not take this drug with aspirin or any other NSAIDs without your doctor's approval. In addition, consult your doctor if you are taking antihypertensives, steroids, anticoagulants, antibiotics, itraconazole or ketoconazole, plicamycin, penicillamine, valproic acid, phenytoin, cyclosporine, digitalis drugs, lithium, methotrexate, probenecid, triamterene, or zidovudine.

FOOD INTERACTIONS
No known food interactions.

DISEASE INTERACTIONS
Consult your doctor if you have any of the following: bleeding problems, inflammation or ulcers of the stomach and intestines, diabetes mellitus, systemic lupus erythematosus (SLE, lupus), anemia, asthma, epilepsy, Parkinson's disease, kidney stones, or a history of heart disease or alcohol abuse. Use of meclofenamate may cause complications in patients with liver or kidney disease, since these organs work together to remove the medication from the body.

Medroxyprogesterone Acetate

Side Effects

SERIOUS
Abnormal menstrual bleeding; unexpected or increased flow of breast milk; mental depression; skin rash; loss of or change in speech, coordination, or vision; severe and sudden shortness of breath. Call your doctor immediately.

COMMON
Stomach pain, swelling of face, ankles, or feet, mild headache, mood changes, unusual fatigue, weight gain.

LESS COMMON
Acne, breast pain or tenderness, hot flashes, insomnia, loss of sexual desire, loss or gain of scalp hair or body hair, brown spots on skin.

PRINCIPAL USES
To treat amenorrhea (cessation of menstrual periods) and abnormal uterine bleeding. It also may be used as a contraceptive.

HOW THE DRUG WORKS
Medroxyprogesterone inhibits secretion of pituitary hormones that in turn regulate menstrual and reproductive cycles. It also alters activity of uterine cells, resulting in, among other changes, thickening of the cervical mucus. These changes make it less likely for a partner's sperm to reach and fertilize an egg.

DOSAGE
For amenorrhea: Tablets, 5 to 10 mg a day for 5 to 10 days. For abnormal uterine bleeding: Tablets, 5 to 10 mg a day for 5 to 10 days beginning on the 16th or 21st day of the menstrual cycle. For contraception: 1 depo (Depo-Provera) injection (150 mg) every 3 months. For use in treating menopause: Tablets, 10 mg a day for 10 to 14 days, together with estrogen in each 25-day cycle.

ONSET OF EFFECT
Varies with mode of delivery. Protection against pregnancy can begin immediately if injection is given within 5 days of the menstrual period.

DURATION OF ACTION
Tablets: 24 hours or more. Injection: More than 3 months.

DIETARY ADVICE
Take it with meals to prevent gastrointestinal upset.

STORAGE
Store in a tightly sealed container away from heat and direct light.

IF YOU MISS A DOSE
Take a missed dose of the tablet as soon as you remember. If it is near the time for the next dose, skip the missed dose and resume your regular dosage schedule. Do not double the next dose.

STOPPING THE DRUG
The decision to stop taking the drug should be made by your doctor.

PROLONGED USE
Consult your doctor about the need for periodic examinations and laboratory tests if you use this drug for a prolonged period.

PRECAUTIONS
Over 60: No special problems are expected in older patients.

Driving and Hazardous Work: Do not drive or engage in hazardous work until you determine how the medicine affects you.

Alcohol: No special problems are expected.

Pregnancy: Before you use medroxyprogesterone, tell your doctor if you are pregnant or plan to become pregnant. This medicine must not be used during pregnancy.

Breast Feeding: Medroxyprogesterone passes into breast milk; avoid or discontinue use while nursing.

Infants and Children: This medication is not recommended for young patients.

Special Concerns: Remember that no contraceptive method is foolproof; 1% of women using the medroxyprogesterone injections have become pregnant.

OVERDOSE
Symptoms: No specific ones have been reported.

What to Do: An overdose of medroxyprogesterone is unlikely to be life-threatening. However, if someone takes a much larger dose than prescribed, call your doctor, emergency medical services (EMS), or the nearest poison control center immediately.

DRUG INTERACTIONS
Consult your doctor for specific advice if you are taking aminoglutethimide, carbamazepine, phenytoin, rifabutin, or rifampin.

FOOD INTERACTIONS
No known food interactions.

DISEASE INTERACTIONS
Do not take medroxyprogesterone if you have: known or suspected breast malignancies or tumors, acute liver disease or liver tumors, or active thrombophlebitis or thromboembolic disease. Consult your doctor if you have any of the following: asthma, epilepsy, migraine headaches, heart or circulation problems, bleeding problems, a history of thrombophlebitis or thromboembolic disease, diabetes mellitus, high blood cholesterol, kidney disease, risk factors for osteoporosis, or central nervous system disorders such as depression.

Medrysone

Side Effects

SERIOUS
Serious side effects are less likely than with ophthalmic dexamethasone, hydrocortisone, or prednisolone, but may include decreased vision or blurring of vision (from cataract); eye pain, nausea, vomiting (from increased eye pressure); and pain, redness, sensitivity to bright light, and discharge (from eye infection). Call your doctor immediately if you experience any of these signs or symptoms. This drug may trigger a recurrence of herpes infection of the eye; mention any previous herpes infection to your doctor.

COMMON
No common side effects are associated with medrysone.

LESS COMMON
Burning, stinging, redness, or watering of eyes.

PRINCIPAL USES
To control inflammation and prevent potentially permanent damage that may result from conditions that involve inflammation in the tissues of the eye. Also used to help relieve redness, irritation, and discomfort in the eye. Medrysone is less effective than ophthalmic dexamethasone, hydrocortisone, or prednisolone but also less likely to cause adverse effects.

HOW THE DRUG WORKS
Medrysone inhibits the release of natural substances that stimulate inflammation and pain in eye tissues.

DOSAGE
1 drop in each eye up to every 4 hours.

ONSET OF EFFECT
Unknown.

DURATION OF ACTION
Unknown.

DIETARY ADVICE
This medication can be used without regard to diet.

STORAGE
Store in a tightly sealed container away from heat, moisture, and direct light. Do not allow it to freeze.

IF YOU MISS A DOSE
Apply it as soon as you remember. If it is near the time for the next dose, skip the missed dose and resume your regular dosage schedule. Do not double the next dose.

STOPPING THE DRUG
Use it as prescribed for the full treatment period, even if your symptoms improve before the scheduled end of therapy.

PROLONGED USE
You should see your doctor regularly for tests and examinations if you take this drug for a prolonged period.

PRECAUTIONS
Over 60: No special problems are expected.

Driving and Hazardous Work: Do not drive or engage in hazardous work until you determine how the medicine affects your vision.

Alcohol: No special precautions are necessary.

Pregnancy: In animal studies, medrysone has caused problems during pregnancy. Reliable human studies have not been done, but no human birth defects have been reported. Before you take medrysone, tell your doctor if you are pregnant or plan to become pregnant.

Breast Feeding: Medrysone has not been reported to cause problems in nursing babies. Consult your doctor for specific advice.

Infants and Children: Children under 2 years of age may be especially sensitive to the effects of medrysone.

Special Concerns: To use the eye drops, first wash your hands. Tilt your head back. Gently apply pressure to the inside corner of the eyelid and with the index finger of the same hand, pull downward on the lower eyelid to make a space. Drop the medicine into this space and close your eye. Apply pressure for 1 or 2 minutes while keeping the eye closed without blinking. Then wash your hands again. Make sure the tip of the dropper does not touch your eye, finger, or any other surface. If your symptoms do not improve in 5 to 7 days or if they become worse, check with your doctor. Wearing contact lenses while using this medication may increase the risk of infection. Your doctor may tell you not to wear contact lenses during and for a day or two after treatment.

OVERDOSE
Symptoms: When used topically, an overdose of medrysone is very unlikely. Inadvertent oral ingestion, however, may cause fever, muscle pain, malaise, loss of appetite, dizziness, fainting, and breathing trouble.

What to Do: An overdose of medrysone is unlikely to be life-threatening. However, if someone applies a much larger dose than prescribed or accidentally ingests the medicine, call your doctor, emergency medical services (EMS), or the nearest poison control center immediately.

DRUG INTERACTIONS
Consult your doctor for specific advice if you are taking any other prescription or over-the-counter medication.

FOOD INTERACTIONS
No known food interactions.

DISEASE INTERACTIONS
Caution is advised when taking medrysone. Consult your doctor if you have any of the following: diabetes, tuberculosis of the eye, glaucoma, cataracts, herpes infection of the eye, or any other eye infection.

Mefenamic Acid

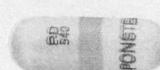

Ponstel 250 mg
(PARKE-DAVIS)

▶ Drug Class: Nonsteroidal anti-inflammatory drug (NSAID)

▶ Available in: Capsules

▶ Available OTC? No

▶ As Generic? No

Side Effects

SERIOUS
Shortness of breath or wheezing, with or without swelling of legs or other signs of heart failure; chest pain; peptic ulcer disease with vomiting of blood; black, tarry stools; decreasing kidney function. Call your doctor immediately.

COMMON
Nausea, vomiting, heartburn, diarrhea, constipation, headache, dizziness, sleepiness.

LESS COMMON
Ulcers or sores in mouth, depression, rashes or blistering of skin, ringing sound in the ears, unusual tingling or numbness of the hands or feet, seizures, blurred vision. Also elevated potassium levels, decreased blood counts; such problems can be detected by your doctor.

PRINCIPAL USES
To treat mild to moderate pain and inflammation caused by tendinitis, arthritis, bursitis, gout, soft tissue injuries, migraine and other vascular headaches, menstrual cramps, and other conditions. When patients fail to respond to one NSAID, another may be tried. The greatest effectiveness often requires trial and error of several different NSAIDs.

HOW THE DRUG WORKS
NSAIDs work by interfering with the formation of prostaglandins, naturally occurring substances in the body that cause inflammation and make nerves more sensitive to pain impulses. NSAIDs also have other modes of action that are less well understood.

DOSAGE
Adults: 250 mg every 6 hours. The drug should not be used for more than 7 days. For children's dose, consult your pediatrician.

ONSET OF EFFECT
Several hours to several days.

DURATION OF ACTION
4 hours or more.

DIETARY ADVICE
Take with food; maintain your usual food and fluid intake.

STORAGE
Store in a tightly sealed container away from heat, moisture, and direct light. Keep away from extremes in temperature.

IF YOU MISS A DOSE
Take it as soon as you remember. If it is near the time for the next dose, skip the missed dose and resume your regular dosage schedule. Do not double the next dose.

STOPPING THE DRUG
The decision to stop taking the drug should be made in consultation with your physician.

PROLONGED USE
Mefenamic acid is not recommended for use longer than 7 days in a course of therapy.

PRECAUTIONS
Over 60: Because of the potentially greater consequences of gastrointestinal side effects, the dose of NSAIDs for older patients, especially those over age 70, is often cut in half.

Driving and Hazardous Work: Avoid such activities until you determine how the medicine affects you.

Alcohol: Avoid alcohol when using this medication because it increases the risk of stomach irritation.

Pregnancy: Avoid or discontinue this drug if you are pregnant or plan to become pregnant.

Breast Feeding: Mefenamic acid passes into breast milk; avoid use while nursing.

Infants and Children: May be used in exceptional circumstances; consult your doctor.

Special Concerns: Because NSAIDs can interfere with blood coagulation, this drug should be stopped at least 3 days prior to any surgery.

OVERDOSE
Symptoms: Severe nausea, vomiting, headache, confusion, seizures.

What to Do: Call your doctor, emergency medical services (EMS), or the nearest poison control center immediately.

DRUG INTERACTIONS
Do not take this drug with aspirin or any other NSAIDs without your doctor's approval. In addition, consult your doctor if you are taking antihypertensives, steroids, anticoagulants, antibiotics, itraconazole or ketoconazole, plicamycin, penicillamine, valproic acid, phenytoin, cyclosporine, digitalis drugs, lithium, methotrexate, probenecid, triamterene, or zidovudine.

FOOD INTERACTIONS
No known food interactions.

DISEASE INTERACTIONS
Consult your doctor if you have any of the following: bleeding problems, inflammation or ulcers of the stomach and intestines, diabetes mellitus, systemic lupus erythematosus (SLE, lupus), anemia, asthma, epilepsy, Parkinson's disease, kidney stones, or a history of heart disease or alcohol abuse. Use of mefenamic acid may cause complications in patients with liver or kidney disease, since these organs work together to remove the medication from the body.

Mefloquine Hydrochloride

Side Effects

SERIOUS
Slowed heartbeat, seizures. Severe anxiety, depression, restlessness, or confusion during preventive therapy may be signs of more serious psychiatric problems. Call your doctor immediately.

COMMON
Treatment-related: dizziness, muscle pain, nausea, fever, headache, vomiting, chills, diarrhea, skin rash, abdominal pain, fatigue, loss of appetite, ringing in the ears. Prevention-related: vomiting, nausea.

LESS COMMON
Treatment-related: hair loss, emotional problems, itching, fatigue. Prevention-related: dizziness, lightheadedness.

PRINCIPAL USES

To treat mild to moderate acute malaria caused by strains of plasmodia (the parasite that causes malaria) that are susceptible to mefloquine—specifically, *Plasmodium falciparum* and *P. vivax*. (The drug may be ineffective against other strains.) Also used to prevent malaria caused by these strains, including chloroquine-resistant *P. falciparum*.

HOW THE DRUG WORKS

Mefloquine is poisonous to the malarial parasite.

DOSAGE

Adults— To treat: 5 tablets (1,250 mg each) taken as a single dose. Patients with acute *P. vivax* malaria are at high risk of relapse. To avoid relapse after the initial treatment, patients should take another antimalarial such as primaquine. To prevent: 250 mg once a week. Begin taking mefloquine one week prior to departure and continue taking the drug for 4 weeks upon return. Children 6 months of age and older— To treat, 20 to 25 mg per 2.2 lbs (1 kg) of body weight. Split the total dose into 2 doses 6 to 8 hours apart in order to reduce the risk and severity of side effects. To prevent: Your pediatrician will determine the appropriate dose.

ONSET OF EFFECT

Unknown.

DURATION OF ACTION

Up to 3 weeks.

DIETARY ADVICE

Do not take on an empty stomach. Take with at least 8 oz of water.

STORAGE

Store in a tightly sealed container away from heat, moisture, and direct light.

IF YOU MISS A DOSE

If taking 1 or more doses a day, take it as soon as you remember. If it is near the time for the next dose, skip the missed dose and resume your regular dosage schedule. Do not double the next dose. If taking 1 weekly dose, take it as soon as possible, then resume regular schedule.

STOPPING THE DRUG

Take it as prescribed for the full treatment period.

PROLONGED USE

If you are taking this drug as a preventive, your doctor may want you to begin at least 1 week before traveling to an area where malaria is prevalent. Keep taking mefloquine while you are in the area and for 4 weeks after you leave. Periodic liver function tests and eye exams are recommended.

PRECAUTIONS

Over 60: Adverse reactions may be more likely and more severe.

Driving and Hazardous Work: Do not drive or engage in hazardous work until you determine how the medicine affects you. Dizziness and coordination difficulties may occur after the drug is discontinued.

Alcohol: No special precautions are necessary.

Pregnancy: The use of mefloquine is discouraged during pregnancy because of the risks it poses to the unborn child. Women of child-bearing age should practice contraception during preventive therapy.

Breast Feeding: Mefloquine passes into breast milk; extreme caution is advised. Consult your physician for specific advice.

Infants and Children: Safety and effectiveness have not been established for children under the age of 6 months. Early vomiting has been associated with mefloquine use in children and with treatment failure. If a second dose is not tolerated, alternative antimalarial measures should be considered.

Special Concerns: If you take mefloquine once a week, take it on the same day every week. Malaria is spread by mosquitoes. Take appropriate precautions, such as using mosquito netting, to guard against being bitten by malaria-carrying mosquitoes.

OVERDOSE

Symptoms: Side effects may be more pronounced. (See Side Effects.)

What to Do: If you have reason to suspect overdose, call your doctor, emergency medical services (EMS), or the nearest poison control center immediately.

DRUG INTERACTIONS

Consult your doctor for more advice if you are taking a beta-blocker, quinidine, quinine, chloroquine, antiarrhythmic drugs, calcium channel blockers, halofantrine, antihistamines, histamine (H1) blockers, tricyclic antidepressants, phenothiazines, anticonvulsants. Also, tell your physician if you are taking any other prescription or over-the-counter drug.

FOOD INTERACTIONS

No known food interactions.

DISEASE INTERACTIONS

Consult your doctor for specific advice if you have a seizure or psychiatric disorder, impaired liver function, any eye condition, or heart disease.

Megestrol Acetate

Generic 20 mg
(PAR)

Additional photographs

▶ Drug Class: Progestin (hormone treatment); antineoplastic (anticancer) agent

▶ Available in: Oral suspension, tablets

▶ Available OTC? No

▶ As Generic? Yes

Side Effects

SERIOUS
Abnormal vaginal discharge or bleeding, changes in menstrual cycle. Less frequently: High blood pressure; palpitations; heart failure; headache; loss of or change in speech, coordination, or vision; numbness or pain in chest, arm, or leg; shortness of breath; high blood sugar causing dry mouth, frequent urination, loss of appetite, and unusual thirst; depression; skin rash. Call your doctor promptly.

COMMON
Diarrhea, nausea, vomiting, impotence, diminished sex drive, abdominal cramps or pain, swollen face, ankles, or feet, mild increase in blood pressure, headache, mood changes, nervousness, fatigue, weight gain.

LESS COMMON
Acne, constipation, breast pain or tenderness, brown spots on skin, hot flashes, loss or gain of hair, insomnia, sweating.

PRINCIPAL USES
To treat cancer of the breast or uterus, and to treat loss of appetite and loss of weight (wasting) caused by AIDS (acquired immunodeficiency syndrome).

HOW THE DRUG WORKS
Megestrol, a synthetic form of the hormone progestin, interferes with the activity of certain other hormones and proteins needed for some types of cancer cells to grow. The mechanism by which megestrol increases weight is unclear. It appears to stimulate the appetite and affect metabolism, resulting in weight gain.

DOSAGE
For breast cancer: 160 mg per day in 1 or several doses for 2 or more months. For uterine cancer: 40 to 320 mg per day for 2 or more months. For loss of weight and appetite associated with AIDS: 800 mg a day for the first month; the dose may be adjusted later.

ONSET OF EFFECT
Unknown.

DURATION OF ACTION
Unknown.

DIETARY ADVICE
No special restrictions..

STORAGE
Store in a tightly sealed container away from heat and direct light.

IF YOU MISS A DOSE
Take it as soon as you remember. If it is near the time for the next dose, skip the missed dose and resume your regular dosage schedule. Do not double the next dose.

STOPPING THE DRUG
The decision to stop taking the drug should be made by your doctor.

PROLONGED USE
You should see your doctor regularly for tests and examinations if you take this drug for a prolonged period.

PRECAUTIONS
Over 60: No special problems are expected in older patients.

Driving and Hazardous Work: Do not drive or engage in hazardous work until you determine how the medicine affects you.

Alcohol: Avoid alcohol while taking this drug.

Pregnancy: Megestrol should never be taken during pregnancy. Consult your doctor immediately if you believe you have become pregnant.

Breast Feeding: Megestrol passes into breast milk; caution is advised. Consult your doctor for specific advice.

Infants and Children: Safety and effectiveness have not been established; consult your pediatrician to weigh risks against benefits.

Special Concerns: If you take any laboratory or diagnostic test, tell the clinician that you are taking megestrol. Megestrol may cause tenderness, swelling, or bleeding of the gums. Brush and floss your teeth carefully and see your dentist regularly.

OVERDOSE
Symptoms: No specific ones have been reported.

What to Do: An overdose of megestrol is unlikely to be life-threatening. However, if someone takes a much larger dose than prescribed, call your doctor, emergency medical services (EMS), or the nearest poison control center.

DRUG INTERACTIONS
Consult your doctor for specific advice if you are taking aminoglutihimide, carbamazepine, phenobarbital, phenytoin, rifabutin, or rifampin.

FOOD INTERACTIONS
No known food interactions.

DISEASE INTERACTIONS
Caution is advised when taking megestrol. Consult your doctor if you have a history of asthma, epilepsy, heart or circulation problems, kidney disease, migraine headaches, bleeding disorders, blood clots, stroke, varicose veins, breast disease, mental depression, high blood cholesterol, diabetes mellitus, or liver disease.

Meloxicam

▶ Drug Class: Nonsteroidal anti-inflammatory drug (NSAID)

▶ Available in: Tablets

▶ Available OTC? No

▶ As Generic? No

Side Effects

SERIOUS
Shortness of breath or wheezing, with or without swelling of legs or other signs of congestive heart failure; chest pain; peptic ulcer disease with vomiting of blood; black, tarry stools; decreasing kidney function. Call your doctor immediately.

COMMON
Diarrhea.

LESS COMMON
Nausea, upper respiratory tract infection, sore throat, dizziness, swelling of the legs.

PRINCIPAL USES
To relieve the pain, inflammation, and stiffness of osteoarthritis.

HOW THE DRUG WORKS
NSAIDs work by interfering with the formation of prostaglandins, naturally occurring substances in the body that cause inflammation and make nerves more sensitive to pain impulses. NSAIDs also have other modes of action that are less well understood.

DOSAGE
Adults: To start, 7.5 mg a day. The dose may be adjusted later to no more than 15 mg a day.

ONSET OF EFFECT
Unknown.

DURATION OF ACTION
Unknown.

DIETARY ADVICE
Meloxicam may be taken with or without food.

STORAGE
Store in a tightly sealed container away from heat, moisture, and direct light.

IF YOU MISS A DOSE
If you do not remember until the next day, skip the missed dose and resume your regular dosage schedule. Do not double the next dose.

STOPPING THE DRUG
The decision to stop taking the drug should be made in consultation with your physician.

PROLONGED USE
The risk of gastrointestinal side effects may be increased with extended use.

PRECAUTIONS
Over 60: Caution should be exercised, as with any NSAID, in using meloxicam. Therapy should be started with the lowest recommended dose.

Driving and Hazardous Work: No special problems are expected.

Alcohol: Avoid alcohol when using this medication because it increases the risk of stomach irritation.

Pregnancy: Discuss with your doctor the relative risks and benefits of using this drug while pregnant. Do not use meloxicam during the last trimester.

Breast Feeding: Meloxicam may pass into breast milk; caution is advised. Consult your doctor for advice on whether to discontinue nursing or discontinue the drug.

Infants and Children: The safety and effectiveness of this drug have not been established for children under the age of 18.

OVERDOSE
Symptoms: Few cases of overdose have been reported. Symptoms may include lethargy, drowsiness, nausea, vomiting, abdominal pain, black, tarry stools, breathing difficulty, and coma.

What to Do: If you suspect an overdose or if someone takes a much larger dose than prescribed, call your doctor, emergency medical services (EMS), or the nearest poison control center immediately.

DRUG INTERACTIONS
Do not take this drug with aspirin or any other NSAIDs without your doctor's approval. In addition, consult your doctor if you are taking furosemide, ACE inhibitors, lithium, cholestyramine, or warfarin.

FOOD INTERACTIONS
No known food interactions.

DISEASE INTERACTIONS
Meloxicam should not be taken by people who have experienced asthma, hives, or allergic-type reactions after taking aspirin or other NSAIDs. People with a history of ulcer disease or gastrointestinal bleeding (especially if elderly or debilitated) should only take meloxicam with extreme caution. Consult your doctor if you have high blood pressure or heart failure. In patients with advanced liver or kidney disease meloxicam is not recommended, since these organs both work to remove the medication from the body.

Melphalan

Alkeran 2 mg
(GLAXO WELLCOME)

▶ Drug Class: Alkylating agent

▶ Available in: Tablets, injection

▶ Available OTC? No

▶ As Generic? No

Side Effects

SERIOUS
Black, tarry, or bloody
stools; blood in the urine;
fever and chills; cough or
hoarseness; pain in lower
back or side; difficult,
decreased, or painful urination; red spots on skin;
unusual bleeding or
bruising; swollen feet or
lower legs. Call your doctor immediately. Some of
these side effects may
recur after you stop tak-
ing melphalan. If so, consult your doctor.

COMMON
There are no common
side effects associated
with melphalan.

LESS COMMON
Nausea and vomiting,
mouth sores, allergic
reaction.

PRINCIPAL USES
To treat multiple myeloma
(a cancer of the bone marrow) and ovarian cancer.

HOW THE DRUG WORKS
Melphalan kills cancer cells
by interfering with the activity of their genetic material,
thus preventing the cells
from reproducing. The drug
may also affect the growth
and development of normal
cells in the body, resulting
in unpleasant side effects.

DOSAGE
For multiple myeloma: 6 mg
(3 tablets) per day for 2 to
3 weeks; the drug is discontinued for up to 4 weeks,
then resumed at a dose of
2 mg a day, depending on
blood counts. For ovarian
cancer: Initial dose is 0.2
mg per 2.2 lbs (1 kg) of
body weight once a day for
5 days. Dosage and duration
of treatment may be altered
to meet the needs of each
patient.

ONSET OF EFFECT
Unknown.

DURATION OF ACTION
Unknown.

DIETARY ADVICE
Melphalan is best taken
with food to minimize stomach upset.

STORAGE
Store in a tightly sealed container away from heat and
direct light.

IF YOU MISS A DOSE
Take it as soon as you
remember. If it is near the
time for the next dose, skip
the missed dose and
resume your regular dosage
schedule. Do not double the
next dose.

STOPPING THE DRUG
The decision to stop taking
the drug should be made by
your doctor.

PROLONGED USE
See your doctor regularly
for tests and examinations if
you must take this medication for a prolonged period.

PRECAUTIONS
Over 60: No special problems are expected.

**Driving and Hazardous
Work:** The use of melphalan should not impair your
ability to perform such
tasks safely.

Alcohol: Avoid alcohol.

Pregnancy: Melphalan can
cause birth defects if taken
by either the father or the
mother. Before you take it,
tell your doctor if you are
pregnant or plan to become
pregnant.

Breast Feeding: Melphalan passes into breast milk;
avoid or discontinue use
while nursing.

Infants and Children:
There is no specific information about the use of
melphalan in children.

Special Concerns: While
taking melphalan, do not
receive any immunizations
without your doctor's
approval. Avoid persons
who have recently had oral
polio vaccine and those with
any infection. Check with
your doctor before having
any dental work done. Consult your doctor or dentist
about appropriate ways to
clean your teeth to avoid
injury. Be careful not to cut
yourself when using sharp
objects such as a safety
razor or nail cutters. Avoid
activities and contact sports
where bruising or injury
could occur. If you vomit
shortly after taking a dose
of melphalan, check with
your doctor. You may be
instructed to take the
dose again.

OVERDOSE
Symptoms: Vomiting,
mouth ulcerations, diarrhea,
gastrointestinal hemorrhage
(causing blood in the stool).

What to Do: Call your
doctor, emergency medical
services (EMS), or the
nearest poison control center immediately.

DRUG INTERACTIONS
Consult your doctor for specific advice if you are taking
amphotericin B, antithyroid
agents, azathioprine, chloramphenicol, colchicine,
flucytosine, interferon, plicamycin, probenecid, or
sulfinpyrazone. Also consult
your doctor if you are taking any over-the-counter
medications.

FOOD INTERACTIONS
No known food interactions.

DISEASE INTERACTIONS
Consult your doctor if you
have any of the following:
shingles, chicken pox, any
infection, kidney disease,
or lung disease.

Meperidine Hydrochloride

BRAND NAME
Demerol

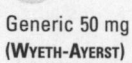

Generic 50 mg
(WYETH-AYERST)

▶ Drug Class: Opioid (narcotic) analgesic

▶ Available in: Syrup, tablets, injection

▶ Available OTC? No

▶ As Generic? Yes

Side Effects

SERIOUS
Meperidine should not be taken for a prolonged period. Serious side effects are indistinguishable from those of overdose: Confusion; slurred speech; extreme sedation, weakness, or dizziness; small, pinpoint pupils; cold, clammy skin; slow breathing; seizures; loss of consciousness.

COMMON
Dizziness or lightheadedness, nausea or vomiting, constipation, mild drowsiness, itching.

LESS COMMON
Mood swings or false sense of well-being (euphoria), redness or flushing of face.

PRINCIPAL USES
To treat moderate to severe pain.

HOW THE DRUG WORKS
Narcotics such as meperidine relieve pain by acting on specific areas of the spinal cord and brain that process pain signals from nerves throughout the body.

DOSAGE
Adults— Syrup or tablets: 50 to 150 mg every 3 or 4 hours as needed. Injection: 50 to 150 mg into a muscle or under the skin every 3 or 4 hours as needed. Children— Syrup, tablet, or injection into a muscle or under the skin: 1.1 to 1.76 mg per 2.2 lbs (1 kg) of body weight every 3 or 4 hours as needed.

ONSET OF EFFECT
Oral forms: 15 minutes. Injection: 10 to 15 minutes.

DURATION OF ACTION
2 to 4 hours.

DIETARY ADVICE
Tablets can be taken with food to lessen stomach upset. Syrup should be taken with a half glass of water.

STORAGE
Store the drug in a tightly sealed container away from heat, moisture, and direct light. Do not allow the liquid form to freeze.

IF YOU MISS A DOSE
If you are taking meperidine on a fixed schedule, take it as soon as you remember. If it is near the time for the next dose, skip the missed dose and resume your regular dosage schedule. Do not double the next dose.

STOPPING THE DRUG
The decision to stop taking the drug should be made by your doctor.

PROLONGED USE
Meperidine should not be taken for a prolonged period. Prolonged use can cause nerve damage and physical dependence. Do not abruptly stop taking meperidine without consulting your doctor.

PRECAUTIONS
Over 60: Adverse reactions may be more likely and more severe in older patients.

Driving and Hazardous Work: Do not drive or engage in hazardous work until you determine how the medicine affects you.

Alcohol: Avoid alcohol.

Pregnancy: Before you use this medication, tell your doctor if you are pregnant or plan to become pregnant. Overuse during pregnancy can cause physical dependence in the unborn baby. Meperidine use just before delivery can cause breathing problems in the newborn.

Breast Feeding: Meperidine passes into breast milk; caution is advised. Consult your doctor for specific advice.

Infants and Children: Adverse reactions may be more likely and more severe in infants and children. Consult your pediatrician for specific advice.

Special Concerns: If you feel the medication is not working properly after a few weeks, do not increase the dose. Consult your doctor. Before having any surgery, tell the doctor or dentist in charge that you are taking meperidine.

OVERDOSE
Symptoms: Confusion; slurred speech; extreme sedation, weakness, or dizziness; small, pinpoint pupils; cold, clammy skin; slow breathing; seizures; loss of consciousness.

What to Do: Call your doctor, emergency medical services (EMS), or the nearest poison control center immediately.

DRUG INTERACTIONS
Consult your doctor for specific advice if you are taking carbamazepine or other medicine for seizures, barbiturates, sedatives, cough medicines, decongestants, antidepressants, other prescription pain medications, MAO inhibitors, naltrexone, rifampin, or zidovudine.

FOOD INTERACTIONS
No known food interactions.

DISEASE INTERACTIONS
Consult your doctor if you have any of the following: history of alcohol or drug abuse; emotional illness; brain disorders or head injury; seizures; lung disease; prostate problems or other problems with urination; gallstones; colitis; heart, kidney, liver, or thyroid disease.

Mephenytoin

BRAND NAME
Mesantoin

▶ Drug Class: Hydantoin anticonvulsant

▶ Available in: Tablets

▶ Available OTC? No

▶ As Generic? No

Side Effects

SERIOUS
Fever, sore throat, swollen glands, red or purple point-like rash on the skin or mucous membranes, blistering or peeling skin lesions, mouth sores or bleeding, easy bruising, paleness, weakness, confusion, lethargy, or seizures may be a sign of a potentially fatal blood disorder or other complication. Call your doctor immediately.

COMMON
Dizziness, drowsiness, fatigue, clumsiness or unsteadiness, double vision, nervousness, nausea, vomiting, insomnia

LESS COMMON
Hair loss, weight gain, swelling, depression, disorientation. Numerous additional side effects are associated with the use of this drug; consult your doctor if you are concerned about any unusual reactions.

PRINCIPAL USES
To control certain kinds of seizures due to epilepsy. It is often given along with another anticonvulsant, such as phenytoin, phenobarbital, or primidone.

HOW THE DRUG WORKS
Mephenytoin is thought to depress the activity of certain parts of the brain and suppress the abnormal firing of neurons that causes seizures.

DOSAGE
Adults: 200 to 800 mg a day, in 3 divided doses. Children: 100 to 400 mg a day, in 3 divided doses. Some patients require higher doses. A low dose is used to start; it may then be gradually increased by your physician.

ONSET OF EFFECT
30 minutes.

DURATION OF ACTION
Maximum effectiveness lasts 24 to 48 hours; effectiveness then gradually decreases.

DIETARY ADVICE
Take with food to minimize stomach upset.

STORAGE
Store in a tightly sealed container away from heat, moisture, and direct light.

IF YOU MISS A DOSE
Take it as soon as you remember. However, if it is near the time for the next dose, skip the missed dose and resume you regular dosage schedule. Do not double the next dose unless advised to do so by your doctor.

STOPPING THE DRUG
Never stop taking this drug abruptly; seizures may ensue. The dose should be tapered gradually over a period of weeks under the supervision of your doctor.

PROLONGED USE
This drug is typically used on a long-term basis. If so, see your doctor regularly for tests and examinations.

PRECAUTIONS
Over 60: Adverse reactions may be more likely and more severe in older patients. A lower dose may be used.

Driving and Hazardous Work: This drug may cause drowsiness or dizziness, particularly in the first few weeks it is used. Do not drive or engage in hazardous work until you determine how the medicine affects you.

Alcohol: Avoid alcohol; it may contribute to excessive drowsiness.

Pregnancy: Anticonvulsants are associated with an increased risk of birth defects, although studies with this drug are incomplete. However, seizures during pregnancy can also increase the risks to the fetus. Discuss with your doctor the potential risks and benefits of using this drug during pregnancy. Folate supplementation is advised starting 1 to 2 months before conception and throughout pregnancy.

Breast Feeding: Mephenytoin may pass into breast milk, although at low levels. Consult your doctor for advice.

Infants and Children: Adverse reactions may be more frequent and more severe in infants and children. Not generally recommended in those younger than age 16.

Special Concerns: See your doctor for regular check-ups to detect the onset of any serious side effects. Your doctor may advise you to carry an ID card or bracelet that says you are taking this drug.

OVERDOSE
Symptoms: Blurred or double vision, difficulty walking, extreme clumsiness or unsteadiness, severe confusion, dizziness or drowsiness.

What to Do: Call your doctor, emergency medical services (EMS), or the nearest poison control center immediately.

DRUG INTERACTIONS
Mephenytoin can interact with many other drugs, including central nervous system depressants, xanthines, amiodarone, antacids, medicines containing calcium, anticoagulants, chloramphenicol, cimetidine, disulfiram, isoniazid, fluconazole, phenylbutazone, sulfonamides, corticosteroids, estrogens or oral contraceptives, corticotropin, oral diazoxide, lidocaine, methadone, phenacemide, rifampin, streptozocin, sucralfate, or other anticonvulsants (such as valproic acid).

FOOD INTERACTIONS
No known food interactions.

DISEASE INTERACTIONS
Special caution is advised in those with a blood disease, porphyria, lupus, coronary artery disease, kidney disease, or liver disease.

Meprobamate

BRAND NAMES
Equanil, Meprospan,
Miltown, Probate, Trancot

▶ Drug Class: Antianxiety drug

▶ Available in: Tablets,
   extended-release capsules

▶ Available OTC? No

▶ As Generic? Yes

Side Effects

SERIOUS
Skin rash, itching, or
hives, confusion, heart-
beat irregularities, sore
throat and fever, unusual
bruising or bleeding,
unusual excitability,
wheezing, shortness of
breath, slowed or labored
breathing. Call your doc-
tor immediately.

COMMON
Drowsiness, loss of coor-
dination, poor balance,
unsteadiness when walk-
ing or standing.

LESS COMMON
Blurred vision or other
vision disturbances, diarrhea, dizziness, lightheadedness, euphoria (false
sense of well-being), nausea, vomiting, headache,
unusual fatigue.

PRINCIPAL USES
To treat anxiety. This drug
is now rarely prescribed;
other drugs are more com-
monly prescribed for this
purpose.

HOW THE DRUG WORKS
The mechanism by which
meprobamate works is
unknown.

DOSAGE
Adults and teenagers—
Tablets: 400 mg, 3 or 4
times a day, or 600 mg,
2 times a day. Extended-
release capsules: 400 to
800 mg, 2 times a day.

ONSET OF EFFECT
Unknown.

DURATION OF ACTION
Unknown.

DIETARY ADVICE
Meprobamate can be taken
with food to prevent gas-
trointestinal upset.

STORAGE
Store in a tightly sealed container away from heat, moisture, and direct light.

IF YOU MISS A DOSE
Take it as soon as you
remember. However, if it is
near the time for the next
dose, skip the missed dose
and resume your regular
dosage schedule. Do not
double the next dose.

STOPPING THE DRUG
Do not stop taking
meprobamate abruptly, as
this may produce with-
drawal symptoms. The
dosage should be reduced
gradually according to your
doctor's instructions.

PROLONGED USE
See your doctor for periodic
evaluation if you must take
this drug for an extended
length of time.

PRECAUTIONS
Over 60: Adverse reactions
may be more likely and
more severe in older
patients.

**Driving and Hazardous
Work:** Meprobamate can
impair mental alertness and
physical coordination. If you
experience such problems,
consult your doctor about
adjusting your dosage.

Alcohol: Alcohol intake
should be extremely moderate or stopped altogether
while taking this drug.

Pregnancy: Meprobamate
may increase the risk of
birth defects if taken early
in pregnancy. Before you
take it, be sure to tell your
doctor if you are pregnant
or plan to become pregnant.

Breast Feeding: Meprobamate passes into breast
milk; do not take it while
nursing.

Infants and Children:
Meprobamate is not recom-
mended for use by children
under the age of 6.

Special Concerns:
Meprobamate use can lead
to psychological or physical
dependence. Short-term
therapy (8 weeks or less)
is typical; do not take the
drug for a longer period
unless advised otherwise by
your physician. Never take
more than the prescribed
daily dose.

OVERDOSE
Symptoms: Severe
confusion, lightheadedness,
dizziness, or drowsiness,
lethargy, shortness of breath,
loss of consciousness.

What to Do: Call your
doctor, emergency medical
services (EMS), or the
nearest poison control
center immediately.

DRUG INTERACTIONS
Consult your doctor for specific advice if you are taking
any drugs that depress the
central nervous system;
these include antihista-
mines, antidepressants or
other psychiatric medica-
tions, barbiturates, sedatives, cough medicines,
decongestants, and
painkillers. Be sure your
doctor knows about any
over-the-counter medication
you may take.

FOOD INTERACTIONS
None reported.

DISEASE INTERACTIONS
Caution is advised when
taking meprobamate. Con-
sult your doctor if you have
a history of alcohol or drug
abuse, epilepsy, or por-
phyria. Use of meprobamate
may cause complications in
patients with impaired liver
or kidney function, since
these organs work together
to remove the medication
from the body.

Mercaptopurine

Purinethol 50 mg
(GLAXO WELLCOME)

▶ Drug Class: Antimetabolite

▶ Available in: Tablets

▶ Available OTC? No

▶ As Generic? No

Side Effects

SERIOUS
Black or tarry stools; blood-tinged urine or stools; cough or hoarseness; fever; chills; lower back pain or pain in flanks; painful, difficult urination; small, red spots on the skin; bleeding from gums, nose, or other unusual places; easy bruising; shortness of breath. See your doctor right away if any of these occur. Other serious side effects include low white blood cell and platelet counts, anemia, and liver damage. Such problems can be detected by your doctor.

COMMON
Unusual fatigue, yellowish tinge to skin and eyes (jaundice). Notify your doctor.

LESS COMMON
Nausea, vomiting, abdominal pain or bloating, mouth sores, darkening of skin, diarrhea, headaches, skin rash and itching, weakness.

PRINCIPAL USES
To treat certain types of leukemia.

HOW THE DRUG WORKS
Mercaptopurine kills cancer cells by interfering with the synthesis of their genetic material, which prevents the cells from reproducing. The drug may also affect the growth and development of other kinds of cells in the body, resulting in unpleasant side effects.

DOSAGE
A variety of dosage schedules and regimens for mercaptopurine, with and without other antitumor drugs, is used. For acute myeloblastic leukemia, acute lymphocytic leukemia, and chronic myelocytic leukemia, the initial dose is 80 to 100 mg per square meter of body surface, once a day. Maintenance dose is 50 to 100 mg per square meter of body surface a day.

ONSET OF EFFECT
2 hours.

DURATION OF ACTION
Variable.

DIETARY ADVICE
Drink plenty of fluids.

STORAGE
Store in a tightly sealed container away from heat and direct light.

IF YOU MISS A DOSE
Take it as soon as you remember. However, if it is near the time for the next dose, skip the missed dose and resume your regular dosage schedule. Do not double the next dose.

STOPPING THE DRUG
The decision to stop taking the drug should be made by your doctor.

PROLONGED USE
See your doctor regularly for tests and examinations if you must take this drug for a prolonged period.

PRECAUTIONS
Over 60: No special problems are expected.

Driving and Hazardous Work: Avoid such activities until you determine how the medicine affects you.

Alcohol: Avoid alcohol.

Pregnancy: Mercaptopurine may cause birth defects if either the father or the mother is taking it at the time of conception. Persons of childbearing years should take steps to prevent pregnancy when taking this medication.

Breast Feeding: Not recommended during therapy.

Infants and Children: No special warnings.

Special Concerns: Your doctor will want to check blood work (liver, kidney, and blood cell function) weekly or monthly while you are taking this medicine. If you vomit after taking a dose, call your doctor to learn if you should take the dose again or wait for the next dose. Do not receive any immunizations while you are taking mercaptopurine, and avoid people with infections. Be careful when brushing your teeth and check with your doctor before having dental work done. Take care not to cut yourself when using sharp objects such as a safety razor. Avoid contact sports.

OVERDOSE
Symptoms: Loss of appetite, nausea, vomiting, diarrhea, gastrointestinal upset.

What to Do: Call your doctor, emergency medical services (EMS), or the nearest poison control center immediately.

DRUG INTERACTIONS
Consult your doctor for specific advice if you are taking acetaminophen, amiodarone, anabolic steroids, androgens, antibiotics, carbamazepine, chloroquine, dantrolene, disulfiram, divalproex, estrogens, etretinate, gold salts, hydroxychloroquine, methyldopa, naltrexone, oral contraceptives, phenothiazines, phenytoin, plicamycin, valproic acid, azathioprine, corticosteroids, cyclosporine, monoclonal antibodies, allopurinol, amphotericin B, antithyroid agents, chloramphenicol, colchicine, flucytosine, ganciclovir, interferon, zidovudine, probenecid, or sulfinpyrazone.

FOOD INTERACTIONS
No known food interactions.

DISEASE INTERACTIONS
Consult your doctor if you have a history of chicken pox, shingles, gout, kidney stones, any infection, kidney disease, or liver disease.

Mesalamine

**Asacol 400 mg
(P&GP)**

▶ Drug Class: Gastrointestinal anti-inflammatory

▶ Available in: Extended-release capsules, delayed-release tablets, enema

▶ Available OTC? No

▶ As Generic? No

Side Effects

SERIOUS
Severe abdominal pains or cramps; bloody diarrhea; fever; severe headache; skin rash and itching; blue or pale skin; severe back or stomach pain, possibly moving to the left arm, neck, or shoulder; chills; rapid heartbeat; nausea or vomiting; shortness of breath; swollen stomach; unusual fatigue; yellow eyes or skin; rectal irritation (with enema). Call your doctor immediately.

COMMON
Mild abdominal cramping, mild diarrhea, dizziness, headache, runny or stuffy nose, sneezing.

LESS COMMON
Acne, back or joint pain, gas or flatulence, loss of appetite, loss of hair.

PRINCIPAL USES
To treat inflammatory bowel diseases such as ulcerative colitis.

HOW THE DRUG WORKS
The exact mechanism of action is uncertain, although it appears that mesalamine inhibits the production of substances known as metabolites of arachidonic acid (leukotrienes and prostaglandins), which produce inflammation in the digestive tract.

DOSAGE
Dosage can differ for different brands. Extended-release capsules— Adults: 1 g, 4 times a day for up to 8 weeks. Delayed-release tablets— Adults: Asacol: 800 mg, 3 times a day for 6 weeks. Enema— 4 g (1 unit) used every night for 3 to 6 weeks.

ONSET OF EFFECT
Unknown.

DURATION OF ACTION
Unknown.

DIETARY ADVICE
Take the oral forms before meals and at bedtime with a full glass of water unless you are directed otherwise by your doctor.

STORAGE
Store in a tightly sealed container away from heat and direct light.

IF YOU MISS A DOSE
Take the oral forms as soon as you remember. If it is near the time for the next dose, skip the missed dose and resume your regular dosage schedule. If you miss a dose of mesalamine enema, take it if you remember the same night. Otherwise, skip the missed dose and resume your regular dosage schedule. In all cases, do not double the next dose.

STOPPING THE DRUG
Take as prescribed for the full treatment period, even if you begin to feel better before the scheduled end of therapy.

PROLONGED USE
You should see your doctor regularly for tests and examinations if you take this drug for a prolonged period.

PRECAUTIONS
Over 60: There is no information comparing the use of mesalamine by older patients with use by other age groups.

Driving and Hazardous Work: Do not drive or engage in hazardous work until you determine how the medicine affects you.

Alcohol: Avoid alcohol.

Pregnancy: Mesalamine has not caused birth defects in animals. Human studies have not been done. Before you take mesalamine, tell your doctor if you are pregnant or plan to become pregnant.

Breast Feeding: Mesalamine may pass into breast milk; caution is advised. Consult your doctor for advice.

Infants and Children: There is no specific information comparing use of mesalamine in infants and children with use in other age groups. Use and dose must be determined by your doctor.

Special Concerns: Do not change to another brand without consulting your doctor. The enema may stain clothing, fabrics, or any surface that it touches.

OVERDOSE
Symptoms: Confusion, severe diarrhea, dizziness or lightheadedness, drowsiness, severe headache, hearing loss, buzzing or ringing in ear, continuing nausea or vomiting.

What to Do: An overdose of mesalamine is unlikely to be life-threatening. However, if someone takes a much larger dose than prescribed, call your doctor, emergency medical services (EMS), or the nearest poison control center.

DRUG INTERACTIONS
Be sure to consult your doctor if you are taking any other prescription or over-the-counter medication.

FOOD INTERACTIONS
No known food interactions.

DISEASE INTERACTIONS
Those with kidney disease should not take mesalamine, as it may make the condition worse. Patients with hypertension should be monitored closely.

Metaproterenol

BRAND NAMES
Alupent, Arm-a-Med
Metaproterenol, Dey-Lute
Metaproterenol, Metaprel

Generic 10 mg
(PAR)

▶ Drug Class: Bronchodilator/
sympathomimetic

▶ Available in: Inhalation
aerosol or solution, syrup,
tablets

▶ Available OTC? No

▶ As Generic? Yes

Side Effects

SERIOUS
Inhaled form: May
become ineffective if
used too often, resulting
in more-severe breathing
difficulty that does not
improve. Signs include
persistent wheezing,
coughing, or shortness of
breath; confusion; bluish
color to lips or finger-
nails; inability to speak.
Ingested form: Chest pain
or heaviness; irregular,
racing, fluttering, or
pounding heartbeat;
lightheadedness; fainting;
severe weakness; severe
headache.

COMMON
Trouble sleeping, dry
mouth, sore throat, ner-
vousness, restlessness.

LESS COMMON
Trembling, sweating,
headache, nausea or
vomiting, flushing or redness to cheeks or other
skin, muscle aches,
unpleasant or unusual
taste in mouth.

PRINCIPAL USES
To dilate air passages in the
lungs that have become narrowed as a result of disease
or inflammation. It is used
in the treatment of asthma
and chronic obstructive pulmonary disease (COPD).

HOW THE DRUG WORKS
Metaproterenol widens
constricted airways by
relaxing the smooth mus-
cles that surround the
bronchial passages.

DOSAGE
Use when needed to relieve
breathing difficulty. Inhalation solution for nebulizers— Adults and children
over 12 years of age: Usual
dose is 10 inhalations, not
to be taken more frequently
than every 3 to 4 hours, for
a usual maximum of 3 to 4
times a day. Infants and children under 12 years of age:
Consult a pediatrician.
Inhalation aerosol— Adults
and children 12 years and
older: 2 to 3 puffs every 3
to 4 hours. Do not exceed
more than 12 puffs per day.
Infants and children under
12 years of age: Not recommended. Syrup and
tablets— Adults and chil-
dren 9 years of age and
older: 20 mg, 3 or 4 times
a day. Infants and children
under 9 years of age:
Consult a pediatrician.

ONSET OF EFFECT
Inhalation: Within 5 min-
utes. Oral: 15 to 30 minutes.

DURATION OF ACTION
Inhalation: 1 to 5 hours.
Oral: Up to 4 hours.

DIETARY ADVICE
Maintain your usual food
and fluid intake.

STORAGE
Store in a tightly sealed container away from heat and
direct light. Do not refrigerate inhalation solutions.

IF YOU MISS A DOSE
Skip the missed dose and
resume your regular dosage
schedule. Do not double the
next dose.

STOPPING THE DRUG
It may not be necessary to
finish the recommended
course of therapy. Consult
your doctor.

PROLONGED USE
Therapy may require
months or years. Excessive
use may result in temporary
loss of effectiveness.

PRECAUTIONS
Over 60: Adverse reactions
may be more likely and
more severe in older
patients.

**Driving and Hazardous
Work:** Avoid such activities
until you determine how the
medicine affects you.

Alcohol: No special precautions are necessary.

Pregnancy: Adequate studies have not been done; the
benefits must be weighed
against potential risks. Consult your doctor for specific
advice.

Breast Feeding: Mothers
who wish to breast feed
while taking this drug
should discuss the matter
with their doctor.

Infants and Children:
Use of the inhalation
aerosol is not recommended
in children younger than 12.

Special Concerns: Pay
heed to any breathing problem that does not improve
after your usual nebulizer
treatment or usual number
of puffs. Seek help immediately if you feel your lungs
are persistently constricted,
if you are using more than
the recommended number
of treatments per day, or if
you feel a recent attack is
somehow different from
others.

OVERDOSE
Symptoms: Chest pain or
heaviness; irregular, racing,
fluttering, or pounding
heartbeat; dizziness; lightheadedness; fainting; severe
weakness; severe headache.

What to Do: Call your
doctor, emergency medical
services (EMS), or the
nearest poison control center immediately.

DRUG INTERACTIONS
Consult your doctor for specific advice if you are taking
a beta-blocker, ergotamine
or ergotamine-like medications, antidepressants, digitalis drugs, or an MAO
inhibitor.

FOOD INTERACTIONS
No known food interactions.

DISEASE INTERACTIONS
Consult your doctor if you
have a history of substance
abuse (especially cocaine),
seizures, brain damage,
heart disease, heartbeat
irregularities, high blood
pressure, anxiety disorders,
or a thyroid condition.

Metformin

Glucophage 850 mg
(Bristol-Myers Squibb)

▶ Drug Class: Antidiabetic
agent/biguanide

▶ Available in: Tablets,
extended-release tablets

▶ Available OTC? No

▶ As Generic? No

Side Effects

SERIOUS
In rare cases, metformin
may lead to lactic acido-
sis, an abnormal and
potentially life-threatening buildup of lactic acid
in the blood. Symptoms
include rapid, shallow
breathing, unusual sleepiness or weakness, mus-
cle pain, and abdominal
distress. Metformin also
occasionally causes
abnormally low blood
glucose levels (hypo-
glycemia); symptoms
include blurred vision,
cold sweats, confusion,
anxiousness, rapid heart-
beat, shakiness, and
nausea. Seek medical
assistance immediately.

COMMON
Diarrhea, nausea, vomit-
ing, abdominal bloating,
gas, diminished appetite.
Usually such symptoms
are mild and transient.
Consult your doctor if the
symptoms persist or
increase in severity.

LESS COMMON
Unpleasant or metallic
taste in mouth.

PRINCIPAL USES
Used to lower abnormally
high blood glucose (sugar)
levels in patients with non-
insulin-dependent (type 2)
diabetes whose blood sugar
levels cannot be adequately
controlled by diet or exercise alone. The drug may
be used alone or in conjunction with sulfonylurea drugs
or insulin.

HOW THE DRUG WORKS
Metformin decreases the
liver's production of glucose, inhibits the break-
down of fatty acids used
to produce glucose, and
increases the removal of
glucose from muscle, the
liver, and other body tissues
where it is stored.

DOSAGE
Available in 500 mg, 850
mg, or 1,000 mg tablets;
extended-release tablets are
available in 500-mg strength
only and should not be used
by patients under the age of
17. Initial dose: 500 mg a
day, taken with dinner. If
tolerated, a second dose can
be added, taken with breakfast. The dose may be
slowly increased (1 tablet
every 1 or 2 weeks) to a
maximum of 2,500 mg a
day. Alternatively, 850 mg
daily, increased by 850 mg
every other week to a maximum of 2,550 mg per day.

ONSET OF EFFECT
Within 2 hours.

DURATION OF ACTION
From 12 to 15 hours.

DIETARY ADVICE
Take with meals to reduce
risk of stomach upset.

STORAGE
Store in a sealed container
at room temperature away
from heat and direct light.

IF YOU MISS A DOSE
Take it with food as soon as
you remember. However, if
it is almost time for the next
dose, skip the missed dose
and resume your regular
dosage schedule. Do not
double the next dose.

STOPPING THE DRUG
Stop taking metformin only
when your doctor advises.

PROLONGED USE
Because metformin helps to
manage diabetes but does
not cure the disease, its use
will be ongoing as long as
your blood glucose levels
are being adequately con-
trolled. If not, the met-
formin dosage may be
adjusted or a different
treatment prescribed.

PRECAUTIONS
Over 60: Because met-
formin is metabolized in the
kidneys, extra caution is
warranted in thin, elderly
patients with mild adrenal
insufficiency (not often
detected by the usual tests
for kidney impairment).

**Driving and Hazardous
Work:** No special precautions are necessary.

Alcohol: Excessive
amounts of alcohol can
increase the effect of metformin, possibly resulting in
abnormally low blood glu-
cose levels.

Pregnancy: Taking metformin is not advised during
pregnancy. Consult your
doctor if you become pregnant or plan to become
pregnant; insulin is usually
the treatment of choice for
pregnant diabetic women.

Breast Feeding: Met-
formin passes into breast
milk, although it has not
been shown to cause harm
to nursing infants. Consult
your doctor for advice.

Infants and Children:
Glucophage may be used in
children 10 years of age and
older; Glucophage XR may
be used in children 17 years
of age and older.

Special Concerns: Do not
take metformin if you have
previously had an allergic
reaction to it.

OVERDOSE
Symptoms: Symptoms of
lactic acidosis or hypo-
glyccmia (see Serious Side
Effects).

What to Do: Seek emergency medical assistance
right away.

DRUG INTERACTIONS
Consult your doctor if you
are taking any of the following: amiloride, calcium
channel blockers, cimeti-
dine, digoxin, furosemide,
morphine, procainamide,
quinidine, quinine, ranitidine, trimethoprim, tri-
amterene, or vancomycin.

FOOD INTERACTIONS
The amount and type of
food you eat affect your
blood glucose levels and
must be taken into account
while you receive met-
formin therapy.

DISEASE INTERACTIONS
Do not take metformin if
you have any condition that
requires careful control of
blood glucose levels, such
as severe infection; any condition contributing to abnormally low blood oxygen
levels, such as congestive
heart failure or emphysema;
metabolic acidosis (buildup
of acid in the blood); a history of alcohol abuse; or
kidney or liver disease.

Methadone Hydrochloride

Generic 5 mg
(ROXANE)

▶ Drug Class: Opioid (narcotic) analgesic

▶ Available in: Oral concentrate, oral solution, tablets, injection

▶ Available OTC? No

▶ As Generic? Yes

Side Effects

SERIOUS
Serious side effects of methadone are indistinguishable from those of overdose: Confusion; severe drowsiness, weakness, or dizziness; slurred speech; small, pinpoint pupils; cold, clammy skin; slow breathing; seizures; loss of consciousness.

COMMON
Dizziness or lightheadedness, nausea or vomiting, constipation, drowsiness, itching.

LESS COMMON
Sweating, swelling of the feet and ankles, redness or flushing of face.

PRINCIPAL USES
To relieve severe pain. It is also used to prevent or ease withdrawal symptoms during detoxification from illegal narcotics, and to serve as maintenance therapy during narcotic addiction treatment programs.

HOW THE DRUG WORKS
Methadone is a long-acting opioid. It binds with natural opiate receptors throughout the central nervous system, thereby altering the perception of and emotional response to pain.

DOSAGE
For pain— Oral solution: 5 to 20 mg every 6 to 8 hours. Tablets: 5 to 10 mg every 6 to 8 hours. For narcotic addiction maintenance therapy— Oral solution or tablets: Up to 120 mg a day, depending on individual needs. Children: Dosages must be determined by your doctor. The injectable form is administered only when patients are unable to take methadone orally.

ONSET OF EFFECT
Oral forms: 30 minutes to 1 hour.

DURATION OF ACTION
Oral forms: 4 to 8 hours.

DIETARY ADVICE
Oral forms can be taken with food to lessen stomach upset. Dispersible tablets should be stirred into water or juice before taking.

STORAGE
Store the medication in a tightly sealed container away from heat, moisture, and direct light. Do not freeze the liquid forms.

IF YOU MISS A DOSE
If you are taking methadone on a fixed schedule, take as soon as you remember. If it is near the time for the next dose, skip the missed dose and resume your regular dosage schedule. Do not double the next dose.

STOPPING THE DRUG
The decision to stop taking the drug should be made by your doctor.

PROLONGED USE
Prolonged use can cause physical dependence.

PRECAUTIONS
Over 60: Adverse reactions may be more likely and more severe in older patients.

Driving and Hazardous Work: Avoid such activities until you determine how the medicine affects you.

Alcohol: Avoid alcohol.

Pregnancy: Adequate human studies have not been done. Before taking methadone, tell your doctor if you are pregnant or plan to become pregnant, and discuss the relative risks and benefits of methadone use during pregnancy.

Breast Feeding: Methadone passes into breast milk; caution is advised. Taking large doses in a maintenance program can cause physical dependence in the baby. Consult your doctor for advice.

Infants and Children: Adverse reactions may be more likely and more severe in children. Consult your doctor for advice.

Special Concerns: If you feel the medication is not working properly after a few weeks, do not increase the dose. Consult your doctor. Before having any surgery, tell the doctor or dentist in charge that you are taking methadone.

OVERDOSE
Symptoms: Confusion; slurred speech; extreme sedation, weakness, or dizziness; small, pinpoint pupils; cold, clammy skin; slow breathing; seizures; loss of consciousness.

What to Do: Call your doctor, emergency medical services (EMS), or the nearest poison control center immediately.

DRUG INTERACTIONS
Consult your doctor for specific advice if you are taking carbamazepine or other medicine for seizures, barbiturates, sedatives, cough medicines, decongestants, antidepressants, other prescription pain medications, MAO inhibitors, naltrexone, rifampin, or zidovudine.

FOOD INTERACTIONS
None are known.

DISEASE INTERACTIONS
Consult your doctor if you have any of the following: history of alcohol or drug abuse; emotional illness; brain disorders or head injury; seizures; lung disease; prostate problems or other problems with urination; gallstones; colitis; heart, kidney, liver, or thyroid disease.

Methamphetamine Hydrochloride

▶ Drug Class: Central
nervous system stimulant/
amphetamine

▶ Available in: Tablets,
extended-release tablets

▶ Available OTC? No

▶ As Generic? No

Side Effects

SERIOUS
Irregular heartbeat, chest
pain, increased blood
pressure, skin rash,
uncontrollable move-
ments of arms and legs,
mental changes, unusual
weakness, very high
fever. Call your doctor
immediately.

COMMON
Mood changes, insomnia,
drowsiness, restlessness.

LESS COMMON
Blurred vision, constipa-
tion, diarrhea, loss of
appetite, headache,
increased sweating,
stomach cramps or
abdominal pain, nausea
or vomiting, changes
in sexual desire or
decreased sexual ability.

PRINCIPAL USES
To treat narcolepsy and
attention-deficit hyperactivity disorder (ADHD) in children and adults.

HOW THE DRUG WORKS
Methamphetamine activates
nerve cells in the brain and
spinal cord to increase
motor activity and alertness,
and lessen drowsiness and
fatigue. In hyperactivity disorders and narcolepsy,
amphetamines improve the
ability to pay attention.

DOSAGE
Children age 6 and older—
To start, regular tablets are
used, 5 mg, 1 or 2 times a
day. The dose is gradually
increased to 20 to 25 mg a
day, either as regular tablets
(in 2 or 3 divided doses) or
extended-release tablets
(once a day). Adults—
Tablets: To start, 5 mg, 2
or 3 times a day. Extended-
release tablets: To start, 10
mg, 1 or 2 times a day. The
dosage may be increased to
a total of 60 mg a day, in 2
or 3 divided doses.

ONSET OF EFFECT
Variable.

DURATION OF ACTION
Variable.

DIETARY ADVICE
This drug can be taken
without regard to food.
Avoid caffeine-containing
beverages like tea, coffee,
and some carbonated colas.
Avoid acidic foods that are
rich in vitamin C, such as
fruit juices and other citrus
products. Avoid vitamin C
tablets.

STORAGE
Store in a tightly sealed container away from heat, moisture, and direct light.

IF YOU MISS A DOSE
Take the missed dose as
soon as you remember. If it
is close to the next dose or
within 6 hours of bedtime,
skip the missed dose and
resume your regular dosage
schedule. Do not double the
next dose.

STOPPING THE DRUG
Take it as prescribed for the
full treatment period, even
if you begin to feel better
before the scheduled end
of therapy. The decision to
stop taking the drug should
be made by your doctor.
The doctor may decrease
your dosage gradually to
reduce the possibility of
withdrawal symptoms.

PROLONGED USE
Amphetamines can be habit-
forming, and prolonged use
may increase the risk of
dependency.

PRECAUTIONS
Over 60: There is no specific information comparing
use of methamphetamine in
older patients with use in
younger persons.

**Driving and Hazardous
Work:** Do not drive or
engage in hazardous work
until you determine how the
medicine affects you.

Alcohol: Avoid alcohol.

Pregnancy: Adequate
human studies have not
been completed. Before taking methamphetamine, tell
your doctor if you are pregnant or plan to become
pregnant.

Breast Feeding: Methamphetamine passes into
breast milk; do not use
it while nursing.

Infants and Children:
This drug is not recom-
mended for use by children
under age 6.

Special Concerns: Take
methamphetamine only as
directed and do not
increase the dose on your
own. Remember that
fatigue, excessive drowsiness, or depression while
taking stimulants may mean
an emergency situation is
developing. Difficulty sleeping may be improved by
taking the last scheduled
dose several hours before
bedtime.

OVERDOSE
Symptoms: Extreme
degrees of restlessness,
agitation, bizarre behavior;
panic; rapid breathing; confusion; high fever; hallucinations; seizures; coma.

What to Do: Call your
doctor, emergency medical
services (EMS), or the
nearest poison control
center immediately.

DRUG INTERACTIONS
Consult your doctor for specific advice if you are taking
tricyclic antidepressants,
caffeine, beta-blockers, digitalis drugs, central nervous
system stimulants, meperidine, MAO inhibitors, sympathomimetic agents, or
thyroid hormones.

FOOD INTERACTIONS
Citrus juices and caffeinated
beverages and foods may
interact with this drug.

DISEASE INTERACTIONS
Consult your doctor if you
have any of the following:
advanced blood vessel disease, heart disease, hyperthyroidism, hypertension,
severe anxiety, Tourette's
syndrome, glaucoma, or a
history of drug abuse.

Methenamine and Methenamine Salts

Generic 500 mg
(JEROME STEVENS)

▶ Drug Class: Anti-infective

▶ Available in: Tablets, enteric-coated tablets, oral suspension, granules for solution

▶ Available OTC? No

▶ As Generic? Yes

Side Effects

SERIOUS
Skin rash, blood in urine, lower back pain, burning or pain while urinating. Call your physician immediately.

COMMON
No common side effects are associated with the use of methenamine.

LESS COMMON
Nausea or vomiting may occur. Contact your doctor if such symptoms persist.

PRINCIPAL USES
To prevent and treat urinary tract infections.

HOW THE DRUG WORKS
Methenamine and methenamine salts kill bacteria in the urinary tract by forming ammonia and formaldehyde, chemicals that are toxic to the microorganisms that cause infection.

DOSAGE
For prevention of infection— Adults and teenagers: 1,000 mg, 2 times a day. Children ages 6 to 12: 500 mg to 1,000 mg, 2 times a day. For treatment of infection— Adults and teenagers: 1,000 mg, 4 times a day. Children ages 6 to 12: 500 mg, 4 times a day. Children up to age 6: 8.3 mg per lb of body weight, 4 times a day.

ONSET OF EFFECT
Within 1 hour.

DURATION OF ACTION
Up to 8 hours.

DIETARY ADVICE
Take it after meals and at bedtime. Drink plenty of liquids, ensuring that your fluid intake is at least 2 quarts a day. This drug works best in highly acidic urine. Maintain a protein-rich diet and consume liberal amounts of cranberries or cranberry juice, plums, or prunes to ensure sufficiently acidic urine. If this cannot be achieved through diet alone, take vitamin C supplements. Avoid citrus fruits and juices.

STORAGE
Store in a tightly sealed container away from heat and direct light.

IF YOU MISS A DOSE
Take it as soon as you remember. However, if it is near the time for the next dose, skip the missed dose and resume your regular dosage schedule. Do not double the next dose.

STOPPING THE DRUG
Take as prescribed for the full treatment period, even if you begin to feel better before the scheduled end of therapy.

PROLONGED USE
Consult your doctor about the need for liver function tests and other tests during prolonged therapy.

PRECAUTIONS
Over 60: Adverse reactions may be more likely and more severe in older patients.

Driving and Hazardous Work: Avoid such activities until you determine how the medication affects you.

Alcohol: No special precautions are necessary.

Pregnancy: It is not known whether methenamine is harmful during pregnancy. Discuss with your physician the relative risks and benefits.

Breast Feeding: Methenamine passes into breast milk but has not been reported to cause problems in nursing babies. Consult your doctor about its use during nursing.

Infants and Children: No special problems are expected.

Special Concerns: If you take the dry granule form of methenamine, dissolve the contents of each packet in 2 to 4 ounces of water and stir well before drinking it. Avoid use of antacids while taking this medicine. Urine pH should be monitored before starting and throughout therapy.

OVERDOSE
Symptoms: No specific ones have been reported.

What to Do: An overdose of methenamine is unlikely to be life-threatening. However, if someone takes a much larger dose than prescribed, call your doctor, emergency medical services (EMS), or the nearest poison control center.

DRUG INTERACTIONS
Consult your doctor for advice if you are taking thiazide diuretics, sodium bicarbonate, methazolamide, sulfamethoxazole, or urinary alkalizers such as acetazolamide.

FOOD INTERACTIONS
While taking methenamine, avoid milk products, citrus fruits and juices, and alkaline foods like vegetables and peanuts.

DISEASE INTERACTIONS
Use of methenamine may cause complications in patients with liver or kidney disease, since these organs work together to remove the medication from the body. Before you take methenamine, tell your doctor if you have ever experienced severe dehydration.

Methimazole

Tapazole 5 mg
(LILLY)

▶ Drug Class: Antithyroid agent

▶ Available in: Tablets

▶ Available OTC? No

▶ As Generic? No

Side Effects

SERIOUS
Cough, continuing or severe fever or chills, hoarseness, mouth sores, pain, swelling, or redness in joints, throat infection, yellow discoloration of the skin or eyes, general feeling of illness. Call your doctor immediately.

COMMON
Mild and temporary fever; rash or itching.

LESS COMMON
Backache; black and tarry stools; blood in urine or stools; shortness of breath; increased or decreased urination; swelling of feet or lower legs; swollen lymph or salivary glands; numbness or tingling of face, fingers, or toes; dizziness; nausea; stomach pain; vomiting.

PRINCIPAL USES
To treat conditions in which the thyroid gland produces too much thyroid hormone.

HOW THE DRUG WORKS
Methimazole interferes with the body's ability to use iodine in the manufacture of thyroid hormone.

DOSAGE
Adults: 15 to 60 mg a day in 1 daily dose or in 2 divided daily doses. Usual maintenance dose is 5 to 15 mg a day. Children: 0.2 mg per 2.2 lbs (1 kg) of body weight a day in 1 daily dose or in 2 divided daily doses. To treat a thyroid crisis: 12 to 20 mg every 4 hours.

ONSET OF EFFECT
5 days or more.

DURATION OF ACTION
Unknown.

DIETARY ADVICE
Methimazole can be taken with or without food. It should be taken consistently in the same way, either with or between meals.

STORAGE
Store in a tightly sealed container away from heat and direct light.

IF YOU MISS A DOSE
Take it as soon as you remember. However, if it is near the time for the next dose, skip the missed dose and resume your regular dosage schedule. Do not double the next dose.

STOPPING THE DRUG
Take it as prescribed for the full treatment period, even if you begin to feel better before the scheduled end of therapy.

PROLONGED USE
No special problems are expected. It may be necessary to take this medication for several years.

PRECAUTIONS
Over 60: Adverse reactions may be more common and more severe in older patients.

Driving and Hazardous Work: The use of this medication should not impair your ability to perform such tasks safely.

Alcohol: Consult your doctor about using alcohol while taking methimazole.

Pregnancy: Too large a dose during pregnancy may cause problems in the fetus. Use of the prescribed dose, with careful monitoring, is not likely to cause problems.

Breast Feeding: Methimazole passes into breast milk, but your doctor may allow you to continue to nurse if the dose is low and the infant is checked regularly.

Infants and Children: No special problems are expected.

Special Concerns: Before undergoing any kind of medical or dental procedure, tell the doctor or dentist in charge that you are taking methimazole. During and after treatment with methimazole, do not receive any immunizations without your doctor's approval, and avoid persons who have taken oral polio vaccine recently.

OVERDOSE
Symptoms: Nausea, vomiting, coldness, constipation, changes in menstrual period, dry and puffy skin, headache, listlessness, swollen neck, sleepiness, muscle aches, unusual weight gain.

What to Do: An overdose of methimazole is unlikely to be life-threatening. However, if someone takes a much larger dose than prescribed, call your doctor, emergency medical services (EMS), or the local poison control center right away.

DRUG INTERACTIONS
Consult your doctor for specific advice if you are taking amiodarone, iodinated glycerol, potassium iodide, anticoagulants, beta-blockers, theophylline, or digitalis drugs.

FOOD INTERACTIONS
Consult your doctor about a special low-iodine diet.

DISEASE INTERACTIONS
Use of methimazole may cause complications in patients with liver disease, since this organ works to remove the medication from the body.

Methocarbamol

Generic 750 mg
(GENEVA)

▶ Drug Class: Muscle relaxant

▶ Available in: Tablets, injection

▶ Available OTC? No

▶ As Generic? Yes

Side Effects

SERIOUS
Fainting; palpitations or
rapid heartbeat; fever;
hives or severe swelling
of face, lips, or tongue
along with shortness of
breath, chest tightness,
or wheezing (indicating a
potentially life-threatening allergic reaction);
seizures; mental depres-
sion. Seek medical help
immediately.

COMMON
Blurred, double, or
altered vision, dizziness
or lightheadedness,
drowsiness, dry mouth.

LESS COMMON
Inability to pass urine;
sores on lips, ulcers in
mouth; abdominal
cramps or pain; clumsi-
ness; unsteady gait; con-
fusion; constipation;
diarrhea; excitability, nervousness, restlessness,
or irritability; flushing
or redness of face; head-
ache; heartburn; hiccups;
muscle weakness; nausea
and vomiting; trembling;
insomnia or fitful sleep;
burning, red eyes;
stuffy nose.

PRINCIPAL USES
Muscle relaxants are used
to relieve stiffness and discomfort caused by severe
sprains and strains, muscle
spasms, or other muscle
problems. They may be prescribed in conjunction with
other treatment methods,
such as physical therapy.

HOW THE DRUG WORKS
Muscle relaxants such as
methocarbamol depress
activity in the central nervous system (brain and
spinal cord), which in turn
interferes with the transmission of nerve impulses from
the spinal cord to the skeletal muscles.

DOSAGE
Adults and teenagers—
Tablets: 1,500 mg, 4 times a
day to start, then the dose
may be reduced. Injection: 1
to 3 g a day, in 1 or several
doses. Children— Consult
your pediatrician.

ONSET OF EFFECT
Immediate after injection;
within 30 minutes after oral
administration.

DURATION OF ACTION
Unknown.

DIETARY ADVICE
Take the tablets with food
to reduce stomach irritation.

STORAGE
Store in a tightly sealed container away from heat and
direct light.

IF YOU MISS A DOSE
Take it as soon as you
remember. However, if it is
near the time for the next
dose, skip the missed dose
and resume your regular
dosage schedule. Do not
double the next dose.

STOPPING THE DRUG
The decision to stop taking
the drug should be made by
your doctor.

PROLONGED USE
You should see your doctor
regularly for tests and
examinations if you take
this drug for a prolonged
period.

PRECAUTIONS
Over 60: No special problems are expected.

**Driving and Hazardous
Work:** Do not drive or
engage in hazardous work
until you determine how the
medicine affects you.

Alcohol: Avoid alcohol
while taking this drug
because it may compound
the sedative effect and may
cause liver damage.

Pregnancy: Adequate studies of methocarbamol dur-
ing pregnancy have not
been done; discuss relative
risks and benefits with your
doctor.

Breast Feeding: Methocarbamol may pass into
breast milk; caution is
advised. Consult your
doctor for advice.

Infants and Children:
No special problems have
been documented; consult
your pediatrician for advice.

Special Concerns:
Methocarbamol can cause
false results in tests of
sugar levels for diabetic
patients. This drug will
intensify the effect that alcohol, sedatives, and other
central nervous system
depressants have on the
brain. Do not take metho-
carbamol if you are allergic
to any skeletal muscle relaxant. Use of this drug should
be accompanied by bed
rest, physical therapy, and
other measures to relieve
discomfort.

OVERDOSE
Symptoms: Nausea, vomiting, diarrhea, loss of
appetite, headache, severe
weakness, fainting, breathing difficulties, irritability,
seizures, feeling of paralysis, profuse sweating, loss
of consciousness.

What to Do: Call your
doctor, emergency medical
services (EMS), or the
nearest poison control
center immediately.

DRUG INTERACTIONS
Consult your doctor for specific advice if you are taking
any drug that depresses the
central nervous system or
any tricyclic antidepressant.

FOOD INTERACTIONS
No known food interactions.

DISEASE INTERACTIONS
Caution is advised when
taking methocarbamol. Consult your doctor if you have
a history of any of the following: alcohol or drug
abuse, allergies, a blood disease caused by an allergy or
another medication, kidney
disease, liver disease, porphyria, or epilepsy.

Methotrexate

BRAND NAMES
Folex, Folex PFS, Mexate, Mexate-AQ, Rheumatrex

Generic 2.5 mg
(MYLAN)

▶ Drug Class: Antineoplastic agent/antimetabolite; antipsoriatic; antirheumatic

▶ Available in: Tablets, injection

▶ Available OTC? No

▶ As Generic? Yes

Side Effects

SERIOUS
Black, tarry stools, bloody vomit, diarrhea, flushing or redness of skin, sores in mouth and on lips, stomach pain, blood in urine or stools, confusion, seizures, cough or hoarseness, fever or chills, pain in lower back or side, painful or difficult urination, red spots on skin, shortness of breath, swollen feet or lower legs, unusual bleeding or bruising, back pain, dark urine, drowsiness, dizziness, headache, joint pain, unusual fatigue, yellow-tinged eyes or skin. Call your doctor immediately.

COMMON
Loss of appetite, nausea and vomiting, minor mouth ulcers.

LESS COMMON
Acne, boils, pale skin, skin rash, or itching.

PRINCIPAL USES
To treat certain kinds of cancer, psoriasis, and rheumatoid arthritis.

HOW THE DRUG WORKS
Methotrexate interferes with the activity of an enzyme needed for the maintenance and replication of cells, especially those that divide and proliferate rapidly. Such cells include many types of cancer cells, as well as those that compose the bone marrow and the cells that line the mouth, intestine, and bladder. Consequently, in addition to its cancer-fighting effects, methotrexate may also harm healthy tissues in the body, causing unpleasant or serious side effects. It is unknown how methotrexate works to ease rheumatoid arthritis, but it appears to modify the function of the immune system, whose activity is believed to play a role in the progression of the disease.

DOSAGE
For psoriasis or rheumatoid arthritis— Tablets: 2.5 to 5 mg every 12 hours for 3 doses in 1 week; or 7.5 to 10 mg once a week. Injection: 10 mg, once a week. For cancer— Use and dose depends on type and stage of disease. Your doctor may alter dosage as needed. Consult pediatrician for children's dose.

ONSET OF EFFECT
Unknown.

DURATION OF ACTION
Unknown.

DIETARY ADVICE
This drug is best taken 1 to 2 hours before meals.

STORAGE
Store in a tightly sealed container away from heat, moisture, and direct light.

IF YOU MISS A DOSE
If you miss a dose, do not take the missed dose and do not double the next dose. Resume your regular schedule and check with your doctor.

STOPPING THE DRUG
The decision to stop taking the drug should be made by your doctor.

PROLONGED USE
See your doctor regularly for tests and examinations.

PRECAUTIONS
Over 60: Adverse reactions may be more likely and more severe in older patients.

Driving and Hazardous Work: Avoid such activities until you determine how the medicine affects you.

Alcohol: Avoid alcohol.

Pregnancy: Methotrexate can cause birth defects and other problems; avoid use during pregnancy.

Breast Feeding: Methotrexate passes into breast milk and may cause serious side effects in the nursing infant; it should not be used during breast feeding.

Infants and Children: Infants are more sensitive to the effects of methotrexate. No special problems are expected in older children.

Special Concerns: Methotrexate may lower your resistance to infection by reducing the number of white blood cells in the blood. Do not have any immunizations without your doctor's approval. Avoid people with infections. Use care when shaving, trimming nails, or using sharp objects. Inform your doctor immediately if you have fever, chills, unusual bleeding or bruising, diarrhea, or a cough. Methotrexate may increase skin sensitivity to sunlight. Limit sun exposure until you see how the medicine affects you. After you stop taking methotrexate, you may experience back pain, blurred vision, confusion, seizures, dizziness, fever, or unusual fatigue; consult your doctor immediately.

OVERDOSE
Symptoms: Severe damage to the liver, kidneys, stomach, intestines, bone marrow, and lungs, causing a wide array of symptoms.

What to Do: If you suspect an overdose, seek medical assistance immediately.

DRUG INTERACTIONS
A number of drugs may interact with methotrexate. Consult your doctor for specific advice if you are taking any drugs that may affect the liver such as azathioprine, retinoids, and sulfasalazine; or any other prescription or over-the-counter medication.

FOOD INTERACTIONS
No known food interactions.

DISEASE INTERACTIONS
Consult your doctor if you have any of the following: a history of alcohol abuse, chicken pox, shingles, colitis, any disease of the immune system, kidney stones, any infection, intestinal blockage, kidney disease, liver disease, mouth sores or inflammation, or stomach ulcers.

Methyldopa

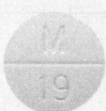

Generic 250 mg
(LEDERLE)

Additional photographs

▶ Drug Class: Centrally acting antihypertensive

▶ Available in: Oral suspension, tablets, injection

▶ Available OTC? No

▶ As Generic? Yes

Side Effects

SERIOUS
Fever shortly after starting to take this medicine, swelling of feet or lower legs, mental depression or anxiety, nightmares, dark or amber urine, stomach cramps, chills, troubled breathing, fast heartbeat, general feeling of discomfort, joint pain, skin rash or itching, yellowish tinge to eyes or skin, continued fatigue, pale stools, nausea and vomiting. Call your doctor immediately.

COMMON
Drowsiness, dry mouth, headache.

LESS COMMON
Diarrhea, dizziness or lightheadedness when getting up, decreased sexual performance, slow heartbeat, stuffy nose, swelling of breasts, unusual milk production, tingling, pain, or weakness in hands or feet.

PRINCIPAL USES
To treat high blood pressure (hypertension).

HOW THE DRUG WORKS
Methyldopa acts upon certain areas of the central nervous system (the brain and spinal cord) that regulate the activity of the heart and the smooth muscle tissue surrounding the arteries. The drug causes blood vessels to relax and widen, which in turn lowers blood pressure.

DOSAGE
Suspension or tablets—Adults: 250 mg to 2 g a day in 2 to 4 doses. Children: 10 mg per 2.2 lbs (1 kg) of body weight in 2 to 4 doses. Injection— Adults: 250 to 500 mg injected into a vein every 6 hours. Children: 20 to 40 mg per 2.2 lbs injected every 6 hours.

ONSET OF EFFECT
Unknown.

DURATION OF ACTION
12 to 24 hours after single oral dose, 24 to 48 hours after multiple oral doses; 10 to 16 hours after injection.

DIETARY ADVICE
Methyldopa can be taken without regard to the timing of meals. Follow a healthy diet (low-salt, low-fat, low-cholesterol) as advised by your doctor to help control blood pressure and prevent heart disease.

STORAGE
Store tablets and injection in a tightly sealed container away from heat, moisture, and direct light. Keep oral suspension refrigerated, but do not allow it to freeze.

IF YOU MISS A DOSE
Take it as soon as you remember. However, if it is near the time for the next dose, skip the missed dose and resume your regular dosage schedule. Do not double the next dose.

STOPPING THE DRUG
Do not stop taking this drug suddenly, as this may cause potentially serious health problems. If therapy is to be discontinued, dosage should be reduced gradually, according to a doctor's instructions.

PROLONGED USE
Lifelong therapy may be required. See your doctor regularly for tests and examinations if you take this medicine for a prolonged period.

PRECAUTIONS
Over 60: Adverse reactions may be more likely and more severe in older patients.

Driving and Hazardous Work: Do not drive or engage in hazardous work until you determine how the medicine affects you.

Alcohol: Avoid alcohol.

Pregnancy: Methyldopa is one of the few antihypertensive medications that can be used by pregnant women. It effectively reduces high blood pressure and has been found in several studies to be safe for both the mother and the unborn child.

Breast Feeding: Methyldopa may pass into breast milk; caution is advised. Consult your doctor for advice.

Infants and Children: No special problems are expected.

Special Concerns: Check your weight frequently and tell your doctor if you gain 5 pounds or more.

OVERDOSE
Symptoms: Weakness, fast heartbeat, dizziness, lightheadedness, constipation or diarrhea, nausea, vomiting, loss of consciousness.

What to Do: Call your doctor, emergency medical services (EMS), or the nearest poison control center immediately.

DRUG INTERACTIONS
Certain drugs may interact with methyldopa. Consult your doctor for specific advice if you are taking an MAO inhibitor.

FOOD INTERACTIONS
No known food interactions.

DISEASE INTERACTIONS
Caution is advised when taking methyldopa. Consult your doctor if you have any of the following: angina, Parkinson's disease, mental depression, or pheochromocytoma. Use of methyldopa may cause complications in patients with kidney disease or liver disease, since these organs work together to remove the medication from the body.

Methylphenidate Hydrochloride

Side Effects

SERIOUS
Fast heartbeat, unusual
bleeding or bruising,
chest pain, fever, joint
pain, increased heartbeat,
skin rash or hives, uncontrolled body movements,
blurred vision or other
vision changes, seizures,
sore throat and fever,
unusual fatigue, weight
loss, mood or mental
changes. Call your doctor
immediately.

COMMON
Loss of appetite, insom-
nia, nervousness.

LESS COMMON
Dizziness, stomach pain,
drowsiness, nausea,
headache.

PRINCIPAL USES
To treat attention-deficit
hyperactivity disorder
(ADHD). It is also used
to treat narcolepsy.

HOW THE DRUG WORKS
Methylphenidate is thought
to stimulate the release of
norepinephrine, a natural
hormone that promotes the
transmission of nerve
impulses in the brain. It
works by decreasing rest-
lessness and increasing
attention in adults and children who cannot concen-
trate for very long, are
easily distracted, or are
unusually impulsive.

DOSAGE
For ADHD— Tablets:
Adults and teenagers: 5 to
20 mg, 2 to 3 times a day,
taken with or after meals.
Children ages 6 to 12: To
start, 5 mg, 2 times a day.
If needed, your doctor may
increase the dose by 5 to
10 mg a week. Extended-
release tablets: Adults,
teenagers and children ages
6 to 12: 20 mg, 1 to 3 times
a day, every 8 hours. For
narcolepsy— Tablets:
Adults and teenagers: 5 to
20 mg, 3 or 4 times a day,
taken with or after meals.
Extended-release tablets:
Adults and teenagers: 20
mg, 2 to 3 times a day.

ONSET OF EFFECT
Tablets: Usually within 30
minutes. Extended-release
tablets: Usually between 30
and 60 minutes.

DURATION OF ACTION
Tablets: 4 to 6 hours.
Extended-release tablets: 6
hours or longer.

DIETARY ADVICE
For ADHD, this medicine
should be taken with or
after meals. For narcolepsy,
it should be taken 30 to 45
minutes before meals.

STORAGE
Store in a tightly sealed container away from heat, moisture, and direct light.

IF YOU MISS A DOSE
Take it as soon as you
remember. If it is near the
time for the next dose, skip
the missed dose and
resume your regular dosage
schedule. Do not double the
next dose.

STOPPING THE DRUG
The decision to stop taking
the drug should be made by
your doctor.

PROLONGED USE
See your doctor regularly
for tests and examinations.

PRECAUTIONS
Over 60: No special problems are expected.

**Driving and Hazardous
Work:** Do not drive or
engage in hazardous work
until you determine how the
medicine affects you.

Alcohol: Avoid alcohol.

Pregnancy: Adequate
human studies have not
been completed. Before taking methylphenidate, tell
your doctor if you are pregnant or plan to become
pregnant.

Breast Feeding: It is not
known whether methyl-
phenidate passes into breast
milk; caution is advised.
Consult your doctor for
advice.

Infants and Children:
This drug is not recom-
mended for use by children
under the age of 6. Older
children may be especially
likely to experience side
effects such as loss of
appetite, stomach pain, and
weight loss.

Special Concerns: To
prevent insomnia, do not
take methylphenidate too
close to bedtime. Your prescription cannot be refilled,
so you must get a new one
from your doctor to obtain
more medication.

OVERDOSE
Symptoms: Agitation, confusion, delirium, seizures,
dry mouth, false sense of
well-being, rapid, pounding,
or irregular heartbeat, fever,
sweating, severe headache,
increased blood pressure,
muscle twitching, trembling
or tremors, vomiting.

What to Do: Call your
doctor, emergency medical
services (EMS), or the
nearest poison control center immediately.

DRUG INTERACTIONS
Call your doctor for specific
advice if you are taking caffeine, amantadine, appetite
suppressants, tricyclic antidepressants, chlophedianol,
pemoline, asthma medicine,
amphetamines, medicine for
colds or sinus problems or
allergies, nabilone, pimozide, or MAO inhibitors.

FOOD INTERACTIONS
Do not drink large amounts
of caffeinated beverages
like coffee, tea, soft drinks,
cocoa, or chocolate milk.

DISEASE INTERACTIONS
Consult your doctor if you
have Tourette's syndrome
or other tics, glaucoma,
epilepsy or another seizure
disorder, high blood pressure, psychosis, severe anxiety, depression, or a history
of alcohol or drug abuse.

Methylprednisolone

Medrol 2 mg
(UPJOHN)

804

Additional photographs

▶ Drug Class: Corticosteroid

▶ Available in: Tablets, injection, enema

▶ Available OTC? No

▶ As Generic? Yes

Side Effects

SERIOUS
Vision problems, frequent urination, increased thirst, rectal bleeding, blistering skin, confusion, hallucinations, paranoia, euphoria, depression, mood swings, redness and swelling at injection site. Call your doctor immedlately.

COMMON
Increased appetite, indigestion, nervousness, insomnia, greater susceptibility to infections, increased blood pressure, slowed wound healing, weight gain, easy bruising, fluid retention.

LESS COMMON
Change in skin color, dizziness, headache, increased sweating, unusual growth of body or facial hair, increased blood sugar, peptic ulcers, adrenal insufficiency, muscle weakness, cataracts, glaucoma, osteoporosis.

PRINCIPAL USES
To treat numerous conditions that involve inflammation (a response by body tissues, producing redness, warmth, swelling, and pain). Such conditions include arthritis, allergic reactions, asthma, some skin diseases, multiple sclerosis flare-ups, and other autoimmune diseases. Also prescribed to treat deficiency of natural steroid hormones.

HOW THE DRUG WORKS
This hormone mimics the effects of the body's natural corticosteroids. It depresses the synthesis, release, and activity of inflammation-producing body chemicals. It also suppresses the activity of the immune system.

DOSAGE
Tablets: 4 to 160 mg a day, depending on condition, in 1 or more doses. Injection: 10 to 160 mg a day injected into a muscle or vein, or 4 to 120 mg as needed, injected into a muscle, joint, or lesion. Enema: 40 mg, 3 to 7 times a week. Consult your pediatrician for children's dose.

ONSET OF EFFECT
Varies widely depending on form used.

DURATION OF ACTION
30 to 36 hours with tablets; 1 to 4 weeks after muscle injection; 1 to 5 weeks after other injections.

DIETARY ADVICE
Take it with food or milk to minimize stomach upset. Your doctor may recommend a low-salt, high-potassium, high-protein diet.

STORAGE
Store in a tightly sealed container away from heat, moisture, and direct light. Do not freeze the liquid form.

IF YOU MISS A DOSE
If you take several doses a day and it is close to the next dose, double the next dose. If you take 1 dose a day and you do not remember until the next day, skip the missed dose and do not double the next dose.

STOPPING THE DRUG
With long-term therapy, do not stop taking the drug abruptly; the dosage should be decreased gradually.

PROLONGED USE
Long-term use may lead to cataracts, diabetes, hypertension, or osteoporosis; see your physician for regular visits.

PRECAUTIONS
Over 60: Adverse reactions may be more likely and more severe in older patients.

Driving and Hazardous Work: Avoid such activities until you determine how the medicine affects you.

Alcohol: May cause stomach problems; avoid it unless your physician approves occasional moderate drinking.

Pregnancy: Overuse during pregnancy can impair growth and development of the child.

Breast Feeding: Do not use this drug while nursing.

Infants and Children: Methylprednisolone may retard the development of bone and other tissues.

Special Concerns: This drug can lower your resistance to infection. Avoid immunizations with live vaccines. Patients undergoing long-term therapy should wear a medical-alert bracelet. Call your doctor if you develop a fever.

OVERDOSE
Symptoms: Fever, muscle or joint pain, nausea, dizziness, fainting, difficulty breathing. Prolonged overuse: Moonface, obesity, unusual hair growth, acne, loss of sexual function, muscle wasting.

What to Do: Seek medical assistance immediately.

DRUG INTERACTIONS
Consult your doctor for specific advice if you are taking aminoglutethimide, antacids, barbiturates, carbamazepine, griseofulvin, mitotane, phenylbutazone, phenytoin, primidone, rifampin, injectable amphotericin B, oral antidiabetes agents, insulin, digitalis drugs, diuretics, or medications containing potassium or sodium.

FOOD INTERACTIONS
Avoid excess sodium.

DISEASE INTERACTIONS
Consult your doctor if you have a history of bone disease, chicken pox, measles, gastrointestinal disorders, diabetes, recent serious infection, glaucoma, heart disease, hypertension, liver or kidney disorders, high blood cholesterol, thyroid problems, myasthenia gravis, or lupus.

Methysergide Maleate

BRAND NAME
Sansert

▶ Drug Class: Antimigraine/antiheadache drug

▶ Available in: Tablets

▶ Available OTC? No

▶ As Generic? No

Side Effects

SERIOUS
Chest pain or tightness; shortness of breath; extreme dizziness; difficult or painful urination; large increase or decrease in urine output; pain in the arms, legs, groin, lower back, or side; swelling of hands, ankles, feet, or lower legs; fever or chills; pale or cold hands or feet; hallucinations. Call your doctor immediately. Contact your doctor as soon as possible if you experience abdominal pain, itching, numbness or tingling of fingers, toes, or face, or weakness in the legs.

COMMON
Diarrhea; mild dizziness or lightheadedness, particularly upon arising from a lying or sitting position; drowsiness; nausea; vomiting.

LESS COMMON
Vision changes, loss of coordination, rapid or slow heartbeat, cough or hoarseness, loss of appetite or weight, raised red spots on your skin, redness or flushing of the face, skin rash.

PRINCIPAL USES
Used to prevent vascular headaches (those that occur in response to changes in normal blood flow within the blood vessels in the brain), such as migraines and cluster headaches. Because of the possible risk of serious, irreversible side effects, methysergide is prescribed only as a last resort for patients with frequent or disabling headaches who are unresponsive to other treatments. This medication is not useful against tension headaches or a vascular headache that has already started.

HOW THE DRUG WORKS
The exact mechanism of action is unknown, although it appears that methysergide eases vascular headaches by causing constriction of the blood vessels in the brain. It is also believed to block the effects of serotonin, a chemical messenger in the nervous system associated with vascular headaches.

DOSAGE
One 2 mg tablet, 2 or 3 times a day, with meals or milk. Do not crush methysergide tablets before taking them.

ONSET OF EFFECT
Within 1 to 2 days.

DURATION OF ACTION
From 1 to 2 days.

DIETARY ADVICE
Take methysergide with meals or milk to prevent stomach upset. A low-salt diet is advised.

STORAGE
Store in a tightly sealed container, away from direct light, moisture, and extremes in temperature.

IF YOU MISS A DOSE
Take it as soon as you remember. However, if it is almost time for the next dose, skip the missed dose and resume your regular dosage schedule. Do not double the next dose.

STOPPING THE DRUG
Stop taking methysergide only when your doctor advises. Methysergide is usually discontinued gradually over 2 to 3 weeks to prevent rebound headaches, which may occur if the drug is discontinued abruptly.

PROLONGED USE
To reduce the risk of serious side effects, after every 4-month course of methysergide therapy, discontinue the drug for 4 weeks before starting the next course.

PRECAUTIONS
Over 60: Adverse reactions may be more likely and more severe in older patients.

Driving and Hazardous Work: Do not drive or engage in hazardous work until you determine how the drug affects you.

Alcohol: Avoid alcohol, which can trigger or exacerbate vascular headaches.

Pregnancy: Avoid use during pregnancy. Consult your doctor if you become or plan to become pregnant.

Breast Feeding: Do not use methysergide while breast feeding.

Infants and Children: Methysergide is not recommended for this age group because of the potential adverse reactions associated with its long-term use.

Special Concerns: Avoid smoking, since it may increase the risk of side effects associated with decreased blood circulation.

OVERDOSE
Symptoms: Cold and pale hands or feet, severe dizziness, excitability.

What to Do: Seek emergency medical assistance right away.

DRUG INTERACTIONS
Consult your physician if you are using or plan to use any other drugs, particularly other types of ergot alkaloids, epinephrine, metaraminol, methoxamine, norepinephrine, phenylephrine, local anesthesia, or tobacco products.

FOOD INTERACTIONS
No known food interactions.

DISEASE INTERACTIONS
Tell your doctor if you have or have had any other medical problems, including arthritis, heart or blood vessel disease, high blood pressure, kidney, liver, or lung disease, stomach ulcer, severe infection, or severe itching.

Metoclopramide Hydrochloride

Generic 10 mg
(SCHEIN)

▶ Drug Class: Gastrointestinal stimulant

▶ Available in: Tablets, syrup, injection

▶ Available OTC? No

▶ As Generic? Yes

Side Effects

SERIOUS
Muscle spasms, aching or crawling sensation in lower legs, stiffness or uncontrolled movements of arms or legs, panicky feeling, unusual nervousness, restlessness, irritability, difficulty speaking or swallowing, dizziness or fainting, fast or irregular heartbeat, general fatigue, shaking of hands and fingers, uncontrolled chewing movements, lip smacking or puckering, loss of balance, severe headache, unusual tongue movements, difficulty walking or shuffling walk. Call your doctor immediately.

COMMON
Diarrhea, restlessness, drowsiness.

LESS COMMON
Breast tenderness and swelling, increased flow of breast milk, menstrual changes, depression, constipation, nausea, skin rash, insomnia, dryness of mouth.

PRINCIPAL USES
To prevent nausea and vomiting caused by anticancer medicines or to treat impaired emptying of food from the stomach (gastroparesis) as a complication of diabetes. Also used as a short-term treatment for heartburn (gastroesophageal reflux, a backflow of stomach acid into the esophagus).

HOW THE DRUG WORKS
Metoclopramide increases the contractions or movements of the stomach and small intestine. It decreases nausea by blocking the effect of the chemical dopamine in the vomiting center of the brain.

DOSAGE
Tablets or syrup— To treat diabetic gastroparesis: Adults and teenagers: 10 mg, 30 minutes before symptoms are likely to begin or before each meal and at bedtime, up to 4 times a day. For heartburn: Adults and teenagers: 10 to 15 mg, 30 minutes before symptoms are likely to begin or before each meal and bedtime. To increase movements of stomach and intestine: Children ages 5 to 14: 2.5 to 5 mg, 3 times a day, 30 minutes before meals. Injection— To increase movements of stomach and intestine: Adults and teenagers: 10 mg into a vein. Children: 0.45 mg per lb of body weight into a vein. Dose may be repeated after 60 minutes. To prevent vomiting and nausea caused by cancer medicines: Adults and teenagers: 1 to 2 mg per 2.2 lbs (1 kg) into a vein 30 minutes before taking cancer medicine. Children: 1 mg per 2.2 lbs (1 kg) into a vein.

ONSET OF EFFECT
Within 3 minutes of intravenous injection; 10 to 15 minutes of intramuscular injection; 30 to 60 minutes after tablets or syrup.

DURATION OF ACTION
1 to 2 hours.

DIETARY ADVICE
Take the drug 30 minutes before meals unless your doctor directs otherwise.

STORAGE
Store in a tightly sealed container away from heat, moisture, and direct light.

IF YOU MISS A DOSE
Take it as soon as you remember. If it is near the time for the next dose, skip the missed dose and resume your regular dosage schedule. Do not double the next dose.

STOPPING THE DRUG
The decision to stop taking the drug should be made by your doctor.

PROLONGED USE
You should see your doctor regularly for tests and examinations if you take this drug for a prolonged period.

PRECAUTIONS
Over 60: Adverse reactions may be more likely and more severe in older patients.

Driving and Hazardous Work: Do not drive or engage in hazardous work until you determine how the medicine affects you.

Alcohol: Avoid alcohol.

Pregnancy: Adequate human studies have not been completed. Before taking metoclopramide, tell your doctor if you are pregnant or plan to become pregnant.

Breast Feeding: Metoclopramide passes into breast milk; caution is advised. Consult your doctor for specific advice.

Infants and Children: The dosage and use should be determined by your doctor. Adverse effects are more likely to occur in infants and children.

Special Concerns: Avoid activities requiring alertness for 2 hours after each dose.

OVERDOSE
Symptoms: Drowsiness, confusion, muscle contractions, irritability, agitation.

What to Do: Call your doctor, emergency medical services (EMS), or the nearest poison control center immediately.

DRUG INTERACTIONS
Consult your doctor for specific advice if you are taking central nervous system depressants such as antihistamines, cold medicines, sleep aids, or tranquilizers.

FOOD INTERACTIONS
No known food interactions.

DISEASE INTERACTIONS
Consult your doctor if you have a history of abdominal or stomach bleeding, asthma, high blood pressure, intestinal blockage, Parkinson's disease, epilepsy, or kidney or liver disease.

Metolazone

Zaroxolyn 5 mg
(FISONS)

Additional photographs

▸ Drug Class: Thiazide-like diuretic

▸ Available in: Tablets, extended-release tablets

▸ Available OTC? No

▸ As Generic? No

Side Effects

SERIOUS
Skin rash, hives, intense itching, swelling of the mouth and throat, breathing difficulty, heart rhythm irregularities, lightheadedness, unusual bleeding or bruising. The powerful combination of metolazone and other diuretics may cause severe dehydration, possibly leading to kidney failure. Call your doctor immediately.

COMMON
Potassium depletion may lead to heart palpitations and weakness. Fluid depletion may lead to dizziness, especially upon arising from a sitting or lying position, as well as thirst, dry mouth, and constipation.

LESS COMMON
Decreased sexual ability, increased sensitivity to sunlight, loss of appetite, gout, increased blood sugar (a problem for diabetic patients), pancreatitis (rare).

PRINCIPAL USES
To treat conditions that cause edema (swelling of body tissues resulting from excess salt and water retention). Many patients are prescribed metolazone in conjunction with other diuretics for particularly resistant fluid retention.

HOW THE DRUG WORKS
Diuretics increase the excretion of salt and water in the urine. Metolazone acts on a part of the kidney that is not affected by loop diuretics such as furosemide or bumetanide. Metolazone and a loop diuretic, when prescribed in combination, thus have a synergistic effect.

DOSAGE
Adults: 2.5 to 10 mg, 1 or 2 times per day.

ONSET OF EFFECT
Approximately 1 hour.

DURATION OF ACTION
From 12 to 24 hours.

DIETARY ADVICE
Take it with food to avoid stomach upset.

STORAGE
Store in a tightly sealed container away from heat and direct light. Keep away from moisture and extremes in temperature.

IF YOU MISS A DOSE
Take it as soon as you remember. If it is near the time for the next dose, skip the missed dose and resume your regular dosage schedule. Do not double the next dose.

STOPPING THE DRUG
The decision to stop taking the drug should be made in consultation with your physician.

PROLONGED USE
See your doctor regularly for examinations and tests if you must take this medicine for an extended period.

PRECAUTIONS
Over 60: Adverse reactions may be more likely and more severe in older patients.

Driving and Hazardous Work: No special precautions are necessary.

Alcohol: No special precautions are necessary.

Pregnancy: Metolazone has caused birth defects in animals. Human studies have not been done. Do not take it during pregnancy unless recommended by your doctor; other diuretics are generally preferred.

Breast Feeding: Metolazone passes into breast milk; avoid or discontinue use during the first month of nursing.

Infants and Children: No unusual side effects are expected in children. The dose must be determined by a pediatrician.

Special Concerns: Metolazone is taken once a day. To prevent it from interfering with sleep, take it in the morning. If you are taking it for high blood pressure, follow the diet and weight control measures recommended by your doctor. Avoid exposure to sunlight, use a sunblock, or wear protective clothing. This medicine may cause your body to lose potassium. Follow your doctor's instructions about eating potassium-rich foods or taking a potassium supplement.

OVERDOSE
Symptoms: Fainting, lethargy, dizziness, drowsiness, gastrointestinal irritation.

What to Do: Call your doctor, emergency medical services (EMS), or the nearest poison control center immediately.

DRUG INTERACTIONS
Consult your doctor for specific advice if you are taking anticoagulants, cholestyramine, colestipol, drugs for diabetes, nonsteroidal anti-inflammatory drugs, digitalis drugs, or lithium.

FOOD INTERACTIONS
No known food interactions.

DISEASE INTERACTIONS
Caution is advised when taking metolazone. Consult your doctor if you have any of the following: diabetes, gout, lupus erythematosus, pancreatitis, heart disease, blood vessel disease, liver disease, or kidney disease.

Metoprolol

BRAND NAMES
Lopressor, Toprol-XL

Generic 50 mg
(MYLAN)

▶ Drug Class: Beta-blocker

▶ Available in: Tablets, extended-release tablets (Injection is for hospital use only.)

▶ Available OTC? No

▶ As Generic? Yes

Side Effects

SERIOUS
Shortness of breath, wheezing; irregular or slow heartbeat (50 beats per minute or less); chest pain or tightness; swelling of the ankles, feet, and lower legs; mental depression. If you experience such symptoms, stop taking metoprolol and call your doctor immediately.

COMMON
Dizziness or lightheadedness, especially when rising suddenly to a standing position; decreased sexual ability; unusual fatigue, weakness, or drowsiness; insomnia.

LESS COMMON
Anxiety, irritability, nervousness; constipation; diarrhea; dry, sore eyes; itching; nausea or vomiting; nightmares or intensely vivid dreams; numbness, tingling, or other unusual sensations in the fingers, toes, or scalp.

PRINCIPAL USES
To treat mild to moderate high blood pressure or angina; to prevent or control heartbeat irregularities (cardiac arrhythmias); to treat congestive heart failure. Injection is used in hospitals for emergency treatment of heart attack, followed by maintenance with oral forms.

HOW THE DRUG WORKS
Metoprolol slows the rate and force of contraction of the heart by blocking certain nerve impulses, thus reducing blood pressure. By modifying nerve impulses to the heart, the drug also helps to stabilize heart rhythm.

DOSAGE
For high blood pressure or angina— Adults: 100 to 400 mg a day in divided doses. Extended-release tablets: Up to 400 mg once a day. For treatment after a heart attack— Initial dose is 50 mg every 6 hours, followed by a maintenance dose of 100 mg or more (up to 400 mg a day), 2 times a day for as long as the physician recommends. For congestive heart failure (Toprol-XL)— The exact dose will be determined by your doctor. Average dose is 25 mg once a day for 2 weeks in people with stable heart failure (NYHA class II) and 12.5 mg once a day in those with more severe heart failure. The dose may then gradually be doubled every 2 weeks to the highest dose the patient can tolerate or up to 200 mg a day.

ONSET OF EFFECT
Within 15 minutes.

DURATION OF ACTION
6 to 12 hours; up to 24 hours with the extended-release tablet.

DIETARY ADVICE
Take it with food. Follow your doctor's dietary restrictions to improve control over high blood pressure and heart disease.

STORAGE
Store in a tightly sealed container away from heat and direct light.

IF YOU MISS A DOSE
Take it as soon as you remember. However, if it is within 4 hours of your next dose (8 hours if using extended-release tablet), skip the missed dose and resume your regular dosage schedule. Do not double the next dose.

STOPPING THE DRUG
This medication should not be stopped suddenly, as this may lead to angina and possibly a heart attack in patients with advanced heart disease. Slow reduction of the dose under doctor's close supervision for 2 to 3 weeks is advised.

PROLONGED USE
Lifelong therapy may be necessary. See your doctor regularly for examinations.

PRECAUTIONS
Over 60: Adverse reactions may be more likely and more severe in older patients.

Driving and Hazardous Work: Use caution until you determine how the medicine affects you.

Alcohol: Drink in careful moderation if at all. Alcohol may interact with the drug and cause a dangerous drop in blood pressure.

Pregnancy: Discuss with your doctor the relative risks and benefits of using this drug while pregnant.

Breast Feeding: Adverse effects in infants have not been documented. Consult your doctor for advice.

Infants and Children: No special problems are expected.

OVERDOSE
Symptoms: Unusually slow or rapid heartbeat, severe dizziness or fainting, poor circulation in the hands (bluish skin), breathing difficulty, seizures.

What to Do: Call your doctor, emergency medical services (EMS), or the nearest poison control center immediately.

DRUG INTERACTIONS
Consult your doctor for specific advice if you are taking amphetamines, oral antidiabetic agents, asthma medication (such as aminophylline or theophylline), calcium channel blockers, clonidine; guanabenz, halothane, immunotherapy for allergies (allergy shots), insulin, MAO inhibitors, reserpine, other beta-blockers, or any over-the-counter medicine.

FOOD INTERACTIONS
None reported.

DISEASE INTERACTIONS
Metoprolol should be used with caution in people with diabetes, especially insulin-dependent diabetes, since the drug may mask symptoms of hypoglycemia. Consult your doctor if you have allergies or asthma, heart or blood vessel disease (including congestive heart failure and peripheral vascular disease), hyperthyroidism, irregular (slow) heartbeat, myasthenia gravis, psoriasis, respiratory problems such as bronchitis or emphysema, kidney or liver disease, or a history of mental depression.

Metronidazole

Generic 250 mg
(SCHEIN/DANBURY)

▸ Drug Class: Antibacterial/
antiprotozoal

▸ Available in: Cream, injection,
topical and vaginal gel,
tablets, extended-release
tablets

▸ Available OTC? No

▸ As Generic? Yes

Side Effects

SERIOUS
Oral and injection forms:
Pain, tingling, numbness,
or weakness in hands or
feet; seizures. Call your
doctor immediately.

COMMON
Oral and injection forms:
Diarrhea, dizziness, lightheadedness, headache,
loss of appetite, nausea,
vomiting, stomach pains
or cramps. Vaginal gel:
Vaginal itching, painful
intercourse, thick, white
vaginal discharge, irritation of sexual partner's
penis, burning urination,
more frequent urination,
redness, stinging, or itching of genital area.

LESS COMMON
Oral and injection forms:
Change in taste, dry
mouth, sharp metallic
taste in mouth. Cream
and gel: Dry skin, skin
irritation, watery eyes
with burning or stinging.
Vaginal gel: Dizziness,
lightheadedness, diar-
rhea, furry tongue, loss
of appetite, metallic taste
in the mouth, nausea,
vomiting.

PRINCIPAL USES
To treat numerous bacterial
infections, including certain
sexually transmitted dis-
eases, gynecological infections, amebiasis (amoeba
infection in the intestine
or liver), brain abscess or
meningitis, pneumonia or
other lung infections, blood
poisoning, bone and joint
infections, infections of the
internal organs (including
liver abscess and peritoni-
tis), and skin infections.

HOW THE DRUG WORKS
Metronidazole kills bacteria
and protozoa, probably by
disrupting the organism's
synthesis of DNA.

DOSAGE
The dose varies greatly
depending on many factors,
including the disorder being
treated, the patient's age,
weight, and general state of
health, and the form of
drug prescribed. Your
doctor will determine the
appropriate dosage regimen
for you.

ONSET OF EFFECT
Unknown.

DURATION OF ACTION
Unknown.

DIETARY ADVICE
Oral forms of metronidazole
can be taken with food to
minimize stomach upset.

STORAGE
Store in a tightly sealed container away from heat, moisture, and direct light. Do
not refrigerate liquid or topical forms.

IF YOU MISS A DOSE
Take it as soon as you
remember. If it is near the
time for the next dose, skip
the missed dose and
resume your regular dosage
schedule. Do not double the
next dose.

STOPPING THE DRUG
Take it as prescribed for the
full treatment period, even if
you feel better before the
scheduled end of therapy.

PROLONGED USE
If your symptoms do not
improve or become worse
after a few days, consult
your doctor.

PRECAUTIONS
Over 60: No special problems are expected.

**Driving and Hazardous
Work:** Do not drive or
engage in hazardous work
until you determine how the
medicine affects you.

Alcohol: A serious reaction, including possible
flushing, rapid heartbeat,
nausea, and vomiting, may
occur if alcohol is con-
sumed while taking this
drug. Alcohol-containing
medications (for example,
cough syrups) should also
be carefully avoided, as
they can cause the same
reaction.

Pregnancy: Metronidazole
has not caused birth defects
in animals. Use of the oral
forms during the first
trimester is not recom-
mended. Before you take
metronidazole, tell your doctor if you are pregnant or
plan to become pregnant.

Breast Feeding: Metronidazole passes into breast
milk; avoid or discontinue
use while nursing.

Infants and Children: In
children, the oral and injection forms are not expected
to cause side effects different from or more severe
than those in older persons.
There is no information on
the use of the topical forms
by children.

Special Concerns: If you
use the vaginal gel, wear
cotton panties, change daily,
and use a sanitary napkin
to prevent leakage. Avoid
using this medicine in or
near the eyes. If it does get
into your eyes, consult your
doctor.

OVERDOSE
Symptoms: No cases of
overdose have been
reported.

What to Do: Emergency
instructions not applicable.

DRUG INTERACTIONS
Consult your doctor for specific advice if you are taking
cimetidine, lithium, anticoagulants, phenytoin, or phenobarbital. If you have
taken disulfiram in the last
2 weeks, then you should
not take metronidazole.
Also tell your doctor if you
are taking any other pre-
scription or over-the-counter
medication.

FOOD INTERACTIONS
No known food interactions.

DISEASE INTERACTIONS
Consult your doctor if you
have a history of blood disease, epilepsy (or other central nervous system dis-
order), heart disease, or
liver disease.

Mexiletine Hydrochloride

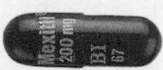

Mexitil 200 mg
(BOEHRINGER INGELHEIM)

Additional photographs

▶ Drug Class: Antiarrhythmic

▶ Available in: Capsules

▶ Available OTC? No

▶ As Generic? Yes

Side Effects

SERIOUS
Chest pain, rapid or irregular heartbeat, shortness of breath, seizures, unusual bleeding or bruising, fever or chills. Call your doctor immediately.

COMMON
Dizziness or lightheadedness; nausea, vomiting, or abdominal pain; heartburn; nervousness; unsteadiness or difficulty in walking; trembling, or shaking of hands.

LESS COMMON
Confusion, blurred vision, constipation or diarrhea, headache, numbness or tingling of hands or toes, ringing in ears, skin rash, slurred speech, difficulty sleeping, unusual fatigue or weakness.

PRINCIPAL USES
To treat irregular heartbeats (cardiac arrhythmias).

HOW THE DRUG WORKS
Mexiletine slows nerve impulses in the heart and makes heart tissue less sensitive to nerve impulses, thus stabilizing heartbeat.

DOSAGE
To start, a 200 to 400 mg dose followed by 200 mg every 8 hours. The dose can be increased to 400 mg every 8 hours.

ONSET OF EFFECT
30 minutes to 2 hours.

DURATION OF ACTION
10 to 12 hours (longer in patients with liver or heart impairment).

DIETARY ADVICE
Mexiletine can be taken with food or an antacid.

STORAGE
Store in a tightly sealed container away from heat and direct light.

IF YOU MISS A DOSE
Take it as soon as you remember. If it is near the time for the next dose, skip the missed dose and resume your regular dosage schedule. Do not double the next dose.

STOPPING THE DRUG
Take it as prescribed for the full treatment period, even if you begin to feel better before the scheduled end of therapy. The decision to stop taking the drug should be made by your doctor.

PROLONGED USE
Lifelong therapy may be necessary. See your doctor regularly for examinations and diagnostic tests if long-term use is required.

PRECAUTIONS
Over 60: There is no specific information comparing use of this medicine in older patients to other age groups.

Driving and Hazardous Work: Do not drive or engage in hazardous work until you determine how the medicine affects you.

Alcohol: No special precautions are necessary.

Pregnancy: In animal studies mexiletine has caused a reduction in successful pregnancies but no birth defects. Before you take mexiletine, tell your physician if you are pregnant or plan to become pregnant.

Breast Feeding: Mexiletine passes into breast milk; you should avoid or discontinue usage while nursing.

Infants and Children: Safety and efficacy of mexiletine in children have not been established. Use and dose must be established by your doctor.

Special Concerns: Your doctor may want you to carry a card or wear a bracelet saying that you are taking mexiletine. Before you have any kind of surgery, tell the doctor or dentist in charge that you are taking this medicine.

OVERDOSE
Symptoms: Severe breathing difficulty, dizziness, drowsiness, burning sensation, nausea, change in mental state, seizures, abnormally slow heartbeat, unconsciousness.

What to Do: Call your doctor, emergency medical services (EMS), or the nearest poison control center immediately.

DRUG INTERACTIONS
Consult your doctor for specific advice if you are taking urinary alkalizers such as antacids, other antiarrhythmics, hepatic enzyme inducers, metoclopramide, theophylline, rifampin, phenytoin, or phenobarbital.

FOOD INTERACTIONS
No known food interactions.

DISEASE INTERACTIONS
Caution is advised when taking mexiletine. Consult your doctor if you have any of the following: low blood pressure, congestive heart failure, a recent heart attack, or a history of seizures. Mexiletine can cause complications in patients with liver disease, since this organ works to remove the medication from the body.

Miconazole

BRAND NAMES
M-Zole 3, Miconazole-7,
Monistat 3, Monistat 7,
Monistat I.V.

▶ Drug Class: Antifungal

▶ Available in: Vaginal cream and suppositories, injection

▶ Available OTC? Yes

▶ As Generic? Yes

Side Effects

SERIOUS
Skin rash or itching; fever or chills; pain at site of injection; vaginal burning, itching, discharge, or irritation not present prior to treatment. Call your doctor immediately.

COMMON
No common side effects are associated with miconazole.

LESS COMMON
Diarrhea, nausea, vomiting, constipation, dizziness, headache, redness or flushing of skin, stomach cramps or pain, burning or irritation of sexual partner's penis.

PRINCIPAL USES
To treat severe fungal infections, including vaginal yeast infections.

HOW THE DRUG WORKS
Miconazole prevents fungal organisms from producing vital substances required for growth and function. This medication is effective only for infections caused by fungal organisms. It will not work for bacterial or viral infections.

DOSAGE
Adults and teenagers—Vaginal cream: At bedtime, insert into the vagina 1 applicatorful for 7 to 14 nights. Vaginal suppositories: At bedtime, insert one 100-mg suppository into the vagina for 7 nights, or one 200-mg or one 400-mg suppository for 3 nights. Injection: 200 to 1,200 mg into a vein 3 times a day for weeks or months. Children ages 1 to 12— Injection: 20 to 40 mg per 2.2 lbs (1 kg) of body weight per day, given in 2 or 3 doses, for weeks or months.

ONSET OF EFFECT
For cream and suppository: Unknown. For injection: Immediate.

DURATION OF ACTION
Unknown.

DIETARY ADVICE
No special restrictions.

STORAGE
Store in a tightly sealed container away from heat, moisture, and direct light. Refrigerate suppositories. Do not allow medication to freeze.

IF YOU MISS A DOSE
Take it as soon as you remember. This will help keep a constant level of medication in your system. If it is near the time for the next dose, skip the missed dose and resume your regular dosage schedule. Do not double the next dose.

STOPPING THE DRUG
Take as directed for the full treatment period, even if you begin to feel better before the scheduled end of therapy. Stopping prematurely increases the risk of reinfection. Some fungal infections take many months to clear up, and some may require continuous treatment.

PROLONGED USE
Therapy with this medication may require months. Prolonged use may increase the risk of adverse effects.

PRECAUTIONS
Over 60: Adverse reactions may be more likely and more severe in older patients.

Driving and Hazardous Work: Do not drive or engage in hazardous work until you determine how the medicine affects you.

Alcohol: Avoid alcohol.

Pregnancy: Adequate studies of miconazole use during pregnancy have not been done. Consult your doctor for advice if you are pregnant or are planning to become pregnant.

Breast Feeding: Miconazole passes into breast milk; caution is advised. Consult your doctor for advice.

Infants and Children: Not recommended for use by children under age 1.

Special Concerns: Sanitary napkins should be used to prevent staining of clothing. The affected area should be kept cool and dry. Do not sit for a long time in a wet bathing suit. Avoid feminine hygiene sprays. Wash daily with unscented soap and dry thoroughly with a clean towel. Tampons should not be used during therapy. The patient's sexual partner should wear a condom during intercourse. Do not stop using this medicine during your menstrual period. After urination or a bowel movement, cleanse by wiping the area from front to back to prevent reinfection.

OVERDOSE
Symptoms: An overdose with miconazole is unlikely.

What to Do: Emergency instructions not applicable.

DRUG INTERACTIONS
Tell your doctor if you are using any other vaginal prescription or over-the-counter medicine when using the vaginal forms. While taking miconazole injection, do not take astemizole or terfenadine. Serious side effects involving the heart may result. Do not take medications containing alcohol, such as cough syrups, elixirs, and tonics. Consult your doctor for specific advice if you are taking cyclosporine, phenytoin, or warfarin.

FOOD INTERACTIONS
No known food interactions.

DISEASE INTERACTIONS
Consult your doctor if you have a history of alcohol abuse. Use of miconazole can cause complications in patients with liver or kidney disease, since these organs work together to remove the medication from the body.

Midodrine Hydrochloride

▶ Drug Class: Alpha-adrenergic agonist

▶ Available in: Tablets

▶ Available OTC? No

▶ As Generic? No

Side Effects

SERIOUS
Very high blood pressure, slow heartbeat, increased dizziness, fainting. Call your doctor immediately.

COMMON
Itching, numbness, or tingling, in the extremities, goose bumps, chills, urinary difficulties.

LESS COMMON
Headache, sinus pressure, redness of face, confusion, dry mouth, nervousness, anxiety, skin rash, vision problems, dizziness, dry skin, backache, gastrointestinal distress, gas, leg cramps.

PRINCIPAL USES
To treat severe cases of orthostatic hypotension (extremely low blood pressure, causing symptoms of dizziness and faintness, especially when rising from a seated or lying position). Used when standard care, such as support stockings, fluid expansion, and lifestyle changes, is ineffective.

HOW THE DRUG WORKS
Midodrine causes constriction of the smooth muscles surrounding the blood vessels. This effect narrows the width of the blood vessels, causing blood pressure to rise, thus helping to correct low blood pressure on standing.

DOSAGE
To start, 10 mg, 3 times a day during waking hours, at intervals of 4 hours. Suggested dosage schedule is to take the medication shortly after rising, then at midday, and then late afternoon (before 6 pm). Blood pressure should be monitored while sitting and lying down at the outset of treatment for possible adjustment of doses.

ONSET OF EFFECT
Within 1 hour.

DURATION OF ACTION
From 2 to 3 hours.

DIETARY ADVICE
No special restrictions.

STORAGE
Store in a tightly sealed container away from heat, moisture, and direct light.

IF YOU MISS A DOSE
Take it as soon as you remember. If it is near the time for the next dose, skip the missed dose and resume your regular dosage schedule. Do not double the next dose.

STOPPING THE DRUG
The decision to stop taking the drug should be made in consultation with your physician.

PROLONGED USE
See your doctor regularly for measurements of blood pressure while sitting and lying down if you must take this drug for a prolonged period. Periodic tests for liver and kidney function will be done.

PRECAUTIONS
Over 60: No special problems are expected.

Driving and Hazardous Work: Do not drive or engage in hazardous work until you determine how the medicine affects you.

Alcohol: Avoid alcohol when using this medication; it may interfere with proper control of blood pressure.

Pregnancy: Adequate studies have not been done. Before taking midodrine, tell your doctor if you are pregnant or plan to become pregnant. Discuss with your doctor the relative benefits and possible risks to the unborn child when using this drug during pregnancy.

Breast Feeding: Midodrine may pass into breast milk; caution is advised. Consult your doctor for specific advice.

Infants and Children: The safety and effectiveness of midodrine in children and infants have not been established.

Special Concerns: The last dose of midodrine should be taken at least 3 hours before bedtime. Use of this drug is not recommended for patients who have persistent and excessively high systolic blood pressure.

OVERDOSE
Symptoms: Goose bumps, sensation of coldness, decreased urine output, rapid heartbeat, ringing in the ears.

What to Do: It is not known whether an overdose of midodrine is life-threatening. However, if someone takes a much larger dose than prescribed, call your doctor, emergency medical services (EMS), or the nearest poison control center immediately.

DRUG INTERACTIONS
Consult your doctor for specific advice if you are taking cardiac glycosides, phenylephrine, pseudoephedrine, beta-blockers, dihydroergotamine, fludrocortisone acetate, prazosin, terazosin, doxazosin, metformin, cimetidine, ranitidine, procainamide, triamterene, flecainide, quinidine, or any other over-the counter or prescription drug.

FOOD INTERACTIONS
No known food interactions.

DISEASE INTERACTIONS
Caution is advised when taking midodrine. Consult your doctor if you have any of the following: urinary retention problems, severe heart disease, diabetes mellitus, vision problems, glaucoma, pheochromocytoma, or thyrotoxicosis. Use of midodrine may cause complications in patients with liver or kidney disease, since these organs work together to remove the medication from the body.

Miglitol

▶ Drug Class: Antidiabetic agent

▶ Available in: Tablets

▶ Available OTC? No

▶ As Generic? No

Side Effects

SERIOUS
No serious side effects are associated with miglitol use.

COMMON
Abdominal pain, diarrhea, and flatulence.

LESS COMMON
Rash. Use in combination with sulfonylureas may cause symptoms of low blood sugar (hypoglycemia), which include sweating, tremor, anxiety, hunger, confusion, seizures, rapid heartbeat, vision changes, dizziness, headache, loss of consciousness. Hypoglycemia must be treated by ingestion of glucose (dextrose). Glucose tablets can be obtained from pharmacies over the counter. Sucrose (table sugar) and foods or drinks containing sugars or starches are ineffective because miglitol prevents their breakdown and absorption.

PRINCIPAL USES
Used as an adjunct (supplemental) therapy to dietary measures and exercise to help control blood sugar levels in patients with type 2 diabetes mellitus. May be used in combination with a sulfonylurea when diet plus either miglitol or a sulfonylurea alone do not adequately control blood sugar levels.

HOW THE DRUG WORKS
Miglitol inhibits the activity of enzymes required to break carbohydrates down into simple sugars within the intestine. This effect delays the digestion of carbohydrates and thus reduces the rise in blood sugar that typically occurs after meals.

DOSAGE
Dosage must be determined for each patient individually, based on blood glucose levels in response to the drug. The recommended starting dosage is 25 mg taken 3 times a day with the first bite of each main meal. Four to eight weeks later, dosage may be increased by your doctor to 50 mg 3 times a day. If, after 3 months, blood sugar levels are not adequately controlled, the dosage may be increased to not more than 100 mg 3 times a day, the maxiumum recommended dose.

ONSET OF EFFECT
Unknown.

DURATION OF ACTION
Unknown.

DIETARY ADVICE
This medicine should be taken with the first bite of breakfast, lunch, and dinner. Follow your doctor's advice regarding diet, weight loss, and exercise.

STORAGE
Store in a tightly sealed container away from heat, moisture, and direct light.

IF YOU MISS A DOSE
If you have finished a meal without taking the medication, skip the missed dose and resume your regular dosing schedule with the next meal. Do not double the next dose.

STOPPING THE DRUG
Do not stop taking the drug without your doctor's approval.

PROLONGED USE
Since type 2 diabetes is a chronic condition, use of miglitol will be ongoing. Blood glucose levels should be checked regularly during treatment so that the dosage may be adjusted if necessary.

PRECAUTIONS
Over 60: No special precautions required.

Driving and Hazardous Work: Miglitol should not impair your ability to perform such tasks safely.

Alcohol: Drink only in moderation when taking miglitol.

Pregnancy: Consult your doctor for advice. Insulin is usually the treatment of choice for pregnant diabetic patients.

Breast Feeding: Miglitol passes into breast milk, although it has not been shown to cause harm to nursing infants. Consult your doctor for advice.

Infants and Children: Safety and effectiveness have not been established for patients under 18 years of age. Consult your doctor for specific advice.

Special Concerns: Follow your doctor's advice about diet, exercise, and weight control. These aspects of treatment are just as essential to the proper control of diabetes as taking medications. Be sure to carry at all times some form of medical identification that indicates you have diabetes and that lists all of the drugs you are taking.

OVERDOSE
Symptoms: Increased gas, diarrhea, and stomach pain.

What to Do: These symptoms usually subside on their own within a short period of time. If not, consult your doctor for advice. Symptoms of hypoglycemia should not occur when taking miglitol alone, but may occur if a patient is also taking a sulfonylurea or insulin for diabetes.

DRUG INTERACTIONS
Consult your doctor if you are taking any of the following drugs that may interact with miglitol: digestive enzyme preparations containing amylase or pancreatin, intestinal absorbents (such as charcoal), insulin, or sulfonylureas (oral antidiabetic agents).

FOOD INTERACTIONS
Avoid foods that contain large amounts of sugar (for example, cake, cookies, candy, acidic fruits). Closely follow the diet your doctor has prescribed.

DISEASE INTERACTIONS
This drug should not be taken by patients with a history of diabetic ketoacidosis, intestinal disorders (including malabsorption or obstruction), inflammatory bowel disease (for example, Crohn's disease or ulcerative colitis), or kidney dysfunction.

Milk of Magnesia (Magnesia; Magnesium Hydroxide)

▶ Drug Class: Antacid/hyperosmotic laxative

▶ Available in: Oral suspension, chewable tablets

▶ Available OTC? Yes

▶ As Generic? Yes

Side Effects

SERIOUS
Dizziness or lightheadedness, continuing feeling of discomfort, irregular heartbeat, loss of appetite, mood or mental changes, muscle weakness, unusual fatigue, unusual weight loss, rectal bleeding. Call your doctor immediately.

COMMON
Nausea, diarrhea.

LESS COMMON
Increased thirst, speckling or whitish color of stools, abdominal cramps.

PRINCIPAL USES
To relieve symptoms of upset stomach; sometimes used for short-term treatment of constipation.

HOW THE DRUG WORKS
As an antacid, milk of magnesia neutralizes stomach acid. As a laxative, it attracts and retains water in the intestine, increasing intestinal movement (peristalsis) and inducing the urge to defecate.

DOSAGE
As an antacid— Adults and teenagers: 5 to 15 ml of liquid form or 650 mg to 1.3 g of tablets 3 or 4 times a day. To relieve constipation— Adults and teenagers: 2.4 to 4.8 g (30 to 60 ml) daily in 1 or more doses. Children ages 6 to 12: 1.2 to 2.4 g (15 to 30 ml) daily in 1 or more doses.

ONSET OF EFFECT
30 minutes to 3 hours.

DURATION OF ACTION
Variable.

DIETARY ADVICE
Take it 1 to 3 hours after meals or at bedtime with a full glass of water.

STORAGE
Store milk of magnesia in a tightly sealed container away from heat, moisture, and direct light.

IF YOU MISS A DOSE
Take it as soon as you remember. If it is near the time for the next dose, skip the missed dose and resume your regular dosage schedule. Do not double the next dose.

STOPPING THE DRUG
You may stop taking the drug whenever you choose.

PROLONGED USE
Do not take milk of magnesia for more than 2 weeks unless your doctor prescribes it.

PRECAUTIONS
Over 60: No special problems are expected.

Driving and Hazardous Work: This medicine should not impair your ability to perform such tasks safely.

Alcohol: Avoid alcohol.

Pregnancy: Extensive human studies have not been done. There have been reports of side effects in babies whose mothers took high doses of antacids for a long time during pregnancy. Before you take milk of magnesia, con-sult your doctor if you are pregnant or plan to become pregnant.

Breast Feeding: Milk of magnesia may pass into breast milk but has not been reported to cause problems in nursing babies. Consult your doctor for specific advice.

Infants and Children: Antacids and other magnesium-containing medications should not be given to children under age 6 unless prescribed by a doctor.

Special Concerns: Take milk of magnesia on a schedule that does not interfere with activities or sleep, as it produces watery stools in 3 to 6 hours. Remember that frequent or protracted use can lead to laxative dependence. Do not take milk of magnesia within 2 hours of taking other medications. Before swallowing, chew tablets well to allow the medicine to work more quickly and effectively.

OVERDOSE
Symptoms: Severe or protracted diarrhea, painful or difficult urination, muscle weakness, continuing loss of appetite, irregular heartbeat, difficulty breathing.

What to Do: An overdose of milk of magnesia is unlikely to be life threatening. However, if someone takes a much larger dose than prescribed, call your doctor, emergency medical services (EMS), or the nearest poison control center immediately.

DRUG INTERACTIONS
Consult your physician for specific advice if you are taking other antacids or laxatives, cellulose sodium phosphate, fluoroquinolones, isoniazid, ketoconazole, sodium polystyrene sulfonate resin, methenamine, mecamylamine, salicylates, or tetracyclines.

FOOD INTERACTIONS
None are known.

DISEASE INTERACTIONS
Do not use this medication if you have any symptoms of appendicitis or inflamed bowel such as lower abdominal or stomach pain, nausea or vomiting, cramping, soreness, or bloating. Consult your physician if you have any of the following: broken bones, colitis, hemorrhoids, intestinal blockage or bleeding, a recent colostomy or ileostomy, swelling of feet or lower legs, heart disease, toxemia of pregnancy, liver disease, or kidney disease.

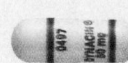

Dynacin 50 mg
(MEDICIS)

▶ Drug Class: Tetracycline antibiotic

▶ Available in: Capsules, oral suspension, tablets, powder, injection

▶ Available OTC? No

▶ As Generic? Yes

Side Effects

SERIOUS
Increased sensitivity of skin to sunlight, abdominal pain, headache, loss of appetite, severe nausea and vomiting, yellow skin, skin discoloration, changes in vision, dizziness or loss of balance, redness, soreness, or swelling at site of injection. Call your doctor immediately.

COMMON
Cramps or burning feeling in stomach, nausea, vomiting, dizziness, light-headedness, unsteadiness, yeast infection or oral thrush (fungal infection of the mouth or throat).

LESS COMMON
Itching in the genital area; sore tongue or mouth.

PRINCIPAL USES
To treat acne or infections caused by bacteria or protozoa (single-celled parasitic organisms).

HOW THE DRUG WORKS
Minocycline kills bacteria and protozoa by inhibiting their manufacture of proteins necessary for their survival.

DOSAGE
Oral forms— Adults and teenagers: 200 mg to start, then 100 mg, 2 times a day, or 100 to 200 mg to start, then 50 mg, 4 times a day. Children age 8 and over: 1.8 mg per lb of body weight to start, then 0.9 mg per lb 2 times a day. Injection— Adults and teenagers: 200 mg to start, then 100 mg, 2 times a day. Children age 8 and over: 1.8 mg per lb to start, then 0.9 mg per lb, 2 times a day.

ONSET OF EFFECT
Immediately after injection; unknown for oral forms.

DURATION OF ACTION
Unknown.

DIETARY ADVICE
Drink extra water when taking capsules or tablets.

STORAGE
Store in a tightly sealed container away from heat, moisture, and direct light.

IF YOU MISS A DOSE
Take it as soon as you remember. If it is near the time for the next dose, skip the missed dose and resume your regular dosage schedule. Do not double the next dose.

STOPPING THE DRUG
Take as prescribed for the full treatment period, even if you begin to feel better before the scheduled end of therapy.

PROLONGED USE
If your symptoms do not improve within a few days (for infection) or a few weeks (for acne), see your doctor. Prolonged use may make you more susceptible to infections caused by microorganisms resistant to antibiotics.

PRECAUTIONS
Over 60: It is not known whether adverse reactions are more likely or more severe in older patients than in younger persons.

Driving and Hazardous Work: Do not drive or engage in hazardous work until you determine how the medicine affects you, since it may cause dizziness.

Alcohol: It is advisable to abstain from alcohol when fighting an infection.

Pregnancy: Use of minocycline during the second half of pregnancy should be avoided because it may discolor the unborn child's teeth, slow growth of teeth and bones, and cause liver problems in the mother.

Breast Feeding: Minocycline passes into breast milk and may be harmful to the nursing infant. The patient must choose between using the drug or breast feeding.

Infants and Children: This drug should not be used by children younger than 8 years old since it can cause permanent tooth staining.

Special Concerns: Oral contraceptives may not work when you take minocycline. Consult your doctor for specific advice. Before having surgery under a general anesthetic, tell the doctor or dentist in charge that you are taking minocycline. If minocycline increases the sensitivity of your skin to the sun, take protective measures and avoid exposure to sunlight. Do not take calcium supplements, magnesium-containing laxatives, sodium bicarbonate, or iron preparations within 2 to 3 hours of taking minocycline. Women predisposed to yeast infections may need treatment with an antifungal while taking minocycline.

OVERDOSE
Symptoms: Severe nausea and vomiting, diarrhea, difficulty swallowing.

What to Do: An overdose is unlikely to be life-threatening. However, if someone takes a much larger dose than prescribed, call your doctor, emergency medical services (EMS), or the nearest poison control center immediately.

DRUG INTERACTIONS
Other drugs may interact with minocycline. Consult your doctor for specific advice if you are taking antacids, calcium supplements, cholestyramine, choline and magnesium salicylates, medicines containing iron, laxatives containing magnesium, or oral contraceptives.

FOOD INTERACTIONS
No known food interactions.

DISEASE INTERACTIONS
Consult your doctor if you have a history of kidney disease or liver disease.

Minoxidil Oral

BRAND NAME
Loniten

Generic 2.5 mg
(SCHEIN/DANBURY)

▶ Drug Class: **Antihypertensive**

▶ Available in: **Tablets**

▶ Available OTC? **No**

▶ As Generic? **Yes**

Side Effects

SERIOUS
Rapid heartbeat (occasionally irregular), rapid weight gain of more than 5 pounds (2 pounds in children), chest pain, shortness of breath. Call your doctor immediately.

COMMON
Swelling of lower legs or feet; increased hair growth, usually on arms, face, and back; flushing or redness of skin.

LESS COMMON
Numbness or tingling of face, hands, or feet, skin rash and itching, breast tenderness in men and women, headache.

PRINCIPAL USES
To treat moderate to severe high blood pressure. Minoxidil is usually used after other medications have failed to achieve satisfactory results.

HOW THE DRUG WORKS
Oral minoxidil acts upon the smooth muscle tissue surrounding the arteries, causing this tissue to relax, which in turn widens the diameter of the blood vessels and thus lowers blood pressure.

DOSAGE
Adults and teenagers: 2.5 to 100 mg daily in a single dose or divided doses. Children up to 12 years of age: 200 micrograms (mcg) to 1 mg per 2.2 lbs (1 kg) of body weight daily in a single dose or divided doses.

ONSET OF EFFECT
30 minutes.

DURATION OF ACTION
2 to 5 days.

DIETARY ADVICE
Take this drug with food to minimize stomach upset. Follow a healthy diet (low-salt, low-fat, low-cholesterol) as advised by your doctor to help control blood pressure and prevent heart disease.

STORAGE
Store in a tightly sealed container away from heat and direct light.

IF YOU MISS A DOSE
Take it as soon as you remember. If it is near the time for the next dose, skip the missed dose and resume your regular dosage schedule. Do not double the next dose.

STOPPING THE DRUG
The decision to stop taking the drug should be made by your doctor. Minoxidil controls your high blood pressure but does not cure it. You may have to take this medicine for the rest of your life.

PROLONGED USE
See your doctor regularly for tests and examinations if you must take this drug for a prolonged period.

PRECAUTIONS
Over 60: Adverse reactions may be more likely and more severe in older patients. Minoxidil may reduce tolerance to cold temperatures in older patients.

Driving and Hazardous Work: The use of minoxidil should not impair your ability to perform such tasks safely.

Alcohol: No special precautions are necessary.

Pregnancy: Minoxidil has not been shown to cause birth defects in animals. Human studies have not been done, but there have been reports of unusual hair growth in newborn babies. High doses in animal studies have caused a reduced rate of pregnancy. Before you take minoxidil, tell your doctor if you are pregnant or are planning to become pregnant.

Breast Feeding: Minoxidil passes into breast milk; caution is advised. Consult your doctor for specific advice.

Infants and Children: Minoxidil is not expected to cause unusual problems in infants and children.

Special Concerns: Minoxidil commonly causes swelling due to fluid retention, so most patients need to take a diuretic with this medication. The drug also raises heart rate and therefore is often prescribed with a drug to stabilize heart rate. While taking minoxidil, weigh yourself every day. Contact your doctor immediately if you suddenly gain 5 pounds or more (2 pounds or more in children); you experience shortness of breath, especially when lying down; or your heart rate increases by 20 or more beats per minute while resting.

OVERDOSE
Symptoms: Very low blood pressure, fast heartbeat, buildup of fluid in the body.

What to Do: An overdose of minoxidil is unlikely to be life-threatening. However, if someone takes a much larger dose than prescribed, call your doctor, emergency medical services (EMS), or the nearest poison control center.

DRUG INTERACTIONS
The following drugs may interact with minoxidil. Consult your doctor for specific advice if you are taking guanethidine, nitrates, or any over-the-counter medicine for appetite control, asthma, colds, cough, hay fever, or sinus problems.

FOOD INTERACTIONS
No known food interactions.

DISEASE INTERACTIONS
Caution is advised when taking minoxidil. Consult your doctor for advice if you have any of the following: angina, heart disease, blood vessel disease, kidney disease, a recent heart attack or stroke, or pheochromocytoma.

BRAND NAME
Rogaine

▶ Drug Class: Hair growth stimulant

▶ Available in: Topical solution

▶ Available OTC? Yes

▶ As Generic? Yes

Side Effects

SERIOUS
Rapid pulse; weakness, dizziness, or lightheaded feeling; chest pain. Notify your doctor immediately. If chest pain is present, call emergency medical services (EMS).

COMMON
Burning, tingling, or mild redness of scalp at application site; mild dryness or flaking of skin; itching.

LESS COMMON
Significant irritation or allergy with redness, itching, flaking, or rash. Tingling of hands or feet; water retention (swelling of face, hands, fingers, or legs); flushing; headache. Stop the drug and notify your doctor immediately.

PRINCIPAL USES
Minoxidil topical solution is prescribed to stimulate hair growth in men and women with a specific type of baldness known as androgenetic alopecia (popularly known as male pattern baldness or female pattern baldness).

HOW THE DRUG WORKS
It is not known how minoxidil works. Although it increases the flow of blood, nutrients, and other important substances to hair follicles, other or additional poorly understood actions are believed responsible for hair growth.

DOSAGE
Adults: Apply 1 ml regardless of the size of the balding area under treatment.

ONSET OF EFFECT
At least 4 months with twice daily therapy.

DURATION OF ACTION
New hair resulting from minoxidil treatments will likely be lost 3 to 4 months following discontinuation of the medication.

DIETARY ADVICE
No special restrictions.

STORAGE
Store in a tightly sealed container away from heat and direct light. Keep away from moisture and extremes in temperature.

IF YOU MISS A DOSE
Apply it as soon as you remember. If it is near the time for the next dose, skip the missed dose and resume your regular dosage schedule. Do not double the next dose.

STOPPING THE DRUG
Use it until you are able to assess changes, if any, in hair growth and cosmetic appearance. This may take at least 4 months. If you decide to abandon efforts to achieve hair regrowth, you may stop the medication at any time.

PROLONGED USE
Ongoing therapy with this medication is required for continued results. Prolonged use may increase the risk of undesirable side effects.

PRECAUTIONS
Over 60: Adverse reactions may be more likely and more severe in older patients.

Driving and Hazardous Work: Do not drive or engage in hazardous work until you determine how the medicine affects you.

Alcohol: No special precautions are necessary.

Pregnancy: Avoid or discontinue topical minoxidil treatment if you are pregnant or trying to become pregnant. Consult your physician.

Breast Feeding: Minoxidil passes into breast milk; do not use it while nursing.

Infants and Children: Topical minoxidil is not recommended for children.

Special Concerns: Anyone with a history of allergy to minoxidil or other components of the product should not use this medication. Minoxidil has potentially serious side effects if absorbed in large amounts into the body. Persons with a history of heart disease should consult their doctor before using this product. Do not apply to irritated, blistered, bleeding, or broken skin. Do not use more than the recommended dose, and do not apply it more frequently than twice a day. Do not use hairdryers to accelerate drying of the medication.

OVERDOSE
Symptoms: Symptoms are similar to those listed under serious side effects: rapid pulse; weakness, dizziness, or a lightheaded feeling; chest pain.

What to Do: If the above symptoms occur or someone ingests the medication, call your doctor, emergency medical services (EMS), or the nearest poison control center immediately.

DRUG INTERACTIONS
Consult your doctor for specific advice if you are taking oral minoxidil, steroids, petrolatum, or acne preparations such as tretinoin. Any person using heart or blood pressure medications should discuss minoxidil use with their doctor before starting treatment.

FOOD INTERACTIONS
No known food interactions.

DISEASE INTERACTIONS
Consult your doctor if you have any disorders affecting your skin or scalp, including rashes, sunburn, or other types of skin eruption or inflammation; heart disease; or high blood pressure.

Mirtazapine

Remeron

Remeron 15 mg
(ORGANON)

▶ Drug Class: Antidepressant

▶ Available in: Tablets

▶ Available OTC? No

▶ As Generic? No

Side Effects

SERIOUS
Mood or mental changes, confusion, breathing difficulties, increased or decreased ability to move limbs, flu-like symptoms, swelling of the lower extremities, skin rash, anxiety, agitation, extreme drowsiness, disorientation, loss of memory, rapid heartbeat. Call your doctor immediately.

COMMON
Dizziness, dry mouth, drowsiness, constipation, increased appetite, weight gain.

LESS COMMON
Muscle pains, unusual dreams, fatigue, back pain, vomiting, increased thirst, nausea, dizziness or fainting when getting up suddenly, sensitivity to touch, tremor, stomach pain, increased urination.

PRINCIPAL USES
To treat symptoms of major depression.

HOW THE DRUG WORKS
While the exact mechanism of action of mirtazapine is not known, it affects levels of brain chemicals (norepinephrine and serotonin) that are thought to be linked to mood, emotions, and mental state.

DOSAGE
To start, 15 mg once a day, at bedtime. The dose may be increased gradually by your doctor to no more than 45 mg a day.

ONSET OF EFFECT
Unknown.

DURATION OF ACTION
Unknown.

DIETARY ADVICE
No special restrictions.

STORAGE
Store in a tightly sealed container away from heat, moisture, and direct light.

IF YOU MISS A DOSE
Take it as soon as you remember. However, if it is near the time for the next day's dose, skip the missed dose and resume your regular dosage schedule. Do not double the next day's dose.

STOPPING THE DRUG
Take as prescribed for the full treatment period, even if you begin to feel better before the scheduled end of therapy. The decision to stop taking the drug should be made in consultation with your doctor.

PROLONGED USE
You should see your doctor regularly for tests and examinations if you take this medicine for a prolonged period. Prolonged use of mirtazapine can decrease the flow of saliva, which can increase the risk of cavities, periodontal disease, and other conditions.

PRECAUTIONS
Over 60: No special problems have been reported.

Driving and Hazardous Work: Exercise caution until you determine how the medicine affects you. Drowsiness or lightheadedness can occur.

Alcohol: Avoid alcohol.

Pregnancy: In animal studies, mirtazapine did not cause birth defects but was shown to cause other problems. Human studies have not been done. Before you take mirtazapine, tell your doctor if you are pregnant or plan to become pregnant.

Breast Feeding: Mirtazapine may pass into breast milk; caution is advised. Consult your doctor for advice.

Infants and Children: The safety and effectiveness of mirtazapine use by infants and children have not been established.

Special Concerns: If dry mouth occurs, use sugarless candy or gum for relief.

OVERDOSE
Symptoms: Severe drowsiness, disorientation, loss of memory, rapid heartbeat.

What to Do: Call your doctor, emergency medical services (EMS), or the nearest poison control center immediately.

DRUG INTERACTIONS
Mirtazapine and MAO inhibitors should not be used within 14 days of each other. Very serious side effects such as myoclonus (uncontrolled muscle jerking), hyperthermia (excessive rise in body temperature), nausea, vomiting, seizures, and extreme stiffness may result. Other drugs may interact with mirtazapine; consult your doctor for specific advice if you are taking central nervous system depressants, high blood pressure medication, diazepam, or kidney medication.

FOOD INTERACTIONS
No known food interactions.

DISEASE INTERACTIONS
Caution is advised when taking mirtazapine. Consult your doctor if you have heart or blood vessel disease; phenylketonuria; or a history of seizures, drug abuse, or mental illness. Use of mirtazapine may cause complications in patients with liver or kidney disease, since these organs work together to remove the medication from the body.

Misoprostol

Cytotec 0.2 mg
(SEARLE)

▶ Drug Class: Prostaglandin

▶ Available in: Tablets

▶ Available OTC? No

▶ As Generic? No

Side Effects

SERIOUS
There are no serious side effects associated with the use of misoprostol.

COMMON
Diarrhea, mild abdominal or stomach pain.

LESS COMMON
Vaginal bleeding, constipation, cramps in lower abdomen, gas, headache, nausea and vomiting.

PRINCIPAL USES
To prevent stomach ulcers in patients taking anti-inflammatory drugs, including aspirin.

HOW THE DRUG WORKS
Ongoing therapy with anti-inflammatory drugs can irritate and damage the stomach lining, increasing the risk of ulcers. Misoprostol helps prevent ulcers and enhances the stomach's natural healing ability by increasing the production of protective mucus, as well as inhibiting the secretion of stomach acid.

DOSAGE
200 to 400 micrograms (mcg), 4 times a day, or 400 mcg, 2 times a day. The dose may be reduced to 100 mcg to prevent side effects. Treatment usually lasts 4 weeks.

ONSET OF EFFECT
30 minutes.

DURATION OF ACTION
3 hours.

DIETARY ADVICE
Misoprostol can be taken with meals to reduce the incidence of diarrhea. The last dose should be taken at bedtime.

STORAGE
Store in a tightly sealed container away from heat and direct light.

IF YOU MISS A DOSE
Take it as soon as you remember. If it is near the time for the next dose, skip the missed dose and resume your regular dosage schedule. Do not double the next dose.

STOPPING THE DRUG
Take the drug as prescribed for the full treatment period, even if you begin to feel better before the scheduled end of therapy.

PROLONGED USE
You should see your doctor regularly for tests and examinations if you take this drug for a prolonged period. You should not take misoprostol for more than 4 weeks unless directed by your doctor.

PRECAUTIONS
Over 60: Misoprostol has not caused side effects or problems in older persons different from those in younger patients.

Driving and Hazardous Work: Do not drive or engage in hazardous work until you determine how the medicine affects you.

Alcohol: Avoid alcohol.

Pregnancy: Misoprostol should not be used during pregnancy, because it may promote contractions and bleeding of the uterus and can cause miscarriage. Before you start taking misoprostol, you must have had a negative pregnancy test within the previous 2 weeks. You must start taking the drug only on the second or third day of your next menstrual period. An effective method of birth control should be used while you are taking misoprostol. If you suspect you are pregnant, stop taking the drug immediately and consult your doctor.

Breast Feeding: Misoprostol may pass into breast milk; avoid or discontinue use while nursing because it may cause diarrhea in nursing babies.

Infants and Children: Use and dosage by anyone under the age of 18 must be determined by your doctor.

OVERDOSE
Symptoms: Tremors, sleepiness, trouble breathing, abdominal pain, severe diarrhea, fever, palpitations, extremely low blood pressure, slow heartbeat.

What to Do: An overdose of misoprostol is unlikely to be life-threatening. However, if someone takes a much larger dose than prescribed, call your doctor, emergency medical services (EMS), or the nearest poison control center.

DRUG INTERACTIONS
Before you take misoprostol, inform your doctor if you are taking any other prescription or over-the-counter medicine. Antacids may be taken with misoprostol to help relieve stomach pain, unless your doctor directs otherwise. Do not take antacids that contain magnesium, since they can cause or worsen the diarrhea that sometimes accompanies misoprostol use.

FOOD INTERACTIONS
No known food interactions.

DISEASE INTERACTIONS
Caution is advised when taking misoprostol. Consult your doctor if you have a history of blood vessel disease or epilepsy.

Mitotane

BRAND NAME
Lysodren

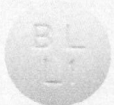

Lysodren 500 mg
(BRISTOL-MYERS SQUIBB)

▶ Drug Class: Antineoplastic (anticancer) agent/antiadrenal

▶ Available in: Tablets

▶ Available OTC? No

▶ As Generic? No

Side Effects

SERIOUS
Darkening of skin, diarrhea, dizziness, drowsiness, loss of appetite, depression, severe nausea and vomiting, skin rash, unusual fatigue, blood in urine, blurred or double vision, shortness of breath, wheezing. Call your doctor immediately.

COMMON
Nausea and vomiting.

LESS COMMON
Aching muscles, dizziness or lightheadedness when rising from a sitting or lying position, fever, flushed or reddened skin, muscle twitching.

PRINCIPAL USES
To treat cancer of the adrenal cortex, the outer part of the adrenal glands, which rest on top of either kidney. The adrenal cortex produces the body's natural corticosteroid hormones.

HOW THE DRUG WORKS
Mitotane appears to suppress activity (steroid production) in the adrenal cortex. For reasons that are unknown, the drug's reduction of steroid production somehow has a destructive effect on cancer cells in the adrenal cortices, and so slows the progression of cancer in that portion of the adrenal gland.

DOSAGE
2 to 6 g daily in 3 or 4 doses. The dosage can be increased to 16 g per day; the usual range is 8 to 10 g per day.

ONSET OF EFFECT
2 to 3 days.

DURATION OF ACTION
Unknown.

DIETARY ADVICE
Can be taken with or without food, according to personal preference. To minimize side effects, the last dose is best taken after the evening meal but before bedtime.

STORAGE
Store in a tightly sealed container away from heat and direct light.

IF YOU MISS A DOSE
Take it as soon as you remember. If it is near the time for the next dose, skip the missed dose and resume your regular dosage schedule. Do not double the next dose.

STOPPING THE DRUG
The decision to stop taking the drug should be made by your doctor.

PROLONGED USE
See your doctor regularly for tests and examinations if you must take this drug for a prolonged period. Neurological assessments are recommended at regular intervals for persons who take mitotane for more than 2 years.

PRECAUTIONS
Over 60: There is no specific information about the use of mitotane in older patients.

Driving and Hazardous Work: Do not drive or engage in hazardous work until you determine how the medicine affects you.

Alcohol: Avoid alcohol.

Pregnancy: Mitotane has not been shown to cause problems during pregnancy. Consult your doctor for specific advice if you are pregnant or plan to become pregnant.

Breast Feeding: It is unknown if mitotane passes into breast milk; caution is advised. Consult your doctor for specific advice.

Infants and Children: There is no specific information about the use of mitotane in infants and children, but it is not expected to cause different side effects or problems than it does in older patients.

Special Concerns: Initial treatment with mitotane often starts in the hospital until the dose is stabilized. Your doctor may want you to carry a card saying that you are taking mitotane. Check with your doctor if you get an infection, illness, or injury of any sort, because mitotane may weaken your body's defenses against infection and inflammation.

OVERDOSE
Symptoms: No specific ones have been reported.

What to Do: An overdose of mitotane is unlikely to be life-threatening. However, if someone takes a much larger dose than prescribed, call your doctor, emergency medical services (EMS), or the nearest poison control center immediately.

DRUG INTERACTIONS
Consult your physician for specific advice if you are taking adrenocorticoids, glucocorticoids, mineralocorticoids, corticotropin, or central nervous system depressants.

FOOD INTERACTIONS
No known food interactions.

DISEASE INTERACTIONS
Caution is advised when taking mitotane. Consult your doctor if you have any infection. Use of mitotane may cause complications in patients with liver disease, since this organ works to remove the medication from the body.

Mitoxantrone Hydrochloride

▶ Drug Class: Antineoplastic (anticancer) agent

▶ Available in: Injection

▶ Available OTC? No

▶ As Generic? No

Side Effects

SERIOUS
Fever, chills, black, tarry stools, cough or shortness of breath, blood in urine or stools, rapid or irregular heartbeat, red spots on skin, swelling of feet and lower legs, unusual bleeding or bruising, sores in mouth and on lips, stomach pain, decreased urination, seizures, blue skin or pain and redness at injection site, skin rash. Call your doctor immediately.

COMMON
Diarrhea, headache, nausea and vomiting, temporary hair loss, bluish green-colored urine.

LESS COMMON
No less-common side effects are associated with mitoxantrone.

PRINCIPAL USES
Mitoxantrone is combined with other chemotherapy agents in the initial first-line of treatment against certain kinds of leukemias. Also used to treat secondary (chronic) progressive, progressive relapsing, or worsening relapsing-remitting multiple sclerosis.

HOW THE DRUG WORKS
It is unknown precisely how mitoxantrone works, but it appears to interfere with the DNA of cancer cells, preventing them from reproducing. The drug may also affect the growth and development of other kinds of cells in the body, resulting in unpleasant side effects, particularly the suppression of bone marrow, which causes anemia and other blood problems.

DOSAGE
Mitoxantrone is administered intravenously in a hospital setting. Dosage will be determined by your doctor.

ONSET OF EFFECT
Unknown.

DURATION OF ACTION
Unknown.

DIETARY ADVICE
Maintain adequate food and fluid intake. Calorie, protein, and vitamin needs increase in patients with cancer. Good nutrition is essential to cope with the demands of chemotherapy.

STORAGE
Not applicable; the dose is administered only at a health care facility.

IF YOU MISS A DOSE
Not applicable, since medication is given by a doctor or other health professional.

STOPPING THE DRUG
The decision to stop taking the drug should be made by your doctor.

PROLONGED USE
You should see your doctor regularly for tests and examinations if you take this drug for a prolonged period.

PRECAUTIONS
Over 60: There is no specific information comparing use of mitoxantrone in older patients with use in younger persons. No special problems are expected.

Driving and Hazardous Work: The use of mitoxantrone should not impair your ability to perform such tasks safely.

Alcohol: Alcohol should be avoided while taking this medication.

Pregnancy: Mitoxantrone may cause birth defects if it is taken by either the father or the mother at the time of conception. It is best to use some kind of birth control while taking mitoxantrone. Tell your doctor immediately if you think you have become pregnant while taking mitoxantrone.

Breast Feeding: Mitoxantrone passes into breast milk; discontinue nursing before beginning treatment.

Infants and Children: There is no specific information that compares use of mitoxantrone in infants and children with use in older persons.

Special Concerns: Do not receive any immunizations without your doctor's approval while you are taking mitoxantrone. Avoid persons with infections. Be careful when using a tooth-brush, dental floss, or toothpick. Take care not to cut yourself when using sharp objects such as a razor. Avoid contact sports. Before having dental work, consult your doctor. Your doctor may want you to drink extra fluids while you are taking this drug.

OVERDOSE
Symptoms: Severe infection as a result of substantial white blood cell suppression (immune system failure).

What to Do: Contact your oncologist, who will closely monitor your blood counts and symptoms and determine the course of your treatment.

DRUG INTERACTIONS
Consult your doctor for specific advice if you are taking amphotericin B, antithyroid agents, azathioprine, chloramphenicol, colchicine, flucytosine, ganciclovir, interferon, plicamycin, zidovudine, probenecid, sulfinpyrazone, or any other cancer medication.

FOOD INTERACTIONS
No known food interactions.

DISEASE INTERACTIONS
Caution is advised when taking mitoxantrone. Consult your doctor if you have a history of any of the following: chicken pox, shingles, gout, kidney stones, heart disease, or any infection. Use of mitoxantrone may cause complications in patients with liver disease, since this organ works to remove the medication from the body.

Moexipril Hydrochloride

BRAND NAME
Univasc

▶ Drug Class: Angiotensin-converting enzyme (ACE) inhibitor

▶ Available in: Tablets

▶ Available OTC? No

▶ As Generic? No

Side Effects

SERIOUS
Fever and chills, sore throat and hoarseness, sudden difficulty breathing or swallowing, swelling of the face, mouth, or extremities, impaired kidney function (ankle swelling, decreased urination), confusion, yellow discoloration of the eyes or skin (indicating liver disorder), intense itching, chest pain or palpitations, abdominal pain. Serious side effects are very rare; contact your doctor immediately.

COMMON
Dry, persistent cough.

LESS COMMON
Dizziness or fainting, skin rash, numbness or tingling in the hands, feet, or lips, unusual fatigue or muscle weakness, nausea, drowsiness, loss of taste, headache.

PRINCIPAL USES
To control high blood pressure; to treat congestive heart failure (CHF); to treat patients with left ventricular dysfunction (damage to the pumping chamber of the heart); and to minimize further kidney damage in diabetics with mild kidney disease.

HOW THE DRUG WORKS
Angiotensin-converting enzyme (ACE) inhibitors block an enzyme that produces angiotensin, a naturally occurring substance that causes blood vessels to constrict and stimulates production of the adrenal hormone, aldosterone, which promotes sodium retention in the body. As a result, ACE inhibitors relax blood vessels (causing them to widen) and reduces sodium retention, which lowers blood pressure and so decreases the workload of the heart.

DOSAGE
To start, 7.5 mg once a day. Dosage may be increased by your doctor up to 30 mg a day, given in 1 or 2 doses.

ONSET OF EFFECT
Within 1 hour.

DURATION OF ACTION
24 hours.

DIETARY ADVICE
Take it on an empty stomach, about 1 hour before mealtime. Follow your doctor's dietary advice (such as low-salt or low-cholesterol restrictions) to improve control over high blood pressure and heart disease. Avoid high-potassium foods like bananas and citrus fruits and juices, unless you are also taking medications, such as diuretics, that lower potassium levels.

STORAGE
Store in a tightly sealed container away from heat and direct light.

IF YOU MISS A DOSE
Take it as soon as you remember. If it is near the time for the next dose, skip the missed dose and resume your regular dosage schedule. Do not double the next dose.

STOPPING THE DRUG
Do not stop taking this drug abruptly, as this may cause potentially serious health problems. Dosage should be reduced gradually, according to your doctor's instructions.

PROLONGED USE
Lifelong therapy may be necessary. See your doctor for regular evaluation.

PRECAUTIONS
Over 60: Smaller doses may be recommended for older patients.

Driving and Hazardous Work: Do not drive or engage in hazardous work until you determine how the medicine affects you.

Alcohol: Consume alcohol only in moderation since it may increase the effect of the drug and cause an excessive drop in blood pressure. Consult your doctor for advice.

Pregnancy: Use of moexipril during the last 6 months of pregnancy may cause severe defects, even death, in the fetus. The drug should be discontinued if you are pregnant or plan to become pregnant.

Breast Feeding: Moexipril may pass into breast milk; caution is advised. Consult your doctor for advice.

Infants and Children:
The safety and efficacy of moexipril for infants and children have not been established. Benefits must be weighed against potential risks; consult your pediatrician for advice.

OVERDOSE
Symptoms: No specific ones have been reported.

What to Do: While overdose is unlikely, call your doctor, emergency medical services (EMS), or the nearest poison control center immediately if you suspect that someone has taken a much larger dose than prescribed.

DRUG INTERACTIONS
Consult your doctor if you are taking diuretics (especially potassium-sparing diuretics), potassium supplements or drugs containing potassium (check ingredient labels), lithium, anticoagulants (such as warfarin), indomethacin or other anti-inflammatory drugs, or any over-the-counter medications (especially cold remedies and diet pills).

FOOD INTERACTIONS
Avoid low-salt milk and salt substitutes. Many of these products contain potassium. Excessive intake of tea, coffee, cola, or other drinks that could create a diuretic effect should be avoided.

DISEASE INTERACTIONS
Consult your doctor if you have systemic lupus erythematosus (SLE) or if you have had a prior allergic reaction to ACE inhibitors. Moexipril should be used with caution by patients with severe kidney disease or renal artery stenosis (narrowing of one or both of the arteries that supply blood to the kidneys).

Moexipril Hydrochloride/Hydrochlorothiazide

▶ Drug Class: Angiotensin-converting enzyme (ACE) inhibitor/diuretic

▶ Available in: Tablets

▶ Available OTC? No

▶ As Generic? No

Side Effects

SERIOUS
Fever and chills, sore throat and hoarseness, sudden difficulty breathing or swallowing, swelling of the face, mouth, or extremities, impaired kidney function (ankle swelling, decreased urination), confusion, yellow discoloration of the eyes or skin (indicating liver disorder), intense itching, chest pain or heartbeat irregularities, abdominal pain. Serious side effects are very rare; contact your doctor immediately.

COMMON
Dry, persistent cough, muscle cramps or pain, heart palpitations, dizziness (especially when rising from a sitting or lying position), dry mouth, unusual thirst, constipation.

LESS COMMON
Fainting, skin rash, numbness or tingling in the hands, feet, or lips, unusual fatigue or muscle weakness, nausea, drowsiness, loss of taste, headache, increased sensitivity to sunlight, loss of appetite, gout.

PRINCIPAL USES
To treat high blood pressure. Used in patients for whom both moexipril and hydrochlorothiazide have been prescribed.

HOW THE DRUG WORKS
This drug combines an angiotensin-converting enzyme (ACE) inhibitor (moexipril hydrochloride) and a thiazide diuretic (hydrochlorothiazide). ACE inhibitors block an enzyme that produces angiotensin, a naturally occurring substance that causes blood vessels to constrict and stimulates production of the adrenal hormone, aldosterone, which promotes sodium retention in the body. As a result, ACE inhibitors relax blood vessels (causing them to widen) and reduces sodium retention, which lowers blood pressure and so decreases the workload of the heart. Hydrochlorothiazide (HCTZ) increases sodium and water in the urine output. By reducing the overall fluid volume in the body, diuretics reduce blood volume and so reduce blood pressure.

DOSAGE
This combination medication comes in two strengths: moexipril/hydrochlorothiazide 7.5/12.5 and 15/25. The dose ranges from 7.5 to 30 mg of moexipril and 12.5 to 50 mg of hydrochlorothiazide per day. Tablets are taken either once a day or in 2 divided doses, 1 hour before meals.

ONSET OF EFFECT
Within 1 hour.

DURATION OF ACTION
Unknown.

DIETARY ADVICE
Take it on an empty stomach, about 1 hour before meals.

STORAGE
Store in a tightly sealed container away from heat, moisture, and direct light.

IF YOU MISS A DOSE
Take it as soon as you remember. If it is near the time for the next dose, skip the missed dose and resume your regular dosage schedule. Do not double the next dose.

STOPPING THE DRUG
Discontinuing this drug abruptly may cause potentially serious problems. The dosage should be reduced gradually, according to your doctor's instructions.

PROLONGED USE
See your doctor regularly for evaluation if you must take this medicine for a prolonged period. Lifelong therapy may be necessary.

PRECAUTIONS
Over 60: Adverse reactions may be more likely and more severe.

Driving and Hazardous Work: No warnings.

Alcohol: Alcohol may increase the effect of the drug and cause an excessive drop in blood pressure; drink only in moderation.

Pregnancy: Before taking this medication, tell your doctor if you are pregnant or plan to become pregnant. Use of this drug during the last 6 months of pregnancy may cause severe defects, even death, in the fetus.

Breast Feeding: Moexipril may pass into breast milk; consult your doctor for specific advice.

Infants and Children: Not recommended for use by children under 18.

Special Concerns: A rare complication is angioedema, characterized by swelling of the lips, tongue, and throat. It may be so severe as to cause obstruction of the airways, which could be fatal.

OVERDOSE
Symptoms: No cases of overdose have been reported; symptoms might include dizziness, faintness, or confusion.

What to Do: While overdose is unlikely, call your doctor, emergency medical services (EMS), or the nearest poison control center immediately if you suspect that someone has taken a much larger dose than prescribed.

DRUG INTERACTIONS
Consult your doctor for specific advice if you are taking cholestyramine, colestipol, corticosteroids, digitalis drugs, antidiabetic drugs, lithium, potassium-containing medications or supplements, or any over-the-counter drug (especially cold remedies and appetite suppressants).

FOOD INTERACTIONS
Avoid low-salt milk and salt substitutes. Many of these products contain potassium.

DISEASE INTERACTIONS
Consult your doctor if you have systemic lupus erythematosus or if you have had a prior allergic reaction to ACE inhibitors. This medication should be used with caution by patients with severe kidney disease or renal artery stenosis (narrowing of one or both of the arteries that supply blood to the kidneys). This medication can increase blood triglycerides and worsen control of blood sugar in people with diabetes.

Molindone

BRAND NAME
Moban

Moban 5 mg
(GATE)

 804
Additional photographs

▶ Drug Class: Neuroleptic; antipsychotic

▶ Available in: Tablets, liquid concentrate

▶ Available OTC? No

▶ As Generic? No

Side Effects

SERIOUS
Restlessness, rigidity and trembling of limbs, involuntary movements of the tongue, face, mouth, or jaw, involuntary movements of the arms or legs, muscle rigidity, irregular pulse, unusually rapid heartbeat, palpitations, or other heartbeat irregularities. Call your doctor immediately.

COMMON
Drowsiness, blurred vision, palpitations, dry mouth or excessive salivation, skin rash, shaking of the hands, stiffness, stooped posture.

LESS COMMON
Increase in sexual desire, menstrual irregularities, discharge of milk from the breast, enlargement of breasts in men and women, prolonged contraction of muscles, liver abnormalities, mental depression, hyperactivity, unusual feeling of well-being (euphoria).

PRINCIPAL USES
To treat psychotic conditions (severe mental disorders characterized by distorted thoughts, perceptions, and emotions), such as schizophrenia.

HOW THE DRUG WORKS
Molindone alters the activity of certain chemicals in the central nervous system, reducing aggressiveness and hyperactivity. It also appears to produce tranquilizing and antipsychotic effects.

DOSAGE
Initial dose is 50 to 75 mg a day; can be increased to 100 mg a day after 3 or 4 days. Maintenance dose may vary from 5 to 15 mg, 3 or 4 times a day, to 10 to 25 mg, 3 or 4 times a day, or 225 mg daily in several divided doses, depending on the severity of the condition being treated. Older and debilitated patients should be started on lower doses.

ONSET OF EFFECT
Sedation may occur within minutes, but onset of antipsychotic effect may take hours to occur or may not occur until days or weeks after the beginning of therapy.

DURATION OF ACTION
24 to 36 hours.

DIETARY ADVICE
No special restrictions.

STORAGE
Store in a tightly sealed container away from heat and direct light.

IF YOU MISS A DOSE
Take it as soon as you remember. If it is near the time for the next dose, skip the missed dose and resume your regular dosage schedule. Do not double the next dose.

STOPPING THE DRUG
The decision to stop taking the drug should be made in consultation with your physician.

PROLONGED USE
Prolonged use may lead to tardive dyskinesia (involuntary movements of the jaw, lips, tongue, and, in rare cases, the arms, legs, hands, or body). Consult your doctor about the need for follow-up evaluations and tests if you must take this drug for an extended period.

PRECAUTIONS
Over 60: Adverse reactions are more likely and more severe in older patients.

Driving and Hazardous Work: Exercise caution until you determine how the medication affects you.

Alcohol: Avoid alcohol.

Pregnancy: Molindone has not been shown to cause birth defects in animals. Human studies have not been done. Before you take molindone, tell your doctor if you are pregnant or plan to become pregnant.

Breast Feeding: It is not known whether molindone passes into breast milk; caution is advised. Discuss potential risks and benefits with your doctor.

Infants and Children: Not recommended for use by children under age 12.

Special Concerns: Molindone is a newer drug very similar to phenothiazines (such as chlorpromazine and perphenazine), but does not appear to cause unexpected weight gain and is not as likely to cause tardive dyskinesia (an irreversible neurological disorder). The liquid concentrate form of molindone contains sulfite and so may cause severe allergic reactions in those who are highly sensitive to sulfites. Persons with asthma are incidentally at increased risk of sulfite sensitivity.

OVERDOSE
Symptoms: Extreme drowsiness, heartbeat irregularities, dry mouth, paradoxical restlessness or agitation, seizures, loss of consciousness.

What to Do: Call your doctor, emergency medical services (EMS), or the nearest poison control center immediately.

DRUG INTERACTIONS
Consult your doctor for advice if you are taking any drugs that depress the central nervous system, including antihistamines, antidepressants or other psychiatric medications, barbiturates, sedatives, cough medicines, decongestants, and painkillers. Be sure your doctor knows about any over-the-counter drugs you may take.

FOOD INTERACTIONS
None reported.

DISEASE INTERACTIONS
Consult your doctor for specific advice if you have any other medical condition.

Mometasone Furoate Nasal

▶ Drug Class: Nasal corticosteroid

▶ Available in: Nasal spray

▶ Available OTC? No

▶ As Generic? No

Side Effects

SERIOUS
No serious side effects are associated with mometasone.

COMMON
Headache, increased susceptibility to viral infection, sore throat, nosebleeds or bloody nasal secretions.

LESS COMMON
Cough, increased susceptibility to upper respiratory infection, menstrual irregularities, bone pain, sinus pain.

PRINCIPAL USES
To prevent and treat the symptoms of allergic rhinitis (seasonal and perennial allergies such as hay fever).

HOW THE DRUG WORKS
Respiratory corticosteroids such as mometasone primarily reduce or prevent inflammation of the lining of the airways, reduce the allergic response to inhaled allergens, and inhibit the secretion of mucus within the airways.

DOSAGE
Adults and teenagers: 2 sprays (50 micrograms [mcg] in each spray) in each nostril once a day, for a maximum daily dose of 200 mcg. To prevent the symptoms of allergic rhinitis from developing, it is recommended that patients with known seasonal allergies begin taking mometasone 2 to 4 weeks before the anticipated start of the pollen season.

ONSET OF EFFECT
From 11 hours to 2 days.

DURATION OF ACTION
Mometasone is effective as long as you continue to take the medication.

DIETARY ADVICE
Mometasone can be used without regard to diet.

STORAGE
Store in a tightly sealed container away from heat, moisture, and direct light.

IF YOU MISS A DOSE
If you miss a dose on one day, resume your regular dosage schedule the next day. Do not double the next dose.

STOPPING THE DRUG
No special instructions.

PROLONGED USE
Consult your doctor about any need for periodic physical examinations and laboratory tests.

PRECAUTIONS
Over 60: No special problems are expected.

Driving and Hazardous Work: Mometasone should not impair your ability to perform such tasks safely.

Alcohol: No special precautions are necessary.

Pregnancy: Nasal steroids have not been reported to cause birth defects if taken during pregnancy. Before using this drug, tell your doctor if you are pregnant or plan to become pregnant.

Breast Feeding: Mometasone may pass into breast milk; caution is advised. Consult your doctor for specific advice.

Infants and Children: Not recommended for use by children under age 12.

Special Concerns: Prior to your initial use of the inhaler, you must prime it by depressing the pump 10 times or until a fine mist appears. You may store the inhaler for up to 1 week without repriming. If it is unused for more than 1 week, reprime it by depressing the pump 2 times or until a fine mist appears. Avoid spraying the medication into the eyes.

OVERDOSE
Symptoms: No cases of overdose have been reported.

What to Do: An overdose with mometasone is unlikely. If someone takes a much larger dose than prescribed, call your doctor.

DRUG INTERACTIONS
Consult your doctor for advice if you are taking systemic corticosteroids, other inhaled corticosteroids, or any drugs that suppress the immune system.

FOOD INTERACTIONS
No known food interactions.

DISEASE INTERACTIONS
Consult your doctor if you have any other medical problem, particularly glaucoma, a herpes infection of the eye, a history of tuberculosis, liver disease, an underactive thyroid, or osteoporosis.

Mometasone Furoate Topical

▶ Drug Class: Antipsoriasis drug; topical corticosteroid

▶ Available in: Cream, lotion, ointment

▶ Available OTC? No

▶ As Generic? No

Side Effects

SERIOUS
No serious side effects are associated with the use of mometasone.

COMMON
Thinning of the skin may occur with prolonged use of mometasone.

LESS COMMON
Burning or discomfort when medication is applied, blisters and pus near hair follicles, unusual bleeding or easy bruising, darkening or prominence of small skin veins, numbness or tingling of affected area, or of hands and fingers, increased susceptibility to infection, cataracts.

PRINCIPAL USES
For topical therapy of skin conditions associated with itching, redness, scaling and peeling, pain, and other signs of inflammation. Topical steroids come in many strengths; your physician will prescribe mometasone, a medium strength steroid, when it is the most appropriate steroid preparation for your particular skin condition.

HOW THE DRUG WORKS
Steroids interfere with the formation of natural substances within your body that are directly responsible for the process of inflammation, which produces swelling, redness, itching, and pain.

DOSAGE
Adults: Apply to the affected areas once daily. Children: Consult your pediatrician.

ONSET OF EFFECT
Soon after application. However, recognizable changes in your condition may take several days or more to develop.

DURATION OF ACTION
Unknown.

DIETARY ADVICE
Maintain your usual food and fluid intake. Increase fluids if you have a fever or diarrhea, in hot weather, or during exercise.

STORAGE
Store in a tightly sealed container away from heat and direct light. Keep away from moisture and extremes in temperature.

IF YOU MISS A DOSE
Apply it as soon as you remember. If it is near the time for the next dose, skip the missed dose and resume your regular dosage schedule.

STOPPING THE DRUG
Apply it as prescribed for the full treatment period, even if you begin to feel better before the scheduled end of the therapy.

PROLONGED USE
Therapy with this medication may require weeks or months. Prolonged use may increase the risk of undesirable side effects (especially thinning of the skin).

PRECAUTIONS
Over 60: Adverse reactions may be more likely and more severe in older patients.

Driving and Hazardous Work: The use of topical mometasone should not impair your ability to perform such tasks safely.

Alcohol: No special precautions are necessary.

Pregnancy: Mometasone should not be used for prolonged periods by pregnant women or by women trying to become pregnant.

Breast Feeding: Mometasone may pass into breast milk; caution is advised. Consult your doctor for advice.

Infants and Children: Not recommended for prolonged use by children. Consult your pediatrician.

Special Concerns: Avoid use of this medication around the eyes. Note that mometasone is not a treatment for acne, burns, infections, or disorders of pigmentation. Do not bandage or wrap the medicated area of skin with any special dressings or coverings unless specifically told to do so by your doctor. Applying special coverings leads to increased absorption of the medication from the skin, and may increase the chance of an undesirable interaction or side effect.

OVERDOSE
Symptoms: No specific ones have been reported.

What to Do: An overdose of mometasone is unlikely to be life-threatening. However, if someone applies a much larger dose than prescribed, call your doctor, emergency medical services (EMS), or the nearest poison control center.

DRUG INTERACTIONS
None are known. Consult your doctor or pharmacist if you are concerned about a particular prescription or nonprescription drug.

FOOD INTERACTIONS
No known food interactions.

DISEASE INTERACTIONS
Consult your doctor if you have any of the following: diabetes, skin infection or skin sores and ulcers, infection at another site in your body, tuberculosis, unusual bleeding or bruising, glaucoma, or cataracts.

Montelukast

BRAND NAME
Singulair

▶ Drug Class: Leukotriene receptor antagonist

▶ Available in: Tablets, chewable tablets

▶ Available OTC? No

▶ As Generic? No

Side Effects

SERIOUS
Skin rash (indicating potentially life-threatening allergic reaction); gastroenteritis (causing loss of appetite, nausea, vomiting, stomach upset, fever, and diarrhea). Call your doctor immediately.

COMMON
Headache.

LESS COMMON
Weakness, fatigue, fever, abdominal pain, indigestion, mouth ulcers, dizziness, nasal congestion, cough, flu-like symptoms.

PRINCIPAL USES
To prevent and treat the symptoms of chronic asthma by preventing bronchospasm (contraction of the smooth muscle tissue surrounding the airways, which results in narrowing and obstruction of the air passages). Montelukast may be used in conjunction with other asthma treatments, such as bronchodilators.

HOW THE DRUG WORKS
Montelukast blocks cell receptors for leukotrienes, naturally formed substances that cause inflammation and constriction of the bronchial airways. Unlike bronchodilators, which relieve the acute symptoms of an asthma attack, montelukast is prescribed to be taken regularly when no symptoms are present, to reduce the chronic inflammation of the airways that is the underlying cause of asthma. This prevents symptomatic asthma attacks.

DOSAGE
Adults and children age 15 and over: One 10 mg tablet per day, taken in the evening. Children ages 6 to 14: One 5 mg chewable tablet per day, taken in the evening. Children ages 2 to 5: One 4 mg chewable tablet per day, taken in the evening.

ONSET OF EFFECT
Unknown.

DURATION OF ACTION
Unknown.

DIETARY ADVICE
Montelukast can be taken without regard to diet.

STORAGE
Store in a tightly sealed container away from heat, moisture, and direct light.

IF YOU MISS A DOSE
If you miss a dose one day, do not double the dose the next day. Resume your regular dosage schedule.

STOPPING THE DRUG
The decision to stop taking the drug should be made in consultation with your physician.

PROLONGED USE
No special problems are expected.

PRECAUTIONS
Over 60: Adverse reactions may be more likely and more severe.

Driving and Hazardous Work: No special precautions are necessary.

Alcohol: No special precautions are necessary.

Pregnancy: Adequate human studies have not been done. Before taking montelukast, tell your doctor if you are pregnant or plan to become pregnant.

Breast Feeding: Montelukast may pass into breast milk; caution is advised. Consult your doctor for specific advice.

Infants and Children: Not recommended for use by children under age 2.

Special Concerns: Montelukast has no effect on an asthma attack that has already started. You should have a fast-acting inhaled bronchodilator on hand to treat an acute asthma attack in progress. Consult your doctor if you need to use inhaled bronchodilators more often than usual, or if you are taking more than the maximum number of inhalations in a 24-hour period. Continue to take montelukast even when you are not experiencing any symptoms, as well as during periods of worsening asthma. In rare cases, if doses of systemic corticosteroids are reduced, montelukast may cause Churg-Strauss syndrome, a tissue disorder that sometimes strikes adult asthma patients and, if untreated, can destroy organs. Early symptoms include fever, muscle aches, and weight loss. Montelukast should not be used as the sole treatment for exercise-induced bronchospasm.

OVERDOSE
Symptoms: No cases of overdose have been reported.

What to Do: An overdose with montelukast is unlikely. If someone takes a much larger dose than prescribed, call your doctor, emergency medical services (EMS), or the nearest poison control center immediately.

DRUG INTERACTIONS
Consult your doctor for specific advice if you are already taking phenobarbital or rifampin. Before you take montelukast, tell your doctor if you are allergic to any other prescription or over-the-counter medicine.

FOOD INTERACTIONS
No known food interactions.

DISEASE INTERACTIONS
If you have phenylketonuria, you should not use the chewable tablet form of montelukast, since it contains phenylalanine. Use of montelukast may cause complications in patients with severe liver disease, since this organ works to remove the medication from the body.

Morphine

M S Contin 15 mg
(PURDUE FREDERICK)

Additional photographs

▶ Drug Class: Opioid (narcotic) analgesic

▶ Available in: Capsules, tablets, oral solution, suppositories, injection

▶ Available OTC? No

▶ As Generic? Yes

Side Effects

SERIOUS
Serious side effects of morphine are indistinguishable from those of overdose: Confusion; severe drowsiness, weakness, or dizziness; slurred speech; small, pinpoint pupils; cold, clammy skin; slow breathing; seizures; loss of consciousness.

COMMON
Dizziness or lightheadedness, nausea or vomiting, constipation, drowsiness, itching.

LESS COMMON
Mood swings, false sense of well-being (euphoria), urinary retention, jerking body movements (myoclonus), hallucinations, sweating.

PRINCIPAL USES
To relieve severe pain.

HOW THE DRUG WORKS
Opioids such as morphine relieve pain by acting on specific areas of the brain and spinal cord that process pain signals from nerves throughout the body.

DOSAGE
Adults— Capsules, tablets, oral solution: To start, 10 to 30 mg every 4 to 6 hours. Dose will be adjusted for individual needs. Extended-release capsules or tablets: Starting dose depends on individual needs and will be adjusted. Suppositories: 10 to 30 mg every 4 to 6 hours. Injection: 5 to 20 mg into a muscle or under the skin every 6 hours. Children— Dosages for all oral forms and suppositories must be determined by your doctor; for injection, 0.1 to 0.2 mg per 2.2 lbs (1 kg) of body weight, to a maximum of 15 mg, under the skin every 4 hours.

ONSET OF EFFECT
Oral forms: Within 60 minutes. Suppositories: 20 to 60 minutes. Injection: 10 to 30 minutes.

DURATION OF ACTION
Immediate-release oral forms: 4 to 5 hours. Extended-release forms: 8 to 12 hours. Suppositories and injection: 4 to 5 hours.

DIETARY ADVICE
Oral forms of morphine can be taken with food to lessen stomach upset. Long-acting tablets must be swallowed whole, without chewing.

STORAGE
Store in a tightly sealed container away from heat, moisture, and direct light. Do not allow liquid forms to freeze.

IF YOU MISS A DOSE
If you are taking morphine on a fixed schedule, take it as soon as you remember. If it is near the time for the next dose, skip the missed dose and resume your regular dosage schedule. Do not double the next dose.

STOPPING THE DRUG
The decision to stop taking the drug should be made in consultation with your physician.

PROLONGED USE
See your doctor regularly for tests and examinations if you must take this medication for a prolonged period. Prolonged use may lead to physical dependence.

PRECAUTIONS
Over 60: Adverse reactions may be more likely and more severe in older patients.

Driving and Hazardous Work: Do not drive or engage in hazardous work until you determine how the medicine affects you.

Alcohol: Avoid alcohol.

Pregnancy: Avoid use during pregnancy if possible.

Breast Feeding: Morphine passes into breast milk; caution is advised. Consult your doctor for specific advice.

Infants and Children: Adverse reactions may be more likely and more severe.

Special Concerns: If you feel the medication is not working adequately after a few weeks, do not increase the dose. Consult your doctor. Before having any surgery, tell the doctor or dentist in charge you are taking morphine. Before

removing the foil wrapper of the suppository, check if it is firm enough to insert. If too soft, put it in the refrigerator for 30 minutes or hold it momentarily under cold water.

OVERDOSE
Symptoms: Confusion; severe drowsiness, weakness, or dizziness; slurred speech; small, pinpoint pupils; cold, clammy skin; slow breathing; seizures; loss of consciousness.

What to Do: Call your doctor, emergency medical services (EMS), or the nearest poison control center immediately.

DRUG INTERACTIONS
Consult your doctor for specific advice if you are taking carbamazepine or other drugs for seizures, barbiturates, sedatives, cough medicines, decongestants, antidepressants, other prescription pain medicine, MAO inhibitors, naltrexone, rifampin, or zidovudine.

FOOD INTERACTIONS
None reported.

DISEASE INTERACTIONS
Consult your physician if you have a history of alcohol or drug abuse; emotional illness; brain disorders or head injury; seizures; lung disease; prostate or other problems with urination; gallstones; colitis; heart, kidney, liver, or thyroid disease.

Moxifloxacin Hydrochloride

▶ Drug Class: Fluoroquinolone antibiotic

▶ Available in: Tablets

▶ Available OTC? No

▶ As Generic? No

Side Effects

SERIOUS
Serious reactions to moxifloxacin are rare and include mental confusion, nightmares, dizziness, hallucinations, anxiety, drowsiness or fainting spells, palpitations, shortness of breath, unusual swelling in the face or extremities, and loss of consciousness. Also skin burning, redness, blisters, rash, or itching on exposure to sunlight; increased risk of tendinitis or tendon rupture. Call your doctor immediately.

COMMON
Nausea, diarrhea, dizziness, headache, abdominal pain, vomiting.

LESS COMMON
Many less common side effects have been associated with moxifloxacin and may include: change in sense of taste, heartburn, weakness, insomnia, cough, dry skin, tinnitus, joint pain, dry mouth, vaginitis.

PRINCIPAL USES
To treat mild to severe bacterial infections, including acute sinusitis, community-acquired pneumonia, and acute bacterial complications due to chronic bronchitis.

HOW THE DRUG WORKS
Moxifloxacin inhibits the activity of a bacterial enzyme (gyrase) that is necessary for proper DNA formation and replication. This fights infection by preventing bacteria from reproducing.

DOSAGE
For acute sinusitis or community-acquired pneumonia: 400 mg once a day for 10 days. For acute bacterial complications due to chronic bronchitis: 400 mg once a day for 5 days.

ONSET OF EFFECT
Varies depending on the infection being treated.

DURATION OF ACTION
Unknown.

DIETARY ADVICE
Can be taken without regard to diet. Drink plenty of fluids.

STORAGE
Store in a tightly sealed container away from heat, moisture, and direct light.

IF YOU MISS A DOSE
Take it as soon as you remember. If it is near the time for the next dose, skip the missed dose and resume regular dosage schedule. Do not double next dose.

STOPPING THE DRUG
It is very important to take this drug as prescribed for the full treatment period, even if you begin to feel better before the scheduled end of therapy.

PROLONGED USE
If your symptoms do not improve or instead become worse after a few days, consult your doctor promptly. Moxifloxacin is typically taken for no more than 5 to 10 days.

PRECAUTIONS

Over 60: No special problems are expected.

Driving and Hazardous Work: Avid such activities until you determine how the medicine affects you.

Alcohol: It is advisable to abstain from alcohol when fighting an infection.

Pregnancy: In some animal tests, moxifloxacin has caused birth defects. Adequate studies in humans have not been done. It should be used during pregnancy only if potential benefits clearly justify the risks. Before you take moxifloxacin, tell your doctor if you are pregnant or plan to become pregnant.

Breast Feeding: Moxifloxacin may pass into breast milk and cause serious side effects in the nursing infant; use of the drug is discouraged when nursing.

Infants and Children: Moxifloxacin is not recommended for use by persons under the age of 18.

Special Concerns: Do not take this medicine if you are allergic to any quinolone antibiotic, such as ciprofloxacin or lomefloxacin.

OVERDOSE
Symptoms: An overdose is unlikely to occur. Possible symptoms after an excessive dose may include decreased activity, drowsiness, vomiting, diarrhea, tremors, and seizures.

What to Do: Call your doctor, emergency medical services (EMS), or the nearest poison control center immediately.

DRUG INTERACTIONS
Because moxifloxacin can affect the function of the heart, it should not be used if you are taking antiarrhythmic drugs such as amiodarone, quinidine, procainamide, or sotalol. It should be used with caution in patients taking erythromycin, antipsychotics, tricylic antidepressants, nonsteroidal anti-inflammatory drugs (NSAIDs; including ibuprofen, aspirin, and naproxen), or digoxin. Moxifloxacin should be taken at least 4 hours before or 8 hours after using ferrous sulfate (iron supplement); dietary supplements containing zinc; didanosine; sucralfate; or antacids containing aluminum salts, magnesium salts, or calcium. Also tell your doctor if you are taking any other prescription or over-the-counter drug.

FOOD INTERACTIONS
No known food interactions.

DISEASE INTERACTIONS
Moxifloxacin should not be taken by people with prolongation of the QT interval on an electrocardiogram, known heart rhythm disturbances, uncorrected hypokalemia (low blood potassium levels), or those taking antiarrhythmic drugs such as amiodarone, quinidine, procainamide, or sotalol. This drug should be used with caution in people with significant bradycardia (slow heart rate), recent myocardial ischemia, known or suspected nervous system disorders, or those who are predisposed to seizures. Use of moxifloxacin is not recommended in people with moderate or severe liver disease.

Mupirocin

▶ Drug Class: Antibiotic

▶ Available in: Ointment, cream

▶ Available OTC? No

▶ As Generic? Yes

Side Effects

SERIOUS
There are no serious side effects associated with the use of mupirocin.

COMMON
Mild stinging or burning sensation with initial application.

LESS COMMON
Persistent irritation or skin allergy with pain or discomfort (stinging or burning) at application site; itching, redness, rash, or dryness of the skin; nausea.

PRINCIPAL USES
Mupirocin is prescribed for topical therapy of certain bacteria-related skin infections. Mupirocin may be used alone or is occasionally used in combination with a second antibiotic (which is usually taken in an oral form).

HOW THE DRUG WORKS
Mupirocin works by preventing bacterial cells from manufacturing vital cell proteins and forming protective cell walls. This ultimately destroys the infecting bacterial organisms.

DOSAGE
Apply to affected skin 3 times a day. The site may be covered with a gauze dressing if desired.

ONSET OF EFFECT
Mupirocin begins antibacterial activity as soon as the ointment or cream is applied. Several days may be required, however, before its full effects become noticeable.

DURATION OF ACTION
Unknown.

DIETARY ADVICE
No special restrictions.

STORAGE
Store in a tightly sealed container away from heat and direct light. Keep away from moisture and extremes in temperature.

IF YOU MISS A DOSE
Apply it as soon as you remember. If it is near the time for the next application, skip the missed one and resume your regular dosage schedule. Do not increase the quantity of medication with the next application.

STOPPING THE DRUG
Apply as prescribed for the full treatment period, even if you begin to feel the affected area is better before the scheduled end of therapy.

PROLONGED USE
Therapy with this medication should not require more than 14 days in most cases. Prolonged use of mupirocin may increase the risk of undesirable side effects.

PRECAUTIONS
Over 60: No special precautions for older patients.

Driving and Hazardous Work: The use of mupirocin should not impair your ability to perform such tasks safely.

Alcohol: No special precautions are necessary.

Pregnancy: Mupirocin has not been evaluated in pregnant women. It is likely that mupirocin is safe for use during pregnancy in certain situations. This should be determined by your doctor.

Breast Feeding: Although not thought to be significantly absorbed into the bloodstream, if excessive amounts of mupirocin were absorbed, the drug could pass into breast milk; consult your doctor for advice.

Infants and Children: Consult your pediatrician.

Special Concerns: Mupirocin should not be used by anyone with a history of allergic reaction to mupirocin or any of the ingredients in the ointment or cream (check the label carefully). As with any other antibiotic, mupirocin is useful only against types of bacteria that are susceptible to its effects. Therefore, it is important to tell your doctor if your condition has not improved—or if it has worsened—within 3 to 5 days of starting mupirocin. The particular bacteria causing your illness may be resistant to mupirocin, and a different antibiotic may be required. Avoid using this drug near or around the eyes.

OVERDOSE
Symptoms: No cases of overdose have been reported.

What to Do: Overapplication of mupirocin is unlikely to be harmful. However, if someone swallows the medication, call your doctor, emergency medical services (EMS), or the nearest poison control center.

DRUG INTERACTIONS
No specific interactions have been reported. Consult your doctor or pharmacist if you are concerned about taking another prescription or nonprescription medication while you are using mupirocin.

FOOD INTERACTIONS
No known food interactions.

DISEASE INTERACTIONS
No disease interactions have been reported.

Muromonab-CD3

▶ Drug Class: Immunosuppressant

▶ Available in: Injection

▶ Available OTC? No

▶ As Generic? No

Side Effects

SERIOUS
Chest pain, wheezing or shortness of breath, rapid or irregular heartbeat, swelling of the face or throat. Call your doctor immediately.

COMMON
Dizziness or faintness, diarrhea, fever and chills, general feeling of illness, headache, nausea, vomiting, muscle or joint pain.

LESS COMMON
Confusion, sensitivity of eyes to light, hallucinations, itching or tingling, stiff neck, skin rash, tremor, weakness, unusual fatigue, seizures.

PRINCIPAL USES
To slow down or reduce the natural tendency of the immune system to reject organ transplants.

HOW THE DRUG WORKS
Muromonab-CD3 suppresses the immune system's reaction against foreign tissue by inhibiting activity of white blood cells, a major component of the immune system's arsenal.

DOSAGE
Adults: 5 mg injected into a vein once a day. This drug should be administered only by or under the direct supervision of your doctor. Children: The dose is determined by your doctor according to body weight.

ONSET OF EFFECT
Within minutes.

DURATION OF ACTION
One week after withdrawal of muromonab-CD3.

DIETARY ADVICE
This drug can be given without regard to meals.

STORAGE
Not applicable. Muromonab-CD3 is administered by a health care professional.

IF YOU MISS A DOSE
Contact your doctor and reschedule your appointment as soon as possible.

STOPPING THE DRUG
The decision to stop taking the drug should be made by your doctor.

PROLONGED USE
See your doctor regularly for tests and examinations if you take this drug for a prolonged period. It may cause effects such as skin cancers or lymphomas that may not occur until years after the medicine is administered.

PRECAUTIONS
Over 60: There is no information comparing use of muromonab-CD3 in older patients with use in younger persons.

Driving and Hazardous Work: Do not drive or engage in hazardous work until you determine how the medicine affects you.

Alcohol: Avoid alcohol.

Pregnancy: Studies of this medication's use during pregnancy have not been done in animals or humans. The drug may cross the placenta, but it is not known whether it harms the fetus. Before you take this drug, tell your doctor if you are pregnant or plan to become pregnant.

Breast Feeding: It is not known whether muromonab-CD3 passes into breast milk; consult your doctor for advice.

Infants and Children: Children are more likely to be dehydrated by the vomiting and diarrhea caused by muromonab-CD3.

Special Concerns: Treatment with muromonab-CD3 may increase the risk of other infections. Avoid persons who have received vaccinations recently or those with colds or other infections. If you think you are getting an infection, inform your doctor at once. Dental work should be done only with great caution during therapy. Practice dental hygiene and be cautious when using toothbrushes, toothpicks, and dental floss. Tell your doctor if you have had any allergic reaction to rodents, such as rats or mice; muromonab-CD3 is extracted from a mouse cell culture.

OVERDOSE
Symptoms: No specific ones have been reported.

What to Do: Call your doctor, emergency medical services (EMS), or the nearest poison control center immediately if you suspect an overdose.

DRUG INTERACTIONS
Consult your doctor for specific advice if you are taking azathioprine, chlorambucil, corticosteroids, cyclophosphamide, cyclosporine, cytarabine, mercaptopurine, or a live-virus vaccine.

FOOD INTERACTIONS
No known food interactions.

DISEASE INTERACTIONS
Caution is advised when taking muromonab-CD3. Consult your doctor if you have any of the following: angina, circulation problems, seizures, a history of recent heart attack, any other heart problem, kidney problems, lung problems, nervous system problems, a history of blood clots, chicken pox, shingles, or any infection.

Mycophenolate Mofetil

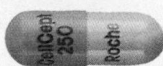

CellCept 250 mg
(ROCHE)

▶ Drug Class: Immunosuppressant

▶ Available in: Capsules, tablets, oral suspension

▶ Available OTC? No

▶ As Generic? No

Side Effects

SERIOUS
Anemia; chest pain; fever or chills; cough or hoarseness; pinpoint red spots on skin; pain in lower back or side; high blood pressure; painful or difficult urination; black, tarry stools; blood in urine or stools; swelling of feet or lower legs; bloody vomit; white patches on mouth, tongue, or throat; unusual bleeding or bruising; tremor. Call your doctor immediately.

COMMON
Abdominal or stomach pain, headache, nausea, vomiting, constipation or diarrhea, heartburn, weakness.

LESS COMMON
Dizziness, skin rash, insomnia, acne.

PRINCIPAL USES
To slow down or reduce the natural tendency of the immune system to reject organ transplants.

HOW THE DRUG WORKS
Mycophenolate suppresses the immune system's reaction against foreign tissue by inhibiting the activity of white blood cells, a major component of the immune system's arsenal.

DOSAGE
Adults: 1 g twice a day in combination with corticosteroids and cyclosporine. Children: Dosage and frequency will be determined by your pediatrician.

ONSET OF EFFECT
Unknown.

DURATION OF ACTION
Unknown.

DIETARY ADVICE
The medication should be taken 30 minutes before or 2 hours after meals. It can be taken with a full glass of water to lessen stomach upset.

STORAGE
Store at room temperature in a tightly sealed container away from heat, moisture, and direct light. Oral suspension may be refrigerated.

IF YOU MISS A DOSE
Take it as soon as you remember. However, if it is near the time for the next dose, skip the missed dose and resume your regular dosage schedule. Do not double the next dose.

STOPPING THE DRUG
The decision to stop taking the drug should be made by your doctor.

PROLONGED USE
You should see your doctor regularly for physical examinations and tests if you must take this drug for an extended period of time.

PRECAUTIONS
Over 60: Information on the effects of mycophenolate in older patients as compared with younger persons is not yet available.

Driving and Hazardous Work: Do not drive or engage in hazardous work until you determine how the medicine affects you.

Alcohol: Avoid alcohol.

Pregnancy: Mycophenolate has caused birth defects in animals. Human studies have not been done, but caution is advised. A pregnancy test should be taken at least 1 week before mycophenolate treatment is started, and reliable methods of contraception should be used before, during, and 6 months after discontinuation of therapy.

Breast Feeding: It is not known whether mycophenolate passes into breast milk, but caution is advised; consult your doctor for advice.

Infants and Children: The safety and efficacy of the use of mycophenolate in infants and children have not been established.

Special Concerns: Patients should avoid contact with persons who may have infections or have recently received a vaccination. They should practice frequent oral hygiene, using a soft toothbrush. The capsules should not be opened, and the powder inside and oral suspension should not be allowed to come in contact with the skin or mucous membranes. If contact occurs, the affected area should be washed thoroughly with soap and water. If the eyes are affected, they should be rinsed with plain water. Discard any unused portion of the oral suspension 60 days after reconstitution.

OVERDOSE
Symptoms: Nausea, diarrhea, vomiting, fatigue.

What to Do: Call your doctor, emergency medical services (EMS), or the nearest poison control center immediately.

DRUG INTERACTIONS
Consult your doctor for specific advice if you are taking azathioprine, chlorambucil, corticosteroids, cyclophosphamide, cyclosporine, mercaptopurine, muromonab-CD3, a live-virus vaccine, or probenecid.

FOOD INTERACTIONS
No known food interactions.

DISEASE INTERACTIONS
Caution is advised when taking mycophenolate. Consult your doctor if you have an active digestive-system disease or kidney disease.

Nabumetone

▶ Drug Class: Nonsteroidal anti-inflammatory drug (NSAID)

▶ Available in: Tablets

▶ Available OTC? No

▶ As Generic? No

Side Effects

SERIOUS
Shortness of breath or wheezing, with or without swelling of legs or other signs of heart failure; chest pain; peptic ulcer disease with vomiting of blood; black, tarry stools; decreasing kidney function. Call your doctor immediately.

COMMON
Nausea, vomiting, heartburn, diarrhea, constipation, headache, dizziness, sleepiness.

LESS COMMON
Ulcers or sores in mouth, depression, rashes or blistering of skin, ringing sound in the ears, unusual tingling or numbness of the hands or feet, seizures, blurred vision. Also elevated potassium levels, decreased blood counts; such problems can be detected by your doctor.

PRINCIPAL USES
To treat mild to moderate pain and inflammation caused by tendinitis, arthritis, bursitis, gout, soft tissue injuries, migraine and other vascular headaches, menstrual cramps, and other conditions. When patients fail to respond to one NSAID, another may be tried. The greatest effectiveness often requires trial and error of several different NSAIDs.

HOW THE DRUG WORKS
NSAIDs work by interfering with the formation of prostaglandins, naturally occurring substances in the body that cause inflammation and make nerves more sensitive to pain impulses. NSAIDs also have other modes of action that are less well understood.

DOSAGE
Adults: 1,000 mg once a day. It may be increased to a maximum of 2,000 mg a day. For children's dose, consult your pediatrician.

ONSET OF EFFECT
From 30 minutes to several hours or longer.

DURATION OF ACTION
Variable.

DIETARY ADVICE
Take with food; maintain your usual food and fluid intake.

STORAGE
Store in a tightly sealed container away from heat, moisture, and direct light.

IF YOU MISS A DOSE
Take it as soon as you remember. However, if it is near the time for the next dose, skip the missed dose and resume your regular dosage schedule. Do not double the next dose.

STOPPING THE DRUG
The decision to stop taking the drug should be made in consultation with your physician.

PROLONGED USE
Prolonged use can cause gastrointestinal problems, including ulceration and bleeding, kidney dysfunction, and liver inflammation. Consult your doctor about the need for medical examinations and lab studies.

PRECAUTIONS
Over 60: Because of the potentially greater consequences of gastrointestinal side effects, the dose of NSAIDs for older patients, especially those over age 70, is often cut in half.

Driving and Hazardous Work: Avoid such activities until you determine how the medicine affects you.

Alcohol: Avoid alcohol when using this medication because it increases the risk of stomach irritation.

Pregnancy: Avoid or discontinue this drug if you are pregnant or plan to become pregnant.

Breast Feeding: Nabumetone passes into breast milk; avoid use while breast feeding.

Infants and Children: May be used in exceptional circumstances; consult your doctor.

Special Concerns: Because NSAIDs can interfere with blood coagulation, this drug should be stopped at least 3 days prior to any surgery.

OVERDOSE
Symptoms: Severe nausea, vomiting, headache, confusion, seizures.

What to Do: Call your doctor, emergency medical services (EMS), or the nearest poison control center immediately.

DRUG INTERACTIONS
Do not take this drug with aspirin or any other NSAIDs without your doctor's approval. In addition, consult your doctor if you are taking antihypertensives, steroids, anticoagulants, antibiotics, itraconazole or ketoconazole, plicamycin, penicillamine, valproic acid, phenytoin, cyclosporine, digitalis drugs, lithium, methotrexate, probenecid, triamterene, or zidovudine.

FOOD INTERACTIONS
No known food interactions.

DISEASE INTERACTIONS
Consult your doctor if you have any of the following: bleeding problems, inflammation or ulcers of the stomach and intestines, diabetes mellitus, systemic lupus erythematosus (SLE, lupus), anemia, asthma, epilepsy, Parkinson's disease, kidney stones, or a history of heart disease or alcohol abuse. Use of nabumetone may cause complications in patients with liver or kidney disease, since these organs work together to remove the medication from the body.

Nadolol

Corgard 20 mg
(**BRISTOL-MYERS SQUIBB**)

Additional photographs

▶ Drug Class: Beta-blocker

▶ Available in: Tablets

▶ Available OTC? No

▶ As Generic? Yes

Side Effects

SERIOUS
Shortness of breath, wheezing; irregular or slow heartbeat (50 beats per minute or less); pain or feelings of tightness or pressure in the chest; swelling of the ankles, feet, and lower legs; mental depression. If you experience any such symptoms, stop taking nadolol and contact your doctor right away.

COMMON
Dizziness or lightheadedness, especially when rising suddenly to a standing position; rapid heartbeat or palpitations; decreased sexual ability; unusual fatigue, weakness, or drowsiness; insomnia.

LESS COMMON
Anxiety, irritability, nervousness; constipation; diarrhea; dry, sore eyes; itching; nausea or vomiting; nightmares or intensely vivid dreams; numbness, tingling, or other unusual sensations in the fingers, toes, or scalp.

PRINCIPAL USES
To treat mild to moderate high blood pressure and angina. It is also used to prevent or control heartbeat irregularities (cardiac arrhythmias).

HOW THE DRUG WORKS
Nadolol slows the rate and force of contraction of the heart by blocking certain nerve impulses, thus reducing blood pressure. By modifying nerve impulses to the heart, the drug also helps to stabilize heart rhythm.

DOSAGE
For high blood pressure: 40 to 320 mg, once a day. For angina: 40 to 240 mg, once a day.

ONSET OF EFFECT
Unknown.

DURATION OF ACTION
Unknown.

DIETARY ADVICE
Follow your doctor's dietary restrictions, such as a low-salt or low-cholesterol diet, to improve control over high blood pressure and heart disease. Take with a full glass of water.

STORAGE
Store in a tightly sealed container away from heat, moisture, and direct light.

IF YOU MISS A DOSE
Take it as soon as you remember. However, if it is within 8 hours of your next dose, skip the missed dose and resume your regular dosage schedule. Do not double the next dose.

STOPPING THE DRUG
This medication should not be stopped suddenly, as this may lead to angina and possibly a heart attack in patients with advanced heart disease. Slow reduction of the dose under a doctor's close supervision for 2 to 3 weeks is advised.

PROLONGED USE
Lifelong therapy may be necessary. See your doctor regularly for examinations and tests if you must take this medicine for a prolonged period.

PRECAUTIONS
Over 60: Adverse reactions may be more likely and more severe in older patients.

Driving and Hazardous Work: May impair alertness, especially in early stages of treatment. Do not drive or engage in hazardous work until you determine how the medicine affects you.

Alcohol: Drink in careful moderation if at all. Alcohol may interact with the drug and cause a dangerous drop in blood pressure.

Pregnancy: Discuss with your doctor the relative risks and benefits of using this drug while pregnant.

Breast Feeding: Trace amounts of nadolol can be found in breast milk, but adverse effects in infants have not been documented. Consult your doctor for advice.

Infants and Children: No special problems.

OVERDOSE
Symptoms: Unusually slow or rapid heartbeat, severe dizziness or fainting, poor circulation in the hands (bluish skin), breathing difficulty, seizures.

What to Do: Call your doctor, emergency medical services (EMS), or the nearest poison control center immediately.

DRUG INTERACTIONS
Consult your doctor for specific advice if you are taking amphetamines, oral antidiabetic agents, asthma medication (such as aminophylline or theophylline), calcium channel blockers, clonidine, guanabenz, halothane, immunotherapy for allergies (allergy shots), insulin, MAO inhibitors, reserpine, other beta-blockers, or any over-the-counter medicine.

FOOD INTERACTIONS
None reported.

DISEASE INTERACTIONS
Nadolol should be used with caution in people with diabetes, especially insulin-dependent diabetes, since the drug may mask symptoms of hypoglycemia. Consult your doctor for special advice if you have allergies or asthma, heart or blood vessel disease (including congestive heart failure and peripheral vascular disease), hyperthyroidism, irregular (slow) heartbeat, myasthenia gravis, psoriasis, respiratory problems such as bronchitis or emphysema, kidney or liver disease, or a history of depression.

Nafarelin Acetate

▶ Drug Class: Gonadotropin-releasing hormone

▶ Available in: Nasal spray

▶ Available OTC? Yes

▶ As Generic? No

Side Effects

SERIOUS
Vaginal bleeding between menstrual periods; longer or heavier menstrual periods; shortness of breath, chest pain, joint pain, and hives caused by an allergic reaction; bloating or tenderness of the lower abdomen; unexpected or excess flow of milk. Call your doctor immediately.

COMMON
Acne, decreased sex drive, dryness of vagina, hot flashes, pain during intercourse, decreased breast size, palpitations, oily skin, cessation of menstrual periods.

LESS COMMON
Breast pain, headache, runny nose, mental depression, mood swings, rash, weight changes.

PRINCIPAL USES
To relieve the pain and discomfort of endometriosis.

HOW THE DRUG WORKS
Nafarelin decreases the production of estrogen by the ovaries. Reduced blood estrogen levels lead to shrinking of endometrial tissue (uterine lining), which eases the painful flare-ups of endometriosis.

DOSAGE
One spray of 200 micrograms into 1 nostril in the morning and 1 spray into the other nostril in the evening, beginning on day 2, 3, or 4 of the menstrual period.

ONSET OF EFFECT
After 4 weeks.

DURATION OF ACTION
3 to 6 months.

DIETARY ADVICE
No special restrictions.

STORAGE
Store container upright away from heat and direct light.

IF YOU MISS A DOSE
Take it as soon as you remember. However, if it is near the time for the next dose, skip the missed dose and resume your regular dosage schedule. Do not double the next dose.

STOPPING THE DRUG
The decision to stop taking the drug should be made by your doctor.

PROLONGED USE
Your doctor should check your progress regularly during prolonged use.

PRECAUTIONS
Over 60: This medicine is generally not used by older patients.

Driving and Hazardous Work: The use of nafarelin should not impair your ability to perform such tasks safely.

Alcohol: Avoid alcohol.

Pregnancy: Nafarelin is not recommended during pregnancy. When taking the drug, women should use nonhormonal contraception (that is, methods other than birth control pills). If you think you are pregnant, stop taking the medicine and call your doctor immediately.

Breast Feeding: Nafarelin may pass into breast milk; caution is advised. Consult your doctor for advice.

Infants and Children: This drug is not recommended for use by children under the age of puberty.

Special Concerns: Tell your doctor if you smoke cigarettes or consume a lot of alcohol or caffeine. When using a new bottle of nafarelin spray, point the bottle away from you and pump about 7 times to prime it. Each time you use the spray, wipe the tip with a clean tissue or cloth. Every 3 or 4 days, rinse the tip with warm water and wipe the tip for about 15 seconds, then dry. To take a dose of nafarelin, first blow your nose gently. Hold your head forward a little, put the spray tip in the nostril, and aim for the back. Close the other nostril by pressing with 1 finger. After the spray, tilt your head back for a few seconds. Do not blow your nose.

OVERDOSE
Symptoms: No specific ones have been reported.

What to Do: An overdose of nafarelin is unlikely to be life-threatening. However, if someone takes a much larger dose than prescribed, call your doctor, emergency medical services (EMS), or the nearest poison control center immediately.

DRUG INTERACTIONS
Consult your doctor for specific advice if you are taking any nasal spray decongestant, adrenocorticoids, or anticonvulsant medication.

FOOD INTERACTIONS
No known food interactions.

DISEASE INTERACTIONS
Caution is advised when taking nafarelin. Consult your doctor if you have any menstrual disorder.

Nalbuphine Hydrochloride

▶ Drug Class: Opioid (narcotic) analgesic

▶ Available in: Injection

▶ Available OTC? No

▶ As Generic? Yes

Side Effects

SERIOUS
Serious side effects of nalbuphine are indistinguishable from those of overdose: Confusion; severe drowsiness, weakness, or dizziness; slurred speech; small, pinpoint pupils; cold, clammy skin; slow breathing; seizures; loss of consciousness.

COMMON
Dizziness or lightheadedness, nausea or vomiting, constipation, drowsiness, itching.

LESS COMMON
Mood swings or false sense of well-being (euphoria), hallucinations.

PRINCIPAL USES
To relieve moderate to severe pain.

HOW THE DRUG WORKS
Opioids such as nalbuphine relieve pain by acting on specific areas of the spinal cord and brain that process pain signals from nerves throughout the body.

DOSAGE
For pain: 10 mg every 3 to 6 hours, into a vein or muscle or under the skin. Children: Dosages must be determined by your doctor.

ONSET OF EFFECT
Into a vein: 2 to 3 minutes. Into a muscle or under the skin: Within 15 minutes

DURATION OF ACTION
3 to 6 hours.

DIETARY ADVICE
This drug can be taken without regard to diet.

STORAGE
Store in a tightly sealed container away from heat, moisture, and direct light. Do not allow it to freeze.

IF YOU MISS A DOSE
If you are taking nalbuphine on a fixed schedule, take it as soon as you remember. If it is near the time for the next dose, skip the missed dose and resume your regular dosage schedule. Do not double the next dose.

STOPPING THE DRUG
The decision to stop taking the drug should be made by your doctor.

PROLONGED USE
See your doctor regularly for tests and examinations if you take this medication for a prolonged period. Prolonged use can cause mental or physical dependence.

PRECAUTIONS
Over 60: Adverse reactions may be more likely and more severe in older patients.

Driving and Hazardous Work: Do not drive or engage in hazardous work until you determine how the medicine affects you.

Alcohol: Avoid alcohol.

Pregnancy: Nalbuphine has not been shown to cause birth defects in animals. Human studies have not been done. Before you use this medication, tell your doctor if you are pregnant or plan to become pregnant. Overuse during pregnancy can cause drug dependence in the fetus.

Breast Feeding: Nalbuphine may pass into breast milk; caution is advised. Consult your doctor for advice.

Infants and Children: Adverse reactions may be more likely and more severe in children. Consult your doctor for advice.

Special Concerns: If you feel the medication is not working properly after a few weeks, do not increase the dose. Consult your doctor. Before having any surgery, tell the doctor or dentist in charge that you are taking this drug.

OVERDOSE
Symptoms: Confusion; severe drowsiness, weakness, or dizziness; slurred speech; small, pinpoint pupils; cold, clammy skin; slow breathing; seizures; loss of consciousness.

What to Do: Call your doctor, emergency medical services (EMS), or the nearest poison control center immediately.

DRUG INTERACTIONS
Consult your physician for specific advice if you are taking carbamazepine or other medicine for seizures, barbiturates, sedatives, cough medicines, decongestants, antidepressants, other prescription pain medications, MAO inhibitors, naltrexone, rifampin, or zidovudine (AZT).

FOOD INTERACTIONS
No known food interactions.

DISEASE INTERACTIONS
Consult your doctor if you have any of the following: history of alcohol or drug abuse; emotional illness; brain disorders or head injury; seizures; lung disease; prostate problems or other problems with urination; gallstones; colitis; heart, kidney, liver, or thyroid disease.

Nalidixic Acid

▶ Drug Class: Anti-infective

▶ Available in: Suspension, tablets

▶ Available OTC? No

▶ As Generic? No

Side Effects

SERIOUS
Blurred, double, or decreased vision, change in color vision, seeing halos around lights, seizures, dark urine, hallucinations, bulging of the fontanel (soft spot) on top of an infant's head, severe headache, mood changes, pale skin, pale stools, skin rash and itching, severe stomach pain, unusual bleeding or bruising, unusual fatigue, yellow eyes or skin. Call your doctor immediately.

COMMON
Dizziness, diarrhea, drowsiness, headache, nausea or vomiting, stomach pain.

LESS COMMON
Increased sensitivity of skin to sunlight.

PRINCIPAL USES
To treat urinary tract infections (UTIs).

HOW THE DRUG WORKS
By interfering with the genetic material of bacteria, nalidixic acid prevents them from reproducing. Eventually the bacteria die out, eliminating the infection.

DOSAGE
Adults and teenagers: 1,000 mg every 6 hours for 1 to 2 weeks, then 500 mg every 6 hours for long-term use. Children 3 months to 12 years: 55 mg per 2.2 lbs (1 kg) of body weight per day in equal doses every 6 hours for 1 to 2 weeks, then 33 mg per 2.2 lbs per day for long-term use.

ONSET OF EFFECT
3 to 4 hours.

DURATION OF ACTION
Unknown.

DIETARY ADVICE
Take nalidixic acid with a full glass of water on an empty stomach, at least 1 hour before or 2 hours after eating. However, if the drug causes stomach upset, nalidixic acid may be taken with food or milk.

STORAGE
Store in a tightly sealed container away from heat and direct light.

IF YOU MISS A DOSE
Take it as soon as you remember. However, if it is near the time for the next dose, skip the missed dose and resume your regular dosage schedule. Do not double the next dose.

STOPPING THE DRUG
Take it as prescribed for the full treatment period, even if you feel better before the scheduled end of therapy.

PROLONGED USE
See your doctor for regular tests and evaluation if you must take this drug for more than 2 weeks.

PRECAUTIONS
Over 60: No special problems are expected.

Driving and Hazardous Work: Avoid such activities until you determine how the medicine affects you.

Alcohol: Drink only in strict moderation.

Pregnancy: Nalidixic acid should not be used during pregnancy because in animal tests it has been shown to cause birth defects.

Breast Feeding: Nalidixic acid passes into breast milk and causes problems in babies with glucose-6-phosphate dehydrogenase (G6PD) deficiency. Problems with other nursing children have not been reported. Consult your doctor for specific individual advice on nursing while you take this medicine.

Infants and Children: This drug is not recommended for use by infants under the age of 3 months.

Special Concerns: Avoid exposure to sunlight until you determine how this medicine affects you. Photosensitivity may last up to 3 months after the last dose. Nalidixic acid may cause false results on tests of blood sugar.

OVERDOSE
Symptoms: Lethargy, psychosis, nausea, vomiting, seizures, severe headache (caused by increased pressure within the skull).

What to Do: Call your doctor, emergency medical services (EMS), or the nearest poison control center immediately.

DRUG INTERACTIONS
Certain drugs may interact adversely with nalidixic acid. Consult your doctor for specific advice, especially if you are taking anticoagulants.

FOOD INTERACTIONS
No known food interactions.

DISEASE INTERACTIONS
Caution is advised when taking nalidixic acid. Consult your doctor if you have any of the following: hardening of the arteries in the brain, G6PD deficiency, or a seizure disorder such as epilepsy. Use of nalidixic acid may cause complications in patients with liver or kidney disease, since these organs work together to remove the medication from the body.

Naltrexone

BRAND NAME
ReVia

▶ Drug Class: Opioid antagonist

▶ Available in: Tablets

▶ Available OTC? No

▶ As Generic? Yes

Side Effects

SERIOUS
Naltrexone may cause liver damage when taken in excess or by people with liver disease due to other causes. Call your doctor immediately if you develop abdominal pain lasting more than a few days, white bowel movements, dark urine, or a yellow discoloration of the eyes or skin.

COMMON
For alcoholism: Nausea, headache, dizziness, nervousness, fatigue. For narcotic addiction: Difficulty sleeping, nervousness, anxiety, abdominal pain or cramps, nausea, vomiting, decreased energy, muscle and joint pain, headache.

LESS COMMON
For alcoholism: Insomnia, vomiting, anxiety, drowsiness. For narcotic addiction: Loss of appetite, constipation, diarrhea, increased thirst, increased energy, depression, irritability, dizziness, skin rash, erectile dysfunction, chills.

PRINCIPAL USES
To aid in the treatment of narcotic and alcohol dependence, in conjunction with psychological and social counseling. Naltrexone is not effective in treating dependency on cocaine or other nonopioid drugs.

HOW THE DRUG WORKS
Naltrexone blocks the euphoric effects of opioid narcotics (such as morphine and heroin) by competitive binding to opioid receptors in the brain. While the precise mechanism of action for alcohol dependence is unclear, naltrexone has been shown to reduce alcohol craving and consumption.

DOSAGE
For alcoholism: 50 mg (1 tablet) once a day. For narcotic dependence: Treatment should not be initiated unless the patient has been opioid-free for at least 7 to 10 days. To start, 25 mg (½ tablet) for the first day. If symptoms of narcotic withdrawal do not appear, dose will be increased to 50 mg once a day. Your doctor may increase or alter the dosage and frequency if necessary.

ONSET OF EFFECT
Within 60 minutes.

DURATION OF ACTION
24 to 72 hours.

DIETARY ADVICE
Naltrexone can be taken without regard to diet.

STORAGE
Store in a tightly sealed container away from heat, moisture, and direct light.

IF YOU MISS A DOSE
What to do if you miss a dose varies by dosage schedule. If you take naltrexone once a day, take the missed dose as soon as possible. However, if you do not remember until the next day, skip the missed dose and resume your regular dosage schedule. Do not double the next dose. If your dosage schedule is different, consult your doctor for advice.

STOPPING THE DRUG
The decision to stop taking the drug should be made in consultation with your physician.

PROLONGED USE
See your doctor regularly for tests of liver function and examinations.

PRECAUTIONS
Over 60: It is not known whether naltrexone causes different or more severe side effects in older patients.

Driving and Hazardous Work: Avoid such activities until you determine how the medicine affects you.

Alcohol: Avoid alcohol.

Pregnancy: Naltrexone has been shown to cause birth defects in animals. Human studies have not been done. This medication should be given during pregnancy only if potential benefits outweigh the risks to the unborn child.

Breast Feeding: Naltrexone may pass into breast milk; caution is advised. Consult your doctor for advice on whether to discontinue nursing or discontinue the drug.

Infants and Children: The safety and effectiveness of this drug have not been established for children under the age of 18.

Special Concerns: Naltrexone will not prevent you from becoming intoxicated upon consumption of alcohol. Carry an identification card indicating you are taking naltrexone. It is of fundamental importance that patients using naltrexone abstain completely from opioid narcotics. If you have not been opioid-free for 7 to 10 days prior to taking naltrexone, it may induce symptoms of acute withdrawal. Also, the effects of naltrexone may be overcome by taking large doses of narcotics, but this poses a serious risk of a fatal narcotic overdose.

OVERDOSE
Symptoms: No cases of overdose have been reported. However, naltrexone may cause liver damage with symptoms including abdominal pain lasting more than a few days, white bowel movements, dark urine, or a yellow discoloration of the eyes or skin.

What to Do: If you suspect an overdose or if someone takes a much larger dose than prescribed, call your doctor, emergency medical services (EMS), or the nearest poison control center immediately.

DRUG INTERACTIONS
Naltrexone should not be used at the same time as narcotic pain relievers such as meperidine, morphine, and methadone. Studies with other types of medications have not be done. Consult your doctor for advice if you are taking any other prescription or over-the-counter drugs.

FOOD INTERACTIONS
No known food interactions.

DISEASE INTERACTIONS
Do not take naltrexone if you have acute hepatitis or liver failure.

Naproxen

Aleve 220 mg
(BAYER)

Additional photographs

▶ Drug Class: Nonsteroidal anti-inflammatory drug (NSAID)

▶ Available in: Tablets, oral suspension, gelcaps

▶ Available OTC? Yes

▶ As Generic? Yes

Side Effects

SERIOUS
Shortness of breath or wheezing, with or without swelling of legs or other signs of heart failure; chest pain; peptic ulcer disease with vomiting of blood; black, tarry stools; decreasing kidney function. Call your doctor immediately.

COMMON
Nausea, vomiting, heartburn, diarrhea, constipation, headache, dizziness, sleepiness.

LESS COMMON
Ulcers or sores in mouth, depression, rashes or blistering of skin, ringing sound in the ears, unusual tingling or numbness of the hands or feet, seizures, blurred vision. Also elevated potassium levels, decreased blood counts; such problems can be detected by your doctor.

PRINCIPAL USES
To relieve minor pain or inflammation associated with headaches, the common cold, toothache, muscle aches, backache, arthritis, gout, tendinitis, bursitis, or menstrual cramps; also, to reduce fever. When patients fail to respond to one NSAID, several others may be tried.

HOW THE DRUG WORKS
NSAIDs work by interfering with the formation of prostaglandins, naturally occurring substances in the body that cause inflammation and make nerves more sensitive to pain impulses. NSAIDs also have other modes of action that are less well understood.

DOSAGE
Adults: 440 to 1,500 mg daily. Maximum dose is 1,500 mg a day, taken in 2 to 3 evenly divided doses.

ONSET OF EFFECT
Rapid; relieves pain within 1 hour. However, it may take up to 2 weeks to suppress inflammation.

DURATION OF ACTION
Up to 12 hours.

DIETARY ADVICE
Take with food; maintain your usual food and fluid intake.

STORAGE
Store tablets in a tightly sealed container away from heat, moisture, and direct light. Store oral suspension in refrigerator, but do not freeze.

IF YOU MISS A DOSE
Take it as soon as you remember. However, if it is near the time for the next dose, skip the missed dose and resume your regular dosage schedule. Do not double the next dose.

STOPPING THE DRUG
If you are taking this drug by prescription, do not stop taking it without first consulting your doctor.

PROLONGED USE
Prolonged use can cause gastrointestinal problems, including ulceration and bleeding, kidney dysfunction, and liver inflammation. Consult your doctor about the need for medical examinations and lab studies.

PRECAUTIONS
Over 60: Because of the potentially greater consequences of gastrointestinal side effects, the dose of NSAIDs for older patients, especially those over age 70, is often cut in half.

Driving and Hazardous Work: Do not drive or engage in hazardous work until you determine how the medication affects you.

Alcohol: Avoid alcohol when taking this drug; the combination of naproxen and alcohol can be highly toxic to the liver.

Pregnancy: Avoid or discontinue this drug if you are pregnant or plan to become pregnant.

Breast Feeding: Naproxen passes into breast milk; avoid or discontinue use while nursing.

Infants and Children: Naproxen may be used in exceptional circumstances; consult your pediatrician for advice.

Special Concerns: Because NSAIDs can interfere with blood coagulation, this drug should be stopped at least 3 days prior to any surgery.

OVERDOSE
Symptoms: Severe nausea, vomiting, headache, confusion, seizures.

What to Do: Call your doctor, emergency medical services (EMS), or the nearest poison control center immediately.

DRUG INTERACTIONS
Do not take this drug with aspirin or any other NSAIDs without your doctor's approval. In addition, consult your doctor if you are taking antihypertensives, steroids, anticoagulants, antibiotics, itraconazole or ketoconazole, plicamycin, penicillamine, valproic acid, phenytoin, cyclosporine, digitalis drugs, lithium, methotrexate, probenecid, triamterene, or zidovudine.

FOOD INTERACTIONS
No known food interactions.

DISEASE INTERACTIONS
Consult your doctor if you have any of the following: bleeding problems, inflammation or ulcers of the stomach and intestines, diabetes mellitus, systemic lupus erythematosus (SLE, lupus), anemia, asthma, epilepsy, Parkinson's disease, kidney stones, or a history of heart disease or alcohol abuse. Use of naproxen may cause complications in patients with liver or kidney disease, since these organs work together to remove the medication from the body.

Naratriptan Hydrochloride

BRAND NAME
Amerge

▶ Drug Class: Antimigraine/ antiheadache drug

▶ Available in: Tablets

▶ Available OTC? No

▶ As Generic? No

Side Effects

SERIOUS
Chest pain or tightness, sudden or severe abdominal pain, shortness of breath, wheezing, heartbeat irregularities or palpitations, skin rash, hives, swelling of the eyelids, face, or lips. Seek emergency medical assistance immediately.

COMMON
Tingling, hot flashes, flushing, weakness, drowsiness or dizziness, fatigue, general feeling of illness.

LESS COMMON
There are no less-common side effects associated with the use of naratriptan.

PRINCIPAL USES
To treat severe, acute migraine headaches. Naratriptan is not intended as a migraine preventive or for use against any other kinds of pain or headache, including basilar and hemiplegic migraines. Your doctor will determine whether this medication is appropriate in your particular case.

HOW THE DRUG WORKS
The exact mechanism of action is unknown.

DOSAGE
A single tablet of 1 or 2.5 mg taken with water is generally effective. If the migraine returns or there is only partial relief, the dose may be repeated once after 4 hours, but no more than 5 mg should be taken in a 24-hour period. Since individuals may vary in response to naratriptan, your experience with the drug will determine the most appropriate initial dosage.

ONSET OF EFFECT
Within 1 to 3 hours.

DURATION OF ACTION
Up to 24 hours.

DIETARY ADVICE
The medication can be taken with or without food.

STORAGE
Store in a tightly sealed container away from heat, moisture, and direct light.

IF YOU MISS A DOSE
Not applicable, since the drug is taken only when necessary.

STOPPING THE DRUG
Consult your doctor before discontinuing naratriptan.

PROLONGED USE
No special problems are expected. However, if you are at risk for coronary artery disease (see Special Concerns), you should undergo periodic medical tests and evaluation.

PRECAUTIONS
Over 60: Naratriptan is not recommended for use in older patients.

Driving and Hazardous Work: Some people feel drowsy or dizzy during or following a migraine attack or after taking naratriptan. Avoid driving or other tasks requiring concentration if you have such symptoms.

Alcohol: No special warnings, although alcohol may trigger or exacerbate migraine headaches.

Pregnancy: Adequate human studies have not been done. Discuss with your doctor the relative risks and benefits of using naratriptan while pregnant.

Breast Feeding: Naratriptan may pass into breast milk; caution is advised. Consult your doctor for specific advice.

Infants and Children: The safety and effectiveness of naratriptan have not been established for patients under age 18. Consult your pediatrician for advice.

Special Concerns: Serious, but rare, heart-related problems may occur after naratriptan use. Anyone at risk for unrecognized coronary artery disease, such as postmenopausal women, men over age 40, or those with risk factors for coronary artery disease (hypertension, high blood cholesterol levels, obesity, diabetes, strong family history of heart disease, or cigarette smoking) should have the first dose of naratriptan administered in a doctor's office. Naratriptan should not be used by anyone with any symptoms of heart disease (chest pain or tightness, shortness of breath).

OVERDOSE
Symptoms: Increase in blood pressure resulting in lightheadedness, tension in the neck, fatigue, and loss of coordination.

What to Do: An overdose with naratriptan is unlikely. If someone takes a much larger dose than prescribed, call your doctor, emergency medical services (EMS), or the nearest poison control center immediately.

DRUG INTERACTIONS
Do not take naratriptan within 24 hours of taking almotriptan, sumatriptan, rizatriptan, zolmitriptan, ergotamine-containing medication, dihydroergotamine mesylate, or methysergide mesylate. Oral contraceptives may interact with naratriptan. Consult your doctor for specific advice.

FOOD INTERACTIONS
No known food interactions.

DISEASE INTERACTIONS
You should not take naratriptan if you have a history of angina, heart disease, stroke, uncontrolled hypertension, heartbeat irregularities, peripheral vascular disease, or severely impaired kidney or liver function.

Natamycin

▶ Drug Class: Antifungal

▶ Available in: Ophthalmic suspension

▶ Available OTC? No

▶ As Generic? No

Side Effects

SERIOUS
Eye redness, swelling or irritation not present before applying natamycin. Call your doctor as soon as possible.

COMMON
No common side effects are associated with natamycin.

LESS COMMON
No less-common side effects are associated with natamycin.

PRINCIPAL USES
To treat several types of fungal infections of the eye, including fungal blepharitis (inflammation of the eyelid), conjunctivitis (inflammation of the mucous membranes that line the inner surface of the eyelids and whites of the eyes), and keratitis (inflammation of the cornea).

HOW THE DRUG WORKS
Natamycin binds to and alters the fungal cell membrane so that vital structures inside the cell pass though the membrane and out of the cell. Without these structures, the fungal cells cannot survive.

DOSAGE
Fungal blepharitis or conjunctivitis: 1 drop every 4 to 6 hours. Fungal keratitis: 1 drop every 1 to 2 hours for the first 3 or 4 days, and 1 drop 6 to 8 times a day thereafter.

ONSET OF EFFECT
Unknown.

DURATION OF ACTION
Unknown.

DIETARY ADVICE
No special restrictions.

STORAGE
Store in a tightly sealed container away from heat, moisture, and direct light. You may store it at room temperature or in the refrigerator, but do not allow it to freeze.

IF YOU MISS A DOSE
Apply natamycin as soon as you remember and then resume your regular dosage schedule. Do not double the next dose.

STOPPING THE DRUG
Use it as prescribed for the full treatment period, even if you begin to feel better before the scheduled end of therapy.

PROLONGED USE
Therapy is generally continued for up to 14 to 21 days, depending on the type and severity of infection, or until the eye infection has been checked. However, no signs of improvement within 7 to 10 days may indicate that a microorganism not susceptible to natamycin is causing the infection; check with your doctor if symptoms do not improve within this amount of time. Your doctor should check your response to natamycin regularly, which may be as often as 3 times a week for certain eye infections.

PRECAUTIONS
Over 60: No special problems are expected.

Driving and Hazardous Work: Avoid such activities until you determine how the medicine affects your vision.

Alcohol: No special precautions are necessary.

Pregnancy: Adequate human studies have not been completed. Before taking natamycin, tell your doctor if you are pregnant or plan to become pregnant.

Breast Feeding: Natamycin may pass into breast milk; caution is advised. Consult your doctor for advice.

Infants and Children: Proper use of natamycin should be determined by your doctor.

Special Concerns: To use the eye drops, first wash your hands. Tilt your head back. Gently apply pressure to the inside corner of the eyelid and with the index finger of the same hand, pull downward on the lower eyelid to make a space. Drop the medicine into this space and close your eye. Apply gentle pressure for 1 or 2 minutes while keeping the eye closed without blinking. Then wash your hands again. Make sure the tip of the dropper does not touch your eye, finger, or any other surface. Shake the container well before each dose.

OVERDOSE
Symptoms: No specific ones have been reported.

What to Do: An overdose of natamycin is unlikely to be life-threatening. However, if someone applies a much larger dose than prescribed or accidentally ingests the medicine, call your doctor, emergency medical services (EMS), or the nearest poison control center immediately.

DRUG INTERACTIONS
None known.

FOOD INTERACTIONS
None known.

DISEASE INTERACTIONS
None known.

Nateglinide

BRAND NAME
Starlix

▶ Drug Class: Antidiabetic agent

▶ Available in: Tablets

▶ Available OTC? No

▶ As Generic? No

Side Effects

SERIOUS
Hypoglycemia (blood sugar levels that are too low), resulting in shakiness, headache, cold sweats, anxiety, and changes in mental state. Immediately ingest sugar-containing food or drink. Inform your doctor about the frequency and timing of hypoglycemic events.

COMMON
None.

LESS COMMON
Increased incidence of upper respiratory infection, flu-like symptoms, dizziness, joint pain.

PRINCIPAL USES
To help control type 2 diabetes mellitus in patients whose blood sugar cannot be adequately controlled by diet and exercise and who have not been chronically treated with other antidiabetic agents. Nateglinide may be used in conjunction with, but not substituted for, the antidiabetic agent metformin to achieve the desired results.

HOW THE DRUG WORKS
Nateglinide stimulates the pancreas to produce more insulin. Increased insulin levels reduce blood glucose by promoting the transport of glucose into muscle cells and other tissues, where it is used as a source of energy. The rapid onset and short duration of nateglinide's action make it effective in controlling glucose levels after a meal.

DOSAGE
The recommended dose is 120 mg 3 times a day (with or without metformin), taken 1 to 30 minutes before meals. If you skip a meal, you should also skip the scheduled dose of nateglinide to reduce the risk of hypoglycemia.

ONSET OF EFFECT
Within 20 minutes.

DURATION OF ACTION
1 to 4 hours.

DIETARY ADVICE
Doses should be taken 1 to 30 minutes before meals. Follow your doctor's advice regarding diet, weight loss, and exercise.

STORAGE
Store in a tightly sealed container away from heat, moisture, and direct light.

IF YOU MISS A DOSE
If you miss a dose, take it just prior to the next meal. Do not double the next dose.

STOPPING THE DRUG
Do not stop taking the drug without your doctor's approval.

PROLONGED USE
Because nateglinide helps to manage diabetes but does not cure the disease, its use will be ongoing as long as your blood glucose levels are being adequately controlled.

PRECAUTIONS
Over 60: Older patients may be more susceptible to hypoglycemia, which may be more difficult to recognize in the elderly.

Driving and Hazardous Work: Do not drive or engage in hazardous work until you determine how the medication affects you.

Alcohol: Limit alcohol intake; hypoglycemia is more likely to occur after the consumption of alcohol.

Pregnancy: Nateglinide should not be used during pregnancy. Insulin is the treatment of choice for pregnant diabetic patients.

Breast Feeding: Nateglinide may pass into breast milk and should not be taken when nursing.

Infants and Children: Safety and effectiveness have not been established for young patients.

Special Concerns: Follow your doctor's advice about diet, exercise, and weight control carefully. These aspects of treatment are just as essential to the proper control of diabetes as taking the medication. Be sure to carry at all times some form of medical identification that indicates you have diabetes and that lists all of the drugs you are taking.

OVERDOSE
Symptoms: Excessive hunger, nausea, anxiety, cold sweats, drowsiness, rapid heartbeat, weakness, changes in mental state, loss of consciousness (indications of hypoglycemia). Overdose is most likely to occur when caloric intake is deficient, following or during more exercise than usual, or after consuming more than a small amount of alcohol.

What to Do: Immediately ingest sugar-containing food or drinks. Call your doctor, emergency medical services (EMS), or local hospital if symptoms persist.

DRUG INTERACTIONS
Consult your doctor if you are taking nonsteroidal anti-inflammatory drugs, (NSAIDs), salicylates, MAO inhibitor antidepressants, beta-blockers, thiazide diuretics, corticosteroids, thyroid hormone, or sympathomimetic drugs.

FOOD INTERACTIONS
A special diet is essential for proper control of blood glucose levels.

DISEASE INTERACTIONS
Do not use nateglinide if you have type 1 diabetes mellitus or diabetic ketoacidosis. Use of nateglinide may cause complications in patients with moderate-to-severe liver disease, since this organ is involved in removing the medication from the body.

Nedocromil Sodium Inhalant

▶ Drug Class: Respiratory inhalant

▶ Available in: Inhalation aerosol

▶ Available OTC? No

▶ As Generic? No

Side Effects

SERIOUS
Increased wheezing, tightness or pain in the chest, or breathing difficulty. Call your doctor right away.

COMMON
There are no common side effects associated with nedocromil.

LESS COMMON
Cough; headache; nausea or vomiting; runny or stuffy nose; throat irritation, soreness, or difficulty swallowing; unpleasant taste.

PRINCIPAL USES

To prevent the symptoms of asthma and to prevent bronchospasm (contraction of the smooth muscle tissue surrounding the airways, which results in narrowing and obstruction of air passages). It cannot relieve an asthma attack once it has started.

HOW THE DRUG WORKS

Nedocromil prevents inflammatory cells in the lungs from releasing substances that cause asthma symptoms or bronchospasm. Unlike bronchodilators that are taken to relieve the acute symptoms of an asthma attack, nedocromil is generally prescribed to be taken on a regular basis when no symptoms are present, to reduce the chronic inflammation of the airways that underlies asthma. Nedocromil may also be used preventively just prior to exposure to certain conditions or substances (cold air, exercise, chemicals, air pollution, or allergens such as pollen or dust mites) that may trigger an acute asthma attack.

DOSAGE

For prevention of asthma symptoms, adults and teenagers: 2 puffs (3.5 to 4 mg) twice a day at regularly spaced times. To prevent bronchospasm, adults and teenagers: 2 puffs up to 30 minutes before exercise or exposure to anything that can trigger bronchospasm. Children: Consult pediatrician for proper dose.

ONSET OF EFFECT

Several days to 4 weeks.

DURATION OF ACTION

6 to 12 hours.

DIETARY ADVICE

This medicine can be taken without regard to diet.

STORAGE

Store in a tightly sealed container away from heat and direct light. Do not allow the medication to freeze. Do not puncture, break, or incinerate the aerosol canister, even if it is empty.

IF YOU MISS A DOSE

Take it as soon as you remember. If it is near the time for the next dose, skip the missed dose and resume your regular dosage schedule. Do not double the next dose.

STOPPING THE DRUG

The decision to stop taking the drug should be made by your doctor.

PROLONGED USE

You should see your doctor regularly for tests and examinations if you take this drug for a prolonged period.

PRECAUTIONS

Over 60: No special problems are expected.

Driving and Hazardous Work: The use of nedocromil should not impair your ability to perform such tasks safely.

Alcohol: No special precautions are necessary.

Pregnancy: Nedocromil has not caused birth defects in animals. Human studies have not been done. Before you take nedocromil, tell your doctor if you are pregnant or plan to become pregnant.

Breast Feeding: Nedocromil may pass into breast milk; caution is advised. Mothers who wish to breast feed while taking nedocromil should consult their doctor for advice.

Infants and Children: No special problems are expected. Use and dose must be determined by your doctor.

Special Concerns: Shake the inhaler well and test before using. Remember to clean the inhaler at least twice a week.

OVERDOSE

Symptoms: No specific ones have been reported.

What to Do: An overdose of nedocromil is unlikely to be life-threatening. However, if someone takes a much larger dose than prescribed, call your doctor, emergency medical services (EMS), or the nearest poison control center.

DRUG INTERACTIONS

Before you take nedocromil, tell your doctor if you are taking any prescription or over-the-counter medicine.

FOOD INTERACTIONS

No known food interactions.

DISEASE INTERACTIONS

No disease interactions have been reported.

Nedocromil Sodium Ophthalmic

▶ Drug Class: Antihistamine

▶ Available in: Ophthalmic solution

▶ Available OTC? No

▶ As Generic? No

Side Effects

SERIOUS
No serious side effects are associated with nedocromil.

COMMON
Headache, temporary burning and stinging of the eye, unpleasant taste, nasal congestion.

LESS COMMON
Asthma, conjunctivitis, eye redness, increased eye sensitivity to light, runny nose.

PRINCIPAL USES
For temporary relief of itching of the eye due to allergic conjunctivitis (inflammation of the mucous membranes that line the inner surface of the eyelids and whites of the eyes).

HOW THE DRUG WORKS
Nedocromil inhibits the release and blocks the effects of histamine, a substance that causes swelling, itching, sneezing, watery eyes, hives, and other symptoms of allergic reaction.

DOSAGE
1 or 2 drops in each affected eye twice a day.

ONSET OF EFFECT
Unknown.

DURATION OF ACTION
Unknown.

DIETARY ADVICE
No special restrictions.

STORAGE
Store in a tightly sealed container away from heat, moisture, and direct light. Do not allow it to freeze.

IF YOU MISS A DOSE
Apply the next dose as needed; do not double the next dose.

STOPPING THE DRUG
This medication is to be used throughout the period of exposure (the duration of the pollen season or until the cause of the conjunctivitis is no longer present), even when symptoms are absent.

PROLONGED USE
See your doctor regularly for tests and examinations if you must take this drug for a prolonged period.

PRECAUTIONS
Over 60: No special problems are expected.

Driving and Hazardous Work: Do not drive or engage in hazardous work until you determine how the medicine affects your vision.

Alcohol: No special precautions.

Pregnancy: In animal studies, large doses of nedocromil did not cause birth defects. Human studies have not been done. Nedocromil should be used by pregnant women only if the potential benefit to the mother justifies the potential risk to the embryo or fetus. Consult your doctor for specific advice.

Breast Feeding: Nedocromil may pass into breast milk; caution is advised. Consult your doctor for advice.

Infants and Children: The safety and effectiveness of nedocromil in infants and children under the age of 3 have not been established.

Special Concerns: To use the eye drops, first wash your hands. Tilt your head back. Gently apply pressure to the inside corner of the eyelid and with the index finger of the same hand, pull downward on the lower eyelid to make a space. Drop the medicine into this space and close your eye. Apply pressure for 1 or 2 minutes while keeping the eye closed without blinking. Then wash your hands again. Make sure the tip of the dropper does not touch your eye, finger, or any other surface. If you use contact lenses, do not wear them while administering nedocromil.

OVERDOSE
Symptoms: No specific ones have been reported. **What to Do:** An overdose of nedocromil is unlikely to be life-threatening. However, if someone applies a much larger dose than prescribed or accidentally ingests the medicine, call your doctor, emergency medical services (EMS), or the nearest poison control center immediately.

DRUG INTERACTIONS
Do not use with any other eye medication. Consult your doctor for specific advice.

FOOD INTERACTIONS
No known food interactions.

DISEASE INTERACTIONS
Caution is advised when taking nedocromil. Consult your doctor if you have any medical condition, especially one affecting the eyes.

Nefazodone Hydrochloride

Serzone 200 mg
(BRISTOL-MYERS SQUIBB)

Additional photographs

▶ Drug Class: Antidepressant

▶ Available in: Tablets

▶ Available OTC? No

▶ As Generic? No

Side Effects

SERIOUS
Blurred, partial loss of, or changes in vision, unsteadiness or clumsiness, skin rash, lightheadedness, ringing in the ears, prolonged or painful erection (lasting more than 4 hours). Call your doctor immediately.

COMMON
Drowsiness or dizziness, agitation, dry mouth, confusion, constipation or diarrhea, unusual dreams, heartburn, fever or chills, insomnia, loss of memory, headache, flushing, nausea or vomiting, increased appetite.

LESS COMMON
Joint pain, increased thirst, breast pain, cough, swelling of lower extremities, sore throat, trembling. Also unusual tingling, burning, or prickling sensations.

PRINCIPAL USES
To treat symptoms of major depression.

HOW THE DRUG WORKS
Nefazodone affects the levels of serotonin and norepinephrine, brain chemicals that are thought to be linked to mood, emotions, and mental state.

DOSAGE
Adults: To start, 100 mg once a day. The dose may be gradually increased by your doctor to a maximum of 600 mg a day. Older adults: To start, 50 mg 1 or 2 times a day. The dose may be gradually increased by your doctor.

ONSET OF EFFECT
The full effect may take several weeks.

DURATION OF ACTION
Unknown.

DIETARY ADVICE
Nefazodone can be taken without regard to diet.

STORAGE
Store in a tightly sealed container away from heat, moisture, and direct light.

IF YOU MISS A DOSE
Take it as soon as you remember. However, if it is near the time for the next dose, skip the missed dose and resume your regular dosage schedule. Do not double the next dose.

STOPPING THE DRUG
Take it as prescribed for the full treatment period, even if you begin to feel better before the scheduled end of therapy. The decision to stop taking the drug should be made in consultation with your doctor.

PROLONGED USE
The usual course of therapy lasts 6 months to 1 year; some patients benefit from additional therapy.

PRECAUTIONS
Over 60: Adverse reactions may be more likely and more severe in older patients. A lower dose may be warranted.

Driving and Hazardous Work: Use caution when driving or engaging in hazardous work until you determine how the medicine affects you. Drowsiness may occur.

Alcohol: Avoid alcohol.

Pregnancy: Nefazodone has not been shown to cause birth defects in animals. Adequate human studies have not been done. Before you take this medication, tell your doctor if you are pregnant or plan to become pregnant.

Breast Feeding: Nefazodone may pass into breast milk; caution is advised.

Infants and Children: The safety and effectiveness of the use of nefazodone in children under age 18 have not been established.

Special Concerns: Use sugarless gum or candy for relief of dry mouth.

OVERDOSE
Symptoms: Lightheadedness, dizziness, confusion, fainting, nausea, vomiting, drowsiness.

What to Do: Call your doctor, emergency medical services (EMS), or the nearest poison control center immediately.

DRUG INTERACTIONS
Do not take nefazodone if you are taking terfenadine or astemizole. Nefazodone and MAO inhibitors should not be used within 14 days of each other. Very serious side effects such as myoclonus (uncontrolled muscle jerking), hyperthermia (excessive rise in body temperature), and extreme stiffness may result. For many patients, especially the elderly, the use of nefazodone in combination with triazolam is not recommended. Other drugs may also interact with nefazodone; consult your doctor if you are taking alprazolam, high blood pressure medication (antihypertensives), atorvastatin, simvastatin, central nervous system depressants (including cold medications, allergy drugs, narcotic pain relievers, and muscle relaxants), or tricyclic antidepressants.

FOOD INTERACTIONS
No known food interactions.

DISEASE INTERACTIONS
Consult your doctor if you have a history of drug or alcohol abuse, any heart condition, a history of seizures, any condition affecting blood vessels of the brain, symptoms of dehydration (confusion, irritability, flushed, dry skin, decreased urine output, extreme thirst), or a history of mental disorders.

Nelfinavir

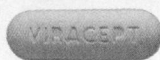

Viracept 250 mg
(AGOURON)

▶ Drug Class: Antiviral/
protease inhibitor

▶ Available in: Oral powder,
tablets

▶ Available OTC? No

▶ As Generic? No

Side Effects

SERIOUS
High blood sugar (diabetes) has occurred in patients taking drugs of this class, although a cause-and-effect relationship has not been established. Contact your doctor if you develop increased thirst or excessive urination.

COMMON
Diarrhea, abdominal pain, low-grade fever, nausea, gas, skin rash.

LESS COMMON
Back pain, headache, loss of appetite, gastrointestinal bleeding, mouth ulcers, vomiting, arthritis, cramps, muscle pain, anxiety, depression, dizziness, insomnia, migraine headache, seizures, drowsiness, breathing difficulty, skin problems, eye disorders, loss of sexual function.

PRINCIPAL USES
To treat HIV (human immunodeficiency virus) infection. While not a cure for HIV, this drug may suppress the replication of the virus and delay the progression of the disease.

HOW THE DRUG WORKS
Nelfinavir blocks the activity of a viral protease, an enzyme that is needed by HIV to reproduce. Blocking the protease causes HIV to make copies that cannot infect new cells.

DOSAGE
Adults: 750 mg, 3 times a day. Children: 20 to 30 mg per 2.2 lbs (1 kg) of body weight, 3 times a day. Instead of tablets, children can be given the oral powder mixed with water, milk, formula, soy milk, or a dietary supplement. Citrus or other acidic foods or juices are not recommended since they may produce a bitter taste when mixed with the medication. Other antiretroviral drugs are prescribed in combination with nelfinavir.

ONSET OF EFFECT
Initial response: Several days. Maximum therapeutic effect: 12 to 16 weeks.

DURATION OF ACTION
Unknown.

DIETARY ADVICE
Nelfinavir should be taken with a light meal or snack.

STORAGE
Store in a tightly sealed container away from heat and direct light. Once oral powder is mixed with liquid, it should not be stored for more than 6 hours; taking the full dose immediately is recommended.

IF YOU MISS A DOSE
Take it as soon as you remember. If it is near the time for the next dose, skip the missed dose and resume your regular dosage schedule. Do not double the next dose.

STOPPING THE DRUG
The decision to stop taking the drug should be made in consultation with your physician.

PROLONGED USE
See your doctor regularly for tests and examinations.

PRECAUTIONS
Over 60: It is not known whether nelfinavir causes different or more severe side effects in older patients.

Driving and Hazardous Work: Avoid such activities until you determine how the medicine affects you.

Alcohol: Avoid alcohol if liver function is impaired.

Pregnancy: Nelfinavir has been shown to cause birth defects in animal studies; however, it is increasingly being used along with other drugs to treat pregnant HIV-infected women.

Breast Feeding: It is unknown whether nelfinavir passes into breast milk; however, to avoid transmitting the virus to an uninfected child, women infected with HIV should not breast feed.

Infants and Children: The safety and effectiveness of nelfinavir have not been established for children under 2 years of age.

Special Concerns: Use of nelfinavir does not eliminate the risk of passing the AIDS virus to other persons. You should take appropriate preventive measures.

OVERDOSE
Symptoms: No cases of overdose have been reported.

What to Do: An overdose of nelfinavir is unlikely to occur. Nonetheless, if you have any reason to suspect an overdose, call your doctor, emergency medical services (EMS), or the nearest poison control center.

DRUG INTERACTIONS
Nelfinavir should not be used concurrently with certain other drugs, because the combination could cause life-threatening heart abnormalities or prolonged loss of consciousness. These drugs include astemizole, midazolam, oral contraceptives, rifampin, amiodarone, quinidine, ergot derivatives (found in certain migraine medications), and triazolam. Other drugs may interact with nelfinavir, requiring some change in your drug regimen. Consult your doctor for specific advice if you are taking any other prescription or over-the-counter medication, especially anticonvulsants (carbamazepine, phenobarbital, phenytoin), indinavir, ritonavir, or rifabutin.

FOOD INTERACTIONS
Food improves the absorption of nelfinavir.

DISEASE INTERACTIONS
Consult your doctor for advice if you have any other medical condition, especially hemophilia. Use of nelfinavir can cause complications in patients with liver disease, as this organ works to remove the drug from the body.

Neomycin/Polymyxin B/Bacitracin Ophthalmic

▶ Drug Class: Antibiotic
combination

▶ Available in: Ophthalmic
ointment

▶ Available OTC? No

▶ As Generic? Yes

Side Effects

SERIOUS
Itching, rash, redness,
swelling, or other eye irritation that was not pre-
sent before therapy. Stop
using the medication and
call your doctor immedi-
ately.

COMMON
Blurred vision for up
to 30 minutes after
application.

LESS COMMON
There are no less-com-
mon side effects associ-
ated with ophthalmic
neomycin/polymyxin B/
bacitracin.

PRINCIPAL USES
To treat or prevent bacterial
infections of the eye.

HOW THE DRUG WORKS
Ophthalmic neomycin/
polymyxin B/bacitracin kills
bacteria by interfering with
the genetic material of bacterial cells, thus preventing
them from multiplying.

DOSAGE
Apply a thin strip of ointment every 3 to 4 hours for
7 to 10 days.

ONSET OF EFFECT
Unknown.

DURATION OF ACTION
Unknown.

DIETARY ADVICE
This medication can be
used without regard to diet.

STORAGE
Store this medication in a
tightly sealed container
away from heat, moisture,
and direct light.

IF YOU MISS A DOSE
Apply it as soon as you
remember. If it is near the
time for the next dose, skip
the missed dose and
resume your regular dosage
schedule. Do not double the
next dose.

STOPPING THE DRUG
Use this drug as prescribed
for the full treatment period,
even if you begin to feel better before the scheduled
end of therapy.

PROLONGED USE
You should see your doctor
regularly for tests and
examinations if you use this
drug for a prolonged period.

PRECAUTIONS
Over 60: No special problems are expected.

**Driving and Hazardous
Work:** Do not drive or
engage in hazardous work
until you determine how the
medicine affects your
vision.

Alcohol: No special precautions are necessary.

Pregnancy: This combination antibiotic has not been
shown to cause birth
defects or other problems
during pregnancy. Before
taking this medication, tell
your doctor if you are pregnant or plan to become
pregnant.

Breast Feeding: This
combination antibiotic has
not been shown to cause
problems in nursing babies.

Infants and Children:
There is no information
comparing the use of this
combination antibiotic in
infants and children with
use in adults.

Special Concerns: To use
the ointment, first wash
your hands. Tilt your head
back. Gently apply pressure
to the inside corner of the
eyelid and with the index
finger of the same hand,
pull downward on the lower
eyelid to make a space. Put
a short strip of ointment
(about ⅓ inch long) into
this space and close your
eye. Apply pressure for 1 or
2 minutes while keeping the
eye closed without blinking.
Then wash your hands
again. Make sure the tip
of the applicator does not
touch your eye, finger, or
any other surface. If your
symptoms do not improve
in a few days or if they
become worse, check with
your doctor. Before you use
this medication, tell your
doctor if you have had an
allergic reaction to
neomycin, polymyxin B,
bacitracin, or any related
antibiotic.

OVERDOSE
Symptoms: No specific
ones have been reported.

What to Do: An overdose
of this combination antibiotic is unlikely to be life-
threatening. If someone
accidentally ingests the
medicine, call your doctor,
emergency medical services
(EMS), or the nearest poison control center.

DRUG INTERACTIONS
Other drugs may interact
with this combination antibiotic. Consult your doctor for
specific advice if you are
taking any other prescription or over-the-counter
medication.

FOOD INTERACTIONS
No known food interactions.

DISEASE INTERACTIONS
Caution is advised when
taking this combination
antibiotic. Consult your doctor if you have any other
medical condition.

Neomycin/Polymyxin B/Bacitracin Topical

BRAND NAMES
Baotino First Aid
Antibiotic, Foille,
Mycitracin, Neosporin
Maximum Strength
Ointment, Neosporin
Ointment, Topisporin

▶ Drug Class: Antibiotic combination

▶ Available in: Ointment

▶ Available OTC? Yes

▶ As Generic? Yes

Side Effects

SERIOUS
Rare, severe allergic reaction that may cause breathing difficulty or, at the extreme, total closure of the airways with potentially fatal anaphylactic shock. Contact emergency medical services (EMS) immediately. In very rare cases hearing loss may occur; if so, call your doctor immediately.

COMMON
No common side effects are associated with this medicine.

LESS COMMON
Irritation or skin allergy with burning, stinging, itching, redness, or rash. Contact your doctor as soon as possible if such side effects persist.

PRINCIPAL USES
To help prevent bacterial skin infections following minor cuts, abrasions, or burns.

HOW THE DRUG WORKS
This is a combination drug containing three distinct antibiotics that each attack and kill bacteria in a different way. Their combined, overlapping effect is capable of warding off infection by a variety of bacterial organisms.

DOSAGE
The usual treatment is to apply the ointment 2 to 5 times a day to areas of the skin that have suffered a minor injury. If you are using the prescription-strength form of the medication, follow your doctor's orders carefully; for over-the-counter forms, follow the directions.

ONSET OF EFFECT
Unknown.

DURATION OF ACTION
Unknown.

DIETARY ADVICE
This medication can be used without regard to diet.

STORAGE
Store in a tightly sealed container away from heat and direct light. Keep away from moisture and extremes in temperature.

IF YOU MISS A DOSE
Apply it as soon as you remember. However, if it is near the time for the next dose, skip the missed dose and resume your regular dosage schedule. Do not apply a double dose.

STOPPING THE DRUG
Use as prescribed for the full treatment period, even if the affected area begins to look and feel better before the scheduled end of therapy. If you stop treatment prematurely, the heartier strains of bacteria are likely to survive, reproduce, and cause a worse infection later (known as a rebound infection).

PROLONGED USE
Consult your physician if you must use this medicine for a prolonged period.

PRECAUTIONS
Over 60: No special precautions for older patients.

Driving and Hazardous Work: No special precautions are necessary.

Alcohol: No special precautions are necessary.

Pregnancy: Clinical studies of the use of this combination antibiotic during pregnancy have not been done. Consult your doctor if you become or are planning to become pregnant.

Breast Feeding: It is not known whether this combination antibiotic passes into breast milk; caution is advised. Consult your doctor for specific advice.

Infants and Children: There is no information about use of this combination antibiotic in infants and children. However, no special problems are expected.

Special Concerns: Do not use this medication if you have a history of allergic reaction to any of the active or inactive ingredients in the ointment. If you use this medicine without a prescription, do not use it to treat puncture wounds, deep wounds, serious burns, or raw areas unless you have first consulted your doctor. Do not use this medicine in the eyes. Before you apply the medication, wash the affected area with soap and water and dry thoroughly. You may cover the treated area with a gauze bandage if you desire.

OVERDOSE
Symptoms: No specific ones have been reported.

What to Do: While no cases of overdose have been reported, if someone accidentally ingests this medicine, call your doctor, emergency medical services (EMS), or the nearest poison control center.

DRUG INTERACTIONS
Do not use other topical medications with this preparation unless otherwise instructed by your doctor.

FOOD INTERACTIONS
No known food interactions.

DISEASE INTERACTIONS
No disease interactions have been reported with the use of this combination antibiotic.

Neomycin/Polymyxin B/Hydrocortisone Ophthalmic and Otic

▶ Drug Class: Antibiotic/corticosteroid combination

▶ Available in: Ophthalmic suspension, otic solution and suspension

▶ Available OTC? No

▶ As Generic? Yes

Side Effects

SERIOUS
Itching, rash, redness, swelling, or other eye or ear irritation that was not present before therapy. Call your doctor immediately.

COMMON
No common side effects are associated with neomycin/ polymyxin B/hydrocortisone.

LESS COMMON
Burning or stinging from the eye drops. There are no less-common side effects associated with the ear preparation.

PRINCIPAL USES
To treat or prevent bacterial infections of the eye or ear and to provide relief from eye or ear irritation and discomfort.

HOW THE DRUG WORKS
Ophthalmic and otic neomycin/polymyxin B/hydrocortisone kills bacteria by interfering with the genetic material of bacterial cells, preventing them from multiplying.

DOSAGE
Ophthalmic suspension—1 drop every 3 to 4 hours. Otic solution and suspension, for ear canal infection— Adults: 4 drops in the ear 3 to 4 times a day. Children: 3 drops in the ear 3 to 4 times a day.

ONSET OF EFFECT
Unknown.

DURATION OF ACTION
Unknown.

DIETARY ADVICE
No special restrictions.

STORAGE
Store in a tightly sealed container away from heat, moisture, and direct light. Do not allow it to freeze.

IF YOU MISS A DOSE
Apply it as soon as you remember. However, if it is near the time for the next dose, skip the missed dose and resume your regular dosage schedule. Do not double the next dose.

STOPPING THE DRUG
Use this drug as prescribed for the full treatment period, even if you begin to feel better before the scheduled end of therapy.

PROLONGED USE
Do not use the ear medication for more than 10 days unless your doctor directs otherwise. If you use the eye medication for a prolonged period, you should see your doctor regularly for tests and examinations.

PRECAUTIONS
Over 60: No special problems are expected.

Driving and Hazardous Work: Do not drive or engage in hazardous work until you determine how the medicine affects your vision.

Alcohol: No special precautions are necessary.

Pregnancy: This medication is not likely to cause problems unless absorbed into the bloodstream; consult your doctor for advice.

Breast Feeding: This combination medication has not been shown to cause problems in nursing babies.

Infants and Children: No special precautions.

Special Concerns: To use the eye drops, first wash your hands. Tilt your head back. Gently apply pressure to the inside corner of the eyelid and with the index finger of the same hand, pull downward on the lower eyelid to make a space. Drop the medicine into this space and close your eye. Apply pressure for 1 or 2 minutes while keeping the eye closed without blinking. To use the ear drops, lie down or tilt your head so the infected ear faces up. Gently pull the earlobe up and back for adults (down and back for children) to straighten the ear canal. Drop the medicine into the ear. Keep the ear facing upward for 5 minutes (2 minutes for children) after inserting the drops to allow the medicine to reach the infection. If necessary, insert a cotton ball to prevent the medicine from leaking out. Make sure the applicator for eye or ear drops does not touch your eye, ear, finger, or any other surface. If your symptoms do not improve in a few days or if they become worse, contact your doctor.

OVERDOSE
Symptoms: No specific ones have been reported.

What to Do: An overdose of this combination medication is unlikely to be life-threatening. If a large volume enters the eye, flush with water. If a large volume enters the ear or someone accidentally ingests the medicine, call your doctor, emergency medical services (EMS), or the nearest poison control center.

DRUG INTERACTIONS
Consult your doctor for specific advice if you are taking any other prescription or over-the-counter medication.

FOOD INTERACTIONS
No known food interactions.

DISEASE INTERACTIONS
Caution is advised when taking this combination antibiotic. Consult your doctor if you have any other eye or ear infection or medical problem.

Neostigmine

BRAND NAME
Prostigmin

▶ Drug Class: Antimyasthenic; muscle stimulant

▶ Available in: Tablets, injection

▶ Available OTC? No

▶ As Generic? Yes

Side Effects

SERIOUS
Skin rash, itching, hives, breathing difficulty, asthmatic wheezing, swelling of the tongue, lips, and throat. Call your doctor right away.

COMMON
Diarrhea, increased sweating, increased watering of mouth, nausea or vomiting, stomach pain or cramps.

LESS COMMON
Increased bronchial secretions, unusual watering of eyes, unusually constricted pupils, gas, increased urination, flushing, weakness.

PRINCIPAL USES
To provide temporary relief of the muscle weakness and fatigability associated with myasthenia gravis. It is also used sometimes to improve bladder or bowel function, particularly after surgery.

HOW THE DRUG WORKS
Neostigmine inhibits the activity of the enzyme cholinesterase, which breaks up acetylcholine, a neurotransmitter involved in muscle activity. Consequently, neostigmine increases the amount of available acetylcholine, which in turn improves muscle strength and endurance in patients with milder forms of myasthenia gravis. The drug's effect also improves the tone of the muscles controlling bladder or bowel activity.

DOSAGE
For myasthenia gravis— Adults and teenagers: Initial dose of tablets (neostigmine bromide) is 15 mg every 3 or 4 hours; maintenance dose is 150 mg every 24 hours in 1 or more doses. Injection (neostigmine methylsulfate): 500 micrograms (mcg) every few hours. Children: With tablets, 2 mg per 2.2 lbs (1 kg) of body weight per day in 6 to 8 doses; or by injection, 10 to 40 mcg per 2.2 lbs every 2 or 3 hours. For bowel and bladder conditions— Adults and teenagers: By injection, 250 to 500 mcg, as needed. Children's use and dosage must be determined by your pediatrician.

ONSET OF EFFECT
From 4 to 30 minutes for injection; 45 to 75 minutes for tablets.

DURATION OF ACTION
2 to 4 hours.

DIETARY ADVICE
Tablets should be taken with food or milk to reduce gastrointestinal upset.

STORAGE
Store in a tightly sealed container away from heat and direct light.

IF YOU MISS A DOSE
Take it as soon as you remember. If it is near the time for the next dose, skip the missed dose and resume your regular dosage schedule. Do not double the next dose.

STOPPING THE DRUG
The decision to stop taking the drug should be made by your doctor.

PROLONGED USE
You should see your doctor regularly for tests and examinations if you take this drug for a prolonged period.

PRECAUTIONS
Over 60: No special problems are expected.

Driving and Hazardous Work: Use of neostigmine should not impair your ability to perform such tasks safely.

Alcohol: No special problems are expected.

Pregnancy: Temporary muscle weakness has occurred in some babies whose mothers took neostigmine during pregnancy. Before you take neostigmine, tell your doctor if you are pregnant or plan to become pregnant.

Breast Feeding: Neostigmine is not believed to pass into breast milk. Consult your doctor for advice.

Infants and Children: No special problems are expected to occur with younger patients.

Special Concerns: Myasthenia gravis patients may be asked to keep a diary of when muscle weakness or other symptoms occur, to allow adjustment of dose size and timing.

OVERDOSE
Symptoms: Abdominal cramps, anxiety, blurred vision, clumsiness or unsteadiness, diarrhea, sweating, excessive salivation, panic attack, progressive muscle weakness leading to paralysis, muscle cramps or twitching, unusual irritability or nervousness, unusual tiredness or weakness, urgent need to urinate.

What to Do: Call your doctor, emergency medical services (EMS), or the nearest poison control center immediately.

DRUG INTERACTIONS
Consult your physician for specific advice if you are taking demecarium, echothiophate, isoflurophate, malathion, guanadrel, guanethidine, procainamide, or trimethaphan.

FOOD INTERACTIONS
No known food interactions.

DISEASE INTERACTIONS
Caution is advised when taking neostigmine. Consult your doctor if you have a history of intestinal blockage, urinary tract blockage, or a current urinary tract infection.

BRAND NAME
Viramune

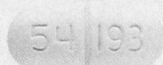

Viramune 200 mg
(BOEHRINGER INGELHEIM)

▶ Drug Class: Antiviral

▶ Available in: Tablets

▶ Available OTC? No

▶ As Generic? No

Side Effects

SERIOUS
Severe skin rash, sometimes with peeling of skin and mucous membranes; yellowish tinge to eyes or skin (indicating liver damage); muscle or joint pain; inflammation of the tissue surrounding the eye. If such symptoms arise, call your doctor immediately.

COMMON
Mild to moderate skin rash (often with itching), abdominal pain or discomfort, diarrhea, nausea, headache.

LESS COMMON
Fever, mouth sores or ulcers, general ill feeling (malaise), inflammation of the tissue surrounding the eye, numbness, tingling, or prickling in the extremities.

PRINCIPAL USES
To treat HIV infection in combination with other drugs. While not a cure for HIV, such drugs may suppress the replication of the virus and delay the progression of the disease.

HOW THE DRUG WORKS
Nevirapine interferes with the activity of enzymes needed for the replication of DNA in viral cells, thus preventing the human immunodeficiency virus (HIV) from reproducing.

DOSAGE
To start, 200 mg once a day, for 14 days; then 200 mg, 2 times a day. Nevirapine should be given in combination with other drugs for HIV, to delay the development of resistant strains of the virus.

ONSET OF EFFECT
Unknown. With most antiretroviral drugs, an early response can be seen within the first few days of therapy, but the maximum effect may take 12 to 16 weeks.

DURATION OF ACTION
Unknown. Effects of the drug may be prolonged if nevirapine is used in combination with other effective drugs and the virus is maximally suppressed.

DIETARY ADVICE
Nevirapine can be taken with or without food. Drink plenty of fluids.

STORAGE
Store in a tightly sealed container away from heat and direct light.

IF YOU MISS A DOSE
Take it as soon as you remember. If it is near the time for the next dose, skip the missed dose and resume your regular dosage schedule. Do not double the next dose.

STOPPING THE DRUG
The decision to stop taking the drug should be made in consultation with your physician.

PROLONGED USE
See your doctor regularly for tests and examinations if you must use this medicine for a prolonged period.

PRECAUTIONS

Over 60: It is not known whether nevirapine causes different or more severe side effects in older patients than it does in younger persons.

Driving and Hazardous Work: Do not drive or engage in hazardous work until you determine how the medicine affects you.

Alcohol: Avoid alcohol if liver function is impaired.

Pregnancy: Nevirapine has been shown to cause birth defects in animals. Adequate human studies have not been done. Nevertheless, nevirapine is increasingly being used in combination with other antiretroviral drugs to treat HIV-infected women who are pregnant.

Breast Feeding: Women infected with HIV should not breast feed, to avoid transmitting the virus to an uninfected child.

Infants and Children: Safety and effectiveness of nevirapine in infants and children have not been established. Use and dose must be determined by your pediatrician.

Special Concerns: Patients who stop nevirapine therapy for more than 7 days should resume with 200 mg once a day for 7 days, then 200 mg once a day for 14 days, then 200 mg, twice a day. Patients taking nevirapine should not use oral contraceptives, but should use another method of birth control, such as condoms.

OVERDOSE
Symptoms: No cases of overdose have been reported.

What to Do: An overdose of nevirapine is unlikely to occur. Nonetheless, if you have any reason to suspect an overdose, call your doctor, emergency medical services (EMS), or the nearest poison control center.

DRUG INTERACTIONS
Consult your doctor for specific advice if you are taking cimetidine, estrogen-containing oral contraceptives, macrolide antibiotics, rifabutin, rifampin, methadone, or any other prescription or over-the-counter medication.

FOOD INTERACTIONS
No known food interactions.

DISEASE INTERACTIONS
Consult your physician if you have any other medical condition. Use of nevirapine may cause complications in patients with liver or kidney disease, since these organs work together to remove the medication from the body.

Nicardipine Hydrochloride Oral

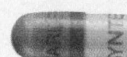

Cardene 30 mg
(SYNTEX)

▶ Drug Class: Calcium channel blocker

▶ Available in: Capsules, sustained-release capsules

▶ Available OTC? No

▶ As Generic? Yes

Side Effects

SERIOUS
Breathing difficulty, coughing, or wheezing; irregular or pounding heartbeat; chest pain; fainting. Call your doctor immediately.

COMMON
Headache, dizziness, skin flushing and feeling of warmth, swelling in the feet, ankles, or calves, palpitations.

LESS COMMON
Constipation or diarrhea, nausea, unusual fatigue and weakness, skin rash, increased urination.

PRINCIPAL USES
To prevent attacks of angina (chest pain associated with heart disease) and to control high blood pressure.

HOW THE DRUG WORKS
Nicardipine interferes with the movement of calcium into heart muscle cells and the smooth muscle cells in the walls of the arteries. This action relaxes blood vessels (causing them to widen), which lowers blood pressure, increases the blood supply to the heart, and decreases the heart's overall workload.

DOSAGE
For angina— Capsules: 20 mg, 3 times a day to start. For high blood pressure— Capsules: 20 to 40 mg, 3 times a day. Sustained-release capsules: 30 mg, 2 times a day. The dose may need to be increased.

ONSET OF EFFECT
Within 20 minutes.

DURATION OF ACTION
Capsules: 6 to 8 hours. Sustained-release capsules: Up to 12 hours.

DIETARY ADVICE
Nicardipine can be taken with or without food.

STORAGE
Store in a tightly sealed container away from heat and direct light.

IF YOU MISS A DOSE
Take it as soon as you remember. If it is near the time for the next dose, skip the missed dose and resume your regular dosage schedule. Do not double the next dose.

STOPPING THE DRUG
Do not stop taking this drug suddenly, as this may cause potentially serious health problems. If therapy is to be discontinued, dosage should be reduced gradually, according to doctor's instructions.

PROLONGED USE
You should see your doctor regularly for examinations and tests if you take this medicine for a prolonged period. Remember that this medication controls your high blood pressure but does not cure it. You may have to take nicardipine for the rest of your life.

PRECAUTIONS
Over 60: Adverse reactions may be more likely and more severe in older patients.

Driving and Hazardous Work: Do not drive or engage in hazardous work until you determine how the medicine affects you.

Alcohol: Avoid alcohol.

Pregnancy: In animal studies, large doses of nicardipine have caused birth defects. Human studies have not been done. Before you take nicardipine, tell your doctor if you are pregnant or plan to become pregnant.

Breast Feeding: Nicardipine may pass into breast milk; caution is advised. Consult your doctor for advice.

Infants and Children: Safety and effectiveness have not been determined for young patients.

Special Concerns: In addition to taking nicardipine, be sure to follow all special instructions on weight control and diet. Your doctor will tell you which specific factors are most important for you.

Check with your doctor before changing your diet.

OVERDOSE
Symptoms: Dizziness, slurred speech, nausea, vomiting, weakness, drowsiness, confusion, heart palpitations, nervousness or excitability.

What to Do: Call your doctor, emergency medical services (EMS), or the nearest poison control center immediately.

DRUG INTERACTIONS
Consult your physician for specific advice if you are taking acetazolamide, amphotericin B, corticosteroids, dichlorphenamide, diuretics, methazolamide, beta-blockers, carbamazepine, cyclosporine, procainamide, quinidine, digitalis drugs, disopyramide or the following eye medicines: betaxolol, levobunolol, metipranolol, or timolol.

FOOD INTERACTIONS
Avoid foods high in sodium.

DISEASE INTERACTIONS
Consult your doctor if you have abnormal heart rhythm or other disorders of the heart and blood vessels, mental depression, or Parkinson's disease. Use of nicardipine may cause complications in patients with liver or kidney disease, since these organs work together to remove the medication from the body.

Nicorette 2 mg
(Hoechst Marion Roussel)

▶ Drug Class: Smoking deterrent

▶ Available in: Chewing gum, skin patch, nasal spray, inhaler

▶ Available OTC? Yes

▶ As Generic? Yes

Side Effects

SERIOUS
With gum: Injury to mouth, dental work, or teeth. Call your dentist. With patch: Hives, itching, skin rash, or swelling. Call your doctor immediately.

COMMON
Mild headache, rapid heartbeat, increased appetite, increased salivation (with gum), sore mouth or throat, pain in jaw or neck, tooth problems (with gum and inhaler), belching (with gum), redness, burning, or itching at site of application (with patch), stinging in the nose (with nasal spray).

LESS COMMON
Constipation, diarrhea, lightheadedness, dry mouth, hiccups (with gum), coughing (with inhaler), hoarseness (with gum and nasal spray), nervousness, irritability, loss of appetite, menstrual pain, joint or muscle pain, stomach upset, sweating, insomnia, unusual dreams, runny nose (with inhaler).

PRINCIPAL USES
To reduce nicotine withdrawal symptoms as part of a comprehensive smoking cessation program.

HOW THE DRUG WORKS
It replaces the nicotine that would otherwise be taken in by tobacco use.

DOSAGE
Used when you have the desire to smoke. Chewing gum: 20 to 24 mg a day; not to exceed 24 pieces of gum a day. Number of sticks is gradually reduced. Skin patch: To start, 1 patch supplying 22 to 24 mg a day. Dose is gradually reduced over 2 to 5 months. Nasal spray: 1 squirt (0.5 mg each, for a total dose of 1 mg) in each nostril as needed, no more than 80 times (40 mg) a day, for 3 to 6 months. Inhaler: Initially (up to 12 weeks), 6 to 16 cartridges a day. The number of cartridges per day is then gradually reduced over the next 6 to 12 weeks.

ONSET OF EFFECT
30 minutes to 2 hours.

DURATION OF ACTION
3 to 6 hours.

DIETARY ADVICE
Gum should be chewed slowly over 30 minutes. Other forms can be used without regard to diet.

STORAGE
Store in a tightly sealed container away from heat and direct light.

IF YOU MISS A DOSE
If you are on a specific regimen, take a missed dose as soon as you remember. If it is near the time for the next dose, skip the missed dose and resume your regular dosage schedule. Otherwise, nicotine is taken as needed.

STOPPING THE DRUG
The decision to stop taking the drug should be made in consultation with your doctor. Dose for the patch should be tapered as directed.

PROLONGED USE
Treatment should generally not exceed 2 to 6 months. If relapse of smoking occurs, treatment may be repeated.

PRECAUTIONS
Over 60: Adverse reactions are not expected to be more severe in older patients than in younger persons.

Driving and Hazardous Work: The use of nicotine should not impair your ability to perform such tasks safely.

Alcohol: No special precautions are necessary.

Pregnancy: Nicotine should not be used during pregnancy. Before you use nicotine, tell your doctor if you are pregnant or plan to become pregnant.

Breast Feeding: Nicotine passes into breast milk; do not use it while nursing.

Infants and Children: Should not be used. Even small amounts of nicotine can cause serious problems in infants and children.

Special Concerns: When disposing of patches, inhaler, or gum, be sure to use a method that keeps them out of the reach of children and animals. You should not smoke while being treated with nicotine. If the gum sticks to dental work, check with your doctor or dentist. Nicotine gum is harder to chew and stickier than ordinary gum and thus is more likely to cause damage. Be careful to follow

directions when applying patch and wash your hands afterward. Do not apply a patch in the same place for at least a week. Do not inhale while spraying the nasal spray.

OVERDOSE
Symptoms: Nausea, vomiting, increased salivation, severe abdominal or stomach pain, diarrhea, severe headache, cold sweats, severe dizziness, hearing and vision disturbances, confusion, weakness, breathing difficulty, heartbeat irregularities, seizures, loss of consciousness.

What to Do: Call your doctor, emergency medical services (EMS), or the nearest poison control center immediately.

DRUG INTERACTIONS
Other drugs may interact with nicotine. Consult your doctor for specific advice if you are taking aminophylline, insulin, oxtriphylline, propoxyphene, or theophylline.

FOOD INTERACTIONS
No known food interactions.

DISEASE INTERACTIONS
Caution is advised when taking nicotine. Consult your doctor if you have a history of diabetes, dental problems (with gum), sinus problems or nasal allergies (with nasal spray), heart or blood vessel disease, inflamed mouth or throat (with gum), skin allergies (with patch), an overactive thyroid, pheochromocytoma, or stomach ulcer.

Nifedipine

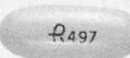

Generic 10 mg
(PUREPAC)

805

Additional photographs

▶ Drug Class: Calcium channel blocker

▶ Available in: Extended-release tablets, capsules

▶ Available OTC? No

▶ As Generic? Yes

Side Effects

SERIOUS
Breathing difficulty, coughing, or wheezing; irregular or pounding heartbeat; chest pain; fainting. Call your doctor immediately.

COMMON
Headache, dizziness, skin flushing and feeling of warmth, swelling in the feet, ankles, or calves, palpitations.

LESS COMMON
Constipation or diarrhea, nausea, unusual fatigue and weakness, skin rash, increased urination, vision problems.

PRINCIPAL USES
To treat high blood pressure and to prevent attacks of angina pectoris (chest pain associated with coronary artery disease).

HOW THE DRUG WORKS
Nifedipine interferes with the movement of calcium into heart muscle cells and the smooth muscle cells in the walls of the arteries. This action relaxes blood vessels (causing them to widen), which lowers blood pressure, increases the blood supply to the heart, and decreases the heart's overall workload.

DOSAGE
Extended-release tablets: 30 or 60 mg once a day. The doses may be increased as determined by your doctor.

ONSET OF EFFECT
Within 20 minutes.

DURATION OF ACTION
Extended-release tablets: 12 to 24 hours.

DIETARY ADVICE
Nifedipine can be taken with or without food.

STORAGE
Store in a tightly sealed container away from heat and direct light.

IF YOU MISS A DOSE
Take it as soon as you remember. If it is near the time for the next dose, skip the missed dose and resume your regular dosage schedule. Do not double the next dose.

STOPPING THE DRUG
Do not stop taking this drug suddenly, as this may cause potentially serious health problems. If therapy is to be discontinued, the dosage should be reduced gradually, according to your doctor's instructions.

PROLONGED USE
You should see your doctor regularly for examinations and tests if you take this medicine for a prolonged period. Remember that this medication controls high blood pressure but does not cure it. You may have to take nifedipine for the rest of your life.

PRECAUTIONS
Over 60: Adverse reactions may be more likely and more severe in older patients.

Driving and Hazardous Work: Do not drive or engage in hazardous work until you determine how the medicine affects you.

Alcohol: Avoid alcohol.

Pregnancy: In animal studies, large doses of nifedipine have been shown to cause birth defects. Human studies have not been done. Before you take nifedipine, tell your doctor if you are pregnant or plan to become pregnant.

Breast Feeding: Nifedipine passes into breast milk but has not been reported to cause problems; caution is advised. Consult your doctor for specific advice.

Infants and Children: While there is no specific information on the use of this medication in younger patients, the use of the capsules is not recommended.

Special Concerns: In addition to taking nifedipine, be sure to follow all special instructions on weight control and diet. Your doctor will tell you which specific factors are most important for you. Check with your doctor before changing your diet.

OVERDOSE
Symptoms: Dizziness, slurred speech, nausea, weakness, drowsiness, confusion, abnormal heartbeat.

What to Do: Call your doctor, emergency medical services (EMS), or the nearest poison control center immediately.

DRUG INTERACTIONS
Consult your physician for specific advice if you are taking acetazolamide, amphotericin B, corticosteroids, dichlorphenamide, diuretics, methazolamide, beta-blockers, carbamazepine, cyclosporine, procainamide, quinidine, digitalis drugs, disopyramide or the following eye medicines: betaxolol, levobunolol, metipranolol, or timolol.

FOOD INTERACTIONS
Avoid foods high in sodium.

DISEASE INTERACTIONS
Caution is advised when taking nifedipine. Consult your doctor if you have any of the following: abnormal heart rhythm, other disorders of the heart and blood vessels, mental depression, or Parkinson's disease. Use of nifedipine may cause complications in patients with liver or kidney disease, since these organs work together to remove the medication from the body.

Nilutamide

▶ Drug Class: Antiandrogen

▶ Available in: Tablets

▶ Available OTC? No

▶ As Generic? No

Side Effects

SERIOUS
Chest pain, difficulty breathing, fever, bone pain, cough, pneumonia. Call your physician immediately.

COMMON
Abdominal pain, headache, loss of appetite, decreased sex drive, nausea, constipation, difficulty of eyes adjusting to darkness, flushing or sensations of warmth.

LESS COMMON
Indigestion, flu-like symptoms, vomiting, dry skin, rash, sweating, loss of body hair, difficulty of eyes adjusting to light, color blindness.

PRINCIPAL USES
Used in conjunction with surgical castration to treat cancer of the prostate.

HOW THE DRUG WORKS
The growth of some types of prostate tumors is stimulated by the hormone testosterone. Nilutamide blocks the activity of testosterone, thus slowing or halting the growth of such tumors. Testosterone is primarily manufactured in the testicles; surgical castration thus further reduces testosterone levels in the body.

DOSAGE
Adult males: To start, 300 mg once a day for 30 days; then 150 mg once a day.

ONSET OF EFFECT
Within hours.

DURATION OF ACTION
Unknown.

DIETARY ADVICE
No special restrictions.

STORAGE
Store in a tightly sealed container away from heat, moisture, and direct light.

IF YOU MISS A DOSE
This drug is prescribed to be taken once a day. If you miss a day, skip the missed dose and resume your regular dosage schedule. Do not double the next dose.

STOPPING THE DRUG
Take it as prescribed for the full treatment period, even if you begin to feel better before the scheduled end of therapy. The decision to stop taking this drug should be made by your doctor.

PROLONGED USE
Nilutamide is not intended to be used on a long-term, ongoing basis. See your physician regularly for evaluation of your condition for the duration of therapy with this drug.

PRECAUTIONS
Over 60: The dosage may be reduced, because the medication takes longer to be eliminated from the body in older patients, but nilutamide is not otherwise expected to cause different side effects or problems in older persons than it does in younger people.

Driving and Hazardous Work: Do not drive or engage in hazardous work until you determine how the medicine affects you.

Alcohol: Avoid alcohol while using this medication.

Pregnancy: Not applicable; prostate cancer occurs only in men.

Breast Feeding: Not applicable; prostate cancer occurs only in men.

Infants and Children: Not applicable.

Special Concerns: Nilutamide treatment must start on the day of or the day after surgical castration is performed.

OVERDOSE
Symptoms: No specific ones have been reported.

What to Do: An overdose with nilutamide is unlikely to occur. If someone takes a much larger dose than prescribed, call your doctor, emergency medical services (EMS), or the nearest poison control center.

DRUG INTERACTIONS
The following drugs may interact with nilutamide. Consult your doctor for specific advice if you are taking vitamin K antagonists, phenytoin, or theophylline. Also tell your doctor if you are taking any other prescription or over-the-counter medication.

FOOD INTERACTIONS
No known food interactions.

DISEASE INTERACTIONS
Caution is advised when taking nilutamide. Consult your doctor for advice if you have severe respiratory problems or any other chronic or significant medical condition. Use of nilutamide may cause complications in patients with liver disease, since this organ works to remove the medication from the body.

Nimodipine

Nimotop 30 mg
(BAYER)

▶ Drug Class: Calcium channel blocker

▶ Available in: Capsules

▶ Available OTC? No

▶ As Generic? No

Side Effects

SERIOUS
Slow or irregular heartbeat, extreme dizziness, fainting, swelling of the extremities, breathing difficulty. Such side effects are rare but serious; call your doctor or emergency medical services (EMS) immediately.

COMMON
Flushing and feeling of warmth, headache.

LESS COMMON
Constipation or diarrhea, dizziness or lightheadedness, nausea, unusual fatigue.

PRINCIPAL USES
To minimize neurological damage in the aftermath of a type of stroke known as subarachnoid hemorrhage (a ruptured blood vessel that spills blood into the space between the protective layers of membranes surrounding the brain).

HOW THE DRUG WORKS
Nimodipine prevents the constriction of smooth muscle tissue that surrounds the blood vessels, especially the arteries in the brain. This helps to keep cerebral arteries open, thus maintaining blood supply to brain tissue, preventing nerve cell death, and preserving function in the areas of the brain affected by the stroke.

DOSAGE
Adults: 60 mg every 4 hours, for 21 consecutive days.

ONSET OF EFFECT
Peak effects within 1 hour.

DURATION OF ACTION
Up to 4 hours.

DIETARY ADVICE
Nimodipine can be taken with or without food.

STORAGE
Store in a tightly sealed container away from heat and direct light.

IF YOU MISS A DOSE
It is imperative to try not to miss a dose of nimodipine. However, if you do miss a dose, take it as soon as you remember. If it is near the time for the next dose, skip the missed dose and resume your regular dosage schedule. Do not double the next dose. If you miss more than one dose, contact your doctor.

STOPPING THE DRUG
Do not stop taking this drug suddenly, as this may cause potentially serious health problems. Therapy with nimodipine typically ends after 21 days, or as determined by your doctor.

PROLONGED USE
Prolonged use is not common; regular medical examinations and tests are necessary if you are required to take this medication for an extended period.

PRECAUTIONS
Over 60: Adverse reactions may be more likely and more severe in older patients.

Driving and Hazardous Work: Do not drive or engage in hazardous work until you determine how the medicine affects you.

Alcohol: Avoid alcohol.

Pregnancy: Large doses of nimodipine have been shown to cause birth defects in animals. Human studies have not been done. Before you take nimodipine, tell your doctor if you are pregnant or plan to become pregnant.

Breast Feeding: Nimodipine may pass into breast milk but has not been reported to cause problems; caution is advised. Consult your doctor for advice.

Infants and Children: While there is no specific information on use of this medication in younger patients, no special problems are expected.

Special Concerns: To be effective, it is crucial to take nimodipine at the regularly scheduled times without fail.

OVERDOSE
Symptoms: Overdose of nimodipine has not been reported. Symptoms would likely be dizziness, confusion, or fainting.

What to Do: If someone takes a much larger dose than prescribed, call your doctor, emergency medical services (EMS), or the nearest poison control center right away.

DRUG INTERACTIONS
Some drugs may interact adversely with nimodipine. Consult your doctor for specific advice if you are taking antihypertensive drugs (beta-blockers or other calcium channel blockers), cimetidine, or fentanyl.

FOOD INTERACTIONS
No known food interactions.

DISEASE INTERACTIONS
Caution is advised when taking nimodipine. Consult your doctor if you have any of the following: abnormal heart rhythm or other disorders of the heart and blood vessels, mental depression, or Parkinson's disease. Use of nimodipine may cause complications in patients with liver or kidney disease, since these organs work together to remove the medication from the body.

Nitrofurantoin

BRAND NAMES
Furadantin, Furalan,
Furatoin, Macrobid,
Macrodantin, Nitrofuracot

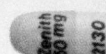

Generic 50 mg
(ZENITH)

▶ Drug Class: Anti-infective

▶ Available in: Capsules, oral
suspension, tablets,
extended-release capsules

▶ Available OTC? No

▶ As Generic? Yes

Side Effects

SERIOUS
Chest pain, chills, cough,
fever, troubled breathing,
dizziness, drowsiness, tingling or burning of face
or mouth, sore throat,
unusual weakness,
unusual fatigue. Call
your doctor immediately.

COMMON
Abdominal pain or stom-
ach upset, diarrhea, nau-
sea, vomiting, loss of
appetite.

LESS COMMON
Dark yellow or brownish
urine.

PRINCIPAL USES
To treat urinary tract infections (UTIs).

HOW THE DRUG WORKS
Nitrofurantoin interferes
with bacterial metabolism
and cell wall formation.
Eventually the bacteria die
out, bringing an end to the
infection.

DOSAGE
Adults and teenagers— Capsules, oral suspension,
tablets: 50 to 100 mg every
6 hours. Extended-rclcase
capsules: 100 mg every 12
hours. Children up to 12
years— Dosage must be
determined by your doctor.

ONSET OF EFFECT
Within 1 hour.

DURATION OF ACTION
Capsules, oral suspension,
tablets: 6 hours. Extended-
release capsules: 24 hours.

DIETARY ADVICE
Nitrofurantoin should be
taken with food or milk.

STORAGE
Store in a tightly sealed container away from heat and
direct light. Keep the oral
suspension from freezing.

IF YOU MISS A DOSE
Take it as soon as you
remember. If it is near the
time for the next dose, skip
the missed dose and
resume your regular dosage
schedule. Do not double the
next dose.

STOPPING THE DRUG
Take as prescribed for the
full treatment period, even if
you begin to feel better
before the scheduled end of
therapy.

PROLONGED USE
See your doctor regularly if
you must take this drug for
a prolonged period.

PRECAUTIONS
Over 60: Adverse reactions
may be more likely and
more severe in older
patients.

**Driving and Hazardous
Work:** Do not drive or
engage in hazardous work
until you determine how the
medicine affects you.

Alcohol: Avoid alcohol.

Pregnancy: Nitrofurantoin
should not be taken within
several weeks of the delivery date or during labor.

Breast Feeding: Nitrofurantoin passes into breast
milk; avoid use while breast
feeding.

Infants and Children:
Nitrofurantoin is not recommended for use by infants
under 1 month old.

Special Concerns: Nitrofurantoin may cause false
results in some urine sugar
tests for diabetes. If your
symptoms do not improve
or instead become worse
within a few days, check
with your doctor. When taking the oral suspension, be
sure to shake the container
forcefully before each dose.
Use a specially marked
measuring spoon or other
device to dispense each
dose. A household teaspoon
might not hold the correct
amount. Tell your doctor if
you have ever had an allergic reaction to nitrofurantoin or any related
medicine, such as furazolidone, or if you are allergic
to any other substance.
When taking the extended-
release capsule, swallow it
whole without chewing.

OVERDOSE
Symptoms: Severe nausea,
vomiting, diarrhea, loss of
appetite.

What to Do: An overdose
of nitrofurantoin is unlikely
to be life-threatening. However, if someone takes a
much larger dose than prescribed, call your doctor,
emergency medical services
(EMS), or the nearest poison control center.

DRUG INTERACTIONS
Consult your doctor for specific advice if you are taking
acetohydroxamine, oral diabetes medicine, dapsone,
furazolidone, methyldopa,
procainamide, quinidine,
sulfonamides, vitamin K,
carbamazepine, chloro-
quine, cisplatin, cytarabine,
vaccine for diphtheria,
tetanus, and pertussis
(DTP), disulfiram, ethotoin,
hydroxychloroquine, lin-
dane, lithium, mephenytoin,
mexiletine, pemoline,
phenytoin, pyridoxine, vincristine, probenecid, sulfinpyrazone, quinine, or any
other anti-infective agent.

FOOD INTERACTIONS
No known food interactions.

DISEASE INTERACTIONS
Consult your doctor if you
have any of the following:
glucose-6-phosphate dehy-
drogenase (G6PD) defi-
ciency, kidney disease, lung
disease, or nerve damage.

Nitroglycerin

Nitrostat 0.4 mg
(PARKE-DAVIS)

▶ Drug Class: Nitrate

▶ Available in: Capsules, tablets, ointment, skin patch, aerosol

▶ Available OTC? No

▶ As Generic? Yes

Side Effects

SERIOUS
Blurred vision, severe or prolonged headache, skin rash, dry mouth. Call your doctor immediately.

COMMON
Flushing of face and neck, headache, nausea or vomiting, dizziness or lightheadedness when getting up, rapid heartbeat, restlessness.

LESS COMMON
Sore, reddened skin.

PRINCIPAL USES
To prevent or relieve attacks of angina (chest pain associated with heart disease).

HOW THE DRUG WORKS
Nitroglycerin relaxes the smooth muscle that surrounds the blood vessels and increases the supply of blood and oxygen to the heart. It also reduces the heart's workload and demand for oxygen.

DOSAGE
Ointment: 15 to 30 mg applied to skin every 6 to 8 hours. Skin patch: 1 patch applied every day, left on for 12 to 14 hours. Aerosol: 1 or 2 doses on or under the tongue at 5-minute intervals to relieve angina attack. Extended-release capsules: 2.5, 6.5, or 9 mg every 12 hours; can be taken every 8 hours. Extended-release tablets: 1.3, 2.6, or 6.5 mg every 12 hours; can be taken every 8 hours. Sublingual (under tongue) or buccal (inside the cheek) tablets: 0.15 to 0.6 mg repeated at 5-minute intervals to treat angina attack. If 3 tablets do not relieve pain, call your doctor.

ONSET OF EFFECT
Sublingual: 2 to 4 minutes. Buccal: 3 minutes. Oral: 20 to 45 minutes. Ointment and skin patch: 30 minutes.

DURATION OF ACTION
Sublingual: 30 to 60 minutes. Buccal: 5 hours. Oral: 8 to 12 hours. Ointment: 4 to 8 hours. Skin patch: Up to 24 hours.

DIETARY ADVICE
Oral forms used as a preventive should be taken 30 minutes before or 1 to 2 hours after meals.

STORAGE
Store in a tightly sealed container away from heat, moisture, and direct light.

IF YOU MISS A DOSE
Take it as soon as you remember. If it is near the time for the next dose, skip the missed dose and resume your regular dosage schedule, as prescribed. Do not double the next dose.

STOPPING THE DRUG
The decision to stop taking nitroglycerin should be made by your doctor.

PROLONGED USE
You should see your doctor regularly for examinations and tests if you take this medicine for a prolonged period.

PRECAUTIONS
Over 60: Adverse reactions may be more likely and more severe in older patients.

Driving and Hazardous Work: Do not drive or engage in hazardous work until you determine how the medicine affects you.

Alcohol: Avoid alcohol.

Pregnancy: Not recommended during pregnancy. Before taking nitroglycerin, be sure to tell your doctor if you are pregnant or plan to become pregnant.

Breast Feeding: Nitroglycerin may pass into breast milk; caution is advised. Consult your doctor for advice.

Infants and Children: No studies in infants and children have been done.

Special Concerns: Skin patch should be applied to different sites to prevent skin irritation.

OVERDOSE
Symptoms: Fast heartbeat, red and perspiring skin, headache, dizziness, palpitations, vision disturbances, nausea, vomiting, confusion, difficulty breathing.

What to Do: Call your doctor, emergency medical services (EMS), or the nearest poison control center immediately.

DRUG INTERACTIONS
Do not take nitroglycerin within 24 hours of taking sildenafil citrate. Sildenafil can enhance the action of nitrates (such as nitroglycerin), causing potentially dangerous decreases in blood pressure. Consult your doctor for specific advice if you are taking other heart medicines or drugs for hypertension.

FOOD INTERACTIONS
No known food interactions.

DISEASE INTERACTIONS
Consult your physician if you have any of the following: anemia, glaucoma, a recent head injury or stroke, a recent heart attack, or an overactive thyroid. Use of nitroglycerin may cause complications in patients with severe liver or kidney disease, since these organs work together to remove the medication from the body.

Nizatidine

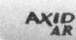

Axid AR 75 mg
(WHITEHALL-ROBINS)

805

Additional photographs

▶ Drug Class: Histamine (H2) blocker

▶ Available in: Capsules, tablets

▶ Available OTC? Yes

▶ As Generic? No

Side Effects

SERIOUS
Irregular heart rhythm (palpitations), slowed heartbeat, severe blood problems, resulting in unusual bleeding, bruising, fever, chills, and increased susceptibility to infection. Call your doctor immediately.

COMMON
Headache, fatigue, drowsiness, dizziness, nausea, vomiting, abdominal pain, diarrhea, constipation.

LESS COMMON
Blurred vision, decreased sexual desire or function, swelling of breasts in males and females, temporary hair loss, hallucinations, depression, insomnia, skin rash, hives, or redness.

PRINCIPAL USES
To treat and prevent the return of ulcers of the stomach and duodenum, as well as conditions that cause increased stomach acid production (such as Zollinger-Ellison syndrome), gastroesophageal reflux (backwash of stomach acid into the esophagus, resulting in heartburn), and minor episodes of heartburn.

HOW THE DRUG WORKS
Nizatidine blocks the action of histamine (a compound produced in the body's cells), which in turn decreases the stomach's secretion of hydrochloric acid. Once stomach acid production has been decreased, the body is better able to heal itself.

DOSAGE
Adults and teenagers— To treat stomach ulcers: 300 mg once a day at bedtime, or 150 mg twice a day. To prevent the recurrence of duodenal ulcers: 150 mg once a day at bedtime. To treat gastroesophageal reflux: 150 mg, 2 times a day. To prevent minor cases of heartburn, acid indigestion, and sour stomach: 75 mg taken 30 to 60 minutes before a meal, once a day.

ONSET OF EFFECT
Within 30 minutes.

DURATION OF ACTION
Up to 12 hours.

DIETARY ADVICE
If you are taking two doses of nizatidine a day, the first dose can be taken after breakfast. Avoid foods that cause stomach irritation.

STORAGE
Store in a tightly sealed container away from heat and direct light.

IF YOU MISS A DOSE
Take it as soon as you remember. If it is near the time for the next dose, skip the missed dose and resume your regular dosage schedule. Do not double the next dose.

STOPPING THE DRUG
Take the prescription-strength form for the full treatment period, even if you begin to feel better before the scheduled end of therapy.

PROLONGED USE
Do not take the maximum daily dosage continually for more than 2 weeks unless directed by your doctor.

PRECAUTIONS
Over 60: Adverse reactions may be more likely and more severe in older patients.

Driving and Hazardous Work: Do not drive or engage in hazardous work until you determine how the medicine affects you.

Alcohol: Avoid alcohol.

Pregnancy: Risks vary, depending on patient and dosage. Consult your physician.

Breast Feeding: Nizatidine passes into breast milk and may pose harm to the child; avoid or discontinue use while nursing.

Infants and Children: Nizatidine is not recommended for young patients, although it has not been shown to cause side effects or problems different from those in adults when used for short periods of time.

Special Concerns: Avoid cigarette smoking because it may increase stomach acid secretion and thus worsen the disease. Do not take nizatidine if you have ever had an allergic reaction to a histamine H2 blocker. If stomach pain becomes worse while using the drug, be sure to tell your doctor right away.

OVERDOSE
Symptoms: No cases of overdose have been reported.

What to Do: Although an overdose is unlikely, if someone takes a much larger dose than prescribed, call your doctor, emergency medical services (EMS), or the nearest poison control center right away.

DRUG INTERACTIONS
No significant drug interactions have been identified. However, nizatidine may increase blood levels of aspirin. Consult your doctor for specific advice if you are taking aspirin.

FOOD INTERACTIONS
Tomato-based mixed vegetable juices, carbonated drinks, citrus fruits and juices, caffeine-containing beverages, and other acidic foods or liquids may irritate the stomach or interfere with the therapeutic action of nizatidine.

DISEASE INTERACTIONS
Patients with kidney disease should not use nizatidine or should use it in smaller, limited doses under careful supervision by a physician.

Norethindrone

▶ Drug Class: Progestin
(hormone)

▶ Available in: Tablets

▶ Available OTC? No

▶ As Generic? No

Side Effects

SERIOUS
Changes in menstrual
bleeding pattern, mental
depression, skin rash,
unexpected or increased
flow of breast milk. Call
your doctor immediately.

COMMON
Abdominal pain or
cramps, swollen face,
ankles, or feet, mood
changes, mild headache,
nervousness, unusual
fatigue, weight gain.

LESS COMMON
Acne, breast pain or ten-
derness, brown spots on
skin, hot flashes, loss or
gain of hair on body or
scalp, loss of sexual
desire, nausea, insomnia.

PRINCIPAL USES
To prevent pregnancy; also
used to treat menstrual disorders such as amenorrhea
(unexpected cessation of
menstrual periods) and
abnormal uterine bleeding,
and to treat endometriosis.

HOW THE DRUG WORKS
Norethindrone prevents
ovulation, probably by
inhibiting secretion of pituitary hormones that in turn
regulate menstrual and
reproductive cycles.
Norethindrone also alters
activity of uterine cells,
resulting in, among other
changes, thickening of the
cervical mucus. These
changes make it less likely
for a partner's sperm to
reach and fertilize an egg.

DOSAGE
For contraception: 0.35 mg
every day at the same time
beginning on the first day of
the menstrual period (28
days from the first day of
the last menstrual period).
For amenorrhea or abnor-
mal uterine bleeding: 2.5 to
10 mg on days 5 through 25
of the menstrual cycle. For
endometriosis: To start, 5
mg a day for 14 days. Your
doctor may gradually
increase your dose up to 15
mg a day for 6 to 9 months.
Contact your physician as
soon as your menstrual
period begins.

ONSET OF EFFECT
Unknown.

DURATION OF ACTION
Unknown.

DIETARY ADVICE
No special restrictions.

STORAGE
Store in a tightly sealed container away from heat and
direct light.

IF YOU MISS A DOSE
When you are 3 hours or
more late or miss 1 day's
dose, take the missed dose
immediately, resume your
regular dosage schedule
and use another method of
contraception for 2 days. If
you miss 2 doses, take 1
tablet immediately and use
another method of birth
control for 7 days. Do not
double the next dose. For
amenorrhea, abnormal
uterine bleeding, and
endometriosis: Take it as
soon as you remember. If it
is near the time for the next
dose, skip the missed dose
and resume your regular
dosage schedule. Do not
double the next dose.

STOPPING THE DRUG
If the medication was given
to treat amenorrhea, abnormal uterine bleeding, or
endometriosis, the decision
to stop taking it should be
made by your doctor.

PROLONGED USE
See your doctor regularly,
usually every 6 to 12
months, for examinations
and tests.

PRECAUTIONS
Over 60: No special problems are expected.

**Driving and Hazardous
Work:** The use of this drug
should not impair your ability to perform such tasks
safely.

Alcohol: No special precautions are necessary.

Pregnancy: This drug
should not be taken during
pregnancy. Problems including genital defects and
smaller-than-normal body
size have been reported in
babies born to women who
took progestins during
pregnancy.

Breast Feeding: Norethindrone passes into breast
milk but has not been
shown to cause problems in
the nursing child. Norethindrone may increase or
decrease the quality or
amount of breast milk. Low-
dose progestins are recommended for contraception
during breast feeding. Consult your doctor for advice.

Infants and Children:
Progestins can been used
for contraception by
teenagers with no unusual
adverse effects.

Special Concerns: Check
with your doctor if vaginal
bleeding continues for an
unusually long time or if
your menstrual period has
not started within 45 days
of the previous one.

OVERDOSE
Symptoms: None are
known; no cases of over-
dose have been reported.

What to Do: An overdose
with norethindrone is
unlikely to occur. Emer-
gency instructions are not
applicable.

DRUG INTERACTIONS
Other drugs may interact
with norethindrone. Consult
your doctor for specific
advice if you are taking
aminoglutethimide, carba-
mazepine, phenobarbital,
phenytoin, rifabutin, or
rifampin.

FOOD INTERACTIONS
No known food interactions.

DISEASE INTERACTIONS
Consult your doctor if you
have a history of any of the
following: breast cancer
(known or suspected), liver
disease, thrombophlebitis,
or thromboembolic disease.

Norfloxacin

BRAND NAMES
Chibroxin, Noroxin

Noroxin 400 mg
(MERCK)

▸ Drug Class: Fluoroquinolone antibiotic

▸ Available in: Eye drops, tablets

▸ Available OTC? No

▸ As Generic? No

Side Effects

SERIOUS
Serious reactions to norfloxacin are rare and include seizures, mental confusion, hallucinations, agitation, nightmares, depression, shortness of breath, unusual swelling in the face or extremities, and loss of consciousness. Also skin burning, redness, blisters, rash, or itching on exposure to sunlight. Call your doctor immediately.

COMMON
Increased sensitivity to sunlight (and increased risk of sunburn) for days following therapy.

LESS COMMON
Diarrhea, nausea and vomiting, stomach pain and upset, gas, headache, dizziness, restlessness, insomnia, changes in taste perception, drowsiness, itching, dry mouth, unusual body aches or pains.

PRINCIPAL USES
To treat urinary tract infections, sexually transmitted diseases, or eye infections caused by bacteria.

HOW THE DRUG WORKS
Norfloxacin inhibits the activity of a bacterial enzyme (gyrase) that is necessary for proper DNA formation and replication. This prevents bacteria cells from reproducing.

DOSAGE
For urinary tract infections: Adults: 400 mg, 2 times a day, for 3 to 21 days. For sexually transmitted diseases: 800 mg in a single one-time dose. For eye infections: 1 drop in each affected eye, 4 times a day, for 7 days.

ONSET OF EFFECT
Varies depending on the infection being treated.

DURATION OF ACTION
Unknown.

DIETARY ADVICE
Tablets should be taken on an empty stomach, 1 hour before or 2 hours after meals, with a full glass of water. Drink plenty of fluids, especially citrus juices or cranberry juice, but avoid milk and dairy derivatives.

STORAGE
Store in a tightly sealed container away from heat, moisture, and direct light.

IF YOU MISS A DOSE
Take it as soon as you remember. If it is near the time for the next dose, skip the missed dose and resume your regular dosage schedule. Do not double the next dose.

STOPPING THE DRUG
It is very important to take this drug as prescribed for the full treatment period, even if you begin to feel better before the scheduled end of therapy.

PROLONGED USE
If your symptoms do not improve or instead become worse after a few days, consult your doctor promptly.

PRECAUTIONS
Over 60: No special problems are expected.

Driving and Hazardous Work: Do not drive or engage in hazardous work until you determine how the medicine affects you.

Alcohol: It is advisable to abstain from alcohol when fighting an infection.

Pregnancy: In some animal tests, norfloxacin has caused birth defects. Adequate studies in humans have not been done. It should be used during pregnancy only if potential benefits clearly justify the risks. Before you take norfloxacin, tell your doctor if you are pregnant or plan to become pregnant.

Breast Feeding: Norfloxacin passes into breast milk and may cause serious side effects in the nursing infant; use of the drug is discouraged when nursing.

Infants and Children: Oral forms of fluoroquinolones such as norfloxacin should not be used by persons under the age of 18. Norfloxacin eye drops should not be used by children under 1 year old.

Special Concerns: If norfloxacin makes your skin or eyes more sensitive to sunlight, wear sunglasses and protective clothing, use a sunscreen with an SPF (sun protection factor) of 15 or higher, and avoid excessive exposure to the sun.

OVERDOSE
Symptoms: Nausea, headache, dizziness, vomiting, drowsiness, seizures.

What to Do: Call your doctor, emergency medical services (EMS), or the nearest poison control center immediately.

DRUG INTERACTIONS
Consult your doctor for specific advice if you are taking aminophylline, antacids, cancer drugs, cyclosporine, didanosine, iron supplements, sucralfate, theophylline, or zinc salts.

FOOD INTERACTIONS
The effects of caffeine may be magnified by this drug. Milk and dairy products can reduce blood levels of norfloxacin by as much as half.

DISEASE INTERACTIONS
Caution is advised when taking norfloxacin. Consult your doctor if you have a disorder of the central nervous system or any other medical condition. Use of norfloxacin may cause complications in patients with kidney disease, since this organ works to remove the medication from the body.

Nortriptyline Hydrochloride

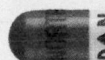

Generic 25 mg
(SCHEIN/DANBURY)

Additional photographs

▶ Drug Class: Tricyclic
antidepressant

▶ Available in: Capsules, oral
solution

▶ Available OTC? No

▶ As Generic? Yes

Side Effects

SERIOUS
Confusion, heartbeat irregularities, hallucinations, seizures, extreme fatigue or drowsiness, blurred or altered vision, breathing difficulty, constipation, staring and absence of facial expression, impaired concentration, difficult urination, fever, extreme and persistent restlessness, loss of coordination and balance, difficulty swallowing or speaking, dilated pupils, eye pain, fainting. Also trembling, shaking, weakness, and stiffness in the extremities; shuffling gait. Call your doctor immediately.

COMMON
Drowsiness or dizziness, headache, dry mouth or unpleasant taste, fatigue, heightened sensitivity to light, weight gain, nausea, increased appetite.

LESS COMMON
Heartburn, sleeping difficulty, diarrhea, increased or profuse sweating, vomiting.

PRINCIPAL USES
To relieve symptoms of major depression, anxiety disorders, panic disorder, or chronic pain.

HOW THE DRUG WORKS
Nortriptyline affects levels of norepinephrine, a brain chemical that is thought to be linked to mood, emotions, and mental state.

DOSAGE
Adults: 25 mg, 3 to 4 times a day; may be increased to a maximum dose of 150 mg a day. Teenagers: 25 to 50 mg a day. Children ages 6 to 12: 10 to 20 mg a day. Older adults: 25 to 100 mg a day; may be increased gradually by your doctor. Dosage is usually determined by blood level monitoring.

ONSET OF EFFECT
1 to 6 weeks.

DURATION OF ACTION
Unknown.

DIETARY ADVICE
To lessen stomach upset, take with food, unless your doctor instructs otherwise. Increase intake of fiber and fluids.

STORAGE
Store in a tightly sealed container away from heat, moisture, and direct light. Do not allow solution to freeze.

IF YOU MISS A DOSE
If you take a one-time daily bedtime dose, do not take the missed dose in the morning because it may cause drowsiness. Call your doctor for specific advice. If you take more than 1 dose a day, take it as soon as you remember. If it is near the time for the next dose, skip the missed dose and resume your regular dosage schedule. Do not double the next dose.

STOPPING THE DRUG
Take as prescribed for the full treatment period, even if you begin to feel better before the scheduled end of therapy. The decision to stop taking the drug should be made in consultation with your doctor.

PROLONGED USE
The usual course of therapy lasts 6 months to 1 year; some patients benefit from additional therapy.

PRECAUTIONS
Over 60: Adverse reactions may be more likely and more severe in older patients. A lower dose may be warranted.

Driving and Hazardous Work: Use caution when driving or engaging in hazardous work until you determine how the medication affects you. Drowsiness or lightheadedness can occur.

Alcohol: Avoid alcohol.

Pregnancy: Adequate human studies have not been done. Consult your doctor for specific advice.

Breast Feeding: Nortriptyline passes into breast milk; do not use it while nursing.

Infants and Children: Not prescribed for children under the age of 6 years.

Special Concerns: This is a potentially dangerous drug, especially if taken in excess. Tricyclic antidepressants should not be within easy reach of suicidal patients. If dry mouth occurs, use candy or sugarless gum for relief.

OVERDOSE
Symptoms: Difficulty breathing, severe fatigue, seizures, confusion, hallucinations, dilated pupils, irregular heartbeat, fever, impaired concentration.

What to Do: Call your doctor, emergency medical services (EMS), or the nearest poison control center immediately.

DRUG INTERACTIONS
Consult your doctor for specific advice if you are taking antithyroid agents, cimetidine, clonidine, guanadrel, guanethidine, metrizamide, appetite suppressants, isoproterenol, ephedrine, epinephrine, amphetamines, phenylephrine, antipsychotic drugs, pimozide, methyldopa, metyrosine, metoclopramide, pemoline, promethazine, trimeprazine, rauwolfia alkaloids, MAO inhibitors, or any drugs that depress the central nervous system.

FOOD INTERACTIONS
No known food interactions.

DISEASE INTERACTIONS
Consult your doctor if you have any of the following: a history of alcohol abuse, difficulty urinating, asthma, bipolar disorder, high blood pressure, stomach or intestinal problems, glaucoma, overactive thyroid, enlarged prostate, schizophrenia, seizures, a blood disorder, or kidney, heart, or liver disease.

Nystatin

Generic 500,000 units
(LEMMON)

▶ Drug Class: Antifungal

▶ Available in: Lozenges, oral suspension, cream, ointment, powder, vaginal tablets

▶ Available OTC? No

▶ As Generic? Yes

Side Effects

SERIOUS
No serious side effects are associated with the use of nystatin.

COMMON
No common side effects are associated with the use of nystatin.

LESS COMMON
Nausea, vomiting, diarrhea, stomach pain, skin or vaginal irritation not present prior to therapy.

PRINCIPAL USES
To treat fungal infections of the skin, mouth, and vagina.

HOW THE DRUG WORKS
Nystatin prevents fungal organisms from producing vital substances required for growth and function. This medication is effective only for infections caused by fungal organisms. It will not work for bacterial or viral infections.

DOSAGE
Lozenges— Adults and children age 5 and older: 1 or 2 lozenges 4 to 5 times a day for up to 14 days. Lozenges should be allowed to dissolve in the mouth, which may take 15 to 30 minutes. Do not swallow. Suspension— Adults and children age 5 and older: 4 to 6 ml (1 teaspoon), 4 times a day. Children up to 5 years: 2 ml, 4 times a day. Premature and low-birth-weight infants: 1 ml, 4 times a day. Follow doctor's instructions for correct use. Cream, ointment, or powder— Adults and children: Apply to the affected area 2 to 3 times a day. Vaginal tablets— Adults and teenagers: Insert one 100,000-unit tablet into the vagina 1 or 2 times a day for 14 days.

ONSET OF EFFECT
Not applicable.

DURATION OF ACTION
Unknown.

DIETARY ADVICE
No special restrictions.

STORAGE
Store in a tightly sealed container away from heat, moisture, and direct light. Lozenges should be kept in the refrigerator, but keep them from freezing.

IF YOU MISS A DOSE
Take it as soon as you remember. However, if it is near the time for the next dose, skip the missed dose and resume your regular dosage schedule. Do not double the next dose.

STOPPING THE DRUG
Take it as prescribed for the full treatment period, even if you begin to feel better before the scheduled end of therapy. The decision to stop taking the drug should be made by your doctor.

PROLONGED USE
Nystatin is generally prescribed for short-term therapy (1 to 3 weeks). Consult your doctor if your condition does not improve, or instead becomes worse, within 1 to 2 weeks of beginning therapy.

PRECAUTIONS
Over 60: There have been no specific studies of the use of nystatin in older patients.

Driving and Hazardous Work: The use of nystatin should not impair your ability to perform such tasks safely.

Alcohol: No special precautions are necessary.

Pregnancy: Adequate studies of use during pregnancy have not been done. Consult your doctor for specific advice if you are pregnant or plan to become pregnant.

Breast Feeding: Nystatin may pass into breast milk; caution is advised. Consult your doctor for specific advice.

Infants and Children: The oral suspension should be used for children up to 5 years of age, rather than the lozenges. There have been no specific studies evaluating the use of the other forms of nystatin in children.

Special Concerns: Patients with dentures may have to soak them each night in nystatin to kill the fungus on the dentures. In some cases new dentures may be necessary.

OVERDOSE
Symptoms: Nausea, vomiting, diarrhea.

What to Do: Call your doctor, emergency medical services (EMS), or the nearest poison control center immediately.

DRUG INTERACTIONS
Other drugs may interact with nystatin. Consult your doctor for specific advice if you are taking any other prescription or over-the-counter drug.

FOOD INTERACTIONS
None known.

DISEASE INTERACTIONS
Consult your doctor for specific advice if you have any other medical condition.

Octreotide Acetate

BRAND NAME
Sandostatin

▶ Drug Class: Hormone

▶ Available in: Injection

▶ Available OTC? No

▶ As Generic? No

Side Effects

SERIOUS

High blood sugar levels causing drowsiness, dry mouth, flushed and dry skin, fruity breath odor, increased urination, loss of appetite, severe stomach pain, nausea, or vomiting, rapid and deep breathing, unusual thirst, unusual fatigue, rapid weight loss. Low blood sugar levels causing anxiety, chills, cool and pale skin, difficulty concentrating, headache, nausea, nervousness, shakiness, sweating, unusual fatigue, weakness. Call your doctor immediately.

COMMON

Stomach or abdominal pain or discomfort; diarrhea, nausea and vomiting; pain, stinging, tingling, or burning at injection site; redness and swelling at the site of injection.

LESS COMMON

Dizziness or lightheadedness, unusual fatigue, headache, red or flushed face, swelling of feet and lower legs.

PRINCIPAL USES

To treat severe, chronic diarrhea that occurs with certain intestinal tumors (carcinoid tumors and vasoactive intestinal peptide tumors). Also used to treat acromegaly, a disease caused by the overproduction of human growth hormone during adulthood, and characterized by thick, bulky overgrowth of the bones in the hands, feet, forehead, and face.

HOW THE DRUG WORKS

Octreotide mimics the activity of the hormone somatostatin, which suppresses the release of certain chemicals that trigger diarrhea. The drug does not attack or cure intestinal cancer, but helps ease symptoms, allowing the patient to lead a more normal life. By suppressing the release of human growth hormone, octreotide slows the progression of acromegaly.

DOSAGE

For carcinoid tumor diarrhea: 100 to 600 micrograms (mcg) a day, administered subcutaneously (under the skin) in 2 to 4 doses. For vasoactive intestinal peptide tumors: 200 to 300 mcg a day in 2 to 4 doses. For acromegaly: From 50 to 300 mcg, 3 times a day. The dose is based on body weight.

ONSET OF EFFECT

Within 30 minutes.

DURATION OF ACTION

Up to 12 hours.

DIETARY ADVICE

No restrictions apply.

STORAGE

Store in a tightly sealed container away from heat and direct light. Keep away from moisture and extremes in temperature.

IF YOU MISS A DOSE

Take it as soon as you remember. If it is near the time for the next dose, skip the missed dose and resume your regular dosage schedule. Do not double the next dose.

STOPPING THE DRUG

The decision to stop taking the drug should be made by your doctor.

PROLONGED USE

You should see your doctor regularly for tests and examinations if you take this drug for a prolonged period.

PRECAUTIONS

Over 60: No special problems are expected.

Driving and Hazardous Work: Do not drive or engage in hazardous work until you determine how the medicine affects you.

Alcohol: Avoid alcohol.

Pregnancy: In animal studies, octreotide has not been shown to cause birth defects, even when given at high doses. Human studies have not been done. Consult your doctor for specific advice if you are pregnant or plan to become pregnant.

Breast Feeding: It is not known whether octreotide passes into breast milk; caution is advised. Consult your doctor for specific advice.

Infants and Children: Octreotide has not been shown to cause different side effects in infants and children than it does in other patients.

Special Concerns: Octreotide can cause either high or low blood sugar levels. Blood sugar should be monitored carefully. Follow your doctor's instructions about selecting and rotating injection sites to help prevent skin problems.

OVERDOSE

Symptoms: Very high or very low blood sugar levels.

What to Do: An overdose of octreotide is unlikely to be life-threatening. However, if someone takes a much larger dose than prescribed, call your doctor, emergency medical services (EMS), or the nearest poison control center.

DRUG INTERACTIONS

Consult your doctor for specific advice if you are taking antidiabetic agents such as glucagon or insulin, or growth hormone.

FOOD INTERACTIONS

No known food interactions.

DISEASE INTERACTIONS

Consult your physician if you have diabetes mellitus, gallbladder disease, or gallstones. Use of octreotide may cause complications in patients with kidney disease, since this organ works to remove the medication from the body.

Ofloxacin Ophthalmic

BRAND NAME
Ocuflox

▶ Drug Class: Antibiotic

▶ Available in: Ophthalmic solution

▶ Available OTC? No

▶ As Generic? No

Side Effects

SERIOUS
Itching, swelling, hives, difficulty breathing. If these signs of allergy develop, stop using the drug and call your doctor immediately.

COMMON
Burning eyes.

LESS COMMON
Increased sensitivity of eyes to light; stinging, itching, tearing, redness, or drying of the eye.

PRINCIPAL USES
To treat bacterial conjunctivitis (infection of the mucous membranes that line the inner surface of the eyelids and whites of the eyes) or bacterial keratitis (infection of the cornea).

HOW THE DRUG WORKS
Ofloxacin kills bacteria by interfering with genetic material of bacterial cells, thus preventing them from multiplying.

DOSAGE
The exact dosing of ophthalmic ofloxacin varies depending on the nature of the infection and its response to treatment. Follow your doctor's instructions precisely. The following dosing example is for conjunctivitis. Adults and children 1 year of age and older: 1 drop in each eye every 2 to 4 hours, while awake, for 2 days, then 1 drop in each eye 4 times a day for up to 5 days.

ONSET OF EFFECT
Unknown.

DURATION OF ACTION
Unknown.

DIETARY ADVICE
No special restrictions.

STORAGE
Store in a tightly sealed container away from heat, moisture, and direct light. Do not refrigerate or allow it to freeze.

IF YOU MISS A DOSE
Apply it as soon as you remember. If it is near the time for the next dose, skip the missed dose and resume your regular dosage schedule. Do not double the next dose.

STOPPING THE DRUG
Use it as prescribed for the full treatment period, even if you feel better before the scheduled end of therapy.

PROLONGED USE
You should see your doctor regularly for tests and examinations if you take this drug for a prolonged period.

PRECAUTIONS
Over 60: No special problems are expected.

Driving and Hazardous Work: Do not drive or engage in hazardous work until you determine how the medicine affects your vision.

Alcohol: No special precautions are necessary.

Pregnancy: Large doses of ophthalmic ofloxacin have caused birth defects and other problems in animals. Human studies have not been done. Before you take ophthalmic ofloxacin, tell your doctor if you are pregnant or plan to become pregnant.

Breast Feeding: Ophthalmic ofloxacin may pass into breast milk; caution is advised. Consult your doctor for advice.

Infants and Children: Not recommended for use on children under age 1.

Special Concerns: To use the eye drops, first wash your hands. Tilt your head back. Gently apply pressure to the inside corner of the eyelid and with the index finger of the same hand, pull downward on the lower eyelid to make a space. Drop the medicine into this space and close your eye. Apply gentle pressure for 1 or 2 minutes while keeping the eye closed without blinking. Then wash your hands again. Make sure the tip of the dropper does not touch your eye, finger, or any other surface. If your symptoms do not improve in a few days or if they become worse, check with your doctor.

OVERDOSE
Symptoms: No specific ones have been reported.

What to Do: An overdose of ophthalmic ofloxacin is unlikely to be life-threatening. If a large volume enters the eye, flush with water. If someone accidentally ingests the medicine, call your doctor, emergency medical services (EMS), or the nearest poison control center immediately.

DRUG INTERACTIONS
Other drugs may interact with ophthalmic ofloxacin. Consult your doctor for specific advice if you are taking any other prescription or over-the-counter medication.

FOOD INTERACTIONS
No known food interactions.

DISEASE INTERACTIONS
Caution is advised when taking ophthalmic ofloxacin. Consult your physician if you have any other medical condition.

Ofloxacin Oral

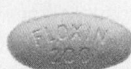

Floxin 200 mg
(ORTHO)

Additional photographs

▶ Drug Class: Fluoroquinolone antibiotic

▶ Available in: Tablets

▶ Available OTC? No

▶ As Generic? No

Side Effects

SERIOUS
Serious reactions to ofloxacin are rare and include seizures, mental confusion, hallucinations, agitation, nightmares, depression, shortness of breath, unusual swelling in the face or extremities, and loss of consciousness. Also skin burning, redness, blisters, rash, or itching on exposure to sunlight. Call your doctor immediately.

COMMON
Increased sensitivity to sunlight (and increased risk of sunburn) for days following therapy.

LESS COMMON
Diarrhea, nausea and vomiting, stomach pain and upset, gas, headache, dizziness, restlessness, insomnia, changes in taste perception, drowsiness, itching, dry mouth, unusual body aches or pains.

PRINCIPAL USES
To treat mild to severe bacterial infections, including those of the urinary tract, lower respiratory tract (such as pneumonia), and the skin. It is also used to treat certain sexually transmitted diseases (chlamydia and gonorrhea) and prostatitis (infection and inflammation of the prostate).

HOW THE DRUG WORKS
Ofloxacin inhibits the activity of a bacterial enzyme (gyrase) that is necessary for proper DNA formation and replication. This fights infection by preventing bacteria cells from reproducing.

DOSAGE
For most infections: 200 to 400 mg, 2 times a day, for 3 to 10 days. For gonorrhea: 400 mg in a single one-time dose.

ONSET OF EFFECT
Varies depending on the infection being treated.

DURATION OF ACTION
Unknown.

DIETARY ADVICE
Take it on an empty stomach, 1 hour before or 2 hours after meals, with a full glass of water. Drink plenty of fluids.

STORAGE
Store in a tightly sealed container away from heat and direct light.

IF YOU MISS A DOSE
Take it as soon as you remember. If it is near the time for the next dose, skip the missed dose and resume your regular dosage schedule. Do not double the next dose.

STOPPING THE DRUG
Take this antibiotic as prescribed for the full treatment period, even if you begin to feel better before the scheduled end of therapy.

PROLONGED USE
See your doctor regularly for tests and examinations if you must take this medicine for a prolonged period. If your symptoms do not improve or instead get worse in a few days, consult your doctor.

PRECAUTIONS

Over 60: No special problems are expected.

Driving and Hazardous Work: Do not drive or engage in hazardous work until you determine how the medicine affects you.

Alcohol: It is advisable to abstain from alcohol when fighting an infection.

Pregnancy: In some animal tests, ofloxacin has caused birth defects. Adequate studies in humans have not been done. It should be used during pregnancy only if potential benefits clearly justify the risks. Before you take ofloxacin, tell your doctor if you are pregnant or plan to become pregnant.

Breast Feeding: Ofloxacin passes into breast milk and may cause serious side effects in the nursing infant; use of the drug is discouraged when nursing.

Infants and Children: Ofloxacin is generally not recommended for use by persons under the age of 18, as it has been shown to interfere with bone development. But ofloxacin may be used by teenagers and younger persons if no alternative treatment is available.

Special Concerns: If ofloxacin causes unusual sensitivity to sunlight, wear protective clothing, use a sunblock and try to avoid exposure to sunlight, especially between 10 am and 3 pm. Do not take any antacid 2 hours before or 2 hours after taking ofloxacin.

OVERDOSE
Symptoms: Nausea, headache, dizziness, vomiting, drowsiness, seizures.

What to Do: Call your doctor, emergency medical services (EMS), or the nearest poison control center immediately.

DRUG INTERACTIONS
Consult your doctor for specific advice if you are taking aminophylline, antacids, didanosine, iron supplements, sucralfate, or zinc salts. Also tell your doctor if you are taking any other prescription or over-the-counter drug.

FOOD INTERACTIONS
No known food interactions.

DISEASE INTERACTIONS
Consult your doctor if you have any disease of the brain or spinal cord. Use of ofloxacin may cause complications in patients with liver or kidney disease, since these organs work together to remove the medication from the body.

Ofloxacin Otic

BRAND NAME
Floxin Otic

▶ Drug Class: Antibiotic

▶ Available in: Otic solution

▶ Available OTC? No

▶ As Generic? No

Side Effects

SERIOUS
No serious side effects are associated with the use of ofloxacin.

COMMON
Bitter taste in the mouth.

LESS COMMON
Earache, itching, skin rash, dizziness or lightheadedness, discomfort upon application.

PRINCIPAL USES
To treat bacterial infections of the ear canal and the middle ear.

HOW THE DRUG WORKS
Ofloxacin inhibits the activity of a bacterial enzyme (gyrase) that is necessary for proper DNA replication and repair. Inhibition of this enzyme fights infection by preventing bacteria cells from reproducing.

DOSAGE
Ear drops should be administered 2 times a day, 12 hours apart, in the affected ear for 10 days (14 days for adults with chronic middle ear infection). Adults and teenagers should receive 10 drops in the affected ear per dose. Children ages 1 to 12 should receive 5 drops in the affected ear per dose.

ONSET OF EFFECT
Unknown.

DURATION OF ACTION
Unknown.

DIETARY ADVICE
The drug can be applied without regard to diet.

STORAGE
Store in a tightly sealed container away from heat, moisture, and direct light.

IF YOU MISS A DOSE
Instill it as soon as you remember. If it is near the time for the next dose, skip the missed dose and resume your regular dosage schedule. Do not double the next dose unless your physician has instructed you to do otherwise.

STOPPING THE DRUG
Take it as prescribed for the full treatment period, even if your symptoms improve before the scheduled end of therapy.

PROLONGED USE
Ofloxacin is prescribed only for short-term use.

PRECAUTIONS
Over 60: No special problems are expected.

Driving and Hazardous Work: No special precautions are necessary.

Alcohol: No special precautions are necessary.

Pregnancy: Adequate human studies have not been done. Before taking ofloxacin, discuss with your doctor the relative risks and benefits of using this drug while pregnant.

Breast Feeding: It is not known whether ofloxacin passes into breast milk after administration to the ear; caution is advised. Consult your doctor for advice.

Infants and Children: Not recommended for use by children under 1 year of age.

Special Concerns: Gently clean any discharge from the outer ear prior to instilling the drops. Do not insert any object or swab into the ear canal. To use the ear drops, lie down or tilt your head so the infected ear faces up. For middle ear infections, the person instilling the drops should gently press the tragus (the small projection of cartilage in front of the ear canal) 4 times in a pumping motion to aid in the passage of the drops through the eardrum and into the middle ear. For ear canal infections, gently pull the earlobe up and back for adults (down and back for children) to straighten the ear canal. Drop the medicine into the ear. Keep the ear facing upward for 5 minutes after inserting the drops to allow the medicine to flow down into the ear canal and reach the infection. You may insert a cotton ball to prevent the medicine from leaking out. Make sure the applicator for the ear drops does not touch your ear, finger, or any other surface. When bathing, avoid getting the affected ear(s) wet. Avoid swimming unless your doctor has given you permission to do so.

OVERDOSE
Symptoms: An overdose with ofloxacin otic is unlikely to occur.

What to Do: If someone instills a much larger dose than prescribed or accidentally swallows ofloxacin otic, call your doctor.

DRUG INTERACTIONS
Do not take ofloxacin otic if you are allergic to ofloxacin or other fluoroquinolone antibiotics.

FOOD INTERACTIONS
None reported.

DISEASE INTERACTIONS
None reported.

Olanzapine

Zyprexa 10 mg
(LILLY)

805

Additional photographs

▶ Drug Class: Neuroleptic; antipsychotic

▶ Available in: Tablets

▶ Available OTC? No

▶ As Generic? No

Side Effects

SERIOUS
Stiffness; shuffling gait; difficulty swallowing or speaking; persistent, uncontrolled chewing, lip-smacking, or tongue movements; fever. Call your doctor immediately.

COMMON
Drowsiness, headache, dizziness, constipation, dry mouth, blurred vision, runny nose.

LESS COMMON
Stomach pain, unclear speech or stuttering, muscle tightness, faintness, increased appetite, increased cough, watering of mouth, insomnia, joint pain, nausea, sore throat, rapid heartbeat, increased thirst, urinary incontinence, vomiting, weight loss.

PRINCIPAL USES
To treat psychotic conditions (severe mental disorders characterized by distorted thoughts, perceptions, and emotions), such as schizophrenia.

HOW THE DRUG WORKS
While the exact mechanism of action of olanzapine is unknown, it appears to alter the activity of certain chemicals in the central nervous system to produce a tranquilizing and antipsychotic effect.

DOSAGE
Initial dose is 5 to 10 mg, once daily. Dose may be increased by your doctor to a maximum of 20 mg a day.

ONSET OF EFFECT
Sedation may occur within minutes, but onset of antipsychotic effect may take hours to occur or may not occur until days or weeks after the beginning of therapy.

DURATION OF ACTION
12 to 24 hours, but effects may persist for several days.

DIETARY ADVICE
No special restrictions.

STORAGE
Store in a tightly sealed container away from heat, moisture, and direct light.

IF YOU MISS A DOSE
Take it as soon as you remember. However, if it is near the time for the next dose, skip the missed dose and resume your regular dosage schedule. Do not double the next dose.

STOPPING THE DRUG
The decision to stop taking the drug should be made in consultation with your physician.

PROLONGED USE
Consult your doctor about the need for follow-up evaluations and tests if you must take this drug for an extended period. Because olanzapine is a recently released drug, its risk of inducing potentially irreversible tardive dyskinesia (involuntary movements of the jaw, lips, tongue, and body) is unknown.

PRECAUTIONS
Over 60: No special problems are expected.

Driving and Hazardous Work: Do not drive or engage in hazardous work until you determine how the medicine affects you.

Alcohol: Avoid alcohol.

Pregnancy: Large doses of olanzapine reduced fetal survival in animal tests. Before you take olanzapine, tell your doctor if you are pregnant or plan to become pregnant.

Breast Feeding: Olanzapine may pass into breast milk; avoid use while breast feeding.

Infants and Children: The safety and effectiveness of olanzapine in children under 18 have not been established.

Special Concerns: Avoid prolonged exposure to high temperatures or hot climates. Drink plenty of fluids and stay cool in the summertime. Avoid overexposure to sunlight until you determine if the drug heightens your skin's sensitivity to ultraviolet light.

OVERDOSE
Symptoms: Extreme drowsiness, slurred speech.

What to Do: Call your doctor, emergency medical services (EMS), or the nearest poison control center immediately.

DRUG INTERACTIONS
The following drugs may interact with olanzapine. Consult your doctor for specific advice if you are taking carbamazepine, omeprazole, rifampin, high blood pressure medication, or any drugs that depress the central nervous system, including antihistamines, antidepressants or other psychiatric medications, barbiturates, sedatives, cough medicines, decongestants, and painkillers. Be sure your doctor knows about any over-the-counter medication you may take.

FOOD INTERACTIONS
No known food interactions.

DISEASE INTERACTIONS
Consult your doctor if you have Parkinson's disease or any movement disorder, glaucoma, epilepsy, liver disease, or kidney disease.

Olopatadine

Side Effects

SERIOUS
No serious side effects are associated with olopatadine.

COMMON
Headache; temporary burning and stinging of the eye.

LESS COMMON
Dry eyes, sensation of something in the eye, vomiting, swollen eyelids, itching of eyes.

PRINCIPAL USES
For temporary relief of itching of the eye due to allergic conjunctivitis (inflammation of the mucous membranes that line the inner surface of the eyelids and whites of the eyes).

HOW THE DRUG WORKS
Olopatadine inhibits the release and blocks the effects of histamine, a substance that causes swelling, itching, sneezing, watery eyes, hives, and other symptoms of allergic reaction.

DOSAGE
1 drop in each affected eye every 6 to 8 hours as needed.

ONSET OF EFFECT
Immediate.

DURATION OF ACTION
6 to 8 hours.

DIETARY ADVICE
No special restrictions.

STORAGE
Store in a tightly sealed container away from heat, moisture, and direct light. Do not allow it to freeze.

IF YOU MISS A DOSE
Apply the next dose as needed; do not double the next dose.

STOPPING THE DRUG
This medication is to be used as needed for relief of itching associated with allergic inflammation. If you are not experiencing symptoms, do not apply the medication.

PROLONGED USE
See your doctor regularly for tests and examinations if you must take this drug for a prolonged period.

PRECAUTIONS
Over 60: No special problems are expected.

Driving and Hazardous Work: Do not drive or engage in hazardous work until you determine how the medicine affects your vision.

Alcohol: Avoid alcohol.

Pregnancy: In animal studies, large doses of olopatadine did not cause birth defects. Human studies have not been done. Olopatadine should be used by pregnant women only if the potential benefit to the mother justifies the potential risk to the embryo or fetus. Consult your doctor for specific advice.

Breast Feeding: Olopatadine may pass into breast milk; caution is advised. Consult your doctor for advice.

Infants and Children: The safety and effectiveness of olopatadine in infants and children under the age of 3 have not been established.

Special Concerns: To use the eye drops, first wash your hands. Tilt your head back. Gently apply pressure to the inside corner of the eyelid and with the index finger of the same hand, pull downward on the lower eyelid to make a space. Drop the medicine into this space and close your eye. Apply pressure for 1 or 2 minutes while keeping the eye closed without blinking. Then wash your hands again. Make sure the tip of the dropper does not touch your eye, finger, or any other surface. If you use contact lenses, you should not wear them while administering olopatadine.

OVERDOSE
Symptoms: No specific ones have been reported.

What to Do: An overdose of olopatadine is unlikely to be life-threatening. However, if someone applies a much larger dose than prescribed or accidentally ingests the medicine, call your doctor, emergency medical services (EMS), or the nearest poison control center immediately.

DRUG INTERACTIONS
Other drugs may interact with olopatadine. Consult your doctor for specific advice if you are taking any other medication.

FOOD INTERACTIONS
No known food interactions.

DISEASE INTERACTIONS
Caution is advised when taking olopatadine. Consult your doctor if you have any medical condition, especially one affecting the eyes.

Olsalazine Sodium

BRAND NAME
Dipentum

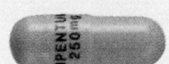

Dipentum 250 mg
(**PHARMACIA**)

▶ Drug Class: Gastrointestinal anti-inflammatory

▶ Available in: Capsules

▶ Available OTC? No

▶ As Generic? No

Side Effects

SERIOUS
Severe pain in the back or stomach, bloody diarrhea, rapid heartbeat, fever, nausea or vomiting, rash, abdominal swelling or stiffness, yellowish tinge to the eyes or skin (jaundice). Call your doctor immediately if such symptoms occur.

COMMON
Abdominal pain or upset; an increase in the number of loose stools; diarrhea; loss of appetite.

LESS COMMON
Joint and muscle pain, acne, depression or anxiety, dizziness, drowsiness, headache, insomnia, skin sensitivity to sunlight, bruising, bleeding in the intestinal tract causing bloody stools.

PRINCIPAL USES
The first line of drug therapy for ulcerative colitis is usually sulfasalazine, but some patients cannot take it because of intolerable side effects. Olsalazine is a chemically similar drug that can be given instead to such patients. It is generally prescribed as maintenance therapy for those who have ulcerative colitis in a state of remission (absence of recent symptom flareups).

HOW THE DRUG WORKS
The exact mechanism of action is uncertain, although it appears that olsalazine inhibits production of substances such as arachidonic acid that produce inflammation in the digestive tract.

DOSAGE
500 mg, 2 times a day.

ONSET OF EFFECT
Unknown.

DURATION OF ACTION
Unknown.

DIETARY ADVICE
Olsalazine should be taken with meals to minimize stomach upset. If stomach or intestinal problems persist, consult your doctor.

STORAGE
Store in a tightly sealed container away from heat and direct light.

IF YOU MISS A DOSE
Take it as soon as you remember, but only with meals. If it is near the time for the next dose, skip the missed dose and resume your regular dosage schedule. Do not double the next dose.

STOPPING THE DRUG
Take it as prescribed for the full treatment period, even if you begin to feel better before the end of therapy.

PROLONGED USE
You should see your doctor regularly for tests and examinations if you must take this drug for a prolonged period.

PRECAUTIONS
Over 60: Olsalazine is not expected to cause different problems in older persons than in younger patients.

Driving and Hazardous Work: Do not drive or engage in hazardous work until you determine how the medicine affects you.

Alcohol: Avoid alcohol when taking this drug.

Pregnancy: Large doses of olsalazine have been shown to cause birth defects in animals. Human studies have not been done. The drug should be used during pregnancy only if its benefits clearly outweigh the potential risks. Before you take olsalazine, be sure to tell your doctor if you are pregnant or plan to become pregnant.

Breast Feeding: Olsalazine may pass into breast milk; caution is advised. In animal studies, olsalazine has been shown to cause slowed growth and other problems during nursing. Consult your doctor for specific advice about stopping breast feeding or switching to another drug.

Infants and Children: There is no information comparing use of olsalazine in infants and children with other age groups. Use and dosage must be determined by your pediatrician.

OVERDOSE
Symptoms: No cases of overdose with olsalazine have been reported.

What to Do: While an overdose is unlikely, call your doctor, emergency medical services (EMS), or the nearest poison control center immediately if you suspect someone has taken a dose much larger than prescribed.

DRUG INTERACTIONS
Consult your doctor for advice if you are taking any other prescription or over-the-counter medication. Olsalazine should not be used by patients who have had prior allergic reactions to aspirin or other salicylate drugs.

FOOD INTERACTIONS
No known food interactions.

DISEASE INTERACTIONS
Caution is advised when taking olsalazine. Consult your doctor if you have high blood pressure or kidney disease.

Omeprazole

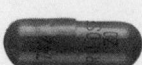

Prilosec 20 mg
(Astra Merck)

▶ Drug Class: Antacid/proton pump inhibitor

▶ Available in: Capsules

▶ Available OTC? No

▶ As Generic? No

Side Effects

SERIOUS
No serious side effects are associated with this medication.

COMMON
Diarrhea, constipation, vomiting, headache, dizziness, stomach pain. Consult your physician if such side effects persist or interfere with daily activities.

LESS COMMON
Bloody or cloudy urine, persistent or recurring sores or ulcers in the mouth, painful or very frequent urination, sore throat, fever, unusual bruising or bleeding, unusual weakness or tiredness, muscle pain, chest pain, nausea. Consult your doctor if such symptoms occur.

PRINCIPAL USES
To treat duodenal (intestinal) ulcers, as well as conditions that cause increased stomach acid production (such as Zollinger-Ellison syndrome), erosive esophagitis (severe, chronic inflammation of the esophagus), and gastroesophageal reflux (backwash of stomach acid into the esophagus, resulting in heartburn).

HOW THE DRUG WORKS
Omeprazole blocks the action of a specific enzyme in the cells that line the stomach, thereby decreasing the production of stomach acid. Reduction of stomach acid promotes healing of ulcers.

DOSAGE
For duodenal ulcer, esophagitis, or gastroesophageal reflux: 20 mg per day. For Zollinger-Ellison syndrome or similar conditions: 60 mg per day.

ONSET OF EFFECT
Within 1 to 3 hours.

DURATION OF ACTION
At least 72 hours.

DIETARY ADVICE
Take omeprazole immediately before a meal. Capsules should be swallowed whole.

STORAGE
Store in a tightly sealed container away from heat and direct light.

IF YOU MISS A DOSE
Take it as soon as you remember. If it is near the time for the next dose, skip the missed dose and resume your regular dosage schedule. Do not double the next dose.

STOPPING THE DRUG
Take it as prescribed for the full treatment period, even if you begin to feel better before the scheduled end of therapy. The decision to stop taking the drug should be made by your doctor.

PROLONGED USE
Omeprazole should not be used indefinitely as maintenance therapy for duodenal ulcer or esophagitis; it is generally taken for a limited period of 4 to 8 weeks. Do not take it for a longer period unless instructed to do so by your doctor. See your doctor regularly for tests and examinations if you must take this drug for an extended period of time.

PRECAUTIONS
Over 60: No specific problems for older people have been reported.

Driving and Hazardous Work: Do not drive or engage in hazardous activities until you determine how the drug affects you.

Alcohol: Avoid alcohol while taking this medication, as it may aggravate your condition.

Pregnancy: In animal tests, omeprazole has not caused problems. Human tests have not been done. Before you take omeprazole, tell your doctor if you are pregnant or plan to become pregnant.

Breast Feeding: Omeprazole may pass into breast milk; caution is advised. Consult your doctor for advice.

Infants and Children: Use and dose for anyone under 18 should be determined by your doctor or pediatrician.

Special Concerns: Tell any doctor or dentist whom you see for treatment that you are taking omeprazole. Do not chew the capsules. If you have trouble swallowing them, you may open them and sprinkle the contents on applesauce or similar food. If your doctor directs, you may take an antacid along with omeprazole.

OVERDOSE
Symptoms: Blurred vision, confusion, profuse sweating, drowsiness, dry mouth, flushing of the face, headache, nausea, palpitations or unusually rapid heartbeat.

What to Do: Call your doctor, emergency medical services (EMS), or the nearest poison control center immediately.

DRUG INTERACTIONS
The following drugs may interact with omeprazole. Consult your doctor for specific advice if you are taking: ampicillin, sucralfate, iron salts or supplements, cyclosporine, diazepam, disulfiram, ketoconazole, phenytoin, or theophylline.

FOOD INTERACTIONS
No significant food interactions have been reported.

DISEASE INTERACTIONS
Caution is advised when taking omeprazole. Consult your doctor if you have liver disease, since it may increase the risk of side effects.

Ondansetron Hydrochloride

▶ Drug Class: Antiemetic

▶ Available in: Tablets, oral solution, injection

▶ Available OTC? No

▶ As Generic? No

Side Effects

SERIOUS
Chest pain, shortness of breath, skin rash, itching or hives, troubled breathing, tightness in chest, wheezing. Call your doctor immediately.

COMMON
Constipation or diarrhea, fever, headache.

LESS COMMON
Abdominal pain, stomach cramps, dizziness or lightheadedness, dry mouth, unusual fatigue or weakness.

PRINCIPAL USES
To prevent nausea and vomiting that may occur after surgery or after treatment with anticancer medicine or radiation.

HOW THE DRUG WORKS
Ondansetron interferes with the chemical receptor sites and nerve pathways involved in the mechanisms that stimulate feelings of nausea and that induce vomiting.

DOSAGE
Tablets and oral solution— To prevent nausea and vomiting after anticancer medicine: Adults and teenagers: 8 mg or 2 teaspoons, 30 minutes before anticancer medicine is given, followed by 8 mg or 2 teaspoons, 8 hours after the first dose, then 8 mg or 2 teaspoons every 12 hours for 1 to 2 days. Children ages 4 to 12: 4 mg or 1 teaspoon, 30 minutes before anticancer medicine is given, followed by 4 mg or 1 teaspoon, 4 and 8 hours later, then 4 mg or 1 teaspoon every 8 hours for 1 to 2 days. To prevent nausea and vomiting after surgery: 16 mg or 4 teaspoons, 1 hour before anesthesia. To prevent nausea and vomiting after radiation treatment: 8 mg or 2 teaspoons, 1 to 2 hours before undergoing treatment; 8 mg or 2 teaspoons every 8 hours each day that radiation treatment is administered. Injection— To prevent nausea and vomiting after anticancer medicine: Adults: 32 mg (or 68 micrograms [mcg] per lb of body weight) into a vein over 15 minutes starting 30 minutes before an anticancer drug is given. Inject again 4 hours and then 8 hours after the initial dose. Children ages 4 to 18: 68 mcg per lb of body weight into a vein over 15 minutes starting 30 minutes before the anticancer medicine is given. To prevent nausea and vomiting after surgery: 4 mg into a vein or muscle from 30 seconds to 5 minutes before anesthesia.

ONSET OF EFFECT
Unknown.

DURATION OF ACTION
Unknown.

DIETARY ADVICE
Take the tablets with food.

STORAGE
Store in a tightly sealed container away from heat, moisture, and direct light.

IF YOU MISS A DOSE
Take it as soon as you remember. If it is near the time for the next dose, skip the missed dose and resume your regular dosage schedule. Do not double the next dose.

STOPPING THE DRUG
The decision to stop taking the drug should be made by your doctor.

PROLONGED USE
You should see your doctor regularly for tests and examinations if you take this medicine for a prolonged period.

PRECAUTIONS
Over 60: This drug has not been shown to cause different side effects or problems in older patients.

Driving and Hazardous Work: Do not drive or engage in hazardous work until you determine how the medicine affects you.

Alcohol: Avoid alcohol.

Pregnancy: Adequate human studies have not been completed. Before taking ondansetron, tell your doctor if you are pregnant or plan to become pregnant.

Breast Feeding: Ondansetron may pass into breast milk; caution is advised. Consult your doctor for advice.

Infants and Children: The dosage for children up to the age of 4 must be determined by your doctor.

OVERDOSE
Symptoms: No specific ones have been reported.

What to Do: An overdose of ondansetron is unlikely to be life-threatening. However, if someone takes a much larger dose than prescribed, call your doctor, emergency medical services (EMS), or the nearest poison control center.

DRUG INTERACTIONS
Consult your doctor for specific advice if you are taking drugs that alter liver function, such as phenobarbital or cimetidine. They may interact with ondansetron.

FOOD INTERACTIONS
No known food interactions.

DISEASE INTERACTIONS
Caution is advised when taking ondansetron. Consult your doctor if you have had recent abdominal surgery or have liver disease.

Orlistat

BRAND NAME
Xenical

▶ Drug Class: Lipase inhibitor

▶ Available in: Capsules

▶ Available OTC? No

▶ As Generic? No

Side Effects

SERIOUS
No serious side effects have yet been reported.

COMMON
Oily spotting, gas with discharge, fecal urgency, oily stool, anal leakage, increased defecation, fecal incontinence.

LESS COMMON
Abdominal pain or discomfort.

PRINCIPAL USES

To achieve weight loss and weight maintenance in the maintenance of obesity when used in conjunction with a reduced-calorie diet and appropriate physical activity. Orlistat is indicated for patients with an initial body mass index (BMI) of 30 or greater and in those with a BMI greater than 27 (see Special Concerns for information on BMI calculation) who also have other risk factors such as high blood pressure, high blood cholesterol, and diabetes.

HOW THE DRUG WORKS

Orlistat inhibits the activity of lipases, intestinal enzymes required for the digestion of dietary fats. Orlistat prevents the breakdown of a portion of ingested fat. The undigested fat cannot be absorbed and is excreted in the feces. Full doses of orlistat reduce the absorption of fat by about 30%.

DOSAGE

120 mg (one capsule) 3 times a day at mealtime.

ONSET OF EFFECT

Within 24 to 48 hours.

DURATION OF ACTION

48 to 72 hours.

DIETARY ADVICE

Take with liquid during or up to one hour after each main meal containing fat. Follow a balanced, reduced-calorie diet. The daily intake of fat (approximately ⅓ of the calories), carbohydrate, and protein should be spread out over the three meals. If a meal is missed or contains no fat, the dose of orlistat can be skipped. Because orlistat can also reduce the absorption of fat-soluble vitamins, a multivitamin supplement (containing vitamins A, D, and E and beta-carotene) should also

be taken once a day at least two hours before or after ingesting orlistat.

STORAGE

Store in a tightly sealed container away from heat, moisture, and direct light.

IF YOU MISS A DOSE

If you miss a dose, take it if you remember within 1 hour of eating. However, if more than 1 hour has passed, skip the missed dose and return to your regular schedule. Do not double the next dose.

STOPPING THE DRUG

The decision to stop taking the drug should be made in consultation with your physician.

PROLONGED USE

The safety and effectiveness of orlistat have not been determined beyond 2 years of use.

PRECAUTIONS

Over 60: No specific studies have been done on older patients.

Driving and Hazardous Work: No special warnings.

Alcohol: No special precautions are necessary.

Pregnancy: Adequate human studies have not been done. Before taking orlistat, tell your doctor if you are pregnant or plan to become pregnant.

Breast Feeding: It is unknown whether orlistat passes into breast milk. However, do not take the drug while nursing. Consult your doctor for advice.

Infants and Children: Safety and effectiveness have not been established for children under age 18.

Special Concerns: A medical cause for obesity (such as hypothyroidism) should be ruled out before taking orlistat. Consult your doctor or a nutritionist for information on a nutritionally-balanced, reduced-calorie diet and an exercise program. The BMI can be calculated by dividing your weight in pounds by your height in inches squared, and then multiplying by 705.

OVERDOSE

Symptoms: No cases of overdose have been reported.

What to Do: An overdose with orlistat is unlikely. If someone takes a much larger dose than prescribed, call your doctor.

DRUG INTERACTIONS

The following drugs may interact with orlistat. Consult your doctor for specific advice if you are taking: cyclosporine, statin (cholesterol-lowering) drugs, warfarin, another weight-loss medication (such as sibutramine or phentermine), or any other prescription or over-the-counter drugs.

FOOD INTERACTIONS

Orlistat reduces the absorption of fat-soluble vitamins A, D, E, and K and beta-carotene. Gastrointestinal side effects may increase following the consumption of high-fat foods or with a diet high in fat (more than 30% of the day's total calories from fat).

DISEASE INTERACTIONS

This drug should not be used if you have chronic malabsorption or gallbladder problems. Consult your doctor if you have an eating disorder (anorexia or bulimia).

Orphenadrine Citrate

BRAND NAMES
Antiflex, Banflex, Flexoject, Mio-Rel, Myolin, Myotrol, Norflex, Orfro, Orphenate

▶ Drug Class: Muscle relaxant

▶ Available in: Extended-release tablets, injection

▶ Available OTC? No

▶ As Generic? Yes

Side Effects

SERIOUS
Fainting; palpitations or rapid heartbeat; fever; hives and severe swelling of face, lips, or tongue along with shortness of breath, chest tightness, or wheezing (indicating a potentially life-threatening allergic reaction); low blood counts. Seek medical help immediately.

COMMON
Dry mouth, drowsiness, dizziness.

LESS COMMON
Inability to pass urine; sores on lips, ulcers in mouth; abdominal cramps or pain; clumsiness; unsteady gait; confusion; constipation; diarrhea; nervousness or irritability; flushing or redness of face; headache; heartburn; hiccups; muscle weakness; nausea and vomiting; trembling; insomnia or fitful sleep; burning, red eyes; stuffy nose.

PRINCIPAL USES
To relieve the stiffness, pain, and discomfort caused by sprains and strains, muscle spasms, or other muscle problems; sometimes used to ease the trembling associated with Parkinson's disease. Orphenadrine may be prescribed in conjunction with other treatment methods, such as physical therapy.

HOW THE DRUG WORKS
Orphenadrine depresses activity in the central nervous system (brain and spinal cord), which in turn interferes with the transmission of nerve impulses from the spinal cord to the muscles.

DOSAGE
Adults and teenagers— Extended-release tablets: 100 mg, 2 times a day, in the morning and evening. Injection: 60 mg injected into a muscle or vein every 12 hours as needed. Children— Use and dosage must be determined by your doctor.

ONSET OF EFFECT
With tablets, 1 hour; with injection, 5 minutes.

DURATION OF ACTION
More than 6 hours.

DIETARY ADVICE
It can be taken with or between meals. To avoid dry mouth, maintain adequate fluid intake and suck on ice chips if desired.

STORAGE
Store in a tightly sealed container away from heat and direct light.

IF YOU MISS A DOSE
Take it as soon as you remember. If it is near the time for the next dose, skip the missed dose and resume your regular dosage schedule. Do not double the next dose.

STOPPING THE DRUG
The decision to stop taking the drug should be made by your doctor.

PROLONGED USE
See your doctor regularly for tests and examinations if you must take this drug for a prolonged period.

PRECAUTIONS
Over 60: There is no specific information comparing use of orphenadrine in older patients with use in younger persons.

Driving and Hazardous Work: Avoid such activities until you determine how the medicine affects you.

Alcohol: Avoid alcohol while taking this drug because it may compound the sedative effect and may cause liver damage.

Pregnancy: Orphenadrine has not been reported to cause problems in pregnancy. Before you take orphenadrine, tell your doctor if you are pregnant or plan to become pregnant.

Breast Feeding: Orphenadrine may pass into breast milk but has not been reported to cause problems in nursing babies. Consult your doctor for advice.

Infants and Children: There is no specific information comparing use of orphenadrine in infants and children with use in older persons.

Special Concerns: If dry mouth occurs, use sugarless candy or gum, bits of ice, or a saliva substitute. If dry mouth persists for more than 2 weeks, consult your dentist. Do not take orphenadrine if you are allergic to any other skeletal muscle relaxant. Orphenadrine will intensify the effect of alcohol, sedatives, and other central nervous system depressants.

OVERDOSE
Symptoms: Heart rhythm disturbances, changes in mental state, drowsiness, seizures, pale or clammy skin, diminished urine output, loss of consciousness.

What to Do: Call your doctor, emergency medical services (EMS), or the nearest poison control center immediately.

DRUG INTERACTIONS
Consult your doctor for specific advice if you are taking tricyclic antidepressants or drugs that depress the central nervous system.

FOOD INTERACTIONS
No known food interactions.

DISEASE INTERACTIONS
Consult your doctor if you have a history of any of the following: disease of the digestive tract, enlarged prostate, rapid or irregular heartbeat, glaucoma, myasthenia gravis, urinary tract blockage, heart disease, or kidney or liver disease.

Oseltamivir Phosphate

▶ Drug Class: Antiviral

▶ Available in: Capsules, oral suspension

▶ Available OTC? No

▶ As Generic? No

Side Effects

SERIOUS
No serious side effects are associated with oseltamivir.

COMMON
Nausea and vomiting.

LESS COMMON
Bronchitis, insomnia, dizziness.

PRINCIPAL USES
To treat and prevent infection from influenza type A or B. Oseltamivir can reduce the severity of symptoms and shorten the duration of flu episodes.

HOW THE DRUG WORKS
Oseltamivir is believed to interfere with the synthesis of the viral enzyme neuraminidase, which is needed in order for the virus to infect cells in the respiratory tract and elsewhere in the body. The drug affects only certain susceptible strains of the influenza type A or B viruses.

DOSAGE
For treatment— Adults and teenagers: 75 mg twice a day for 5 days. Treatment should be initiated as soon as possible, and no longer than 2 days after the onset of signs or symptoms of the flu. Children 12 and under: Consult your pediatrician. For prevention— Adults and teenagers: 75 mg once a day for 7 days. Therapy should be initiated within 2 days of exposure. For prevention during a community outbreak, 75 mg once a day for up to 6 weeks.

ONSET OF EFFECT
Unknown.

DURATION OF ACTION
Unknown.

DIETARY ADVICE
No special restrictions.

STORAGE
Store in a tightly sealed container away from heat, moisture, and direct light. Do not allow oral suspension to freeze.

IF YOU MISS A DOSE
Take it as soon as you remember. If it is near (within 2 hours) the time for the next dose, skip the missed dose and resume your regular dosage schedule. Do not double the next dose.

STOPPING THE DRUG
It is important to take oseltamivir for the full treatment period as prescribed. Do not stop taking the drug before the scheduled end of therapy even if you begin to feel better, as this may lead to a relapse.

PROLONGED USE
If your symptoms do not improve or if they become worse in a few days, consult your doctor.

PRECAUTIONS
Over 60: No special problems are expected.

Driving and Hazardous Work: Do not drive or engage in hazardous work until you determine how the medicine affects you.

Alcohol: No special precautions are necessary.

Pregnancy: Adequate studies have not been completed. Discuss with your doctor the relative risks and benefits of using this drug while pregnant.

Breast Feeding: Oseltamivir may pass into breast milk, although it is unknown if this poses any risks to the nursing infant. Consult your doctor for specific advice.

Infants and Children: The safety and effectiveness of this drug for treatment have not been established for children under the age of 1. The safety and effectiveness of this drug for prevention have not been established for children under the age of 13.

Special Concerns: This medication is not a substitute for a flu shot. Continue to receive your annual flu shot. Shake the oral suspension well before use.

OVERDOSE
Symptoms: No cases have been reported. However, nausea and vomiting are likely symptoms.

What to Do: If you have any reason to suspect an overdose, call your doctor, emergency medical services (EMS), or the nearest poison control center.

DRUG INTERACTIONS
No drug interactions have been reported.

FOOD INTERACTIONS
No known food interactions.

DISEASE INTERACTIONS
The dose of oseltamivir should be lowered in patients with significant kidney disease. Safety has not been determined in people with liver disease.

Oxacillin

BRAND NAMES
Bactocill, Prostaphlin

▶ Drug Class: Penicillin antibiotic

▶ Available in: Capsules, oral suspension, injection

▶ Available OTC? No

▶ As Generic? Yes

Side Effects

SERIOUS
Irregular or fast breathing, fever, joint pain, lightheadedness, fainting, severely decreased urination, severe or bloody diarrhea, puffiness of face, redness of skin, shortness of breath, severe rash, hives, and itching, depression, unusual bleeding or bruising, yellow discoloration of the eyes or skin. Call your doctor immediately.

COMMON
Rash, mild diarrhea, nausea, vomiting, headache, sore tongue, sore mouth, vaginal discharge and itching, white patches in mouth.

LESS COMMON
Diminished urine output, chills, weakness, fatigue.

PRINCIPAL USES
To treat a variety of bacterial infections, especially those caused by staphylococcus bacteria. Oxacillin is effective only against infections caused by bacteria; it is ineffective against those caused by viruses, fungi, or other microorganisms.

HOW THE DRUG WORKS
Oxacillin blocks the formation of bacterial cell walls, rendering bacteria unable to multiply and spread.

DOSAGE
Oral forms— Adults and children weighing more than 88 lbs: 500 to 1,000 mg every 4 to 6 hours. Children up to 88 lbs: 5.7 to 11.4 mg per lb of body weight every 6 hours. Injection— Adults and children weighing more than 88 lbs: 250 to 1,000 mg every 4 to 6 hours. Children under 88 lbs: 5.7 to 11.4 mg per lb of body weight every 4 to 6 hours. Infants: 2.8 mg per lb of body weight every 6 hours.

ONSET OF EFFECT
Immediate after I.V. injection; unknown for other forms.

DURATION OF ACTION
Unknown.

DIETARY ADVICE
Oral doses should be given at least 1 hour before or 2 hours after meals.

STORAGE
Store in a tightly sealed container away from heat and direct light. Liquid forms can be refrigerated but not frozen.

IF YOU MISS A DOSE
Take it as soon as you remember. If it is near the time for the next dose, skip the missed dose and resume your regular dosage schedule. Do not double the next dose.

STOPPING THE DRUG
Take it as prescribed for the full treatment period, even if you begin to feel better before the scheduled end of therapy. Stopping the drug prematurely may slow your recovery or lead to a rebound infection, also known as superinfection, in which the heartier strains of bacteria survive and multiply, leading to a more serious and drug-resistant infection.

PROLONGED USE
Prolonged use of any antibiotic increases the risk of superinfection; caution is advised.

PRECAUTIONS
Over 60: Oxacillin is not expected to cause different or more severe side effects in older patients than it does in younger persons.

Driving and Hazardous Work: The use of oxacillin should not impair your ability to perform such tasks safely.

Alcohol: No special precautions are necessary.

Pregnancy: Oxacillin and other penicillins have not caused birth defects in animals. Human studies have not been done. Before you take oxacillin, tell your doctor if you are pregnant or plan to become pregnant.

Breast Feeding: Oxacillin passes into breast milk; avoid or discontinue use while nursing.

Infants and Children: No special problems are expected.

Special Concerns: Before you have any medical test, tell the doctor in charge that you are taking oxacillin. It can cause false results on some urine sugar tests for diabetics. Oral contraceptives may not be effective while you are taking oxacillin. Use other methods of contraception to avoid an unplanned pregnancy.

OVERDOSE
Symptoms: Unusual muscle excitability, agitation, confusion, hallucinations, seizures, loss of consciousness, coma.

What to Do: Call your doctor, emergency medical services (EMS), or the nearest poison control center immediately.

DRUG INTERACTIONS
Consult your physician for specific advice if you are taking aminoglycosides, ACE inhibitors, diuretics, potassium supplements or potassium-containing medications, anticoagulants or other anticlotting drugs, nonsteroidal anti-inflammatory drugs, sulfinpyrazone, cholestyramine, colestipol, oral contraceptives, methotrexate, probenecid, or rifampin.

FOOD INTERACTIONS
No known food interactions.

DISEASE INTERACTIONS
Consult your doctor if you have a history of allergies, congestive heart failure, gastrointestinal disorders (especially colitis associated with the use of antibiotics), or impaired kidney function.

Oxaprozin

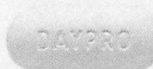

DayPro 600 mg
(SEARLE)

▶ Drug Class: Nonsteroidal anti-inflammatory drug (NSAID)

▶ Available in: Caplets

▶ Available OTC? No

▶ As Generic? No

Side Effects

SERIOUS
Shortness of breath or wheezing, with or without swelling of legs or other signs of heart failure; chest pain; peptic ulcer disease with vomiting of blood; black, tarry stools; decreasing kidney function. Call your doctor immediately.

COMMON
Nausea, vomiting, heartburn, diarrhea, constipation, headache, dizziness, sleepiness.

LESS COMMON
Ulcers or sores in mouth, depression, rashes or blistering of skin, ringing sound in the ears, unusual tingling or numbness of the hands or feet, seizures, blurred vision. Also elevated potassium levels, decreased blood counts; such problems can be detected by your doctor.

PRINCIPAL USES
To treat mild to moderate pain and inflammation caused by tendinitis, arthritis, bursitis, gout, soft tissue injuries, migraine and other vascular headaches, menstrual cramps, and other conditions. When patients fail to respond to one NSAID, another may be tried. The greatest effectiveness often requires trial and error of several different NSAIDs.

HOW THE DRUG WORKS
NSAIDs work by interfering with the formation of prostaglandins, naturally occurring substances in the body that cause inflammation and make nerves more sensitive to pain impulses. NSAIDs also have other modes of action that are less well understood.

DOSAGE
Adults: 1,200 mg once a day. Maximum daily dose is 1,800 mg divided into smaller amounts taken 2 or 3 times a day. Children: Consult your pediatrician.

ONSET OF EFFECT
From 30 minutes to several hours or longer.

DURATION OF ACTION
Varies.

DIETARY ADVICE
Take with food; maintain your usual food and fluid intake.

STORAGE
Store in a tightly sealed container away from heat, moisture, and direct light.

IF YOU MISS A DOSE
Take it as soon as you remember. If it is near the time for the next dose, skip the missed dose and resume your regular dosage schedule. Do not double the next dose.

STOPPING THE DRUG
The decision to stop taking the drug should be made in consultation with your physician.

PROLONGED USE
Prolonged use can cause gastrointestinal problems, including ulceration and bleeding, kidney dysfunction, and liver inflammation. Consult your doctor about the need for medical examinations and laboratory tests.

PRECAUTIONS
Over 60: Because of the potentially greater consequences of gastrointestinal side effects, the dose of NSAIDs for older patients, especially those over age 70, is often cut in half.

Driving and Hazardous Work: Avoid such activities until you determine how the medicine affects you.

Alcohol: Avoid alcohol when using this medication because it increases the risk of stomach irritation.

Pregnancy: Avoid or discontinue this drug if you are pregnant or plan to become pregnant.

Breast Feeding: Oxaprozin passes into breast milk; avoid use while nursing.

Infants and Children: May be used in exceptional circumstances; consult your doctor.

Special Concerns: Because NSAIDs can interfere with blood coagulation, this drug should be stopped at least 3 days prior to any surgery.

OVERDOSE
Symptoms: Severe nausea, vomiting, headache, confusion, seizures.

What to Do: Call your doctor, emergency medical services (EMS), or the nearest poison control center immediately.

DRUG INTERACTIONS
Do not take this drug with aspirin or any other NSAIDs without your doctor's approval. In addition, consult your doctor if you are taking antihypertensives, steroids, anticoagulants, antibiotics, itraconazole or ketoconazole, plicamycin, penicillamine, valproic acid, phenytoin, cyclosporine, digitalis drugs, lithium, methotrexate, probenecid, triamterene, or zidovudine.

FOOD INTERACTIONS
No known food interactions.

DISEASE INTERACTIONS
Consult your doctor if you have any of the following: bleeding problems, inflammation or ulcers of the stomach and intestines, diabetes mellitus, systemic lupus erythematosus (SLE, lupus), anemia, asthma, epilepsy, Parkinson's disease, kidney stones, or a history of heart disease or alcohol abuse. Use of oxaprozin may cause complications in patients with liver or kidney disease, since these organs work together to remove the medication from the body.

Oxazepam

BRAND NAME
Serax

Generic 10 mg
(PUREPAC)

▶ Drug Class: Benzodiazepine tranquilizer; antianxiety agent

▶ Available in: Capsules, tablets

▶ Available OTC? No

▶ As Generic? Yes

Side Effects

SERIOUS
Difficulty concentrating, outbursts of anger, other behavior problems, depression, hallucinations, low blood pressure (causing faintness or confusion), memory impairment, muscle weakness, skin rash or itching, sore throat, fever and chills, sores or ulcers in throat or mouth, unusual bruising or bleeding, extreme fatigue, yellowish tinge to eyes or skin. Call your doctor immediately.

COMMON
Drowsiness, loss of coordination, unsteady gait, dizziness, lightheadedness, slurred speech.

LESS COMMON
Change in sexual desire or ability, constipation, false sense of well-being, nausea and vomiting, urinary problems, unusual fatigue.

PRINCIPAL USES
To treat anxiety and panic disorder. Also used to prevent alcohol withdrawal symptoms.

HOW THE DRUG WORKS
In general, oxazepam produces mild sedation by depressing activity in the central nervous system. In particular, oxazepam appears to enhance the effect of gamma-aminobutyric acid (GABA), a natural chemical that inhibits the firing of neurons and dampens the transmission of nerve signals, thus decreasing nervous excitation.

DOSAGE
For anxiety— Adults: 10 to 30 mg, 3 or 4 times a day. Older adults: Initial dose of 10 mg, 3 times a day. The dose may be increased to a maximum of 15 mg, 4 times a day. For alcohol withdrawal symptoms— Dosage will be adjusted by your doctor on an individual basis.

ONSET OF EFFECT
30 minutes to 2 hours.

DURATION OF ACTION
8 to 12 hours.

DIETARY ADVICE
Oxazepam can be taken with food to prevent gastrointestinal upset.

STORAGE
Store in a tightly sealed container away from heat, moisture, and direct light.

IF YOU MISS A DOSE
Take it as soon as you remember. If it is near the time for the next dose, skip the missed dose and resume your regular dosage schedule. Do not double the next dose.

STOPPING THE DRUG
Discontinuing the drug abruptly may produce withdrawal symptoms. The dosage should be reduced gradually according to your doctor's instructions.

PROLONGED USE
Short-term therapy (8 weeks or less) is typical; do not take it for a longer period unless so advised by your doctor.

PRECAUTIONS
Over 60: A lower dose may be warranted.

Driving and Hazardous Work: Oxazepam can impair mental alertness and physical coordination. Adjust your activities accordingly.

Alcohol: Avoid alcohol.

Pregnancy: Use during pregnancy should be avoided if possible. Be sure to tell your doctor if you are pregnant or plan to become pregnant.

Breast Feeding: Oxazepam passes into breast milk; do not take it while nursing.

Infants and Children: Oxazepam should be used by children only under close medical supervision.

Special Concerns: Oxazepam use can lead to psychological or physical dependence. Never take more than the prescribed daily dose.

OVERDOSE
Symptoms: Extreme drowsiness, confusion, slurred speech, slow reflexes, poor coordination, staggering gait, tremor, slowed breathing, loss of consciousness.

What to Do: Call your doctor, emergency medical services (EMS), or the nearest poison control center immediately.

DRUG INTERACTIONS
Other drugs may interact with oxazepam. Consult your doctor for specific advice if you are taking any drugs that depress the central nervous system; these include antihistamines, antidepressants or other psychiatric medications, barbiturates, sedatives, cough medicines, decongestants, and painkillers. Be sure your doctor knows about any over-the-counter medication you may take.

FOOD INTERACTIONS
None known.

DISEASE INTERACTIONS
Consult your doctor if you have a history of alcohol or drug abuse, stroke or other brain disease, any chronic lung disease, hyperactivity, depression or other mental illness, myasthenia gravis, sleep apnea, epilepsy, porphyria, kidney disease, or liver disease.

Oxcarbazepine

BRAND NAME
Trileptal

▶ Drug Class: Anticonvulsant

▶ Available in: Tablets

▶ Available OTC? No

▶ As Generic? No

Side Effects

SERIOUS
No serious side effects are associated with the use of oxcarbazepine.

COMMON
Dizziness, drowsiness, fatigue, nausea, vomiting, indigestion, abdominal pain, double vision or other visual disturbances, coordination difficulties, abnormal gait, tremor.

LESS COMMON
Muscle weakness, insomnia, nervousness, speech and language difficulties, impaired hand-eye coordination, impaired concentration, acne.

PRINCIPAL USES
To control partial seizures, either alone (monotherapy) or in conjunction with other anticonvulsants, in adults with epilepsy. Oxcarbazine is also used in conjunction with other anticonvulsants in the treatment of partial seizures in children ages 4 to 16 with epilepsy.

HOW THE DRUG WORKS
The mechanism of action is unclear. It is believed that oxcarbazepine inhibits activity in certain parts of the brain and suppresses the abnormal firing of neurons that causes seizures.

DOSAGE
Adults— The drug should be taken in 2 equal doses per day. Monotherapy (use of oxcarbazepine alone): To start, 600 mg a day; dose should be increased by 300 mg a day every third day to a dose of 1,200 mg a day. Adjunctive therapy (use with other anticonvulsants): To start, 600 mg a day. If necessary, dose may be increased at weekly intervals by an additional 600 mg a day, up to 1,200 mg a day. Converting to monotherapy: This should be done in close consultation with your doctor. To start, 600 mg a day while simultaneously initiating the reduction of the other anticonvulsant. If necessary, oxcarbazepine's dose may be increased by a maximum of 600 mg a day at weekly intervals, up to 2,400 mg a day. Children ages 4 to 16— The drug should be taken in 2 equal doses per day. To start, 8 to 10 mg per 2.2 lbs (1 kg), but no more than 600 mg a day. The maintenance dose is dependent upon body weight. Your doctor will determine the appropriate dosage.

ONSET OF EFFECT
At least 2 to 3 days.

DURATION OF ACTION
Unknown.

DIETARY ADVICE
Can be taken without regard to meals.

STORAGE
Store in a tightly sealed container away from heat, moisture, and direct light.

IF YOU MISS A DOSE
Take it as soon as you remember. If it is near the time for the next dose, skip the missed dose and resume your regular dosage schedule. Do not double the next dose.

STOPPING THE DRUG
The decision to stop taking the drug should be made by your doctor. Never stop this drug abruptly because this may cause seizures. The dose is typically tapered over a period of weeks.

PROLONGED USE
This drug is often taken for prolonged periods. See your doctor for periodic checkups.

PRECAUTIONS
Over 60: Adverse reactions may be more likely and more severe.

Driving and Hazardous Work: This drug may cause drowsiness or dizziness, particularly in the first few weeks it is used. Do not drive or engage in hazardous work until you determine how the medicine affects you.

Alcohol: Avoid alcohol; it may contribute to excessive drowsiness.

Pregnancy: Oxcarbazepine has caused birth defects in animal studies. Human studies with this drug have not been done, but other anticonvulsants are known to increase the risk of birth defects. However, seizures during pregnancy can also increase the risks to the fetus. Discuss with your doctor the potential risks and benefits of using this drug during pregnancy.

Breast Feeding: Oxcarbazepine passes into breast milk. Consult your doctor for specific advice concerning the relative risks and benefits of using this drug while breast feeding.

Infants and Children: Not recommended for use by children under age 4.

Special Concerns: See your doctor for regular check-ups to detect the onset of any serious side effects. Periodic measurements of serum sodium may be required because the drug can lower sodium levels in the blood. Your doctor may advise you to carry an ID card or bracelet that says you are taking this drug. Oxcarbazepine may reduce the effectiveness of oral contraceptives; other means of contraception should be considered.

OVERDOSE
Symptoms: Few overdoses have been reported.

What to Do: If an excessive dose is taken, seek emergency medical attention immediately.

DRUG INTERACTIONS
During combination therapy, it may be necessary to lower the dose of phenytoin.

FOOD INTERACTIONS
No known food interactions.

DISEASE INTERACTIONS
A lower dose of oxcarbazepine may be needed in patients with decreased kidney function or severe liver disease.

Oxybutynin Chloride

BRAND NAMES
Ditropan, Ditropan XL

Generic 5 mg
(SIDMAK)

▶ Drug Class: Antispasmodic

▶ Available in: Syrup, tablets, extended-release tablets

▶ Available OTC? No

▶ As Generic? Yes

Side Effects

SERIOUS
Eye pain, skin rash or hives. Call your doctor immediately.

COMMON
Constipation; decreased sweating; drowsiness; dry mouth, nose, and throat.

LESS COMMON
Blurred vision, decreased sexual ability, difficulty urinating, difficulty swallowing, headache, increased sensitivity of eyes to light, nausea or vomiting, insomnia, unusual fatigue, reduced flow of breast milk.

PRINCIPAL USES
To decrease muscle spasms of the bladder and the frequent urination caused by the spasms.

HOW THE DRUG WORKS
Oxybutynin relaxes the muscle cells of the urinary tract and increases urinary bladder capacity.

DOSAGE
Syrup or tablets— Adults: 5 mg, 2 or 3 times a day. Children ages 5 to 12: 5 mg, 2 times a day. Dose may be gradually increased by your doctor to a maximum dose of 20 mg a day. Extended-release tablets— Adults: 5 mg once a day. Dose may be gradually increased by your doctor to a maximum dose of 30 mg a day.

ONSET OF EFFECT
30 to 60 minutes.

DURATION OF ACTION
6 to 10 hours. Extended-release: up to 24 hours.

DIETARY ADVICE
Take it with water on an empty stomach. It can, however, be taken with food to prevent stomach upset.

STORAGE
Store in a tightly sealed container away from heat and direct light. Keep the syrup form refrigerated, but do not allow it to freeze.

IF YOU MISS A DOSE
Take it as soon as you remember. If it is near the time for the next dose, skip the missed dose and resume your regular dosage schedule. Do not double the next dose.

STOPPING THE DRUG
The decision to stop taking the drug should be made by your doctor.

PROLONGED USE
See your doctor periodically if you must take this drug for a prolonged period.

PRECAUTIONS
Over 60: Adverse reactions may be more likely and more severe.

Driving and Hazardous Work: Avoid such activities until you determine how the medicine affects you.

Alcohol: Avoid alcohol.

Pregnancy: Oxybutynin has not been shown to cause birth defects in animals. Adequate human studies have not been done. Consult your doctor for advice.

Breast Feeding: Oxybutynin has not been reported to affect nursing infants. However, nursing may be difficult since the medication can reduce the flow of breast milk.

Infants and Children: The proper dose for children under the age of 5 has not been determined. The safety and effectiveness of the extended-release form have not been established in children under the age of 18.

Special Concerns: Wear sunglasses and avoid exposure to bright light if the drug increases your sensitivity to sunlight. Use extra care not to become overheated during warm weather or exercise, since oxybutynin may interfere with the ability to sweat, increasing the risk of heat stroke. Use sugarless gum, candy, or ice chips to relieve dryness in the mouth, nose, and throat. If dryness persists for more than 2 weeks, check with your doctor or dentist.

OVERDOSE
Symptoms: Flushing, fever, confusion, clumsiness, severe drowsiness, rapid heartbeat, hallucinations, breathing difficulty, unusual nervousness, restlessness or irritability.

What to Do: An overdose of oxybutynin is unlikely to be life-threatening. However, if someone takes a much larger dose than prescribed, call your doctor, emergency medical services (EMS), or the nearest poison control center.

DRUG INTERACTIONS
Consult your doctor for specific advice if you are taking amantadine, anticholinergics, antidepressants, antidyskinetics (such as medication for Parkinson's disease or other movement disorders), antihistamines, antipsychotics, buclizine, carbamazepine, cyclizine, cyclobenzaprine, disopyramide, flavoxate, ipratropium, meclizine, methylphenidate, orphenadrine, procainamide, promethazine, quinidine, or trimeprazine.

FOOD INTERACTIONS
No known food interactions.

DISEASE INTERACTIONS
Consult your doctor if you have any of the following: severe bleeding, colitis, enlarged prostate, glaucoma, heart disease, severe and constant dryness of the mouth, hiatal hernia, high blood pressure, any intestinal or stomach problem, myasthenia gravis, toxemia of pregnancy, any problem with urination, or an overactive thyroid. Use of oxybutynin may cause complications in patients with liver or kidney disease, since these organs work together to remove the medication from the body.

BRAND NAMES
OxyContin, Roxicodone,
Roxicodone Intensol

Oxycontin 20 mg
(PURDUE)

Additional photographs

▶ Drug Class: Opioid (narcotic)
analgesic

▶ Available in: Oral solution,
tablets, controlled-release
tablets

▶ Available OTC? No

▶ As Generic? No

Side Effects

SERIOUS
Serious side effects of
oxycodone are indistin-
guishable from those of
overdose: Confusion;
severe drowsiness,
weakness, or dizziness;
slurred speech; small,
pinpoint pupils; cold,
clammy skin; slow
breathing; seizures;
loss of consciousness.

COMMON
Dizziness or lightheaded-
ness, nausea or vomiting,
drowsiness, constipation,
itching.

LESS COMMON
Swelling in the feet,
sweating, false sense
of well-being (euphoria),
urinary retention.

PRINCIPAL USES
To relieve moderate to
severe pain.

HOW THE DRUG WORKS
Opioids such as oxycodone
relieve pain by acting on
specific areas of the spinal
cord and brain that process
pain signals from nerves
throughout the body.

DOSAGE
5 mg every 3 to 6 hours, or
10 mg, 3 to 4 times a day as
needed. Children: Dosages
must be determined by
your pediatrician. Con-
trolled-release tablets: Your
doctor will determine the
proper dosage.

ONSET OF EFFECT
10 to 15 minutes.

DURATION OF ACTION
3 to 6 hours.

DIETARY ADVICE
This medication can be
taken with food or milk to
lessen stomach upset.

STORAGE
Store in a tightly sealed container away from heat, moisture, and direct light. Do
not freeze the liquid form.

IF YOU MISS A DOSE
If you are taking oxycodone
on a fixed schedule, take it
as soon as you remember. If
it is near the time for the
next dose, skip the missed
dose and resume your regular dosage schedule. Do not
double the next dose.

STOPPING THE DRUG
The decision to stop taking
the drug should be made by
your doctor.

PROLONGED USE
You should see your doctor
regularly for tests and
examinations if you must
take this medication for an
extended period. Prolonged

use can cause physical
dependence.

PRECAUTIONS
Over 60: Adverse reactions
may be more likely and
more severe in older
patients.

**Driving and Hazardous
Work:** Do not drive or
engage in hazardous work
until you determine how
the medicine affects you.

Alcohol: Avoid alcohol.

Pregnancy: Human studies have not been done.
Before using this drug, tell
your doctor if you are pregnant or plan to become
pregnant. Overuse during
pregnancy can cause drug
dependence in the fetus.

Breast Feeding: Oxy-
codone may pass into breast
milk; caution is advised.
Consult your doctor for
specific advice.

Infants and Children:
Adverse reactions to oxy-
codone may be more likely
and more severe in chil-
dren. Consult your doctor
for specific advice.

Special Concerns: If you
feel the medication is not
working properly after a few
weeks, do not increase the
dose. Consult your doctor.
Before having any surgery,
tell the doctor or dentist in
charge that you are taking
this drug. The controlled-
release tablets are pre-
scribed for use only in
opioid-tolerant patients
requiring daily doses of
160 mg or more.

OVERDOSE
Symptoms: Confusion;
severe drowsiness, weak-
ness, or dizziness; slurred
speech; small, pinpoint
pupils; cold, clammy skin;

slow breathing; seizures;
loss of consciousness.

What to Do: Call your
doctor, emergency medical
services (EMS), or the
nearest poison control
center immediately.

DRUG INTERACTIONS
Consult your doctor for specific advice if you are taking
carbamazepine or other
medicine for seizures, barbiturates, sedatives, cough
medicines, decongestants,
antidepressants, other prescription pain medications,
MAO inhibitors, naltrexone,
rifampin, or zidovudine.

FOOD INTERACTIONS
No known food interactions.

DISEASE INTERACTIONS
Consult your doctor if you
have any of the following: a
history of alcohol or drug
abuse; emotional illness;
brain disorders or head
injury; seizures; lung disease; prostate problems or
other problems with urination; gallstones; colitis;
heart, kidney, liver, or
thyroid disease.

Oxycodone/Acetaminophen

Percocet 5/325 mg
(DUPONT)

▶ Drug Class: Opioid (narcotic)
  analgesic

▶ Available in: Capsules, oral
  solution, tablets

▶ Available OTC? No

▶ As Generic? Yes

Side Effects

SERIOUS
Bloody, dark, or cloudy
urine; severe pain in
lower back or side; pale
or black, tarry stools; yellowish tinge to the eyes
or skin; hallucinations;
frequent urge to urinate;
painful or difficult urination; sudden decrease in
amount of urine; unusual
bleeding or bruising;
irregular heartbeat; skin
rash, hives, or itching;
unusual excitement;
swelling of face; confu-
sion; trembling or
uncontrolled muscle
movements; redness or
flushing of face. Call your
doctor immediately.

COMMON
Dizziness, lightheaded-
ness, nausea or vomiting,
drowsiness, constipation.

LESS COMMON
Allergic reaction, false
sense of well-being
(euphoria), depression,
loss of appetite, blurring
or change in vision,
headache, sweating.

PRINCIPAL USES
To relieve moderate to
severe pain when nonpre-
scription pain relievers
prove inadequate. A nar-
cotic analgesic such as oxycodone, in combination with
acetaminophen, may pro-
vide better pain relief than
either medicine used alone.
Used together, relief may be
achieved at lower doses of
the two drugs.

HOW THE DRUG WORKS
Opioids such as oxycodone
relieve pain by acting on
specific areas of the central
nervous system (brain and
spinal cord) that process
pain signals from nerves
throughout the body. Acetaminophen appears to interfere with the action of
prostaglandins, naturally
occurring substances in the
body that cause inflamma-
tion and make nerves more
sensitive to pain impulses.

DOSAGE
Adults: 1 capsule or tablet
every 4 to 6 hours, or 1 teaspoon of the oral solution
every 4 to 6 hours.

ONSET OF EFFECT
Unknown.

DURATION OF ACTION
Unknown.

DIETARY ADVICE
This medication can be
taken with food or milk to
lessen stomach irritation.

STORAGE
Store in a tightly sealed container away from heat, moisture, and direct light.

IF YOU MISS A DOSE
If you are taking the drug
on a fixed schedule, take it
as soon as you remember.
However, if it is near the
time for the next dose,
skip the missed dose and
resume your regular
dosage schedule. Do not
double the next dose.

STOPPING THE DRUG
The decision to stop taking
the drug should be made by
your doctor.

PROLONGED USE
See your doctor regularly
for examinations and laboratory tests if long-term therapy is required. Prolonged
use of narcotics can cause
physical dependence; pro-
longed use of aceta-
minophen at high doses
can cause liver damage.

PRECAUTIONS
Over 60: Adverse reactions
may be more likely and
more severe in older
patients.

**Driving and Hazardous
Work:** Do not drive or
engage in hazardous work
until you determine how the
medicine affects you.

Alcohol: Avoid alcohol.

Pregnancy: Human studies have not been done.
Before you use this drug,
tell your doctor if you are
pregnant or plan to become
pregnant. Overuse of the
medication during preg-
nancy can cause drug
dependence in the fetus.

Breast Feeding: It is not
known whether this medication passes into breast milk;
caution is advised. Consult
your doctor for advice.

Infants and Children:
Adverse reactions may be
more likely and more
severe in children.

Special Concerns: If you
feel the medication is not
working properly after a few
weeks, do not increase the
dose. Consult your doctor.

OVERDOSE
Symptoms: Severe dizziness or drowsiness; cold,
clammy skin; difficult or
slow breathing or shortness
of breath; severe confusion;
seizures; stomach cramps
or pain; diarrhea; low blood
pressure; increased sweating; constricted pupils of
eyes; nausea or vomiting;
irregular heartbeat; severe
weakness.

What to Do: Call your
doctor, emergency medical
services (EMS), or the
nearest poison control center immediately.

DRUG INTERACTIONS
Consult your doctor for specific advice if you are taking
any prescription or over-the-
counter drugs, especially
drugs with acetaminophen;
central nervous system
depressants such as antihistamines or medicine for hay
fever, allergies, or colds;
barbiturates; seizure medicine; muscle relaxants;
anesthetics; tranquilizers,
sedatives, or sleep aids.

FOOD INTERACTIONS
No known food interactions.

DISEASE INTERACTIONS
Consult your physician if
you have a head injury or
brain disease, an underactive thyroid, an enlarged
prostate, seizures, kidney
or liver disease, gallbladder
problems, a blood disorder,
or a history of alcohol or
drug abuse.

Oxycodone/Aspirin

▸ Drug Class: Opioid (narcotic) analgesic

▸ Available in: Tablets

▸ Available OTC? No

▸ As Generic? Yes

Side Effects

SERIOUS
Serious side effects are indistinguishable from those of overdose. See Overdose.

COMMON
Lightheadedness, dizziness, drowsiness, nausea and vomiting.

LESS COMMON
Euphoric feeling, depression, constipation, itching.

PRINCIPAL USES
To relieve moderate to severe pain when nonprescription pain relievers fail. A narcotic analgesic such as oxycodone, combined with aspirin, may provide superior pain relief than either medicine alone, and in lower dosages.

HOW THE DRUG WORKS
Opioids such as oxycodone relieve pain by acting on specific areas of the central nervous system (brain and spinal cord) that process pain signals from nerves throughout the body. Nonsteroidal anti-inflammatory drugs (NSAIDs) such as aspirin inhibit the release of chemicals in the body called prostaglandins, which play a role in inflammation.

DOSAGE
Adults: 1 or 2 half-strength tablets or 1 full-strength tablet every 4 to 6 hours as needed. Teenagers: ½ half-strength tablet every 6 hours as needed. Children age 6 to 12: ¼ half-strength tablet every 6 hours as needed.

ONSET OF EFFECT
Unknown.

DURATION OF ACTION
Unknown.

DIETARY ADVICE
This drug can be taken with food or a full glass of water to lessen stomach irritation.

STORAGE
Store in a tightly sealed container away from heat, moisture, and direct light.

IF YOU MISS A DOSE
If you are taking the drug on a fixed schedule, take it as soon as you remember. However, if it is near the time for the next dose, skip the missed dose and resume regular dosage schedule. Do not double the next dose.

STOPPING THE DRUG
The decision to stop the drug should be made in consultation with your doctor.

PROLONGED USE
See your doctor regularly for examinations and laboratory tests if long-term therapy is required.

PRECAUTIONS
Over 60: Adverse reactions may be more likely and more severe.

Driving and Hazardous Work: Avoid such activities until you determine how the medicine affects you.

Alcohol: Avoid alcohol.

Pregnancy: Human studies have not been done. Before you use this drug, tell your doctor if you are pregnant or plan to become pregnant. Overuse of the medication during pregnancy can cause drug dependence in the fetus.

Breast Feeding: It is not known whether this drug passes into breast milk; consult your doctor for advice.

Infants and Children: Adverse reactions may be more likely and more severe. This drug should not be given to children with a current or recent viral infection such as chickenpox or the flu. Aspirin has been linked to a rare, but potentially fatal illness called Reye's syndrome. Consult your doctor for more information.

Special Concerns: If you feel the medication is not working properly after a few weeks, do not increase the dose. Consult your doctor. Prolonged use can cause psychological and physical dependence, whichcan lead to abuse of the drug.

OVERDOSE
Symptoms: Loss of hearing, blood in urine, cold, clammy skin, confusion, seizures, diarrhea, severe dizziness or lightheadedness, severe drowsiness, extreme excitement, nervousness, or restlessness, fever, hallucinations, severe or ongoing headache, increased sweating or thirst, severe or continuing nausea or vomiting, pinpoint pupils of eyes, tinnitus (ringing or buzzing in the ears), shortness of breath or breathing difficulty, slowed heartbeat, abdominal pain, vision problems, severe weakness.

What to Do: Call your doctor, emergency medical services (EMS), or the nearest poison control center immediately.

DRUG INTERACTIONS
Consult your doctor for specific advice if you are taking any prescription or over-the-counter drugs, especially medications containing aspirin or other NSAIDs (such as ibuprofen, ketoprofen, or naproxen); acetaminophen; central nervous system depressants such as antihistamines or medicine for hay fever, allergies, or colds; barbiturates; seizure medicine; muscle relaxants; anesthetics; tranquilizers, sedatives, or sleep aids.

FOOD INTERACTIONS
No known food interactions.

DISEASE INTERACTIONS
Consult your physician if you have a head injury or brain disease, an underactive thyroid, an enlarged prostate, seizures, kidney or liver disease, gallbladder problems, asthma, diarrhea caused by antibiotics or poisoning, a blood disorder, or a history of alcohol or drug abuse.

Oxymetazoline Nasal

BRAND NAMES
4-Way Long Lasting Nasal Spray, Afrin, Allerest 12-Hour Nasal Spray, Cheracol, Dristan 12-Hr Nasal Spray, Duramist Up To 12 Hours Decongestant Nasal Spray, Duration 12 Hour Nasal Spray, Neo-Synephrine 12 Hour Nasal Spray, Nostrilla Long-Acting Nasal Decongestant, NTZ Long Acting Decongestant Nose Drops, Sinarest 12 Hour Nasal Spray, Vicks Sinex Long-Acting 12-Hour Formula

▶ Drug Class: Decongestant

▶ Available in: Nasal drops, nasal spray

▶ Available OTC? Yes

▶ As Generic? Yes

Side Effects

SERIOUS
No serious side effects have been reported.

COMMON
Burning, dryness, or stinging inside the nose. An increase in nasal discharge or congestion may occur after 3 to 5 days of continuous use.

LESS COMMON
Headache, rapid or irregular heartbeat, excitability, restlessness.

PRINCIPAL USES
To relieve nasal congestion caused by allergies, colds, or sinus conditions.

HOW THE DRUG WORKS
Oxymetazoline constricts blood vessels to reduce the blood flow to swollen nasal passages and other tissues, which reduces nasal secretions and improves nasal airflow.

DOSAGE
Adults and children 6 years of age and older: 2 or 3 drops or sprays of 0.05% solution in each nostril 2 times a day, in the morning and evening. Children ages 2 to 6: 2 or 3 drops of 0.025% solution in each nostril 2 times a day, in the morning and evening.

ONSET OF EFFECT
Rapid.

DURATION OF ACTION
Unknown.

DIETARY ADVICE
Drink plenty of fluids.

STORAGE
Store in a tightly sealed container away from heat and direct light.

IF YOU MISS A DOSE
Take it as soon as you remember. If it is near the time for the next dose, skip the missed dose and resume your regular dosage schedule. Do not double the next dose.

STOPPING THE DRUG
Do not use this medicine for more than 3 days without consulting your doctor.

PROLONGED USE
Using this medicine for more than 3 days may lead to rebound congestion (more severe congestion caused by the body's adaptation to the drug).

PRECAUTIONS

Over 60: Although no studies have specifically examined the use of this drug in older patients, no special problems are expected.

Driving and Hazardous Work: Do not drive or engage in hazardous work until you determine how the medicine affects you.

Alcohol: Avoid alcohol.

Pregnancy: Oxymetazoline has not been shown to cause birth defects or other problems if taken during pregnancy.

Breast Feeding: It is not known whether oxymetazoline passes into breast milk; caution is advised. Consult your doctor for advice.

Infants and Children: This drug is not recommended for children under the age of 2.

Special Concerns: Each container of medicine should be used by only one person to avoid spread of infection. Blow your nose gently before using this medicine. To use the nose drops, tilt your head back or lie down on a bed and hang your head over the side. Keep your head tilted back for a few minutes after instilling the drops. To use the nasal spray, keep your head upright and sniff briskly while spraying. For best results, spray again in 3 to 5 minutes.

OVERDOSE
Symptoms: Rapid, irregular, or pounding heartbeat; headache or dizziness; increased sweating; nervousness; trembling; paleness; insomnia. Such symptoms are more likely to be observed in young children.

What to Do: If someone takes a much larger dose than recommended, call your doctor, emergency medical services (EMS), or the nearest poison control center immediately.

DRUG INTERACTIONS
Before you take oxymetazoline, tell your doctor if you are taking maprotiline or tricyclic antidepressants.

FOOD INTERACTIONS
No known food interactions.

DISEASE INTERACTIONS
Consult your doctor if you have a history of any of the following: high blood pressure, diabetes mellitus, heart disease, blood vessel disease, or an overactive thyroid gland.

Oxymetazoline Ophthalmic

BRAND NAMES
OcuClear, Visine L.R.

▶ Drug Class: Ophthalmic decongestant

▶ Available in: Ophthalmic solution

▶ Available OTC? Yes

▶ As Generic? No

Side Effects

SERIOUS
No serious side effects have been reported.

COMMON
No common side effects have been reported.

LESS COMMON
Headache, rapid or irregular heartbeat, excitability, restlessness, increase in redness of the eye.

PRINCIPAL USES
To reduce redness of the eye caused by minor irritation.

HOW THE DRUG WORKS
Ophthalmic oxymetazoline reduces redness by constricting the superficial blood vessels in the whites (sclera) of the eye.

DOSAGE
Adults and children age 6 and older: 1 drop in the affected eye every 6 hours, as needed.

ONSET OF EFFECT
Rapid, within 5 minutes.

DURATION OF ACTION
About 6 hours.

DIETARY ADVICE
This medication can be used without regard to diet.

STORAGE
Store in a tightly sealed container away from heat, moisture, and direct light. Do not allow the medicine to freeze.

IF YOU MISS A DOSE
Apply it as soon as you remember. However, if it is near the time for the next dose, skip the missed dose and resume your regular dosage schedule. Do not double the next dose.

STOPPING THE DRUG
Do not use this medicine for more than 3 days without consulting your doctor.

PROLONGED USE
Consult your doctor if you intend to use this medicine for more than 3 days.

PRECAUTIONS
Over 60: Although no studies have specifically examined the use of this drug in older patients, no special problems are expected.

Driving and Hazardous Work: Do not drive or engage in hazardous work until you determine how the medicine affects you.

Alcohol: No special precautions are necessary.

Pregnancy: No problems are expected, but studies of effects in pregnancy have not been done in humans. Consult your physician.

Breast Feeding: No problems are expected, but studies of effects in breast feeding have not been done in humans. Consult your doctor.

Infants and Children: Dosage for children under the age of 6 should be determined by a pediatrician.

Special Concerns: To use the eye drops, first wash your hands. Tilt your head back. Gently apply pressure to the inside corner of the eyelid and with the index finger of the same hand, pull downward on the lower eyelid to make a space. Drop the medicine into this space and close your eye. Apply pressure for 1 or 2 minutes while keeping the eye closed without blinking. Then wash your hands again. Make sure the tip of the dropper does not touch your eye, finger, or any other surface.

OVERDOSE
Symptoms: Dizziness; headache; rapid, irregular, or pounding heartbeat; trembling; insomnia.

What to Do: Call your doctor, emergency medical services (EMS), or the nearest poison control center immediately.

DRUG INTERACTIONS
Before you take oxymetazoline, tell your doctor if you are taking maprotiline or tricyclic antidepressants.

FOOD INTERACTIONS
No known food interactions.

DISEASE INTERACTIONS
Caution is advised when taking oxymetazoline. Consult your doctor if you have a history of any of the following: high blood pressure; eye disease, infection, or injury; narrow-angle glaucoma; heart disease; blood vessel disease; or an overactive thyroid gland.

Paclitaxel Injection

▶ Drug Class: Antineoplastic (anticancer) agent

▶ Available in: Injection

▶ Available OTC? No

▶ As Generic? No

Side Effects

SERIOUS
Black, tarry, or bloody stools; blood-tinged (pink or maroon) urine; cough or hoarseness; fever and chills; lower back or flank pain; painful, difficult urination; tiny bright red spots on skin; bleeding from gums, nose, other unusual places; easy bruising, shortness of breath. These side effects may mean that normal blood cells and special blood-clotting cells have been affected, or that normal immune cells have been affected and an infection is developing somewhere in your body. See your doctor as soon as possible if any of these side effects occur.

COMMON
Diarrhea, nausea, and vomiting; numbness, burning, or tingling in hands or feet; pain in the joints and muscles, especially in the limbs; total but temporary loss of body hair (hair begins to regrow after therapy is discontinued).

LESS COMMON
Dizziness or lightheadedness, slowed heartbeat.

PRINCIPAL USES
To treat cancers of the ovary, breast, lung, head, and neck, and to treat melanoma (a type of skin cancer that can spread to other organs). Paclitaxel is also used as secondary treatment for AIDS-related Kaposi's sarcoma.

HOW THE DRUG WORKS
Paclitaxel interferes with essential phases of cell division in cancer cells, preventing them from multiplying. The drug may also affect the health and development of other kinds of cells in the body, resulting in unpleasant side effects.

DOSAGE
135 to 175 mg per square meter of body surface, either as a 24-hour infusion or as a 3-hour infusion administered every 3 to 4 hours. AIDS-related Kaposi's sarcoma: 135 mg per square meter of body surface as a 3-hour infusion administered every 3 weeks or 100 mg per square meter of body surface as a 3-hour infusion every 2 weeks. Your oncologist will determine the proper dosage schedule.

ONSET OF EFFECT
Unknown.

DURATION OF ACTION
Unknown.

DIETARY ADVICE
Maintain adequate food and fluid intake. Calorie, protein, and vitamin needs increase in patients with cancer. Good nutrition is essential to cope with the demands of chemotherapy.

STORAGE
Not applicable; the dose is administered only at a health care facility.

IF YOU MISS A DOSE
Not applicable, since it is given by a doctor or other health care professional.

STOPPING THE DRUG
The decision to stop taking the drug should be made by your doctor.

PROLONGED USE
You should see your doctor regularly for tests and examinations if you must take this drug for a prolonged period.

PRECAUTIONS
Over 60: No special age-related problems are expected.

Driving and Hazardous Work: Do not drive or engage in hazardous work until you determine how the medicine affects you.

Alcohol: Avoid alcohol.

Pregnancy: Paclitaxel has caused fetal death and miscarriage in animals. Tell your doctor at once if you become pregnant while taking paclitaxel.

Breast Feeding: Paclitaxel may pass into breast milk; avoid or discontinue usage while nursing.

Infants and Children: There is no specific information comparing the use of paclitaxel in infants and children with its use in older persons.

Special Concerns: While taking paclitaxel, do not receive any immunizations without consulting your doctor. Avoid persons with infections. Be careful when using a toothbrush, dental floss, or toothpick. Check with your doctor before having any dental work. Do not touch your eyes or the inside of your nose unless you have just washed your hands. Be careful not to cut yourself when using sharp objects such as a razor. Avoid contact sports and other activities during which bruising could occur.

OVERDOSE
Symptoms: Excessive dosages over an extended period of time may cause weakness, fatigue, and low resistance to infections (due to anemia), numbness or tingling in the extremities (due to peripheral nerve damage), and increased inflammation of the mucous membranes.

What to Do: Notify your doctor right away if you develop such symptoms.

DRUG INTERACTIONS
Consult your doctor for specific advice if you are taking amphotericin B, antithyroid agents, azathioprine, chloramphenicol, colchicine, flucytosine, ganciclovir, ketoconazole, interferon, plicamycin, or zidovudine.

FOOD INTERACTIONS
No known food interactions.

DISEASE INTERACTIONS
Caution is advised when taking paclitaxel. Consult your doctor if you have a history of any of the following: chicken pox, shingles, heart rhythm problems, or any recent infection.

Pancrelipase

Viokase 30,000/8,000/30,000 units
(A.H. ROBINS)

▶ Drug Class: Pancreatic
enzyme

▶ Available in: Capsules,
delayed-release capsules,
powder, tablets

▶ Available OTC? No

▶ As Generic? Yes

Side Effects

SERIOUS
Serious side effects are
not likely with normal
doses. With high doses,
side effects may include
diarrhea, intestinal blockage, nausea, and stom-
ach cramps or pain. Very
high doses may cause
blood in urine, joint pain,
or swelling of feet or
lower legs. If the powder
form is accidentally
inhaled, breathing prob-
lems, tightness in the
chest, and wheezing may
occur. Call your doctor
immediately.

COMMON
No common side effects
have been reported with
the recommended
dosage.

LESS COMMON
Skin rash or hives.

PRINCIPAL USES
The pancreas secretes various substances—including
digestive enzymes, insulin,
and glucagon—that are
essential to good health.
Pancrelipase is prescribed
to replace the enzymes
needed for digestion in
patients for whom the pancreas is not functioning
properly.

HOW THE DRUG WORKS
Pancrelipase contains the
enzymes that would other-
wise be manufactured by
the pancreas to digest proteins, starches, and fats.

DOSAGE
Capsules— Adults and
teenagers: 1 to 3 capsules
before or with meals and
snacks. Children: Contents
of 1 to 3 capsules sprinkled
on food with each meal.
Delayed-release capsules—
Adults and teenagers: 1 to
2 capsules before or with
meals and snacks. Children:
1 to 2 capsules with meals.
Powder— Adults and teen-
agers: ¼ teaspoon (0.7
gram) with meals and
snacks. Children: ¼ tea-
spoon with meals. Tablets—
Adults and teenagers: 1 to 3
tablets before or with meals
and snacks. Children: 1 to 2
tablets with meals. Doses
may be altered as deter-
mined by your doctor.

ONSET OF EFFECT
Variable.

DURATION OF ACTION
Variable.

DIETARY ADVICE
Take before or with meals
and snacks as directed.

STORAGE
Store in a tightly sealed container away from heat, moisture, and direct light.

IF YOU MISS A DOSE
Take it as soon as you
remember. However, if it is
near the time for the next
dose, skip the missed dose
and resume your regular
dosage schedule. Do not
double the next dose.

STOPPING THE DRUG
The decision to stop taking
the drug should be made by
your doctor.

PROLONGED USE
You should see your doctor
regularly for tests and
examinations while taking
this medicine. Lifetime therapy with pancrelipase may
be required.

PRECAUTIONS
Over 60: No special problems are expected in older
patients.

**Driving and Hazardous
Work:** The use of this medication should not impair
your ability to perform such
tasks safely.

Alcohol: No special precautions are necessary.

Pregnancy: Animal and
human studies have not
been done. Before you take
pancrelipase, tell your doctor if you are pregnant or
plan to become pregnant.

Breast Feeding: It is not
known whether pancreli-
pase passes into breast
milk. Problems have not
been reported. Consult your
doctor for specific advice.

Infants and Children:
The dosage for children
under 6 months of age has
not been established.

Special Concerns: Be
careful not to inhale the
powder form or powder
from capsules; it may cause
stuffy nose, shortness of
breath, troubled breathing,

wheezing, or tightness in
the chest. Do not change
brands or forms of pancrelipase without consulting
your physician; different
products may work in different ways. If your physician
prescribes a personal diet
for you, be careful to
observe it.

OVERDOSE
Symptoms: Nausea or
vomiting, abdominal
cramps, diarrhea.

What to Do: Call your
doctor, emergency medical
services (EMS), or the
nearest poison control
center immediately.

DRUG INTERACTIONS
Consult your doctor for specific advice if you are taking
any prescription or over-the-
counter medication.

FOOD INTERACTIONS
No known food interactions.

DISEASE INTERACTIONS
Consult your doctor if you
have any other medical
problem, especially pancreatitis, which is sudden and
severe inflammation of the
pancreas.

Pantoprazole Sodium

▶ Drug Class: Antacid/proton pump inhibitor

▶ Available in: Delayed-release tablets

▶ Available OTC? No

▶ As Generic? No

Side Effects

SERIOUS
No serious side effects are associated with the use of pantoprazole.

COMMON
Diarrhea.

LESS COMMON
Rash, raised blood sugar levels. Many additional side effects can occur; consult your doctor if you are concerned about any adverse or unusual reactions you experience while taking this drug.

PRINCIPAL USES
For the short-term treatment of erosive esophagitis (severe, chronic inflammation or ulceration of the esophagus) associated with gastroesophageal reflux disease (GERD; backwash of stomach acid into the esophagus).

HOW THE DRUG WORKS
Pantoprazole blocks the action of a specific enzyme in the cells that line the stomach, thereby decreasing the production of stomach acid.

DOSAGE
Adults: 40 mg once a day for up to 8 weeks.

ONSET OF EFFECT
Within 1 to 3 hours.

DURATION OF ACTION
Unknown.

DIETARY ADVICE
Pantoprazole may be taken without regard to meals. Tablets should be swallowed whole.

STORAGE
Store in a tightly sealed container away from heat, moisture, and direct light.

IF YOU MISS A DOSE
Take it as soon as you remember. However, if it is near the time for the next dose, skip the missed dose and resume your regular dosage schedule. Do not double the next dose.

STOPPING THE DRUG
Take as prescribed for the full treatment period, even if your symptoms improve before the scheduled end of therapy. The decision to stop taking the drug should be made by your doctor.

PROLONGED USE
Pantoprazole should not be used indefinitely as mainte-nance therapy for esophagitis; it is generally taken for a limited period of up to 8 weeks. For those who have not healed within this period, an additional 8 weeks of therapy may be considered by your doctor.

PRECAUTIONS
Over 60: No special problems are expected.

Driving and Hazardous Work: No special precautions are necessary.

Alcohol: Avoid alcohol while taking this medication, as it may aggravate your condition.

Pregnancy: In animal tests, pantoprazole has not caused problems. Human tests have not been done. Before you take pantoprazole, tell your doctor if you are pregnant or plan to become pregnant.

Breast Feeding: Pantoprazole may pass into breast milk; caution is advised. Consult your doctor for advice. Discuss with your doctor the relative risks and benefits of using this drug while nursing.

Infants and Children: Safety and effectiveness have not been established for patients under age 18.

Special Concerns: Do not chew, crush, or split the tablets. If your doctor directs, you may take an antacid along with pantoprazole.

OVERDOSE
Symptoms: Few cases of overdose have been reported.

What to Do: An overdose is unlikely to be life-threatening. However, if someone takes a much larger dose than prescribed, call your doctor, emergency medical services (EMS), or the nearest poison control center immediately.

DRUG INTERACTIONS
Drug interactions are unlikely. Consult your doctor for specific advice if you are taking: ampicillin, iron salts or supplements, or ketoconazole.

FOOD INTERACTIONS
No significant food interactions have been reported.

DISEASE INTERACTIONS
Consult your doctor if you have severe liver disease, which may increase the risk of side effects.

Papaverine Hydrochloride

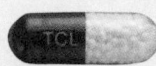
Side Effects

SERIOUS
Oral forms: Blurred or
double vision, drowsi-
ness, fatigue. Injection
for erectile dysfunction:
Lumps in penis, painful
or prolonged erection
(lasting more than 4
hours). Call your doctor
immediately.

COMMON
Oral forms: None. Injec-
tion for erectile dysfunction: Mild pain or burning
along the penis.

LESS COMMON
Oral forms: Dizziness,
rapid heartbeat, flushing
of face, difficult breathing. Injection: Bruising,
bleeding, or tingling at
injection site; impaired
ejaculation; dizziness.

PRINCIPAL USES
To treat problems caused
by poor blood circulation.
The injectable form of
papaverine has recently
been approved to treat erectile dysfunction (impotence)
in men.

HOW THE DRUG WORKS
Papaverine causes dilation
of blood vessels, improving
blood flow to the tissues
supplied by the affected vessels. When injected into the
penis, papaverine causes the
penile arteries to dilate,
thus promoting erection.

DOSAGE
To treat poor blood circulation (average adult dose)—
Tablets: 100 to 300 mg, 3 to
5 times a day. Extended-
release capsules: 150 mg
every 12 hours. May be
increased by your doctor to
150 mg every 8 hours, or
300 mg every 12 hours.
Injection: 30 to 120 mg into
a vein or muscle every 3
hours. (Dose for children
will be determined by pediatrician.) For erectile dysfunction— Injection: 30 mg,
self-administered at the
base of penis as needed,
just prior to sexual activity.
Patients with erectile dysfunction due to nerve
damage (as opposed to
circulatory problems) may
require lower doses. It
should not be administered
more than once per day,
more than 2 days in a row,
or more than 3 times a
week. Dose may be
increased to 60 mg a day
based on patient response.

ONSET OF EFFECT
For circulation: Rapid.
For erectile dysfunction:
Variable; usually 10 to 15
minutes.

DURATION OF ACTION
Call your doctor immedi-
ately if erection persists for
more than 4 hours.

DIETARY ADVICE
Oral forms can be taken
with meals, milk, or
antacids to minimize
stomach upset.

STORAGE
Store in a tightly sealed container away from heat, moisture, and direct light. Do
not refrigerate or freeze
injectable forms of pure
papaverine. Various mix-
tures of papaverine with
other agents may require
refrigeration.

IF YOU MISS A DOSE
Oral forms: Take the medicine as soon as you remember. If it is near the time for
the next dose, skip the
missed dose and resume
your regular dosage schedule. Do not double the next
dose. Injection: Use as
needed.

STOPPING THE DRUG
The decision to stop taking
the drug should be made in
consultation with your
physician.

PROLONGED USE
See your doctor regularly
for tests and examinations
to evaluate your condition
and make any necessary
adjustments in therapy.

PRECAUTIONS
Over 60: Oral forms may
reduce older patients' tolerance to cold temperatures.

**Driving and Hazardous
Work:** No special precautions are necessary.

Alcohol: Avoid alcohol.

Pregnancy: Adequate studies on the use of oral
papaverine during preg-
nancy have not been done;
consult your doctor for
advice.

Breast Feeding: Oral
papaverine may pass into
breast milk; caution is
advised. Consult a doctor.

Infants and Children:
Lower doses of oral
papaverine are needed; consult your pediatrician.

Special Concerns: Oral
forms: Papaverine may
cause dizziness; get up
slowly from a seated or
prone position. If you have
glaucoma, you should have
regular eye examinations. If
you have difficulty swallowing the whole capsule, you
can mix its contents with
jelly or jam and swallow the
mixture without chewing.
Avoid smoking. Injection:
Your doctor should instruct
you on how to administer
the papaverine before you
attempt to do it yourself.

OVERDOSE
Symptoms: Oral forms:
Blurred or double vision,
drowsiness, fatigue. Injection: Painful erection or
erection that persists for
more than 4 hours. This
may cause permanent dam-
age to the tissues of the
penis and may result in the
inability to achieve subsequent erections.

What to Do: Seek medical
assistance immediately.

DRUG INTERACTIONS
Consult your doctor for specific advice if you are taking
any other prescription or
over-the-counter drug.

FOOD INTERACTIONS
No known food interactions.

DISEASE INTERACTIONS
Consult your doctor if you
have had heart disease,
glaucoma, or a recent heart
attack or stroke.

Paroxetine Hydrochloride

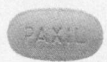

Paxil 20 mg
(SMITHKLINE BEECHAM)

▶ Drug Class: Selective serotonin reuptake inhibitor (SSRI)
antidepressant

▶ Available in: Tablets, oral
suspension

▶ Available OTC? No

▶ As Generic? No

Side Effects

SERIOUS
Muscle pain or fatigue,
lightheadedness or
fainting, rash, agitation
or irritability, severe
drowsiness, dilated
pupils, severe dry
mouth, rapid heartbeat,
trembling, severe nausea
or vomiting. Call your
doctor immediately.

COMMON
Insomnia, dizziness, sex-
ual dysfunction, unusual
fatigue, loss of initiative,
nausea or vomiting, con-
stipation, difficulty urinating, headache, trembling.

LESS COMMON
Decreased sexual desire,
blurred vision, increased
or decreased appetite,
weight gain or loss,
heartbeat irregularities,
change in sense of taste.
Also tingling, prickling,
or burning feeling.

PRINCIPAL USES
To treat symptoms of major
depression, obsessive-compulsive disorder, panic disorder, and social anxiety
disorder.

HOW THE DRUG WORKS
Paroxetine affects levels of
serotonin, a brain chemical
that is thought to be linked
to mood, emotions, and
mental state.

DOSAGE
Adults: To start, 20 mg once
a day, usually taken in the
morning; dose may be gradually increased by your doctor to 50 mg a day. Older
adults: To start, 10 mg once
a day; may be gradually
increased by your doctor
to 40 mg a day.

ONSET OF EFFECT
From 1 to 4 weeks.

DURATION OF ACTION
Unknown.

DIETARY ADVICE
This drug can be taken
without regard to diet.

STORAGE
Store in a tightly sealed container away from heat, moisture, and direct light.

IF YOU MISS A DOSE
Take it as soon as you
remember. If it is near the
time for the next dose, skip
the missed dose and
resume your regular dosage
schedule. Do not double the
next dose.

STOPPING THE DRUG
Take as prescribed for the
full treatment period even
if you begin to feel better
before the scheduled end
of therapy. The decision to
stop taking the drug should
be made in consultation
with your doctor. Dosage
should be gradually tapered
over 1 to 2 weeks.

PROLONGED USE
Usual course of therapy for
depression lasts 6 months
to 1 year; some patients
may benefit from additional
therapy.

PRECAUTIONS
Over 60: Adverse reactions
may be more likely and
more severe in older
patients. A lower dose may
be warranted.

**Driving and Hazardous
Work:** Exercise caution
until you determine how the
medicine affects you.

Alcohol: Avoid alcohol.

Pregnancy: Adequate studies of paroxetine use during
pregnancy have not been
done. Before you take
paroxetine, tell your doctor
if you are pregnant or plan
to become pregnant.

Breast Feeding: Paroxetine passes into breast milk;
caution is advised. Consult
your doctor for advice.

Infants and Children:
The safety and effectiveness
of the use of paroxetine in
children have not been
established.

Special Concerns: Take
paroxetine at least 6 hours
before bedtime to prevent
insomnia, unless it causes
drowsiness.

OVERDOSE
Symptoms: Agitation or
irritability, severe drowsiness, dizziness, coma,
dilated pupils, severe dry
mouth, rapid heartbeat,
trembling, severe nausea
and vomiting.

What to Do: Call your
doctor, emergency medical
services (EMS), or the
nearest poison control center immediately.

DRUG INTERACTIONS
Paroxetine and MAO
inhibitors should not be
used within 14 days of each
other. Very serious side
effects such as myoclonus
(uncontrolled muscle
spasms), hyperthermia
(excessive rise in body
temperature), and extreme
stiffness may result. Do
not take paroxetine with
thioridazine; dangerous
heart rhythm irregularities
may result. Tryptophan,
warfarin, sumatriptan,
naratriptan, rizatriptan, and
zolmitriptan may also interact with paroxetine; consult
your doctor for advice.

FOOD INTERACTIONS
No known food interactions.

DISEASE INTERACTIONS
Caution is advised when
taking paroxetine. Consult
your doctor if you have a
history of alcohol or drug
abuse or a seizure disorder.
Use of paroxetine may
cause complications in
patients with liver or kidney
disease, since these organs
work together to remove
the drug from the body.

Pemoline

Cylert 18.75 mg
(ABBOTT)

Additional photographs

▶ Drug Class: Central nervous system stimulant

▶ Available in: Tablets, chewable tablets

▶ Available OTC? No

▶ As Generic? No

Side Effects

SERIOUS
The most serious potential side effect is liver toxicity, which can cause jaundice (characterized by yellowish discoloration of the skin and eyes), nausea, vomiting, abdominal pain, fatigue, loss of appetite, and dark urine. Call your doctor immediately.

COMMON
Insomnia, loss of appetite, weight loss.

LESS COMMON
Dizziness, stomachache, drowsiness, mental depression, increased irritability, nausea, skin rash.

PRINCIPAL USES
To treat attention-deficit hyperactivity disorder (ADHD) in children and adults. Because of the risk of serious side effects, pemoline is generally not considered appropriate as first-line therapy.

HOW THE DRUG WORKS
Pemoline is thought to stimulate the release of norepinephrine, a natural hormone that promotes the transmission of nerve impulses in the central nervous system. It works by decreasing restlessness and increasing attention in adults and children who cannot concentrate for very long, are easily distracted, or are impulsive.

DOSAGE
Adults and children age 6 and older: To start, 37.5 mg every morning. Dose may be increased by your doctor in increments of 18.75 mg weekly, up to a maximum of 112.5 mg a day.

ONSET OF EFFECT
Significant benefit may not be evident until the third or fourth week of therapy.

DURATION OF ACTION
8 to 12 hours.

DIETARY ADVICE
No special restrictions.

STORAGE
Store in a tightly sealed container away from heat, moisture, and direct light.

IF YOU MISS A DOSE
Pemoline is generally prescribed for once-daily use in the morning. If you are unable to take it on a particular day, resume your regular scheduled dose the following morning.

STOPPING THE DRUG
The decision to stop taking the drug should be made in consultation with your physician.

PROLONGED USE
Liver function tests should be performed every 2 weeks after starting pemoline for as long as you remain on the medication. The drug should be discontinued if no clinical benefit is observed 3 weeks after dosage has been increased to 112.5 mg daily.

PRECAUTIONS
Over 60: No special problems are expected.

Driving and Hazardous Work: Avoid such activities until you determine how the medicine affects you.

Alcohol: Avoid alcohol.

Pregnancy: In animal studies, pemoline has been shown to cause stillbirths and decreased survival; however, it has not been shown to cause birth defects in humans. Before you take pemoline, tell your doctor if you are pregnant or plan to become pregnant, so that you may weigh the potential risks and benefits.

Breast Feeding: Pemoline may pass into breast milk; caution is advised. Consult your doctor for advice.

Infants and Children: There have been reports of slowed growth in children who have taken pemoline for long periods. Consult your doctor for advice.

Special Concerns: Your doctor should be thoroughly familiar with pemoline and should ask you to sign a patient consent form that helps spell out the risks of taking this medication. After you stop taking pemoline, you may exhibit unusual behavior and experience severe mental depression or unusual fatigue. Consult your doctor if you develop these symptoms. Pemoline can cause physical or mental dependence if taken for a long time. Signs of dependence include a strong desire to continue taking the medicine, a need to increase the dose to attain the same effect, and withdrawal symptoms when you stop taking the drug. Check with your doctor if you have such symptoms.

OVERDOSE
Symptoms: Agitation, muscle trembling or twitching, confusion, high blood pressure, seizures, false sense of well-being, rapid heartbeat, hallucinations, enlarged pupils, restlessness, vomiting, high fever with sweating, uncontrolled movements of the eyes or parts of the body, severe headache.

What to Do: Call your doctor, emergency medical services (EMS), or the nearest poison control center immediately.

DRUG INTERACTIONS
Consult your doctor for specific advice if you are taking any other prescription or over-the-counter medication.

FOOD INTERACTIONS
Avoid coffee, tea, cola, and other drinks that are high in caffeine.

DISEASE INTERACTIONS
Pemoline should not be used by patients with liver disease. Use of pemoline may cause complications in patients with kidney disease. Consult your doctor if you have Tourette's syndrome or other tic disorders.

Penbutolol Sulfate

▶ Drug Class: Beta-blocker

▶ Available in: Tablets

▶ Available OTC? No

▶ As Generic? No

Side Effects

SERIOUS
Shortness of breath, wheezing; irregular or slow heartbeat (50 beats per minute or less); pain or feelings of tightness or pressure in the chest; swelling of the ankles, feet, and lower legs; mental depression. If you experience such symptoms, stop taking penbutolol sulfate and call your doctor immediately.

COMMON
Dizziness or lightheadedness, especially when rising suddenly to a standing position; decreased sexual ability; unusual fatigue, weakness, or drowsiness; insomnia.

LESS COMMON
Anxiety, irritability, nervousness; constipation; diarrhea; dry, sore eyes; itching; nausea; vomiting; nightmares or intensely vivid dreams; numbness, tingling, or other unusual sensations in the fingers, toes, or scalp.

PRINCIPAL USES
To treat mild to moderate high blood pressure.

HOW THE DRUG WORKS
Penbutolol sulfate slows the rate and force of contraction of the heart by blocking certain nerve impulses, thus reducing blood pressure.

DOSAGE
20 mg once a day.

ONSET OF EFFECT
Within 1 hour.

DURATION OF ACTION
Up to 24 hours.

DIETARY ADVICE
Follow your doctor's dietary restrictions, such as a low-salt or low-cholesterol diet, to improve control over high blood pressure and heart disease.

STORAGE
Store in a tightly sealed container away from heat and direct light.

IF YOU MISS A DOSE
Take the medicine as soon as you remember. If it is within 8 hours of your next dose, skip the missed dose and resume your regular schedule. Do not double the next dose.

STOPPING THE DRUG
This drug should not be stopped suddenly, as this may lead to angina and possibly a heart attack in patients with advanced heart disease. Slow reduction of the dose under your doctor's close supervision for 2 to 3 weeks is advised.

PROLONGED USE
Regular visits to your doctor are needed to evaluate the drug's ongoing, long-term effectiveness.

PRECAUTIONS
Over 60: Adverse reactions may be more likely and more severe in older patients.

Driving and Hazardous Work: Do not drive or engage in hazardous work until you determine how the medicine affects you.

Alcohol: Drink in careful moderation if at all. Alcohol may interact with the drug and cause a dangerous drop in blood pressure.

Pregnancy: Discuss with your doctor the relative risks and benefits of using this drug while pregnant.

Breast Feeding: Trace amounts of penbutolol sulfate can be found in breast milk, but adverse effects in infants have not been documented. Consult your doctor for specific advice.

Infants and Children: No special problems.

OVERDOSE
Symptoms: Unusually slow or rapid heartbeat, severe dizziness or fainting, poor circulation in the hands (bluish skin), breathing difficulty, seizures.

What to Do: Call your doctor, emergency medical services (EMS), or the nearest poison control center immediately.

DRUG INTERACTIONS
Consult your doctor for specific advice if you are taking amphetamines, oral antidiabetic agents, asthma medication (such as aminophylline or theophylline), calcium channel blockers, clonidine, guanabenz, halothane, immunotherapy for allergies (allergy shots), insulin, MAO inhibitors, reserpine, other beta-blockers, or any over-the-counter medicine.

FOOD INTERACTIONS
None reported.

DISEASE INTERACTIONS
Penbutolol sulfate should be used with caution in people with diabetes, especially insulin-dependent diabetes, since the drug may mask symptoms of hypoglycemia. Consult your doctor if you have allergies or asthma, heart or blood vessel disease (including congestive heart failure and peripheral vascular disease), hyperthyroidism, irregular (slow) heartbeat, myasthenia gravis, psoriasis, respiratory problems such as bronchitis or emphysema, kidney or liver disease, or a history of mental depression.

Penciclovir

▶ Drug Class: Antiviral

▶ Available in: Topical cream

▶ Available OTC? No

▶ As Generic? No

Side Effects

SERIOUS
No serious side effects have been reported.

COMMON
Headache, allergic reaction at site of application.

LESS COMMON
Numbness or deadening of feeling in skin at application sites, skin rash, odd taste or changes in taste perception.

PRINCIPAL USES
To treat herpes labialis infection (cold sores) of the lips and face in adults with healthy immune systems. (Other treatments are recommended for those with impaired immune function.)

HOW THE DRUG WORKS
Penciclovir interferes with the activity of enzymes needed for the replication of viral DNA in cells, thus preventing the virus from multiplying.

DOSAGE
Apply it every 2 hours during waking hours, for 4 days. Start treatment as early as possible, when the first lesions appear on the face.

ONSET OF EFFECT
Unknown.

DURATION OF ACTION
Unknown.

DIETARY ADVICE
There are no special dietary recommendations, but before eating, be sure to wash your hands thoroughly after applying penciclovir.

STORAGE
Store in a tightly sealed container away from heat and direct light.

IF YOU MISS A DOSE
Apply it as soon as you remember. If it is near the time for the next dose, skip the missed dose and resume your regular dosage schedule. Do not double the next dose.

STOPPING THE DRUG
The decision to stop using this medication should be made in consultation with your doctor.

PROLONGED USE
See your doctor regularly for tests and examinations if you must use this medicine for a prolonged period.

PRECAUTIONS
Over 60: In human tests penciclovir did not cause more side effects in older patients than it did in younger users.

Driving and Hazardous Work: The use of penciclovir should not impair your ability to perform such tasks safely.

Alcohol: No special precautions are necessary.

Pregnancy: Penciclovir has not been shown to cause birth defects in animals. Human studies have not been done. Before you take penciclovir, tell your doctor if you are pregnant or planning to become pregnant. Use this medication during pregnancy only if its benefits clearly outweigh potential risks.

Breast Feeding: In animal studies, penciclovir given orally was shown to pass into breast milk, and in fact to be present in higher concentrations than those found in the blood. While there is no information on whether penciclovir passes into human breast milk after topical application, you should consult your doctor to help you decide whether to discontinue breast feeding (if the drug is determined to be necessary to the mother) or to discontinue the drug.

Infants and Children: The safety and effectiveness of penciclovir in infants and children have not been established. This medication should be used only under close medical supervision.

Special Concerns: Be careful not to apply penciclovir to the mucous membranes of the mouth and nose. Apply it with care near the eyes, since it can cause pain and irritation if it enters them. You should not use penciclovir if you are allergic to it or to any of its chemical components.

OVERDOSE
Symptoms: No specific ones have been reported.

What to Do: An overdose of penciclovir is very unlikely to occur. However, if someone accidentally ingests a large quantity of the medicine, call your doctor, emergency medical services (EMS), or the nearest poison control center.

DRUG INTERACTIONS
Other drugs may interact with penciclovir. Consult your doctor for specific advice if you are taking any other prescription or over-the-counter medication.

FOOD INTERACTIONS
No known food interactions.

DISEASE INTERACTIONS
Consult your doctor for advice if you have any other medical condition.

Penicillamine

Cuprimine 125 mg
(MERCK)

▶ Drug Class: Chelating agent; antirheumatic; antiurolithic

▶ Available in: Capsules, tablets

▶ Available OTC? No

▶ As Generic? No

Side Effects

SERIOUS
Joint pain, wheezing or tightness in chest, hives, skin rash or itching, cloudy or bloody urine, shortness of breath, unusual fatigue, sore throat and fever, painful or swollen glands, weight gain, unusual bleeding. Also white spots, sores, or ulcers in mouth; swollen face, feet, or lower legs. Call your doctor immediately.

COMMON
Diarrhea, nausea or vomiting, loss of taste, mild stomach pain, loss of appetite.

LESS COMMON
No less-common side effects are associated with this drug.

PRINCIPAL USES
To treat Wilson's disease (excessive accumulation of copper in the body tissues) and rheumatoid arthritis, and to prevent or treat kidney stones in patients with excessive amounts of the amino acid cystine in the urine or who have a history of recurrent cystine kidney stones. It can also be used to treat heavy metal (mercury, lead) poisoning.

HOW THE DRUG WORKS
Penicillamine is a chelating (chemical binding) agent that removes excess copper (the underlying problem in Wilson's disease), mercury, and lead from the body. It is not clear how penicillamine improves rheumatoid arthritis, but it may suppress the body's release of certain chemicals that cause inflammation. Penicillamine also binds with cystine and eliminates it from the body; high concentrations of cystine can cause kidney stone formation.

DOSAGE
For Wilson's disease— Adults and teenagers: To start, 250 mg, 4 times a day; may be increased to 500 mg, 4 times a day. Children: To start, 250 mg once a day; may be increased. For rheumatoid arthritis— Adults: To start, 125 to 250 mg once a day; may be increased to 500 mg, 3 times a day. To prevent cystine kidney stones— Adults: To start, 500 mg, 4 times a day; may be increased to 1,000 mg, 4 times a day. Children: To start, 3.5 mg per lb of body weight, 4 times a day; may be increased. To treat heavy metal poisoning— 500 mg to 1.5 g a day in adults for 1 to 2 months.

ONSET OF EFFECT
For Wilson's disease: Within 1 to 3 months. For rheumatoid arthritis: Within 2 to 3 months. For kidney stones: Unknown.

DURATION OF ACTION
Unknown.

DIETARY ADVICE
For Wilson's disease or rheumatoid arthritis: Take it on an empty stomach. For rheumatoid arthritis, take it at least 1 hour before or after any other food, milk, or medicine. For prevention or treatment of kidney stones: Drink at least 2 full glasses of water at bedtime and another 2 glasses of water during the night.

STORAGE
Store in a tightly sealed container away from heat, moisture, and direct light.

IF YOU MISS A DOSE
Take it as soon as you remember. If you take 2 or more doses a day and it is near the time for the next dose, skip the missed dose and resume your regular dosage schedule. If you take 1 dose a day, simply skip the missed dose and resume your schedule the next day. In either case, do not double the next dose.

STOPPING THE DRUG
Take it as prescribed for the full treatment period.

PROLONGED USE
See your doctor regularly for tests and examinations.

PRECAUTIONS
Over 60: Adverse reactions may be more likely and more severe.

Driving and Hazardous Work: The use of penicillamine should not impair your ability to engage in such tasks safely.

Alcohol: No special precautions are necessary.

Pregnancy: Penicillamine may cause birth defects if taken during pregnancy.

Breast Feeding: Penicillamine may pass into breast milk; do not use it while nursing.

Infants and Children: No special warnings.

Special Concerns: Do not take any iron-containing medication or supplement within 2 hours of taking penicillamine. Patients should take 25 mg a day of vitamin B6 during therapy, since the drug increases the need for this vitamin. Patients may also take a multivitamin, but those with Wilson's disease must ensure it is copper-free.

OVERDOSE
Symptoms: None known.

What to Do: If someone takes a much larger dose than prescribed, seek medical assistance immediately.

DRUG INTERACTIONS
Do not take gold compounds or phenylbutazone if you are taking penicillamine. Also, tell your doctor if you are taking any other prescription or over-the-counter medication.

FOOD INTERACTIONS
Patients with Wilson's disease should not eat foods high in copper such as chocolate, nuts, shellfish, mushrooms, liver, molasses, and broccoli.

DISEASE INTERACTIONS
Consult your doctor if you have a history of blood problems or kidney disease. Persons sensitive to penicillin may have allergic reactions to penicillamine.

Penicillin G

BRAND NAMES
Bicillin L-A, Crysticillin 300 AS, Pentids, Permapen, Pfizerpen

▶ Drug Class: Penicillin antibiotic

▶ Available in: Capsules, oral solution, injection

▶ Available OTC? No

▶ As Generic? No

Side Effects

SERIOUS
Irregular, rapid, or labored breathing, light-headedness or sudden fainting, joint pain, fever, severe abdominal pain and cramping with watery or bloody stools, severe allergic reaction (marked by sudden swelling of the lips, tongue, face, or throat; breathing difficulty; skin rash, itching, or hives), unusual bleeding or bruising, yellowish tinge to eyes or skin. Call your doctor immediately.

COMMON
Mild rash, mild diarrhea, nausea, vomiting, headache, vaginal discharge and itching, pain or white patches in the mouth or on the tongue.

LESS COMMON
Diminished urine output, chills, weakness, fatigue.

PRINCIPAL USES
To treat a variety of bacterial infections, including those of the ear, nose, and throat, skin and soft tissues, genitourinary tract, and the respiratory tract. It is also prescribed preventively before surgery or dental work in patients at risk for endocarditis (infection of the interior lining of the heart, which may damage the heart's valves). May also be given to treat meningitis and syphilis. Penicillin G is also approved for prophylactic use following known exposure to anthrax bacteria and for treating anthrax infections.

HOW THE DRUG WORKS
Penicillin G blocks the formation of bacterial cell walls, rendering bacteria unable to multiply and spread.

DOSAGE
Oral forms— Adults and teenagers: 200,000 to 500,000 units every 4 to 6 hours. Children: 189 to 13,636 units per lb of body weight every 4 to 8 hours. Injection (benzathine form)— Adults and teenagers: 1,200,000 to 2,400,000 units in 1 dose. Children: 300,000 to 1,200,000 units in 1 dose. Injection (procaine form)— Adults and teenagers: 600,000 to 1,200,000 units once a day. Children: 22,727 units per lb of body weight once a day. Other injection forms— Adults and teenagers: 1,000,000 to 5,000,000 units injected every 4 to 6 hours. Children: 3,788 to 11,363 units per lb of body weight every 4 to 6 hours. Infants: 13,636 units per lb of body weight every 12 hours.

ONSET OF EFFECT
Immediate after intravenous injection; unknown for other forms.

DURATION OF ACTION
Unknown.

DIETARY ADVICE
Oral doses should be given at least 1 hour before or 2 hours after meals.

STORAGE
Store in a tightly sealed container away from heat and direct light. Liquid forms can be refrigerated, but not frozen.

IF YOU MISS A DOSE
Take it as soon as you remember. If it is near the time for the next dose, skip the missed dose and resume your regular dosage schedule. Do not double the next dose.

STOPPING THE DRUG
Take this drug as prescribed for the full treatment period, even if you feel better before the scheduled end of therapy.

PROLONGED USE
See your doctor regularly for tests and examinations if you must take this medicine for a prolonged period.

PRECAUTIONS
Over 60: No special problems are expected.

Driving and Hazardous Work: Use of this drug should not impair ability to perform such tasks safely.

Alcohol: No special precautions are necessary.

Pregnancy: Adequate studies of use of this drug during pregnancy have not been done; however, no problems have been reported.

Breast Feeding: Penicillin G may pass into breast milk and cause problems in the nursing infant; avoid use while nursing.

Infants and Children: No special problems are expected.

Special Concerns: Penicillin G can cause false results on some urine sugar tests for patients with diabetes. Those who are prone to asthma, hay fever, hives, or allergies may be more likely to have an allergic reaction to a penicillin antibiotic. If severe diarrhea occurs as a side effect of this drug, do not take antidiarrheal medications; call your doctor.

OVERDOSE
Symptoms: Severe nausea, vomiting, diarrhea, seizures.

What to Do: Call your doctor, emergency medical services (EMS), or the nearest poison control center immediately.

DRUG INTERACTIONS
Consult your physician for specific advice if you are taking aminoglycosides, ACE inhibitors, diuretics, potassium supplements or potassium-containing medications, anticoagulants or other anticlotting drugs, nonsteroidal anti-inflammatory drugs, sulfinpyrazone, cholestyramine, colestipol, oral contraceptives, methotrexate, probenecid, or rifampin.

FOOD INTERACTIONS
No known food interactions.

DISEASE INTERACTIONS
Consult your doctor if you have a history of allergies, asthma, bleeding disorders (such as hemophilia), congestive heart failure, cystic fibrosis, gastrointestinal disorders (especially colitis associated with the use of antibiotics), infectious mononucleosis, or impaired kidney function.

Penicillin V

Generic 500 mg
(BIOCRAFT)

Additional photographs

▶ Drug Class: Penicillin antibiotic

▶ Available in: Tablets, delayed-release tablets, liquid

▶ Available OTC? No

▶ As Generic? Yes

Side Effects

SERIOUS
Irregular, rapid, or labored breathing, light-headedness or sudden fainting, joint pain, fever, severe abdominal pain and cramping with watery or bloody stools, severe allergic reaction (marked by sudden swelling of the lips, tongue, face, or throat; breathing difficulty; skin rash, itching, or hives), unusual bleeding or bruising, yellowish tinge to eyes or skin. Call your doctor immediately.

COMMON
Mild rash, mild diarrhea, nausea, vomiting, headache, vaginal discharge and itching, pain or white patches in the mouth or on the tongue.

LESS COMMON
Diminished urine output, chills, weakness, fatigue.

PRINCIPAL USES
To treat a variety of bacterial infections, including those of the ear, nose, and throat, skin and soft tissues, genitourinary tract, and the respiratory tract. It is also prescribed before surgery or dental work in patients at risk for endocarditis (infection of the lining of the heart, which may damage the heart's valves).

HOW THE DRUG WORKS
Penicillin V destroys susceptible bacteria by interfering with their ability to produce cell walls as they multiply.

DOSAGE
Adults: 500 to 2,000 mg a day for infections; 2,000 mg to prevent bacterial endocarditis; or as ordered by physician. Children: 15 to 50 mg per 2.2 lbs (1 kg) of body weight per day in divided doses to treat infections. To prevent infection after dental surgery, 2 g (1 g for children), 30 to 60 minutes before procedure, then 1 g (500 mg for children) 6 hours afterward.

ONSET OF EFFECT
Unknown.

DURATION OF ACTION
Up to 6 hours.

DIETARY ADVICE
Take it on an empty stomach, 1 to 2 hours before or 3 to 4 hours after a meal.

STORAGE
Store in a tightly sealed container away from heat and direct light.

IF YOU MISS A DOSE
Take it as soon as you remember. If it is near the time for the next dose, skip the missed dose and resume your regular dosage schedule. Do not double the next dose.

STOPPING THE DRUG
It is very important to take this drug as prescribed for the full treatment period. Stopping the drug prematurely may lead to serious complications.

PROLONGED USE
Prolonged use of any antibiotic increases the risk of superinfection (a more severe and drug-resistant infection); caution is advised.

PRECAUTIONS
Over 60: No special problems are expected.

Driving and Hazardous Work: The use of penicillin should not impair your ability to perform such tasks safely.

Alcohol: No special precautions are necessary.

Pregnancy: Adequate studies of penicillin antibiotic use during pregnancy have not been done; however, no problems have been reported.

Breast Feeding: Penicillin V may pass into breast milk and cause problems in the nursing infant; avoid use while nursing.

Infants and Children: No special problems are expected.

Special Concerns: Penicillin V can cause false results on some urine sugar tests for patients with diabetes. If severe diarrhea occurs as a side effect of this drug, do not take antidiarrheal medications; call your doctor. Oral contraceptives may not be effective while you are taking penicillin; consider other methods of birth control. Those who are prone to asthma, hay fever, hives, or allergies may be more likely to have an allergic reaction to a penicillin antibiotic.

OVERDOSE
Symptoms: Severe nausea, vomiting, diarrhea, seizures.

What to Do: An overdose of penicillin is unlikely to be life-threatening. However, if someone takes a much larger dose than prescribed, call your doctor or emergency medical services (EMS) right away.

DRUG INTERACTIONS
Consult your physician for specific advice if you are taking aminoglycosides, ACE inhibitors, diuretics, potassium supplements or potassium-containing medications, anticoagulants or other anticlotting drugs, nonsteroidal anti-inflammatory drugs, sulfinpyrazone, cholestyramine, colestipol, oral contraceptives, methotrexate, probenecid, or rifampin.

FOOD INTERACTIONS
Acidic foods or juices can reduce the antibiotic effect.

DISEASE INTERACTIONS
Consult your doctor if you have a history of allergies, asthma, congestive heart failure, gastrointestinal disorders (especially colitis associated with the use of antibiotics), or impaired kidney function.

Pentamidine Isethionate

▶ Drug Class: Anti-infective; antiprotozoal

▶ Available in: Inhalation, injection

▶ Available OTC? No

▶ As Generic? Yes

Side Effects

SERIOUS
Inhalation: Chest pain or congestion, difficulty breathing or swallowing, wheezing, skin rash, burning pain, dryness or feeling of lump in throat, cough. Injection: Decreased urination, unusual bruising or bleeding due to reduced number of platelets (clotting agents) in the blood, sore throat and fever; symptoms of high blood sugar or diabetes mellitus (flushed, dry skin, drowsiness, fruity breath, increased urination and thirst, loss of appetite); symptoms of low blood sugar (nausea, headache, anxiety, cold sweats or chills, shakiness, cool, pale skin, increased appetite); signs of low blood pressure (dizziness, confusion, fatigue, blurred vision, fainting or lightheadedness); dry, red, or itchy skin; vomiting or nausea; fast or irregular pulse; abdominal pain; pain or redness at injection site. Serious side effects occur commonly; call your doctor immediately.

COMMON
Injection: Loss of appetite, diarrhea, unpleasant metallic taste, nausea and vomiting.

LESS COMMON
There are no less-common side effects.

PRINCIPAL USES
To prevent and treat Pneumocystis carinii pneumonia (PCP). This serious type of pneumonia is prevalent among AIDS patients. The inhalation form is used to attempt to prevent PCP. The injection form is used to treat PCP. It may also be used for other types of infection as determined by your doctor.

HOW THE DRUG WORKS
The exact way in which pentamidine works is unknown.

DOSAGE
To prevent PCP— Inhalation (using the Respirgard II nebulizer by Marquest), adults and children age 5 and older: 300 mg once every 4 weeks. To treat PCP— Injection: 3 to 4 mg per 2.2 lbs (1 kg) of body weight into a vein over a period of 1 to 2 hours once a day for 21 days.

ONSET OF EFFECT
Unknown.

DURATION OF ACTION
Unknown.

DIETARY ADVICE
No special restrictions.

STORAGE
Not applicable; the dose is administered only at a health care facility.

IF YOU MISS A DOSE
Be sure to receive treatment as soon as possible. Contact your doctor.

STOPPING THE DRUG
Take it as prescribed for the full treatment period. The decision to stop taking the drug should be made in consultation with your physician.

PROLONGED USE
See your doctor regularly for tests and examinations if you must take this medicine for a prolonged period.

PRECAUTIONS
Over 60: No studies have been done specifically on older patients.

Driving and Hazardous Work: Do not drive or engage in hazardous work until you determine how the medicine affects you.

Alcohol: Avoid alcohol.

Pregnancy: Adequate human studies have not been done. Before taking this drug, tell your doctor if you are currently pregnant or plan to become pregnant.

Breast Feeding: Pentamidine may pass into breast milk; avoid use while breast feeding.

Infants and Children: Adequate studies on the use of pentamidine in children younger than 4 months have not been done. Consult your doctor for more information.

Special Concerns: Do not mix the inhalation solution with any other drugs or use any other drug in the nebulizer. Injectable pentamidine can cause a sudden drop in blood pressure. Lie down while taking it. The drug may also increase the chance of infection because it can lower the number of white blood cells in your blood. Consult your doctor at once if you detect signs of an infection (fever, sore throat). Use an electric shaver rather than a razor, as pentamidine may increase the risk of uncontrolled bleeding. Consult your dentist about ways to safely clean your teeth.

OVERDOSE
Symptoms: See Serious Side Effects.

What to Do: An overdose is unlikely. However, if you suspect an overdose, call your doctor, emergency medical services (EMS), or the nearest control center immediately.

DRUG INTERACTIONS
Other drugs may interact with pentamidine. Consult your doctor if you are taking bone marrow depressants, didanosine, macrolide antibiotics, foscarnet, or any drugs that may damage the kidney. Also consult your doctor if you are undergoing radiation therapy.

FOOD INTERACTIONS
No known food interactions.

DISEASE INTERACTIONS
Consult your doctor if you have heart, kidney, or liver disease, tuberculosis, a bleeding disorder, low blood pressure, diabetes mellitus, or low blood sugar. PCP prevention by inhalation may be less effective in those with chronic obstructive pulmonary disease (emphysema).

Pentazocine

BRAND NAME
Talwin

▶ Drug Class: Opioid agonist-antagonist analgesic

▶ Available in: Injection

▶ Available OTC? No

▶ As Generic? No

Side Effects

SERIOUS
Serious side effects of pentazocine are indistinguishable from those of overdose: Confusion; severe drowsiness, weakness, or dizziness; slurred speech; small, pinpoint pupils; cold, clammy skin; slow breathing; seizures; loss of consciousness.

COMMON
Dizziness or lightheadedness, nausea or vomiting, constipation, itching.

LESS COMMON
Mood swings or false sense of well-being and euphoria; hallucinations; nightmares.

PRINCIPAL USES
To relieve moderate to severe pain.

HOW THE DRUG WORKS
Opioids such as pentazocine relieve pain by acting on areas of the brain that process pain signals from nerves throughout the body.

DOSAGE
Adults: 25 to 50 mg every 3 or 4 hours. Maximum dose is 360 mg a day. Children: The dose must be determined by your pediatrician.

ONSET OF EFFECT
Into a vein: Within 2 to 3 minutes. Into a muscle: Within 15 to 20 minutes.

DURATION OF ACTION
From 2 to 3 hours.

DIETARY ADVICE
Drink 2 to 3 quarts of fluid a day, if possible, to help prevent constipation.

STORAGE
Not applicable; the dose is administered only in a health care facility.

IF YOU MISS A DOSE
Not applicable; the dose is administered by a health care professional.

STOPPING THE DRUG
The decision to stop taking the drug should be made by your doctor.

PROLONGED USE
You should see your doctor regularly for tests and examinations if you take this medication for a prolonged period. Prolonged use can cause physical dependence.

PRECAUTIONS
Over 60: Adverse reactions may be more likely and more severe in older patients.

Driving and Hazardous Work: Do not drive or engage in hazardous work until you determine how the medicine affects you.

Alcohol: Avoid alcohol while using this medication.

Pregnancy: In animal studies, pentazocine has not been shown to cause birth defects; adequate human studies have not been done. Before using this drug, tell your doctor if you are pregnant or plan to become pregnant. Overuse during pregnancy can cause drug dependence in the fetus.

Breast Feeding: Pentazocine may pass into breast milk; caution is advised. Consult your doctor for specific advice.

Infants and Children: Adverse reactions may be more likely and more severe in children. Consult your doctor for specific advice. Not recommended for use by children under the age of 12.

Special Concerns: If you feel the medication is not working properly after a few weeks, consult your doctor about other treatment options. Before undergoing any surgical procedure (including dental surgery), be sure to tell the doctor or dentist in charge that you are taking pentazocine.

OVERDOSE
Symptoms: Confusion; severe drowsiness, weakness, or dizziness; slurred speech; small, pinpoint pupils; cold, clammy skin; slow breathing; seizures; loss of consciousness.

What to Do: Call your doctor, emergency medical services (EMS), or the nearest poison control center immediately.

DRUG INTERACTIONS
Consult your physician for specific advice if you are taking carbamazepine or other medicine for seizures, barbiturates, sedatives, cough medicines, decongestants, antidepressants, other prescription pain medications, MAO inhibitors, naltrexone, rifampin, or zidovudine (AZT).

FOOD INTERACTIONS
No known food interactions.

DISEASE INTERACTIONS
Consult your doctor if you have any of the following: a history of alcohol or drug abuse, emotional illness, brain disorders or head injury, seizures, lung disease, prostate disorders or other problems with urination, gallstones, colitis, or heart, kidney, liver, or thyroid disease.

Pentobarbital Sodium

BRAND NAME
Nembutal

▶ Drug Class: Barbiturate

▶ Available in: Capsules, elixir, injection, suppositories

▶ Available OTC? No

▶ As Generic? Yes

Side Effects

SERIOUS
Excitability, confusion, or excessive sedation to the point you cannot be awakened. Also yellowish tinge to the eyes or skin; swollen eyelids, face, or lips, wheezing, or rash (these may be signs of drug allergy); sores on lips or mouth. Call your doctor immediately.

COMMON
Clumsiness, unsteadiness, persistent drowsiness, dizziness or lightheadedness.

LESS COMMON
Anxiety or nervousness, nightmares, insomnia, constipation, feeling faint, irritability, headache, nausea or vomiting.

PRINCIPAL USES
Primarily for sedation before surgery and to control certain types of seizures. With the availability of newer sleep-inducing drugs, pentobarbital is now rarely used for short-term treatment of insomnia.

HOW THE DRUG WORKS
Barbiturates such as pentobarbital act as powerful sedatives by reducing activity in the central nervous system.

DOSAGE
Sedation before surgery— Adult oral dosage: 100 mg. Children's oral dosage: 0.9 mg to 2.7 mg per lb of body weight, usually not more than 100 mg. To control seizures— Usually given intravenously by a doctor. Pentobarbital injection (into a vein or muscle) is only done under the direction of a physician. For insomnia— Adult oral dosage: 100 mg taken at bedtime.

ONSET OF EFFECT
Within 30 minutes.

DURATION OF ACTION
1 to 4 hours for oral or rectal forms, 15 minutes for injection.

DIETARY ADVICE
Oral forms can be taken with fluid or food.

STORAGE
Store in a tightly sealed container away from heat, moisture, and direct light.

IF YOU MISS A DOSE
Take it as soon as you remember. If it is near the time for the next dose, skip the missed dose and resume your regular dosage schedule. Do not double the next dose.

STOPPING THE DRUG
The decision to stop taking the drug should be made by your doctor. There is a risk of withdrawal side effects when the drug is stopped suddenly.

PROLONGED USE
Barbiturates may be habit-forming, and prolonged use may increase the risk of dependency. Pentobarbital, as well as other barbiturates, when used for insomnia, is only prescribed on a short-term basis. It is not usually effective when used for longer than 2 weeks.

PRECAUTIONS
Over 60: Adverse reactions may be more likely and more severe in older patients and may require that smaller doses be used.

Driving and Hazardous Work: Because of sedative effects, do not drive or engage in hazardous work until you determine how the medicine affects you.

Alcohol: Avoid alcohol; its sedative effects are additive to those of the drug.

Pregnancy: Pentobarbital can cause birth defects and problems during pregnancy. Before taking pentobarbital, be sure to tell your doctor if you are pregnant or plan to become pregnant.

Breast Feeding: Pentobarbital passes into breast milk in small amounts and can cause side effects in breast-feeding infants. Consult your doctor for advice.

Infants and Children: As with older patients, infants and children are more sensitive to the effects of pentobarbital. A lower dose may be warranted.

Special Concerns: Pentobarbital may cause physical or mental dependence. Check with your doctor at once if you feel overly sedated or if you suffer withdrawal side effects when you stop the drug.

OVERDOSE
Symptoms: Severe sedation or excessive drowsiness, confusion, irritability, shortness of breath or troubled breathing, slurred speech, staggering walk, severe weakness.

What to Do: Call your doctor, emergency medical services (EMS), or the nearest poison control center immediately.

DRUG INTERACTIONS
Consult your doctor for specific advice if you are taking other seizure medicines, central nervous system depressants, warfarin (blood thinner), or oral contraceptives. Pentobarbital may make oral contraceptives less effective.

FOOD INTERACTIONS
No known food interactions.

DISEASE INTERACTIONS
Caution is advised when taking pentobarbital. Consult your doctor if you have any of the following: kidney disease, liver disease, porphyria, hyperactivity, mental depression, or a history of alcohol or drug abuse.

Pentosan Polysulfate Sodium

BNP 7600   BNP 7600

Elmiron 100 mg
(BAKER NORTON)

▶ Drug Class: Synthetic sulfated polysaccharide

▶ Available in: Capsules

▶ Available OTC? No

▶ As Generic? No

Side Effects

SERIOUS
Fever, unusual tiredness or fatigue, chills, itching, skin rash or hives, difficulty breathing, sore throat, unusual bleeding or bruising. Call your doctor immediately.

COMMON
No common side effects are associated with the use of pentosan.

LESS COMMON
Abdominal pain, hair loss, diarrhea, nausea, stomach distress, dizziness, rash, headache.

PRINCIPAL USES
To relieve bladder pain or discomfort caused by interstitial cystitis, an inflammatory bladder condition predominantly affecting women, marked by frequent and painful urination.

HOW THE DRUG WORKS
The exact mechanism of action is unknown, but pentosan is believed to adhere to the mucosal lining of the bladder, acting as a coating to prevent irritating substances in the urine from reaching the bladder wall.

DOSAGE
100 mg, 3 times a day.

ONSET OF EFFECT
Unknown.

DURATION OF ACTION
Unknown.

DIETARY ADVICE
Should be taken with a full glass of water on an empty stomach, at least 1 hour before or 2 hours after meals, and at least 1 hour before or after any other food, milk or milk-based product, or medication.

STORAGE
Store in a tightly sealed container away from heat, moisture, and direct light.

IF YOU MISS A DOSE
Take it as soon as you remember. If it is near the time for the next dose, skip the missed dose and resume your regular dosage schedule. Do not double the next dose.

STOPPING THE DRUG
Take it as prescribed for the full treatment period, even if you begin to feel better before the scheduled end of therapy. The decision to stop taking the drug should be made by your doctor.

PROLONGED USE
Therapy generally lasts for 3 months. You should be reassessed by your doctor at that time. If your condition has not improved and there are few side effects, your doctor may continue therapy for an additional 3 months.

PRECAUTIONS
Over 60: Adverse reactions may be more likely and more severe in older patients.

Driving and Hazardous Work: Do not drive or engage in hazardous work until you determine how the medicine affects you.

Alcohol: Avoid alcohol when taking this medication, since it may provoke further bladder irritation.

Pregnancy: Adequate studies of the use of this drug during pregnancy have not been done. Before taking pentosan, tell your doctor if you are pregnant or plan to become pregnant.

Breast Feeding: Pentosan may pass into breast milk; caution is advised. Consult your doctor for advice.

Infants and Children: The safety and effectiveness of pentosan use by patients under age 16 have not been established.

Special Concerns: This drug may increase your susceptibility to sunburn. Use measures to protect your skin from ultraviolet light until you determine how the medicine affects you.

OVERDOSE
Symptoms: An overdose of pentosan is unlikely; no cases of overdose have been reported.

What to Do: Emergency instructions not applicable.

DRUG INTERACTIONS
The following drugs may interact with pentosan. Consult your doctor for specific advice if you are taking alteplase, aspirin, warfarin or any other anticoagulant, heparin, or streptokinase.

FOOD INTERACTIONS
No known food interactions.

DISEASE INTERACTIONS
Caution is advised when taking pentosan. Consult your doctor if you have any of the following conditions: hemophilia, low platelet count or any bleeding problems, blockage or obstruction of the intestine, stomach or intestinal ulcers, polyps, liver disease, or blood vessel disease.

Pentoxifylline

Trental 400 mg
(HOECHST MARION ROUSSEL)

▶ Drug Class: Hemorheologic agent

▶ Available in: Extended-release tablets

▶ Available OTC? No

▶ As Generic? Yes

Side Effects

SERIOUS
Chest pain, heartbeat irregularities. Call your doctor or emergency medical services (EMS) immediately.

COMMON
No common side effects have been reported.

LESS COMMON
Dizziness, headache, stomach pain or upset, nausea or vomiting.

PRINCIPAL USES
To improve blood flow and reduce leg pain in patients with poor circulation.

HOW THE DRUG WORKS
It decreases the viscosity (or thickness) of blood, permitting easier red blood cell movement throughout the circulatory system.

DOSAGE
400 mg, 2 or 3 times a day.

ONSET OF EFFECT
Unknown. The full effect may take 2 to 4 weeks or longer.

DURATION OF ACTION
Unknown.

DIETARY ADVICE
Pentoxifylline should be taken with meals to lessen the risk of stomach upset. Taking an antacid may also help.

STORAGE
Store in a tightly sealed container away from heat and direct light.

IF YOU MISS A DOSE
Take a missed dose as soon as you remember. If it is near the time for the next dose, skip the missed dose and resume your regular dosage schedule, as prescribed. Do not double the next dose.

STOPPING THE DRUG
The decision to stop taking the drug should be made by your doctor. Take as prescribed for the full treatment period, even if you are feeling better before the scheduled end of therapy.

PROLONGED USE
You should see your doctor regularly for tests and physical examinations if you must take this drug for a prolonged period of time.

PRECAUTIONS
Over 60: Adverse reactions may be more likely and more severe in older patients.

Driving and Hazardous Work: Do not drive or engage in hazardous work until you determine how the medicine affects you.

Alcohol: Alcohol should be avoided while taking this medication.

Pregnancy: Pentoxifylline has not been shown to cause birth defects, but in animal studies it has caused other harmful effects. Human studies have not been done. Before you take pentoxifylline, be sure to tell your doctor if you are pregnant or plan to become pregnant.

Breast Feeding: Pentoxifylline passes into breast milk; caution is advised. Consult your doctor for specific advice.

Infants and Children: There is no specific information comparing use of pentoxifylline in infants and children with other age groups. Use and dosage must be determined by your doctor.

Special Concerns: In addition to taking pentoxifylline, you should practice such measures as weight control and exercise. Bathe your feet daily in lukewarm water, applying lanolin afterward, and wear clean cotton socks. Do not smoke cigarettes, since smoking can make your condition worse by narrowing blood vessels; indeed, tobacco of all types must be avoided. Tablets should be swallowed whole, without breaking, crushing, or chewing.

OVERDOSE
Symptoms: Flushing, very low blood pressure, nervousness, agitation, tremors, seizures, fever, agitation, loss of consciousness, very slow heartbeat. Symptoms usually appear 4 to 5 hours following an overdose.

What to Do: Discontinue the medication and call your doctor, emergency medical services (EMS), or the nearest poison control center right away.

DRUG INTERACTIONS
Consult your doctor for specific advice if you are taking anticoagulants, theophylline, drugs for hypertension, or any other prescription or over-the-counter drugs.

FOOD INTERACTIONS
No known food interactions.

DISEASE INTERACTIONS
Caution is advised when taking pentoxifylline. Consult your doctor if you have any condition in which there is a risk of bleeding, such as a recent stroke. Use of pentoxifylline may cause complications in patients with liver or kidney disease, since these organs work together to remove the medication from the body.

Pergolide Mesylate

Permax 0.05 mg
(ATHENA)

▶ Drug Class: Antiparkinsonism drug

▶ Available in: Tablets

▶ Available OTC? No

▶ As Generic? No

Side Effects

SERIOUS
Confusion, hallucinations, unusual or abnormal muscle movements, low blood pressure (causing dizziness, lightheadedness, fainting, or confusion) pain or burning while urinating (symptoms of a urinary tract infection).

COMMON
Dizziness or lightheadedness when standing or sitting up suddenly is particularly common when the drug is first started but usually subsides with continued use.

LESS COMMON
High blood pressure, diarrhea, dry mouth, facial swelling.

PRINCIPAL USES
Pergolide is used in conjunction with levodopa/carbidopa to treat Parkinson's disease or Parkinson-like syndromes, which can occur following injury to or infection of the nervous system, damage to the blood vessels in the brain, or exposure to certain toxins.

HOW THE DRUG WORKS
Pergolide directly stimulates receptor cells that act with the brain chemical dopamine to initiate and enhance smooth control of voluntary muscle movement.

DOSAGE
Adults: Initial dose is 0.05 mg, once a day. This is gradually increased over the course of 12 days to 0.25 mg a day. The dose can then be increased every 3 days until the ideal therapeutic response is achieved. The usual adult maintenance dose is 3 mg a day, usually given in 3 divided doses. The maximum dose is 5 mg a day. Children: This medication is generally not prescribed for children.

ONSET OF EFFECT
Unknown.

DURATION OF ACTION
Unknown.

DIETARY ADVICE
No special restrictions.

STORAGE
Store in a tightly sealed container away from heat, moisture, and direct light.

IF YOU MISS A DOSE
Take it as soon as you remember. If it is near the time for the next dose, skip the missed dose and resume your regular dosage schedule. Do not double the next dose.

STOPPING THE DRUG
Consult your doctor before stopping the drug. The dosage should be tapered gradually over the course of 7 to 14 days.

PROLONGED USE
It is not known whether long-term use of pergolide presents any special problems; study of the drug's long-term effects is very limited.

PRECAUTIONS
Over 60: No special problems are expected, but use this drug with caution.

Driving and Hazardous Work: Pergolide may cause drowsiness or confusion. Do not drive or engage in hazardous work until you determine how the medicine affects you.

Alcohol: Avoid alcohol.

Pregnancy: Adequate human studies have not been done. This drug should not be used in pregnant women.

Breast Feeding: Pergolide may inhibit the secretion of breast milk and so should not be used by nursing mothers.

Infants and Children: The safety and effectiveness of this medication for infants and children have not been established; consult your pediatrician.

Special Concerns: This drug should be used with special caution by those with any gastrointestinal disorders or any urinary difficulty, for example, problems when urinating, pain with urination, or urinary tract infection.

OVERDOSE
Symptoms: There have been very few reports of pergolide mesylate overdose. Signs and symptoms include low blood pressure and agitation.

What to Do: Call your doctor, emergency medical services (EMS), or the nearest poison control center immediately.

DRUG INTERACTIONS
Pergolide may interact with phenothiazine antipsychotic drugs such as chlorpromazine hydrochloride, thioridazine hydrochloride, or prochlorperazine. Consult your doctor for advice.

FOOD INTERACTIONS
No known food interactions.

DISEASE INTERACTIONS
Consult your doctor if you have any of the following: a gastrointestinal disorder, a urinary tract disorder, or heart disease (especially a condition associated with heart rhythm abnormalities).

Perindopril Erbumine

▶ Drug Class: Angiotensin-converting enzyme (ACE) inhibitor

▶ Available in: Tablets

▶ Available OTC? No

▶ As Generic? No

Side Effects

SERIOUS
Fever and chills, sore throat and hoarseness, sudden difficulty breathing or swallowing, swelling of the face, mouth, or extremities, impaired kidney function (ankle swelling, decreased urination), confusion, yellow discoloration of the eyes or skin (indicating liver dysfunction), intense itching, chest pain or palpitations, abdominal pain. Serious side effects are very rare; contact your doctor immediately.

COMMON
Dry, persistent cough.

LESS COMMON
Dizziness or fainting, skin rash, numbness or tingling in the hands, feet, or lips, unusual fatigue or muscle weakness, nausea, drowsiness, loss of taste, headache.

PRINCIPAL USES
To control high blood pressure (hypertension).

HOW THE DRUG WORKS
Angiotensin-converting enzyme (ACE) inhibitors block an enzyme that produces angiotensin, a naturally occurring substance that causes blood vessels to constrict and stimulates production of the adrenal hormone, aldosterone, which promotes sodium retention in the body. As a result, ACE inhibitors relax blood vessels (causing them to widen) and reduces sodium retention, which lowers blood pressure and so decreases the workload of the heart.

DOSAGE
To start, 4 mg once a day. Doses may be increased to a maximum of 16 mg a day in 1 or 2 doses. The usual maintenance dose is 4 to 8 mg a day. Patients over the age of 65 should start with a dose of 2 mg and not take more than 8 mg a day without consulting their doctor.

ONSET OF EFFECT
Within 1 to 2 hours.

DURATION OF ACTION
Up to 24 hours.

DIETARY ADVICE
Perindopril can be taken without regard to meals. Follow your doctor's dietary advice (such as low-salt or low-cholesterol restrictions) to improve control over high blood pressure and heart disease. Avoid high-potassium foods like bananas and citrus fruits and juices, unless you are also taking medications, such as diuretics, that lower potassium levels.

STORAGE
Store in a tightly sealed container away from heat, moisture, and direct light.

IF YOU MISS A DOSE
Take it as soon as you remember. If it is near the time for the next dose, skip the missed dose and resume your regular dosage schedule. Do not double the next dose.

STOPPING THE DRUG
Do not stop taking this drug abruptly, as this may cause potentially serious health problems. Dosage should be reduced gradually, according to your doctor's instructions.

PROLONGED USE
See your doctor regularly for examinations and tests if you must take this medicine for a prolonged period. Remember that perindopril helps control high blood pressure but does not cure it. Lifelong therapy may be necessary.

PRECAUTIONS
Over 60: Some elderly patients may be more sensitive to the effects of this drug; smaller doses may be warranted.

Driving and Hazardous Work: Do not drive or engage in hazardous work until you determine how the medicine affects you.

Alcohol: Consume alcohol only in moderation since it may increase the effect of the drug and cause an excessive drop in blood pressure. Consult your doctor for advice.

Pregnancy: Use of perindopril during the last six months of pregnancy may cause severe defects, even death, in the fetus. The drug should be discontinued if you are pregnant or plan to become pregnant.

Breast Feeding: Perindopril may pass into breast milk; caution is advised. Consult your doctor for advice.

Infants and Children: Safety and effectiveness have not been established for patients under age 18.

Special Concerns: Perindopril has to be stopped if blood liver enzymes become markedly elevated.

OVERDOSE
Symptoms: Dizziness or fainting due to extremely low blood pressure.

What to Do: Few cases of overdose have been reported. However, call your doctor, emergency medical services (EMS), or the nearest poison control center immediately if you suspect that someone has taken a much larger dose than prescribed.

DRUG INTERACTIONS
Consult your doctor if you are taking diuretics (especially potassium-sparing diuretics), potassium supplements or drugs containing potassium (check ingredient labels), lithium, or gentamicin.

FOOD INTERACTIONS
Avoid low-salt milk and salt substitutes. Many of these products contain potassium.

DISEASE INTERACTIONS
Consult your doctor if you have had a prior allergic reaction to an ACE inhibitor, congestive heart failure, other types of heart disease, liver disease, or kidney failure.

Permethrin

BRAND NAMES
Elimite, Nix

▶ Drug Class: Topical antiparasitic

▶ Available in: Lotion

▶ Available OTC? Yes

▶ As Generic? Yes

Side Effects

SERIOUS
No serious side effects have been reported.

COMMON
Burning, itching, numbness, rash, redness, stinging, swelling, or tingling of scalp. In most cases such symptoms are mild and temporary; notify your doctor if they are more troublesome or if they persist.

LESS COMMON
No less-common side effects have been reported.

PRINCIPAL USES
To treat infestations of head lice.

HOW THE DRUG WORKS
Permethrin is absorbed into the bodies of lice, where it blocks nerve activity, ultimately causing paralysis and death of the lice. (The drug has no such toxic effect on humans.)

DOSAGE
For treatment of head lice (pediculus humanus capitus): After the hair has been washed with shampoo, rinsed with water, and dried with a towel, apply a sufficient amount (approximately 25 ml) of liquid. Allow it to remain on the hair for 10 minutes, then rinse off with water. Rinse thoroughly and dry with a clean towel. Use a fine-tooth comb to remove any remaining nits or nit shells. If lice are found after 7 days, repeat the treatment.

ONSET OF EFFECT
Within 10 minutes.

DURATION OF ACTION
Up to 10 days.

DIETARY ADVICE
Permethrin can be used without regard to diet.

STORAGE
Store in a tightly sealed container away from heat and direct light.

IF YOU MISS A DOSE
If a second dose is needed and you do not administer it after 7 days, do so as soon as you remember.

STOPPING THE DRUG
You need not take the second dose if no lice are found after 7 days.

PROLONGED USE
If lice recur, consult your doctor.

PRECAUTIONS
Over 60: There is no information comparing the use of permethrin in older patients with use in younger persons; no special problems are expected.

Driving and Hazardous Work: The use of permethrin should not impair your ability to perform such tasks safely.

Alcohol: No special problems are expected.

Pregnancy: In animal studies, permethrin has not caused problems or birth defects. Human studies have not been done. Before you use permethrin, tell your doctor if you are pregnant or plan to become pregnant.

Breast Feeding: Permethrin may pass into breast milk; caution is advised. Consult your doctor for advice.

Infants and Children: Use and dosage in children up to 2 years of age must be determined by your doctor.

Special Concerns: All members of your household should be examined for lice and given treatment if necessary. Any sexual partner should be examined and treated if necessary. Clothing, household linen, hairbrushes, combs, and bedding should be thoroughly cleaned by machine washing with hot water and machine drying for at least 20 minutes, using the hot cycle. Seal nonwashable items in a plastic bag for at least 2 weeks or spray them with a product designed to eliminate lice and their nits. You should not use this drug if you are hypersensitive to chrysanthemums. Treatment with permethrin may temporarily worsen the itching and other symptoms of head lice infestation.

OVERDOSE
Symptoms: No cases of overdose have been reported.

What to Do: Although overdose is unlikely, if someone accidentally ingests the drug, call your doctor, emergency medical services (EMS), or the nearest poison control center immediately.

DRUG INTERACTIONS
Before you use this medicine, tell your doctor if you are using any other prescription or over-the-counter medication that is to be applied to the scalp.

FOOD INTERACTIONS
No known food interactions.

DISEASE INTERACTIONS
Consult your doctor if you have severe inflammation of the skin.

Generic 8 mg
(GENEVA)

805

Additional photographs

▶ Drug Class: Neuroleptic;
antipsychotic

▶ Available in: Oral solution,
tablets, injection

▶ Available OTC? No

▶ As Generic? Yes

Side Effects

SERIOUS
Rapid heartbeat, profuse
sweating, seizures, difficulty breathing, neck stiffness, swelling of the
tongue, difficulty swal-
lowing. Also a rare condition can develop called
neuroleptic malignant
syndrome, characterized
by stiffness or spasms of
the muscles, high fever,
and confusion or disori-
entation. Call your doctor
immediately.

COMMON
Nausea, reduced sweat-
ing, dry mouth, blurred
vision, drowsiness, shak-
ing of hands, stiffness,
stooped posture.

LESS COMMON
Difficult urination, men-
strual irregularities,
breast pain or swelling,
unexpected weight gain,
uncontrolled movements
of the tongue, fever,
chills, sore throat,
unusual bruising or
bleeding, heart palpita-
tions, skin rash, itching,
increased sensitivity of
the skin to sunlight.

PRINCIPAL USES
To treat psychotic condi-
tions (severe mental disorders characterized by
distorted thoughts, perceptions, and emotions), such
as schizophrenia.

HOW THE DRUG WORKS
Perphenazine blocks receptors of dopamine (a chemical that aids in the
transmission of nerve
impulses) in the central nervous system. Presumably,
this produces a tranquilizing
or antipsychotic effect.

DOSAGE
Usual adult dose: Initially,
4 to 8 mg a day. Your physician may gradually increase
the dose as needed and tolerated, not to exceed 64 mg
a day.

ONSET OF EFFECT
Sedation may occur within
minutes, but onset of
antipsychotic effect may
take hours to occur or may
not occur until days or
weeks after the beginning
of therapy.

DURATION OF ACTION
12 to 24 hours, but effects
may persist for several days.

DIETARY ADVICE
Can be taken with food or a
full glass of milk or water.

STORAGE
Store in a tightly sealed container away from heat, moisture, and direct light.

IF YOU MISS A DOSE
Take it as soon as you
remember. However, if it is
near the time for the next
dose, skip the missed dose
and resume your regular
dosage schedule. Do not
double the next dose.

STOPPING THE DRUG
The decision to stop taking
the drug should be made in
consultation with your
physician.

PROLONGED USE
Consult your doctor about
the need for follow-up evaluations and tests if you must
take this drug for an
extended period.

PRECAUTIONS
Over 60: Adverse reactions
are more likely and more
severe in older patients.

**Driving and Hazardous
Work:** Avoid such activities
until you determine how the
medicine affects you.

Alcohol: Avoid alcohol.

Pregnancy: Avoid using
perphenazine if you are
pregnant or plan to become
pregnant.

Breast Feeding: Either
avoid taking the drug if possible or refrain from breast
feeding.

Infants and Children:
Adverse reactions may be
more likely and more
severe in children.

Special Concerns: Avoid
prolonged exposure to high
temperatures or hot cli-
mates. Drink plenty of fluids
and stay cool in the sum-
mertime. Avoid overexpo-
sure to sunlight until you
determine if the drug
heightens your skin's sensitivity to ultraviolet light.

OVERDOSE
Symptoms: Extreme
drowsiness, heartbeat irregularities, dry mouth, paradoxical restlessness or
agitation, seizures, loss
of consciousness.

What to Do: Call your
doctor, emergency medical
services (EMS), or the
nearest poison control
center immediately.

DRUG INTERACTIONS
Consult your doctor for
specific advice if you are
taking amantadine, high
blood pressure medication,
bromocriptine, deferoxam-
ine, diuretics, levobunolol,
heart medication, metipranolol, nabilone, other psychiatric drugs, pentamidine,
pimozide, promethazine,
trimeprazine, a thyroid
agent, central nervous system depressants, epineph-
rine, lithium, levodopa,
methyldopa, metoclo-
pramide, mctyrosine,
pemoline, a rauwolfia
alkaloid, or metrizamide.

FOOD INTERACTIONS
No known food interactions.

DISEASE INTERACTIONS
Consult your doctor if you
have Parkinson's disease or
any movement disorder,
glaucoma, epilepsy, liver
disease, or kidney disease.

Phenazopyridine Hydrochloride

Generic 100 mg
(ABLE)

▶ Drug Class: Urinary analgesic

▶ Available in: Tablets

▶ Available OTC? Yes

▶ As Generic? Yes

Side Effects

SERIOUS
Serious side effects are rare. Call your doctor immediately if you experience any of the following: difficulty breathing, swelling of the face, fingers, feet, or lower legs, blue or purple-blue skin color, unusual fatigue, fever, confusion, sudden decrease in urine output, shortness of breath, tightness in the chest, skin rash, yellow discoloration of the eyes or skin, unusual weight gain.

COMMON
Reddish orange urine.

LESS COMMON
Indigestion, dizziness, stomach cramps or pain, headache.

PRINCIPAL USES
For short-term relief of symptoms caused by irritation of the urinary tract. Such symptoms include burning, pain, and discomfort during urination, as well as an increased urge to urinate with only small amounts of urine passed on each occasion. Irritation of the urinary tract commonly occurs as a result of bladder infection; phenazopyridine can ease symptoms but will not cure such an infection.

HOW THE DRUG WORKS
Phenazopyridine passes through—and has a local anesthetic effect upon the lining of—the urinary tract, thus relieving the discomfort associated with infection or inflammation.

DOSAGE
Adults: 200 mg, 3 times a day. Children: 1.8 mg per lb of body weight, 3 times a day.

ONSET OF EFFECT
Unknown.

DURATION OF ACTION
Unknown.

DIETARY ADVICE
This medication is best taken with or after meals to minimize stomach upset.

STORAGE
Store in a tightly sealed container away from heat, moisture, and direct light.

IF YOU MISS A DOSE
Take it as soon as you remember. If it is near the time for the next dose, skip the missed dose and resume your regular dosage schedule. Do not double the next dose.

STOPPING THE DRUG
The decision to stop taking the drug should be made by your doctor. If it is being taken with an antibiotic, it should be taken for only 2 days (6 doses).

PROLONGED USE
Phenazopyridine is intended only for short-term use.

PRECAUTIONS
Over 60: No special problems are expected.

Driving and Hazardous Work: Do not drive or engage in hazardous work until you determine how the medicine affects you.

Alcohol: No special precautions are necessary.

Pregnancy: Adequate human studies have not been done. Before taking phenazopyridine, tell your doctor if you are pregnant or plan to become pregnant.

Breast Feeding: Phenazopyridine may pass into breast milk; caution is advised. Consult your doctor for advice.

Infants and Children: No special problems are expected.

Special Concerns: Phenazopyridine causes the urine to turn reddish orange. This is harmless, but it may stain clothing. The drug may also cause permanent staining or discoloration of soft contact lenses; it is best to wear glasses while taking the drug. For diabetic patients, phenazopyridine may cause false test results with sugar and urine ketone tests. Do not chew the tablets; chewing may cause permanent discoloration of teeth. Do not use any leftover medicine for future urinary tract infections without consulting your doctor.

OVERDOSE
Symptoms: Fatigue, paleness, shortness of breath, heart palpitations, bloody or cloudy urine, decreased urine output, swelling of the ankles and calves, lower back or flank pain, nausea or vomiting.

What to Do: While an overdose is unlikely, call your doctor, emergency medical services (EMS), or the nearest poison control center immediately if symptoms of overdose occur.

DRUG INTERACTIONS
Some drugs may interact with phenazopyridine. Consult your doctor for specific advice if you are taking any prescription or over-the-counter medication.

FOOD INTERACTIONS
No known food interactions.

DISEASE INTERACTIONS
Caution is advised when taking phenazopyridine. Consult your doctor if you have any of the following: glucose-6-phosphate dehydrogenase deficiency (G6PD), hepatitis, uremia, pyelonephritis (kidney infection) during pregnancy, or other kidney disease.

Phenelzine Sulfate

Nardil 15 mg
(PARKE-DAVIS)

▶ Drug Class: Monoamine oxidase (MAO) inhibitor antidepressant

▶ Available in: Tablets

▶ Available OTC? No

▶ As Generic? No

Side Effects

SERIOUS
Severe headache, high blood pressure, severe chest pain, dilated pupils, irregular heartbeat, sensitivity of eyes to light (photophobia), fever and sweating, nausea and vomiting, stiff neck, extreme dizziness. Call your doctor immediately.

COMMON
Blurring of vision, decreased urination, sexual dysfunction, dizziness or lightheadedness, mild headache, appetite changes including cravings for sweets, weight gain, increase in sweating, muscle twitching during sleep, restlessness, shakiness, fatigue, insomnia.

LESS COMMON
Chills, constipation, decrease in appetite, dry mouth, swelling in the lower extremities.

PRINCIPAL USES
To treat symptoms of major mental depression.

HOW THE DRUG WORKS
Phenelzine inhibits the activity of monoamine oxidase, an enzyme that renders certain brain chemicals (epinephrine, norepinephrine, and dopamine) inactive. Consequently, this drug increases the availability of these chemicals in the nervous system; this is thought to have an antidepressant effect.

DOSAGE
Adults: To start, 15 mg, 3 times a day; may be increased to 90 mg a day. Older adults: To start, 15 mg once a day; may be increased to 60 mg a day.

ONSET OF EFFECT
7 to 10 days; it may take up to 8 weeks for full effect.

DURATION OF ACTION
Up to 10 days after treatment stops.

DIETARY ADVICE
See Food Interactions.

STORAGE
Store in a tightly sealed container away from heat and direct light.

IF YOU MISS A DOSE
Take it as soon as you remember. If it is near the time for the next dose, skip the missed dose and resume your regular dosage schedule. Do not double the next dose.

STOPPING THE DRUG
The decision to stop taking the drug should be made in consultation with your physician.

PROLONGED USE
The usual course of therapy lasts 6 months to 1 year; some patients benefit from additional therapy. See your doctor regularly for tests and examinations if long-term therapy is required.

PRECAUTIONS
Over 60: Adverse reactions may be more likely and more severe in older patients.

Driving and Hazardous Work: Use caution when driving or engaging in hazardous work until you determine how the medicine affects you.

Alcohol: Avoid alcohol.

Pregnancy: Using this drug during pregnancy may increase the risk of birth defects.

Breast Feeding: Phenelzine may pass into breast milk; caution is advised. Consult your doctor for specific advice.

Infants and Children: Phenelzine is not recommended for children 16 years of age and under.

Special Concerns: Before having any surgery, emergency treatment, or dental treatment, tell the doctor or dentist in charge that you are taking phenelzine. Your doctor may advise you to carry a card saying that you use phenelzine.

OVERDOSE
Symptoms: Profound anxiety, confusion, seizures, cold, clammy skin, severe drowsiness, irregular pulse, hallucinations, severe headache, fainting, stiff muscles, sweating, breathing difficulty.

What to Do: Call your doctor, emergency medical services (EMS), or the nearest poison control center immediately.

DRUG INTERACTIONS
Consult your doctor for specific advice if you are taking or have recently taken amphetamines, blood pressure medications, diet pills, cyclobenzaprine, fluoxetine, levodopa, maprotiline, asthma medication, cold or allergy medication, meperidine, methylphenidate, another MAO inhibitor, paroxetine, sertraline, a tricyclic antidepressant, an oral diabetes drug, insulin, bupropion, buspirone, carbamazepine, any central nervous system depressant, dextromethorphan, trazodone, or tryptophan.

FOOD INTERACTIONS
Do not eat foods with a high tyramine content, such as cheeses; yeast or meat extracts; pickled or smoked meat, poultry, or fish; processed meats like bologna, salami, and pepperoni; and sauerkraut. Do not drink red wine or alcohol-free or reduced-alcohol beer. Do not drink beverages or eat food with a high caffeine content, such as coffee and chocolate.

DISEASE INTERACTIONS
Caution is advised when taking phenelzine. Consult your doctor if you have any of the following: a history of alcohol abuse, angina, frequent headaches, asthma, bronchitis, diabetes, epilepsy, heart disease or a recent heart attack, blood vessel disease, liver disease, Parkinson's disease, a recent stroke, kidney disease, an overactive thyroid, or pheochromocytoma.

Phenobarbital

Generic 30 mg
(ROXANE)

▶ Drug Class: Barbiturate

▶ Available in: Capsules, elixir, tablets, injection

▶ Available OTC? No

▶ As Generic? Yes

Side Effects

SERIOUS
Excitability, confusion, or excessive sedation to the point you cannot be awakened. Also yellow discoloration of eyes or skin; swollen eyelids, face, or lips, wheezing, or rash (may be signs of drug allergy); sores on the lips or mouth. Call your doctor immediately.

COMMON
Clumsiness, unsteadiness, persistent drowsiness, dizziness or lightheadedness.

LESS COMMON
Anxiety or nervousness, nightmares, insomnia, constipation, feeling faint, irritability, headache, nausea or vomiting.

PRINCIPAL USES
Primarily used for sedation before surgery and to control certain types of seizures. With the availability of newer sleep-inducing drugs, it is now rarely used for the short-term treatment of insomnia.

HOW THE DRUG WORKS
Barbiturates such as phenobarbital act as powerful sedatives by reducing activity in the central nervous system (the brain and spinal cord).

DOSAGE
For sedation— Adult oral dose: 30 to 120 mg, 2 or 3 times a day (not to exceed 400 mg a day). Children's oral dose: 2 mg per 2.2 lbs (1 kg) of body weight, 3 times a day. For seizures— Adult oral dose: 60 to 250 mg a day. Children's oral dose: 1 to 6 mg per 2.2 lbs of body weight per day. For insomnia— Adult oral dose: 100 to 320 mg at bedtime. Dosages for injectable forms of the drug will be determined by your doctor.

ONSET OF EFFECT
About 1 hour.

DURATION OF ACTION
10 to 12 hours.

DIETARY ADVICE
Tablets may be crushed and taken with fluid or food.

STORAGE
Store in a tightly sealed container away from heat, moisture, and direct light.

IF YOU MISS A DOSE
If you are taking phenobarbital regularly, take the missed dose as soon as you remember. If it is near the time for the next dose, skip the missed dose and resume your regular dosage schedule. Do not double the next dose.

STOPPING THE DRUG
The decision to stop taking the drug should be made by your doctor. There is a risk of withdrawal side effects when the drug is stopped suddenly.

PROLONGED USE
Barbiturates may be habit-forming, and prolonged use may increase the risk of dependency. Phenobarbital, as well as other barbiturates, is used only for short-term treatment of insomnia. It is not usually effective when used for longer than 14 days.

PRECAUTIONS
Over 60: Adverse reactions may be more likely and more severe in older patients and may require that smaller doses be used.

Driving and Hazardous Work: Because of sedative effects, do not drive or engage in hazardous work until you determine how the medicine affects you.

Alcohol: Avoid alcohol; its sedative effects are additive to those of the drug.

Pregnancy: Phenobarbital can cause birth defects and problems during pregnancy. Before you take phenobarbital, tell your doctor if you are pregnant or plan to become pregnant.

Breast Feeding: Phenobarbital passes into breast milk in small amounts and can cause side effects in breast-feeding infants. Consult your doctor for advice.

Infants and Children: As with older patients, infants and children are sensitive to the effects of phenobarbital.

Special Concerns: Phenobarbital may cause physical or mental dependence.

Check with your doctor if you feel overly sedated or if you suffer withdrawal side effects when you stop taking the drug.

OVERDOSE
Symptoms: Severe sedation or excessive drowsiness, confusion, severe weakness, slurred speech, staggering walk, shortness of breath or troubled breathing.

What to Do: Call your doctor, emergency medical services (EMS), or the nearest poison control center immediately.

DRUG INTERACTIONS
Consult your doctor for specific advice if you are taking other seizure medications, central nervous system depressants, warfarin (blood thinner), or oral contraceptives. Phenobarbital may make oral contraceptives less effective.

FOOD INTERACTIONS
No known food interactions.

DISEASE INTERACTIONS
Caution is advised when taking phenobarbital. Consult your doctor if you have any of the following: kidney disease, liver disease, porphyria, anemia, hyperactivity, mental depression, or a history of alcohol or drug abuse.

Phenoxybenzamine Hydrochloride

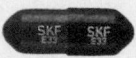

Dibenzyline 10 mg
(SMITHKLINE BEECHAM)

▶ Drug Class: Centrally acting antihypertensive

▶ Available in: Capsules

▶ Available OTC? No

▶ As Generic? No

Side Effects

SERIOUS
In laboratory animals, high and repeated doses of phenoxybenzamine have caused tumors. Whether such effects occur in humans is unknown.

COMMON
Dizziness or lightheadedness, especially when getting up from a sitting or lying position, rapid heartbeat, constricted pupils, stuffy nose.

LESS COMMON
Drowsiness, confusion, dry mouth, headache, lack of energy, male sexual problems, unusual fatigue.

PRINCIPAL USES
To treat high blood pressure caused by pheochromocytoma, a rare type of tumor that develops inside the adrenal glands, small hormone-producing glands located atop the kidneys.

HOW THE DRUG WORKS
Phenoxybenzamine acts upon certain areas of the central nervous system (the brain and spinal cord) that regulate the activity of the heart and the smooth muscle tissue surrounding the arteries. The drug causes the blood vessels to relax and widen, which lowers blood pressure.

DOSAGE
Adults: To start, 10 mg, 2 times a day. It may be increased to 20 to 40 mg, 2 or 3 times a day. Children: To start, 0.2 mg per 2.2 lbs (1 kg) of body weight once a day. It may be increased to 0.4 to 1.2 mg per 2.2 lbs in 3 or 4 daily doses.

ONSET OF EFFECT
Several hours.

DURATION OF ACTION
3 to 4 days.

DIETARY ADVICE
Take it with milk to avoid gastrointestinal irritation. Follow a healthy diet (low-salt, low-fat, low-cholesterol) as advised by your doctor to help control blood pressure and prevent heart disease.

STORAGE
Store in a tightly sealed container away from heat and direct light.

IF YOU MISS A DOSE
Take it as soon as you remember. If it is near the time for the next dose, skip the missed dose and resume your regular dosage schedule. Do not double the next dose.

STOPPING THE DRUG
The decision to stop taking the drug should be made by your doctor.

PROLONGED USE
You should see your doctor regularly for tests and examinations if you take this drug for a prolonged period.

PRECAUTIONS
Over 60: Adverse reactions, especially dizziness and lightheadedness, may be more likely and more severe in older patients. Phenoxybenzamine may reduce tolerance to cold temperatures in older patients.

Driving and Hazardous Work: Do not drive or engage in hazardous work until you determine how the medicine affects you.

Alcohol: Alcohol should be avoided while taking this medication.

Pregnancy: Animal and human studies of phenoxybenzamine have not been done. Before you take phenoxybenzamine, tell your doctor if you are pregnant or plan to become pregnant.

Breast Feeding: It is not known if phenoxybenzamine passes into breast milk. It has not been reported to cause problems in breast-fed babies. Consult your doctor about its use while nursing.

Infants and Children: No special problems expected.

Special Concerns: Before you have any kind of dental or surgical procedure, be sure to tell the doctor or dentist in charge that you take phenoxybenzamine. If dryness of the mouth continues for more than 2 weeks, consult your doctor or dentist. Be cautious in hot weather, as well as during exercise, or if you must stand for long periods of time, since these situations may increase the chances that you will become dizzy or lightheaded.

OVERDOSE
Symptoms: Dizziness, faintness, rapid heartbeat, vomiting, lethargy, loss of consciousness.

What to Do: Call your doctor, emergency medical services (EMS), or the nearest poison control center immediately.

DRUG INTERACTIONS
Consult your doctor for specific advice if you are taking diazoxide, dopamine, guanadrel, guanethidine, epinephrine, metaraminol, methoxamine, phenylephrine, or any over-the-counter medicines for appetite control, asthma, colds, hay fever, cough, or sinus problems.

FOOD INTERACTIONS
No known food interactions.

DISEASE INTERACTIONS
Caution is advised when taking phenoxybenzamine. Consult your doctor if you have cerebrovascular insufficiency, coronary artery disease, congestive heart failure, kidney disease, or a lung infection, or if you have had a recent heart attack or stroke.

Phentermine

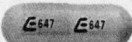

Generic 30 mg
(EON)

▶ Drug Class: Appetite suppressant

▶ Available in: Tablets, capsules

▶ Available OTC? No

▶ As Generic? Yes

Side Effects

SERIOUS
Confusion or mental depression, skin rash or hives, high blood pressure, sore throat and fever, unusual bleeding or bruising. Call your doctor immediately.

COMMON
Irritability, nervousness, restlessness, insomnia.

LESS COMMON
Blurred vision, change in sexual desire, constipation or diarrhea, difficult or painful urination, dizziness, lightheadedness, drowsiness, dry mouth, rapid heartbeat, increased urination, headache, increased sweating, nausea or vomiting, stomach cramps, unpleasant taste in the mouth.

PRINCIPAL USES
To suppress appetite in obese patients. It should be used in conjunction with a strict diet and should not be prescribed as the sole method for achieving weight loss.

HOW THE DRUG WORKS
Researchers believe that the appetite-control center for the body may be found in a part of the brain called the hypothalamus. Phentermine probably affects the transmission of nerve impulses in this area.

DOSAGE
15 to 37.5 mg once a day.

ONSET OF EFFECT
Within 1 hour.

DURATION OF ACTION
12 to 14 hours.

DIETARY ADVICE
Phentermine can be taken before breakfast or 1 to 2 hours after breakfast.

STORAGE
Store in a tightly sealed container away from heat and direct light.

IF YOU MISS A DOSE
Take it as soon as you remember. If it is near the time for the next dose, skip the missed dose and resume your regular dosage schedule. Do not double the next dose.

STOPPING THE DRUG
Take as prescribed for the full treatment period, even if you begin to observe favorable results before the scheduled end of therapy.

PROLONGED USE
Prolonged use of phentermine may result in drug tolerance or occasionally drug dependence.

PRECAUTIONS
Over 60: Adverse reactions may be more likely and more severe in older patients, especially when taken in combination with drugs that act on the central nervous system.

Driving and Hazardous Work: Do not drive or engage in hazardous work until you determine how the medicine affects you.

Alcohol: Avoid alcohol.

Pregnancy: Phentermine has not been shown to cause birth defects in humans. Before you take this drug, tell your doctor if you are pregnant or planning to become pregnant.

Breast Feeding: Phentermine may pass into breast milk; caution is advised. Consult your doctor for advice.

Infants and Children: Not recommended for use by children under age 16.

Special Concerns: After you stop taking this drug, your body may need time to adjust. Phentermine may affect blood sugar levels; consult your doctor if you have any concern. Notify your doctor if you experience mental depression, nausea or vomiting, unusual fatigue, or trembling after you stop taking phentermine. Before you have medical or dental treatment, be sure to tell your doctor or dentist that you are taking phentermine.

OVERDOSE
Symptoms: Stomach cramps, severe diarrhea, fever, hallucinations, unusual high or low blood pressure, irregular heartbeat, severe nausea or vomiting, feeling of panic, restlessness, tremor.

What to Do: An overdose of phentermine is unlikely to be life-threatening. However, if someone takes a much larger dose than recommended, call your doctor, emergency medical services (EMS), or the nearest poison control center immediately.

DRUG INTERACTIONS
The following drugs may interact with phentermine. Consult your doctor for specific advice if you are taking amantadine, amphetamines, chlophenadiol, medicine for asthma, colds, sinus problems, or allergies, methyl-phenidate, nabilone, pemoline, selective serotonin reuptake inhibitors (SSRIs), or MAO inhibitors.

FOOD INTERACTIONS
Avoid caffeine-containing beverages.

DISEASE INTERACTIONS
Caution is advised when taking phentermine. Consult your doctor if you have any of the following: a history of drug or alcohol abuse, diabetes, epilepsy, glaucoma, heart disease, blood vessel disease, high blood pressure, an overactive thyroid, or kidney disease.

Phenylephrine Hydrochloride Ophthalmic

BRAND NAMES
Ak-Dilate, Ak-Nefrin, Dilatair, I-Phrine, Isopto Frin, Mydfrin, Neo-Synephrine Ophthalmic, Ocu-Phrin, Ocugestrin, Phenoptic, Prefrin Liquifilm, Relief Eye Drops for Red Eyes

▶ Drug Class: Adrenergic agent

▶ Available in: Ophthalmic solution

▶ Available OTC? Yes

▶ As Generic? Yes

Side Effects

SERIOUS
Dizziness; paleness; rapid, irregular, or pounding heartbeat; trembling; increased sweating. Call your doctor immediately.

COMMON
Unusually large pupils; burning, stinging, or watering of eyes; sensitivity of eyes to light; headache or brow ache.

LESS COMMON
Eye irritation not present prior to therapy.

PRINCIPAL USES
The 2.5% and 10% solutions are used to dilate the pupil of the eye (prior to eye exams or ophthalmologic procedures) and to treat certain eye conditions. The 0.12% solution is used to reduce redness of the eye caused by minor irritation.

HOW THE DRUG WORKS
Ophthalmic phenylephrine affects the muscles that control the pupils, causing them to dilate, which helps the doctor view the interior structures of the eye. The drug reduces redness by constricting the superficial blood vessels in the whites of the eye.

DOSAGE
For redness— Adults and children: 1 drop of 0.12% solution every 3 or 4 hours as needed. For certain eye conditions— Adults and teenagers: 1 drop of 2.5% or 10% solution from 1 to 3 times a day. Children: 1 drop of 2.5% solution from 1 to 3 times a day.

ONSET OF EFFECT
Rapid.

DURATION OF ACTION
From 2 to 7 hours depending on the strength of the solution.

DIETARY ADVICE
This medication can be used without regard to diet.

STORAGE
Store in a tightly sealed container away from heat, moisture, and direct light. Do not allow the medicine to freeze.

IF YOU MISS A DOSE
Apply it as soon as you remember. However, if it is near the time for the next dose, skip the missed dose and resume your regular dosage schedule. Do not double the next dose.

STOPPING THE DRUG
The decision to stop using the drug should be made by your doctor.

PROLONGED USE
You should see your doctor regularly for tests and examinations if you must use this drug for an extended period of time.

PRECAUTIONS
Over 60: No special problems are expected.

Driving and Hazardous Work: Do not drive or engage in hazardous work until you determine how the medicine affects your vision.

Alcohol: No special precautions are necessary.

Pregnancy: No problems are expected, but studies of effects in pregnancy have not been done in humans. Consult your physician.

Breast Feeding: No problems are expected, but studies of effects in breast feeding have not been done in humans. Consult your doctor.

Infants and Children: Adverse reactions may be more likely and more severe in infants and children. The 10% solution should not be used on infants. The other strengths should not be used on low-birth-weight infants.

Special Concerns: To use the eye drops, first wash your hands. Tilt your head back. Gently apply pressure to the inside corner of the eyelid and with the index finger of the same hand, pull downward on the lower eyelid to make a space. Drop the medicine into this space and close your eye. Apply pressure for 1 or 2 minutes while keeping the eye closed without blinking. Then wash your hands again. Make sure the tip of the dropper does not touch your eye, finger, or any other surface. Phenylephrine will make your eyes more sensitive to sunlight. If this occurs, wear sunglasses or avoid bright light as comfort dictates. If this effect continues for more than 12 hours after you have stopped using the medicine, consult your doctor. Ophthalmic phenylephrine is available over the counter only in the 0.12% solution. The 2.5% and 10% solutions are by doctor's prescription only.

OVERDOSE
Symptoms: Dizziness; paleness; rapid, irregular, or pounding heartbeat; trembling; profuse sweating; vomiting; coma; shock.

What to Do: Call your doctor, emergency medical services (EMS), or the nearest poison control center immediately.

DRUG INTERACTIONS
Be sure to tell your doctor if you are using any other prescription or over-the-counter medication.

FOOD INTERACTIONS
No known food interactions.

DISEASE INTERACTIONS
Consult your doctor if you have a history of heart disease, blood vessel disease, diabetes mellitus, high blood pressure, or idiopathic orthostatic hypotension (low blood pressure). This drug should not be used by those with a history of closed-angle glaucoma.

Phenylephrine Hydrochloride Systemic

BRAND NAMES
Alconefrin, Doktors, Duration, Neo-Synephrine, Nostril Spray Pump, Rhinall, Vicks Sinex

▶ Drug Class: Decongestant

▶ Available in: Nasal jelly, nasal drops, nasal spray

▶ Available OTC? Yes

▶ As Generic? Yes

Side Effects

SERIOUS
No serious side effects have been reported.

COMMON
Burning, dryness, or stinging inside the nose. An increase in nasal discharge or congestion may occur after 3 to 5 days of continuous use.

LESS COMMON
Headache, rapid or irregular heartbeat, excitability, restlessness.

PRINCIPAL USES
To relieve nasal congestion caused by allergies, colds, or sinus conditions; to relieve congestion associated with ear infections.

HOW THE DRUG WORKS
Phenylephrine constricts blood vessels to reduce the blood flow to swollen nasal passages and other tissues, which reduces nasal secretions and improves nasal airflow.

DOSAGE
Adults and children 12 and over: 2 to 3 drops of 0.25% to 0.5% solution, or 1 to 2 sprays, or a small amount of jelly in each nostril every 4 hours. Children 6 to 12 years: 2 to 3 drops or 1 to 2 sprays of a 0.25% solution in each nostril every 4 hours. Children under 6 years: 2 to 3 drops of 0.125% solution every 4 hours.

ONSET OF EFFECT
Rapid.

DURATION OF ACTION
From 30 minutes to 4 hours.

DIETARY ADVICE
Drink plenty of fluids.

STORAGE
Store in a tightly sealed container away from heat and direct light.

IF YOU MISS A DOSE
Take it as soon as you remember. If it is near the time for the next dose, skip the missed dose and resume your regular dosage schedule. Do not double the next dose.

STOPPING THE DRUG
Do not use this medicine for more than 3 days without consulting your doctor.

PROLONGED USE
Using this medicine for more than 3 days may lead to rebound congestion (more severe congestion caused by the body's adaptation to the drug).

PRECAUTIONS
Over 60: Although no studies have specifically examined the use of this drug in older patients, no special problems are expected.

Driving and Hazardous Work: Do not drive or engage in hazardous work until you determine how the medicine affects you.

Alcohol: Avoid alcohol.

Pregnancy: Phenylephrine hydrochloride has not been shown to cause birth defects or other problems if taken during pregnancy.

Breast Feeding: It is not known whether phenylephrine passes into breast milk; caution is advised. Consult your doctor for specific advice.

Infants and Children: Adverse reactions may be more likely and more severe in infants and children.

Special Concerns: Each container of medicine should be used by only one person to avoid spread of infection. Blow your nose gently before using this medicine. To use the nose drops, tilt your head back or lie down on a bed and hang your head over the side. Keep your head tilted back for a few minutes after instilling the drops. To use the nasal spray, keep your head upright and sniff briskly while spraying. For best results, spray again in 3 to 5 minutes. To use the nasal jelly, first wash your hands, then place an amount of jelly about the size of a pea into each nostril and sniff it well back into the nose.

OVERDOSE
Symptoms: Rapid, irregular, or pounding heartbeat; headache or dizziness; increased sweating; nervousness; trembling; paleness; insomnia. Such symptoms are more likely to be seen in young children.

What to Do: If someone takes a much larger dose than recommended, call your doctor, emergency medical services (EMS), or the nearest poison control center immediately.

DRUG INTERACTIONS
Before you take phenylephrine, tell your doctor if you are taking any other prescription or over-the-counter drug.

FOOD INTERACTIONS
No known food interactions.

DISEASE INTERACTIONS
Consult your doctor if you have a history of any of the following: high blood pressure, diabetes mellitus, heart disease, blood vessel disease, or an overactive thyroid gland.

Phenytoin

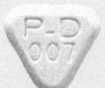

Dilantin 50 mg
(PARKE-DAVIS)

Additional photographs

▸ Drug Class: Anticonvulsant

▸ Available in: Prompt and
extended capsules, chewable
tablets, oral suspension

▸ Available OTC? No

▸ As Generic? Yes

Side Effects

SERIOUS
Fever, sore throat,
swollen glands, point-
like rash on the skin or
mucous membranes, blis-
tering or peeling, mouth
sores or bleeding gums,
easy bruising, pallor,
weakness, confusion, or
seizures may be a sign of
a potentially fatal blood
disorder or other compli-
cation. Call your doctor
immediately.

COMMON
Sedation, lethargy,
nervousness, dizziness,
thickened gums, exces-
sive growth of body and
facial hair. High doses
may cause abnormal
movements of the eyes,
mouth, tongue, or limbs.
Prolonged use may cause
mild nerve impairment in
the arms or legs.

LESS COMMON
Constipation, acne, mild
skin rash, incoordination.
There are numerous
additional possible side
effects; consult your doctor if you are concerned
about any adverse or
unusual reactions.

PRINCIPAL USES
To prevent or control
seizures in the treatment of
certain types of epilepsy
and other conditions.

HOW THE DRUG WORKS
Phenytoin is thought to
depress the activity of certain parts of the brain and
suppress the irregular and
uncontrolled firing of neurons that causes seizures.

DOSAGE
Adults: 200 to 500 mg a day,
as a single dose or in 2
divided doses. Children: 5
to 300 mg a day, as a single
dose or in 2 divided doses.
Some patients require
higher doses. A low dose is
used to start, then gradually
increased by your doctor.

ONSET OF EFFECT
Several hours.

DURATION OF ACTION
Maximum effect lasts for 24
hours or longer; effectiveness then gradually
decreases.

DIETARY ADVICE
Take with food to minimize
stomach upset. Tablets may
be crushed, chewed, or
swallowed whole.

STORAGE
Store in a tightly sealed container away from heat, moisture, and direct light.

IF YOU MISS A DOSE
Take it as soon as you
remember. Be especially
attentive about not missing
a dose if you are taking this
drug only once daily.

STOPPING THE DRUG
This medication should
never be stopped abruptly
because this may cause
seizures. The dose is typically tapered over a period
of weeks under the supervision of your doctor.

PROLONGED USE
This drug is often taken for
prolonged periods. See your
physician for periodic
checkups.

PRECAUTIONS
Over 60: Older patients
may require lower doses to
minimize side effects.

**Driving and Hazardous
Work:** Do not drive or
engage in hazardous work
until you determine how the
medicine affects you.

Alcohol: May contribute to
excessive drowsiness.

Pregnancy: Anticonvulsants are associated with
an increased risk of birth
defects. However, seizures
during pregnancy can also
increase the risks to the
unborn child. Discuss with
your doctor the potential
risks and benefits of using
this drug during pregnancy.
Folate supplementation is
recommended beginning
1 to 2 months before con-
ception and throughout
pregnancy.

Breast Feeding: Phenytoin passes into breast milk,
although at low levels. Consult your doctor for advice.

Infants and Children:
No special problems are
expected.

Special Concerns: The
generic version of this drug
is not recommended. Do
not change the brand of
phenytoin you are taking
without consulting your doctor. The suspension form of
phenytoin should be shaken
well before you take it. Your
doctor may advise you to
wear a medical bracelet or
carry an identification card
saying that you are taking
this medication.

OVERDOSE
Symptoms: Blurred or
double vision, difficulty
walking, severe clumsiness
or unsteadiness, severe
confusion, dizziness or
drowsiness.

What to Do: Call your
doctor, emergency medical
services (EMS), or the
nearest poison control
center immediately.

DRUG INTERACTIONS
Many other drugs may
interact with phenytoin,
including other anticonvulsants (carbamazepine, phenobarbital, primidone,
valproic acid), allopurinol,
amiodarone, anticancer
drugs, chloramphenicol,
chlorpheniramine, cimeti-
dine, diazoxide, dicumarol,
disulfiram, isoniazid, loxapine, phenylbutazone,
rifampin, sulfonamides,
trazodone, trimethoprim.

FOOD INTERACTIONS
No known food interactions.

DISEASE INTERACTIONS
Caution is advised in those
with liver or kidney disease,
since these organs work
together to remove the
medication from the body.

Pilocarpine Ophthalmic

BRAND NAMES
Adsorbocarpine,
Akarpine, Isopto Carpine,
Ocu-Carpine, Ocusert
Pilo-20, Ocusert Pilo-40,
Pilagan, Pilocar, Pilopine
HS, Piloptic, Pilostat

▶ Drug Class: Antiglaucoma
agent

▶ Available in: Ophthalmic solution and gel, ocular system

▶ Available OTC? No

▶ As Generic? Yes

Side Effects

SERIOUS
Increased sweating,
muscle tremors, nausea,
vomiting, or diarrhea,
troubled breathing or
wheezing, watering of
mouth, eye pain. Call
your doctor immediately.

COMMON
Decreased night vision,
blurred vision, change in
near or far vision, eye-
brow pain (usually disap-
pears within a week).

LESS COMMON
Headache, eye irritation.

PRINCIPAL USES
To treat glaucoma and to
constrict the pupil.

HOW THE DRUG WORKS
Glaucoma, a sight-threatening disorder, occurs when
aqueous humor (the fluid
inside the eye) cannot drain
properly, causing an
increase in pressure within
the eyeball (intraocular
pressure). This can damage
the optic nerve and lead to
a gradually progressive loss
of vision. Pilocarpine con-
tracts the muscles that constrict the pupil; this action
appears to help open the
structures that allow
drainage of the aqueous
humor, thereby decreasing
eye pressure.

DOSAGE
Ophthalmic solution—
Adults and children:
Chronic glaucoma: 1 drop
into the eye 1 to 4 times a
day. Acute closed-angle
glaucoma: 1 drop into the
eye every 5 to 10 minutes
for 3 to 6 doses, then 1 drop
every 1 to 3 hours. Oph-
thalmic gel— Adults and
teenagers: Once a day at
bedtime. Children: Use and
dosage must be determined
by your doctor. Ocular system: Adults and children: 1
insert every 7 days. Infants:
Use and dosage must be
determined by your doctor.

ONSET OF EFFECT
10 to 60 minutes.

DURATION OF ACTION
Ophthalmic solution: 4 to 14
hours. Ophthalmic gel: Up
to 24 hours; Ocular system:
Up to 7 days.

DIETARY ADVICE
No special restrictions.

STORAGE
Store in a tightly sealed container away from heat, moisture, and direct light. Store
the ophthalmic solution and
the 3.5 g size of the ophthalmic gel at room temperature. The 5 g size of the
ophthalmic gel and the ocular system should be refrigerated until used, but do not
allow either to freeze.

IF YOU MISS A DOSE
Apply it as soon as you
remember. If it is near the
time for the next dose, skip
the missed dose and
resume your regular dosage
schedule. Do not double the
next dose.

STOPPING THE DRUG
The decision to stop using
the drug should be made
by your doctor.

PROLONGED USE
See your doctor regularly
for tests and examinations if
you take this medication for
a prolonged period.

PRECAUTIONS
Over 60: No special problems are expected.

**Driving and Hazardous
Work:** Do not drive or
engage in hazardous work
until you determine how
the medicine affects your
vision.

Alcohol: No special precautions are necessary.

Pregnancy: No specific
studies in humans have
been done. Consult your
doctor for specific advice.

Breast Feeding: No specific studies in humans have
been done. Consult your
doctor for advice.

Infants and Children:
No special precautions.

Special Concerns: To use
the eye drops or the gel,
first wash your hands. Tilt
your head back. Gently
apply pressure to the inside
corner of the eyelid and
with your index finger, pull
downward on the lower eyelid to make a space. Drop
the medicine or put a short
strip of gel (about ½ inch
long) into this space and
close your eye. Apply pressure for 1 or 2 minutes
while keeping the eye
closed without blinking.
Wash hands again. Make
sure the tip of the dropper
or the applicator does not
touch your eye, finger, or
any other surface. To use
the eye insert, follow the
package directions carefully.
The unit should be inserted
at bedtime unless your doctor instructs otherwise.

OVERDOSE
Symptoms: Sweating, nausea, vomiting, diarrhea,
trouble breathing.

What to Do: An overdose
of ophthalmic pilocarpine is
unlikely to be life-threatening. If a large volume enters
the eye, flush with water.
If someone accidentally
ingests the medicine, call
your doctor, emergency
medical services (EMS), or
the nearest poison control
center immediately.

DRUG INTERACTIONS
Consult your doctor for specific advice if you are taking
any other prescription or
over-the-counter medication.

FOOD INTERACTIONS
No known food interactions.

DISEASE INTERACTIONS
Consult your doctor if you
have asthma or any other
eye disease or problem.
This medicine should not
be used if iritis (inflammation in the eye) is present
or develops.

Pilocarpine Systemic

BRAND NAME
Salagen

▶ Drug Class: Cholinergic parasympathomimetic agent

▶ Available in: Tablets

▶ Available OTC? No

▶ As Generic? No

Side Effects

SERIOUS
Serious side effects of pilocarpine are indistinguishable from those of overdose and include chest pain, heartbeat irregularities, severe or ongoing diarrhea, confusion, nausea or vomiting, headache, stomach pain or cramps, difficulty breathing, severe or persistent vision problems, severe trembling or shaking, and fatigue. Call your doctor immediately.

COMMON
Increased sweating.

LESS COMMON
Bloating or fluid retention, chills, nausea or vomiting, diarrhea, runny nose, dizziness, rapid heartbeat, headache, indigestion, frequent urination, redness of face or feeling of warmth, trembling or shaking, difficulty swallowing, excessive tearing, change in voice.

PRINCIPAL USES
To treat dryness of the mouth and throat that occurs after radiation therapy for cancer of the head and neck.

HOW THE DRUG WORKS
Pilocarpine stimulates the activity of salivary glands.

DOSAGE
Adults: 5 mg, 3 times a day. If needed, the dose may be increased to 10 mg, 3 times a day.

ONSET OF EFFECT
Unknown.

DURATION OF ACTION
Unknown.

DIETARY ADVICE
Take it with food to reduce stomach upset. Otherwise, no special restrictions.

STORAGE
Store in a tightly sealed container away from heat, moisture, and direct light.

IF YOU MISS A DOSE
Take it as soon as you remember. If it is near the time for the next dose, skip the missed dose and resume your regular dosage schedule. Do not double the next dose.

STOPPING THE DRUG
Take it as prescribed for the full treatment period, even if you begin to feel better before the scheduled end of therapy. The decision to stop taking the drug should be made by your doctor.

PROLONGED USE
See your physician and your dentist regularly for tests and examinations if you must take this drug for a prolonged period. A dry mouth condition increases the likelihood of dental cavities or other mouth problems.

PRECAUTIONS
Over 60: No special problems have been reported.

Driving and Hazardous Work: Do not drive or engage in hazardous work until you determine how the medicine affects you.

Alcohol: Moderate alcohol intake is acceptable.

Pregnancy: Adequate human studies have not been done. Before taking pilocarpine, tell your physician if you are pregnant or plan to become pregnant.

Breast Feeding: Pilocarpine may pass into breast milk; avoid or discontinue use while nursing, unless approved by your doctor.

Infants and Children: The safety and effectiveness of pilocarpine for infants and children have not been established.

Special Concerns: See your dentist regularly while taking pilocarpine. If the drug causes increased sweating, consume more fluids to prevent dehydration. Consult your doctor if you have any concerns about the proper amount of fluid intake.

OVERDOSE
Symptoms: Chest pain, heartbeat irregularities, severe or ongoing diarrhea, confusion, nausea or vomiting, severe headache, stomach pain or cramps, difficulty breathing, vision problems, severe trembling or shaking, severe fatigue.

What to Do: Call your doctor, emergency medical services (EMS), or the nearest poison control center immediately.

DRUG INTERACTIONS
Other drugs may interact with pilocarpine. Consult your doctor for specific advice if you are taking anticholinergics, antiglaucoma agents, bethanecol, cholinergics, or beta-blockers.

FOOD INTERACTIONS
No known food interactions.

DISEASE INTERACTIONS
Pilocarpine should not be used if you have uncontrolled asthma, narrow-angle closure glaucoma, acute iritis, or major heart, blood vessel, or lung disease. Consult your doctor if you have any of the following: controlled asthma, chronic bronchitis or any other breathing problem, gallbladder problems, heart or blood vessel disease, psychological disorders, detached retina, or another retinal disease.

Pindolol

Visken 10 mg
(NOVARTIS)

▶ Drug Class: Beta-blocker

▶ Available in: Tablets

▶ Available OTC? No

▶ As Generic? Yes

Side Effects

SERIOUS
Shortness of breath, wheezing; irregular or slow heartbeat (50 beats per minute or less); pain or feelings of tightness or pressure in the chest; swelling of the ankles, feet, and lower legs; mental depression. If you experience any such symptoms, stop taking pindolol and contact your doctor right away.

COMMON
Dizziness or lightheadedness, especially when rising suddenly to a standing position; decreased sexual ability; unusual fatigue, weakness, or drowsiness; insomnia.

LESS COMMON
Anxiety, irritability, nervousness; constipation; diarrhea; dry, sore eyes; itching; nausea or vomiting; nightmares or intensely vivid dreams; numbness, tingling, or other unusual sensations in the fingers, toes, or scalp.

PRINCIPAL USES
To treat mild to moderate high blood pressure.

HOW THE DRUG WORKS
Pindolol slows the rate and force of contraction of the heart by blocking certain nerve impulses, thus reducing blood pressure.

DOSAGE
Adults: 5 mg, 2 times a day. Dosage may be increased to a maximum of 30 mg, 2 times a day.

ONSET OF EFFECT
Within 1 hour.

DURATION OF ACTION
Up to 12 hours.

DIETARY ADVICE
Pindolol can be taken without regard to diet.

STORAGE
Store in a tightly sealed container away from heat and direct light.

IF YOU MISS A DOSE
Take it as soon as you remember. If it is near the time for the next dose, skip the missed dose and resume your regular dosage schedule. Do not double the next dose.

STOPPING THE DRUG
The decision to stop taking the drug should be made by your doctor. Slow reduction of the dose under doctor's close supervision for 2 to 3 weeks is advised.

PROLONGED USE
Lifelong therapy with pindolol may be necessary; prolonged use may be associated with a greater incidence of side effects. Regular monitoring and evaluation by your doctor is advised.

PRECAUTIONS
Over 60: Adverse reactions may be more likely and more severe in older patients. Resistance to cold temperatures may be decreased in older patients.

Driving and Hazardous Work: Use caution when driving or engaging in hazardous work until you determine how the medicine affects you.

Alcohol: Drink in careful moderation if at all. Alcohol may interact with the drug and cause a dangerous drop in blood pressure.

Pregnancy: Pindolol was shown to cause fetal harm in some animal studies. Before you take it, tell your doctor if you are pregnant or plan to become pregnant.

Breast Feeding: Pindolol passes into breast milk; consult your doctor about its use during nursing.

Infants and Children: The dosage must be determined by your pediatrician.

Special Concerns: Take extra care during exercise or hot weather, as taking this drug may contribute to dizziness. Check your pulse regularly while taking pindolol. If it is slower than your usual rate or less than 50 beats a minute, check with your doctor.

OVERDOSE
Symptoms: Unusually slow or rapid heartbeat, severe dizziness or fainting, poor circulation in the hands (bluish skin), breathing difficulty; seizures.

What to Do: An overdose of pindolol is unlikely to be life-threatening. However, if someone takes a much larger dose than prescribed, call your doctor, emergency medical services (EMS), or the nearest poison control center immediately.

DRUG INTERACTIONS
Consult your doctor for specific advice if you are taking allergy shots, aminophylline, caffeine, oxtriphylline, theophylline, oral antidiabetics, insulin, calcium channel blockers, clonidine, guanabenz, or MAO inhibitors.

FOOD INTERACTIONS
No known food interactions.

DISEASE INTERACTIONS
Pindolol should be used with caution in people with diabetes, especially insulin-dependent diabetes, since the drug may mask symptoms of hypoglycemia. Use of pindolol may cause complications in patients with liver or kidney disease, since these organs work together to remove the medication from the body. Also consult your doctor if you have any of the following: any allergy (including hay fever), bronchitis, emphysema, heart disease, blood vessel disease, mental depression, myasthenia gravis, psoriasis, or hyperthyroidism.

Pioglitazone Hydrochloride

▶ Drug Class: Thiazolidine-dione/antidiabetic agent

▶ Available in: Tablets

▶ Available OTC? No

▶ As Generic? No

Side Effects

SERIOUS
No serious side effects have been associated with pioglitazone.

COMMON
Upper respiratory tract infection, sore throat.

LESS COMMON
Headache, sinusitis, muscle pain, tooth disorder, edema (swelling).

PRINCIPAL USES
As a single therapeutic agent or as an adjunct (supplemental) therapy to a sulfonylurea, metformin, or insulin to control blood glucose (sugar) levels in patients with non-insulin-dependent (type 2) diabetes.

HOW THE DRUG WORKS
Pioglitazone increases the body's sensitivity and response to insulin.

DOSAGE
To start, 15 to 30 mg once a day. For people taking only pioglitazone and who do not respond adequately, the dose may be increased by a doctor to no more than 45 mg once a day. If monotherapy does not control blood glucose, combination therapy should be considered. If hypoglycemia occurs when taking pioglitazone in combination with a sulfonylurea or insulin, it may be necessary to decrease the dose of the sulfonylurea or insulin.

ONSET OF EFFECT
Within 1 week.

DURATION OF ACTION
Unknown.

DIETARY ADVICE
Pioglitazone may be taken with or without food.

STORAGE
Store in a tightly sealed container away from heat, moisture, and direct light.

IF YOU MISS A DOSE
If it is the same day, take the missed dose as soon as you remember. If you miss an entire day's dose, resume your regular dosage schedule the following day and do not double the next dose.

STOPPING THE DRUG
The decision to stop taking the drug should be made in consultation with your physician.

PROLONGED USE
See your doctor regularly for liver function tests if you take pioglitazone for an extended period.

PRECAUTIONS
Over 60: No special problems are expected.

Driving and Hazardous Work: Pioglitazone should not impair your ability to perform such tasks safely.

Alcohol: Drink only in moderation.

Pregnancy: Adequate studies of pioglitazone use during pregnancy have not been done. In general, insulin is the treatment of choice for controlling blood glucose levels during pregnancy. Pioglitazone should not be used during pregnancy unless your doctor believes the potential benefit justifies the potential risk to the fetus. Pioglitazone may stimulate ovulation in premenopausal women who have stopped ovulating. Contraception may be advised.

Breast Feeding: Pioglitazone may pass into breast milk; do not use it while nursing.

Infants and Children: Safety and effectiveness of pioglitazone have not been established in children.

Special Concerns: Another thiazolidinedione drug, troglitazone, has been associated with rare, serious, and sometimes fatal, liver-related side effects. Although no similar side effects have been reported for pioglitazone, liver function tests are recommended just prior to treatment, every two months for the first year, and periodically thereafter. If you develop unexplained symptoms of liver dysfunction, such as nausea, vomiting, abdominal pain, fatigue, loss of appetite, or dark urine, call your doctor immediately. It is important to follow your doctor's advice on diet, exercise, and other measures to help control diabetes.

OVERDOSE
Symptoms: No specific ones have been reported.

What to Do: While no cases of overdose have been reported, if someone takes a much larger dose than prescribed, call your doctor, emergency medical services (EMS), or the nearest poison control center immediately.

DRUG INTERACTIONS
No known drug interactions.

FOOD INTERACTIONS
No known food interactions.

DISEASE INTERACTIONS
Pioglitazone should not be taken by those with type 1 diabetes or for the treatment of diabetic ketoacidosis. Caution is advised if you have edema or heart failure. Consult your doctor prior to using pioglitazone if you have any type of liver abnormality.

Piperazine

BRAND NAME
Piperazine is available in generic form only.

▶ Drug Class: Anthelmintic

▶ Available in: Tablets

▶ Available OTC? No

▶ As Generic? Yes

Side Effects

SERIOUS
Joint pain, skin rash, fever, itching. Call your physician as soon as possible.

COMMON
No common side effects are associated with the use of piperazine.

LESS COMMON
Headache, diarrhea, stomach cramps or pain, dizziness, muscle fatigue, trembling, drowsiness, nausea or vomiting.

PRINCIPAL USES
To treat various worm infections, including ascariasis (common roundworm) and enterobiasis (pinworm), as an alternative to more standard lines of therapy. It is also used to treat partial intestinal obstruction by the common roundworm, a condition primarily occurring in children.

HOW THE DRUG WORKS
Piperazine paralyzes the worm; it is then expelled from the body in the stool.

DOSAGE
For common roundworms— Adults: 3.5 g a day for 2 days. Treatment may be repeated after a week. Children: 75 mg per 2.2 lbs (1 kg) of body weight a day for 2 days. Treatment may be repeated after 2 weeks. For pinworms— Adults and children: 65 mg per 2.2 lbs for 7 days. Treatment may be repeated after a week.

ONSET OF EFFECT
Unknown.

DURATION OF ACTION
Unknown.

DIETARY ADVICE
No special restrictions.

STORAGE
Store in a tightly sealed container away from heat, moisture, and direct light.

IF YOU MISS A DOSE
Take it as soon as possible. If it is near the time for the next dose, skip the missed dose and resume your regular dosage schedule. Do not double the next dose.

STOPPING THE DRUG
Take as prescribed for the full treatment period, even if you begin to feel better before the scheduled end of therapy.

PROLONGED USE
See your doctor regularly for tests and examinations if you take this medicine for a prolonged period.

PRECAUTIONS
Over 60: Adverse reactions may be more likely and more severe.

Driving and Hazardous Work: No special precautions are necessary.

Alcohol: No special precautions are necessary.

Pregnancy: Adequate studies of piperazine use during pregnancy have not been done. Consult your doctor for specific advice if you are pregnant or plan to become pregnant.

Breast Feeding: Piperazine may pass into breast milk; caution is advised. Consult your doctor for specific advice.

Infants and Children: Adverse reactions may be more likely and more severe in children.

Special Concerns: For pinworm infection, clothing, bedding, and towels should be washed daily. All members of the family may have to be treated to eradicate the infestation. A second treatment for all household members may be necessary after 2 or 3 weeks. All bedding and nightclothes should be washed after treatment. To prevent reinfection, you should wash the anal region daily, change your underwear and bedding every day, and wash your hands and fingernails before each meal and after bowel movements. If your symptoms do not improve after a full course of treatment, consult your doctor.

OVERDOSE
Symptoms: Muscle fatigue, seizures, difficulty breathing.

What to Do: An overdose of piperazine is unlikely to be life-threatening. However, if someone takes a much larger dose than prescribed, call your doctor, emergency medical services (EMS), or the nearest poison control center.

DRUG INTERACTIONS
Other drugs may interact with piperazine. Consult your doctor for specific advice if you are taking phenothiazines or pyrantel. Also tell your doctor if you are taking any other prescription or over-the-counter medication.

FOOD INTERACTIONS
No known food interactions.

DISEASE INTERACTIONS
Caution is advised when taking piperazine. This drug should not be used if you have a seizure disorder, especially a history of epilepsy. Use of piperazine may cause complications in patients with kidney disease, since this organ works to remove the medication from the body.

Pirbuterol Acetate

▶ Drug Class: Bronchodilator/
sympathomimetic

▶ Available in: Inhalation
aerosol

▶ Available OTC? No

▶ As Generic? No

Side Effects

SERIOUS
Pirbuterol may become
ineffective if used too
often, resulting in more-
severe breathing diffi-
culty that does not
improve. Signs include
persistent wheezing,
coughing, or shortness of
breath; confusion; bluish
color to lips or finger-
nails; inability to speak.
Other side effects include
chest pain or heaviness;
irregular, racing, fluttering, or pounding heart-
beat; lightheadedness;
fainting; severe weak-
ness; severe headache.

COMMON
Sleeping difficulty, dry
mouth, sore throat, ner-
vousness, excitability,
restlessness.

LESS COMMON
Trembling, sweating,
headache, nausea or
vomiting, flushing or redness to cheeks or other
skin, mood changes,
unusual bruising, numb-
ness, tingling, or other
change in sensation of
hands and feet, loss of
appetite, changes in
sense of smell and taste.

PRINCIPAL USES
To dilate air passages in the
lungs that have become narrowed as a result of disease
or inflammation. It is used
in the treatment of asthma
and chronic obstructive pulmonary disease (COPD).

HOW THE DRUG WORKS
Pirbuterol widens con-
stricted airways in the lungs
by relaxing the smooth
muscles that surround the
bronchial passages.

DOSAGE
May be used when needed
to relieve breathing difficulty. Adults and children 12
years and older, by inhalation aerosol: 1 to 2 inhalations every 4 to 6 hours. Do
not exceed more than 12
inhalations per day. Infants
and children less than 12
years of age: Consult your
pediatrician.

ONSET OF EFFECT
Within 5 minutes.

DURATION OF ACTION
5 hours.

DIETARY ADVICE
Maintain your usual food
and fluid intake.

STORAGE
Store in a tightly sealed container away from heat and
direct light. Do not refrigerate inhalation solutions.

IF YOU MISS A DOSE
Skip the missed dose and
resume your regular dosage
schedule. Do not double the
next dose.

STOPPING THE DRUG
It may not be necessary to
finish the recommended
course of therapy. Consult
your doctor.

PROLONGED USE
Therapy may require
months or years. Excessive
use may result in temporary
loss of effectiveness.

PRECAUTIONS
Over 60: Adverse reactions
may be more likely and
more severe in older
patients.

**Driving and Hazardous
Work:** Do not drive or
engage in hazardous work
until you determine how the
medicine affects you.

Alcohol: No special precautions are necessary.

Pregnancy: Adequate studies have not been done; the
benefits must be weighed
against potential risks. Consult your doctor for advice.

Breast Feeding: It is not
known if pirbuterol passes
into breast milk. Mothers
who wish to breast-feed
while taking this drug
should discuss the matter
with their doctor.

Infants and Children:
Use of the inhalation
aerosol requires special
coordination skills and is
not recommended in young
children. Dosage in children
younger than 12 has not
been established.

Special Concerns: Pay
heed to any asthma attack
or other breathing problem
that does not improve after
your usual nebulizer treatment or usual number of
puffs. Seek help immedi-
ately if you feel your lungs
are persistently constricted,
if you are using more than
the recommended number
of treatments or puffs per
day, or if you feel a recent
attack is somehow different
from others. Do not use
with other mouthpieces
or canisters.

OVERDOSE
Symptoms: Chest pain or
heaviness; irregular, racing,
fluttering, or pounding
heartbeat; dizziness; lightheadedness; fainting; severe
weakness; severe headache.

What to Do: Call your
doctor, emergency medical
services (EMS), or the
nearest poison control center immediately.

DRUG INTERACTIONS
Consult your doctor for specific advice if you are taking
a beta-blocker, ergotamine
or ergotamine-like medications, antidepressants, digitalis drugs, or an MAO
inhibitor.

FOOD INTERACTIONS
No known food interactions.

DISEASE INTERACTIONS
Consult your doctor if you
have a history of substance
abuse (especially cocaine),
seizures, brain damage,
heart disease, heartbeat
irregularities, high blood
pressure, anxiety disorders,
or a thyroid condition.

Piroxicam

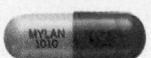

Generic 10 mg
(MYLAN)

Additional photographs

▶ Drug Class: Nonsteroidal anti-inflammatory drug (NSAID)

▶ Available in: Capsules

▶ Available OTC? No

▶ As Generic? Yes

Side Effects

SERIOUS
Shortness of breath or wheezing, with or without swelling of legs or other signs of heart failure; chest pain; peptic ulcer disease with vomiting of blood; black, tarry stools; decreasing kidney function. Call your doctor immediately.

COMMON
Nausea, vomiting, heartburn, diarrhea, constipation, headache, dizziness, sleepiness.

LESS COMMON
Ulcers or sores in mouth, depression, rashes or blistering of skin, ringing sound in the ears, unusual tingling or numbness of the hands or feet, seizures, blurred vision. Also elevated potassium levels, decreased blood counts; such problems can be detected by your doctor.

PRINCIPAL USES
To treat mild to moderate pain and inflammation caused by tendinitis, arthritis, bursitis, gout, soft tissue injuries, migraine and other vascular headaches, menstrual cramps, and other conditions. When patients fail to respond to one NSAID, another may be tried. The greatest effectiveness often requires trial and error of several different NSAIDs.

HOW THE DRUG WORKS
NSAIDs work by interfering with the formation of prostaglandins, naturally occurring substances in the body that cause inflammation and make nerves more sensitive to pain impulses. NSAIDs also have other modes of action that are less well understood.

DOSAGE
Adults: 20 mg once a day. The dose may be increased to 20 mg, 2 times a day. For children's dose, consult your pediatrician.

ONSET OF EFFECT
Several hours for analgesic relief; up to 2 weeks for anti-inflammatory effects.

DURATION OF ACTION
Varies.

DIETARY ADVICE
Take with food; maintain your usual food and fluid intake.

STORAGE
Store in a tightly sealed container away from heat, moisture, and direct light.

IF YOU MISS A DOSE
Take it as soon as you remember. If it is near the time for the next dose, skip the missed dose and resume your regular dosage schedule. Do not double the next dose.

STOPPING THE DRUG
The decision to stop taking the drug should be made in consultation with your physician.

PROLONGED USE
Prolonged use can cause gastrointestinal problems, including ulceration and bleeding, kidney dysfunction, and liver inflammation. Consult your doctor about the need for medical examinations and lab tests.

PRECAUTIONS
Over 60: Because of the potentially greater consequences of gastrointestinal side effects, the dose of NSAIDs for older patients, especially those over age 70, is often cut in half.

Driving and Hazardous Work: Avoid such activities until you determine how the medicine affects you.

Alcohol: Avoid alcohol when using this medication because it increases the risk of stomach irritation.

Pregnancy: Avoid or discontinue this drug if you are pregnant or plan to become pregnant.

Breast Feeding: Piroxicam passes into breast milk; avoid use while nursing.

Infants and Children: May be used in exceptional circumstances; consult your doctor.

Special Concerns: Because NSAIDs can interfere with blood coagulation, this drug should be stopped at least 3 days prior to any surgery.

OVERDOSE
Symptoms: Severe nausea, vomiting, headache, confusion, seizures.

What to Do: Call your doctor, emergency medical services (EMS), or the nearest poison control center immediately.

DRUG INTERACTIONS
Do not take this drug with aspirin or any other NSAIDs without your doctor's approval. In addition, consult your doctor if you are taking antihypertensives, steroids, anticoagulants, antibiotics, itraconazole or ketoconazole, plicamycin, penicillamine, valproic acid, phenytoin, cyclosporine, digitalis drugs, lithium, methotrexate, probenecid, triamterene, or zidovudine.

FOOD INTERACTIONS
No known food interactions.

DISEASE INTERACTIONS
Caution is advised when taking piroxicam. Consult your doctor if you have any of the following: bleeding problems, inflammation or ulcers of the stomach and intestines, diabetes mellitus, systemic lupus erythematosus (SLE, lupus), anemia, asthma, epilepsy, Parkinson's disease, kidney stones, or a history of heart disease or alcohol abuse. Use of piroxicam may cause complications in patients with liver or kidney disease, since these organs work together to remove the medication from the body.

Pneumococcal Vaccine

BRAND NAMES
Pneumovax 23,
Pnu-Imune 23

▶ Drug Class: Vaccine

▶ Available in: Injection

▶ Available OTC? No

▶ As Generic? No

Side Effects

SERIOUS
Serious allergic reaction involving difficulty swallowing or breathing; reddened skin, especially around the ears; itching, particularly of the hands or feet; hives; unusual and severe fatigue; swollen face, eyes, or nasal passages; and fever over 102°F. Call your doctor immediately.

COMMON
Pain, redness, swelling, or the formation of a hard lump at the site of the injection.

LESS COMMON
Fever, aches and pains in the joints or muscles, skin rash, unusual fatigue, general feeling of illness or discomfort, swollen glands.

PRINCIPAL USES
To prevent pneumococcal bacteria infections such as pneumonia, meningitis, and bacteremia (a severe bacterial blood infection).

HOW THE DRUG WORKS
Pneumococcal vaccine stimulates the body's immune system to produce its own protective antibodies against the bacteria.

DOSAGE
Adults and children age 2 and older: A single injection under the skin or into a muscle of the upper arm or midthigh.

ONSET OF EFFECT
2 to 3 weeks.

DURATION OF ACTION
5 to 10 years.

DIETARY ADVICE
No special restrictions.

STORAGE
Not applicable; the dose is administered only at a health care facility.

IF YOU MISS A DOSE
Not applicable.

STOPPING THE DRUG
Not applicable.

PROLONGED USE
Not applicable.

PRECAUTIONS
Over 60: Pneumococcal vaccine is particularly recommended for persons over the age of 50. It is not expected to cause different or more severe side effects in older persons than it does in younger people.

Driving and Hazardous Work: Do not drive or engage in hazardous work until you determine how the medicine affects you.

Alcohol: No special precautions are necessary.

Pregnancy: Studies on the effects of pneumococcal vaccine in pregnant women have not been done. However, if needed, it should be given only after the first trimester of pregnancy. It should be given only to women who have a condition that makes them more vulnerable to infection or more likely to develop serious problems from a pneumococcal infection. Before you receive pneumococcal vaccine, tell your doctor if you are pregnant or plan to become pregnant.

Breast Feeding: Pneumococcal vaccine may pass into breast milk; caution is advised. Consult your doctor for specific advice.

Infants and Children: This vaccine is not recommended for use by children under the age of 2.

Special Concerns: If you have more than one doctor, be sure they all know that you have received this vaccine. In general, only one shot of the vaccine is needed for protection. Revaccination is recommended for persons who received the pneumococcal vaccine that was distributed between 1977 and 1983 if they are at high risk for infection. A second vaccination, 3 to 5 years after the first, may be necessary for children under age 10 with nephrotic syndrome, asplenia, or sickle-cell anemia.

OVERDOSE
Symptoms: An overdose with this vaccine is unlikely.

What to Do: No cases of overdose have been reported.

DRUG INTERACTIONS
Other drugs may interact with pneumococcal vaccine. Consult your doctor for advice if you are taking any prescription or over-the-counter medication. Tell your doctor if you have had any pneumococcal vaccine in the past.

FOOD INTERACTIONS
No known food interactions.

DISEASE INTERACTIONS
Consult your doctor if you have any severe illness that is causing fever. The vaccine should be given with caution to patients receiving anticoagulant therapy. Patients who have received extensive chemotherapy or radiation treatment for Hodgkin's disease should not receive the pneumococcal vaccine.

Podofilox

BRAND NAME
Condylox

▶ Drug Class: Antimitotic

▶ Available in: Topical gel, solution

▶ Available OTC? No

▶ As Generic? No

Side Effects

SERIOUS
No serious side effects are associated with the use of podofilox.

COMMON
Burning, inflammation, pain, itching, sores, stinging, redness at the application sites.

LESS COMMON
Local tingling, blisters, dryness, crusting, swelling, scarring, bleeding, or chafing at the application sites. Vomiting, headache, insomnia, painful intercourse.

PRINCIPAL USES
To treat external condylomata acuminata (genital and perianal warts) in adults. Genital and perianal warts are caused by the human papillomavirus (HPV).

HOW THE DRUG WORKS
The exact mechanism of action is unknown.

DOSAGE
Apply a thin layer with the supplied cotton-tipped applicator (topical solution) or with the applicator tip or finger (topical gel) to the affected area(s) 2 times a day, in the morning and evening, for 3 consecutive days. Then discontinue treatment for 4 consecutive days. This cycle of treatment may be repeated until there are no more visible warts or for a maximum of 4 cycles. Your doctor should demonstrate the proper technique prior to the initial application.

ONSET OF EFFECT
Unknown.

DURATION OF ACTION
Unknown.

DIETARY ADVICE
Podofilox can be used without regard to diet.

STORAGE
Store in a tightly sealed container away from moisture, direct light, and extremes in temperature.

IF YOU MISS A DOSE
Apply it as soon as you remember. If it is near the time for the next dose, skip the missed dose and resume your regular dosage schedule. Do not apply more than directed. It will not make the medicine work better and may increase side effects.

STOPPING THE DRUG
Apply podofilox in one-week cycles until there is no visible wart tissue or for a maximum of 4 cycles. Consult your doctor for specific advice if further treatment is needed.

PROLONGED USE
Safety and effectiveness beyond 4 weeks have not been determined. If response to therapy is incomplete after 4 one-week cycles, discontinue treatment and contact your physician.

PRECAUTIONS
Over 60: No special problems are expected.

Driving and Hazardous Work: The use of podofilox should not impair your ability to perform such tasks safely.

Alcohol: No special precautions are necessary.

Pregnancy: Adequate human studies have not been done. Before taking podofilox, discuss with your doctor the relative risks and benefits of using this drug while pregnant.

Breast Feeding: Podofilox may pass into breast milk; caution is advised. Consult your doctor for advice.

Infants and Children: The safety and effectiveness of podofilox in children under the age of 12 have not been established. Genital and perianal warts are contracted by people who are sexually active.

Special Concerns: Let the treated areas dry before allowing contact with unaffected skin. Wash your hands before and after each application. Podofilox is for external use only; do not apply to the urethra, rectum, or vagina. Do not apply the topical solution to the perianal (around the anus) area. Avoid getting podofilox into your eyes. If eye contact occurs, flush the eye at once with large quantities of water, and contact your doctor. Do not have sexual intercourse during the 3 days you are applying podofilox. Condoms may help protect new sexual partners from contracting HPV as well as other sexually transmitted diseases such as herpes and HIV. However, they are not 100% effective. If the warts reappear, contact your doctor.

OVERDOSE
Symptoms: An overdose with podofilox is unlikely.

What to Do: If someone applies a much larger dose than prescribed or accidentally ingests podofilox, call your doctor.

DRUG INTERACTIONS
None reported.

FOOD INTERACTIONS
None reported.

DISEASE INTERACTIONS
None reported.

Poliovirus Vaccine

BRAND NAMES
Ipol, Orimune

▶ Drug Class: Vaccine

▶ Available in: Injection, oral solution

▶ Available OTC? No

▶ As Generic? Yes

Side Effects

SERIOUS
Serious allergic reaction involving difficulty swallowing or breathing; reddened skin, especially around the ears; itching, particularly of the hands or feet; hives; unusual and severe fatigue; and swollen face, eyes, or nasal passages. Call your doctor immediately.

COMMON
No common side effects are associated with the poliovirus vaccine.

LESS COMMON
Injection: Fever; soreness, rash, tenderness, or pain at injection site. There are no less-common side effects associated with the oral suspension.

PRINCIPAL USES
To prevent poliomyelitis (polio).

HOW THE DRUG WORKS
Poliovirus vaccine stimulates the body's immune system to produce its own protective antibodies against the virus that causes polio.

DOSAGE
Injection (inactivated vaccine)— All doses are given under the skin, in either the upper arm (adults) or mid-thigh (infants and children). First dose is given at initial visit. For children, this is usually at 6 to 8 weeks of age. Second dose is given 8 weeks later. Third dose is given 8 weeks to 12 months after the second dose. Fourth dose, when needed, is given 6 to 12 months after the third dose. First booster dose, for children, is usually administered upon entering school, usually between ages 4 and 6. Oral solution (live vaccine)— Follow the same dosage schedule as used for the injection form.

ONSET OF EFFECT
Within 7 to 10 days.

DURATION OF ACTION
Up to 12 years.

DIETARY ADVICE
No special restrictions.

STORAGE
Not applicable; the dose is administered only at a health care facility.

IF YOU MISS A DOSE
If your child misses a scheduled vaccination, contact your pediatrician.

STOPPING THE DRUG
The full schedule of vaccinations should be followed unless a medical problem intervenes.

PROLONGED USE
No special problems are expected.

PRECAUTIONS
Over 60: Poliovirus vaccine is not expected to cause different or more severe side effects in older patients than it does in younger persons. Inactivated poliovirus vaccine is preferred in adults.

Driving and Hazardous Work: No special precautions are necessary.

Alcohol: No special precautions are necessary.

Pregnancy: Studies on the effects of poliovirus vaccine in pregnant women have not been done. However, if needed, it should be given only to pregnant women at great risk of acquiring polio. Consult your doctor for advice.

Breast Feeding: Poliovirus vaccine has not been reported to cause problems during breast feeding. Consult your doctor for advice. If your child has taken the oral solution, refrain from breast feeding for 2 to 3 hours before and after immunization.

Infants and Children: This vaccine is not recommended for use by infants under the age of 6 weeks.

Special Concerns: Immunization with inactivated polio vaccine is recommended for any adult at risk of the disease, such as those traveling to countries where polio is not under control, those who have not had the complete series of immunizations, those who work in medical facilities or day-care centers, and those working in laboratories where poliovirus samples may be handled.

OVERDOSE
Symptoms: An overdose of poliovirus vaccine is unlikely.

What to Do: No cases of overdose have been reported.

DRUG INTERACTIONS
Consult your doctor for specific advice if you are undergoing chemotherapy for cancer or if you are taking corticosteroids.

FOOD INTERACTIONS
No known food interactions.

DISEASE INTERACTIONS
Except under special circumstances, you should not receive the poliovirus vaccine if you have ongoing diarrhea, any moderate or severe illness causing fever or vomiting, any immune deficiency condition, such as HIV, a family history of immune deficiency, or a household member with an immunodeficiency. Consult your doctor.

Polyethylene Glycol Solution (PEG)

Co-Lav, Culavage, Colyte, Go-Evac, GoLYTELY, NuLYTELY, OCL

▶ Drug Class: Stimulant laxative

▶ Available in: Oral solution, powder for oral solution

▶ Available OTC? No

▶ As Generic? No

Side Effects

SERIOUS
Skin rash. Call your doctor immediately should this occur.

COMMON
Bloating, nausea.

LESS COMMON
Stomach upset or abdominal cramps, vomiting, irritation of the anal region.

PRINCIPAL USES
To clean the colon and rectum prior to diagnostic tests or surgical procedures involving the colon.

HOW THE DRUG WORKS
Polyethylene glycol (PEG) solution induces mild diarrhea to flush solid material from the colon.

DOSAGE
Adults and teenagers: Drink 1 full glass (8 oz) of PEG rapidly every 10 minutes until at least 4 liters have been consumed. Children: 11.3 to 18.2 ml per pound of body weight per hour.

ONSET OF EFFECT
Within 1 hour.

DURATION OF ACTION
Variable.

DIETARY ADVICE
Consume no food for 4 hours before taking PEG. Afterward, drink only clear fluids like water, ginger ale, decaffeinated cola, decaffeinated tea, or broth.

STORAGE
Store in a tightly sealed container away from heat, moisture, and direct light. Refrigerate the solution but do not allow it to freeze.

IF YOU MISS A DOSE
Take it as soon as you remember. If it is near the time for the next dose, skip the missed dose and resume your regular dosage schedule. Do not double the next dose.

STOPPING THE DRUG
Continue drinking the solution until your stools are watery, clear and free of solid material. The decision to stop taking the drug should be made by your doctor.

PROLONGED USE
PEG is not intended for prolonged use.

PRECAUTIONS
Over 60: No special problems are expected in older patients.

Driving and Hazardous Work: Do not drive or engage in hazardous work until you determine how the medicine affects you.

Alcohol: Avoid alcohol.

Pregnancy: Adequate human studies have not been completed. Before taking PEG, tell your doctor if you are pregnant or plan to become pregnant.

Breast Feeding: PEG may pass into breast milk; caution is advised. Consult your doctor for specific advice.

Infants and Children: There is no specific information comparing use of PEG in children with use in other age groups. However, no special problems are expected.

Special Concerns: It will take up to 3 hours to consume the full recommended dose of PEG. The first bowel movement may start in 1 hour. Patients using the powder form of PEG should first mix the powder with water and add enough lukewarm water to reach the fill mark on the bottle. Shake well until all the ingredients are dissolved. Do not add any flavorings or other ingredients to the solution. Do not drink the solution chilled. Cases of hypothermia have been reported following ingestion of chilled solutions. Use the mixed solution within 48 hours.

OVERDOSE
Symptoms: Diarrhea, abdominal pain, bloating.

What to Do: An overdose of PEG is unlikely to occur. However, if you are concerned about the possibility of an overdose, call a doctor, emergency medical services (EMS), or the nearest poison control center.

DRUG INTERACTIONS
Any other oral medication taken within 1 hour of PEG may be flushed from the body. Consult your doctor for advice if you are taking any other medication.

FOOD INTERACTIONS
Do not consume any food for at least 4 hours before taking PEG.

DISEASE INTERACTIONS
Caution is advised when taking PEG. Consult your doctor if you have a history of any of the following: blockage or obstruction of the intestine, paralytic ileus, perforated bowel, toxic colitis, or toxic megacolon.

Potassium Chloride

K-Dur 10 750 mg
(KEY)

Additional photographs

▶ Drug Class: Electrolyte

▶ Available in: Liquid, soluble granules, powder, tablets, sustained-release capsules

▶ Available OTC? No

▶ As Generic? Yes

Side Effects

SERIOUS
Numbness or tingling in the hands, feet, or lips; slowed or irregular heartbeat; breathing difficulty; unusual fatigue or weakness; confusion. Stop taking the drug and consult your doctor at once.

COMMON
Diarrhea, abdominal discomfort, gas, nausea and vomiting.

LESS COMMON
Black or bloody stools, pain when swallowing. Consult your doctor if such symptoms persist.

PRINCIPAL USES
To restore or maintain proper potassium levels in the body. Potassium is an electrolyte, a mineral that helps maintain proper fluid balance. It is also vital in the transmission of nerve impulses.

HOW THE DRUG WORKS
Potassium chloride is absorbed in the body fluids and taken into the cells where it is part of a number of metabolic actions, especially those that involve the release of energy. It also aids in the conduction of nerve impulses responsible for muscle movement and heart contraction.

DOSAGE
20 milliequivalents (mEq) to 100 mEq daily in divided doses. A single dose should not exceed 20 mEq.

ONSET OF EFFECT
Unknown.

DURATION OF ACTION
Unknown.

DIETARY ADVICE
Must be taken after meals or with food and a glass of water or other liquid. Follow all special dietary guidelines as outlined by your doctor.

STORAGE
Store in a tightly sealed container away from heat and direct light. Keep liquid forms of potassium refrigerated, but do not allow to freeze.

IF YOU MISS A DOSE
If you remember within 2 hours, take the missed dose with food or liquids and resume your regular dosage schedule. If you remember after 2 hours, skip the missed dose and return to your regular dosage schedule. Do not double the next dose.

STOPPING THE DRUG
Do not stop taking potassium without first consulting your physician. Be especially careful not to stop taking potassium abruptly if you are also taking digitalis drugs (digoxin).

PROLONGED USE
Requires periodic testing of blood potassium levels by your doctor.

PRECAUTIONS
Over 60: Elderly people may be at greater risk of retaining too much potassium owing to age-related changes in the ability of the kidneys to excrete it. Older patients should have their potassium levels checked regularly.

Driving and Hazardous Work: No special problems are expected.

Alcohol: No special problems are expected.

Pregnancy: Potassium supplements are considered safe during pregnancy if used exactly as prescribed.

Breast Feeding: Potassium may pass into breast milk. Consult your doctor for specific advice.

Infants and Children: Although the safety and effectiveness of potassium use by children have not been established, no specific problems have been documented.

Special Concerns: Remember that the foods in your diet must also be considered when calculating your total intake of potassium. Be certain to read all labels carefully, especially on all products labeled "low-sodium," such as canned foods and some breads, many of which contain

potassium. Do not crush sustained-release forms. Swallow tablets without chewing, sucking, or crushing. Be sure the powder form is completely dissolved before ingesting.

OVERDOSE
Symptoms: Irregular heartbeat; muscle weakness, which may progress to paralysis of the diaphragm and interfere with breathing.

What to Do: Call your doctor, emergency medical services (EMS), or the nearest poison control center immediately.

DRUG INTERACTIONS
The following drugs may interact adversely with potassium chloride. Consult your doctor for advice if you are taking digitalis drugs, potassium-sparing diuretics, thiazide diuretics, NSAIDs, beta-blockers, heparin, triamterene, anticholinergics, or ACE inhibitors.

FOOD INTERACTIONS
To prevent ingestion of too much potassium, discuss your diet with your doctor. Foods high in potassium include avocados, bananas, broccoli, dried fruits, grapefruit, beans, meats, nuts, spinach, low-salt milk, squash, melon, brussels sprouts, zucchini, frozen orange juice, and tomatoes.

DISEASE INTERACTIONS
Consult your doctor if you have any of the following: intestinal obstruction, dehydration, severe diarrhea, compression of the esophagus, delayed gastric emptying, peptic ulcer, heart block, or a predisposition to retaining potassium.

Pramipexole Dihydrochloride

BRAND NAME
Mirapex

- ▶ Drug Class: Dopamine agonist
- ▶ Available in: Tablets
- ▶ Available OTC? No
- ▶ As Generic? No

Side Effects

SERIOUS
Excessively low blood pressure (orthostatic hypotension), causing extreme dizziness, confusion, nausea, fainting, or blackouts, especially when rising from a seated or lying position; hallucinations; impaired control over voluntary movements (dyskinesia).

COMMON
Mild to moderate dizziness or faintness (caused by a less severe drop in blood pressure) upon standing or sitting up; drowsiness; dry mouth.

LESS COMMON
Increased sweating, vision abnormalities, joint pain, increased urine output, weakness, pneumonia, increased incidence of accidental injury, tooth disease, leg cramps.

PRINCIPAL USES
To treat the symptoms of Parkinson's disease.

HOW THE DRUG WORKS
The exact mechanism of action is unknown, but pramipexole is believed to help increase the release of certain neurological chemicals that improve control over movement.

DOSAGE
Initial dose (for first week of therapy): 0.125 mg, 3 times a day. The dose is gradually increased (usually once a week for 7 weeks) up to 1.5 mg, taken 3 times a day, for a total dose of 4.5 mg a day.

ONSET OF EFFECT
Unknown.

DURATION OF ACTION
Unknown.

DIETARY ADVICE
Pramipexole may be taken with meals, if desired, to minimize the incidence of nausea or stomach upset.

STORAGE
Store in a tightly sealed container away from heat and direct light. Keep away from moisture and extremes in temperature.

IF YOU MISS A DOSE
Take it as soon as you remember. If it is near the time for the next dose, skip the missed dose and resume your regular dosage schedule. Do not double the next dose.

STOPPING THE DRUG
The decision to stop taking the drug should be made in consultation with your doctor. Do not stop taking pramipexole suddenly; it is recommended that the dose be reduced gradually over a period of at least 1 week, according to your doctor's instructions.

PROLONGED USE
Lifetime therapy with pramipexole may be necessary; prolonged use may be associated with a greater incidence of side effects. Regular monitoring and evaluation by your doctor is advised.

PRECAUTIONS
Over 60: Adverse reactions (especially hallucinations) may be more likely and more severe in older patients. Lower doses may be advised.

Driving and Hazardous Work: Pramipexole may cause sudden and extreme drowsiness. Do not drive or engage in hazardous work until you determine how the medicine affects you.

Alcohol: Avoid alcohol.

Pregnancy: Pramipexole should not be used by pregnant women.

Breast Feeding: Pramipexole should not be taken while nursing. The patient must choose between using the drug or breast feeding.

Infants and Children: Pramipexole should not be taken by children.

Special Concerns: This drug may cause dizziness and faintness, especially when getting up out of a chair or sitting up after lying down (a condition known as postural orthostatic hypertension, characterized by temporary episodes of excessively low blood pressure). Be cautious and move slowly when arising.

OVERDOSE
Symptoms: No cases of overdose have been reported.

What to Do: An overdose of pramipexole is unlikely to occur. However, if someone takes a much larger dose than prescribed, call your doctor, emergency medical services (EMS), or the nearest poison control center right away.

DRUG INTERACTIONS
Consult your doctor for specific advice if you are taking antiulcer drugs (specifically, histamine H2 blockers such as cimetidine and ranitidine), calcium channel blockers (such as diltiazem and verapamil), potassium-sparing diuretics (such as triamterene), or other dopamine agonists (such as phenothiazines, butyrophenones, thioxanthenes, and metoclopramide).

FOOD INTERACTIONS
No known food interactions.

DISEASE INTERACTIONS
Use of pramipexole may cause complications in patients with a history of kidney disease, since this medication is eliminated from the body through the kidneys.

Pravastatin

BRAND NAME
Pravachol

▶ Drug Class: Antilipidemic
(cholesterol-lowering agent)

▶ Available in: Tablets

▶ Available OTC? No

▶ As Generic? No

Side Effects

SERIOUS
Fever, unusual or unexplained muscle aches and tenderness. Call your doctor right away.

COMMON
Side effects occur in only 1% to 2% of patients. These include constipation or diarrhea, dizziness, gas, headache, heartburn, nausea, skin rash, stomach pain, rise in liver enzymes (detectable by your doctor).

LESS COMMON
Insomnia.

PRINCIPAL USES
To treat high cholesterol. Usually prescribed after first lines of treatment—including diet, weight loss, and exercise—fail to reduce total and low-density lipoprotein (LDL) cholesterol to acceptable levels.

HOW THE DRUG WORKS
Pravastatin blocks the action of an enzyme required for the manufacture of cholesterol, thereby interfering with its formation. By lowering the amount of cholesterol in the liver cells, pravastatin increases the formation of receptors for LDL, and thereby reduces blood levels of total and LDL cholesterol. In addition to lowering LDL cholesterol, pravastatin also modestly reduces triglyceride levels and raises HDL (the so-called "good") cholesterol.

DOSAGE
Initial dose is 10 to 20 mg once a day. The dose may be increased to a maximum of 40 mg per day. The drug is most effective when taken in the evening.

ONSET OF EFFECT
2 to 4 weeks.

DURATION OF ACTION
The effect persists for the duration of therapy.

DIETARY ADVICE
Cholesterol-lowering drugs are only one part of a total program that should include regular exercise and a healthy diet. The American Heart Association publishes a "Healthy Heart" diet, which is recommended.

STORAGE
Store in a tightly sealed container away from heat and direct light.

IF YOU MISS A DOSE
Take it as soon as you remember. Take the next scheduled dose at the proper time and resume your regular dosage schedule, as prescribed. Do not double the next dose.

STOPPING THE DRUG
The decision to stop taking the drug should be made in consultation with your doctor. Once the medication is discontinued, blood cholesterol is likely to return to original elevated levels.

PROLONGED USE
Side effects are more likely with prolonged use. As you continue with pravastatin, your doctor will periodically order blood tests to evaluate liver function.

PRECAUTIONS
Over 60: No special problems are expected.

Driving and Hazardous Work: The use of pravastatin should not impair your ability to perform such tasks safely.

Alcohol: No special precautions are necessary.

Pregnancy: Pravastatin should not be used during pregnancy or by women who plan to become pregnant in the near future.

Breast Feeding: This drug is not recommended for women who are nursing.

Infants and Children: Long-term effects of pravastatin in children have not been determined. Rarely used in young patients; consult your doctor.

Special Concerns: Important elements of treatment for high cholesterol include proper diet, weight loss, regular moderate exercise, and the avoidance of certain medications that may increase cholesterol levels. Because pravastatin has potential side effects, it is important that you maintain a recommended healthy diet and cooperate with other treatments your physician may suggest.

OVERDOSE
Symptoms: Overdose is unlikely to occur.

What to Do: Emergency instructions not applicable.

DRUG INTERACTIONS
Consult your doctor if you are taking cyclosporine, gemfibrozil, niacin, antibiotics, especially erythromycin, or medications for fungus infections. All of these drugs may increase the risk of myositis (muscle inflammation) when taken with pravastatin and may lead to kidney failure.

FOOD INTERACTIONS
No known food interactions.

DISEASE INTERACTIONS
Consult your doctor if you have any of the following problems: liver, kidney, or muscle disease, or a medical history involving organ transplant or recent surgery.

Praziquantel

BRAND NAME
Biltricide

Biltricide 600 mg
(BAYER)

▶ Drug Class: Anthelmintic

▶ Available in: Tablets

▶ Available OTC? No

▶ As Generic? No

Side Effects

SERIOUS
No serious side effects are associated with the use of praziquantel.

COMMON
Stomach pain or cramps, dizziness, drowsiness, bloody diarrhea, fever, nausea or vomiting, headache, increased sweating, loss of appetite, general discomfort. These symptoms are likely to occur as allergic reactions to dead worms and usually resolve on their own.

LESS COMMON
Hives, skin rash, itching.

PRINCIPAL USES
To treat trematode (fluke) infections such as clonorchiasis caused by *Clonorchis sinensis* (Chinese or Oriental liver fluke), opisthorchiasis caused by *Opisthorchis viverrini* and *O. felineus* (liver flukes), and schistosomiasis caused by *Schistosoma mekongi,* *S. japonicum, S. mansoni,* and *S. hematobium* (blood flukes). Praziquantel may be prescribed to treat other types of parasite-related disease as determined by your physician.

HOW THE DRUG WORKS
Praziquantel works by causing severe spasms and paralysis of the worm's muscles. The body's immune system can then better attack and expel the worm.

DOSAGE
For clonorchiasis, opisthorchiasis, and lung or intestinal fluke infection— Adults and children age 4 and older: 25 mg per 2.2 lbs (1 kg) of body weight, 3 times a day for 1 day. For schistosomiasis— Adults and children age 4 and older: 20 mg per 2.2 lbs, 2 to 3 times for 1 day. (Different doses may be prescribed in conjunction with corticosteroids to treat certain other parasite-related diseases.)

ONSET OF EFFECT
Unknown.

DURATION OF ACTION
Unknown.

DIETARY ADVICE
Praziquantel is best taken during meals with liquid. Do not chew the tablets.

STORAGE
Store in a tightly sealed container away from heat, moisture, and direct light.

IF YOU MISS A DOSE
Take it as soon as you remember. However, if it is near the time for the next dose, skip the missed dose and resume your regular dosage schedule. Do not double the next dose.

STOPPING THE DRUG
Take it as prescribed for the full treatment period.

PROLONGED USE
See your doctor regularly for tests and examinations if you must take this medicine for a prolonged period. If your condition has not improved by the end of the course of therapy, consult your doctor.

PRECAUTIONS
Over 60: Adverse reactions may be more likely and more severe in older patients.

Driving and Hazardous Work: Avoid such activities until you determine how the medicine affects you. If it does cause problems, do not drive or engage in hazardous activities the day you take praziquantel and for 24 hours after treatment.

Alcohol: No special precautions are necessary.

Pregnancy: Adequate human studies have not been done. Before taking praziquantel, tell your doctor if you are pregnant or plan to become pregnant.

Breast Feeding: Praziquantel passes into breast milk. Stop nursing the day you start therapy. Do not restart breast feeding until 72 hours after therapy is completed. All breast milk during this time should be extracted with a breast pump or squeezed out and thrown away.

Infants and Children: Use and dosage for children under age 4 must be determined by your pediatrician.

Special Concerns: Praziquantel has a bitter taste that can cause gagging or vomiting, especially if the pills are chewed. Swallow the pills whole with a small amount of liquid during meals.

OVERDOSE
Symptoms: An overdose with praziquantel is unlikely.

What to Do: An overdose with praziquantel is unlikely to be life-threatening. However, if you take a much larger dose than prescribed, take a fast-acting laxative and call your doctor.

DRUG INTERACTIONS
Consult your doctor for advice if you are taking any other prescription or over-the-counter medication, especially corticosteroids (used concurrently with praziquantel in the treatment of some parasite-related diseases), cimetidine, ketoconazole, or miconazole.

FOOD INTERACTIONS
No known food interactions.

DISEASE INTERACTIONS
Praziquantel should not be used when Taenia solium worm cysts are present in the eye. The death of the worm cysts by praziquantel may cause irreparable damage to the eyes. Caution is advised when taking praziquantel. If you have liver disease, you may be at greater risk for side effects. Consult your doctor for specific advice.

Prazosin

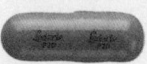

Side Effects

SERIOUS
Dizziness or lightheaded-
ness, especially when
getting up from a sitting
or lying position, fainting,
loss of bladder control,
pounding heartbeat,
swelling of feet and
lower legs, chest pain,
continuing inappropriate
and painful erections,
shortness of breath. Call
your doctor immediately.

COMMON
Drowsiness, headache,
lack of energy.

LESS COMMON
Dry mouth, unusual
fatigue, nervousness,
nausea, frequent urge
to urinate.

PRINCIPAL USES
To treat high blood pres-
sure (hypertension).

HOW THE DRUG WORKS
Prazosin causes the blood
vessels to relax and widen,
which in turn lowers blood
pressure.

DOSAGE
Adults: To start, 0.5 to 1
mg, 2 or 3 times a day. The
dose may be increased
slowly to 6 to 15 mg a day
divided into 2 or 3 doses.
Children: 50 to 400 micrograms (mcg) per 2.2 lbs (1
kg) of body weight divided
into 2 or 3 doses.

ONSET OF EFFECT
30 to 90 minutes. The full
effect may not be realized
for 3 to 4 weeks.

DURATION OF ACTION
7 to 10 hours.

DIETARY ADVICE
Follow a healthy diet (low-
salt, low-fat, low-cholesterol)
as advised by your doctor to
help control blood pressure
and prevent heart disease.

STORAGE
Store in a tightly sealed container away from heat and
direct light.

IF YOU MISS A DOSE
Take it as soon as you
remember. If it is near the
time for the next dose, skip
the missed dose and
resume your regular dosage
schedule. Do not double the
next dose.

STOPPING THE DRUG
The decision to stop taking
the drug should be made by
your doctor. Prazosin controls high blood pressure
but does not cure it.

PROLONGED USE
Lifelong therapy may be
necessary. See your doctor
regularly for tests and
examinations if you take
this drug for a prolonged
period.

PRECAUTIONS
Over 60: Adverse reactions, particularly dizziness,
lightheadedness, and fainting, may be more likely and
more severe in older
patients. This medication
may reduce tolerance to
cold temperatures in older
patients.

**Driving and Hazardous
Work:** Do not drive or
engage in hazardous work
until you determine how the
medicine affects you.

Alcohol: Avoid alcohol.

Pregnancy: In animal studies and limited human studies, prazosin has not caused
birth defects. High doses in
animal studies have caused
reduced birth weight.
Before you take prazosin,
tell your doctor if you are
pregnant or plan to become
pregnant.

Breast Feeding: Prazosin
passes into breast milk; caution is advised. Consult your
doctor for advice.

Infants and Children:
There is no information
comparing use of prazosin
by infants and children with
use by older patients. Consult your doctor for specific
advice.

Special Concerns: Be
careful when you start
using this medication or
when the dose is increased,
since you may be more
likely to experience dizziness or lightheadedness at
these times. For the same
reason, as you continue to
take prazosin use extra care
in hot weather, as well as
during exercise or if you
must stand for a long time.

OVERDOSE
Symptoms: Drowsiness,
slowed reflexes, extremely
low blood pressure.

What to Do: An overdose
of prazosin is unlikely to be
life-threatening. However,
if someone takes a much
larger dose than prescribed,
call your doctor, emergency
medical services (EMS), or
the nearest poison control
center immediately.

DRUG INTERACTIONS
Consult your doctor for
advice if you are taking nonsteroidal anti-inflammatory
drugs (NSAIDs), estrogens,
sympathomimetics, propranolol or other beta-blockers,
or any over-the-counter
drug for appetite control,
asthma, colds, cough, hay
fever, or sinus problems.

FOOD INTERACTIONS
No known food interactions.

DISEASE INTERACTIONS
Caution is advised when
taking prazosin. Consult
your doctor if you have
angina, severe heart dis-
ease, or kidney disease.

Prednisolone Ophthalmic

▶ Drug Class: Corticosteroid

▶ Available in: Ophthalmic solution, suspension

▶ Available OTC? No

▶ As Generic? Yes

Side Effects

SERIOUS
Decreased vision or blurring of vision (from cataract); eye pain, nausea, vomiting (from increased eye pressure); pain, redness, sensitivity to bright light, discharge (from eye infection). Call your doctor immediately if you experience any of these signs or symptoms. The drug may trigger a recurrence of herpes infection of the eye; mention any previous herpes infection to your doctor.

COMMON
Increased eye pressure (especially with the topical prednisolone acetate form); this is usually reversed once the drug is stopped.

LESS COMMON
Burning, stinging, redness, or watering of eyes.

PRINCIPAL USES
To control inflammation and prevent potentially permanent damage that may result from eye problems such as conjunctivitis, herpes of the eye, and cornea injuries. It is also used to help relieve redness, irritation, and discomfort in the eye, and may be used after eye surgery to control any inflammatory response.

HOW THE DRUG WORKS
Ophthalmic prednisolone inhibits the release of natural substances that stimulate an inflammatory reaction and pain in eye tissues.

DOSAGE
Solution or suspension: 1 or 2 drops in each eye up to 16 times a day.

ONSET OF EFFECT
Unknown.

DURATION OF ACTION
Unknown.

DIETARY ADVICE
No special restrictions.

STORAGE
Store in a tightly sealed container away from heat, moisture, and direct light. Do not allow it to freeze.

IF YOU MISS A DOSE
Apply it as soon as you remember. If it is near the time for the next dose, skip the missed dose and resume your regular dosage schedule. Do not double the next dose.

STOPPING THE DRUG
It is very important to use this drug as prescribed for the full treatment period, even if symptoms improve before the scheduled end of therapy.

PROLONGED USE
You should see your doctor regularly for tests and examinations if you use this drug for a prolonged period.

PRECAUTIONS
Over 60: No special problems are expected.

Driving and Hazardous Work: Do not drive or engage in hazardous work until you determine how the medicine affects your vision.

Alcohol: No special precautions are necessary.

Pregnancy: Adequate human studies have not been done, though no birth defects have been reported. Before taking ophthalmic prednisolone, tell your doctor if you are pregnant or plan to become pregnant.

Breast Feeding: Ophthalmic prednisolone has not been reported to cause problems in nursing babies. Consult your doctor for advice.

Infants and Children: Children under 2 years of age may be especially sensitive to the effects of ophthalmic prednisolone.

Special Concerns: To use the eye drops, first wash your hands. Tilt your head back. Gently apply pressure to the inside corner of the eyelid and with the index finger of the same hand, pull downward on the lower eyelid to make a space. Drop the medicine into this space and close your eye. Apply pressure for 1 or 2 minutes while keeping the eye closed without blinking. Then wash your hands again. Make sure the tip of the dropper does not touch your eye, finger, or any other surface. If your symptoms do not improve in 5 to 7 days or if they become worse, check with your doctor. Wearing contact lenses while using this medication may increase the risk of infection. Your doctor may tell you not to wear contact lenses during and for a day or two after treatment.

OVERDOSE
Symptoms: When used topically, an overdose is very unlikely. Inadvertent oral ingestion, however, may cause fever, muscle pain, loss of appetite, dizziness, fainting, and trouble breathing.

What to Do: An overdose of this drug is unlikely to be life-threatening. However, if someone applies a much larger dose than prescribed or accidentally ingests the medicine, call your doctor, emergency medical services (EMS), or the nearest poison control center.

DRUG INTERACTIONS
Consult your doctor for specific advice if you are taking any other prescription or over-the-counter medication.

FOOD INTERACTIONS
No known food interactions.

DISEASE INTERACTIONS
Consult your doctor if you have any of the following: cataracts, diabetes, glaucoma, herpes infection of the eye, tuberculosis of the eye, or any other eye infection.

Prednisolone Systemic

Side Effects

SERIOUS
Vision problems, frequent urination, increased thirst, rectal bleeding, blistering skin, confusion, hallucinations, paranoia, euphoria, depression, mood swings, redness and swelling at injection site. Call your doctor immediately.

COMMON
Increased appetite, indigestion, nervousness, insomnia, greater susceptibility to infections, increased blood pressure, slowed wound healing, weight gain, easy bruising, fluid retention.

LESS COMMON
Change in skin color, dizziness, headache, increased sweating, unusual growth of body or facial hair, increased blood sugar, peptic ulcers, adrenal insufficiency, muscle weakness, cataracts, glaucoma, osteoporosis.

PRINCIPAL USES
To treat numerous conditions that involve inflammation (a response by body tissues, producing redness, warmth, swelling, and pain). Such conditions include arthritis, allergic reactions, asthma, some skin diseases, multiple sclerosis flare-ups, and other autoimmune diseases. Also prescribed to treat deficiency of natural steroid hormones.

HOW THE DRUG WORKS
This hormone mimics the effects of the body's natural corticosteroids. It depresses the synthesis, release, and activity of inflammation-producing body chemicals. It also suppresses the activity of the immune system.

DOSAGE
Oral dosage: 5 to 200 mg a day, depending on condition, in 1 or several doses. Injection: 2 to 100 mg a day injected into a muscle, joint, vein, or lesion depending on condition. Consult pediatrician for children's dose.

ONSET OF EFFECT
Within 1 hour of taking oral forms or after injection into a muscle or vein; 1 to 2 days after injection into a lesion.

DURATION OF ACTION
30 to 36 hours for tablets; 3 to 4 days for injection.

DIETARY ADVICE
It can be taken with food or milk to minimize stomach upset. Your doctor may recommend a special diet.

STORAGE
Store in a tightly sealed container away from heat, moisture, and direct light. Do not allow liquid forms to freeze.

IF YOU MISS A DOSE
If you take several doses a day and it is close to the next dose, double the next dose. If you take 1 dose a day and you do not remember until the next day, skip the missed dose and do not double the next dose.

STOPPING THE DRUG
With long-term therapy, do not stop taking the drug abruptly; the dosage should be decreased gradually.

PROLONGED USE
Long-term use may lead to cataracts, diabetes, hypertension, or osteoporosis; see your doctor for regular examinations.

PRECAUTIONS
Over 60: Adverse reactions may be more likely and more severe.

Driving and Hazardous Work: Avoid such activities until you determine how the medicine affects you.

Alcohol: May cause stomach problems; avoid it unless your physician approves occasional moderate drinking.

Pregnancy: Overuse during pregnancy can impair growth and development of the child.

Breast Feeding: Do not use this drug while nursing.

Infants and Children: Prednisolone may retard the development of bone and other tissues.

Special Concerns: This drug can lower resistance to infection. Avoid immunizations with live vaccines. Patients undergoing long-term therapy should wear a medical-alert bracelet. Call your doctor if you develop a fever.

OVERDOSE
Symptoms: Fever, muscle or joint pain, nausea, dizziness, fainting, difficulty breathing. Prolonged overuse: Moonface, obesity, unusual hair growth, acne, loss of sexual function, muscle wasting.

What to Do: Call your doctor, emergency medical services (EMS), or the nearest poison control center immediately.

DRUG INTERACTIONS
Consult your doctor for advice if you are taking aminoglutethimide, antacids, barbiturates, carbamazepine, griseofulvin, mitotane, phenylbutazone, phenytoin, primidone, rifampin, injectable amphotericin B, oral antidiabetes agents, insulin, digitalis drugs, diuretics or drugs containing potassium or sodium.

FOOD INTERACTIONS
Avoid excess sodium.

DISEASE INTERACTIONS
Consult your doctor if you have a history of bone disease, chicken pox, measles, gastrointestinal disorders, diabetes, recent serious infection, glaucoma, heart disease, hypertension, liver or kidney disorders, high blood cholesterol, thyroid problems, myasthenia gravis, or lupus.

Prednisone

BRAND NAMES
Deltasone, Liquid Pred,
Meticorten, Orasone,
Prednicen-M, Prednisone
Intensol, Sterapred

Generic 20 mg
(SCHEIN)

Additional photographs

▶ Drug Class: Corticosteroid

▶ Available in: Oral suspension, syrup, tablets

▶ Available OTC? No

▶ As Generic? Yes

Side Effects

SERIOUS
Vision problems, frequent urination, increased thirst, rectal bleeding, blistering skin, confusion, hallucinations, paranoia, euphoria, depression, mood swings, redness and swelling at injection site. Call your doctor immediately.

COMMON
Increased appetite, indigestion, nervousness, insomnia, greater susceptibility to infections, increased blood pressure, slowed wound healing, weight gain, easy bruising, fluid retention.

LESS COMMON
Change in skin color, dizziness, headache, increased sweating, unusual growth of body or facial hair, increased blood sugar, peptic ulcers, adrenal insufficiency, muscle weakness, cataracts, glaucoma, osteoporosis.

PRINCIPAL USES
To treat numerous conditions that involve inflammation (a response by body tissues, producing redness, warmth, swelling, and pain). Such conditions include arthritis, allergic reactions, asthma, some skin diseases, multiple sclerosis flare-ups, and other autoimmune diseases. Also prescribed to treat deficiency of natural steroid hormones.

HOW THE DRUG WORKS
Prednisone mimics the effects of the body's natural corticosteroid hormones. It depresses the synthesis, release, and activity of inflammation-producing body chemicals. It also suppresses the activity of the immune system.

DOSAGE
Adults and teenagers— For severe inflammation or to suppress the immune system: 5 to 100 mg a day in divided doses. For multiple sclerosis: 200 mg daily for 1 week, then 80 mg every other day for 1 month. Children— Consult your pediatrician.

ONSET OF EFFECT
Variable.

DURATION OF ACTION
Variable.

DIETARY ADVICE
It can be taken with food or milk to minimize stomach upset. Your doctor may recommend a low-salt, high-potassium, high-protein diet.

STORAGE
Store in a tightly sealed container away from heat, moisture, and direct light. Do not allow liquid forms to freeze.

IF YOU MISS A DOSE
Take it as soon as you remember. If you take several doses a day and it is close to the next dose, double the next dose. If you take 1 dose a day and you do not remember until the next day, skip the missed dose and do not double the next dose.

STOPPING THE DRUG
With long-term therapy, do not stop taking the drug abruptly; the dosage should be decreased gradually.

PROLONGED USE
Long-term use may lead to cataracts, diabetes, hypertension, or osteoporosis; see your doctor for regular examinations.

PRECAUTIONS
Over 60: Adverse reactions may be more likely and more severe.

Driving and Hazardous Work: Avoid such activities until you determine how the medicine affects you.

Alcohol: May cause stomach problems; avoid it unless your physician approves occasional moderate drinking.

Pregnancy: Overuse during pregnancy can retard the child's growth and cause other developmental problems.

Breast Feeding: Do not use this drug while nursing.

Infants and Children: Prednisone may retard the growth and development of bone and other tissues.

Special Concerns: This drug can lower resistance to infection. Avoid immunizations with live vaccines. Patients undergoing long-term therapy should wear a medical-alert bracelet. Call your doctor if you develop a fever.

OVERDOSE
Symptoms: Fever, muscle or joint pain, nausea, dizziness, fainting, difficulty breathing. Prolonged overuse: Moonface, obesity, unusual hair growth, acne, loss of sexual function, muscle wasting.

What to Do: Call your doctor, emergency medical services (EMS), or the nearest poison control center immediately.

DRUG INTERACTIONS
Consult your doctor for specific advice if you are taking aminoglutethimide, antacids, barbiturates, carbamazepine, griseofulvin, mitotane, phenylbutazone, phenytoin, primidone, rifampin, injectable amphotericin B, oral antidiabetes agents, insulin, digitalis drugs, diuretics, or medications containing potassium or sodium.

FOOD INTERACTIONS
Avoid excess sodium.

DISEASE INTERACTIONS
Consult your doctor if you have a history of bone disease, chicken pox, measles, gastrointestinal disorders, diabetes, recent serious infection, glaucoma, heart disease, hypertension, liver or kidney disorders, high blood cholesterol, thyroid problems, myasthenia gravis, or lupus.

Primaquine

Generic 26.3 mg
(SANOFI WINTHROP)

▶ Drug Class: Anti-
  infective/antimalarial

▶ Available in: Tablets

▶ Available OTC? No

▶ As Generic? Yes

Side Effects

SERIOUS
Discontinue taking pri-
maquine and consult
your doctor immediately
if your urine is markedly
darker than usual. Other
serious side effects
include unusual fatigue;
pain in the back, legs, or
stomach; loss of appetite;
pale skin; fever; blue
fingernails, lips, or skin;
difficulty breathing;
dizziness or lightheaded-
ness. Call your doctor
immediately.

COMMON
Stomach cramps or pain,
nausea and vomiting.

LESS COMMON
Low white blood cell
counts causing sore
throat, fever, or other
signs of infection (rare).

PRINCIPAL USES
To prevent relapses of
malaria caused by the proto-
zoans Plasmodium vivax
and Plasmodium ovale. It is
used after chloroquine treatment has been completed,
or following preventive therapy with chloroquine in people who have had heavy
exposure to these forms
of malaria.

HOW THE DRUG WORKS
Primaquine alters the DNA
and interferes with the
energy-producing biological
processes of the protozoa.

DOSAGE
Adults and teenagers: One
26.3 mg tablet (15 mg base)
once a day for 14 days; in
patients with mild G6PD
deficiency, 3 tablets (45 mg
base) weekly for 8 weeks; in
patients with severe G6PD
deficiency, 2 tablets (30 mg
base) weekly for 30 weeks.
Some strains of Plasmodium
vivax (particularly those
from Southeast Asia), may
require a higher dose of
39.4 to 52.6 mg once a day
for 14 days. Consult your
doctor. Children age 12 and
under: 0.68 mg (0.39 mg
base) per 2.2 lbs (1 kg) of
body weight once a day for
14 days.

ONSET OF EFFECT
Unknown.

DURATION OF ACTION
Unknown.

DIETARY ADVICE
Primaquine can be taken
with food or juice to minimize stomach upset. Notify
your doctor if you experience persistent stomach
upset with pain, nausea,
or vomiting.

STORAGE
Store in a tightly sealed container away from heat, moisture, and direct light.

IF YOU MISS A DOSE
Take it as soon as you
remember. However, if it is
near the time for the next
dose, skip the missed dose
and resume your regular
dosage schedule. Do not
double the next dose.

STOPPING THE DRUG
Take it as prescribed for the
full treatment period, even if
you begin to feel better
before the scheduled end of
therapy.

PROLONGED USE
See your doctor regularly
for blood tests and examinations if you must take this
medicine for a prolonged
period.

PRECAUTIONS
Over 60: Adverse reactions
may be more likely and
more severe in older
patients.

**Driving and Hazardous
Work:** Do not drive or
engage in hazardous work
until you determine how the
medicine affects you.

Alcohol: No special precautions are necessary.

Pregnancy: Primaquine
should not be used during
pregnancy. Before you take
primaquine, tell your doctor
if you are pregnant or plan
to become pregnant.

Breast Feeding: Primaquine may pass into breast
milk; caution is advised.
Consult your doctor for
advice.

Infants and Children:
Adverse reactions may be
more likely and more
severe in children.

Special Concerns: You
should not take primaquine
if you are taking or have
taken quinacrine within the
previous 3 months. If you
are of Mediterranean,
African, or East Asian
ancestry, you may be at
higher risk for side effects
due to a deficiency of the
enzyme glucose-6-phosphate
dehydrogenase (G6PD);
consult your doctor.

OVERDOSE
Symptoms: Weakness,
pale, sickly appearance,
shortness of breath, severe
abdominal cramps, vomit-
ing, heartbeat irregularities.

What to Do: Call your
doctor, emergency medical
services (EMS), or the
nearest poison control center immediately.

DRUG INTERACTIONS
Consult your physician for
specific advice if you are
taking quinacrine or any
drugs that may cause ane-
mia (such as sulfonamides
and nitrofurans) or bone
marrow suppression
(including methotrexate,
phenylbutazone, and chlo-
ramphenicol). Also, tell your
physician if you are taking
any other prescription or
over-the-counter drug.

FOOD INTERACTIONS
No known food interactions.

DISEASE INTERACTIONS
You should not take pri-
maquine if you are acutely
ill with a disease that may
reduce white blood cell
counts, such as rheumatoid
arthritis or lupus erythematosus. Consult your doctor if you have a family
history of favism or
hemolytic anemia, G6PD
deficiency, or a deficiency of
nicotinamide adenine dinu-
cleotide (NADH).

Primidone

BRAND NAMES
Myidone, Mysoline

Mysoline 250 mg
(**Wyeth-Ayerst**)

▶ Drug Class: Anticonvulsant

▶ Available in: Tablets, suspension

▶ Available OTC? No

▶ As Generic? Yes

Side Effects

SERIOUS
Fever, sore throat, swollen glands, red or purple point-like rash on the skin or mucous membranes, blistering or peeling skin lesions, mouth sores, easy bruising, paleness, weakness, confusion, lethargy, or seizures may be a sign of a potentially fatal blood reaction or other complication. Call your doctor immediately.

COMMON
Drowsiness, dizziness, loss of coordination, double vision, hyperactivity (in children).

LESS COMMON
Loss of appetite, mental or mood changes, nausea or vomiting, impotence, mild rash, lethargy followed by insomnia. There are numerous additional side effects associated with this drug; consult your doctor if you are concerned about any adverse or unusual reactions.

PRINCIPAL USES
To control certain types of seizures due to epilepsy.

HOW THE DRUG WORKS
Primidone is thought to depress the activity of certain parts of the brain and suppress the abnormal firing of neurons that causes seizures.

DOSAGE
Adults: 500 to 1,000 mg (or more) a day, in 3 or 4 divided doses. Children: 10 to 20 mg a day, in 3 or 4 divided doses. A low dose is used to start, and gradually increased.

ONSET OF EFFECT
Several hours.

DURATION OF ACTION
Maximum effectiveness:12 hours or longer; effectiveness then gradually decreases.

DIETARY ADVICE
Take with food to help avoid stomach upset.

STORAGE
Store in a tightly sealed container away from heat, moisture, and direct light. Do not freeze the liquid form.

IF YOU MISS A DOSE
Take it as soon as you remember. If it is near the time for the next dose, skip the missed dose and resume regular dosage schedule. Do not double the next dose, unless so advised by your doctor.

STOPPING THE DRUG
Never stop this drug abruptly; seizures may ensue. Your doctor will taper the dose gradually over a period of weeks to months.

PROLONGED USE
This drug is typically taken for prolonged periods. See your doctor regularly for tests and examinations.

PRECAUTIONS
Over 60: Older patients may require lower doses to minimize side effects.

Driving and Hazardous Work: This drug may cause drowsiness or dizziness. Do not drive or engage in hazardous work until you determine how it affects you.

Alcohol: May contribute to excessive drowsiness.

Pregnancy: Birth defects and bleeding problems in the mother have been reported in association with primidone use during pregnancy. Scientific studies are incomplete. However, seizures during pregnancy also increase the risks to the fetus. Discuss with your doctor the potential risks and benefits of using this drug during pregnancy. Folate supplementation is recommended beginning 1 to 2 months before conception and throughout the course of pregnancy.

Breast Feeding: Primidone passes into breast milk, although at low levels. Consult your doctor for advice.

Infants and Children: Adverse reactions may be more likely and more severe in children.

Special Concerns: The generic version of this drug is not recommended. Do not change the brand of primidone you are taking without consulting your doctor. The suspension form of primidone should be shaken well before you take it. Your doctor may want you to carry an ID card or bracelet saying that you are taking this drug.

OVERDOSE
Symptoms: Drowsiness, breathing problems, loss of consciousness.

What to Do: Call your doctor, emergency medical services (EMS), or the nearest poison control center immediately.

DRUG INTERACTIONS
Primidone may interact with other drugs, including other anticonvulsants (phenytoin, carbamazepine, clonazepam, valproic acid), benzodiazepines, caffeine, calcium channel blockers, corticosteroids, corticotropin, cyclophosphamide, cyclosporine, dacarbazine, digitoxin, disopyramide, doxycycline, general anesthetics, griseofulvin, H1 blockers, haloperidol, isoniazid, ketamine, levothyroxine, loxapine, maprotiline, metoprolol, mexiletine, phenytoin, propranolol, quinidine, theophylline, tricyclic antidepressants, vitamin D, and warfarin. May decrease the effectiveness of oral contraceptives, causing contraceptive failure.

FOOD INTERACTIONS
No known food interactions.

DISEASE INTERACTIONS
Caution is advised if you have asthma, chronic lung disease, hyperactivity (in children), kidney or liver disease, or porphyria.

Probenecid

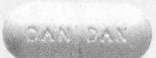

Generic 500 mg
(Schein)

▸ Drug Class: Antigout drug;
adjunct to antibiotic therapy

▸ Available in: Tablets

▸ Available OTC? No

▸ As Generic? Yes

Side Effects

SERIOUS
Rapid or irregular heartbeat; puffiness or swelling around eyes; trouble breathing; tightness in chest; changes in skin color; rash, hives, or itching; bloody or cloudy urine; difficult urination; lower back or side pain; sores, ulcers, or white spots on lips or in mouth; sore throat and fever; sudden decrease in urine; swollen face, fingers, feet, or lower legs; swollen or painful glands; unusual bleeding or bruising; unusual fatigue; yellow discoloration of the eyes or skin; unusual weight gain. Call your doctor immediately.

COMMON
Headache, redness, pain or swelling in joints, loss of appetite, nausea or vomiting.

LESS COMMON
Dizziness, reddened face, frequent urge to urinate, sore gums.

PRINCIPAL USES
To treat chronic gout and gouty arthritis—specifically, to lower the uric acid level in hopes of preventing future gout attacks. Probenecid is also prescribed to enhance the action of certain antibiotics when treating infections.

HOW THE DRUG WORKS
Gout occurs when excessive amounts of uric acid build up in the blood. This leads to the formation of uric-acid-based crystals that are deposited in the joints, causing inflammation and leading to the sharp, excruciating pain of a gout attack. Probenecid promotes excretion of excess uric acid from the body and so eases or prevents gout attacks. Probenecid also slows the body's removal of antibiotics, thus increasing their levels in the blood and prolonging their duration of action.

DOSAGE
For gout— 250 mg, 2 times a day for first week, then 500 mg, 2 times a day, to maximum of 2,000 mg per day. For antibiotic therapy with penicillin— 500 mg, 4 times a day. Children ages 2 to 14: 25 mg per 2.2 lbs (1 kg) of body weight to start, then 25 mg per 2.2 lbs in 4 daily doses. To treat gonorrhea— 1 g of probenecid with or before 3.5 mg of ampicillin or 4.8 million units of injected penicillin.

ONSET OF EFFECT
To ease gout: Several months of therapy may be required before probenecid begins to prevent gout attacks. To suppress the excretion of antibiotics: 2 hours.

DURATION OF ACTION
For gout: Unknown. For enhancement of antibiotic therapy: 2 hours.

DIETARY ADVICE
It can be taken with food or antacids to reduce stomach upset. Drink 8 to 10 full glasses of water a day.

STORAGE
Store in a tightly sealed container away from heat and direct light.

IF YOU MISS A DOSE
Take it as soon as you remember. If it is near the time for the next dose, skip the missed dose and resume your regular dosage schedule. Do not double the next dose.

STOPPING THE DRUG
The decision to stop taking the drug should be made by your doctor.

PROLONGED USE
See your doctor regularly for tests and examinations if you take this drug for a prolonged period. Gout attacks may continue for a while after you start taking probenecid.

PRECAUTIONS
Over 60: No special problems are expected.

Driving and Hazardous Work: Avoid such activities until you determine how the medicine affects you.

Alcohol: Avoid alcohol.

Pregnancy: Probenecid has not been shown to cause problems during pregnancy.

Breast Feeding: Probenecid may pass into breast milk; caution is advised. Consult your doctor for advice.

Infants and Children: Not recommended for use by children under age 2.

Special Concerns: Before you have any medical tests, be sure to tell the doctor you are taking probenecid.

OVERDOSE
Symptoms: Nausea, vomiting, diarrhea, seizures.

What to Do: Call your doctor, emergency medical services (EMS), or the nearest poison control center immediately.

DRUG INTERACTIONS
Consult your doctor for specific advice if you are taking anticancer (chemotherapy) medications, aspirin or other salicylates, heparin, indomethacin, ketoprofen, methotrexate, medicine for any type of infection, nitrofurantoin, or zidovudine.

FOOD INTERACTIONS
None are likely, but a low-purine diet is recommended to reduce the risk of gout attacks. Foods high in purines include anchovies, sardines, legumes, poultry, sweetbreads, liver, kidneys, and other organ meats.

DISEASE INTERACTIONS
Caution is advised when taking probenecid. Consult your doctor if you have a blood disease, cancer, kidney disease or kidney stones, or a stomach ulcer.

Procainamide Hydrochloride

Generic 500 mg
(ZENITH)

Additional photographs

▶ Drug Class: Antiarrhythmic

▶ Available in: Capsules, tablets, extended-release tablets, injection

▶ Available OTC? No

▶ As Generic? Yes

Side Effects

SERIOUS
Fainting; rapid or irregular heartbeat (palpitations); fever and chills; joint pain or swelling; painful breathing; skin rash or itching; confusion; sore mouth, gums, or throat; hallucinations; depression; unusual bleeding or bruising; unusual fatigue. Call your doctor immediately.

COMMON
Diarrhea, abdominal pain, nausea, vomiting, loss of appetite.

LESS COMMON
Dizziness, lightheadedness, weakness, dry mouth.

PRINCIPAL USES
To treat irregular heartbeats (cardiac arrhythmias).

HOW THE DRUG WORKS
Procainamide hydrochloride slows nerve impulses in the heart and reduces the sensitivity of heart tissue to certain nerve impulses, thus stabilizing the heartbeat.

DOSAGE
Tablets and capsules— Adults: 500 to 1,000 mg every 4 to 6 hours. Children: 12.5 mg per 2.2 lbs (1 kg) of body weight 4 times a day. Extended-release tablets— 1,000 to 2,000 mg every 12 hours.

ONSET OF EFFECT
Oral: 60 to 90 minutes. Injection: immediate.

DURATION OF ACTION
From 3 to 8 hours (longer in patients with kidney disease or heart failure).

DIETARY ADVICE
Procainamide should be taken with a glass of water on an empty stomach 1 hour before or 2 hours after meals.

STORAGE
Store in a tightly sealed container away from heat and direct light.

IF YOU MISS A DOSE
Take a missed dose as soon as you remember. If it is near the time for the next dose, skip the missed dose and resume your regular dosage schedule. Do not double the next dose.

STOPPING THE DRUG
Take as prescribed for the full treatment period, even if you begin to feel better before the scheduled end of therapy. The decision to stop taking the drug should be made by your doctor.

PROLONGED USE
Lifelong therapy may be necessary. See your doctor regularly for examinations and diagnostic tests if you must take this medicine for a prolonged period.

PRECAUTIONS
Over 60: Adverse reactions may be more likely and more severe in older patients.

Driving and Hazardous Work: Do not drive or engage in hazardous work until you determine how the medicine affects you.

Alcohol: Avoid alcohol.

Pregnancy: Procainamide has not been shown to cause problems during pregnancy. In any case, if you are taking this drug, be sure to tell your doctor if you are pregnant or plan to become pregnant.

Breast Feeding: Procainamide passes into breast milk. Consult your doctor for specific advice.

Infants and Children: Procainamide has not been shown to cause problems in limited use in children.

Special Concerns: Your doctor may want you to carry a medical identification card or bracelet saying you use procainamide. Before having any kind of surgical procedure or medical test, tell the doctor or dentist in charge that you are taking procainamide.

OVERDOSE
Symptoms: Confusion, severe dizziness, fainting, rapid or irregular heartbeat, decrease in urination, nausea or vomiting.

What to Do: Call your doctor, emergency medical services (EMS), or the nearest poison control center immediately.

DRUG INTERACTIONS
Consult your doctor for specific advice if you are taking other antiarrhythmics, drugs for high blood pressure, antimyasthenics, pimozide, or antihistamines.

FOOD INTERACTIONS
No known food interactions.

DISEASE INTERACTIONS
Consult your doctor if you have any of the following: heart block, asthma, myasthenia gravis, or systemic lupus erythematosus. Use of procainamide may cause complications in patients with liver or kidney disease, since these organs work together to remove the medication from the body.

Procarbazine Hydrochloride

▶ Drug Class: Antineoplastic (anticancer) agent

▶ Available in: Capsules

▶ Available OTC? No

▶ As Generic? No

Side Effects

SERIOUS

Severe chest pain; dilated pupils; rapid or slowed heartbeat; severe headache; sensitivity of eyes to light; increased sweating; stiff neck; black, tarry stools; blood in urine or stools; bloody vomit; cough or hoarseness; fever and chills; pain in lower back or flanks; painful or difficult urination; tiny bright red spots on skin; unusual bleeding or bruising; confusion; seizures; hallucinations; absent menstrual periods; shortness of breath; thickened bronchial (lung) secretions; diarrhea; sores in mouth and on the lips; tingling or numbness of fingers or toes; incoordination or unsteady gait; yellowish tinge to eyes or skin. Such side effects may mean that normal blood cells and special blood-clotting cells have been affected, or that the immune system has been affected and an infection is developing. See your doctor immediately.

COMMON

Drowsiness, muscle or joint pain, muscle twitching, nausea or vomiting, nervousness, restlessness, nightmares, insomnia, unusual fatigue.

LESS COMMON

Constipation, darkened skin, difficulty swallowing, lightheadedness when arising, dry mouth, loss of appetite, depression, flushing of the face.

PRINCIPAL USES

To treat Hodgkin's disease (a cancer affecting the spleen and lymph nodes). Procarbazine is usually only one drug of several given in combination with other chemotherapy agents to fight cancer.

HOW THE DRUG WORKS

Procarbazine kills cancer cells by interfering with the activity of their genetic material, which prevents the cells from reproducing. The drug may also affect the growth and development of other kinds of cells in the body, resulting in unpleasant side effects. Procarbazine is also a weak inhibitor of the enzyme known as monoamine oxidase (MAO); MAO inhibitors are routinely prescribed to treat depression, although this has no impact on procarbazine's function as a cancer-fighting drug.

DOSAGE

Adults: 2 to 4 mg per 2.2 lbs (1 kg) of body weight per day for first week. Then 4 to 6 mg per 2.2 lbs per day until the blood cell count falls substantially. Then 1 to 2 mg per 2.2 lbs per day. Children: 50 mg per square meter of body surface per day for first week, then 100 mg per square meter of body surface per day until toxicity occurs, then 50 mg per square meter of body surface per day.

ONSET OF EFFECT

Unknown.

DURATION OF ACTION

Unknown.

DIETARY ADVICE

Maintain adequate food and fluid intake. Calorie, protein, and vitamin needs increase in patients with cancer. Good nutrition is essential to cope with the demands of chemotherapy. Foods high in the substance tyramine must be eliminated from the diet during therapy; see Special Concerns and Food Interactions for further information.

STORAGE

Store in a tightly sealed container away from heat and direct light. Unopened vials should be refrigerated but not allowed to freeze.

IF YOU MISS A DOSE

If you miss a dose, take it as soon as you remember. If it is near the time for the next dose, skip the missed dose and resume your regular dosage schedule. Do not double the next dose.

STOPPING THE DRUG

The decision to stop taking the drug should be made by your doctor.

PROLONGED USE

You should see your doctor regularly for tests and examinations if you take this drug for a prolonged period.

PRECAUTIONS

Over 60: Adverse reactions may be more likely and more severe in older patients.

Driving and Hazardous Work: Do not drive or engage in hazardous work until you determine how the medicine affects you.

Alcohol: Avoid alcohol.

Pregnancy: Procarbazine can cause birth defects if either the father or mother takes it. Consult your doctor for specific advice if you are pregnant or plan to become pregnant. Use of a reliable method of birth control is recommended throughout the duration of therapy with procarbazine.

Breast Feeding: Procarbazine passes into breast milk; avoid or discontinue use of this drug while breast feeding.

Infants and Children: Procarbazine is not expected to cause different problems in infants and children than it does in older persons.

Special Concerns: Like all drugs categorized as MAO inhibitors, procarbazine prevents the liver and other body tissues from neutralizing a substance called tyramine, which, in the bloodstream, causes a sudden increase in blood pressure. Therefore, foods high in tyramines must be avoided while undergoing therapy with procarbazine. Such foods include aged cheeses, processed meats, many varieties of dried or preserved foods, as well as certain kinds of liquor and wine (especially red wine). See Food Interactions for a more complete list of foods and beverages high in tyramines. While taking procarbazine, do not receive any immunizations without consulting your doctor. Avoid people with infections and those who have recently had oral polio vaccine. Be careful when using a toothbrush, dental floss, or toothpick. Check with your doctor before having any dental work done. If you are going to have surgery, tell the doctor or dentist in charge that you are taking procarbazine. Do not touch your eyes or the inside of your nose unless you have just washed your hands. Be careful not to cut yourself when using sharp objects such as a razor. Avoid contact sports and other activities during which bruising could occur.

Procarbazine Hydrochloride (continued)

OVERDOSE

Symptoms: Nausea, vomiting, diarrhea, tremors, seizures, loss of consciousness, very low blood pressure, coma.

What to Do: Call your doctor, emergency medical services (EMS), or the nearest poison control center immediately.

DRUG INTERACTIONS

Consult your doctor for specific advice if you are taking amantadine, anticholinergics, diabetes medicine, antidyskinetics, antihistamines, antipsychotics, buclizine, central nervous system depressants, cyclizine, disopyramide, flavoxate, ipratropium, meclizine, orphenadrine, oxybutynin, procainamide, promethazine, quinidine, trimeprazine, amphetamines, diet pills, dextromethorphan, levodopa, asthma or cold medicine, methyldopa, methylphenidate, narcotic pain medicine, amphotericin B, antithyroid agents, azathioprine, chloramphenicol, colchicine, flucytosine, interferon, plicamycin, zidovudine, buspirone, carbamazepine, cyclobenzaprine, maprotiline, other MAO inhibitors, antidepressants, fluoxetine, guanadrel, guanethidine, or rauwolfia alkaloids.

FOOD INTERACTIONS

Avoid tyramine-rich foods, which include aged cheeses, avocados, banana skins, bean curd, bologna and other processed lunch meats, chicken livers, chocolate, figs, canned or dried fish, pickled herring, meat extracts, pepperoni, raisins, raspberries, unpasteurized beer, Chianti, sherry, vermouth, and red wines in general. Also avoid caffeine-rich beverages or foods.

DISEASE INTERACTIONS

Caution is advised when taking procarbazine. Consult your doctor if you have a history of any of the following: alcoholism, angina, recent heart attack or stroke, chicken pox, shingles, epilepsy, frequent headaches, infection, kidney disease, liver disease, mental illness, overactive thyroid, Parkinson's disease, or pheochromocytoma.

Prochlorperazine

BRAND NAMES
Compa-Z, Compazine,
Compazine Spansule,
Contrazine

Compazine 5 mg
(SMITHKLINE BEECHAM)

▶ Drug Class: Neuroleptic;
antiemetic

▶ Available in: Extended-
release capsules, syrup,
tablets, suppositories,
injection

▶ Available OTC? No

▶ As Generic? Yes

Side Effects

SERIOUS
Rapid heartbeat, profuse
sweating, seizures, difficulty breathing, neck stiffness, swelling of the
tongue, difficulty swal-
lowing. Also a rare condition can develop called
neuroleptic malignant
syndrome, characterized
by stiffness or spasms of
the muscles, high fever,
and confusion or disori-
entation. Call your doctor
immediately.

COMMON
Nausea, reduced sweat-
ing, dry mouth, blurred
vision, drowsiness, shak-
ing of hands, stiffness,
stooped posture.

LESS COMMON
Difficult urination, men-
strual irregularities,
breast pain or swelling,
unexpected weight gain,
uncontrolled movements
of the tongue, fever,
chills, sore throat,
unusual bruising or
bleeding, heart palpita-
tions, skin rash, itching,
increased sensitivity of
the skin to sunlight.

PRINCIPAL USES
To treat severe nausea and
vomiting.

HOW THE DRUG WORKS
Prochlorperazine sup-
presses activity in the trigger zones of the brain and
gastrointestinal tract that
govern the vomiting reflex.

DOSAGE
Usual adult dose: Initially,
5 to 10 mg, 3 or 4 times a
day. Injection: 10 to 20 mg
injected into a muscle every
4 to 6 hours. Your doctor
may increase the dose as
needed and tolerated.

ONSET OF EFFECT
30 to 40 minutes for oral
forms; 60 minutes for suppository; 10 to 20 minutes
after injection.

DURATION OF ACTION
3 to 4 hours; 12 hours for
extended-release capsules.

DIETARY ADVICE
Can be taken with food or a
full glass of milk or water.

STORAGE
Store in a tightly sealed container away from heat and
direct light.

IF YOU MISS A DOSE
Take it as soon as you
remember. If it is near the
time for the next dose, skip
the missed dose and
resume your regular dosage
schedule. Do not double the
next dose.

STOPPING THE DRUG
The decision to stop taking
the drug should be made by
your doctor.

PROLONGED USE
See your doctor regularly
for tests and examinations if
you must take this medicine
for a prolonged period.

PRECAUTIONS
Over 60: Adverse reactions
are more common in elderly
patients. A lower dose may
be warranted.

**Driving and Hazardous
Work:** Do not drive or
engage in hazardous work
until you determine how the
medicine affects you.

Alcohol: Avoid alcohol.

Pregnancy: Avoid using
this drug if you are pregnant or plan to become
pregnant.

Breast Feeding: Either
avoid taking the drug if possible or refrain from breast
feeding.

Infants and Children:
Adverse reactions may be
more likely and more
severe in children.

Special Concerns: Avoid
prolonged exposure to high
temperatures or hot cli-
mates while taking prochlorperazine. Drink plenty of
fluids and try to stay cool
in the summertime. Avoid
overexposure to sunlight
until you determine if the
drug heightens your skin's
sensitivity to ultraviolet radiation and increases your
risk of sunburn.

OVERDOSE
Symptoms: Extreme
drowsiness, heartbeat irregularities, dry mouth, paradoxical restlessness or
agitation, seizures, loss
of consciousness.

What to Do: Call your
doctor, emergency medical
services (EMS), or the
nearest poison control center immediately.

DRUG INTERACTIONS
Consult your doctor for specific advice if you are taking
anticholinergics, anticonvulsants, antidepressants, antihistamines, antihyperten-
sives, bupropion, central
nervous system depressants
such as barbiturates, clozapine, dronabinol, ethinamate,
fluoxetine, guanethidine,
guanfacine, lithium, methyldopa, carbamazepine,
rifampin, or trihexyphenidyl.

FOOD INTERACTIONS
None known.

DISEASE INTERACTIONS
Consult your doctor if you
have a history of alcohol
abuse, any blood disorder,
breast cancer, benign prostatic hyperplasia (BPH),
epilepsy or seizures, glaucoma, heart, lung, or blood
vessel disease, liver disease,
Parkinson's disease, peptic
ulcer, or urinary difficulty.

Procyclidine

BRAND NAME
Kemadrin

Kemadrin 5 mg
(GLAXO WELLCOME)

▶ Drug Class: Antiparkinsonism drug

▶ Available in: Tablets

▶ Available OTC? No

▶ As Generic? No

Side Effects

SERIOUS
Confusion, severe drowsiness, rapid heartbeat, hallucinations, glaucoma.

COMMON
Blurred vision; constipation; dry mouth, nose, and throat.

LESS COMMON
Dizziness and lightheadedness, loss of memory, nausea.

PRINCIPAL USES
To treat Parkinson's disease and Parkinson-like syndromes, which can occur as a result of injury to or infection of the central nervous system, damage to blood vessels in the brain, or exposure to certain toxins.

HOW THE DRUG WORKS
Procyclidine promotes the release of dopamine in the brain. Dopamine is a chemical that is necessary for both the initiation and smooth control of voluntary muscle movement.

DOSAGE
Adults: To start, 2.5 mg, 3 times a day. The dosage is increased gradually to 5 mg, 3 times a day. Children: This drug has not been extensively studied in children; consult a pediatrician.

ONSET OF EFFECT
Within 1 hour.

DURATION OF ACTION
From 6 to 12 hours.

DIETARY ADVICE
Procyclidine should be taken after meals to prevent nausea.

STORAGE
Store in a tightly sealed container away from heat, moisture, and direct light.

IF YOU MISS A DOSE
Take it as soon as you remember, unless the time for your next scheduled dose is within the next 2 hours. If so, skip the missed dose and resume your regular dosage schedule. Do not double the next dose.

STOPPING THE DRUG
The decision to stop taking the drug should be made in consultation with your doctor. The dosage should be decreased gradually.

PROLONGED USE
No special difficulties are expected with long-term use of procyclidine.

PRECAUTIONS
Over 60: Adverse reactions may be more likely and more severe in older patients. Procyclidine should be used cautiously in patients in this age group. If higher doses are needed, it is best to increase the dose very gradually.

Driving and Hazardous Work: Procyclidine can cause drowsiness or confusion. Do not drive or engage in hazardous work until you determine how it affects you.

Alcohol: Avoid alcohol; combined with the medication, alcohol is likely to cause or worsen confusion.

Pregnancy: This medication should not be used in pregnant women.

Breast Feeding: It is not known to what degree procyclidine passes into breast milk. Nursing mothers should avoid use of this medication.

Infants and Children: There is little known about the safety and effectiveness of procyclidine in infants and children. Consult your pediatrician to discuss the use of this drug in children.

Special Concerns: Procyclidine can cause or worsen glaucoma (the buildup of excessive pressure within the eye, and a leading cause of blindness). See your ophthalmologist regularly for periodic monitoring of eye pressure.

OVERDOSE
Symptoms: Clumsiness, seizures, severe mouth dryness, drowsiness, hallucinations, loss of consciousness.

What to Do: Call your doctor, emergency medical services (EMS), or the nearest poison control center immediately.

DRUG INTERACTIONS
Procyclidine may interact with many drugs, in particular drugs that depress the central nervous system (such as alcohol, barbiturates, and other sleep-inducing drugs) and MAO inhibitor antidepressants (such as phenelzine sulfate and tranylcypromine sulfate). Consult your doctor if you are taking these drugs.

FOOD INTERACTIONS
No known food interactions.

DISEASE INTERACTIONS
Caution is advised when taking procyclidine. Consult your doctor if you have any of the following: irregular heartbeat or heart rhythm abnormalities, glaucoma, intestinal obstruction, urinary retention or trouble urinating, or enlarged prostate (benign prostatic hyperplasia).

Progesterone Intrauterine System

▶ Drug Class: Progestin (hormone)

▶ Available in: Intrauterine device

▶ Available OTC? No

▶ As Generic? Yes

Side Effects

SERIOUS
Severe abdominal pain or cramping; faintness, dizziness, or sharp pain at time of IUD insertion; heavy or unexpected uterine bleeding between periods; fever; odorous discharge; unusual fatigue; any unusual uterine bleeding. Call your doctor immediately.

COMMON
No common side effects are associated with use of the progesterone IUD.

LESS COMMON
There are no less-common side effects associated with use of the progesterone IUD.

PRINCIPAL USES
As a contraceptive (birth control method).

HOW THE DRUG WORKS
Progesterone inhibits the secretion of pituitary hormones that in turn regulate menstrual and reproductive cycles; it also alters the activity of uterine cells.

DOSAGE
1 intrauterine device (IUD) is inserted into the vagina by a health professional and replaced within 12 months.

ONSET OF EFFECT
Within days.

DURATION OF ACTION
1 year.

DIETARY ADVICE
The IUD can be used without regard to diet.

STORAGE
Not applicable.

IF YOU MISS A DOSE
Not applicable; the IUD remains implanted in the body for the entire duration of use.

STOPPING THE DRUG
Consult your gynecologist if you decide you no longer wish to use the IUD.

PROLONGED USE
You should check for the IUD thread every month, especially after each menstrual period. Wash your hands thoroughly before checking. Use your middle fingers to find the thread inside the cervix. Do not pull on the thread. If you cannot find the thread, call your gynecologist.

PRECAUTIONS
Over 60: Not applicable to patients over 60.

Driving and Hazardous Work: The use of a progesterone IUD should not impair your ability to perform such tasks safely.

Alcohol: No special precautions are necessary.

Pregnancy: This IUD should not be used during pregnancy or by a woman who has had an ectopic pregnancy.

Breast Feeding: The progesterone IUD has not been shown to cause problems in nursing babies. Its use is recommended for women who require contraception while breast-feeding.

Infants and Children: Sexually active teenagers are urged to use a contraceptive method (for example, condoms) that protects them against sexually transmitted diseases; this IUD does not. Teenagers who have not given birth generally have more side effects than teenagers or adults who have. The IUD may move out of place, harming the uterus or cervix. Abdominal pain and increased menstrual bleeding are more common in teenagers than in older women.

Special Concerns: It is possible for pregnancy to occur while using the progesterone-containing IUD. Notify your doctor immediately if you feel the changes that can occur with pregnancy, such as enlarged or tender breasts, lack of menstrual period, unusual uterine bleeding, or pain and cramping in the lower abdomen. Until your doctor can see you, use another birth control method, such as condoms. If you think that the IUD has moved out of place, call your doctor immediately. If you think you are pregnant, do a home pregnancy test. Do not try to put the IUD in place inside the uterus yourself, nor try to remove it yourself.

OVERDOSE
Symptoms: Not applicable.

What to Do: Emergency instructions not applicable.

DRUG INTERACTIONS
The following drugs may interact with progesterone. Consult your doctor for specific advice if you are taking aminoglutethimide, carbamazepine, phenytoin, rifabutin, or rifampin.

FOOD INTERACTIONS
No known food interactions.

DISEASE INTERACTIONS
Caution is advised when using the progesterone IUD. Consult your doctor if you have any of the following conditions: uterine abnormalities or bleeding problems, acquired immunodeficiency syndrome (AIDS), a blood disorder, a heart defect, insulin-dependent diabetes, a recent sexually transmitted disease, abnormally slow heartbeat, or any recent surgery involving the uterus or fallopian tubes.

Progesterone Systemic and Topical

▶ Drug Class: Progestin (hormone)

▶ Available in: Injection, vaginal gel, capsules, suppositories

▶ Available OTC? No

▶ As Generic? Yes

Side Effects

SERIOUS
Changes in or cessation of menstrual bleeding; unexpected or increased flow of breast milk; mental depression; skin rash; loss of or change in speech, coordination, or vision; severe and sudden shortness of breath; severe headache. Call your doctor immediately.

COMMON
Stomach pain or cramping, swelling of face, ankles, or feet, mild headache, mood changes, unusual fatigue, weight gain, pain or irritation at site of injection.

LESS COMMON
Acne, breast pain or tenderness, hot flashes, insomnia, loss of sexual desire, loss or gain of scalp hair or body hair, brown spots on skin.

PRINCIPAL USES

To treat amenorrhea (cessation of menstruation) and abnormal uterine bleeding in the absence of structural pathology (such as uterine fibroids or uterine cancer). The vaginal gel is used as part of Assisted Reproductive Technology for infertile women with progesterone deficiency, and to promote menstruation in women with premature amenorrhea.

HOW THE DRUG WORKS

Progesterone inhibits the secretion of pituitary hormones that in turn regulate a woman's menstrual and reproductive cycles; it also alters the activity of cells in the uterine lining.

DOSAGE

Injection— For amenorrhea and abnormal uterine bleeding: 5 to 10 mg injected into a muscle daily for 6 to 10 days, or 150 mg injected into a muscle as a single dose. Your doctor may tell you to take estrogen for 2 weeks prior to receiving the injection. (Progesterone vaginal suppositories may be provided by a pharmacist in lieu of injections.) Vaginal gel— For amenorrhea: 45 mg (Crinone 4%) every other day, up to 6 doses. For progesterone supplementation: 90 mg (Crinone 8%), once a day. For progesterone replacement: 90 mg, 2 times a day. Capsules— For secondary amenorrhea: 400 mg once in the evening for 10 days.

ONSET OF EFFECT

Injection— For amenorrhea: 48 to 70 hours after the last injection. For uterine bleeding: Within 6 days. Treatment will be stopped if bleeding continues or recurs. Vaginal gel and capsules— Unknown.

DURATION OF ACTION

Unknown.

DIETARY ADVICE

Progesterone can be taken without regard to diet.

STORAGE

Store in a tightly sealed container away from heat and direct light. Do not allow gel to freeze.

IF YOU MISS A DOSE

Injection: Inject the drug as soon as you remember. However, if it is near the time for the next dose, skip the missed dose and resume your regular dosage schedule. Do not double the next dose. Vaginal gel: If you miss a dose, do not apply an excessive amount the next day. Resume regular dosage schedule. Capsules: If you miss a dose on one day, skip the missed dose and resume regular schedule. Do not double the next dose.

STOPPING THE DRUG

Consult your doctor.

PROLONGED USE

Consult your doctor about the need for periodic examinations and laboratory tests.

PRECAUTIONS

Over 60: No special problems are expected.

Driving and Hazardous Work: No special precautions are necessary.

Alcohol: No special precautions are necessary.

Pregnancy: This hormone should not be used during pregnancy. If you suspect a pregnancy, stop taking progesterone immediately and call your doctor. Before using injected progesterone, tell your doctor if you are pregnant or plan to become pregnant. The vaginal gel may be used safely as part of Assisted Reproductive Technology in progesterone-deficient women.

Breast Feeding: Progesterone passes into breast milk and may change the quality or quantity of milk. Discuss with your doctor the risks and benefits of using it while nursing.

Infants and Children: Safety and effectiveness have not been determined.

Special Concerns: You should have a Pap test at least every 6 months while receiving progesterone. Be alert for signs of excessive fluid retention in your body.

OVERDOSE

Symptoms: None.

What to Do: An overdose is unlikely to be life-threatening. However, if someone takes a much larger dose than prescribed or accidentally ingests the gel, seek emergency medical attention right away

DRUG INTERACTIONS

Consult your doctor for specific advice if you are taking aminoglutethimide, carbamazepine, phenytoin, rifabutin, or rifampin.

FOOD INTERACTIONS

Do not take the capsules if you are allergic to peanuts; they contain peanut oil.

DISEASE INTERACTIONS

Consult your doctor if you have any of the following: asthma, epilepsy, heart problems, circulation problems, migraine headaches, breast disease, bleeding problems, diabetes, high blood cholesterol, or central nervous system disorders such as depression. Use of progesterone may cause complications in patients with liver or kidney disease, since these organs work together to remove drugs and other substances from the body.

Promethazine Hydrochloride

Phenergan 25 mg
(Wyeth-Ayerst)

▶ Drug Class: Antihistamine

▶ Available in: Tablets, syrup, injection, suppositories

▶ Available OTC? No

▶ As Generic? Yes

Side Effects

SERIOUS
Sore throat and fever, unusual fatigue, unusual bleeding or bruising. Call your doctor immediately.

COMMON
Drowsiness, thickening of mucus.

LESS COMMON
Blurred vision; confusion; difficult or painful urination; dizziness; dry mouth, nose, or throat; increased sensitivity of skin to sunlight; faintness; increased sweating; stinging or burning of rectum (suppository form); loss of appetite; ringing or buzzing in ears; skin rash; fast heartbeat; unusual excitement or irritability.

PRINCIPAL USES
To relieve the symptoms of hay fever and other allergies, to prevent motion sickness, and to treat nausea and vomiting. Promethazine may also be used in some patients for its sedative effect.

HOW THE DRUG WORKS
Promethazine interferes with, but does not block, the release and action of histamine, a naturally occurring substance in the body that causes swelling, itching, sneezing, watery eyes, hives, and other symptoms of allergic reaction. Promethazine also has an anticholinergic effect, meaning it blocks the transmission of certain nerve impulses, which in turn relaxes the smooth muscle tissue controlling activity in the bladder, stomach, intestine, lungs, and other organ systems. This effect thereby helps to ease the symptoms of motion sickness, nausea, gastrointestinal upset, and anxiety.

DOSAGE
Tablets or syrup— For allergies: Adults and teenagers: 10 to 12.5 mg, 4 times a day before meals and at bedtime, or 25 mg at bedtime. Children 2 and older: 5 to 12.5 mg, 3 times a day, or 25 mg at bedtime. For nausea and vomiting: Adults and teenagers: 25 mg for first dose, then 10 to 25 mg every 4 to 6 hours as needed. Children 2 and older: 10 to 25 mg every 4 to 6 hours. To prevent motion sickness: Adults and teenagers: 25 mg taken 30 to 60 minutes before traveling. Children 2 and older: 10 to 25 mg, 30 to 60 minutes before traveling. For dizziness: Adults and teenagers: 25 mg, 2 times a day. Children 2 and older: 10 to 25, mg 2 times a day. As a

sedative: Adults and teenagers: 25 to 50 mg. Children 2 and older: 10 to 25 mg. Injection— For allergies: Adults and teenagers: 25 mg into a vein or muscle. Children 2 and older: 6.25 to 12.5 mg, 3 times a day into a muscle, or 25 mg at bedtime. For nausea and vomiting: Adults and teenagers: 12.5 to 25 mg every 4 hours into a vein or muscle. Children 2 and older: 12.5 to 25 mg every 4 to 6 hours into a muscle. As a sedative: Adults and teenagers: 25 to 50 mg injected into a vein or muscle. Children 2 and older: 12.5 to 25 mg into a muscle. Suppositories— For allergies: Adults and teenagers: 25 mg at first; 25 mg, 2 hours later if needed. Children 2 and older: 6.25 to 12.5 mg, 3 times a day, or 25 mg at bedtime. For nausea and vomiting: Adults and teenagers: 25 mg at first, then 12.5 to 25 mg every 4 to 6 hours if needed. Children 2 and older: 12.5 to 25 mg every 4 to 6 hours. For dizziness: Adults and teenagers: 25 mg, 2 times a day. Children 2 and older: 12.5 to 25 mg, 2 times a day. As a sedative: Adults and teenagers: 25 to 50 mg. Children 2 and older: 12.25 to 25 mg.

ONSET OF EFFECT
15 to 60 minutes orally or by suppository; 20 minutes after injection.

DURATION OF ACTION
Up to 12 hours.

DIETARY ADVICE
Take it with food or milk to lessen stomach irritation.

STORAGE
Store in a tightly sealed container away from heat and direct light at room temperature. Do not store the tablets in a place with

excessive moisture, such as the bathroom medicine cabinet. Do not allow the syrup or injection to freeze.

IF YOU MISS A DOSE
Take it as soon as you remember. If it is near the time for the next dose, skip the missed dose and resume your regular dosage schedule. Do not double the next dose.

STOPPING THE DRUG
You should take it as prescribed for the full treatment period, but you may stop taking the drug if you are feeling better before the scheduled end of therapy.

PROLONGED USE
See your doctor regularly if you take this medicine for a prolonged period. Prolonged use of this antihistamine may decrease salivary flow, which may lead to thrush (white, furry patches in the mouth caused by fungal infection), periodontal disease (disease and decay of the teeth, gums, jaw, and other supportive structures in the mouth), dental caries (cavities), and gingivitis (gum disease). Practice good oral hygiene to prevent these disorders.

PRECAUTIONS
Over 60: Adverse reactions may be more likely and more severe in older patients.

Driving and Hazardous Work: Do not drive or engage in hazardous work until you determine how the medicine affects you.

Alcohol: Avoid alcohol.

Pregnancy: Promethazine has not been shown to cause birth defects in animals. Thorough human studies have not been done. However, if the mother

Promethazine Hydrochloride (continued)

takes the drug within 2 weeks of delivery, the baby may have jaundice or problems with blood clotting. Before you take it, tell your doctor if you are pregnant or plan to become pregnant.

Breast Feeding: Promethazine passes into breast milk; avoid or discontinue use while nursing. The flow of breast milk may be decreased as a result of the medication.

Infants and Children: Adverse reactions, such as seizures, may be more common and more severe in infants and children. It is not recommended for children with a history of

breathing difficulty while sleeping or with a family history of sudden infant death syndrome (SIDS). Children and adolescents with signs of Reye's syndrome should not take promethazine, especially by injection. Promethazine's side effects may be mistaken for symptoms of Reye's syndrome.

Special Concerns: If you have an allergy test, stop taking promethazine 4 days before the test and tell the doctor that you were taking promethazine.

OVERDOSE

Symptoms: Clumsiness; insomnia; seizures; severe dryness of mouth, nose, or throat; redness of face; hallucinations; muscle spasms; trouble breathing; jerky movements of head and face; dizziness; trembling and shaking of hands.

What to Do: Call your doctor, emergency medical services (EMS), or the nearest poison control center immediately.

DRUG INTERACTIONS

Consult your doctor for specific advice if you are taking amoxapine, antipsychotics, medications containing alcohol, barbiturates, methyl-

dopa, metoclopramide, metyrosine, epinephrine, metrizamide, pemoline, pimozide, rauwolfia alkaloids, anticholinergics, central nervous system depressants, maprotiline, other antihistamines, tricyclic antidepressants, levodopa, or MAO inhibitors.

FOOD INTERACTIONS

No known food interactions.

DISEASE INTERACTIONS

Consult your doctor if you have any of the following: blood disease, heart or blood vessel disease, enlarged prostate, urinary tract blockage, epilepsy, glaucoma, Reye's syndrome, jaundice, or liver disease.

Propafenone

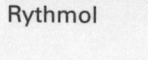

Rythmol 150 mg
(Knoll)

▶ Drug Class: Antiarrhythmic

▶ Available in: Tablets

▶ Available OTC? No

▶ As Generic? No

Side Effects

SERIOUS
Fast or irregular heartbeat, chest pain, shortness of breath, swelling of feet or lower legs. Call your doctor immediately.

COMMON
Dizziness, change in taste, bitter or metallic taste.

LESS COMMON
Blurred vision, headache, constipation or diarrhea, skin rash, dry mouth, nausea or vomiting, unusual fatigue.

PRINCIPAL USES
To correct heartbeat irregularities (cardiac arrhythmias).

HOW THE DRUG WORKS
Propafenone slows the conduction of nerve impulses in the heart and reduces the sensitivity of heart tissue to specific nerve impulses, which helps to stabilize heartbeat. It also has weak beta-blocking properties.

DOSAGE
Adults: 150 mg every 8 hours. It may be increased after 3 or 4 days to 225 mg every 8 hours, or 300 mg every 12 hours, up to a maximum of 300 mg every 8 hours. The maintenance dose will be determined by careful follow-up, including ECG and blood pressure monitoring. Lower doses may be required for the elderly and those with liver or heart disease.

ONSET OF EFFECT
1 hour.

DURATION OF ACTION
8 to 12 hours.

DIETARY ADVICE
Propafenone can be taken with food to minimize stomach upset.

STORAGE
Store in a tightly sealed container away from heat, moisture, and direct light.

IF YOU MISS A DOSE
Take it as soon as you remember, unless the time for your next scheduled dose is within the next 4 hours. If so, skip the missed dose and resume your regular dosage schedule. Do not double the next dose.

STOPPING THE DRUG
The decision to stop taking the drug should be made in conjunction with your doctor.

PROLONGED USE
Lifelong therapy may be necessary. See your doctor regularly for examinations and diagnostic tests if you must take this medicine for a prolonged period.

PRECAUTIONS
Over 60: The dose may need to be reduced.

Driving and Hazardous Work: Avoid such activities until you determine how the medication affects you.

Alcohol: Avoid alcohol.

Pregnancy: Adequate studies on the use of this drug during pregnancy have not been done. Before taking propafenone, tell your doctor if you are pregnant or plan to become pregnant.

Breast Feeding: Propafenone passes into breast milk; caution is advised. Consult your doctor for advice.

Infants and Children: The safety and efficacy of propafenone in infants and children have not been established. Limited use in young patients indicates that the incidence of side effects in younger persons is the same as for older patients. Consult your pediatrician for advice.

Special Concerns: Wearing a medical bracelet or carrying an identification card saying that you take this medication is recommended. Before having any kind of surgery, tell the doctor or dentist in charge that you use this drug.

OVERDOSE
Symptoms: Dizziness or faintness, drowsiness, slow heartbeat, seizures, heart palpitations.

What to Do: Call your doctor, emergency medical services (EMS), or the nearest poison control center immediately.

DRUG INTERACTIONS
Consult your doctor for specific advice if you are taking warfarin, local anesthetics, other antiarrhythmic agents, digitalis drugs, beta-blockers, ritonavir, rifampin, cimetidine, or quinidine.

FOOD INTERACTIONS
No known food interactions.

DISEASE INTERACTIONS
Consult your doctor if you have had a recent heart attack or if you have any of the following: asthma, bronchitis, emphysema, slow heartbeat, or congestive heart failure. Use of propafenone may cause complications in patients with liver or kidney disease, since these organs work together to remove the medication from the body.

Propantheline Bromide

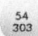
▶ Drug Class: Anticholinergic; antispasmodic

▶ Available in: Tablets

▶ Available OTC? No

▶ As Generic? Yes

Side Effects

SERIOUS
Confusion, persistent lightheadedness, dizziness, fainting, eye pain, skin rash or hives. Call your doctor immediately.

COMMON
Constipation; decreased sweating; dry mouth, nose, throat, or skin.

LESS COMMON
Blurred vision, bloated feeling, difficult urination, drowsiness, headache, sensitivity of eyes to light, memory loss, nausea or vomiting, unusual fatigue.

PRINCIPAL USES
To help treat peptic (stomach and intestinal) ulcers, usually in conjunction with other forms of therapy.

HOW THE DRUG WORKS
Propantheline inhibits nerve receptor sites that stimulate both the secretion of stomach acid and the smooth muscle activity in the digestive tract. This, in turn, promotes healing of ulcers.

DOSAGE
Adults and teenagers: 7.5 to 15 mg, 3 times a day 30 minutes before meals, and 30 mg at bedtime. The dose may be changed. Older adults: 7.5 mg, 3 times a day before meals. Children: 170 micrograms per lb of body weight 4 times a day. The dose may be changed.

ONSET OF EFFECT
Unknown.

DURATION OF ACTION
6 hours.

DIETARY ADVICE
Take it 30 minutes before meals unless your doctor advises otherwise.

STORAGE
Store in a tightly sealed container away from heat and direct light.

IF YOU MISS A DOSE
Take it as soon as you remember. If it is near the time for the next dose, skip the missed dose and resume your regular dosage schedule. Do not double the next dose.

STOPPING THE DRUG
The decision to stop taking the drug should be made by your doctor. Your doctor may reduce the dosage gradually; stopping abruptly can cause withdrawal side effects.

PROLONGED USE
See your doctor regularly for tests and examinations if you use it for a prolonged period.

PRECAUTIONS
Over 60: Adverse reactions may be more likely and more severe in older patients.

Driving and Hazardous Work: Do not drive or engage in hazardous work until you determine how the medicine affects you.

Alcohol: Avoid alcohol.

Pregnancy: Studies of propantheline in animals or humans have not been done. Before you take propantheline, tell your doctor if you are pregnant or plan to become pregnant.

Breast Feeding: Propantheline may pass into breast milk; caution is advised. Consult your doctor for advice.

Infants and Children: Use and dosage for infants and children should be determined by your doctor.

Special Concerns: Propantheline increases the risk of heat prostration; take special care not to become overheated by exercise or during hot weather.

OVERDOSE
Symptoms: Dry mouth; thirst; difficulty swallowing; muscular weakness or paralysis; restlessness; vomiting; fever; dizziness; headache; anxiety; rapid pulse and respiration; shallow breathing; abnormal heartbeat; increased need to urinate; blurred vision; flushed, hot, and dry skin; skin rash; decreased level of consciousness or loss of consciousness.

What to Do: Call your doctor, emergency medical services (EMS), or the nearest poison control center immediately.

DRUG INTERACTIONS
Consult your doctor for specific advice if you are taking antacids, diarrhea medicine containing kaolin or attapulgite, ketoconazole, other anticholinergics, tricyclic antidepressants, or potassium chloride.

FOOD INTERACTIONS
No known food interactions.

DISEASE INTERACTIONS
Caution is advised when taking propantheline. Consult your doctor if you have any of the following: bleeding problems, glaucoma, colitis, severe dryness of mouth, enlarged prostate, glaucoma, heart disease, hiatal hernia, high blood pressure, any intestinal problem, chronic lung disease, myasthenia gravis, toxemia of pregnancy, urinary difficulty, Down's syndrome, overactive thyroid, or, in children, spastic paralysis. Use of propantheline may cause complications in patients with liver or kidney disease, since these organs work together to remove the drug from the body.

Propoxyphene

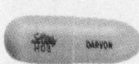

Darvon 65 mg
(LILLY)

▶ Drug Class: Opioid (narcotic)
analgesic

▶ Available in: Capsules, oral
suspension, tablets

▶ Available OTC? No

▶ As Generic? Yes

Side Effects

SERIOUS
Some serious side effects
of propoxyphene are
indistinguishable from
those of overdose: Confu-
sion; sleepiness; slurred
speech; unconsciousness;
small, pinpoint pupils;
cold, clammy skin; slow
breathing; seizures;
severe drowsiness, weak-
ness, or dizziness. Other
serious side effects
include dark urine, yellow
discoloration of eyes or
skin, and pale stools.

COMMON
Dizziness or lightheaded-
ness, nausea or vomiting,
constipation, itching.

LESS COMMON
Mood swings or false
sense of well-being
(euphoria), hallucinations.

PRINCIPAL USES
To relieve mild to moderate
pain.

HOW THE DRUG WORKS
Opioids such as propoxy-
phene relieve pain by acting
on specific areas of the
spinal cord and brain that
process pain signals from
nerves throughout the body.

DOSAGE
There are two forms of
propoxyphene: propoxy-
phene hydrochloride and
propoxyphene napsylate,
which is less powerful.
Adults— Propoxyphene
hydrochloride: 65 mg every
4 hours; no more than 390
mg a day. Propoxyphene
napsylate: 100 mg every 4
hours; no more than 600
mg a day. Children— Dose
will be determined by a
pediatrician.

ONSET OF EFFECT
15 to 60 minutes.

DURATION OF ACTION
4 to 6 hours.

DIETARY ADVICE
It can be taken with food to
lessen stomach upset.

STORAGE
Store in a tightly sealed container away from heat, moisture, and direct light. Do
not freeze the liquid form.

IF YOU MISS A DOSE
If you are taking propoxyphene on a fixed schedule,
take it as soon as you
remember. If it is near the
time for the next dose, skip
the missed dose and
resume your regular dosage
schedule. Do not double the
next dose.

STOPPING THE DRUG
The decision to stop taking
the drug should be made by
your doctor.

PROLONGED USE
You should see your doctor
regularly for tests and
examinations if you take
this medication for an
extended period. Prolonged
use can cause nerve dam-
age or physical dependence.

PRECAUTIONS
Over 60: Adverse reactions
may be more likely and
more severe in older
patients.

**Driving and Hazardous
Work:** Do not drive or
engage in hazardous work
until you determine how the
medicine affects you.

Alcohol: Avoid alcohol.

Pregnancy: Propoxyphene
has not caused birth defects
in animals. Human studies
have not been done. Before
you use this medication, tell
your doctor if you are pregnant or plan to become
pregnant. Overuse during
pregnancy can cause drug
dependence in the fetus.

Breast Feeding:
Propoxyphene passes into
breast milk; caution is
advised. Consult your doctor for specific advice.

Infants and Children:
Adverse reactions may be
more likely and more
severe in children. Consult
your doctor for advice.

Special Concerns: If you
feel the medication is not
working properly after a few
weeks, do not increase the
dose. Consult your doctor.
Before having any surgery,
tell the doctor or dentist in
charge that you are taking
this drug.

OVERDOSE
Symptoms: Confusion;
sleepiness; slurred speech;
unconsciousness; small, pinpoint pupils; cold, clammy

skin; slow breathing;
seizures; severe drowsiness,
weakness, or dizziness.

What to Do: Call your
doctor, emergency medical
services (EMS), or the
nearest poison control center immediately.

DRUG INTERACTIONS
Consult your doctor for specific advice if you are taking
carbamazepine or other
medicine for seizures, barbiturates, sedatives, cough
medicines, decongestants,
antidepressants, other prescription pain medications,
MAO inhibitors, naltrexone,
rifampin, or zidovudine.

FOOD INTERACTIONS
No known food interactions.

DISEASE INTERACTIONS
Consult your doctor if you
have any of the following: a
history of alcohol or drug
abuse; emotional illness;
brain disorders or a head
injury; seizures; lung disease; prostate problems or
other problems with urination; gallstones; colitis;
heart, kidney, liver, or
thyroid disease.

Propoxyphene/Acetaminophen

Generic 65/650 mg
(MYLAN)

▶ Drug Class: Opioid (narcotic) analgesic

▶ Available in: Tablets

▶ Available OTC? No

▶ As Generic? Yes

Side Effects

SERIOUS
Bloody, dark, or cloudy urine; severe pain in the lower back or side; pale or black, tarry stools; yellow discoloration of eyes or skin (jaundice); hallucinations; frequent urge to urinate; painful or difficult urination; sudden decrease in urine output; increased sweating; unusual bleeding or bruising; irregular heartbeat; skin rash, hives, or itching; exciteability; ringing or buzzing in the ears; pinpoint red spots on skin; sore throat and fever; confusion; trembling or uncontrolled muscle movements; redness, flushing, or swelling of the face. Call your doctor immediately.

COMMON
Dizziness, lightheadedness, constipation, nausea, vomiting, drowsiness, unusual fatigue.

LESS COMMON
Stomach pain, false sense of well-being (euphoria), depression, loss of appetite, blurred vision, nightmares or unusual dreams, dry mouth, headache, nervousness, insomnia.

PRINCIPAL USES
To relieve mild to moderate pain.

HOW THE DRUG WORKS
Opioids such as propoxyphene relieve pain by acting on specific areas of the spinal cord and brain that process pain signals from nerves throughout the body. Acetaminophen appears to interfere with the action of prostaglandins, naturally occurring substances in the body that cause inflammation and make nerves more sensitive to pain impulses.

DOSAGE
Adults: 1 or 2 tablets, depending on strength, every 4 to 6 hours. Children: Dose must be determined individually by your pediatrician.

ONSET OF EFFECT
Within 2 hours.

DURATION OF ACTION
Unknown.

DIETARY ADVICE
It can be taken with food to lessen stomach irritation.

STORAGE
Store in a tightly sealed container away from heat, moisture, and direct light.

IF YOU MISS A DOSE
If you are taking the drug on a fixed schedule, take it as soon as you remember. If it is near the time for the next dose, skip the missed dose and resume your regular dosage schedule. Do not double the next dose.

STOPPING THE DRUG
The decision to stop taking the drug should be made by your doctor.

PROLONGED USE
You should see your doctor regularly for tests and examinations if you take this medication for a prolonged period. Prolonged use can cause nerve damage as well as physical dependence.

PRECAUTIONS
Over 60: Adverse reactions may be more likely and more severe in older patients.

Driving and Hazardous Work: Do not drive or engage in hazardous work until you determine how the medicine affects you.

Alcohol: Avoid alcohol.

Pregnancy: Propoxyphene has not caused birth defects in animals. Human studies have not been done. Before you use this medication, tell your doctor if you are pregnant or plan to become pregnant. Overuse of the medication during pregnancy can cause physical dependence in the newborn.

Breast Feeding: Propoxyphene and acetaminophen pass into breast milk and may cause sedation in the nursing infant; caution is advised. Consult your doctor for advice.

Infants and Children: Adverse reactions may be more likely and more severe in children. Consult your pediatrician for advice.

Special Concerns: If you feel the medication is not working properly after a few weeks, do not increase the dose. Consult your doctor.

OVERDOSE
Symptoms: Severe dizziness or drowsiness; cold, clammy skin; difficult or slow breathing or shortness of breath; severe confusion; seizures; stomach cramps or pain; diarrhea; low blood pressure; increased sweating; constricted pupils; nausea or vomiting; irregular heartbeat; severe weakness.

What to Do: Call your doctor, emergency medical services (EMS), or the nearest poison control center immediately.

DRUG INTERACTIONS
Consult your doctor for specific advice if you are taking any prescription or over-the-counter drugs, especially other drugs containing acetaminophen, or central nervous system depressants which include: antihistamines or decongestants for hay fever, allergies, or colds; barbiturates; seizure medication; muscle relaxants; anesthetics; tranquilizers, sedatives, or sleep-inducing medications.

FOOD INTERACTIONS
No known food interactions.

DISEASE INTERACTIONS
Consult your doctor if you have a head injury or brain disease, an underactive thyroid, an enlarged prostate, seizures, kidney or liver disease, gall bladder problems, a blood disorder, or a history of alcohol or drug abuse.

Propranolol Hydrochloride

Generic 40 mg
(SCHEIN/DANBURY)

Additional photographs

▸ Drug Class: Beta-blocker

▸ Available in: Extended-
release capsules, oral
solution, tablets, injection

▸ Available OTC? No

▸ As Generic? Yes

Side Effects

SERIOUS
Shortness of breath,
wheezing; irregular or
slow heartbeat (50 beats
per minute or less); pain
or feelings of tightness
or pressure in the chest;
swelling of the ankles,
feet, and lower legs;
depression. Call your
doctor immediately.

COMMON
Dizziness or lightheaded-
ness, especially when
rising suddenly to a
standing position;
decreased sexual ability;
unusual fatigue, weak-
ness, or drowsiness;
insomnia.

LESS COMMON
Anxiety, irritability; constipation; diarrhea; dry
eyes; itching; nausea or
vomiting; nightmares or
intensely vivid dreams;
numbness, tingling, or
prickling in the fingers,
toes, or scalp.

PRINCIPAL USES
To treat angina, mild to
moderate high blood pres-
sure, irregular heartbeat
(cardiac arrhythmias),
hypertrophic cardiomyopa-
thy (weakness of the heart
muscle), heart attack,
pheochromocytoma,
tremors, and migraine
headaches.

HOW THE DRUG WORKS
Propranolol blocks nerve
impulses to various parts
of the body, which accounts
for its many effects. For
example, it slows the heart's
rate and force of the contraction (which helps lower
blood pressure), decreases
the heart's oxygen requirement (which helps prevent
angina), and helps stabilize
heart rhythm.

DOSAGE
Adults— For angina: 80 to
320 mg a day in 2, 3, or 4
doses. For high blood pressure: 40 mg, 2 times a day;
may be increased up to 640
mg a day. For irregular
heartbeat: 10 to 30 mg, 3 or
4 times a day. For cardiomy-
opathy: 20 to 40 mg, 3 or 4
times a day. For pheochromocytoma: 30 to 160 mg a
day in divided doses. For
preventing migraine
headache: 20 mg, 4 times
a day; may be increased to
240 mg a day. For trem-
bling: 40 mg, 2 times a day;
may be increased to 320 mg
a day. Children— For high
blood pressure: 0.5 mg to
4 mg per 2.2 lbs (1 kg) of
body weight a day. For
irregular heartbeat: 0.5 to
4 mg per 2.2 lbs of body
weight a day in divided
doses.

ONSET OF EFFECT
Within 30 minutes.

DURATION OF ACTION
Up to 12 hours.

DIETARY ADVICE
Mix the concentrated oral
solution with water, juice, or
a carbonated drink.

STORAGE
Store in a tightly sealed container away from heat and
direct light.

IF YOU MISS A DOSE
Take it as soon as you
remember. If it is near the
time for the next dose, skip
the missed dose and
resume your regular dosage
schedule. Do not double the
next dose.

STOPPING THE DRUG
Do not stop taking this drug
suddenly; the dosage must
be slowly tapered under
your physician's close
supervision.

PROLONGED USE
Lifelong therapy with propranolol may be necessary;
prolonged use may be associated with a greater incidence of side effects.
Regular monitoring and
evaluation by your doctor
is advised.

PRECAUTIONS
Over 60: Adverse reactions
may be more likely and
more severe in older
patients.

**Driving and Hazardous
Work:** Do not drive or
engage in hazardous work
until you determine how the
drug affects you.

Alcohol: Avoid alcohol.

Pregnancy: Consult your
doctor to weigh the risks
and benefits of using propranolol during pregnancy.

Breast Feeding: Propranolol passes into breast
milk; caution is advised.

Infants and Children:
Dosage will be determined
by your pediatrician.

Special Concerns: Take
extra care during exercise
or hot weather to avoid
dizziness and fainting.
Check your pulse often;
if it is slower than usual or
less than 50 beats a minute,
call your doctor.

OVERDOSE
Symptoms: Unusually slow
or rapid heartbeat, severe
dizziness or fainting, poor
circulation in the hands
(bluish skin), breathing
difficulty; seizures.

What to Do: Call your
doctor, emergency medical
services (EMS), or the
nearest poison control
center immediately.

DRUG INTERACTIONS
Consult your doctor for specific advice if you are taking
allergy shots, amino-
phylline, caffeine, oxtriphylline, theophylline, oral
antidiabetics, insulin, calcium channel blockers,
clonidine, guanabenz,
or MAO inhibitors.

FOOD INTERACTIONS
No known food interactions.

DISEASE INTERACTIONS
Must be used with caution
in people with diabetes,
especially insulin-dependent
diabetes, since the drug
may mask symptoms of
hypoglycemia. Consult your
doctor if you have allergies,
bronchitis, emphysema,
heart or blood vessel disease (including congestive
heart failure and peripheral
vascular disease), mental
depression, myasthenia
gravis, psoriasis, hyperthyroidism, kidney disease,
or liver disease.

Propranolol/Hydrochlorothiazide

BRAND NAMES
Inderide, Inderide LA

Generic 40/25 mg
(PUREPAC)

▶ Drug Class: Beta-blocker/
thiazide diuretic; antihypertensive

▶ Available in: Extended-
release capsules, tablets

▶ Available OTC? No

▶ As Generic? Yes

Side Effects

SERIOUS
Slow heartbeat, difficulty
breathing, mental depres-
sion, cold hands and feet,
swelling of ankles, feet,
or lower legs. Call your
doctor immediately.

COMMON
Dizziness or lightheaded-
ness, decreased sexual
ability, drowsiness,
insomnia.

LESS COMMON
Anxiety, loss of appetite,
upset stomach, nervous-
ness or excitability, constipation or diarrhea,
increased sensitivity
of the skin to sunlight,
numbness and tingling
in the fingers and toes,
stuffy nose.

PRINCIPAL USES
To control hypertension
(high blood pressure).

HOW THE DRUG WORKS
Propranolol, a beta-blocker,
blocks nerve impulses to
various parts of the body,
which accounts for its many
effects. For example, it
reduces the heart rate and
force of the heart's contractions (which helps to lower
blood pressure), decreases
the heart's oxygen requirement (which helps prevent
angina) and helps stabilize
heart rhythm. Hydro-
chlorothiazide, a diuretic,
increases the excretion of
salt and water in the urine.
By reducing the overall
amount of fluid in the body,
diuretics reduce pressure
within the blood vessels.

DOSAGE
Adults— Extended-release
capsules: 1 capsule a day.
Tablets: 1 or 2 tablets, 2
times a day.

ONSET OF EFFECT
Unknown.

DURATION OF ACTION
Unknown.

DIETARY ADVICE
No special restrictions.

STORAGE
Store in a tightly sealed container away from heat, moisture, and direct light.

IF YOU MISS A DOSE
Take it as soon as you
remember. If it is near the
time for the next dose, skip
the missed dose and
resume your regular dosage
schedule. Do not double the
next dose.

STOPPING THE DRUG
The decision to stop taking
the drug should be made in
consultation with your
physician. Do not stop taking this drug abruptly; your

doctor will gradually
decrease your dose before
stopping completely.

PROLONGED USE
Propranolol/hydrochloro-
thiazide is used to control
high blood pressure, but it
cannot cure it. Lifelong therapy may be necessary. See
your doctor regularly for
tests and examinations if
you must take this drug for
a prolonged period of time.

PRECAUTIONS
Over 60: Adverse reactions, especially dizziness,
lightheadedness, and
reduced tolerance to cold,
may be more likely and
more severe in older
patients.

**Driving and Hazardous
Work:** Do not drive or
engage in hazardous work
until you determine how the
medicine affects you.

Alcohol: Avoid alcohol.

Pregnancy: Beta-blockers
and thiazide diuretics may
cause problems during
pregnancy. Before taking
this medication, tell your
doctor if you are pregnant
or plan to become pregnant.

Breast Feeding: This
drug passes into breast
milk; caution is advised.
Consult your doctor for specific advice.

Infants and Children:
Adequate studies of the use
of this drug by children
have not been done. No special problems are expected.
Consult your pediatrician
for advice.

Special Concerns: In
addition to taking this medicine, follow your doctor's
instructions on weight control and diet for reduction of
blood pressure. Protect
yourself from sunlight until

you determine how this
medicine affects you.

OVERDOSE
Symptoms: Slow heart-
beat, severe dizziness or
fainting, difficulty breathing,
bluish colored fingernails or
palms of hands, seizures.

What to Do: Call your
doctor, emergency medical
services (EMS), or the
nearest poison control
center immediately.

DRUG INTERACTIONS
Consult your doctor for specific advice if you are receiving allergy shots or skin
tests, or are taking oral diabetes medications, insulin,
calcium channel blockers,
digitalis drugs, clonidine,
lithium, MAO inhibitors,
xanthines, or guanabenz.

FOOD INTERACTIONS
Avoid foods high in sodium.

DISEASE INTERACTIONS
Consult your doctor if you
have any of the following:
any allergic condition,
bronchial asthma, emphy-
sema, slow heartbeat, heart
or blood vessel disease, diabetes mellitus, congestive
heart failure, kidney disease, liver disease, depression, or an overactive
thyroid (hyperthyroidism).

Propylthiouracil

Generic 50 mg
(LEDERLE)

▶ Drug Class: Antithyroid agent

▶ Available in: Tablets

▶ Available OTC? No

▶ As Generic? Yes

Side Effects

SERIOUS
Cough, continuing or severe fever or chills; hoarseness; mouth sores; pain, swelling, or redness in joints; throat infection; yellowish tinge (jaundice) in skin or eyes; general feeling of discomfort, weakness, or illness. Call your doctor immediately.

COMMON
Mild and temporary fever; rash or itching.

LESS COMMON
Backache, black and tarry stools, blood in urine or stools, shortness of breath, increased or decreased urination, swelling of feet or lower legs, swollen lymph or salivary glands, numbness or tingling of face, fingers, or toes, dizziness, nausea, stomach pain, vomiting.

PRINCIPAL USES
To treat conditions in which the thyroid gland produces too much thyroid hormone (hyperthyroidism).

HOW THE DRUG WORKS
Propylthiouracil interferes with the body's ability to use iodine in the manufacture of thyroid hormone.

DOSAGE
Adults: To start, 300 to 900 mg a day, with doses every 8 hours. Maximum dose: 1,200 mg a day. Usual maintenance dose is 50 to 600 mg a day. Children ages 6 to 10: To start, 50 to 150 mg a day in 3 doses. The dose can be adjusted later. Children ages 10 and older: 50 to 300 mg per day, in 3 doses. To treat a thyroid crisis: 400 mg or more (up to 900 mg a day) for the first day, reduced gradually over subsequent days.

ONSET OF EFFECT
5 days or more.

DURATION OF ACTION
Unknown.

DIETARY ADVICE
Take it with meals to minimize stomach upset.

STORAGE
Store in a tightly sealed container away from heat and direct light.

IF YOU MISS A DOSE
Take it as soon as you remember. If it is near the time for the next dose, skip the missed dose and resume your regular dosage schedule. Do not double the next dose.

STOPPING THE DRUG
The decision to stop taking the drug should be made by your doctor.

PROLONGED USE
No special problems are expected. It may be necessary to take this medication for several years.

PRECAUTIONS
Over 60: Adverse reactions may be more common and more severe in older patients.

Driving and Hazardous Work: The use of propylthiouracil should not impair your ability to perform such tasks safely.

Alcohol: Consult your doctor about consuming alcohol while taking this drug.

Pregnancy: Too large a dose during pregnancy may cause problems in the fetus. The prescribed dose, with careful monitoring, is not likely to cause problems.

Breast Feeding: Although propylthiouracil passes into breast milk, your doctor may allow you to continue breast feeding if the dose is kept low and the infant is checked regularly.

Infants and Children: This medicine has not been shown to cause different side effects or problems in children than it does in adults.

Special Concerns: Before undergoing any kind of medical or dental procedure, be sure to tell the doctor or dentist in charge that you are taking propylthiouracil. During and after treatment, do not receive any immunizations without your doctor's approval, and avoid persons who have recently taken oral polio vaccine.

OVERDOSE
Symptoms: Nausea, vomiting, coldness, constipation, changes in menstrual period, dry and puffy skin, headache, listlessness, muscle aches, sleepiness, swollen neck, unusual weight gain.

What to Do: An overdose of propylthiouracil is unlikely to be life-threatening. However, if someone takes a much larger dose than prescribed, call your doctor, emergency medical services (EMS), or local poison control center.

DRUG INTERACTIONS
Consult your doctor for advice if you are taking amiodarone, iodinated glycerol, potassium iodide, anticoagulants, or digitalis drugs.

FOOD INTERACTIONS
Consult your doctor about the need for a special low-iodine diet.

DISEASE INTERACTIONS
Use of propylthiouracil may cause complications in patients who have liver disease, since this organ works to remove medications from the body.

Protriptyline Hydrochloride

Generic 5 mg
(SIDMAK)

▶ Drug Class: Tricyclic antidepressant

▶ Available in: Tablets

▶ Available OTC? No

▶ As Generic? Yes

Side Effects

SERIOUS
Confusion, heartbeat irregularities, hallucinations, seizures, extreme fatigue or drowsiness, blurred or altered vision, breathing difficulty, constipation, staring and absence of facial expression, impaired concentration, difficult urination, fever, extreme and persistent restlessness, loss of coordination and balance, difficulty swallowing or speaking, dilated pupils, eye pain, fainting. Also trembling, shaking, weakness, and stiffness in the extremities; shuffling gait. Call your doctor immediately.

COMMON
Drowsiness or dizziness, headache, dry mouth or unpleasant taste, fatigue, heightened sensitivity to light, weight gain, increased appetite, nausea, excitability.

LESS COMMON
Heartburn or indigestion, sleeping difficulty, diarrhea, increased sweating, vomiting.

PRINCIPAL USES
To relieve symptoms of major depression.

HOW THE DRUG WORKS
Protriptyline affects levels of norepinephrine, a brain chemical that is thought to be linked to mood, emotions, and mental state.

DOSAGE
Adults: To start, 5 to 10 mg, 3 to 4 times a day; may be increased to 60 mg a day. Teenagers: To start, 5 mg, 3 times a day; may be increased gradually by your doctor. Older adults: To start, 5 mg, 3 times a day; may be increased gradually by your doctor.

ONSET OF EFFECT
1 to 6 weeks.

DURATION OF ACTION
Unknown.

DIETARY ADVICE
To lessen stomach upset, take with food, unless your doctor instructs otherwise. Increase intake of fiber and fluids.

STORAGE
Store in a tightly sealed container away from heat, moisture, and direct light.

IF YOU MISS A DOSE
If you take a one-time daily bedtime dose, do not take the missed dose in the morning because it may cause drowsiness. Call your doctor. If you take more than 1 dose a day, take it as soon as you remember. However, if it is near the time for the next dose, skip the missed dose and resume your regular dosage schedule. Do not double the next dose.

STOPPING THE DRUG
Take as prescribed for the full treatment period, even if you begin to feel better before the scheduled end of therapy. The decision to stop taking the drug should be made in consultation with your doctor.

PROLONGED USE
The usual course of therapy lasts 6 months to 1 year; some patients benefit from additional therapy.

PRECAUTIONS
Over 60: Adverse reactions may be more likely and more severe in older patients. A lower dose may be warranted.

Driving and Hazardous Work: Use caution when driving or engaging in hazardous work until you know how the medication affects you. Drowsiness or lightheadedness can occur.

Alcohol: Avoid alcohol.

Pregnancy: Adequate human studies have not been done. Consult your doctor for specific advice.

Breast Feeding: Protriptyline passes into breast milk; do not use it while nursing.

Infants and Children: This drug is not prescribed for children under age 6.

Special Concerns: This is a potentially dangerous drug, especially if taken in excess. Tricyclic antidepressants should not be within easy reach of suicidal patients. If dry mouth occurs, use candy or sugarless gum for relief.

OVERDOSE
Symptoms: Difficulty breathing, severe fatigue, seizures, confusion, hallucinations, dilated pupils, irregular heartbeat, fever, impaired ability to concentrate.

What to Do: Call your doctor, emergency medical services (EMS), or the nearest poison control center immediately.

DRUG INTERACTIONS
Consult your doctor for specific advice if you are taking antithyroid agents, cimetidine, clonidine, guanadrel, guanethidine, metrizamide, appetite suppressants, isoproterenol, ephedrine, epinephrine, amphetamines, phenylephrine, antipsychotic drugs, pimozide, methyldopa, metyrosine, metoclopramide, pemoline, promethazine, trimeprazine, rauwolfia alkaloids, MAO inhibitors, or any drugs that depress the central nervous system.

FOOD INTERACTIONS
No known food interactions.

DISEASE INTERACTIONS
Consult your doctor if you have any of the following: a history of alcohol abuse, difficulty urinating, asthma, bipolar disorder, high blood pressure, stomach or intestinal problems, glaucoma, overactive thyroid, enlarged prostate, schizophrenia, seizures, a blood disorder, or kidney, heart, or liver disease.

Pseudoephedrine

BRAND NAMES
Cenafed, Decofed, Dorcol
Children's Decongestant
Liquid, Drixoral Non-
Drowsy Formula,
Efidac/24, Genaphed,
Halofed, Myfedrine,
Novafed, Pedia/Care
Infants' Oral
Decongestant Drops,
Pseudo, Pseudogest,
Sudafed, Sufedrin

Sudafed 12 Hour 120 mg
(GLAXO WELLCOME)

806

Additional photographs

▶ Drug Class: Decongestant/
cough drug

▶ Available in: Extended-
release capsules, oral
solution, syrup, tablets

▶ Available OTC? Yes

▶ As Generic? Yes

Side Effects

SERIOUS
Seizures, irregular or
slowed heartbeat, short-
ness of breath, breathing
difficulty, hallucinations.
Stop taking the medica-
tion and call your doctor
right away.

COMMON
Nervousness, restless-
ness, insomnia.

LESS COMMON
Difficult or painful urination, dizziness or light-
headedness, rapid or
pounding heartbeat,
increased sweating, nau-
sea or vomiting, trem-
bling, trouble breathing,
paleness, weakness.

PRINCIPAL USES
To relieve nasal or sinus
congestion caused by colds,
sinus infection, hay fever, or
other respiratory allergies.

HOW THE DRUG WORKS
Pseudoephedrine narrows
and constricts blood vessels
to reduce the blood flow to
swollen nasal passages and
other tissues, which
reduces nasal secretions,
shrinks swollen nasal
mucous membranes, and
improves airflow in nasal
passages.

DOSAGE
Short-acting forms— Adults
and teenagers: 60 mg every
4 to 6 hours; not more than
240 mg in 24 hours. Chil-
dren 6 to 12 years of age: 30
mg every 4 to 6 hours; not
more than 120 mg in 24
hours. Children 2 to 6 years
of age: 15 mg every 4
hours; not more than 60 mg
in 24 hours. Extended-
release form— Adults and
teenagers: 120 mg every 12
hours or 240 mg every 24
hours. No more than 240
mg in 24 hours.

ONSET OF EFFECT
15 to 30 minutes.

DURATION OF ACTION
3 to 4 hours for short-acting
forms, 8 to 12 hours for
extended-release form.

DIETARY ADVICE
Be sure to drink plenty of
fluids.

STORAGE
Store in a tightly sealed container away from heat and
direct light. Do not allow
the liquid form to freeze.

IF YOU MISS A DOSE
Take it as soon as you
remember. If it is near the
time for the next dose, skip
the missed dose and
resume your regular dosage
schedule. Do not double the
next dose.

STOPPING THE DRUG
Do not take this drug
longer than recommended
on the label unless directed
to do so by your doctor.

PROLONGED USE
Consult your doctor about
taking pseudoephedrine for
more than 5 to 7 days.

PRECAUTIONS
Over 60: Side effects may
be more likely and more
severe in elderly patients.

**Driving and Hazardous
Work:** Avoid such activities
until you determine how the
medicine affects you.

Alcohol: No special precautions are necessary.

Pregnancy: Safety has not
been established; it should
be used only if clearly necessary. Consult your doctor
for specific advice.

Breast Feeding: Pseudoephedrine passes into
breast milk; avoid or discontinue use while nursing.

Infants and Children:
Use of extended-release
forms of pseudoephedrine is
not recommended for chil-
dren under the age of 12.

Special Concerns: If your
symptoms do not improve
within 7 days, check with
your doctor. To help prevent
insomnia, take the last dose
at least 2 hours before your
bedtime.

OVERDOSE
Symptoms: Drowsiness,
sedation, profuse sweating,
pale or clammy skin, low
blood pressure, diminished
urine output, dizziness,
changes in mental state, hallucinations, seizures, loss of
consciousness.

What to Do: In some
cases an overdose can be
fatal, especially among
elderly patients. At the first
sign of overdose, call your
doctor, emergency medical
services (EMS), or the
nearest poison control
center immediately.

DRUG INTERACTIONS
Consult your doctor for specific advice if you are taking
beta-blockers or MAO
inhibitors.

FOOD INTERACTIONS
No known food interactions.

DISEASE INTERACTIONS
Caution is advised when
taking pseudoephedrine.
Consult your doctor if you
have any of the following:
diabetes, enlarged prostate,
heart disease, blood vessel
disease, high blood pres-
sure, or an overactive thyroid gland.

Pseudoephedrine/Guaifenesin

BRAND NAMES
Deconsal II, Deconsal LA, Entex PSE

▶ Drug Class: Decongestant/ cough drug

▶ Available in: Capsules, oral solution, syrup, tablets, extended-release forms

▶ Available OTC? Yes

▶ As Generic? No

Side Effects

SERIOUS
Skin rash, hives, itching, rapid or irregular heartbeat, persistent headache, nervousness or restlessness, shortness of breath or breathing difficulty, seizures, unusual fear and anxiety. Call your doctor or emergency medical services (EMS) right away.

COMMON
Constipation; decreased sweating; difficult urination; dizziness or lightheadedness; drowsiness; dry mouth, nose, or throat; increased sensitivity of skin to sun; nausea or vomiting; nightmares; stomach pain; thickened mucus; insomnia; unusual excitement or restlessness; unusual tiredness or weakness. Contact your doctor if these symptoms persist or interfere with your daily activities.

LESS COMMON
There are no less-common side effects associated with this drug.

PRINCIPAL USES
To relieve nasal or sinus congestion caused by colds, influenza (flu), hay fever, and other respiratory allergies. Also intended to break up congestion in the lungs to promote better breathing.

HOW THE DRUG WORKS
Pseudoephedrine narrows and constricts blood vessels to reduce the blood flow to swollen nasal passages and other tissues, which reduces nasal secretions, shrinks swollen nasal mucous membranes, and improves airflow. Guaifenesin purportedly breaks up, liquefies, and loosens mucus secretions in the respiratory tract, making it easier to cough up phlegm and thus breathe easier. (There is some debate however as to whether guaifenesin is actually effective in this regard.)

DOSAGE
Take the drug as directed to relieve symptoms.

ONSET OF EFFECT
Within 1 hour.

DURATION OF ACTION
Unknown.

DIETARY ADVICE
No special restrictions.

STORAGE
Store in a tightly sealed container away from heat and direct light.

IF YOU MISS A DOSE
Take it as soon as you remember. If it is near the time for the next dose, skip the missed dose and resume your regular dosage schedule. Do not double the next dose.

STOPPING THE DRUG
The decision to stop taking the drug should be made by your doctor or when you note improvement.

PROLONGED USE
Check with your doctor if symptoms do not improve within 5 days.

PRECAUTIONS
Over 60: Adverse reactions may be more likely and more severe in older patients.

Driving and Hazardous Work: Do not drive or engage in hazardous work until you determine how the medicine affects you.

Alcohol: Avoid alcohol.

Pregnancy: Before taking pseudoephedrine and guaifenesin, tell your doctor if you are pregnant or plan to become pregnant.

Breast Feeding: Pseudoephedrine passes into breast milk; avoid or discontinue use while nursing.

Infants and Children: Check the package label or with your doctor before giving it to infants or children.

Special Concerns: If you have trouble sleeping, take the last dose of pseudoephedrine and guaifenesin a few hours before bedtime. Before having any surgery, tell your doctor or dentist that you are taking this drug. Be sure your doctor knows if you have high blood pressure.

OVERDOSE
Symptoms: Rapid, pounding, or irregular heartbeat, continuing and severe headache, severe nausea or vomiting, severe nervousness or restlessness, severe shortness of breath or troubled breathing.

What to Do: Call your doctor, emergency medical services (EMS), or the nearest poison control center immediately.

DRUG INTERACTIONS
Consult your doctor if you are taking any prescription or nonprescription medication. Do not take any drug for diet or appetite control unless you have checked with your doctor first.

FOOD INTERACTIONS
No known food interactions.

DISEASE INTERACTIONS
Caution is advised when taking pseudoephedrine and guaifenesin. Consult your doctor if you have any of the following: anemia, gout, hemophilia, stomach problems, brain disease, colitis, seizures, diarrhea, gallbladder disease or gallstones, cystic fibrosis, diabetes mellitus, any chronic lung disease, enlarged prostate, difficult urination, glaucoma, heart or blood vessel disease, thyroid disease, or high blood pressure. Use of pseudoephedrine and guaifenesin may cause complications in persons with liver or kidney disease, since these organs work together to remove the medication from the body.

Psyllium

BRAND NAMES
Cillium, Konsyl, Naturacil, Perdiem Fiber, Syllact

- ▶ Drug Class: Bulk-forming laxative
- ▶ Available in: Caramels, granules, powder
- ▶ Available OTC? Yes
- ▶ As Generic? Yes

Side Effects

SERIOUS
Difficulty breathing, intestinal blockage (resulting in severe, painful constipation), skin rash or itching, difficulty swallowing. Call your doctor immediately.

COMMON
No common side effects have been reported.

LESS COMMON
Nausea, vomiting, partial intestinal obstruction, abdominal pain or cramping.

PRINCIPAL USES
To relieve constipation. It also may be prescribed for treatment of diarrhea.

HOW THE DRUG WORKS
Psyllium is a natural soluble fiber derived from the husks of a seed grain. It absorbs liquid in the intestines and swells to form a soft, bulky stool. The increased bulk of the stool stimulates bowel activity and triggers the urge to defecate. Psyllium has also been shown in studies to improve the ratio of HDL ("good") cholesterol to LDL ("bad") cholesterol in the blood. For this reason, it is sometimes prescribed as part of a program to reduce high cholesterol levels before resorting to drug therapy.

DOSAGE
Adults: 1 to 2 rounded teaspoons or 1 packet dissolved in water, 1, 2, or 3 times a day, followed by a second glass of liquid. Children over 6: 1 level teaspoon in half a glass of water.

ONSET OF EFFECT
Usually, 12 to 24 hours. In some cases, up to 3 days.

DURATION OF ACTION
Variable.

DIETARY ADVICE
Take psyllium with a full glass of cold liquid, such as fruit juice or water, and follow with another full glass.

STORAGE
Store in a tightly sealed container away from heat, moisture, and direct light.

IF YOU MISS A DOSE
Take it as soon as you remember. If it is near the time for the next dose, skip the missed dose and resume your regular dosage schedule. Do not double the next dose.

STOPPING THE DRUG
Take it as prescribed for the full treatment period. However, you may stop taking it if you are feeling better before the scheduled end of therapy.

PROLONGED USE
Do not take psyllium for more than 1 week unless your doctor has ordered a special schedule for you.

PRECAUTIONS
Over 60: No special problems are expected.

Driving and Hazardous Work: The use of psyllium should not impair your ability to perform such tasks safely.

Alcohol: Avoid alcohol; it can irritate the gastrointestinal tract and interfere with proper digestion.

Pregnancy: Discuss with your doctor the relative risks and benefits of using psyllium while pregnant.

Breast Feeding: Psyllium may pass into breast milk; caution is advised. Consult your doctor for advice.

Infants and Children: Not recommended for use by children under age 6.

Special Concerns: You should have an adequate amount of fiber-containing food in your diet, such as cereals, fresh fruit, and vegetables. Before taking psyllium, tell your doctor if you have had any unusual or allergic reaction to laxatives. Make sure that your doctor knows if you are on any special diet. Do not take any other medicine within 2 hours of taking psyllium. Drink from 6 to 8 eight-ounce glasses of water every day.

OVERDOSE
Symptoms: Intestinal blockage.

What to Do: An overdose of psyllium is unlikely. However, if someone takes a much larger dose than prescribed, seek medical help promptly.

DRUG INTERACTIONS
Consult your doctor for advice if you are taking oral tetracyclines.

FOOD INTERACTIONS
Psyllium may interfere with the absorption of certain minerals, especially in high doses or with regular use.

DISEASE INTERACTIONS
Consult your doctor if you have any of the following: heart disease, a colostomy or ileostomy, diabetes mellitus, high blood pressure, kidney disease, rectal bleeding of unknown cause, difficulty swallowing, or any signs of appendicitis.

Pyrantel Pamoate

BRAND NAMES
Antiminth, Reese's
Pinworm Medicine

▶ Drug Class: Anthelmintic

▶ Available in: Oral suspension

▶ Available OTC? Yes

▶ As Generic? Yes

Side Effects

SERIOUS
Skin rash. Stop using the drug and call your doctor as soon as possible.

COMMON
No common side effects are associated with the use of pyrantel.

LESS COMMON
Pain or cramps in abdomen or stomach, headache, dizziness, diarrhea, drowsiness, insomnia, nausea or vomiting, loss of appetite.

PRINCIPAL USES
To treat various worm infections, including ascariasis (common roundworm) and enterobiasis or oxyuriasis (pinworm). It may be used to treat more than one worm infection at a time. It may also be used for other types of infection as determined by your doctor.

HOW THE DRUG WORKS
Pyrantel paralyzes the worm. While it is paralyzed, the worm is expelled from the body in the stool.

DOSAGE
Adults and children age 2 and older— For roundworms: 1 dose of 11 mg per 2.2 lbs (1 kg) of body weight. Maximum dose is 1,000 mg. If necessary, the dose may be repeated in 2 to 3 weeks. For pinworms: 1 dose of 11 mg per 2.2 lbs of body weight. Maximum dose is 1,000 mg. Repeat the dose in 2 to 3 weeks.

ONSET OF EFFECT
Variable.

DURATION OF ACTION
Variable.

DIETARY ADVICE
Pyrantel can be taken with fruit juice, milk, or food.

STORAGE
Store in a tightly sealed container away from heat, moisture, and direct light. Do not allow it to freeze.

IF YOU MISS A DOSE
Take a missed dose as soon as you remember.

STOPPING THE DRUG
Consult your physician.

PROLONGED USE
Pyrantel is generally prescribed for one-time use (two-time use for pinworms).

PRECAUTIONS
Over 60: Adverse reactions may be more likely and more severe in older patients.

Driving and Hazardous Work: Do not drive or engage in hazardous work until you determine how the medicine affects you.

Alcohol: No special precautions are necessary.

Pregnancy: Pyrantel is not recommended for use in pregnant women. Consult your doctor for specific advice if you are pregnant or plan to become pregnant.

Breast Feeding: Pyrantel may pass into breast milk; caution is advised. Consult your doctor for advice.

Infants and Children: Use and dosage for children under the age of 2 should be determined by your doctor. Not recommended for use by children under the age of 1.

Special Concerns: For pinworm infection, clothing, bedding, and towels should be washed daily. All members of the family may have to be treated to eradicate the infestation. A second treatment for all household members may be necessary after 2 or 3 weeks. All bedding and nightclothes should be washed after treatment. To prevent reinfection, you should wash the anal region daily, change your underwear and bedding every day, and wash your hands and fingernails before each meal and after bowel movements. Consult your doctor if your condition has not improved upon completion of therapy.

OVERDOSE
Symptoms: An overdose with pyrantel is unlikely.

What to Do: If someone takes a much larger dose than prescribed, call your doctor, emergency medical services (EMS), or the nearest poison control center right away.

DRUG INTERACTIONS
Do not take piperazine when taking pyrantel. The effectiveness of both drugs may be reduced. Consult your doctor for specific advice. Also tell your doctor if you are taking any other prescription or over-the-counter medication.

FOOD INTERACTIONS
No known food interactions.

DISEASE INTERACTIONS
Caution is advised when taking pyrantel. Consult your doctor for specific advice if you have any other medical condition.

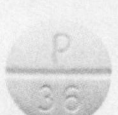

Generic 500 mg
(LEDERLE)

▸ Drug Class: Anti-
infective/antitubercular agent

▸ Available in: Tablets

▸ Available OTC? No

▸ As Generic? Yes

Side Effects

SERIOUS
Joint pain or swelling,
especially in leg and foot
joints; nausea, vomiting,
weakness, fatigue, yellow
discoloration of the eyes
or skin (may be signs of
hepatitis). Call your doctor immediately.

COMMON
Joint pain, hepatitis (see
above).

LESS COMMON
Skin rash, itching, stom-
ach upset.

PRINCIPAL USES
To treat active tuberculosis;
it must be used in conjunction with other antitubercular agents such as isoniazid,
streptomycin, and rifampin.

HOW THE DRUG WORKS
Pyrazinamide kills the
tuberculosis bacteria.

DOSAGE
Adults: 1.5 to 2.5 g (6.8 to
13.6 mg per lb of body
weight) per day. Children:
6.8 to 13.6 mg per lb once
a day; not more than 2,000
mg daily. It may also be
given to adults or children
2 to 3 times a week in a
dose of 22.7 to 31.8 mg per
lb. If the schedule is twice
a week, adults should take
no more than 4,000 mg per
dose; if the schedule is 3
times a week, no more than
2,500 mg per dose. Children
should receive not more
than 2,000 mg per day,
even if it is taken only 2
or 3 times a week.

ONSET OF EFFECT
Unknown.

DURATION OF ACTION
Unknown.

DIETARY ADVICE
Take it with food to minimize stomach irritation.

STORAGE
Store in a tightly sealed container away from heat, moisture, and direct light.

IF YOU MISS A DOSE
Take it as soon as you
remember. This will help
keep a constant level of
medication in your system.
If it is near the time for the
next dose, skip the missed
dose and resume your regular dosage schedule. Do not
double the next dose.

STOPPING THE DRUG
Take it as prescribed for the
full treatment period, even if

you begin to feel better
before the scheduled end of
therapy. Treatment may
continue for months or
years. The decision to stop
taking the drug should be
made by your doctor.

PROLONGED USE
Consult your doctor about
the need for periodic medical examinations and laboratory tests. If your
symptoms do not improve
or instead become worse in
2 to 3 weeks, consult your
doctor.

PRECAUTIONS
Over 60: Adverse reactions
may be more likely and
more severe in older
patients.

**Driving and Hazardous
Work:** The use of pyrazinamide should not impair
your ability to perform
such tasks safely.

Alcohol: Avoid alcohol.

Pregnancy: Adequate
human studies have not
been done. Before taking
pyrazinamide, tell your doctor if you are pregnant or
are planning to become
pregnant.

Breast Feeding: Pyrazinamide passes into breast
milk; caution is advised.
Consult your doctor for
specific advice.

Infants and Children:
Pyrazinamide has not been
shown to cause different or
more severe side effects in
children. However, owing to
the serious nature of the
side effects, it should be
used only under the strict
supervision of your doctor.
Discuss with your pediatrician the relative risks and
benefits of your child's
using this drug.

Special Concerns: Pyrazinamide may cause false
results on urine ketone
tests for diabetes. Check
with your doctor before
adjusting your medication
dosage or diet. Patients with
HIV may require a longer
period of treatment.

OVERDOSE
Symptoms: Abnormal
results on tests of liver function. This problem can be
detected by your doctor.

What to Do: An overdose
of pyrazinamide is unlikely
to be life-threatening. However, if someone takes a
much larger dose than prescribed, call your doctor,
emergency medical services
(EMS), or the nearest poison control center.

DRUG INTERACTIONS
Consult your doctor for specific advice if you are taking
any other prescription or
over-the-counter medication.

FOOD INTERACTIONS
No known food interactions.

DISEASE INTERACTIONS
Consult your doctor if you
have a history of alcohol
abuse, diabetes, or gout.
The use of pyrazinamide
may cause complications in
patients who have liver disease, since this organ works
to remove the medication
from the body.

Pyrethrins/Piperonyl Butoxide

▶ Drug Class: Topical antiparasitic

▶ Available in: Gel, solution shampoo, topical solution

▶ Available OTC? Yes

▶ As Generic? Yes

Side Effects

SERIOUS
Skin irritation not present before use of the medicine, skin rash or infection, sudden attacks of sneezing, stuffy or runny nose, wheezing or difficulty breathing. Call your doctor immediately.

COMMON
No common side effects are associated with pyrethrins and piperonyl butoxide.

LESS COMMON
No less-common side effects are associated with pyrethrins and piperonyl butoxide.

PRINCIPAL USES
To treat head, body, and pubic lice infestations. Although this drug is available without a prescription, your doctor may have special instructions regarding its proper use.

HOW THE DRUG WORKS
Pyrethrins and piperonyl butoxide are a combination of active ingredients. The medication is absorbed into the bodies of lice, where it blocks nerve activity, ultimately causing paralysis and death of the lice. (The drug has no such toxic effect on humans.)

DOSAGE
Use 1 time, then repeat one more time in 7 to 10 days. Gel or solution: Apply enough medicine to thoroughly wet hair, scalp, or skin. Allow the medicine to remain on the affected areas for 10 minutes, then wash with warm water and soap or regular shampoo. Rinse thoroughly and dry with a clean towel. Shampoo: Apply enough medicine to wet the hair, scalp, or skin. Allow the medicine to remain on the affected areas for 10 minutes, then use a small amount of water to work shampoo more thoroughly into affected area. Rinse and dry with a clean towel. With either method, use a nit-removal comb to remove dead lice and eggs from hair.

ONSET OF EFFECT
Within 10 minutes.

DURATION OF ACTION
Up to 10 days.

DIETARY ADVICE
This medication can be used without regard to diet.

STORAGE
Store in a tightly sealed container away from heat and direct light, and away from children.

IF YOU MISS A DOSE
If you do not administer the second dose within 10 days after the initial dose, do so as soon as you remember.

STOPPING THE DRUG
Take both recommended doses, even if you are feeling better before the scheduled end of therapy.

PROLONGED USE
If lice recur, consult your doctor.

PRECAUTIONS
Over 60: No special problems are expected in older patients.

Driving and Hazardous Work: The use of pyrethrins and piperonyl butoxide should not impair your ability to perform such tasks safely.

Alcohol: No special precautions are necessary.

Pregnancy: This drug has not been shown to cause birth defects or other problems during pregnancy. Before you use pyrethrins and piperonyl butoxide, tell your doctor if you are pregnant or plan to become pregnant.

Breast Feeding: Pyrethrins and piperonyl butoxide may pass into breast milk; caution is advised. Consult your doctor for specific information.

Infants and Children: No special problems are expected in younger patients.

Special Concerns: All members of your household should be examined for lice and given treatment if necessary. Clothing, household linen, hairbrushes, combs, and bedding should be thoroughly cleaned. Furniture, rugs, and floors should be vacuumed thoroughly. Toilet seats should be scrubbed frequently. If you use this medicine for pubic lice, your sexual partner may also need to be treated. Keep this medicine away from the mouth and do not inhale it. Apply it in a well-ventilated room to help prevent inhalation. Keep the medicine away from the eyes and other mucous membranes, such as the inside of the nose or vagina.

OVERDOSE
Symptoms: If accidentally ingested, pyrethrins and piperonyl butoxide can cause nausea, vomiting, muscle paralysis, and central nervous system depression.

What to Do: Call your doctor, emergency medical services (EMS), or the nearest poison control center immediately.

DRUG INTERACTIONS
Before you use this medicine, tell your doctor if you are using any other prescription or over-the-counter medications.

FOOD INTERACTIONS
No known food interactions.

DISEASE INTERACTIONS
Consult your doctor if you have any severe inflammation of the skin.

Quazepam

BRAND NAME
Doral

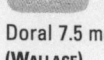

Doral 7.5 mg
(WALLACE)

▶ Drug Class: Benzodiazepine tranquilizer

▶ Available in: Tablets

▶ Available OTC? No

▶ As Generic? No

Side Effects

SERIOUS
Difficulty concentrating, outbursts of anger, other behavior problems, depression, hallucinations, low blood pressure (causing faintness or confusion), memory impairment, muscle weakness, skin rash or itching, sore throat, fever and chills, sores or ulcers in throat or mouth, unusual bruising or bleeding, extreme fatigue, yellowish tinge to eyes or skin. Call your doctor immediately.

COMMON
Drowsiness, loss of coordination, unsteady gait, dizziness, lightheadedness, slurred speech.

LESS COMMON
Change in sexual desire or ability, constipation, false sense of well-being, nausea and vomiting, urinary problems, unusual fatigue.

PRINCIPAL USES
To treat insomnia.

HOW THE DRUG WORKS
In general, quazepam produces mild sedation by depressing activity in the central nervous system. In particular, quazepam appears to enhance the effect of gamma-aminobutyric acid (GABA), a natural chemical that inhibits the firing of neurons and dampens the transmission of nerve signals, thus decreasing nervous excitation.

DOSAGE
Adults: 7.5 to 15 mg in 1 dose at bedtime. Use and dose for children under the age of 18 must be determined by your doctor.

ONSET OF EFFECT
Unknown.

DURATION OF ACTION
Unknown.

DIETARY ADVICE
Quazepam should be taken 30 to 60 minutes before bedtime with a full glass of water. It can be taken with food to prevent gastrointestinal upset.

STORAGE
Store in a tightly sealed container away from heat and direct light.

IF YOU MISS A DOSE
Take it as soon as you remember, unless it is late at night. Do not take the medicine unless your schedule allows a full night's sleep.

STOPPING THE DRUG
Discontinuing the drug abruptly may produce withdrawal symptoms (sleep disruption, nervousness, irritability, diarrhea, abdominal cramps, muscle aches, memory impairment).

Dosage may need to be reduced gradually.

PROLONGED USE
Do not take quazepam for more than 8 weeks without consulting your doctor.

PRECAUTIONS
Over 60: Adverse reactions are more likely and more severe. A lower dose may be warranted.

Driving and Hazardous Work: Quazepam can impair mental alertness and physical coordination. Adjust your activities accordingly.

Alcohol: Avoid alcohol.

Pregnancy: Use during pregnancy should be avoided if possible. Be sure to tell your doctor if you are pregnant or plan to become pregnant.

Breast Feeding: Quazepam passes into breast milk; do not take it while nursing.

Infants and Children: Safety and effectiveness have not been established for children under age 18.

Special Concerns: Quazepam use can lead to psychological or physical dependence. Never take more than the prescribed daily dose. Never stop taking the drug abruptly.

OVERDOSE
Symptoms: Extreme drowsiness, confusion, slurred speech, slow reflexes, poor coordination, staggering gait, tremor, slowed breathing, loss of consciousness.

What to Do: Call your doctor, emergency medical services (EMS), or the nearest poison control center immediately.

DRUG INTERACTIONS
Other drugs may interact with quazepam. Consult your doctor for specific advice if you are taking any drugs that depress the central nervous system; these include antihistamines, antidepressants or other psychiatric medications, barbiturates, sedatives, cough medicines, decongestants, and painkillers. Be sure your doctor knows about any over-the-counter medication you may take.

FOOD INTERACTIONS
None reported.

DISEASE INTERACTIONS
Caution is advised when taking quazepam. Consult your doctor if you have a history of alcohol or drug abuse, stroke or other brain disease, any chronic lung disease, hyperactivity, depression or other mental illness, myasthenia gravis, sleep apnea, epilepsy, porphyria, kidney disease, or liver disease.

Quetiapine Fumarate

BRAND NAME
Seroquel

▶ Drug Class: Antipsychotic

▶ Available in: Tablets

▶ Available OTC? No

▶ As Generic? No

Side Effects

SERIOUS
Tardive dyskinesia (involuntary movements of the jaw, lips, and tongue), amnesia, psychosis, hallucinations, paranoia, delusions, manic episodes, suicidal impulses, catatonic reaction, stroke, shortness of breath, asthma, paralysis of one side of the body. Call your doctor immediately. Neuroleptic malignant syndrome, characterized by high fever, muscle rigidity, altered mental status, and heart rhythm abnormalities, is a potentially fatal condition.

COMMON
Drowsiness, headache, dizziness, constipation.

LESS COMMON
Dry mouth, lightheadedness when rising from a sitting or lying position (orthostatic hypotension), rapid heartbeat, indigestion, weakness, abdominal pain, skin rash, unexpected weight gain.

PRINCIPAL USES
To treat psychotic conditions (severe mental disorders characterized by distorted thoughts, perceptions, and emotions), such as schizophrenia.

HOW THE DRUG WORKS
While the exact mechanism of action of quetiapine is unknown, it appears to interfere with receptors for certain critical natural substances (neurotransmitters) in the brain to produce a tranquilizing and antipsychotic effect.

DOSAGE
Initial dose is 25 mg twice a day. On the second and third days, the dose should be increased by 25 to 50 mg, 2 to 3 times a day, if tolerated. On the fourth day, the dosage should be 300 to 400 mg a day in 2 or 3 divided doses. If needed, further adjustments in dose should occur at least 2 days apart in increments or decrements of 25 to 50 mg, 2 times a day. Clinical trials have not evaluated daily doses greater than 800 mg.

ONSET OF EFFECT
Unknown.

DURATION OF ACTION
Unknown.

DIETARY ADVICE
Quetiapine can be taken without regard to food intake.

STORAGE
Store in a tightly sealed container away from heat, moisture, and direct light.

IF YOU MISS A DOSE
Take it as soon as you remember. If it is near the time for the next dose, skip the missed dose and resume your regular dosage schedule. Do not double the next dose.

STOPPING THE DRUG
Take it as prescribed for the full treatment period. The decision to stop taking the drug should be made in consultation with your physician.

PROLONGED USE
Prolonged use may lead to a potentially irreversible condition called tardive dyskinesia (involuntary movements of the jaw, lips, and tongue). Your doctor must periodically evaluate the drug's effectiveness if it is used for an extended period. Examinations of the eyes for possible development of cataracts are recommended at the onset of treatment and at 6-month intervals during chronic treatment.

PRECAUTIONS
Over 60: Adverse reactions are more likely and more severe. A lower dose may be warranted.

Driving and Hazardous Work: The use of quetiapine may impair your ability to perform such tasks safely. Do not drive or engage in hazardous work until you determine how the medicine affects you.

Alcohol: Avoid alcohol.

Pregnancy: Adequate human studies have not been done. Discuss with your doctor the relative risks and benefits of using this drug while pregnant.

Breast Feeding: Quetiapine may pass into breast milk; avoid or discontinue breast feeding while taking this drug.

Infants and Children: Not recommended for use by children under age 18.

Special Concerns: Avoid prolonged exposure to high temperatures or hot climates. Drink plenty of fluids and stay cool in the summertime.

OVERDOSE
Symptoms: Few cases of overdose have been reported. In clinical studies, excessive doses appear to exacerbate quetiapine's known side effects.

What to Do: Call your doctor, emergency medical services (EMS), or the nearest poison control center immediately.

DRUG INTERACTIONS
Consult your doctor for specific advice if you are taking phenytoin, ketoconazole, itraconazole, fluconazole, erythromycin, antihypertensives, antiparkinsonism drugs, central nervous system depressants, or any other prescription or over-the-counter drug.

FOOD INTERACTIONS
No known food interactions.

DISEASE INTERACTIONS
Caution is advised when taking quetiapine if you have a history of liver disease, severe kidney dysfunction, symptomatic reactions to low blood pressure (dizziness, lightheadedness, or fainting, especially when rising from a sitting or lying position), heart disease, stroke, or seizures.

Quinacrine Hydrochloride

▶ Drug Class: Anti-infective/antimalarial/anthelmintic

▶ Available in: Tablets

▶ Available OTC? No

▶ As Generic? No

Side Effects

SERIOUS
Hallucinations; mental or mood changes; irritability; nervousness; skin rash; reddening, itching or peeling of skin; nightmares. Call your doctor immediately.

COMMON
Yellow color of the skin and urine, stomach or abdominal cramps, loss of appetite, dizziness, headache, nausea or vomiting, diarrhea.

LESS COMMON
No less-common side effects are associated with the use of quinacrine.

PRINCIPAL USES
Used as a primary agent in the treatment of giardiasis (traveler's diarrhea), a protozoal infection of the intestinal tract, usually contracted by consuming water that is contaminated with Giardia lamblia cysts.

HOW THE DRUG WORKS
The exact way in which quinacrine works is unknown. It appears to interfere with the parasite's metabolism.

DOSAGE
Adults and teenagers: 100 mg, 3 times a day for 5 to 7 days. Children under age 12: 2 mg per 2.2 lbs (1 kg) of body weight 3 times a day, not to exceed 300 mg daily, for 5 to 7 days.

ONSET OF EFFECT
Unknown.

DURATION OF ACTION
Unknown.

DIETARY ADVICE
This medication is best taken after meals with a full glass of water, fruit juice, or tea, unless your doctor instructs otherwise. Tablets may be crushed and mixed with chocolate syrup, honey, or jam for persons who cannot stand the bitter taste or have difficulty swallowing tablets.

STORAGE
Store in a tightly sealed container away from heat, moisture, and direct light.

IF YOU MISS A DOSE
Take it as soon as you remember. If it is near the time for the next dose, skip the missed dose and resume your regular dosage schedule. Do not double the next dose.

STOPPING THE DRUG
Take it as prescribed for the full treatment period, even if you feel better before the scheduled end of therapy.

PROLONGED USE
See your doctor regularly for tests and examinations to check the medication's effectiveness. The dosage may need to be adjusted.

PRECAUTIONS
Over 60: Adverse reactions may be more likely and more severe. A lower dose may be warranted.

Driving and Hazardous Work: The use of quinacrine may impair your ability to perform such tasks safely. Exercise caution until you determine how this medication affects you.

Alcohol: Avoid all forms of alcohol, including medications such as cough syrup.

Pregnancy: Do not take quinacrine while pregnant; treatment should be delayed until after childbirth. If you are planning to become pregnant, consult your physician.

Breast Feeding: Quinacrine passes into breast milk and may be harmful to the nursing infant; caution is advised. Consult your doctor for specific advice.

Infants and Children: Adverse reactions may be more likely and more severe. Quinacrine's bitter taste may cause vomiting in children. Tablets may be crushed and mixed with chocolate syrup, honey, or jam to cover the taste. Discuss with your pediatrician the relative risks and benefits of your child using this medication.

OVERDOSE
Symptoms: Fainting, seizures, heart rhythm irregularities.

What to Do: Stop taking the drug and call your doctor, emergency medical services (EMS), or the nearest poison control center.

DRUG INTERACTIONS
Other drugs may interact with quinacrine. Do not take primaquine for up to 3 months after taking quinacrine. Also tell your doctor if you are taking any other prescription or over-the-counter medication.

FOOD INTERACTIONS
No known food interactions.

DISEASE INTERACTIONS
Consult your doctor for specific advice if you have any of the following: a history of mental illness or alcoholism, porphyria, or psoriasis. Also tell your doctor if you have any other medical condition.

Quinapril Hydrochloride

Accupril 10 mg
(PARKE-DAVIS)

Additional photographs

▶ Drug Class: Angiotensin-converting enzyme (ACE) inhibitor

▶ Available in: Tablets

▶ Available OTC? No

▶ As Generic? No

Side Effects

SERIOUS
Fever and chills, sore throat and hoarseness, sudden difficulty breathing or swallowing, swelling of the face, mouth, or extremities, impaired kidney function (ankle swelling, decreased urination), confusion, yellow discoloration of the eyes or skin (indicating liver disorder), intense itching, chest pain or palpitations, abdominal pain. Serious side effects are very rare; contact your doctor immediately.

COMMON
Dry, persistent cough.

LESS COMMON
Dizziness or fainting, skin rash, numbness or tingling in the hands, feet, or lips, unusual fatigue or muscle weakness, nausea, drowsiness, loss of taste, headache.

PRINCIPAL USES
To control high blood pressure (hypertension); to treat congestive heart failure (CHF); to treat patients with left ventricular dysfunction (damage to the pumping chamber of the heart); and to minimize further kidney damage in diabetics with mild kidney disease.

HOW THE DRUG WORKS
Angiotensin-converting enzyme (ACE) inhibitors block an enzyme that produces angiotensin, a naturally occurring substance that causes blood vessels to constrict and stimulates production of the adrenal hormone, aldosterone, which promotes sodium retention in the body. As a result, ACE inhibitors relax blood vessels (causing them to widen) and reduces sodium retention, which lowers blood pressure and so decreases the workload of the heart.

DOSAGE
10 mg once a day. Dose may be increased to 20 to 80 mg a day, taken in 1 or 2 doses.

ONSET OF EFFECT
Within 1 hour.

DURATION OF ACTION
24 hours.

DIETARY ADVICE
Take quinapril on an empty stomach, about 1 hour before mealtime. Follow your doctor's dietary advice (such as low-salt or low-cholesterol restrictions) to improve control over high blood pressure and heart disease. Avoid high-potassium foods like bananas and citrus fruits and juices, unless you are also taking drugs such as diuretics that lower potassium levels.

STORAGE
Store in a tightly sealed container away from heat and direct light.

IF YOU MISS A DOSE
Take it as soon as you remember. If it is near the time for the next dose, skip the missed dose and resume your regular dosage schedule. Do not double the next dose.

STOPPING THE DRUG
Do not stop taking this drug abruptly, as this may cause potentially serious health problems. Dosage should be reduced gradually, according to your doctor's instructions.

PROLONGED USE
Lifelong therapy may be necessary. See your doctor regularly for examinations and tests if you must take this drug for a prolonged period.

PRECAUTIONS
Over 60: No special problems are expected.

Driving and Hazardous Work: Avoid such activities until you determine how the medicine affects you.

Alcohol: Consume alcohol only in moderation since it may increase the effect of the drug and cause an excessive drop in blood pressure. Consult your doctor for advice.

Pregnancy: Use of quinapril during the last 6 months of pregnancy may cause severe defects, even death, to the fetus. The drug should be discontinued if you are pregnant or plan to become pregnant.

Breast Feeding: Quinapril may pass into breast milk; caution is advised. Consult your doctor for advice.

Infants and Children:
The safety and efficacy of quinapril use by infants and children have not been established. Benefits must be weighed against potential risks; consult your pediatrician for specific advice.

OVERDOSE
Symptoms: No specific ones have been reported.

What to Do: While overdose is unlikely, call your doctor, emergency medical services (EMS), or the nearest poison control center immediately if you suspect that someone has taken a much larger dose than prescribed.

DRUG INTERACTIONS
Consult your doctor if you are taking diuretics (especially potassium-sparing diuretics), potassium supplements or drugs containing potassium (check ingredient labels), lithium, anticoagulants (such as warfarin), indomethacin or other anti-inflammatory drugs, or any over-the-counter medications (especially cold remedies and diet pills).

FOOD INTERACTIONS
Avoid low-salt milk and salt substitutes. Many of these products contain potassium. Avoid consuming large servings of high-potassium foods like bananas and citrus fruits or juices.

DISEASE INTERACTIONS
Consult your doctor if you have systemic lupus erythematosus (SLE) or if you have had a prior allergic reaction to ACE inhibitors. Quinapril should be used with caution by patients with severe kidney disease or renal artery stenosis (narrowing of one or both of the arteries that supply blood to the kidneys).

Quinapril Hydrochloride/Hydrochlorothiazide

▶ Drug Class: Angiotensin-converting enzyme (ACE) inhibitor/diuretic

▶ Available in: Tablets

▶ Available OTC? No

▶ As Generic? No

Side Effects

SERIOUS
Fever and chills, sore throat and hoarseness, sudden difficulty breathing or swallowing, swelling of the face, mouth, or extremities, impaired kidney function (ankle swelling, decreased urination), confusion, yellow discoloration of the eyes or skin (indicating liver disorder), intense itching, chest pain or heartbeat irregularities, abdominal pain. Serious side effects are very rare; contact your doctor immediately.

COMMON
Dry, persistent cough, drowsiness.

LESS COMMON
Dizziness or fainting, skin rash, numbness or tingling in the hands, feet, or lips, change in color of the hands from white to blue to red (Raynaud's phenomenon) in cold weather, unusual fatigue or muscle weakness, nausea, loss of taste, headache, unusual dreams.

PRINCIPAL USES
To treat high blood pressure (hypertension). Used in patients for whom both quinapril and hydrochlorothiazide have been prescribed.

HOW THE DRUG WORKS
Angiotensin-converting enzyme (ACE) inhibitors such as quinapril block an enzyme that produces angiotensin, a naturally occurring substance that causes blood vessels to constrict and stimulates production of the adrenal hormone, aldosterone, which promotes sodium retention in the body. As a result, ACE inhibitors relax blood vessels (causing them to widen) and reduces sodium retention, which lowers blood pressure and so decreases the workload of the heart. Hydrochlorothiazide (HCTZ), a diuretic, increases sodium and water in the urine output. By reducing the overall fluid volume in the body, diuretics reduce blood volume and so reduce blood pressure.

DOSAGE
This combination medication comes in three strengths: quinapril/hydrochlorothiazide 10/12.5, 20/12.5, and 20/25. Your doctor will determine the appropriate dose.

ONSET OF EFFECT
Within 1 hour for quinapril; within 2 hours for HCTZ.

DURATION OF ACTION
24 hours for quinapril; 6 to 12 hours for HCTZ.

DIETARY ADVICE
Follow your doctor's dietary advice (such as low-salt or low-cholesterol restrictions) to improve control over high blood pressure and prevent heart disease.

STORAGE
Store in a tightly sealed container away from heat, moisture, and direct light.

IF YOU MISS A DOSE
If you do not remember until the next day, skip the missed dose and resume your regular dosage schedule. Do not double the next dose.

STOPPING THE DRUG
Discontinuing this drug abruptly may cause potentially serious problems. The dosage should be reduced gradually, according to your doctor's instructions.

PROLONGED USE
See your doctor regularly for evaluation if you must take this medicine for a prolonged period. Lifelong therapy may be necessary.

PRECAUTIONS
Over 60: Adverse reactions may be more likely and more severe.

Driving and Hazardous Work: Avoid such activities until you determine how the medicine affects you.

Alcohol: Consume alcohol only in moderation since it may increase the effect of the drug and cause an excessive drop in blood pressure. Consult your doctor for advice.

Pregnancy: Before taking this medication, tell your doctor if you are pregnant or plan to become pregnant. Use of this drug during the last 6 months of pregnancy may cause severe defects, even death, in the fetus.

Breast Feeding: Quinapril and hydrochlorothiazide may pass into breast milk; caution is advised. Consult your doctor for specific advice.

Infants and Children: Not recommended for use by children under 18.

Special Concerns: A rare complication is angioedema, characterized by swelling of the lips, tongue, and throat. It may be so severe as to cause obstruction of the airways, which could be fatal.

OVERDOSE
Symptoms: Overdose has not been reported; symptoms might include dizziness, faintness, or confusion.

What to Do: While overdose is unlikely, seek emergency medical attention immediately if you suspect that someone has taken a much larger dose than prescribed.

DRUG INTERACTIONS
Consult your doctor for specific advice if you are taking cholestyramine, colestipol, corticosteroids, digitalis drugs, antidiabetic drugs, lithium, potassium-containing medications or supplements, or any over-the-counter drug (especially cold remedies and appetite suppressants).

FOOD INTERACTIONS
Avoid low-salt milk and salt substitutes. Many of these products contain potassium.

DISEASE INTERACTIONS
Consult your doctor if you have systemic lupus erythematosus or if you have had a prior allergic reaction to ACE inhibitors. This medication should be used with caution by patients with abnormal liver function and is not recommended for those with severe kidney disease. This medication can increase blood triglycerides and worsen control of blood sugar in people with diabetes.

Quinidine

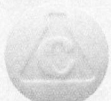

Quinaglute 324 mg
(BERLEX)

Additional photographs

▶ Drug Class: Antiarrhythmic

▶ Available in: Capsules,
tablets, extended-release
tablets

▶ Available OTC? No

▶ As Generic? Yes

Side Effects

SERIOUS
Dizziness, lightheaded-
ness, or fainting, any
change in vision, fever,
severe headache, ringing
or buzzing in the ears,
hearing loss, skin rash
or hives, shortness of
breath or wheezing, rapid
heartbeat, unusual bleed-
ing or bruising, unex-
plained fatigue. Call your
doctor immediately.

COMMON
Diarrhea, loss of appetite,
bitter taste, flushing and
itching skin, nausea,
vomiting, stomach pain
or cramps.

LESS COMMON
Mental confusion, rash.

PRINCIPAL USES
To correct irregular heartbeats (cardiac arrhythmias).

HOW THE DRUG WORKS
Quinidine slows nerve
impulses in the heart and
reduces the sensitivity of
heart tissue to certain nerve
impulses, thus stabilizing
heartbeat.

DOSAGE
Capsules and tablets—
Adults: 300 to 600 mg, 4
times a day. Children: 6 to
8.5 mg per 2.2 lbs (1 kg) of
body weight, 5 times a day.
Extended-release tablets—
Adults: 300 to 660 mg every
6 to 12 hours.

ONSET OF EFFECT
Oral forms, 1 to 2 hours.

DURATION OF ACTION
6 to 8 hours.

DIETARY ADVICE
Oral forms are usually
taken with a full glass of
water 1 hour before or 2
hours after meals. The
medication can be taken
with food or milk to lessen
stomach upset.

STORAGE
Store in a tightly sealed container away from heat and
direct light.

IF YOU MISS A DOSE
If you miss a dose, take it
as soon as you remember. If
it is close to the next dose,
skip the missed dose and
resume your regular dosage
schedule, as prescribed. Do
not double the next dose.

STOPPING THE DRUG
Take as prescribed for the
full treatment period, even if
you begin to feel better
before the scheduled end of
therapy. The decision to
stop taking the drug should
be made by your doctor.

PROLONGED USE
Lifelong therapy may be
necessary. See your doctor
regularly for examinations
and diagnostic tests if you
must take this medicine for
a prolonged period.

PRECAUTIONS
Over 60: Adverse reactions
may be more likely and
more severe in older
patients.

**Driving and Hazardous
Work:** Do not drive or
engage in hazardous work
until you determine how the
medicine affects you.

Alcohol: No special precautions are required.

Pregnancy: In animal studies, quinine, a closely
related drug, has caused
birth defects. Tests of quinidine have not been done.
Before you take quinidine,
tell your doctor if you are
pregnant or plan to become
pregnant.

Breast Feeding: Quinidine
passes into breast milk; caution is advised. Consult your
doctor for specific advice.

Infants and Children:
The long-acting oral dosage
form is not recommended
for use in children.

Special Concerns: You
may have to wear dark
glasses both indoors and
outside if quinidine makes
you sensitive to light.

OVERDOSE
Symptoms: Lethargy, confusion, headache, seizures,
dizziness, vomiting, stomach pain, hearing and vision
disturbances, fainting,
severe weakness or fatigue,
breathing difficulty, loss of
consciousness.

What to Do: Call your
doctor, emergency medical
services (EMS), or the
nearest poison control
center immediately.

DRUG INTERACTIONS
Avoid diuretics if possible
to prevent lowering of blood
potassium levels. Consult
your doctor for specific
advice if you are taking
digoxin, phenobarbital,
phenytoin, anticoagulants,
other heart medications,
antacids, acetazolamide,
or pimozide.

FOOD INTERACTIONS
No known food interactions.

DISEASE INTERACTIONS
Consult your doctor if you
have any of the following:
asthma, emphysema, an
infection of any kind, myasthenia gravis, hyperthyroidism, or psoriasis. Use of
quinidine may cause complications in patients with liver
or kidney disease, since
these organs work together
to remove the medication
from the body.

Rabeprazole Sodium

BRAND NAME
AcipHex

▶ Drug Class: Antacid/proton pump inhibitor

▶ Available in: Delayed-release tablets

▶ Available OTC? No

▶ As Generic? No

Side Effects

SERIOUS
No serious side effects are associated with the use of rabeprazole.

COMMON
Headache.

LESS COMMON
Weakness, fever, chills, allergic reaction, diarrhea, nausea, vomiting, abdominal pain, dry mouth, change in appetite, difficulty swallowing, muscle or joint pain. Many additional side effects can occur; consult your doctor if you are concerned about any adverse or unusual reactions you experience while taking this drug.

PRINCIPAL USES
To treat duodenal (intestinal) ulcers, as well as conditions that cause extreme increases in stomach acid production (such as Zollinger-Ellison syndrome), erosive esophagitis (severe, chronic inflammation or ulceration of the esophagus), and heartburn due to gastroesophageal reflux (backwash of stomach acid into the esophagus).

HOW THE DRUG WORKS
Rabeprazole blocks the action of a specific enzyme in the cells that line the stomach, thereby decreasing the production of stomach acid. Reduction of stomach acid promotes healing of ulcers.

DOSAGE
For duodenal ulcer, esophagitis, or gastroesophageal reflux: 20 mg a day. For Zollinger-Ellison syndrome or similar conditions: 60 to 100 mg a day, up to 60 mg twice a day.

ONSET OF EFFECT
Within 1 hour.

DURATION OF ACTION
At least 24 hours.

DIETARY ADVICE
Take rabeprazole after the morning meal. Tablets should be swallowed whole.

STORAGE
Store in a tightly sealed container away from heat, moisture, and direct light.

IF YOU MISS A DOSE
Take it as soon as you remember. However, if it is near the time for the next dose, skip the missed dose and resume your regular dosage schedule. Do not double the next dose.

STOPPING THE DRUG
Take as prescribed for the full treatment period, even if your symptoms improve before the scheduled end of therapy. The decision to stop taking the drug should be made in consultation with your doctor.

PROLONGED USE
Rabeprazole should not be used indefinitely as maintenance therapy for esophagitis; it is generally taken for a limited period of 4 to 8 weeks. For those who have not healed within this period, an additional 8 weeks of therapy may be considered by your doctor. People with duodenal ulcer generally heal within 4 weeks of therapy. Some people with Zollinger-Ellison syndrome have been treated for up to one year. See your doctor regularly for tests and examinations if you must take this drug for an extended period of time.

PRECAUTIONS
Over 60: No specific problems for older people have been reported.

Driving and Hazardous Work: Avoid such activities until you determine how the drug affects you.

Alcohol: Avoid alcohol while taking this medication, as it may aggravate your condition.

Pregnancy: In animal tests, rabeprazole has not caused problems. Human tests have not been done. Before you take rabeprazole, tell your doctor if you are pregnant or plan to become pregnant.

Breast Feeding: Rabeprazole may pass into breast milk; caution is advised. Consult your doctor for advice.

Infants and Children: Safety and effectiveness have not been established for patients under age 18.

Special Concerns: Do not chew, crush, or split the tablets. If your doctor directs, you may take an antacid along with rabeprazole.

OVERDOSE
Symptoms: Few cases of overdose have been reported.

What to Do: An overdose is unlikely to be life-threatening. However, if someone takes a much larger dose than prescribed, call your doctor, emergency medical services (EMS), or the nearest poison control center immediately.

DRUG INTERACTIONS
Consult your doctor for specific advice if you are taking ketoconazole or digoxin.

FOOD INTERACTIONS
No significant food interactions have been reported.

DISEASE INTERACTIONS
Consult your doctor if you have severe liver disease, since it may increase the risk of side effects.

Raloxifene Hydrochloride

▶ Drug Class: Selective estrogen receptor modulator (SERM)

▶ Available in: Tablets

▶ Available OTC? No

▶ As Generic? No

Side Effects

SERIOUS
No serious side effects are associated with the use of raloxifene.

COMMON
Increased incidence of infections, flu-like symptoms, hot flashes, joint pain, sinusitis, unexpected weight gain.

LESS COMMON
Leg cramps, mild chest pain, fever, migraine, indigestion, vomiting, flatulence, stomach upset, swelling of the legs and feet, muscle pain, insomnia, sore throat, increased cough, pneumonia, laryngitis, rash, sweating, yeast infection, urinary tract infection, white vaginal discharge.

PRINCIPAL USES
For the treatment and prevention of osteoporosis in postmenopausal women. Unlike estrogen, raloxifene does not stimulate overgrowth of the endometrium (the tissue lining the uterus) and thus does not increase the risk of uterine cancer.

HOW THE DRUG WORKS
Healthy bone tissue is continuously remodeled (broken down and then reformed); the minerals and other components of bone are reabsorbed by certain cells and then replaced by new bone formation. Raloxifene suppresses the activity of the cells that resorb bone; consequently, the breakdown of bone tissue occurs more slowly than the laying down of new bone. This action preserves bone density and strength.

DOSAGE
One 60 mg tablet a day.

ONSET OF EFFECT
Unknown.

DURATION OF ACTION
Unknown.

DIETARY ADVICE
Raloxifene may be taken at any time of day without regard to meal schedule. Patients are generally advised to take calcium and vitamin D supplements to aid bone formation.

STORAGE
Store in a tightly sealed container away from heat, moisture, and direct light.

IF YOU MISS A DOSE
If you miss a dose on one day, do not double the dose the next day.

STOPPING THE DRUG
The decision to stop taking the drug should be made in consultation with your physician.

PROLONGED USE
Safety and effectiveness beyond three years of use have not been determined.

PRECAUTIONS
Over 60: No special problems are expected.

Driving and Hazardous Work: No special problems are expected.

Alcohol: Alcohol should be restricted in high-risk women because it is a risk factor for osteoporosis.

Pregnancy: Raloxifene is normally not used in premenopausal women. The drug should not be given to pregnant women.

Breast Feeding: Raloxifene should not be used by nursing mothers.

Infants and Children: Raloxifene should not be used by children.

Special Concerns: Patients taking raloxifene are encouraged to engage in regular weight-bearing exercise and should avoid cigarettes and limit alcohol, which inhibit healthy bone production. Unlike estrogen replacement therapy, raloxifene does not reduce hot flashes in postmenopausal women.

OVERDOSE
Symptoms: No cases of overdose have been reported.

What to Do: An overdose with raloxifene is unlikely. If someone takes a much larger dose than prescribed, call your doctor.

DRUG INTERACTIONS
Estrogen should not be taken concurrently with raloxifene. Since cholestyramine reduces absorption of raloxifene, the two drugs should not be taken at the same time of day. Consult your doctor if you are taking any of the following drugs that may interact with raloxifene: warfarin, clofibrate, indomethacin, naproxen, ibuprofen, diazepam, or diazoxide.

FOOD INTERACTIONS
No known food interactions.

DISEASE INTERACTIONS
You should not take raloxifene if you have a history of thromboembolic disease, including deep vein thrombosis, pulmonary embolism, and retinal vein thrombosis. Raloxifene must be used with caution by patients with impaired liver function; consult your doctor for specific advice.

Ramipril

Altace 5 mg
(Hoechst Marion Roussel)

▶ Drug Class: Angiotensin-converting enzyme (ACE) inhibitor

▶ Available in: Tablets

▶ Available OTC? No

▶ As Generic? No

Side Effects

SERIOUS
Fever and chills, sore throat and hoarseness, sudden difficulty breathing or swallowing, swelling of the face, mouth, or extremities, impaired kidney function (ankle swelling, decreased urination), confusion, yellow discoloration of the eyes or skin (indicating liver disorder), intense itching, chest pain or palpitations, abdominal pain. Serious side effects are very rare; contact your doctor immediately.

COMMON
Dry, persistent cough.

LESS COMMON
Dizziness or fainting, skin rash, numbness or tingling in the hands, feet, or lips, unusual fatigue or muscle weakness, nausea, drowsiness, loss of taste, headache.

PRINCIPAL USES
To control high blood pressure (hypertension); to treat congestive heart failure; to treat patients with left ventricular dysfunction (damage to the pumping chamber of the heart); to reduce risk of heart attack, stroke, and death from cardiovascular causes; and to minimize further kidney damage in diabetics with mild kidney disease.

HOW THE DRUG WORKS
Angiotensin-converting enzyme (ACE) inhibitors block an enzyme that produces angiotensin, a naturally occurring substance that causes blood vessels to constrict and stimulates production of the adrenal hormone, aldosterone, which promotes sodium retention in the body. As a result, ACE inhibitors relax blood vessels (causing them to widen) and reduces sodium retention, which lowers blood pressure and so decreases the workload of the heart.

DOSAGE
2.5 mg to 20 mg per day, taken in 1 or 2 doses.

ONSET OF EFFECT
Within 1 to 2 hours.

DURATION OF ACTION
24 hours.

DIETARY ADVICE
Take it on an empty stomach, about 1 hour before mealtime. Follow your doctor's dietary advice (such as low-salt or low-cholesterol restrictions) to improve control over high blood pressure and heart disease. Avoid high-potassium foods like bananas and citrus fruits and juices, unless you are also taking medications, such as diuretics, that lower potassium levels.

STORAGE
Store in a tightly sealed container away from heat and direct light.

IF YOU MISS A DOSE
Take it as soon as you remember. If it is near the time for the next dose, skip the missed dose and resume your regular dosage schedule. Do not double the next dose.

STOPPING THE DRUG
Do not stop taking this drug abruptly, as this may cause potentially serious health problems. Dosage should be reduced gradually, according to your doctor's instructions.

PROLONGED USE
Lifelong therapy may be necessary. See your doctor regularly for examinations and tests if you must take this medicine for a prolonged period of time.

PRECAUTIONS
Over 60: No special problems are expected.

Driving and Hazardous Work: Do not drive or engage in hazardous work until you determine how the medicine affects you.

Alcohol: Consume alcohol only in moderation since it may increase the effect of the drug and cause an excessive drop in blood pressure. Consult your doctor for advice.

Pregnancy: Use of ramipril during the last 6 months of pregnancy may cause severe defects, even death, in the fetus. The drug should be discontinued if you are pregnant or plan to become pregnant.

Breast Feeding: Ramipril may pass into breast milk;

caution is advised. Consult your doctor for advice.

Infants and Children: Children may be especially sensitive to the effects of ramipril. Benefits must be weighed against potential risks; consult your pediatrician for advice.

OVERDOSE
Symptoms: Dizziness or fainting due to extremely low blood pressure.

What to Do: Call your doctor, emergency medical services (EMS), or the nearest poison control center immediately.

DRUG INTERACTIONS
Consult your doctor if you are taking diuretics (especially potassium-sparing diuretics), potassium supplements or drugs containing potassium (check ingredient labels), lithium, anticoagulants (such as warfarin), indomethacin or other anti-inflammatory drugs, or any over-the-counter medications (especially cold remedies and diet pills).

FOOD INTERACTIONS
Avoid low-salt milk and salt substitutes. Many of these products contain potassium. Avoid consuming large servings of high-potassium foods like bananas and citrus fruits or juices.

DISEASE INTERACTIONS
Consult your doctor if you have systemic lupus erythematosus (SLE) or if you have had a prior allergic reaction to ACE inhibitors. Ramipril should be used with caution by patients with severe kidney disease or renal artery stenosis (narrowing of one or both of the arteries that supply blood to the kidneys).

Ranitidine

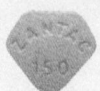

Zantac 150 mg
(**GLAXO WELLCOME**)

Additional photographs

▶ Drug Class: **Histamine (H2) blocker**

▶ Available in: Capsules, tablets, injection, syrup, granules

▶ Available OTC? **Yes**

▶ As Generic? **Yes**

Side Effects

SERIOUS
Irregular heart rhythm (palpitations), slowed heartbeat, severe blood problems resulting in unusual bleeding, bruising, fever, chills, and increased susceptibility to infection. Call your doctor immediately.

COMMON
Headache, fatigue, drowsiness, dizziness, nausea, vomiting, abdominal pain, diarrhea, constipation.

LESS COMMON
Blurred vision, decreased sexual desire or function, swelling of breasts in males or females, temporary hair loss, hallucinations, depression, insomnia, skin rash, hives, or redness.

PRINCIPAL USES
To treat ulcers of the stomach and duodenum, conditions that cause increased stomach acid production (such as Zollinger-Ellison syndrome), erosive esophagitis (severe, chronic inflammation of the esophagus), and gastroesophageal reflux (backwash of stomach acid into the esophagus, resulting in heartburn).

HOW THE DRUG WORKS
Ranitidine blocks the action of histamine (a compound produced in the body's cells), which in turn decreases the stomach's secretion of hydrochloric acid. Once stomach acid production is decreased, the body is better able to heal itself.

DOSAGE
Adults— Oral dose: 150 mg, 2 times a day, in the morning and at bedtime, or 300 mg once daily before bedtime. Injection: 50 mg every 6 to 8 hours. Patients with Zollinger-Ellison syndrome may require up to 6 g per day, taken orally. For treatment of heartburn with the over-the-counter form: 75 mg, as needed, not to exceed 150 mg a day. Children— Consult your pediatrician for appropriate individual dosage.

ONSET OF EFFECT
30 to 60 minutes.

DURATION OF ACTION
Up to 13 hours.

DIETARY ADVICE
Avoid foods that cause stomach irritation.

STORAGE
Store away from heat and direct light. Keep liquid form from freezing.

IF YOU MISS A DOSE
Take it as soon as you remember. If it is near the time for the next dose, skip the missed dose and resume your regular dosage schedule. Do not double the next dose.

STOPPING THE DRUG
Take the prescription-strength medication for the full treatment period, even if you begin to feel better before the scheduled end of therapy.

PROLONGED USE
Do not take nonprescription-strength ranitidine for more than 2 weeks unless you have been otherwise instructed by your doctor.

PRECAUTIONS
Over 60: Adverse reactions may be more likely and more severe in older patients.

Driving and Hazardous Work: Do not drive or engage in hazardous work until you determine how the medicine affects you.

Alcohol: Avoid alcohol. Ranitidine may increase blood alcohol levels.

Pregnancy: Risks vary, depending on the patient and dosage. Consult your doctor.

Breast Feeding: Ranitidine passes into breast milk and may pose harm to the child; avoid or discontinue use while nursing.

Infants and Children: Ranitidine is not recommended for young patients, although it has not been shown to cause any side effects or problems different from those in adults when used for short periods of time.

Special Concerns: Avoid cigarette smoking because it may increase stomach acid secretion and thus worsen the disease. Do not take ranitidine if you have ever had an allergic reaction to a histamine (H2) blocker. If stomach pain becomes worse while using the drug, be sure to tell your doctor right away.

OVERDOSE
Symptoms: Vomiting, diarrhea, breathing problems, slurred speech, rapid heartbeat, delirium.

What to Do: Call your doctor, emergency medical services (EMS), or the nearest poison control center immediately.

DRUG INTERACTIONS
Consult your doctor for specific advice if you are taking antacids, antidepressants, aspirin, beta-blockers, caffeine, diazepam, glipizide, ketoconazole, lidocaine, phenytoin, procainamide, theophylline, or warfarin.

FOOD INTERACTIONS
Carbonated drinks, citrus fruits and juices, caffeine-containing beverages, and other acidic foods or liquids may irritate the stomach or interfere with the therapeutic action of ranitidine.

DISEASE INTERACTIONS
Patients with kidney disease should not use ranitidine or should use it in smaller, limited doses under careful supervision by a physician.

Ranitidine Bismuth Citrate

BRAND NAME
Tritec

▶ Drug Class: Antiulcer drug

▶ Available in: Tablets

▶ Available OTC? No

▶ As Generic? No

Side Effects

SERIOUS
No serious side effects have been reported.

COMMON
Diarrhea, nausea and vomiting, headache, changes in taste perception, sleep disorders, chest symptoms, skin itching.

LESS COMMON
Abdominal discomfort, tremors.

PRINCIPAL USES
To treat duodenal ulcers caused by infection with *Helicobacter pylori* bacteria. Therapy with ranitidine bismuth citrate is done in combination with the antibiotic clarithromycin.

HOW THE DRUG WORKS
Research has shown that the majority of peptic ulcers are caused by infection with a bacterium known as *Helicobacter pylori*. Clarithromycin kills bacteria; ranitidine bismuth citrate enhances clarithromycin's antibiotic effect to help eradicate *Helicobacter pylori*. Ranitidine bismuth citrate also inhibits the secretion of stomach acid, thereby facilitating the healing of ulcers.

DOSAGE
400 mg of ranitidine bismuth citrate 2 times a day for 4 weeks with 500 mg of clarithromycin, 3 times a day for the first 2 weeks. Ranitidine bismuth citrate should never be taken alone for treatment of active duodenal ulcers.

ONSET OF EFFECT
Unknown.

DURATION OF ACTION
Unknown.

DIETARY ADVICE
This drug is best taken at least 30 minutes after meals.

STORAGE
Store in a tightly sealed container away from heat and direct light.

IF YOU MISS A DOSE
Take it as soon as you remember. If it is near the time for the next dose, skip the missed dose and resume your regular dosage schedule. Do not double the next dose.

STOPPING THE DRUG
Take it as prescribed for the full treatment period, even if you begin to feel better before the scheduled end of therapy.

PROLONGED USE
This drug is not intended for prolonged use. Healing of the ulcer should occur within 4 weeks, and a second course of therapy is not warranted if the first proves ineffective.

PRECAUTIONS
Over 60: Ranitidine bismuth citrate does not cause more side effects and problems in older patients than it does in younger people.

Driving and Hazardous Work: The use of this drug should not impair your ability to perform such tasks safely.

Alcohol: Avoid alcohol.

Pregnancy: In animal studies, ranitidine bismuth citrate has not caused problems; human studies have not been done. However, ranitidine bismuth citrate taken with clarithromycin may cause problems during pregnancy. Before you take this drug combination, tell your doctor if you are pregnant or plan to become pregnant.

Breast Feeding: It is not known whether ranitidine bismuth citrate passes into breast milk; caution is advised. Consult your doctor for specific advice.

Infants and Children: The safety and effectiveness of ranitidine bismuth citrate and clarithromycin for use by infants and children have not been established.

Special Concerns: Patients whose *Helicobacter pylori* infections are not eradicated after treatment with ranitidine bismuth citrate and clarithromycin should be considered to be infected with bacteria that are resistant to clarithromycin. They should not be treated with clarithromycin again. The bismuth component of this drug may cause a temporary and harmless darkening of the tongue and the stools.

OVERDOSE
Symptoms: No specific ones have been reported.

What to Do: An overdose of ranitidine bismuth citrate is unlikely to be life-threatening. However, if someone takes a much larger dose than prescribed, call your doctor, emergency medical services (EMS), or the nearest poison control center immediately.

DRUG INTERACTIONS
Drug interactions with ranitidine bismuth citrate have not been established. Before you take the medication, tell your doctor if you are taking any prescription or over-the-counter drug.

FOOD INTERACTIONS
No known food interactions.

DISEASE INTERACTIONS
Caution is advised when taking ranitidine bismuth citrate. Tell your doctor if you have any other medical condition. Use of this drug may cause problems in patients with kidney disease, because this organ works to remove the medication from the body.

Repaglinide

BRAND NAME
Prandin

▶ Drug Class: Antidiabetic agent

▶ Available in: Tablets

▶ Available OTC? No

▶ As Generic? No

Side Effects

SERIOUS
Hypoglycemia (blood sugar levels that are too low), resulting in shakiness, headache, cold sweats, anxiety, and changes in mental state. Immediately ingest sugar-containing food or drink. Inform your doctor about the frequency and timing of hypoglycemic events.

COMMON
Increased incidence of upper respiratory or sinus infection, headache, back pain, joint pain, diarrhea.

LESS COMMON
Constipation, indigestion, urinary tract infection, mild allergic reaction.

PRINCIPAL USES
Used as an adjunct (supplemental) therapy to dietary measures and exercise to help control blood sugar levels in patients with type 2 diabetes mellitus. Repaglinide is the first in a new class of oral antidiabetic drugs designed to control blood glucose levels following meals.

HOW THE DRUG WORKS
Repaglinide stimulates the pancreas to produce more insulin. Increased insulin levels reduce blood glucose by promoting the transport of glucose into muscle cells and other tissues, where it is used as a source of energy. The rapid onset and short duration of repaglinide's action make it effective in controlling glucose levels after a meal.

DOSAGE
Dosage must be determined for each patient individually, based on blood glucose levels and response to the drug. The recommended dosage range is 0.5 to 4 mg taken 15 to 30 minutes before meals. Repaglinide may be taken before meals 2, 3, or 4 times a day depending on the patient's meal pattern. The maximum recommended daily dose is 16 mg.

ONSET OF EFFECT
30 to 60 minutes.

DURATION OF ACTION
1 to 2 hours.

DIETARY ADVICE
Doses should be taken 15 to 30 minutes before meals. Follow the dietary guidelines given by your doctor.

STORAGE
Store in a tightly sealed container away from heat, moisture, and direct light.

IF YOU MISS A DOSE
If you miss a dose, take it with the next meal. Do not double the next dose.

STOPPING THE DRUG
Do not stop taking the drug without your doctor's approval.

PROLONGED USE
Prolonged use increases the risk of adverse effects. Periodic physical examinations and blood tests to monitor glucose levels are needed.

PRECAUTIONS
Over 60: Older patients may be more susceptible to adverse effects, especially hypoglycemia, which may be more difficult to recognize in the elderly.

Driving and Hazardous Work: Caution is advised until you have reached a stable dosing regimen that does not produce episodes of hypoglycemia.

Alcohol: Limit alcohol intake; hypoglycemia is more likely to occur after the consumption of alcohol.

Pregnancy: Repaglinide is not usually given during pregnancy. Insulin is the treatment of choice for pregnant diabetic patients.

Breast Feeding: Repaglinide may pass into breast milk; consult your doctor for advice if you are considering breast feeding.

Infants and Children: Safety and effectiveness have not been established for young patients.

Special Concerns: Follow your doctor's advice about diet, exercise, and weight control carefully. These aspects of treatment are just as essential to the proper control of diabetes as taking the medication. Be sure to carry at all times some form of medical identification that indicates you have diabetes and that lists all of the drugs you are taking.

OVERDOSE
Symptoms: Excessive hunger, nausea, anxiety, cold sweats, drowsiness, rapid heartbeat, weakness, changes in mental state, loss of consciousness (indications of hypoglycemia). Overdose is most likely to occur when caloric intake is deficient, following or during more exercise than usual, or after consuming more than a small amount of alcohol.

What to Do: Call your doctor, emergency medical services (EMS), or local hospital immediately.

DRUG INTERACTIONS
Consult your doctor if you are taking antifungal agents such as ketoconazole or miconazole; also, antibiotics, rifampin, barbiturates, carbamazepine, aspirin or other NSAIDs, sulfonamides, chloramphenicol, probenecid, MAO inhibitors, beta-blockers, diuretics, corticosteroids, phenothiazines, estrogens, oral contraceptives, phenytoin, calcium channel blockers, sympathomimetics, or isoniazid.

FOOD INTERACTIONS
A special diet is essential for proper control of blood glucose levels.

DISEASE INTERACTIONS
Do not use repaglinide if you have type 1 diabetes mellitus. Use of repaglinide may cause complications in patients with impaired liver or kidney function, since these organs are both involved in removing the medication from the body.

Resorcinol

▶ Drug Class: Acne drug

▶ Available in: Lotion, cream, stick

▶ Available OTC? Yes

▶ As Generic? Yes

Side Effects

SERIOUS
No serious side effects are associated with resorcinol during normal use (as prescribed).

COMMON
Mild redness and peeling of the skin. Such side effects tend to occur at the beginning of therapy and diminish as your body adjusts to the medication; notify your doctor if such symptoms persist or interfere with daily activities.

LESS COMMON
More-severe irritation or allergy with redness, peeling, burning, stinging, itching, or rash. Call your doctor.

PRINCIPAL USES
To treat acne and seborrheic dermatitis. Resorcinol is also infrequently used to treat eczema, psoriasis, corns, calluses, warts, and other skin conditions.

HOW THE DRUG WORKS
Resorcinol fights fungal and bacterial organisms and promotes softening, dissolution, and peeling of the skin.

DOSAGE
For acne and seborrheic dermatitis: Apply once or twice daily as recommended or as tolerated. Wash your hands thoroughly after applying resorcinol.

ONSET OF EFFECT
Unknown.

DURATION OF ACTION
Unknown.

DIETARY ADVICE
No special restrictions.

STORAGE
Store in a tightly sealed container away from heat and direct light.

IF YOU MISS A DOSE
Skip the missed application and resume your regular dosage schedule. Do not double the next dose.

STOPPING THE DRUG
If you are using resorcinol by prescription, the decision to stop using the drug should be made by your doctor. If you are using it without a prescription, you may stop using it whenever your acne clears; however, it is likely that discontinuing use of the drug will lead to a recurrence of acne.

PROLONGED USE
Do not use resorcinol for longer than prescribed.

PRECAUTIONS
Over 60: No special problems are expected.

Driving and Hazardous Work: No special precautions are necessary.

Alcohol: No special precautions are necessary.

Pregnancy: Resorcinol has not been shown to cause birth defects or other problems during pregnancy. However, it may be absorbed through the skin. Consult your doctor for specific advice if you are pregnant or plan to become pregnant.

Breast Feeding: Resorcinol may be absorbed into the body through the skin; caution is advised. Consult your doctor for advice.

Infants and Children: Resorcinol should not be used on large areas of the body of children.

Special Concerns: Anyone with a history of allergy to resorcinol or any other ingredients in the specific product should not use this medication. Resorcinol should not be used on wounds, because it may cause methemoglobinemia, a blood disorder. It should not be applied over large areas of the body, especially when used in high concentrations. Avoid contact of resorcinol with the eyes. This medication is generally not recommended for black persons, since it may significantly darken treated areas of skin. Resorcinol may darken light-colored hair.

OVERDOSE
Symptoms: If ingested, diarrhea, nausea, abdominal pain, vomiting, drowsiness, dizziness, severe or persistent headache, breathing difficulty, unusual tiredness or weakness, slow heartbeat, and profuse sweating may occur.

What to Do: In case of ingestion, call your doctor, emergency medical services (EMS), or the nearest poison control center.

DRUG INTERACTIONS
The following drugs or other products may irritate the skin and therefore should not be used with resorcinol unless recommended by your doctor: abrasive soaps or cleansers, alcohol-containing preparations (including astringents, aftershave lotions, other perfumed toiletries), any other acne agent, any preparation containing a peeling agent such as benzoyl peroxide, salicylic acid, alpha hydroxy acids, sulfur, or vitamin A, and soaps, medicated cosmetics, or other cosmetics that dry the skin.

FOOD INTERACTIONS
No known food interactions.

DISEASE INTERACTIONS
You should not use resorcinol if you have had a prior allergic reaction to it.

Rifabutin

BRAND NAME
Mycobutin

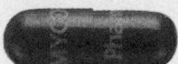

Mycobutin 150 mg
(PHARMACIA)

▶ Drug Class: Anti-infective

▶ Available in: Capsules

▶ Available OTC? No

▶ As Generic? No

Side Effects

SERIOUS
No serious side effects are associated with the use of rifabutin.

COMMON
Reddish orange or brown discoloration of urine, saliva, phlegm, stools, sweat, skin, and tears; skin rash; nausea and vomiting; low white blood cell count.

LESS COMMON
Joint aches, eye irritation, blurred or decreased vision.

PRINCIPAL USES
A tuberculosis-like disease known as Mycobacterium avium complex (MAC) is common in people with advanced AIDS. Rifabutin is used to prevent MAC and can be used with other drugs to treat MAC infection. It is occasionally used to treat tuberculosis.

HOW THE DRUG WORKS
Rifabutin interferes with the activity of enzymes needed for the replication of RNA (ribonucleic acid) in bacterial cells, thus preventing the bacteria from reproducing.

DOSAGE
Adults and teenagers: 300 mg once a day, or 150 mg, 2 times a day.

ONSET OF EFFECT
Unknown.

DURATION OF ACTION
Unknown.

DIETARY ADVICE
Take it on an empty stomach, 1 hour before or 2 hours after meals. If nausea and vomiting develop or you are unable to swallow the pills, the contents of the capsules can be mixed with food such as applesauce.

STORAGE
Store in a tightly sealed container away from heat, moisture, and direct light.

IF YOU MISS A DOSE
Take the drug as soon as you remember. This will help keep a constant level of medication in your system. If it is near the time for the next dose, skip the missed dose and resume your regular dosage schedule. Do not double the next dose.

STOPPING THE DRUG
Take it as prescribed for the full treatment period, even if you begin to feel better before the scheduled end of therapy. Treatment may continue for months or years. The decision to stop taking the drug should be made by your doctor.

PROLONGED USE
Consult your doctor about the need for periodic medical examinations and laboratory tests. Long-term therapy is usually required.

PRECAUTIONS
Over 60: No special problems are expected.

Driving and Hazardous Work: Do not drive or engage in hazardous work until you determine how the medicine affects you.

Alcohol: Avoid alcohol.

Pregnancy: Adequate studies of rifabutin use during pregnancy have not been done. This drug should be given during pregnancy only if potential benefits clearly outweigh the risks to the unborn child. There is no evidence that the drug will reduce the risk of transmitting the virus from the mother to the fetus.

Breast Feeding: It is not known whether rifabutin passes into breast milk; caution is advised. Women who are infected with HIV should not breast feed, to avoid transmitting the virus to an uninfected child.

Infants and Children: Use and dose for infants and children must be determined by your doctor. It is not known whether rifabutin causes different or more severe side effects in infants and children than it does in older persons.

Special Concerns: Soft contact lenses may become permanently discolored. If you have been using oral contraceptives, you should use a different method of birth control while taking rifabutin.

OVERDOSE
Symptoms: An overdose with rifabutin is unlikely.

What to Do: If someone takes a much larger dose than prescribed, call your doctor, emergency medical services (EMS), or the nearest poison control center right away.

DRUG INTERACTIONS
Rifabutin should not be taken if you are also taking the protease inhibitor ritonavir, and it should be used with caution if you are taking other protease inhibitors (a class of drugs used to treat AIDS). Consult your doctor for specific advice if you are taking ketoconazole, phenytoin, prednisone, propranolol, quinidine, oral contraceptives, sulfonylureas (oral antidiabetics), warfarin, or zidovudine. Also tell your doctor if you are taking any other prescription or over-the-counter medication.

FOOD INTERACTIONS
No known food interactions.

DISEASE INTERACTIONS
Caution is advised when taking rifabutin. Consult your doctor if you have active tuberculosis (TB). If you have to take rifabutin and have active TB, you must take other medications to cure TB. Rifabutin, if used alone, may cause drug-resistant strains of the TB bacterium to thrive, resulting in a TB infection that is very hard to treat.

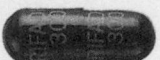

Rifadin 300 mg
(Hoechst Marion Roussel)

▶ Drug Class: Anti-infective/
antitubercular agent

▶ Available in: Capsules,
injection

▶ Available OTC? No

▶ As Generic? Yes

Side Effects

SERIOUS
Difficulty breathing, chills, pain in muscles and bones, dizziness, headache, itching, fever, shivering, skin rash and redness, nausea and vomiting, diarrhea, yellow discoloration of the skin or eyes. Call your doctor immediately.

COMMON
Reddish orange or brown discoloration of urine, saliva, phlegm, stools, sweat, skin, and tears; stomach cramps.

LESS COMMON
There are no less-common side effects associated with the use of rifampin.

PRINCIPAL USES
To treat all forms of tuberculosis (TB); must be used in conjunction with other antitubercular agents. Also to prevent the spread of TB by people who are carriers of it but who do not have active disease, and to treat other bacterial infections and persons who have been exposed to certain types of meningitis-causing bacteria.

HOW THE DRUG WORKS
Rifampin interferes with the activity of enzymes needed for the replication of RNA (ribonucleic acid) in bacterial cells, preventing the bacteria from reproducing.

DOSAGE
To treat tuberculosis—
Adults and teenagers: 600 mg once a day. Children ages 5 to 12: 4.5 to 9 mg per lb of body weight once a day (not more than 600 mg a day). Older adults: 4.5 mg per lb once a day. It may be decreased to twice a week. To prevent meningitis—Adults and teenagers: 600 mg twice a day for 2 days. Children 1 month to 12 years: 9 mg per lb twice a day for 2 days, or 9 to 18 mg per lb once a day for 4 days. Newborns: 2.3 mg per lb twice a day for 2 days.

ONSET OF EFFECT
Unknown.

DURATION OF ACTION
Unknown.

DIETARY ADVICE
Take the capsules on an empty stomach at least 1 hour before or 2 hours after meals. If you experience nausea and vomiting from taking the medication, or you have trouble swallowing the pills, mix the contents of the capsules in with food such as applesauce.

STORAGE
Store in a tightly sealed container away from heat, moisture, and direct light.

IF YOU MISS A DOSE
Take the drug as soon as you remember. This will help keep a constant level of medication in your system. However, if it is near the time for the next dose, skip the missed dose and resume your regular dosage schedule. Do not double the next dose.

STOPPING THE DRUG
Take it as prescribed for the full treatment period, even if you feel better before the scheduled end of therapy. Treatment may continue for months or years. The decision to stop taking it should be made by your doctor.

PROLONGED USE
Consult your doctor about the need for periodic medical examinations and laboratory tests. If symptoms do not improve or instead become worse in 2 to 3 weeks, consult your doctor.

PRECAUTIONS
Over 60: No special problems are expected.

Driving and Hazardous Work: Do not drive or engage in hazardous work until you determine how the medicine affects you.

Alcohol: Avoid alcohol.

Pregnancy: Rifampin, in conjunction with other antitubercular agents, can be used to treat tuberculosis in pregnant women. Before you take it, tell your doctor if you are pregnant or plan to become pregnant.

Breast Feeding: Rifampin passes into breast milk; caution is advised. Consult your doctor for specific advice.

Infants and Children: No special problems are expected.

Special Concerns: Rifampin can lower your white blood cell count and the number of platelets in your blood, temporarily increasing the risk of infection, slowing healing, and making your gums more susceptible to bleeding. Try to delay dental work until after therapy. Soft contact lenses may become permanently discolored. Oral contraceptives containing estrogen may be ineffective during use.

OVERDOSE
Symptoms: Whole-body itching, facial swelling, changes in mental state, reddish orange discoloration of skin, eyes, and mouth.

What to Do: Call your doctor, emergency medical services (EMS), or the nearest poison control center immediately.

DRUG INTERACTIONS
Consult your doctor for advice if you are taking theophylline, anticoagulants, oral antidiabetics, azole antifungal agents, anticancer agents, estrogens, corticosteroids, digitalis drugs, antiarrhythmics, antitubercular agents, methadone, phenytoin, verapamil, protease inhibitors, cyclosporine, or tacrolimus (FK506).

FOOD INTERACTIONS
No known food interactions.

DISEASE INTERACTIONS
Consult your doctor if you have a history of alcohol abuse. Use of rifampin may cause complications in patients with liver disease, since this organ works to remove the medication from the body.

Rifapentine

BRAND NAME
Priftin

▶ Drug Class: Anti-infective/ antitubercular agent

▶ Available in: Tablets

▶ Available OTC? No

▶ As Generic? No

Side Effects

SERIOUS
Pain or swelling in joints, fever, dizziness, headache, itching, skin rash and redness, loss of appetite, nausea, vomiting, diarrhea, yellow discoloration of the skin or eyes, dark urine. Call your doctor immediately.

COMMON
Reddish orange or brown discoloration of urine, saliva, phlegm, stools, sweat, skin, tears, and breast milk; stomach cramps.

LESS COMMON
There are no less-common side effects associated with the use of rifapentine.

PRINCIPAL USES
To treat active pulmonary tuberculosis; must be used in conjunction with other antitubercular agents (such as isoniazid, pyrazinamide, ethambutol, and streptomycin) to which the bacteria is susceptible.

HOW THE DRUG WORKS
Rifapentine interferes with the activity of enzymes needed for the formation of RNA (ribonucleic acid) in the bacteria that causes tuberculosis, preventing them from reproducing.

DOSAGE
For first 2 months of treatment: 600 mg (four 150 mg tablets) twice a week (with no more than 3 days between doses) in combination with other antitubercular agents. For the next 4 months of treatment: 600 mg once a week in conjunction with other antitubercular agents.

ONSET OF EFFECT
Unknown.

DURATION OF ACTION
Unknown.

DIETARY ADVICE
Take with liquid or food to minimize stomach irritation.

STORAGE
Store in a tightly sealed container away from heat, moisture, and direct light.

IF YOU MISS A DOSE
It is critical to take each dose to prevent the development of bacteria resistant to the drug's action. If you do miss a dose, take it as soon as you remember. This will help keep a constant level of medication in your system. However, if it is near the time for the next dose, skip the missed dose and resume regular dosage schedule. Do not double the next dose.

STOPPING THE DRUG
Take it as prescribed for the full treatment period. Treatment may continue for months or years. The decision to stop taking it should be made by your doctor.

PROLONGED USE
Tuberculosis bacteria must be tested for sensitivity to the drug (and other tuberculosis medications) before starting treatment and throughout the course of therapy. If symptoms do not improve or instead become worse in 2 to 3 weeks, consult your doctor.

PRECAUTIONS
Over 60: No special problems are expected.

Driving and Hazardous Work: No special problems are expected.

Alcohol: Avoid alcohol.

Pregnancy: Adequate studies of rifapentine use during pregnancy have not been done. This drug should be taken during pregnancy only if potential benefits clearly outweigh the risks to the unborn child.

Breast Feeding: It is not known whether rifapentine passes into breast milk; caution is advised. Consult your doctor for advice. Rifapentine may produce a redish orange or brown discoloration of body fluids, including breast milk.

Infants and Children: Safety and effectiveness for use by children under the age of 12 have not been determined.

Special Concerns: Rifapentine can lower your white blood cell count and the number of platelets in your blood, temporarily increasing the risk of infection, slowing healing, and making your gums more susceptible to bleeding. Try to delay dental work until after therapy. Soft contact lenses or dentures may become permanently discolored. Oral hormone contraceptives may be ineffective during treatment with rifapentine.

OVERDOSE
Symptoms: No overdoses have been reported.

What to Do: If someone takes a much larger dose than prescribed, seek medical attention right away.

DRUG INTERACTIONS
Rifapentine should be used with extreme caution, if at all, with protease inhibitors such as indinavir. Consult your doctor for advice if you are taking hormonal contraceptives, anticonvulsants, antiarrythmics, antibiotics, theophylline, anticoagulants, oral antidiabetic drugs, azole antifungal agents, barbiturates, benzodiazepines, beta-blockers, calcium channel blockers, clofibrate, haloperidol, estrogens and progestins, corticosteroids, digitalis drugs, other antitubercular agents, levothyroxine, narcotic analgesics, quinine, zidovudine, delavirdine, lamivudine, sildenafil citrate, tricyclic antidepressants, cyclosporine, or tacrolimus (FK506).

FOOD INTERACTIONS
No known food interactions.

DISEASE INTERACTIONS
Rifapentine should not be used if you have porphyria. Consult your doctor if you have a history of alcohol abuse. Use of rifapentine may cause complications in patients with liver disease, since this organ works to remove the medication from the body.

Riluzole

Rilutek 50 mg
(RHONE-POLENC RORER)

▶ Drug Class: Neuroprotective

▶ Available in: Tablets

▶ Available OTC? No

▶ As Generic? No

Side Effects

SERIOUS
No serious side effects are known to be associated with the use of riluzole.

COMMON
Elevated liver enzymes (detectable by your doctor); occurrence of some of the symptoms of ALS, including weakness, muscle fatigue, lack of energy, nausea, vomiting.

LESS COMMON
Dizziness, numbness or tingling around the mouth, drowsiness, loss of appetite, diarrhea.

PRINCIPAL USES
To treat amyotrophic lateral sclerosis (ALS, more commonly known as Lou Gehrig's disease). Riluzole is not a cure for the disease, but it is the first and currently only drug approved for the treatment of ALS. It can extend the life of the patient in the early stages of the disease and delay the time before a tracheostomy (surgical opening of the throat) is required to permit breathing.

HOW THE DRUG WORKS
ALS is a disease marked by degeneration of the motor nerve cells of the spinal cord, lower brain stem, and cortex, resulting in gradual loss of muscle control; the senses and mental faculties are not affected. The deterioration of the muscles governing crucial body functions—especially swallowing and breathing—eventually proves fatal. The exact way in which riluzole works is unclear, but it appears to protect nerve tissue against degenerative changes, which slows the course of ALS.

DOSAGE
Usual adult dose: 50 mg every 12 hours. It should be taken at the same time each day. Do not change the dosage on your own without consulting your doctor.

ONSET OF EFFECT
Unknown.

DURATION OF ACTION
Unknown.

DIETARY ADVICE
Riluzole works best when taken at the same time each day, with a full glass of water, at least 1 hour before or 2 hours after eating.

STORAGE
Store in a tightly sealed container away from heat, moisture, and direct light.

IF YOU MISS A DOSE
Skip the missed dose and resume your regular dosage schedule the next day. Do not double the next dose.

STOPPING THE DRUG
No special problems are expected.

PROLONGED USE
Prolonged use of riluzole is often necessary.

PRECAUTIONS
Over 60: No special problems are expected.

Driving and Hazardous Work: Do not drive or engage in hazardous work until you determine how this medication affects you.

Alcohol: Avoid alcohol.

Pregnancy: Adequate studies of the use of riluzole during pregnancy have not been done. Consult your doctor for specific advice.

Breast Feeding: It is not known if riluzole passes into breast milk, but in light of the potentially serious risks to nursing infants, it is recommended that women using this medication refrain from breast feeding.

Infants and Children: Riluzole is generally not prescribed for children; safety and effectiveness for patients in this age group have not been established.

OVERDOSE
Symptoms: No cases of overdose have been reported.

What to Do: Emergency instructions not applicable.

DRUG INTERACTIONS
Consult your doctor for specific advice if you are taking any other prescription or over-the-counter medication.

FOOD INTERACTIONS
No known food interactions.

DISEASE INTERACTIONS
No disease interactions have been reported.

Rimantadine Hydrochloride

Flumadine 100 mg
(FOREST)

▶ Drug Class: Antiviral

▶ Available in: Syrup, tablets

▶ Available OTC? No

▶ As Generic? No

Side Effects

SERIOUS
No serious side effects are associated with rimantadine.

COMMON
Nausea and vomiting, mild diarrhea.

LESS COMMON
Dizziness, trouble concentrating, nervousness, dry mouth, loss of appetite, stomach pain, unusual fatigue, insomnia.

PRINCIPAL USES
To prevent or treat influenza type A.

HOW THE DRUG WORKS
Rimantadine interferes with the activity of the virus's genetic material, blocking an essential step in the the process of viral replication. The drug affects only certain susceptible strains of the influenza type A virus.

DOSAGE
Adults and children age 10 and older: 100 mg, 2 times a day, or 200 mg once a day. Children up to age 10: 2.3 mg per lb of body weight, once a day; the dose should not exceed a total of 150 mg daily. Frail, older adults or those with impaired liver or kidney function: 100 mg once a day. The drug should be continued for about 7 days.

ONSET OF EFFECT
Unknown. For prevention of flu, take rimantadine prior to or immediately after exposure to others with influenza.

DURATION OF ACTION
Unknown.

DIETARY ADVICE
Take it on an empty stomach at least 1 hour before or 2 hours after a meal.

STORAGE
Store in a tightly sealed container away from heat and direct light. Do not allow the syrup to freeze.

IF YOU MISS A DOSE
Take it as soon as you remember. If it is near the time for the next dose, skip the missed dose and resume your regular dosage schedule. Do not double the next dose.

STOPPING THE DRUG
It is important to take rimantadine for the full treatment period as prescribed, whether for treatment or prevention of influenza. If you have the flu, do not stop taking the drug before the scheduled end of therapy even if you begin to feel better, as this may lead to a relapse.

PROLONGED USE
If your symptoms do not improve or if they become worse in a few days, you should consult your doctor. You should see your doctor regularly for tests and examinations if you take this medicine for a prolonged period.

PRECAUTIONS
Over 60: Adverse reactions may be more likely and more severe; a smaller dose is commonly prescribed.

Driving and Hazardous Work: Do not drive or engage in hazardous work until you determine how the medicine affects you.

Alcohol: Avoid alcohol.

Pregnancy: Rimantadine has been shown to cause birth defects in animals. Human studies have not been done. Before you take rimantadine, tell your physician if you are pregnant or plan to become pregnant.

Breast Feeding: Rimantadine may pass into breast milk, although it is unknown if this poses any risks to the nursing infant. Consult your doctor for specific advice.

Infants and Children: In tests, rimantadine was not demonstrated to cause unusual side effects or problems in children over 1 year of age. Tests in children under 1 year of age have not been done. Consult your pediatrician for advice.

Special Concerns: Ask your doctor about receiving an influenza vaccine (flu shot) if you have not yet had one. If you are taking the syrup form of rimantadine, use a special measuring spoon to dispense the dose accurately. If the medicine causes insomnia, take it several hours before going to bed.

OVERDOSE
Symptoms: Agitation, heart rhythm abnormalities.

What to Do: An overdose of rimantadine is unlikely to be life-threatening. However, if someone takes a much larger dose than prescribed, call your doctor, emergency medical services (EMS), or the nearest poison control center.

DRUG INTERACTIONS
Other drugs may interact with rimantadine; consult your doctor for specific advice if you are taking any other prescription or over-the-counter medication.

FOOD INTERACTIONS
No known food interactions.

DISEASE INTERACTIONS
Consult your doctor if you have a history of epilepsy or other seizures. Use of rimantadine may cause complications in patients with liver or kidney disease, since these organs work together to remove the medication from the body.

Rimexolone

BRAND NAME
Vexol

▶ Drug Class: Corticosteroid

▶ Available in: Ophthalmic suspension

▶ Available OTC? No

▶ As Generic? No

Side Effects

SERIOUS
Decreased or blurred vision (from cataract); eye pain, nausea, vomiting (from increased eye pressure); pain, redness, sensitivity to bright light, discharge (from eye infection). Call your doctor immediately if you experience any of these signs or symptoms. This drug may trigger a recurrence of herpes infection of the eye; mention any previous herpes infection to your doctor.

COMMON
Increased eye pressure; this is usually reversed once the drug is stopped.

LESS COMMON
Burning, stinging, redness, or watering of eyes.

PRINCIPAL USES
To control inflammation and prevent potentially permanent damage that may result from conditions involving inflammation in the tissues of the eye. Such conditions may occur in the aftermath of eye surgery or in association with uveitis (inflammation of the uvea, the central portion of the eye).

HOW THE DRUG WORKS
Rimexolone inhibits the release of natural substances that stimulate an inflammatory reaction and pain or scarring in eye tissues.

DOSAGE
For treatment of postoperative eye inflammation: Instill 1 or 2 drops into affected eye(s) 4 times a day or as directed by your doctor. For uveitis: Instill 1 or 2 drops every hour during waking hours for the first week. The dose is then gradually tapered according to the doctor's instructions until uveitis resolves. Always shake the medicine well before using it.

ONSET OF EFFECT
Unknown.

DURATION OF ACTION
Unknown.

DIETARY ADVICE
No special restrictions.

STORAGE
Store in a tightly sealed container away from heat, moisture, and direct light. Do not allow it to freeze.

IF YOU MISS A DOSE
Apply it as soon as you remember. If it is near the time for the next dose, skip the missed dose and resume your regular dosage schedule. Do not double the next dose.

STOPPING THE DRUG
Take this drug as prescribed for the full treatment period, even if symptoms begin to improve before the scheduled end of therapy.

PROLONGED USE
See your doctor regularly for tests and examinations if you must take this drug for a prolonged period.

PRECAUTIONS
Over 60: No special problems are expected.

Driving and Hazardous Work: Do not drive or engage in hazardous work until you determine how the medicine affects your vision.

Alcohol: No special precautions are necessary.

Pregnancy: Adequate human studies have not been done; rimexolone should be used during pregnancy only if benefits clearly outweigh potential risks.

Breast Feeding: It is unknown if rimexolone passes into breast milk; caution is advised. Consult your doctor for specific advice.

Infants and Children: Safety and effectiveness have not been established for children.

Special Concerns: To use the eye drops, first wash your hands. Tilt your head back. Gently apply pressure to the inside corner of the eyelid and with the index finger of the same hand, pull downward on the lower eyelid to make a space. Drop the medicine into this space and close your eye. Apply pressure for 1 or 2 minutes while keeping the eye closed without blinking.

Then wash your hands again. Make sure the tip of the dropper does not touch your eye, finger or any other surface. If your symptoms do not improve in 5 to 7 days or if they become worse, check with your doctor. Wearing contact lenses while using this medication may increase the risk of infection. Your doctor may tell you not to wear contact lenses during treatment and for a day or two afterward.

OVERDOSE
Symptoms: When used topically, an overdose of rimexolone is very unlikely. Inadvertent oral ingestion, however, may cause fever, muscle pain, loss of appetite, dizziness, fainting, and breathing trouble.

What to Do: In case of accidental ingestion, call your doctor, emergency medical services (EMS), or the nearest poison control center right away.

DRUG INTERACTIONS
No drug interactions have been reported. Nonetheless, it is wise to consult your doctor before taking any other prescription or over-the-counter eye medication.

FOOD INTERACTIONS
No food interactions have been reported.

DISEASE INTERACTIONS
Consult your doctor if you have a history of cataracts, diabetes mellitus, glaucoma, herpes infection of the eye, fungal infection of the eye, or any other eye infection.

Risedronate Sodium

BRAND NAME
Actonel

▶ Drug Class: Bisphosphonate inhibitor of bone resorption

▶ Available in: Tablets

▶ Available OTC? No

▶ As Generic? No

Side Effects

SERIOUS
Serious side effects are rare and may include chest pain, swelling of the arms, legs, face, lips, tongue, or throat.

COMMON
Flu-like symptoms, diarrhea, abdominal pain, nausea, constipation, joint pain, headache, dizziness, skin rash.

LESS COMMON
Weakness, growth of tumors, belching, bone pain, leg cramps, muscle weakness, bronchitis, sinus infection, ringing in the ears, dry eye.

PRINCIPAL USES

To treat and prevent osteoporosis in postmenopausal women. Also used to prevent and treat steroid-induced osteoporosis in men and women who are either beginning or continuing treatment with steroids (such as prednisone) for chronic diseases. To treat Paget's disease, a disorder characterized by rapid breakdown and reformation of bone, which can lead to fragility and malformation of bones.

HOW THE DRUG WORKS

Healthy bones are continuously remodeled (broken down and then reformed); the minerals and other components of bones are reabsorbed by one set of cells (osteoclasts) and replaced by another set of cells to form new bone. Risedronate suppresses the activity of osteoclasts; consequently, the breakdown of bone tissue occurs more slowly than the laying down of new bone. As a result, bone density and strength are preserved.

DOSAGE

For treatment and prevention of osteoporosis (postmenopausal and steroid-induced): 5 mg a day. For Paget's disease: 30 mg once a day for 2 months.

ONSET OF EFFECT

Unknown.

DURATION OF ACTION

Unknown.

DIETARY ADVICE

Take it with a full glass of plain water. Taking risedronate with food or beverages (including mineral water) other than plain water is likely to reduce the absorption of the drug from the intestine. Take the tablets at least 30 minutes before the first food or drink of the day (other than plain water). The drug must be taken in an upright position. Maintain adequate vitamin D and calcium intake; however, vitamin or mineral supplements should be taken no sooner than 2 hours after taking the drug.

STORAGE

Store in a tightly sealed container away from heat, moisture, and direct light.

IF YOU MISS A DOSE

If you miss a dose on one day, do not double the dose the next day. Resume your regular dosage schedule.

STOPPING THE DRUG

Take it as prescribed for the full treatment period. The decision to stop taking the drug should be made in consultation with your physician.

PROLONGED USE

For Paget's disease: Risedronate is generally prescribed for a 2-month course of therapy. A second round of treatment may be considered after this 2 month period. Consult your doctor.

PRECAUTIONS

Over 60: No special problems are expected.

Driving and Hazardous Work: Do not drive or engage in hazardous work until you determine how the medicine affects you.

Alcohol: No special precautions are necessary.

Pregnancy: Consult your doctor about whether the benefits of taking the medicine outweigh the potential risks to the unborn child.

Breast Feeding: Risedronate may pass into breast milk; caution is advised. Consult your doctor for specific advice.

Infants and Children: Safety and effectiveness have not been established for children under age 18.

Special Concerns: Remain upright for at least 30 minutes after taking this medication. If you develop symptoms of esophageal disease (such as difficulty or pain when swallowing; chest pain, specifically behind the sternum; or severe or persistent heartburn), contact your doctor before continuing risedronate.

OVERDOSE

Symptoms: No cases of overdose have been reported.

What to Do: If someone takes a much larger dose than prescribed, call your doctor, emergency medical services (EMS), or a poison control center.

DRUG INTERACTIONS

Aluminum-, calcium-, or magnesium-containing antacids, if needed, should be taken no sooner than 2 hours after taking risedronate.

FOOD INTERACTIONS

No known food interactions, although risedronate works best when taken on an empty stomach.

DISEASE INTERACTIONS

Kidney impairment or a gastrointestinal disease may increase the risk of side effects. Low blood calcium levels and vitamin D deficiency must be treated before using risedronate.

Risperidone

Risperdal 1 mg
(JANSSEN)

▶ Drug Class: Antipsychotic

▶ Available in: Tablets, oral solution

▶ Available OTC? No

▶ As Generic? No

Side Effects

SERIOUS
Rapid heartbeat, profuse sweating, seizures, difficulty breathing, neck stiffness, swelling of the tongue, difficulty swallowing. Also a rare condition can develop called neuroleptic malignant syndrome, characterized by stiffness or spasms of the muscles, high fever, and confusion or disorientation. Call your doctor immediately.

COMMON
Nausea, reduced perspiration, dry mouth, blurred vision, drowsiness, shaking of the hands, muscle stiffness, stooped posture.

LESS COMMON
Difficult urination, menstrual irregularities, breast pain or swelling, unexpected weight gain, uncontrolled movements of the tongue, fever, chills, sore throat, unusual bruising or bleeding, heart palpitations, skin rash, itching, increased sensitivity of the skin to sunlight.

PRINCIPAL USES
To treat psychotic conditions (severe mental disorders characterized by distorted thoughts, perceptions, and emotions), such as schizophrenia.

HOW THE DRUG WORKS
While the exact mechanism of action of risperidone is unknown, it appears to alter the activity of certain chemicals in the central nervous system to produce a tranquilizing and antipsychotic effect.

DOSAGE
Adults and teenagers— 2 to 6 mg a day in 1 or 2 divided doses. Dosage may be adjusted by your doctor, if needed, at intervals of not less than one week. Older adults— To start, 0.5 mg, 2 times a day; may be increased to 3 mg a day.

ONSET OF EFFECT
Sedation may occur within minutes, but onset of antipsychotic effect may take hours to occur or may not occur until days or weeks after the beginning of therapy.

DURATION OF ACTION
At least 12 to 24 hours, although effects may persist for several days.

DIETARY ADVICE
No special restrictions.

STORAGE
Store in a tightly sealed container away from heat, moisture, and direct light.

IF YOU MISS A DOSE
Take it as soon as you remember. However, if it is near the time for the next dose, skip the missed dose and resume your regular dosage schedule. Do not double the next dose.

STOPPING THE DRUG
The decision to stop taking the drug should be made in consultation with your physician.

PROLONGED USE
Prolonged use may lead to tardive dyskinesia (involuntary movements of the jaw, lips, tongue, and, in rare cases, the arms, legs, hands, or body). Consult your doctor about the need for follow-up evaluations and tests if you must take this drug for an extended period.

PRECAUTIONS
Over 60: Adverse reactions may be more likely and more severe in older patients.

Driving and Hazardous Work: Do not drive or engage in hazardous work until you determine how the medicine affects you.

Alcohol: Avoid alcohol.

Pregnancy: Adequate studies have not been done. Before you take risperidone, tell your doctor if you are pregnant or plan to become pregnant.

Breast Feeding: It is not known if risperidone passes into breast milk; caution is advised. Consult your doctor for specific advice.

Infants and Children: Risperidone is not commonly prescribed for patients under age 18.

Special Concerns: Avoid prolonged exposure to high temperatures or hot climates. Drink plenty of fluids and stay cool in the summertime. Avoid overexposure to sunlight until you determine if the drug heightens your skin's sensitivity to ultraviolet light.

OVERDOSE
Symptoms: Drowsiness, rapid heartbeat, low blood pressure, seizures.

What to Do: Call your doctor, emergency medical services (EMS), or the nearest poison control center immediately.

DRUG INTERACTIONS
Other drugs may interact with risperidone. Consult your doctor for advice if you are taking an antidepressant, bromocriptine, carbamazepine, clozapine, high blood pressure medication, levodopa, pergolide, or any medications that depress the central nervous system, including antihistamines, cold remedies, decongestants, and tranquilizers.

FOOD INTERACTIONS
No known food interactions.

DISEASE INTERACTIONS
Consult your doctor if you have Parkinson's disease or any movement disorder, glaucoma, epilepsy, liver disease, kidney disease, heart disease.

Ritonavir

BRAND NAME
Norvir

Norvir 100 mg
(ABBOTT)

▶ Drug Class: Antiviral/protease inhibitor

▶ Available in: Capsules, oral solution

▶ Available OTC? No

▶ As Generic? No

Side Effects

SERIOUS
High blood sugar (diabetes) has occurred in patients taking drugs of this class, although a cause-and-effect relationship has not been established. Contact your doctor if you develop increased thirst or excessive urination.

COMMON
Diarrhea, abdominal pain, low-grade fever, nausea, gas, skin rash, fatigue, numbness or tingling around the mouth or in the arms and legs. Treat diarrhea with over-the-counter fiber supplements or antidiarrheal drugs. Side effects are most common during the first weeks of therapy.

LESS COMMON
Back pain, fever, headache or migraines, loss of appetite, gastrointestinal bleeding, mouth ulcers, vomiting, joint pain, muscle pain or cramps, anxiety, depression, dizziness, insomnia, seizures, drowsiness, breathing difficulty, skin problems, eye disorders, impaired sexual function.

PRINCIPAL USES
To treat HIV (human immunodeficiency virus), often in combination with other drugs. While not a cure for HIV, this drug may suppress replication of the virus and delay the progression of the disease.

HOW THE DRUG WORKS
Ritonavir blocks the activity of a viral protease, an enzyme that is needed by HIV to reproduce. Blocking the protease causes HIV to make copies that cannot infect new cells.

DOSAGE
Adults and children 12 and over: 600 mg, 2 times a day. Dose should be started lower and increased gradually, starting with 300 mg, 2 times a day for 1 to 2 days, then 400 mg, 2 times a day for 1 to 3 days, then 500 mg, 2 times a day for 1 to 8 days, then 600 mg, 2 times a day thereafter. The full dose should be reached in no later than 14 days. Lower doses (400 to 500 mg, 2 times a day) are sometimes used when ritonavir is combined with other drugs such as saquinavir. Children ages 2 to 12: 400 mg per square meter of body mass 2 times a day, not to exceed 600 mg 2 times a day. Dose should be started lower and increased gradually, starting with 250 mg per square meter and increased at 2- to 3-day intervals by 50 mg per square meter 2 times a day.

ONSET OF EFFECT
Unknown. Maximum effect may take 12 to 16 weeks.

DURATION OF ACTION
Unknown. Effects of the drug may be prolonged if it is used with other drugs and the virus is maximally suppressed.

DIETARY ADVICE
Take it with food. The solution can be mixed with chocolate milk to improve taste; take it within 1 hour after mixing.

STORAGE
Store oral solution at room temperature in a tightly sealed container. Refrigerate capsules.

IF YOU MISS A DOSE
Take it as soon as you remember. If it is near the time for the next dose, skip the missed dose and resume regular dosage schedule. Do not double the next dose.

STOPPING THE DRUG
Consult your physician.

PROLONGED USE
See your doctor regularly for tests and examinations.

PRECAUTIONS
Over 60: No special advice.

Driving and Hazardous Work: Avoid such activities until you determine how the medicine affects you.

Alcohol: Avoid alcohol if liver function is impaired.

Pregnancy: Adequate studies of use during pregnancy have not been done; consult your doctor for specific advice. There is no evidence that the drug will reduce the risk of transmitting the virus from the mother to the fetus.

Breast Feeding: Women infected with HIV should not breast feed, to avoid transmitting the virus to an uninfected child.

Infants and Children: Not recommended for use by children under age 2.

Special Concerns: Do not switch between the capsules and solution without consulting your doctor; the body absorbs them at different rates. Taking ritonavir does not eliminate the risk of passing the AIDS virus to other persons. Take appropriate preventive measures.

OVERDOSE
Symptoms: Temporary numbness, tingling, or prickling.

What to Do: An overdose is unlikely to occur or be life-threatening. If, however, someone takes a much larger dose than prescribed, seek medical assistance right away.

DRUG INTERACTIONS
You should not take ritonavir with the following drugs because serious or life-threatening adverse effects such as heartbeat irregularities, breathing difficulties, or excessive sedation could occur: amiodarone, astemizole, bepridil, , flecainide, propafenone, quinidine, terfenadine, midazolam, triazolam, pimozide, ergotamine, or dihydroergotamine. Use of ritonavir with the cholesterol-lowering statin medications (such as simvastatin, lovastatin, atorvastatin, fluvastatin, pravastatin, and nystatin) is not recommended. Consult your doctor for specific advice if you are taking any other prescription or over-the-counter medication.

FOOD INTERACTIONS
Increasing the amount of fat in the diet can help to reduce side effects.

DISEASE INTERACTIONS
Consult your doctor if you have liver disease or any other medical condition.

Rivastigmine Tartrate

BRAND NAME
Exelon

▶ Drug Class: Reversible cholinesterase inhibitor

▶ Available in: Capsules, oral solution

▶ Available OTC? No

▶ As Generic? No

Side Effects

SERIOUS
Possible gastrointestinal bleeding. No other serious side effects are associated with the use of rivastigmine.

COMMON
Significant nausea, vomiting, loss of appetite, and weight loss. Other common side effects include heartburn, weakness, dizziness, diarrhea, abdominal pain.

LESS COMMON
Increased sweating, fatigue, malaise, headache, drowsiness, tremor, flatulence, insomnia, depression, anxiety.

PRINCIPAL USES
To treat mild to moderate Alzheimer's disease.

HOW THE DRUG WORKS
The exact mechanism of action is unknown. However, rivastigmine is believed to work by inhibiting acetylcholinesterase enzymes, which reduces the breakdown of acetylcholine, a brain chemical crucial to memory. Acetylcholine deficiency is thought to result in memory loss associated with Alzheimer's disease.

DOSAGE
To start, 1.5 mg twice a day. After two weeks of treatment, your doctor may increase the dose to 3 mg twice a day. The dose may be further increased at no less than 2-week intervals to 4.5 mg twice a day and then to the maximum dose of 6 mg twice a day, if tolerated.

ONSET OF EFFECT
Unknown.

DURATION OF ACTION
Unknown.

DIETARY ADVICE
Rivastigmine should be taken with meals in the morning and evening. The oral solution may be swallowed directly from the syringe or mixed with a small glass of water, cold fruit juice, or soda.

STORAGE
Store in a tightly sealed container away from heat, moisture, and direct light. Do not freeze the oral solution.

IF YOU MISS A DOSE
Take it as soon as you remember, unless the time for your next scheduled dose is within the next 2 hours. If so, do not take the missed dose. Take your next scheduled dose at the proper time and resume your regular dosage schedule. Do not double the next dose. If therapy has been interrupted for several days or longer, consult your physician.

STOPPING THE DRUG
The decision to stop taking the drug should be made in consultation with your physician.

PROLONGED USE
No problems are expected with long-term use.

PRECAUTIONS
Over 60: No special problems are expected.

Driving and Hazardous Work: Do not drive or engage in hazardous work until you determine how the medicine affects you.

Alcohol: Avoid alcohol while using this medication.

Pregnancy: In some animal studies, large doses of rivastigmine were shown to cause problems. Before you take rivastigmine, tell your doctor if you are pregnant or plan to become pregnant.

Breast Feeding: It is not known whether rivastigmine passes into breast milk; caution is advised. Consult your doctor for specific advice.

Infants and Children: Rivastigmine is not intended for use in children.

Special Concerns: Before you have any surgery or dental or emergency treatment, tell the doctor or dentist in charge that you are taking rivastigmine. Rivastigmine will not cure Alzheimer's disease and will not stop the disease from getting worse, but it will improve cognitive ability of some patients. Caretakers should be instructed in the correct way to administer the oral solution of rivastigmine.

OVERDOSE
Symptoms: Severe nausea, vomiting, increased salivation, sweating, slow heartbeat, low blood pressure, irregular breathing, unconsciousness, increased muscle weakness, death.

What to Do: Call your doctor, emergency medical services (EMS), or the nearest poison control center immediately.

DRUG INTERACTIONS
Nonsteroidal anti-inflammatory drugs (NSAIDs) may increase the risk of peptic ulcer or gastrointestinal bleeding when taken with rivastigmine.

FOOD INTERACTIONS
No known food interactions.

DISEASE INTERACTIONS
Caution is advised when taking rivastigmine. Consult your doctor if you have any of the following: asthma, epilepsy or a history of seizures, heart problems, intestinal blockage, stomach or duodenal ulcer, liver disease, or urinary problems.

Rizatriptan Benzoate

▶ Drug Class: Antimigraine/
   antiheadache drug

▶ Available in: Tablets, orally
   disintegrating wafers

▶ Available OTC? No

▶ As Generic? No

Side Effects

SERIOUS
Serious side effects with rizatriptan are rare. However, rizatriptan may cause a heart attack, chest pain or tightness, sudden or severe abdominal pain, shortness of breath, wheezing, heartbeat irregularities, swelling of eyelids, face, or lips, skin rash, or hives. Seek emergency medical assistance immediately.

COMMON
Sensations of cold or warmth, dizziness, drowsiness, fatigue, hot flashes, diarrhea, vomiting, flushing, difficulty concentrating, tremor, false sense of well-being, prickling or tingling sensations.

LESS COMMON
Chills, sensitivity to heat, weakness, stiffness, muscle pain, spasms, and cramps, bone and joint pain, indigestion, increased thirst, flatulence, nervousness, insomnia, anxiety, mental depression, confusion, sore throat, nasal irritation, nose bleeds, ringing in the ears, vision difficulties, increased sweating, itching, mild rash, frequent urination.

PRINCIPAL USES
To treat severe, acute migraine headaches. Rizatriptan is not intended as a migraine preventive or for use against any other kinds of pain or headache, including basilar and hemiplegic migraines. Your doctor will determine whether this medication is appropriate in your particular case.

HOW THE DRUG WORKS
The exact mechanism of rizatriptan's action is unknown.

DOSAGE
A single dose ranging from 5 to 10 mg is generally effective. If the migraine returns or there is only partial relief, the dose may be repeated once after 2 hours, but no more than 30 mg should be taken in a 24-hour period. Since individual response to rizatriptan may vary, your doctor will determine the appropriate dosage. A general recommendation is to take one 5 mg tablet as the initial dose.

ONSET OF EFFECT
Within 2 hours.

DURATION OF ACTION
Up to 24 hours.

DIETARY ADVICE
The medication can be taken with or without food.

STORAGE
Store in a tightly sealed container away from heat, moisture, and direct light.

IF YOU MISS A DOSE
Not applicable, since the drug is taken only when necessary.

STOPPING THE DRUG
Consult your doctor before discontinuing rizatriptan.

PROLONGED USE
No special problems are expected. Patients at risk for heart disease should undergo periodic medical tests and evaluation.

PRECAUTIONS
Over 60: This drug should not be used unless the presence of coronary heart disease has been ruled out through appropriate diagnostic tests.

Driving and Hazardous Work: Some people feel drowsy or dizzy during or following a migraine attack or after taking rizatriptan. Avoid driving or other tasks requiring concentration if you have such symptoms.

Alcohol: No special warnings, although alcohol may trigger or exacerbate migraine headaches.

Pregnancy: Adequate human studies have not been done. Discuss with your doctor the relative risks and benefits of using rizatriptan while pregnant.

Breast Feeding: Rizatriptan may pass into breast milk; consult your doctor for specific advice.

Infants and Children: Safety and effectiveness have not been established for children under age 18.

Special Concerns: Serious, but rare, heart-related problems may occur after taking rizatriptan. Rizatriptan should not be used by anyone with any symptoms of coronary artery disease (chest pain or tightness, shortness of breath). Anyone at risk for unrecognized CAD—such as postmenopausal women, men over the age of 40, or those with known risk factors for heart disease (hypertension, high

blood cholesterol levels, obesity, diabetes, strong family history of heart disease, or cigarette smoking)—should have the first dose of rizatriptan administered in a doctor's office, and then only after tests show they are probably free of coronary artery disease.

OVERDOSE
Symptoms: No overdoses have been reported.

What to Do: Although overdose is unlikely, if you take a much larger dose than prescribed, call your doctor, emergency medical services (EMS), or the nearest poison control center immediately.

DRUG INTERACTIONS
Do not take rizatriptan within 24 hours of taking almotriptan, naratriptan, sumatriptan, zolmitriptan, ergotamine-containing medication, dihydroergotamine mesylate, or methysergide mesylate. Rizatriptan and MAO inhibitors such as phenelzine, tranylcypromine, procarbazine, and selegiline should not be used within 14 days of each other. Rizatriptan should be used with caution in patients taking SSRIs (selective serotonin reuptake inhibitors), which include fluoxetine, fluvoxamine, paroxetine, and sertraline.

FOOD INTERACTIONS
No known food interactions.

DISEASE INTERACTIONS
You should not take rizatriptan if you have a history of angina, heart disease, stroke, uncontrolled hypertension, heartbeat irregularities, or peripheral vascular disease. Rizatriptan should be used with caution in patients with liver disease or severely impaired kidney function.

Rofecoxib

▶ Drug Class: Nonsteroidal anti-inflammatory drug (NSAID)/COX-2 inhibitor

▶ Available in: Tablets, oral suspension

▶ Available OTC? No

▶ As Generic? No

Side Effects

SERIOUS
Stomach ulcers. Black, tarry stools may signal stomach bleeding. Symptoms of liver disease (nausea, fatigue, lethargy, itching, yellowish discoloration of the eyes or skin, fluid retention). Call your doctor immediately.

COMMON
Indigestion, mild swelling, heartburn, nausea, increased blood pressure.

LESS COMMON
Flatulence, sore throat, upper respiratory tract infection, back pain, and mild abdominal pain.

PRINCIPAL USES
For the management of chronic osteoarthritis pain. Rofecoxib is also used in the short-term relief of acute general and menstrual pain.

HOW THE DRUG WORKS
By inhibiting the activity of the enzyme cyclooxygenase-2 (COX-2), rofecoxib reduces the synthesis of prostaglandins that play a role in causing arthritis pain and inflammation. It does not inhibit the activity of COX-1, the enzyme involved in the synthesis of prostaglandins that help protect against stomach ulcers and other health problems.

DOSAGE
For osteoarthritis: To start, 12.5 mg once a day. Your doctor may increase the dose to 25 mg once a day if adequate relief is not achieved with the lower dose. For acute or menstrual pain: 50 mg once a day. To minimize potential gastrointestinal side effects, the lowest effective dose should be used for the shortest possible time. Use of rofecoxib for more than 5 days for relief of acute pain has not been studied.

ONSET OF EFFECT
For acute pain: Within 45 minutes. For osteoarthritis: Unknown.

DURATION OF ACTION
Unknown.

DIETARY ADVICE
Rofecoxib may be taken with or without food.

STORAGE
Store in a tightly sealed container away from heat, moisture, and direct light. Do not refrigerate the oral suspension.

IF YOU MISS A DOSE
If you do not remember until the next day, skip the missed dose and resume your regular dosage schedule. Do not double the next dose.

STOPPING THE DRUG
The decision to stop taking the drug should be made in consultation with your physician.

PROLONGED USE
The risk of gastrointestinal side effects may be increased with extended use.

PRECAUTIONS
Over 60: No special problems are expected. Therapy should be started with the lowest recommended dose.

Driving and Hazardous Work: No special problems are expected.

Alcohol: Avoid alcohol when using this medication because it increases the risk of stomach irritation.

Pregnancy: Discuss with your doctor the relative risks and benefits of using this drug while pregnant. Do not use rofecoxib during the last trimester.

Breast Feeding: Rofecoxib may pass into breast milk; caution is advised. Consult your doctor for advice on whether to discontinue nursing or discontinue the drug.

Infants and Children: The safety and effectiveness of this drug have not been established for children under the age of 18.

OVERDOSE
Symptoms: No cases of overdose have been reported. Symptoms may include lethargy, drowsiness, nausea, vomiting, abdominal pain, black, tarry stools, breathing difficulty, and coma.

What to Do: If you suspect an overdose or if someone takes a much larger dose than prescribed, call your doctor, emergency medical services (EMS), or the nearest poison control center immediately.

DRUG INTERACTIONS
Do not take this drug with aspirin or any other NSAIDs without your doctor's approval. In addition, consult your doctor if you are taking furosemide, ACE inhibitors, methotrexate, lithium, rifampin, or warfarin.

FOOD INTERACTIONS
No known food interactions.

DISEASE INTERACTIONS
Rofecoxib should not be taken by people who have experienced asthma, hives, or allergic-type reactions after taking aspirin or other NSAIDs. Consult your doctor if you have any of the following: bleeding problems, inflammation or ulcers of the stomach and intestines, asthma, high blood pressure, or heart failure. Use of rofecoxib may cause complications in patients with liver or kidney disease, since these organs both work to remove the medication from the body.

Ropinirole Hydrochloride

▶ Drug Class: Antiparkinsonism drug

▶ Available in: Tablets

▶ Available OTC? No

▶ As Generic? No

Side Effects

SERIOUS
Chest pain, heart rhythm irregularities, confusion, hallucinations. Call your doctor immediately.

COMMON
Nausea, dizziness, faintness, sweating, or loss of consciousness, caused by a significant drop in blood pressure that occurs when rising from a seated or lying position (orthostatic hypotension). Also unusual drowsiness, fatigue, indigestion, vomiting, increased susceptibility to viral infection, headache, impaired ability to execute voluntary movements.

LESS COMMON
Flushing, dry mouth, increased sweating, weakness, swelling of the legs or feet, general feeling of illness, pain, decreased reflexes, abdominal pain, loss of appetite, flatulence, amnesia, impaired concentration, yawning, erectile dysfunction, bronchitis, sore throat, shortness of breath, vision abnormalities, increased incidence of accidental injury, tremor, constipation, diarrhea, joint pain, arthritis, anxiety, nervousness.

PRINCIPAL USES
To treat signs and symptoms of Parkinson's disease.

HOW THE DRUG WORKS
Ropinirole is believed to act by stimulating specific dopamine receptors in the brain, enhancing control over voluntary movements.

DOSAGE
Week 1: 0.25 mg, 3 times a day. Doses may be gradually increased on an individual basis to achieve maximal benefit with the least side effects. Week 2: 0.5 mg, 3 times a day. Week 3: 0.75 mg, 3 times a day. Week 4: 1 mg, 3 times a day. After week 4, if necessary, daily dosage may be increased by 1.5 mg per day on a weekly basis up to a dose of 9 mg a day, and then by 3 mg per day weekly to a total dose of 24 mg a day.

ONSET OF EFFECT
Unknown.

DURATION OF ACTION
Unknown.

DIETARY ADVICE
Ropinirole can be taken without regard to meals. However, taking it with food may help to reduce the risk of stomach upset.

STORAGE
Store in a tightly sealed container away from heat, moisture, and direct light.

IF YOU MISS A DOSE
Take it as soon as you remember. If it is near the time for the next dose, skip the missed dose and resume your regular dosage schedule. Do not double the next dose.

STOPPING THE DRUG
Ropinirole should be discontinued gradually over a 7-day period. The frequency of dosage should be reduced from 3 times a day to 2 times a day for 4 days. For the remaining 3 days, the frequency should be reduced to once a day before completely discontinuing the drug.

PROLONGED USE
Side effects are more likely with prolonged use.

PRECAUTIONS
Over 60: Adverse effects such as hallucinations are more likely and may be more severe in older patients. A reduced dose may be necessary.

Driving and Hazardous Work: Do not drive or engage in dangerous work until you determine how ropinirole affects you.

Alcohol: Alcohol should be avoided because this medicine increases its effects.

Pregnancy: Adequate human studies have not been done. Before taking ropinirole, tell your doctor if you are or plan to become pregnant. Discuss with your doctor the relative risks and benefits of using this drug while pregnant.

Breast Feeding: Ropinirole may pass into breast milk; caution is advised. Consult your doctor for specific advice.

Infants and Children: Ropinirole is not recommended for children under the age of 18.

Special Concerns: This drug may cause dizziness and faintness, especially when getting up out of a chair or sitting up after lying down (a condition known as postural or orthostatic hypertension, characterized by temporary episodes of excessively low blood pressure). Be cautious and move slowly when arising.

OVERDOSE
Symptoms: An overdose is unlikely to occur. Possible symptoms after an excessive dose may include mild facial paralysis or spasticity, nausea, agitation, drowsiness, sedation, orthostatic hypotension, chest pain, confusion, and vomiting.

What to Do: If someone takes a much larger dose than prescribed, call your doctor, emergency medical services (EMS), or the nearest poison control center immediately.

DRUG INTERACTIONS
Consult your doctor if you are taking any of the following drugs that may interact with ropinirole: ciprofloxacin, metoclopramide, or any sedatives, tranquilizers, or analgesics.

FOOD INTERACTIONS
None reported.

DISEASE INTERACTIONS
None reported.

Ropivacaine Hydrochloride Monohydrate

BRAND NAME
Naropin

▶ Drug Class: Local anesthetic

▶ Available in: Injection

▶ Available OTC? No

▶ As Generic? No

Side Effects

SERIOUS
Dizziness, nausea, back pain, fever, headache, burning or prickling sensation, vomiting, anxiety, blurred vision, drowsiness, incoherent speech, metallic taste, numbness or tingling of mouth or lips, itching, restlessness, tremors, twitching, difficulty urinating. Call your doctor immediately.

COMMON
No common side effects have been reported.

LESS COMMON
No less-common side effects have been reported.

PRINCIPAL USES
As a local (site specific) anesthetic to help manage pain during or after surgery and during childbirth (both conventional childbirth and cesarean section).

HOW THE DRUG WORKS
Ropivacaine interferes with the ability of certain nerves to conduct electrical signals, thereby blocking the transmission of nerve impulses that carry pain messages.

DOSAGE
Dosage range and frequency vary considerably based on the reason the drug is being used and the status of the individual patient. Your doctor will determine the proper dose accordingly.

ONSET OF EFFECT
1 to 30 minutes, depending on the concentration and dose of the drug, as well as the site of administration.

DURATION OF ACTION
Depends on the concentration and dose of the drug, as well as the site of administration. Duration ranges from 30 minutes to 8 hours.

DIETARY ADVICE
No special restrictions.

STORAGE
Not applicable; this drug is administered only in a hospital setting.

IF YOU MISS A DOSE
Not applicable; your doctor will decide when to administer doses.

STOPPING THE DRUG
The decision to stop taking the drug should be made by your doctor.

PROLONGED USE
Ropivacaine is not intended for prolonged use.

PRECAUTIONS
Over 60: Adverse reactions may be more likely and more severe in older patients.

Driving and Hazardous Work: Not applicable; this drug is used only in a hospital setting.

Alcohol: Not applicable; this drug is used exclusively in a hospital setting.

Pregnancy: Ropivacaine has been shown in scientific study to cross the placenta, although sufficient studies of whether this poses harm to the fetus have not been done. Use of ropivacaine during the first phase of labor may delay or prolong the second stage by interfering with the mother's reflex urge to push or by reducing the mother's ability to push. If ropivacaine is to be used for surgical purposes (that is, other than childbirth), be sure to tell your doctor if you are pregnant or plan to become pregnant.

Breast Feeding: Ropivacaine may pass into breast milk; however, no problems have been documented. Consult your doctor for advice.

Infants and Children: Safety and efficacy of ropivacaine in children under the age of 12 have not been established.

Special Concerns: Blood pressure, heart rate, neurological status, and respiratory status should be monitored carefully during therapy.

OVERDOSE
Symptoms: Bluish lips or skin, dizziness, seizures.

What to Do: Since ropivacaine is generally used in hospital situations only, emergency procedures will be carried out by hospital personnel if an accidental overdose were to occur.

DRUG INTERACTIONS
Consult your doctor for specific advice if you are taking other local anesthetics, fluvoxamine, imipramine, theophylline, or verapamil.

FOOD INTERACTIONS
No known food interactions.

DISEASE INTERACTIONS
Caution is advised when taking ropivacaine. Consult your doctor if you have heart disease. Use of ropivacaine may cause complications in patients with liver or kidney disease, since these organs work together to remove the medication from the body.

Rosiglitazone Maleate

BRAND NAME
Avandia

▶ Drug Class: Thiazolidine-dione/antidiabetic agent

▶ Available in: Tablets

▶ Available OTC? No

▶ As Generic? No

Side Effects

SERIOUS
No serious side effects have been associated with rosiglitazone.

COMMON
Weight gain.

LESS COMMON
Upper respiratory tract infection, headache, edema (swelling).

PRINCIPAL USES
As a single therapeutic agent or as an adjunct (supplemental) therapy to metformin to control blood glucose (sugar) levels in patients with non-insulin-dependent (type 2) diabetes.

HOW THE DRUG WORKS
Rosiglitazone increases the body's sensitivity and response to its own insulin.

DOSAGE
To start, 4 mg, once a day (in the morning) or in two divided doses (in the morning and evening). Patients not responding adequately to 4 mg a day after 12 weeks may have their dose increased by their doctor to 8 mg once a day or in two divided doses.

ONSET OF EFFECT
Within 2 to 4 weeks.

DURATION OF ACTION
Unknown.

DIETARY ADVICE
Rosiglitazone may be taken with or without food.

STORAGE
Store in a tightly sealed container away from heat, moisture, and direct light.

IF YOU MISS A DOSE
Take it as soon as you remember. If it is near the time for the next dose, skip the missed dose and resume your regular dosage schedule. Do not double the next dose.

STOPPING THE DRUG
The decision to stop taking the drug should be made in consultation with your physician.

PROLONGED USE
See your doctor regularly for liver function tests if you take rosiglitazone for an extended period.

PRECAUTIONS
Over 60: No special problems are expected.

Driving and Hazardous Work: The use of rosiglitazone should not impair your ability to perform such tasks safely.

Alcohol: Drink only in moderation.

Pregnancy: Adequate studies of rosiglitazone use during pregnancy have not been done. In general, insulin is the treatment of choice for controlling blood glucose levels during pregnancy. Rosiglitazone should not be used during pregnancy unless your doctor believes the potential benefit justifies the potential risk to the fetus. Rosiglitazone may stimulate ovulation in premenopausal women who have stopped ovulating. Contraception may be advised.

Breast Feeding: Rosiglitazone may pass into breast milk; do not use it while nursing.

Infants and Children: Safety and effectiveness of rosiglitazone have not been established in children.

Special Concerns: Another thiazolidinedione drug, troglitazone, has been associated with rare, serious, and sometimes fatal, liver-related side effects. Although no similar side effects have been reported for rosiglitazone, liver function tests are recommended just prior to treatment, every two months for the first year, and periodically thereafter. If you develop unexplained symptoms of liver dysfunction, such as nausea, vomiting, abdominal pain, fatigue, loss of appetite, or dark urine, call your doctor immediately. It is important to follow your doctor's advice on diet, exercise, and other measures to help control diabetes.

OVERDOSE
Symptoms: No specific ones have been reported.

What to Do: While no cases of overdose have been reported, if someone takes a much larger dose than prescribed, call your doctor, emergency medical services (EMS), or the nearest poison control center immediately.

DRUG INTERACTIONS
No known drug interactions.

FOOD INTERACTIONS
No known food interactions.

DISEASE INTERACTIONS
Rosiglitazone should not be taken by those with type 1 diabetes or for the treatment of diabetic ketoacidosis. Caution is advised if you have edema or heart failure. Consult your doctor prior to using rosiglitazone if you have any type of liver abnormality.

Salmeterol Xinafoate

BRAND NAME
Serevent

▶ Drug Class: Bronchodilator/
sympathomimetic

▶ Available in: Inhalation
aerosol, inhalation powder

▶ Available OTC? No

▶ As Generic? No

Side Effects

SERIOUS
Salmeterol may become
ineffective if used too
often, resulting in more-
severe breathing diffi-
culty that does not
improve. Signs include
persistent wheezing,
coughing, or shortness of
breath; confusion; bluish
color to lips or finger-
nails; inability to speak.
Other side effects include
chest pain or heaviness;
irregular, racing, fluttering, or pounding heart-
beat; lightheadedness;
fainting; severe weak-
ness; severe headache.

COMMON
Headache, sore throat,
runny or stuffy nose.

LESS COMMON
Abdominal pain, diar-
rhea, nausea, cough,
muscle aches.

PRINCIPAL USES
Salmeterol is used to dilate
air passages in the lungs
that have become narrowed
as a result of disease or
inflammation. It is used in
the treatment of asthma and
chronic obstructive pul-
monary disease (COPD).

HOW THE DRUG WORKS
Salmeterol widens con-
stricted airways in the lungs
by relaxing the smooth
muscles that surround the
bronchial passages.

DOSAGE
This drug may be used
when needed to relieve
breathing difficulty. Adults
and children 12 years and
older— By inhalation
aerosol: Two inhalations
twice daily, approximately
12 hours apart. By inhalation powder: One inhalation
twice a day, approximately
12 hours apart.

ONSET OF EFFECT
Within 15 minutes.

DURATION OF ACTION
Up to 12 hours.

DIETARY ADVICE
Maintain your usual food
and fluid intake. Increase
fluids if you have a fever or
diarrhea, in hot weather, or
during exercise.

STORAGE
Store in a tightly sealed container away from heat, moisture, and direct light.

IF YOU MISS A DOSE
Take it as soon as you
remember. If it is near the
time for the next dose, skip
the missed dose and
resume your regular dosage
schedule. Do not double the
next dose.

STOPPING THE DRUG
The decision to stop taking
the drug should be made by
your doctor.

PROLONGED USE
It may not be necessary to
finish the recommended
course of therapy. Consult
your doctor.

PRECAUTIONS
Over 60: Adverse reactions
may be more likely and
more severe in older
patients.

**Driving and Hazardous
Work:** Do not drive or
engage in hazardous work
until you determine how the
medicine affects you.

Alcohol: No special precautions are necessary.

Pregnancy: Safety of use
during pregnancy has not
been established. Consult
your doctor.

Breast Feeding: It is not
known if salmeterol passes
into breast milk. Mothers
who wish to breast-feed
while taking this drug
should discuss the matter
with their doctor.

Infants and Children:
Use of salmeterol inhalation
aerosol is not recommended
in children younger than 12.

Special Concerns: This
medication takes 15 minutes
to work. Do not use salmeterol for acute or sudden
attacks, or for worsening
asthma. Pay heed to any
asthma attack or other
breathing difficulty that
does not improve after your
usual rescue treatment.
Seek help immediately if
you feel your lungs are persistently constricted, if you
are using more than the
recommended number of
treatments or puffs per day,
or if you feel a recent attack
is somehow different from
others. Do not wash the
device for the inhalation
powder. Keep it dry.

OVERDOSE
Symptoms: Chest pain or
heaviness; irregular, racing,
fluttering, or pounding
heartbeat; dizziness; lightheadedness; severe weak-
ness; fainting; severe
headache; muscle tremors
or shaking.

What to Do: Call your
doctor, emergency medical
services (EMS), or the
nearest poison control
center immediately.

DRUG INTERACTIONS
Consult your doctor for specific advice if you are taking
beta-blockers.

FOOD INTERACTIONS
No known food interactions.

DISEASE INTERACTIONS
Consult your doctor if you
have a history of any of the
following: heart disease or
heartbeat irregularities,
high blood pressure, anxiety disorders, or a thyroid
condition.

Salsalate

Generic 500 mg
(SIDMAK)

Additional photographs

▶ Drug Class: Salicylate/nonsteroidal anti-inflammatory drug (NSAID)

▶ Available in: Capsules, tablets

▶ Available OTC? No

▶ As Generic? Yes

Side Effects

SERIOUS
Hearing loss, blood in the urine, severe diarrhea, difficulty swallowing, dizziness, lightheadedness, severe drowsiness, extreme nervousness or excitability, confusion, seizures, change in skin color, hallucinations, increased sweating and thirst, severe nausea or vomiting, shortness of breath, tightness in the chest, severe stomach pain, swollen eyelids, face, or lips, fever, bloody or black, tarry stools, severe headache, buzzing or ringing in the ears, vomiting of blood or dark material. Call your doctor immediately.

COMMON
Mild stomach or abdominal cramps, pains, or discomfort; indigestion, heartburn, nausea or vomiting; skin rash, hives, or itching.

LESS COMMON
None reported.

PRINCIPAL USES
To treat rheumatoid arthritis, osteoarthritis, and other rheumatic (joint) disorders.

HOW THE DRUG WORKS
Salsalate appears to work by interfering with the action of prostaglandins, naturally occurring substances in the body that cause inflammation and make nerves more sensitive to pain impulses.

DOSAGE
Adults and teenagers: To start, 500 to 1,000 mg, 2 or 3 times a day. The dose may be adjusted later.

ONSET OF EFFECT
Unknown.

DURATION OF ACTION
Unknown.

DIETARY ADVICE
Salsalate should be taken with food or milk, to minimize stomach upset, and a large glass of water.

STORAGE
Store in a tightly sealed container away from heat, moisture, and direct light.

IF YOU MISS A DOSE
Take it as soon as you remember. If it is near the time for the next dose, skip the missed dose and resume your regular dosage schedule. Do not double the next dose.

STOPPING THE DRUG
Take as directed for the full treatment period, even if you begin to feel better before the scheduled end of therapy.

PROLONGED USE
See your doctor regularly for tests and examinations if you must take this medicine for a prolonged period.

PRECAUTIONS
Over 60: Adverse reactions may be more likely and more severe in older patients.

Driving and Hazardous Work: Do not drive or engage in hazardous work until you determine how the medicine affects you.

Alcohol: Avoid alcohol.

Pregnancy: Adequate studies have not been done. Consult your doctor if you are pregnant or plan to become pregnant.

Breast Feeding: Salsalate passes into breast milk; caution is advised.

Infants and Children: Do not give salsalate to a child or teenager with a fever or other signs of a viral infection like the flu or chicken pox without consulting your doctor.

Special Concerns: Salsalate may cause false urine-sugar-test results for diabetics if you are taking 4 or more 500 mg doses, or 3 or more 750 mg doses, per day.

OVERDOSE
Symptoms: Confusion, dizziness, ringing or buzzing in the ears, severe drowsiness or fatigue, excitability or nervousness, rapid or heavy breathing, sweating, diarrhea, vomiting, fever, dehydration, loss of consciousness.

What to Do: Call your doctor, emergency medical services (EMS), or the nearest poison control center immediately. To prevent further absorption of salsalate, take ipecac syrup.

DRUG INTERACTIONS
Consult your doctor for advice if you are taking NSAIDs, carbonic anhydrase inhibitors, citrates, sodium bicarbonate, antacids, anticoagulants, heparin, thrombolytic agents, oral antidiabetic agents or insulin, cefamandole, cefoperazone, cefotetan, plicamycin, valproic acid, methotrexate, vancomycin, probenecid, or sulfinpyrazone.

FOOD INTERACTIONS
No known food interactions.

DISEASE INTERACTIONS
Caution is advised when taking salsalate. Consult your doctor if you have any of the following: anemia, stomach ulcer or other stomach problems, hyperthyroidism, glucose-6-phosphate dehydrogenase (G6PD) deficiency, high blood pressure, gout, heart disease, any bleeding problems, or a history of asthma or allergies. Use of this drug may cause complications in patients with liver or kidney disease, since these organs work together to remove the medication from the body.

Saquinavir

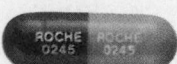

Invirase 200 mg
(ROCHE)

▶ Drug Class: Antiviral/protease inhibitor

▶ Available in: Capsules

▶ Available OTC? No

▶ As Generic? No

Side Effects

SERIOUS
High blood sugar (diabetes) has occurred in patients taking drugs of this class, although a cause-and-effect relationship has not been established. Contact your doctor if you develop increased thirst or excessive urination. Other serious side effects include: psychosis, thoughts of suicide, and lung disease.

COMMON
Burning, prickling, numbness, or tingling sensations in various parts of the body, confusion, seizures, headache, loss of muscle coordination, diarrhea, abdominal discomfort, nausea, skin rash, increased skin sensitivity to light, general weakness.

LESS COMMON
Loss of appetite, kidney stones, urinary tract bleeding, hair loss, swelling of the eyelid, nail problems, night sweats, small bump-like growths on the skin, impotence, anxiety attack, leg cramps.

PRINCIPAL USES
To treat HIV (human immunodeficiency virus) infection in combination with other drugs. While not a cure for HIV infection, saquinavir may suppress the replication of the virus and delay progression of the disease.

HOW THE DRUG WORKS
Saquinavir blocks the activity of a viral protease, an enzyme that is needed by HIV to reproduce. Blocking the protease causes HIV to make copies that cannot infect new cells.

DOSAGE
Adults and teenagers 16 and over: 600 mg, 3 times a day, in combination with other antiretroviral drugs. Higher doses (up to 1,200 mg, 3 times a day) are sometimes used. Lower doses (400 mg, 2 times a day) are used when saquinavir is combined with ritonavir, a similar drug.

ONSET OF EFFECT
Unknown. With most antiretroviral drugs, an early response can be seen within the first few days of therapy, but the maximum effect may take 12 to 16 weeks.

DURATION OF ACTION
Unknown.

DIETARY ADVICE
It should be taken within 2 hours after a full meal.

STORAGE
Capsules should be refrigerated. If brought to room temperature, store in a tightly sealed container away from heat and direct light and use within 3 months.

IF YOU MISS A DOSE
Take it as soon as you remember. However, if it is near the time for the next dose, skip the missed dose and resume your regular dosage schedule. Do not double the next dose.

STOPPING THE DRUG
The decision to stop taking the drug should be made in consultation with your physician.

PROLONGED USE
See your doctor regularly for tests and examinations.

PRECAUTIONS
Over 60: No special studies have been done on older patients.

Driving and Hazardous Work: Avoid such activities until you determine how the medicine affects you.

Alcohol: Avoid alcohol if liver function is impaired.

Pregnancy: Saquinavir has been shown to cause birth defects in animal studies. Human studies have not been done. Nevertheless, the drug is being used increasingly in combination with other antiretroviral drugs to treat pregnant HIV-infected women.

Breast Feeding: It is unknown whether saquinavir passes into breast milk; however, women infected with HIV should not breast-feed, to avoid transmitting the virus to an uninfected child.

Infants and Children: The safety and effectiveness of saquinavir in children under the age of 16 have not been established.

Special Concerns: Use of saquinavir does not eliminate the risk of passing the AIDS virus to other persons. You should take appropriate preventive measures. If saquinavir increases skin sensitivity to sunlight, wear tightly woven clothing and use sunscreen when outdoors. Do not substitute one brand of saquinavir for another without consulting your doctor. They are not equal in strength.

OVERDOSE
Symptoms: No cases of overdose have been reported.

What to Do: An overdose of saquinavir is unlikely to occur. Nonetheless, if you have any reason to suspect an overdose, call your doctor, emergency medical services (EMS), or the nearest poison control center.

DRUG INTERACTIONS
Saquinavir should not be used at the same time as triazolam, midazolam, "statins" (cholesterol-lowering drugs), or ergotamine/belladonna alkaloids. Consult your doctor for specific advice if you are taking any other prescription or over-the-counter medication, especially rifampin, rifabutin, nevirapine, or sildenafil. Some drugs, such as ketoconazole, delavirdine, ritonavir, and nelfinavir, are used in combination with saquinavir because they increase its blood levels and, possibly, its effectiveness.

FOOD INTERACTIONS
Fatty foods and grapefruit juice enhance the body's absorption of saquinavir. Food may reduce side effects.

DISEASE INTERACTIONS
Consult your doctor if you have any other medical condition. Use of saquinavir may cause complications in patients with liver disease, because this organ works to remove the medication from the body.

Scopolamine Ophthalmic

BRAND NAME
Isopto Hyoscine

▶ Drug Class: Eye muscle relaxant, pupil enlarger

▶ Available in: Ophthalmic solution

▶ Available OTC? No

▶ As Generic? No

Side Effects

SERIOUS
If absorbed into the bloodstream: Clumsiness or unsteadiness, flushing or redness of face, confusion or unusual behavior, hallucinations, slurred speech, fever, unusual tiredness or weakness, dizziness, rapid or irregular heartbeat, unusually dry skin, skin rash, dry mouth, swollen stomach (in infants). Seek medical assistance immediately.

COMMON
Blurred vision, increased sensitivity to light.

LESS COMMON
Eye irritation not present or not as severe as before use, swelling of eyelids.

PRINCIPAL USES
Used for eye examinations, before and after eye surgery, and to treat certain eye conditions, including uveitis (inflammation of the uvea, or the central portion of the eye) and posterior synechiae (a potentially blinding eye disorder).

HOW THE DRUG WORKS
Scopolamine relaxes the muscles that control the lens and pupil. This prevents the lens from focusing and widens the pupil to allow the doctor to view the interior structures of the eye. It immobilizes tiny structures within the eye, which prevents scarring of eye tissue and may alleviate pain somewhat.

DOSAGE
Uveitis: 1 drop up to 4 times a day for adults and children, depending on the severity of the condition and the size and weight of the patient. Posterior synechiae: 1 drop every 10 minutes for 3 doses for adults. Use in children must be determined by your pediatrician.

ONSET OF EFFECT
In less than 1 hour.

DURATION OF ACTION
Up to 1 week.

DIETARY ADVICE
No special restrictions.

STORAGE
Store in a tightly sealed container away from heat, moisture, and direct light. Keep refrigerated, but do not allow it to freeze.

IF YOU MISS A DOSE
Apply it as soon as you remember. If it is near the time for the next dose, skip the missed dose and resume your regular dosage schedule. Do not double the next dose.

STOPPING THE DRUG
Use it as prescribed for the full treatment period, even if you feel better before the scheduled end of therapy.

PROLONGED USE
Prolonged use may produce eye irritation, including redness, swelling, oozing of fluid, or skin inflammation. Call your doctor if such symptoms persist for more than 7 days.

PRECAUTIONS
Over 60: Adverse reactions may be more likely and more severe in older patients.

Driving and Hazardous Work: Do not drive or engage in hazardous work until you determine how the medicine affects your vision. Extreme caution should be observed for activities that require sharp vision for close objects (less than an arm's length away).

Alcohol: No special precautions are necessary.

Pregnancy: Adequate studies have not been done. Inform your doctor if you are pregnant or plan to become pregnant.

Breast Feeding: Use extreme caution. Ophthalmic scopolamine is absorbed systemically and passes into breast milk in small amounts. Breast-fed infants may exhibit a rapid pulse, fever, or dry skin.

Infants and Children: Infants and children with blond hair or blue eyes may be more sensitive to scopolamine ophthalmic and may have an increased risk of side effects. Use with extreme caution.

Special Concerns: To use the eye drops, first wash your hands. Tilt your head back. Gently apply pressure to the inside corner of the eyelid and with the index finger of the same hand, pull downward on the lower eyelid to make a space. Drop the medicine into this space and close your eye. Apply pressure for 1 or 2 minutes while keeping the eye closed without blinking. Wash your hands again. Make certain that the tip of the dropper does not touch your eye, finger, or any other surface.

OVERDOSE
Symptoms: Drowsiness, hallucinations, memory problems, dry mouth, dry skin, restlessness, palpitations, dizziness and disorientation, delirium.

What to Do: Call your doctor, emergency medical services (EMS), or the nearest poison control center immediately.

DRUG INTERACTIONS
If absorbed into the body, it may interact with the following: anticholinergics; certain antiglaucoma agents, such as demecarium, echothiophate, or pilocarpine; antimyasthenics; potassium citrate or supplements; or medications producing central nervous system depression, such as antiemetic agents, phenothiazines, or barbiturates.

FOOD INTERACTIONS
No known food interactions.

DISEASE INTERACTIONS
Consult your doctor for advice if you have glaucoma or another eye problem, or if a child has Down's syndrome, spastic paralysis, or brain damage.

Scopolamine Systemic

▶ Drug Class: Anticholinergic; antispasmodic

▶ Available in: Transdermal patch, injection

▶ Available OTC? No

▶ As Generic? Yes

Side Effects

SERIOUS
Confusion, lightheadedness, dizziness, skin rash or hives, fainting, eye pain. Call your doctor immediately.

COMMON
Constipation; dryness of mouth, nose, throat, or skin; decreased sweating.

LESS COMMON
Blurred vision, decreased breast milk flow, unusual fatigue, difficulty swallowing, drowsiness, false sense of well-being, headache, increased sensitivity of eyes to light, loss of memory, difficulty with urination, nausea, vomiting, bloated feeling, irritation at injection site, insomnia.

PRINCIPAL USES
To treat urinary, stomach, or intestinal cramps, or motion sickness.

HOW THE DRUG WORKS
Acetylcholine is a naturally occurring chemical in the body involved in the activity of nerves, muscles, glands, and other physiological processes. Scopolamine interferes with the action of acetylcholine, leading to a variety of effects, including the drying of secretions (saliva, perspiration), relief of intestinal muscle spasm, and changing the size of the pupils. Scopolamine may relieve nausea, vomiting, and motion sickness by acting on nerves affecting balance in the inner ear.

DOSAGE
To treat urinary problems or intestinal problems—Injection: 10 to 20 mg, 3 or 4 times a day. The dose may be changed by your doctor. To treat motion sickness—Transdermal patch: Apply a 1.5 mg patch behind the ear at least 4 to 12 hours before travel. Use of scopolamine in children is not recommended.

ONSET OF EFFECT
Injection: Within 30 minutes. Transdermal patch: Unknown.

DURATION OF ACTION
Injection: 4 hours. Transdermal patch: Up to 72 hours.

DIETARY ADVICE
No special restrictions.

STORAGE
Store in a tightly sealed container away from heat and direct light.

IF YOU MISS A DOSE
Take it as soon as you remember. However, if it is near the time for the next dose, skip the missed dose and resume your regular dosage schedule. Do not double the next dose.

STOPPING THE DRUG
The decision to stop taking the drug should be made by your doctor.

PROLONGED USE
See your doctor regularly for tests and examinations if you take this medicine for a prolonged period.

PRECAUTIONS
Over 60: Adverse reactions may be more likely and more severe.

Driving and Hazardous Work: Do not drive or engage in hazardous work until you determine how the medicine affects you.

Alcohol: Avoid alcohol.

Pregnancy: Adequate human studies have not been completed. Before taking scopolamine, tell your doctor if you are pregnant or plan to become pregnant.

Breast Feeding: Scopolamine may pass into breast milk; caution is advised. Consult your doctor for specific advice.

Infants and Children: Adverse reactions may be more common and more severe in children and infants. Consult your doctor for specific advice.

Special Concerns: Do not touch the adhesive area of the patch. Wash hands thoroughly before and after application. If patch is dislodged, place a new patch behind the other ear. Do not reapply a dislodged patch. If you use the patch for more than 72 hours, you may experience nausea, vomiting, headache, or dizziness.

OVERDOSE
Symptoms: Dry mouth, dilated pupils, delirium, disorientation, memory disturbances, dizziness, restlessness, hallucinations, drowsiness.

What to Do: Call your doctor, emergency medical services (EMS), or the nearest poison control center immediately.

DRUG INTERACTIONS
Consult your doctor for specific advice if you are taking antacids, diarrhea medicines, digoxin, ketoconazole, central nervous system depressants (such as antihistamines, sleep aids, or tranquilizers), other cholinergics, tricyclic antidepressants, potassium chloride.

FOOD INTERACTIONS
No known food interactions.

DISEASE INTERACTIONS
Caution is advised when taking scopolamine. Consult your doctor if you have a history of bleeding disorders, colitis, severe mouth dryness, enlarged prostate, fever, glaucoma, heart disease, hiatal hernia, high blood pressure, any intestinal problem, lung disease, myasthenia gravis, toxemia of pregnancy, urinary tract blockage, difficulty urinating, kidney or liver disease, or an overactive thyroid; or if a child has brain damage, Down syndrome, or spastic paralysis.

Selegiline Hydrochloride (L-Deprenyl)

Eldepryl 5 mg
(SOMERSET)

▶ Drug Class: Antiparkinsonism drug

▶ Available in: Tablets

▶ Available OTC? No

▶ As Generic? Yes

Side Effects

SERIOUS
Dizziness, low blood pressure (causing dizziness, lightheadedness, fainting, or confusion), involuntary muscle movements, heart rhythm abnormalities.

COMMON
Nausea, dry mouth.

LESS COMMON
Palpitations, drowsiness.

PRINCIPAL USES
To treat Parkinson's disease, in conjunction with levodopa/carbidopa. Also used to treat Parkinson-like syndromes, which may occur following infection of or injury to the central nervous system (brain and spinal cord), because of damage to blood vessels in the brain, or after exposure to certain toxins. Without levodopa/carbidopa, this drug has no known benefit.

HOW THE DRUG WORKS
When used with levodopa/carbidopa, selegiline allows more levodopa/carbidopa to be available for use in the body by inhibiting a nervous system enzyme called monoamine oxidase (MAO). MAO, which is found in the brain and intestinal tract, acts to break down certain chemicals that play a role in the initiation and control of muscle movement.

DOSAGE
Adults: 5 mg twice daily. Children: This drug should not be used by children.

ONSET OF EFFECT
Approximately 1 to 2 hours.

DURATION OF ACTION
Approximately 4 hours.

DIETARY ADVICE
On rare occasions, patients taking the recommended dose of selegiline have had reactions with foods that contain tyramines. (See Food Interactions for more information.)

STORAGE
Store in a tightly sealed container away from heat, moisture, and direct light.

IF YOU MISS A DOSE
Take it as soon as you remember, unless the time for your next scheduled dose is within the next 2 hours. If so, skip the missed dose and resume your regular dosage schedule. Do not double the next dose.

STOPPING THE DRUG
Consult with your physician before stopping this drug. The dose should be tapered gradually—from 2 tablets to a single tablet for 7 days—before the drug is completely discontinued.

PROLONGED USE
Selegiline may be taken for prolonged periods. There are no known untoward effects specifically associated with long-term use.

PRECAUTIONS
Over 60: Adverse reactions may be more likely and more severe in older people. The medication should be used with caution by patients in this age group.

Driving and Hazardous Work: This drug may cause confusion or drowsiness. Do not drive or engage in hazardous work until you determine how it affects you.

Alcohol: Avoid alcohol.

Pregnancy: Adequate human studies have not been done to determine the safety of this drug during pregnancy. It should not be used by pregnant women.

Breast Feeding: The extent to which selegiline passes through breast milk is unknown. It should therefore be avoided by nursing mothers.

Infants and Children: This drug has not been tested in infants and children; safety and effectiveness have not been established. It should therefore not be used by patients in this age group.

OVERDOSE
Symptoms: Dizziness, fainting, confusion, delirium, abdominal pain.

What to Do: Call your doctor, emergency medical services (EMS), or the nearest poison control center immediately.

DRUG INTERACTIONS
Other drugs may interact with selegiline. Consult your doctor for specific advice if you are taking meperidine hydrochloride or other opioid (narcotic) analgesics, or MAO inhibitor antidepressants such as phenelzine sulfate or tranylcypromine sulfate.

FOOD INTERACTIONS
Consult your doctor before eating tyramine-rich foods, which include aged cheeses, avocados, banana skins, bean curd, bologna and other processed lunch meats, chicken livers, chocolate, figs, canned or dried fish, pickled herring, meat extracts, pepperoni, raisins, raspberries, unpasteurized beer, Chianti, sherry, vermouth, red wines in general, and caffeine-rich beverages or foods.

DISEASE INTERACTIONS
Caution is advised when taking selegiline hydrochloride. Consult your doctor if you have any of the following: a change in your mental state, significant heart disease, peptic ulcer disease, or wheezing or feelings of tightness or pressure in the chest.

Senna

Senokot 8.6 mg
(PURDUE FREDERICK)

Additional photographs

▶ Drug Class: Laxative

▶ Available in: Tablets, granules, oral solution, syrup

▶ Available OTC? Yes

▶ As Generic? No

Side Effects

SERIOUS
Confusion, irregular
heartbeat, muscle
cramps, pink to red or
yellow to brown coloration of urine and
stools, unusual tiredness
or weakness, laxative
dependence. Call your
doctor immediately.

COMMON
Belching, cramping, diarrhea, nausea.

LESS COMMON
No less-common side
effects have been
reported.

PRINCIPAL USES
For short-term treatment of
constipation.

HOW THE DRUG WORKS
Senna stimulates water and
electrolyte (mineral salt)
secretion in the intestine
to induce defecation.

DOSAGE
Adults and teenagers: 2
tablets, or 1 teaspoon of
granules, or 10 to 15 ml of
syrup. Children ages 6 to
12: 1 tablet or 1/2 teaspoon
of granules. The medicine
should be given at bedtime.

ONSET OF EFFECT
Within 6 to 10 hours.

DURATION OF ACTION
Variable.

DIETARY ADVICE
Each dose of senna should
be taken on an empty stomach with a full glass (8 oz)
of water or fruit juice.

STORAGE
Store in a tightly sealed container away from heat, moisture, and direct light.

IF YOU MISS A DOSE
Take it as soon as you
remember. If it is near the
time for the next dose, skip
the missed dose and
resume your regular dosage
schedule. Do not double the
next dose.

STOPPING THE DRUG
Take senna as prescribed
for the full treatment period.
However, you may stop taking the drug if you are feeling better before the
scheduled end of therapy.

PROLONGED USE
If regular bowel movement
does not resume in 1 week,
discontinue use of senna
and consult your doctor.

PRECAUTIONS
Over 60: Adverse reactions
may be more likely and
more severe in older
patients.

**Driving and Hazardous
Work:** Do not drive or
engage in hazardous work
until you determine how the
medicine affects you.

Alcohol: Avoid alcohol.

Pregnancy: Senna may
cause unwanted effects during pregnancy if not used
properly. Consult your doctor for specific advice.

Breast Feeding: Senna
may pass into breast milk;
caution is advised. Consult
your doctor for advice.

Infants and Children:
Senna is not recommended
for use by children under
the age of 6 unless it has
been prescribed by a doctor.

Special Concerns: You
should increase your intake
of foods containing vitamin
D, such as milk products,
and maintain an adequate
intake of foods containing
folic acid, such as fresh
vegetables, fruits, whole
grains, and liver, while
taking senna. Do not take
any other medicine within
2 hours of taking senna.
Senna is one of the most
effective laxatives for relieving constipation caused by
narcotic analgesics like morphine and codeine.

OVERDOSE
Symptoms: Sudden vomiting, nausea, diarrhea, or
cramping.

What to Do: An overdose
of senna is unlikely to be
life-threatening. However,
if someone takes a much
larger dose than prescribed,
call your doctor, emergency
medical services (EMS), or
the nearest poison control
center immediately.

DRUG INTERACTIONS
Consult your doctor for specific advice if you are taking
anticoagulants, digitalis
drugs, ciprofloxacin,
etidronate, sodium polystyrene sulfonate, or oral
tetracyclines.

FOOD INTERACTIONS
No known food interactions.

DISEASE INTERACTIONS
Caution is advised when
taking senna. Consult your
doctor if you have a history
of any of the following:
appendicitis, rectal bleeding
of unknown cause,
colostomy, intestinal blockage, ileostomy, diabetes,
heart disease, high blood
pressure, kidney disease,
or difficulty swallowing.

Sertraline Hydrochloride

BRAND NAME
Zoloft

Zoloft 50 mg
(ROERIG)

▶ Drug Class: Selective serotonin reuptake inhibitor (SSRI) antidepressant

▶ Available in: Capsules, tablets

▶ Available OTC? No

▶ As Generic? No

Side Effects

SERIOUS
Skin rash, hives, or itching; unusually fast speech, fever, extreme agitation. Call your doctor immediately.

COMMON
Insomnia, diarrhea, sexual dysfunction, decrease in appetite, weight loss, drowsiness, headache, dry mouth, stomach cramps, abdominal pain, gas, trembling, fatigue, loss of initiative.

LESS COMMON
Anxiety, agitation, increased appetite, blurred or altered vision, constipation, heartbeat irregularities, flushing, unusual feeling of warmth, vomiting.

PRINCIPAL USES
To treat symptoms of major depression, obsessive-compulsive disorder, and panic disorder.

HOW THE DRUG WORKS
Sertraline affects levels of serotonin, a brain chemical that is thought to be linked to mood, emotions, and mental state.

DOSAGE
Adults: To start, 50 mg once a day, in the morning or evening. Dose may be gradually increased by your doctor to 200 mg a day. Older adults: To start, 12.5 to 25 mg once a day. Dose may be gradually increased by your doctor to 200 mg a day. Children ages 6 to 12: To start, 25 mg once a day. Children ages 13 to 17: To start, 50 mg once a day. Dose may be gradually increased by pediatrician.

ONSET OF EFFECT
1 to 4 weeks.

DURATION OF ACTION
Unknown.

DIETARY ADVICE
No special restrictions.

STORAGE
Store in a tightly sealed container away from heat, moisture and direct light.

IF YOU MISS A DOSE
Take it as soon as you remember. If it is near the time for the next dose, skip the missed dose and resume your regular dosage schedule. Do not double the next dose.

STOPPING THE DRUG
Take it as prescribed for the full treatment period. When it is time to stop therapy, your dosage will be tapered gradually by your doctor.

PROLONGED USE
Usual course of therapy lasts 6 months to 1 year; some patients benefit from additional therapy.

PRECAUTIONS
Over 60: No special problems have been reported.

Driving and Hazardous Work: Use caution when driving or engaging in hazardous work until you determine how the medicine affects you.

Alcohol: Avoid alcohol.

Pregnancy: Adequate studies of sertraline use during pregnancy have not been done. Before you take sertraline, tell your doctor if you are currently pregnant or plan to become pregnant.

Breast Feeding: It is not known whether sertraline passes into breast milk; caution is advised. Consult your doctor for specific advice.

Infants and Children: The safety and effectiveness of the use of sertraline in children under age 6 have not been established.

Special Concerns: Take sertraline at least 6 hours before bedtime to prevent insomnia, unless the drug causes drowsiness.

OVERDOSE
Symptoms: Sleepiness, nausea, vomiting, rapid heartbeat, anxiety, dilated pupils.

What to Do: Call your doctor, emergency medical services (EMS), or the nearest poison control center immediately.

DRUG INTERACTIONS
Sertraline and MAO inhibitors should not be used within 14 days of each other. Very serious side effects such as myoclonus (uncontrolled muscle spasms), hyperthermia (excessive rise in body temperature), and extreme stiffness may result. The following drugs may also interact with sertraline; consult your doctor for advice if you are taking cimetidine, digitoxin, warfarin, sumatriptan, naratriptan, zolmitriptan, oral antidiabetic agents (such as tolbutamide), tricyclic antidepressants, or any prescription or over-the-counter drugs that depress the central nervous system (including antihistamines, barbiturates, sedatives, cough medicines, and decongestants).

FOOD INTERACTIONS
No known food interactions.

DISEASE INTERACTIONS
Consult your doctor if you have a history of alcohol or drug abuse. Use of sertraline may cause complications in patients with liver or kidney disease, since these organs work together to remove the medication from the body.

Sibutramine Hydrochloride Monohydrate

BRAND NAME
Meridia

▶ Drug Class: Inhibitor of neurotransmitter reuptake

▶ Available in: Capsules

▶ Available OTC? No

▶ As Generic? No

Side Effects

SERIOUS
No serious side effects have yet been reported. However, if you experience symptoms such as shortness of breath or chest pain that were not present before taking the medication, call your doctor.

COMMON
Dry mouth, constipation, insomnia.

LESS COMMON
Headache, increased sweating, increased blood pressure and heart rate.

PRINCIPAL USES
To aid in the medical management of obesity in conjunction with a carefully supervised diet and exercise program. The drug is only recommended for overweight people with a body mass index (BMI) greater than 30 or greater than 27 in people with other risk factors such as diabetes or high blood pressure.

HOW THE DRUG WORKS
Sibutramine affects the appetite control center in the brain by inhibiting the reuptake of neurotransmitters like serotonin. The resulting increase in their availability suppresses appetite.

DOSAGE
To start, 10 mg once a day. Dose may be increased up to 15 mg once a day.

ONSET OF EFFECT
Significant weight changes may take several weeks or months to develop.

DURATION OF ACTION
When taking sibutramine regularly, most people lose weight within the first six months. Weight loss is maintained for the duration of therapy.

DIETARY ADVICE
Can be taken with a meal or on an empty stomach.

STORAGE
Store in a tightly sealed container away from heat, moisture, and direct light.

IF YOU MISS A DOSE
If you miss a dose one day, do not double the dose the next day. Resume your regular dosage schedule.

STOPPING THE DRUG
The decision to stop taking the drug should be made in consultation with your physician.

PROLONGED USE
The safety and effectiveness of sibutramine have not been determined beyond 2 years of use.

PRECAUTIONS
Over 60: No specific studies have been done on older patients.

Driving and Hazardous Work: Do not drive or engage in hazardous work until you determine how the medicine affects you.

Alcohol: Sibutramine may increase the sedative effects of alcohol. Consult you doctor for specific advice.

Pregnancy: Sibutramine should not be used by pregnant women. Before taking sibutramine, tell your doctor if you are pregnant or plan to become pregnant.

Breast Feeding: Sibutramine should not be used by nursing mothers.

Infants and Children: Children under the age of 16 should not use sibutramine.

Special Concerns: Although no serious adverse reactions have been reported with sibutramine (at the time of publication), other diet drugs have been associated with an increased risk of potentially grave cardiovascular and cardiopulmonary problems. If you experience any unusual or disturbing adverse effects, stop taking sibutramine and call your physician immediately.

OVERDOSE
Symptoms: No cases of overdose have been reported.

What to Do: If someone takes a much larger dose than prescribed or a child swallows the drug, call your doctor, emergency medical services (EMS), or the nearest poison control center immediately.

DRUG INTERACTIONS
You should not take sibutramine if you take MAO inhibitors, other weight loss medications, medications for depression, migraine medications, dihydroergotamine, meperidine, fentanyl, pentazocine, dextromethorphan (found in many cough medicines), lithium, or tryptophan. Sibutramine may interact with ketoconazole, erythromycin, over-the-counter cough and cold medications, allergy medicines, and decongestants. Consult your doctor for specific advice.

FOOD INTERACTIONS
No known food interactions.

DISEASE INTERACTIONS
You should not take sibutramine if you have coronary artery disease, angina, cardiac arrhythmia, history of heart attack, congestive heart failure, history of stroke, anorexia nervosa, history of seizures, or narrow angle glaucoma. Sibutramine can substantially raise blood pressure in some patients. Use of sibutramine may cause complications in patients with liver or kidney disease, since these organs work together to remove the medication from the body. Consult your doctor if you have a history of migraines, mental depression, Parkinson's disease, thyroid disorders, osteoporosis, gallbladder disease, a major eating disorder (anorexia nervosa or bulimia nervosa), or any other medical problem.

Sildenafil Citrate

BRAND NAME
Viagra

▶ Drug Class: Phosphodi-
esterase type 5 inhibitor

▶ Available in: Tablets

▶ Available OTC? No

▶ As Generic? No

Side Effects

SERIOUS
Rarely, a painful or pro-
longed erection (lasting
more than 4 hours) may
occur. If erection does
not resolve on its own in
a reasonable amount of
time, seek medical help
promptly. If erection does
resolve on its own, con-
sult your doctor for spe-
cific guidelines. Serious
cardiovascular events
such as heart attack,
sudden cardiac death,
cardiac arrhythmias, cerebral hemorrhage, and
transient ischemic attack
have been reported fol-
lowing the use of silde-
nafil. However, it is
unclear whether these
events are due to the
consumption of sildenafil,
the presence of preexist-
ing cardiovascular risk
factors, to sexual activity,
or a combination of these
factors.

COMMON
Headache, flushing, indi-
gestion. Such side effects
are generally mild to
moderate and usually
short-lived.

LESS COMMON
Nasal congestion, vision
abnormalities, bloodshot
or burning eyes, diarrhea,
blood in the urine.

PRINCIPAL USES
To treat erectile dysfunction
(impotence), which may
occur in association with
atherosclerosis, vascular
disease or other circulatory
problems, diabetes, kidney
disease, hormonal abnor-
malities, neurological disease or injury, severe
depression or other psychological difficulties.

HOW THE DRUG WORKS
Sildenafil, the first drug in
a new class of medications,
works by increasing the
blood flow to the penis necessary for establishing and
maintaining an erection. The
drug accomplishes this by
selectively inhibiting the
action of an enzyme (phos-
phodiesterase type 5) that
breaks down a substance
that relaxes smooth muscles
and permits blood flow that
engorges the columns of
erectile tissue in the penis.
Unlike other treatments for
erectile dysfunction, which
produce erections with or
without sexual arousal, sildenafil allows the patient to
respond naturally to sexual
stimulation. In clinical trials,
over 70% of attempts at sexual intercourse were suc-
cessful among men who
took the drug.

DOSAGE
The recommended dose for
most patients is 50 mg,
taken approximately 1 hour
before sexual activity. The
dose may be increased to
no more than 100 mg, or
may be decreased to 25 mg.
Your doctor will help to
determine the correct dose
for you. Do not take the
drug more than once in a
24-hour period.

ONSET OF EFFECT
Within 30 minutes to 4
hours.

DURATION OF ACTION
Unknown.

DIETARY ADVICE
Sildenafil can be taken without regard to meals.

STORAGE
Store in a tightly sealed container away from heat, moisture, and direct light.

IF YOU MISS A DOSE
Not applicable. Sildenafil is
taken only as needed.

STOPPING THE DRUG
Not applicable.

PROLONGED USE
Sildenafil treats but does
not cure erectile dysfunction. Patients must continue
using sildenafil to maintain
its benefit; lifelong therapy
may be warranted.

PRECAUTIONS
Over 60: No special problems are expected.

**Driving and Hazardous
Work:** This drug should
not impair your ability to
perform such tasks safely.

Alcohol: No special precautions are necessary.
However, alcohol is known
to decrease sexual function.

Pregnancy: Not applicable;
sildenafil is not approved for
use by women.

Breast Feeding: Not
applicable; sildenafil is not
approved for use by women.

Infants and Children:
Not applicable; sildenafil is
not to be used by children.

Special Concerns: Sildenafil does not offer any protection against sexually
transmitted diseases. Appro
priate measures (for example, using condoms) should
be taken to ensure adequate
protection against sexually
transmitted diseases, including infection with the
human immunodeficiency

virus (HIV). Sildenafil
should be taken only by
men who have been clini-
cally evaluated for and
diagnosed with erectile
dysfunction by a doctor.

OVERDOSE
Symptoms: No cases
of overdose have been
reported.

What to Do: An overdose
with sildenafil is unlikely.
If someone takes a much
larger dose than prescribed,
call your doctor.

DRUG INTERACTIONS
Sildenafil can enhance the
action of nitrates (such as
nitroglycerin, which is used
to treat episodes of angina),
causing potentially dangerous decreases in blood pressure. Therefore, sildenafil
should not be used by
patients taking nitrates of
any kind. Use of sildenafil in
conjunction with other erec-
tile-dysfunction medications
is not recommended. Con-
sult your doctor if you are
taking protease inhibitors
such as ritonavir and
saquinavir, which may
affect levels of sildenafil
in the blood.

FOOD INTERACTIONS
No known food interactions.

DISEASE INTERACTIONS
Caution is advised when
taking sildenafil. Consult
your doctor if you have a
history of any of the following: high or very low blood
pressure; structural deformity of the penis; a bleeding
disorder; heart attack,
stroke, or life-threatening
arrhythmia within the past
six months; heart failure;
coronary heart disease;
retinitis pigmentosa; peptic
ulcer; sickle cell anemia;
multiple myeloma; or
leukemia.

Simethicone

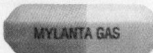

Mylanta Gas Relief 62.5 mg
(JOHNSON & JOHNSON/MERCK)

Additional photographs

▶ Drug Class: Antacid;
antiflatulant

▶ Available in: Tablets, chewable tablets, capsules, drops

▶ Available OTC? Yes

▶ As Generic? Yes

Side Effects

SERIOUS
No serious side effects
have been reported.

COMMON
Expulsion of excess gas
causing belching and
flatulence.

LESS COMMON
No less-common side
effects have been
reported.

PRINCIPAL USES
To relieve pain caused by
excess gas in stomach and
intestines. It may also be
employed in a clinical setting to decrease gas before
diagnostic radiography of
the stomach or intestines,
or prior to endoscopy.

HOW THE DRUG WORKS
Simethicone disperses and
prevents the formation of
gas bubbles in the gastrointestinal tract.

DOSAGE
Tablets or capsules: 60 to
125 mg, 4 times a day, after
meals and at bedtime.
Chewable tablets: 40 to 125
mg, 4 times a day after
meals and at bedtime, or
150 mg, 3 times a day after
meals. Drops: 40 to 95 mg,
4 times a day after meals
and at bedtime. The liquid
form should be taken by
mouth even if it comes in
a dropper bottle. The dose
should not exceed 500 mg
a day for all forms unless
your doctor advises otherwise. (In some cases your
doctor may wish to double
the dose.)

ONSET OF EFFECT
Immediate.

DURATION OF ACTION
Unknown.

DIETARY ADVICE
This medicine should be
taken after meals and at
bedtime for optimal results.

STORAGE
Store in a tightly sealed
container away from heat,
moisture, and direct light.
Store the liquid form at
room temperature.

IF YOU MISS A DOSE
Take it as soon as you
remember. However, if it is
near the time for the next
dose, skip the missed dose
and resume your regular
dosage schedule. Do not
double the next dose.

STOPPING THE DRUG
Take simethicone as prescribed for the full treatment period. However, you
may stop taking the drug
if you are feeling better
before the scheduled
end of therapy.

PROLONGED USE
Consult your doctor if you
take simethicone for a prolonged period.

PRECAUTIONS
Over 60: There is no specific information comparing
use of simethicone in older
persons with use in younger
persons. However, no special problems are expected.

**Driving and Hazardous
Work:** The use of simethicone should not impair
your ability to perform
such tasks safely.

Alcohol: No special problems are expected.

Pregnancy: Simethicone is
not absorbed into the body
and is not expected to cause
problems during pregnancy.

Breast Feeding: Simethicone has not been
reported to cause problems
in nursing babies.

Infants and Children:
Use of simethicone for the
treatment of infant colic is
not recommended because
of limited information on its
safety in infants. Simethicone should not be dispensed to children unless a
doctor instructs otherwise.

Special Concerns: If you
take the chewable tablets,
chew them thoroughly
before swallowing for more
complete and faster results.
Shake the liquid form well
before using. You should
change position frequently
and walk about to help eliminate gas. Tell your doctor if
you are on a low-sodium,
low-sugar or other special
diet. You should exercise
regularly and develop regular bowel habits. Do not
smoke before meals.

OVERDOSE
Symptoms: No specific
ones have been reported.

What to Do: An overdose
of simethicone is not life-threatening. However, if
someone takes a much
larger dose than recommended, call your doctor
or the nearest poison control center.

DRUG INTERACTIONS
None known.

FOOD INTERACTIONS
Avoid any foods that
increase gas formation.
Chew your food slowly and
thoroughly. Avoid carbonated drinks.

DISEASE INTERACTIONS
None known.

Simvastatin

Side Effects

SERIOUS
Fever, unusual or unexplained muscle aches and tenderness. Call
your doctor right away.

COMMON
Side effects occur in only 1% to 2% of patients. They may include constipation or diarrhea, dizziness or lightheadedness, bloating or gas, heartburn, nausea, skin rash, stomach pain, rise in liver enzymes.

LESS COMMON
Insomnia.

PRINCIPAL USES
To treat high cholesterol. Also used to reduce the risk of stroke or transient ischemic attack ("ministroke") in patients with high cholesterol and heart disease. Usually prescribed after first lines of treatment—including diet, weight loss, and exercise—fail to reduce total and low-density lipoprotein (LDL) cholesterol to acceptable levels.

HOW THE DRUG WORKS
Simvastatin blocks the action of an enzyme required for the manufacture of cholesterol, thereby interfering with its formation. By lowering the amount of cholesterol in the liver cells, simvastatin increases the formation of receptors for LDL, and thereby reduces blood levels of total and LDL cholesterol. In addition to lowering LDL cholesterol, simvastatin also modestly reduces triglyceride levels and raises HDL (the so-called "good") cholesterol.

DOSAGE
Initial dose is 10 to 40 mg once a day. It may be increased to a maximum of 80 mg per day. Simvastatin is most effective when taken in the evening.

ONSET OF EFFECT
2 to 4 weeks.

DURATION OF ACTION
The effect persists for the duration of therapy.

DIETARY ADVICE
Cholesterol-lowering drugs are only one part of a total program that should include regular exercise and a healthy diet. The American Heart Association publishes a "Healthy Heart" diet, which is recommended.

STORAGE
Store in a tightly sealed container away from heat and direct light.

IF YOU MISS A DOSE
Take it as soon as you remember. Take your next dose at the proper time and resume your regular dosage schedule. Do not double the next dose.

STOPPING THE DRUG
The decision to stop taking the drug should be made in consultation with your doctor. Once the medication is discontinued, blood cholesterol is likely to return to original elevated levels.

PROLONGED USE
Side effects are more likely with prolonged use. As you continue with simvastatin, your doctor will periodically order blood tests to evaluate liver function.

PRECAUTIONS
Over 60: No special problems are expected in older patients.

Driving and Hazardous Work: The use of simvastatin should not impair your ability to perform such tasks safely.

Alcohol: No special precautions are necessary.

Pregnancy: Should not be used during pregnancy or by women who plan to become pregnant in the near future.

Breast Feeding: This drug is not recommended for women who are nursing.

Infants and Children: The long-term effects of simvastatin in children have not been determined. It is rarely used in children; consult your pediatrician.

Special Concerns: Important elements of treatment for high cholesterol include proper diet, weight loss, regular moderate exercise, and the avoidance of certain medications that may increase cholesterol levels. Because simvastatin has potential side effects, it is important that you maintain a recommended healthy diet and cooperate with other treatments your physician may suggest.

OVERDOSE
Symptoms: No specific ones have been reported; overdose is unlikely.

What to Do: Emergency instructions not applicable.

DRUG INTERACTIONS
Consult your doctor if you are taking cyclosporine, gemfibrozil, niacin, antibiotics, especially erythromycin, HIV protease inhibitors, or medications for fungus infections. All of these drugs may increase the risk of myositis (muscle inflammation) when taken with simvastatin and may lead to kidney failure.

FOOD INTERACTIONS
No known food interactions.

DISEASE INTERACTIONS
Consult your doctor if you have liver, kidney, or muscle disease, or a medical history involving organ transplant or recent surgery.

Sodium Bicarbonate

BRAND NAMES
Alka-Seltzer, Arm
and Hammer Pure
Baking Soda, Bell/ans,
Citrocarbonate, Soda Mint

Generic 324 mg
(CONCORD)

▶ Drug Class: Antacid

▶ Available in: Effervescent
powder, powder, tablets

▶ Available OTC? Yes

▶ As Generic? Yes

Side Effects

SERIOUS
Frequent urge to urinate,
nervousness or restless-
ness, mental or mood
changes, muscle twitch-
ing or pain, nausea or
vomiting, slow breathing,
continuing headache, loss
of appetite, swelling of
feet or lower legs,
unpleasant taste, unusual
fatigue. Call your doctor
immediately.

COMMON
No common side effects
are associated with
sodium bicarbonate.

LESS COMMON
Stomach cramps,
increased thirst.

PRINCIPAL USES
To relieve heartburn, sour
stomach, or acid indiges-
tion. It may also be pre-
scribed to treat metabolic
acidosis (excess acid
buildup in the body fluids),
to prevent urinary stones,
and as part of the treatment
of gout.

HOW THE DRUG WORKS
Sodium bicarbonate neutralizes stomach acid and
reduces the action of
pepsin, a digestive enzyme.
This provides symptomatic
relief from excess stomach
acid. Also, the bicarbonate
is a base, meaning it can
help correct the pH balance
(reduce the acidity) of
blood and urine.

DOSAGE
Effervescent powder— For
heartburn or sour stomach:
3.9 to 10 g (1 to 2 ½ teaspoons) in a glass of cold
water. Usually not more
than 19.5 g a day (5 tea-
spoons). Children ages 6 to
12: 1 to 1.9 g (¼ to ½ teaspoon) in a glass of cold
water. Powder— For heart-
burn or sour stomach: ½
teaspoon in a glass of water
every 2 hours. Dose may be
changed if needed. To make
the urine less acidic: 1 teaspoon (1.9 g) in a glass of
water every 4 hours; usually
not more than 4 teaspoons a
day. Dose may be changed
by your doctor. Tablets—
For heartburn or sour stomach: 325 mg to 2 g, 1 to 4
times a day. Children ages 6
to 12: 520 mg. Dose may be
repeated in 30 minutes. To
make the urine less acidic—
To start, 4 g; then 1 to 2 g
every 4 hours. Maximum
adult dose usually not more
than 16 g a day. Children:
23 to 230 mg per 2.2 lbs
(1 kg) of body weight a
day. Dose may be changed
if needed.

ONSET OF EFFECT
Rapid when used as an
antacid for heartburn and
sour stomach.

DURATION OF ACTION
Unknown.

DIETARY ADVICE
Sodium bicarbonate should
be taken after meals. Be
sure to account for the large
amount of sodium in this
medication if you are on a
salt-restricted diet.

STORAGE
Store in a tightly sealed container away from heat, moisture, and direct light.

IF YOU MISS A DOSE
Take it as soon as you
remember. If it is near
the time for the next dose,
skip the missed dose and
resume your regular dosage
schedule. Do not double the
next dose.

STOPPING THE DRUG
Take as directed if taking it
by prescription.

PROLONGED USE
Do not take sodium bicar-
bonate for more than 2
weeks or on a routine basis
without consulting your
physician.

PRECAUTIONS
Over 60: See Dietary
Advice.

**Driving and Hazardous
Work:** No special precautions are necessary.

Alcohol: Avoid alcohol.

Pregnancy: No problems
have been reported.

Breast Feeding: No problems have been reported.

Infants and Children:
Use and dosage for infants
and children under 6 years
of age should be deter-
mined by your doctor.

OVERDOSE
Symptoms: See Serious
Side Effects.

What to Do: An overdose
of sodium bicarbonate is
unlikely to be life-threatening. However, if someone
takes a much larger dose
than recommended, call
your doctor, emergency
medical services (EMS), or
the nearest poison control
center immediately.

DRUG INTERACTIONS
Do not take any other over-
the-counter medications
containing sodium bicarbonate such as Alka-Seltzer.
Consult your doctor for specific advice if you are taking
ketoconazole, tetracyclines,
mecamylamine, methena-
mine, urinary acidifiers,
amphetamines, anticholinergics, quinidine, citrates,
enteric-coated medications,
ephedrine, flecainide, fluoroquinolones, iron, lithium,
methotrexate, mexiletine,
sucralfate, or salicylates.

FOOD INTERACTIONS
Do not take sodium bicar-
bonate with milk or milk
products.

DISEASE INTERACTIONS
Do not take sodium bicar-
bonate if you have any sign
of appendicitis (stomach
pain, bloating, nausea, and
vomiting). If you have kidney problems, use sodium
bicarbonate only on advice
of your doctor. Consult your
doctor if you have intestinal
or rectal bleeding, edema
(swelling of the hands or
feet), heart, liver, or kidney
disease, hypertension, urination problems, or toxemia
of pregnancy.

Sodium Phosphate/Sodium Biphosphate

BRAND NAMES
Fleet, Fleet Phospho-Soda

► Drug Class: Hyperosmotic laxative

► Available in: Oral solution, effervescent powder, enema

► Available OTC? Yes

► As Generic? Yes

Side Effects

SERIOUS
Confusion, dizziness or lightheadedness, irregular heartbeat, muscle cramps, unusual tiredness or weakness. Call your doctor immediately.

COMMON
Cramping, diarrhea, gas, increased thirst.

LESS COMMON
No less-common side effects have been reported.

PRINCIPAL USES
To treat short-term constipation or for rapid emptying of the colon prior to bowel or rectal examination.

HOW THE DRUG WORKS
This medication attracts and retains water in the intestine, increasing peristalsis (bowel activity) and the urge to defecate.

DOSAGE
Oral— Adults and teenagers: 20 to 30 ml (4 to 6 teaspoons) mixed with ½ glass cool water. Children ages 10 to 12: 10 ml (2 teaspoons). Children ages 6 to 10: 5 ml (1 teaspoon). Enema— Adults and teenagers: 118 ml (contents of 1 disposable adult enema) given rectally. Children over 2: ½ adult dose (contents of 1 disposable pediatric enema).

ONSET OF EFFECT
30 minutes to 3 hours after oral administration, 3 to 5 minutes after enema.

DURATION OF ACTION
Variable with oral use; upon evacuation with enema.

DIETARY ADVICE
Sodium phosphate/sodium biphosphate should not be used with food. The unpleasant taste that may occur when you take the medicine can be lessened by taking it with citrus fruit juice or a citrus-flavored soft drink.

STORAGE
Store in a tightly sealed container away from heat and direct light.

IF YOU MISS A DOSE
Oral forms: If you are taking this laxative on a fixed schedule, take the missed dose as soon as you remember. If it is near the time for the next dose, skip the missed dose and resume your regular dosage schedule. Do not double the next dose. Enema: Not applicable.

STOPPING THE DRUG
Take it as prescribed for the full treatment period. However, you may stop taking the drug if you feel better before the scheduled end of therapy.

PROLONGED USE
Do not use any laxative for longer than 2 weeks without consulting your doctor.

PRECAUTIONS
Over 60: Adverse reactions may be more likely and more severe in older patients.

Driving and Hazardous Work: Do not drive or engage in hazardous work until you determine how the medicine affects you.

Alcohol: Avoid alcohol.

Pregnancy: This laxative contains a large amount of sodium, which may have unwanted effects during pregnancy, such as higher blood pressure. If you have to take a laxative during pregnancy, consult your doctor for specific advice.

Breast Feeding: Sodium phosphate may pass into breast milk; caution is advised. Consult your doctor for specific advice.

Infants and Children: Do not give sodium phosphate/sodium biphosphate to children under the age of 6 without consulting your doctor.

Special Concerns: Chilling the oral form of the medication or taking it with ice or following it with citrus fruit juice or citrus-fla-vored carbonated beverages may make it more palatable. Remember that chronic use of sodium phosphate or any laxative can lead to laxative dependence. You should consume adequate amounts of bulk (fiber) in your diet, such as bran, whole-grain cereals, fruit, and vegetables. This laxative should be taken on a schedule that does not interfere with activities or sleep; it produces watery stools within 3 to 6 hours. It should not be taken within 2 hours of taking other medications.

OVERDOSE
Symptoms: Excessive bowel activity, dehydration causing low blood pressure and abnormal heartbeat, metabolic acidosis, blood chemistry abnormalities.

What to Do: An overdose of sodium phosphate/sodium biphosphate is unlikely to be life-threatening. However, if someone takes a much larger dose than prescribed, call your doctor, emergency medical services (EMS), or the nearest poison control center immediately.

DRUG INTERACTIONS
Consult your doctor for advice if you are taking anticoagulants, digitalis drugs, ciprofloxacin, etidronate, sodium polystyrene sulfonate, or oral tetracyclines.

FOOD INTERACTIONS
No known food interactions.

DISEASE INTERACTIONS
Consult your doctor if you have a history of appendicitis, rectal bleeding of unknown cause, colostomy, intestinal blockage, ileostomy, diabetes, heart disease, high blood pressure, kidney disease, or swallowing difficulties.

Sodium Polystyrene Sulfonate

BRAND NAMES
Kayexalate, SPS

▶ Drug Class: Potassium-removing resin

▶ Available in: Powder for suspension, suspension

▶ Available OTC? No

▶ As Generic? Yes

Side Effects

SERIOUS
Severe stomach pain with nausea and vomiting (fecal impaction), heartbeat irregularities, abdominal and muscle cramps, weight gain, irritability, difficulty thinking, confusion, decreased urination, severe muscle fatigue, swelling of hands, feet, or lower legs. Call your doctor immediately.

COMMON
Loss of appetite, constipation, nausea, vomiting.

LESS COMMON
There are no less-common side effects associated with sodium polystyrene sulfonate.

PRINCIPAL USES
To treat abnormally high blood levels of potassium (hyperkalemia) caused by acute kidney failure.

HOW THE DRUG WORKS
Sodium polystyrene sulfonate is a resin that lowers potassium levels by exchanging sodium present in the medication with potassium present in the body. This process occurs within the intestines.

DOSAGE
The powder for suspension and the suspension can be taken either orally or rectally. Adults— Oral: 15 g (4 level tablespoons of powder), 1 to 4 times a day; may be increased to 40 g, 4 times a day. Rectal: 25 to 100 g as needed, given as an enema or in a dialysis bag. Children— Oral: 1 g per 2.2 lbs (1 kg) of body weight, as needed. Rectal: 1 g per 2.2 lbs, as needed, given as an enema or in a dialysis bag. Oral dosage is preferred because the drug should remain in the intestine for at least 6 hours.

ONSET OF EFFECT
Unknown.

DURATION OF ACTION
Unknown.

DIETARY ADVICE
The oral medication should not be mixed with orange juice (orange juice is high in potassium).

STORAGE
Store in a tightly sealed container away from heat, moisture, and direct light. Liquid form can be refrigerated, but do not allow it to freeze.

IF YOU MISS A DOSE
Take it as soon as you remember. However, if it is near the time for the next dose, skip the missed dose and resume your regular dosage schedule. Do not double the next dose.

STOPPING THE DRUG
The decision to stop taking the drug should be made in consultation with your physician.

PROLONGED USE
See your doctor regularly for tests and examinations if you must take this medication for a prolonged period.

PRECAUTIONS
Over 60: Side effects, especially fecal impaction, may be more likely in older patients.

Driving and Hazardous Work: Do not drive or engage in hazardous work until you determine how the medicine affects you.

Alcohol: Avoid alcohol.

Pregnancy: Adequate studies of the use of sodium polystyrene sulfonate during pregnancy have not been done. Before taking it, consult your doctor if you are pregnant or plan to become pregnant.

Breast Feeding: It is not known whether sodium polystyrene sulfonate passes into breast milk; consult your doctor for advice.

Infants and Children: No special problems are expected.

Special Concerns: If you are taking the suspension made from the powder, shake it well before using. Do not use mineral oil when administering this drug rectally. The suspension should be used within 24 hours of preparation.

OVERDOSE
Symptoms: Severe nausea, vomiting, fecal impaction, swelling of hands, feet, or lower legs, decreased urination, severe muscle fatigue, confusion.

What to Do: Call your doctor, emergency medical services (EMS), or the nearest poison control center immediately.

DRUG INTERACTIONS
The following drugs may interact with sodium polystyrene sulfonate. Consult your doctor for specific advice if you are taking antacids, digitalis drugs, laxatives, diuretics, potassium supplements, or any other prescription or over-the-counter medication.

FOOD INTERACTIONS
Orange juice can increase blood levels of potassium.

DISEASE INTERACTIONS
Caution is advised when taking sodium polystyrene sulfonate. Consult your doctor for advice if you have a history of congestive heart failure, severe high blood pressure, or severe edema (swelling of body tissues caused by fluid retention).

Somatrem

BRAND NAME
Protropin

▶ Drug Class: Growth hormone

▶ Available in: Injection

▶ Available OTC? No

▶ As Generic? No

Side Effects

SERIOUS
Pain and swelling at the site of injection; pain in hip or knee (possibly causing a limp); skin rash or itching. Call your doctor right away.

COMMON
No common side effects are associated with somatrem.

LESS COMMON
No uncommon side effects are associated with somatrem.

PRINCIPAL USES
To replace growth hormone if it is not produced sufficiently by the pituitary gland.

HOW THE DRUG WORKS
Somatrem stimulates growth in the same manner as natural growth hormone.

DOSAGE
0.136 mg per lb of body weight weekly, in multiple doses as determined by your doctor.

ONSET OF EFFECT
Within 1 hour.

DURATION OF ACTION
12 to 48 hours.

DIETARY ADVICE
None.

STORAGE
Keep the liquid refrigerated, but do not allow it to freeze. Use it within 7 days.

IF YOU MISS A DOSE
Take it as soon as you remember. If it is near the time for the next dose, skip the missed dose and resume your regular dosage schedule. Do not double the next dose.

STOPPING THE DRUG
The decision to stop taking the drug should be made by your doctor.

PROLONGED USE
After 2 years of use, growth rate generally decreases. If this occurs, the patient should be checked for compliance with therapy or the presence of other medical problems or the presence of antibodies to the medicine. Prolonged use of somatrem may cause a condition known as acromegaly (overgrowth of face, hands, and feet, organ enlargement, diabetes, atherosclerosis, high blood pressure, and carpal tunnel syndrome), resulting from excess quantities of pituitary hormone.

PRECAUTIONS
Over 60: Somatrem can be used to replace deficient growth hormone levels in people of any age. Though not approved for this use, growth hormone has been administered to elderly patients to increase muscle strength. Such use can result in edema (swelling of tissues due to excess fluid retention) and high blood pressure.

Driving and Hazardous Work: The use of somatrem should not impair the ability to perform such tasks safely.

Alcohol: No special precautions are necessary.

Pregnancy: It is unknown whether somatrem causes fetal harm; the drug should be used by pregnant women only if absolutely necessary. Consult your doctor for specific advice.

Breast Feeding: It is unknown whether somatrem passes into breast milk or causes harm to a nursing infant; the drug should be used by nursing mothers only if clearly needed. Consult your doctor.

Infants and Children: Somatrem should not be given to a child whose bone ends (epiphyses) have closed, signaling the end of bone growth.

Special Concerns: If somatrem is given to adults or children with normal growth hormone production, serious unwanted effects may occur, such as diabetes, high blood pressure, atherosclerosis, and abnormal growth of bone and internal organs including the heart, kidneys, and liver. If growth with somatrem is not satisfactory, some patients may be given low doses of sex hormones to improve their response to the medication. Annual tests of bone age are recommended. Periodic tests of thyroid function should be done, since low thyroid function interferes with the response to human growth hormone. If low growth hormone production is due to a lesion in the cranium, the lesion should be monitored at frequent intervals. If somatrem is injected into muscle, the needle used for injections should be at least 1 inch long to ensure that the medicine reaches the muscle.

OVERDOSE
Symptoms: No specific ones have been reported.

What to Do: An overdose of somatrem is unlikely to be life-threatening. However, if someone receives a much larger dose than prescribed, call your doctor, emergency medical services (EMS), or local poison control center immediately.

DRUG INTERACTIONS
Consult your doctor for specific advice if you (or your child) are also taking the following drugs that may interact with somatrem: anabolic steroids, estrogens, androgens, thyroid hormones, corticosteroids, or corticotropin.

FOOD INTERACTIONS
No known food interactions.

DISEASE INTERACTIONS
Caution is advised when taking somatrem. Consult your doctor if you have low thyroid function or any malignancy (cancerous growth).

▶ Drug Class: Growth hormone

▶ Available in: Injection

▶ Available OTC? No

▶ As Generic? No

Side Effects

SERIOUS
Pain and swelling at the site of injection; pain in hip or knee (possibly causing a limp); skin rash or itching. Call your doctor right away.

COMMON
No common side effects are associated with somatropin.

LESS COMMON
No uncommon side effects are associated with somatropin.

PRINCIPAL USES
To replace growth hormone if it is not produced sufficiently by the pituitary gland.

HOW THE DRUG WORKS
Somatropin stimulates growth in the same manner as natural growth hormone.

DOSAGE
Adults: To start, not more than 0.006 mg per kg (2.2 lbs) of body weight given daily as an injection under the skin. The dosage may be increased by your doctor to no more than 0.025 mg per kg in patients under 35 years and 0.0125 mg per kg in patients over 35 years. Children: Up to 0.3 mg per kg weekly, divided into daily injections under the skin as determined by the doctor.

ONSET OF EFFECT
Within 1 hour.

DURATION OF ACTION
12 to 48 hours.

DIETARY ADVICE
No special restrictions.

STORAGE
Keep the liquid refrigerated, but do not allow it to freeze. Use it within 7 days.

IF YOU MISS A DOSE
Take it as soon as you remember. If it is near the time for the next dose, skip the missed dose and resume your regular dosage schedule. Do not double the next dose.

STOPPING THE DRUG
The decision to stop taking the drug should be made by your doctor.

PROLONGED USE
After 2 years of use, growth rate generally decreases. If this occurs, the patient should be checked for compliance with therapy or the presence of other medical problems or the presence of antibodies to the medicine. Prolonged use of somatropin may cause a condition known as acromegaly (overgrowth of face, hands, and feet, organ enlargement, diabetes, atherosclerosis, high blood pressure, and carpal tunnel syndrome), resulting from excess quantities of pituitary hormone.

PRECAUTIONS
Over 60: Somatropin can be used to replace deficient growth hormone levels in people of any age. Though not approved for this use, growth hormone has been administered to elderly patients to increase muscle strength. Such use can result in edema (swelling of tissues due to excess fluid retention) and high blood pressure.

Driving and Hazardous Work: The use of somatropin should not impair the ability to perform such tasks safely.

Alcohol: No special precautions are necessary.

Pregnancy: It is unknown whether somatropin causes fetal harm; the drug should be used by pregnant women only if absolutely necessary. Consult your doctor for specific advice.

Breast Feeding: It is not known whether somatropin passes into breast milk or causes harm to a nursing infant; the drug should be used by nursing mothers only if clearly needed. Consult your doctor.

Infants and Children: Somatropin should not be given to a child whose bone ends (epiphyses) have closed, signaling the end of bone growth.

Special Concerns: If somatropin is given to adults or children with normal growth hormone production, serious unwanted effects may occur, such as diabetes, high blood pressure, atherosclerosis, and abnormal growth of bone and internal organs including the heart, kidneys, and liver. If growth is not satisfactory, some patients may be given low doses of sex hormones to improve their response to somatropin. Annual tests of bone age are recommended. Periodic tests of thyroid function should be done, since low thyroid function interferes with response to human growth hormone. If low growth hormone production is due to a lesion in the cranium, the lesion should be monitored frequently. If somatropin is injected into muscle, the needle used for injections should be at least 1 inch long.

OVERDOSE
Symptoms: None.

What to Do: An overdose is unlikely to be life-threatening. However, if someone receives a much larger dose than prescribed, seek medical assistance immediately.

DRUG INTERACTIONS
Consult your doctor for specific advice if you (or your child) are also taking the following drugs that may interact with somatropin: anabolic steroids, estrogens, androgens, thyroid hormones, corticosteroids, or corticotropin.

FOOD INTERACTIONS
No known food interactions.

DISEASE INTERACTIONS
Consult your doctor if you have low thyroid function or any malignancy (cancerous growth).

Sotalol Hydrochloride

Side Effects

SERIOUS
Severe, occasionally life-threatening arrhythmias, shortness of breath, wheezing; irregular or slow heartbeat (50 beats per minute or less); pain or feelings of tightness or pressure in the chest; swelling of the ankles, feet, and lower legs; mental depression. If you experience such symptoms, stop taking sotalol and call your doctor immediately.

COMMON
Dizziness or lightheadedness, especially when rising suddenly to a standing position; rapid heartbeat or palpitations; decreased sexual ability; unusual fatigue, weakness, or drowsiness; insomnia. Notify your doctor.

LESS COMMON
Anxiety, irritability, nervousness; constipation; diarrhea; dry, sore eyes; itching; nausea or vomiting; nightmares or intensely vivid dreams; numbness, tingling, or other unusual sensations in the fingers, toes, or scalp. Call your doctor if such symptoms persist.

PRINCIPAL USES
This drug is used only to treat or prevent life-threatening heart rhythm disturbances (cardiac arrhythmias). It requires close monitoring by a physician.

HOW THE DRUG WORKS
Beta-blockers such as sotalol work by preventing—or blocking—nerve impulses from exerting an accelerating or intensifying effect on specific parts of the body, especially the blood vessels and heart. In this way, sotalol slows and stabilizes heartbeat.

DOSAGE
Adults: 80 mg, 2 times a day. The dosage may be increased to 320 mg a day in 2 or 3 divided doses.

ONSET OF EFFECT
Unknown.

DURATION OF ACTION
Up to 12 hours.

DIETARY ADVICE
Should be taken on an empty stomach, 1 hour before or 2 hours after meals.

STORAGE
Store in a tightly sealed container away from heat and direct light.

IF YOU MISS A DOSE
Take it as soon as you remember. However, if it is near the time for the next dose, skip the missed dose and resume your regular dosage schedule. Do not double the next dose.

STOPPING THE DRUG
Do not discontinue the drug abruptly, as this may cause serious health problems. Dosage must be gradually tapered in accordance with your doctor's instructions.

PROLONGED USE
Your doctor should check your progress in regular visits if you take sotalol for a prolonged period.

PRECAUTIONS
Over 60: Adverse reactions may be more likely and more severe. Resistance to cold temperatures may be decreased in older patients

Driving and Hazardous Work: Do not drive or engage in hazardous work until you determine how the medicine affects you.

Alcohol: Avoid alcohol.

Pregnancy: Before taking sotalol, tell your doctor if you are pregnant or plan to become pregnant.

Breast Feeding: Sotalol passes into breast milk; consult your doctor about its use during nursing.

Infants and Children: Dosage for infants and children must be determined by your pediatrician.

Special Concerns: To avoid dizziness and fainting, take extra care during exercise or hot weather. Check your pulse regularly while taking sotalol. If it is slower than your usual rate, or less than 50 beats per minute, check with your doctor; a slow pulse rate may indicate circulation problems.

OVERDOSE
Symptoms: Unusually slow or rapid heartbeat, confusion, severe dizziness or fainting, poor circulation in the hands (bluish skin), breathing difficulty.

What to Do: Call your doctor, emergency medical services (EMS), or the nearest poison control center immediately.

DRUG INTERACTIONS
Consult your doctor for specific advice if you are taking amphetamines, oral antidiabetic agents, asthma medication (such as aminophylline or theophylline), calcium channel blockers, clonidine, guanabenz, halothane, immunotherapy for allergies (allergy shots), insulin, MAO inhibitors, reserpine, other beta-blockers, or any over-the-counter medicine.

FOOD INTERACTIONS
No known food interactions.

DISEASE INTERACTIONS
People with the following conditions should consult their doctor before using sotalol: allergies or asthma; diabetes mellitus; heart or blood vessel disease (including congestive heart failure and peripheral vascular disease); hyperthyroidism; irregular (slow) heartbeat; a history of mental depression; myasthenia gravis; psoriasis; respiratory problems such as bronchitis or emphysema; kidney or liver disease.

Sparfloxacin

▶ Drug Class: Fluoroquinolone antibiotic

▶ Available in: Tablets

▶ Available OTC? No

▶ As Generic? No

Side Effects

SERIOUS
Serious reactions to sparfloxacin are rare and include seizures, mental confusion, hallucinations, agitation, nightmares, depression, shortness of breath, unusual swelling in the face or extremities, and loss of consciousness. Also skin burning, redness, blisters, rash, or itching on exposure to sunlight; increased risk of tendinitis or tendon rupture. Call your doctor immediately.

COMMON
Increased sensitivity to sunlight (and increased risk of sunburn) for days following therapy.

LESS COMMON
Diarrhea, nausea and vomiting, stomach pain and upset, gas, headache, dizziness, restlessness, insomnia, changes in taste perception, drowsiness, itching, dry mouth, unusual body aches or pains.

PRINCIPAL USES
To treat pneumonia, chronic bronchitis, and other bacterial infections.

HOW THE DRUG WORKS
Sparfloxacin inhibits the activity of a bacterial enzyme (gyrase) that is necessary for proper DNA formation and replication. This fights infection by preventing bacteria cells from reproducing.

DOSAGE
Adults: To start, 400 mg in 1 dose on the first day, then take 200 mg, once a day for 9 days. For patients with kidney impairment, 400 mg to start, wait 2 days, then take 200 mg every other day for 9 days.

ONSET OF EFFECT
Varies depending on the infection being treated.

DURATION OF ACTION
Unknown.

DIETARY ADVICE
Drink plenty of fluids.

STORAGE
Store in a tightly sealed container away from heat and direct light.

IF YOU MISS A DOSE
Take it as soon as you remember. If it is near the time for the next dose, skip the missed dose and resume your regular dosage schedule. Do not double the next dose.

STOPPING THE DRUG
It is very important to take this drug as prescribed for the full treatment period, even if you begin to feel better before the scheduled end of therapy (unless you experience intolerable side effects, including increased sensitivity to sunlight, in which case, discontinue taking the drug and call your physician right away).

PROLONGED USE
See your doctor regularly for tests and examinations if you must take this medicine for a prolonged period.

PRECAUTIONS
Over 60: No special problems are expected.

Driving and Hazardous Work: Do not drive or engage in hazardous work until you determine how the medicine affects you.

Alcohol: It is advisable to abstain from alcohol when fighting an infection.

Pregnancy: In some animal tests, sparfloxacin has caused birth defects. Adequate studies in humans have not been done. It should be used during pregnancy only if the potential benefit justifies the risk. Before you take sparfloxacin, tell your doctor if you are pregnant or plan to become pregnant.

Breast Feeding: Sparfloxacin passes into breast milk and may cause serious side effects in the nursing infant; use of the drug is discouraged when nursing.

Infants and Children: Not recommended for use by persons under age 18, as it has been shown to interfere with bone development.

Special Concerns: If this drug causes increased sensitivity to sunlight, stop taking the medicine and try to avoid exposure to sunlight for the next week; also wear protective clothing and use a sunblock. Sparfloxacin should not be taken by a patient whose work makes it impossible to avoid exposure to sunlight. It is important to drink plenty of fluids while taking this antibiotic.

OVERDOSE
Symptoms: No specific ones have been reported.

What to Do: If you have any reason to suspect an overdose, call your doctor, emergency medical services (EMS), or the nearest poison control center.

DRUG INTERACTIONS
The following drugs may interact with sparfloxacin. Consult your doctor for specific advice if you are taking aminophylline, antacids, didanosine, iron supplements, sucralfate, or zinc salts. Also tell your doctor if you are taking any other prescription or over-the-counter drug.

FOOD INTERACTIONS
No known food interactions.

DISEASE INTERACTIONS
Caution is advised when taking sparfloxacin. Consult your doctor if you have any other medical condition. Use of sparfloxacin can cause complications in patients with kidney disease, since this organ works to remove the medication from the body.

Spironolactone

BRAND NAME
Aldactone

Generic 25 mg
(**MYLAN**)

▶ Drug Class: Potassium-
  sparing diuretic

▶ Available in: Tablets

▶ Available OTC? No

▶ As Generic? Yes

Side Effects

SERIOUS
Skin rash or itching, shortness of breath, cough or hoarseness, fever or chills, pain in lower back or side, painful or difficult urination. Call your doctor immediately.

COMMON
Nausea, vomiting, diarrhea.

LESS COMMON
Dizziness, headache, sweating, decreased sexual ability, breast tenderness, breast enlargement in men, increased hair growth in females, irregular menstrual periods.

PRINCIPAL USES
As adjunctive (supplementary) treatment with other diuretics to increase excretion of sodium and water in the urine while conserving potassium. Spironolactone may be used on its own in patients with liver disease or primary hyperaldosteronism, a life-threatening disorder that occurs when the adrenal glands secrete too much of the hormone aldosterone.

HOW THE DRUG WORKS
Spironolactone blocks the effect of aldosterone in the kidneys to increase excretion of sodium and water in the urine while conserving potassium. In conjunction with thiazide or loop diuretics, spironolactone reduces the overall fluid volume in the body, which helps to control symptoms of liver disease, heart disease, and kidney disease.

DOSAGE
Adults: 100 to 400 mg a day in 2 to 4 doses. Children: 1 to 3 mg per 2.2 lbs (1 kg) of body weight, in 1 to 4 doses a day.

ONSET OF EFFECT
1 to 2 days.

DURATION OF ACTION
2 to 3 days.

DIETARY ADVICE
Take it with meals to enhance absorption.

STORAGE
Store in a tightly sealed container away from heat and direct light.

IF YOU MISS A DOSE
Take it as soon as you remember. If it is near the time for the next dose, skip the missed dose and resume your regular dosage schedule. Do not double the next dose.

STOPPING THE DRUG
The decision to stop taking the drug should be made by your doctor.

PROLONGED USE
You should see your doctor periodically for tests if you take this medicine for a prolonged period.

PRECAUTIONS
Over 60: No special precautions are warranted.

Driving and Hazardous Work: The use of spironolactone should not impair your ability to perform such tasks safely.

Alcohol: No special precautions are necessary.

Pregnancy: This drug has not been shown to cause birth defects in animals; human tests have not been done. In any case, spironolactone is not usually prescribed during pregnancy.

Breast Feeding: Spironolactone passes into breast milk but has not been reported to cause problems. Consult your doctor for advice about its use while nursing.

Infants and Children: No special problems are expected in children.

OVERDOSE
Symptoms: Acute electrolyte imbalance causing central nervous system disturbances.

What to Do: An overdose of spironolactone is unlikely to be life-threatening. However, if someone takes a much larger dose than prescribed, call your doctor, emergency medical services (EMS), or the nearest poison control center.

DRUG INTERACTIONS
Consult your doctor for specific advice if you are taking cyclosporine, potassium-containing medicines or supplements, digoxin, or lithium. Also, since angiotensin-converting enzyme (ACE) inhibitors block aldosterone production, spironolactone is not useful in patients taking this type of medication.

FOOD INTERACTIONS
Avoid consuming large servings of high-potassium foods, which include bananas, melons, prunes, citrus fruits and juices (and most fruits in general), avocados, potatoes, nuts, baked beans, brussels sprouts, and skim milk.

DISEASE INTERACTIONS
Caution is advised when taking spironolactone. Consult your doctor if you have any of the following: kidney stones, menstrual problems, breast enlargement, liver disease, or kidney disease.

BRAND NAMES
Aldactazide, Spirozide

Generic 25/25 mg
(MYLAN)

▶ Drug Class: Diuretic combination

▶ Available in: Tablets

▶ Available OTC? No

▶ As Generic? Yes

Side Effects

SERIOUS
Skin rash, hives, palpitations, lightheadedness, unusual bleeding. Call your doctor immediately.

COMMON
Fluid depletion leading to dizziness, especially when rising from a sitting or lying position.

LESS COMMON
Gout, increased blood sugar levels, breast enlargement in men, decreased sexual ability, increased sensitivity of the skin to sunlight.

PRINCIPAL USES
To treat edema (swelling of body tissues resulting from excess salt and water retention) and to control high blood pressure.

HOW THE DRUG WORKS
Spironolactone, a potassium-sparing diuretic, blocks the effect of aldosterone—a hormone that regulates sodium and potassium levels in the body—in the kidneys to increase excretion of sodium and water in the urine while conserving potassium. Hydrochlorothiazide, a thiazide diuretic, increases the excretion of sodium and water in the urine. By reducing the overall fluid volume in the body, diuretics reduce pressure within the blood vessels.

DOSAGE
Adults: 1 to 4 tablets a day, usually taken as a single dose.

ONSET OF EFFECT
Within 2 hours.

DURATION OF ACTION
24 hours.

DIETARY ADVICE
Take it in the morning after breakfast.

STORAGE
Store in a tightly sealed container away from heat, moisture, and direct light.

IF YOU MISS A DOSE
Take it as soon as you remember. However, if it is near the time for the next dose, skip the missed dose and resume your regular dosage schedule. Do not double the next dose.

STOPPING THE DRUG
Take it as prescribed for the full treatment period. The decision to stop taking the drug should be made in consultation with your physician.

PROLONGED USE
See your doctor regularly for tests and examinations if you must take this medication for a prolonged period. If you are taking this medication for high blood pressure, lifelong therapy may be necessary.

PRECAUTIONS
Over 60: No special problems are expected.

Driving and Hazardous Work: The use of this drug should not impair your ability to perform such tasks safely.

Alcohol: No special precautions are necessary.

Pregnancy: This medication should not be taken during pregnancy unless recommended by your physician. Other diuretics are preferred.

Breast Feeding: Spironolactone and hydrochlorothiazide pass into breast milk; avoid or discontinue usage during the first month of breast feeding.

Infants and Children: This medication is seldom prescribed for children and infants.

Special Concerns: If you are taking this medicine to control high blood pressure, you should also follow your doctor's advice on weight control, diet, and exercise. Avoid exposure to sunlight until you determine how the medicine affects you. Spironolactone sometimes causes enlarged breasts in men and irregular menstrual periods in women.

OVERDOSE
Symptoms: Acute electrolyte imbalance causing central nervous system disturbances, fainting, lethargy, dizziness, drowsiness, confusion, gastrointestinal irritation.

What to Do: Call your doctor, emergency medical services (EMS), or the nearest poison control center immediately.

DRUG INTERACTIONS
Consult your doctor for specific advice if you are taking ACE inhibitors, cyclosporine, any potassium-containing medicines or supplements, cholestyramine, colestipol, digitalis drugs, or lithium.

FOOD INTERACTIONS
Avoid potassium-rich foods and beverages such as apple, orange, or other citrus fruit juices.

DISEASE INTERACTIONS
Consult your doctor if you have diabetes mellitus, a history of gout or kidney stones, heart or blood vessel disease, systemic lupus erythematosus, liver disease, kidney disease, or pancreatitis.

Stavudine (d4T)

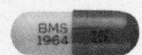

Zerit 15 mg
(BRISTOL-MYERS SQUIBB)

Additional photographs

▶ Drug Class: Antiviral

▶ Available in: Capsules

▶ Available OTC? No

▶ As Generic? No

Side Effects

SERIOUS
Burning, tingling, pain, or numbness in hands or feet. Also fever, muscle aches, joint pain, skin rash, nausea, vomiting, severe abdominal pain, unusual fatigue. Call your doctor immediately.

COMMON
No common side effects are associated with the use of stavudine.

LESS COMMON
Diarrhea, insomnia, headache, loss of appetite, general weakness and loss of energy.

PRINCIPAL USES
To treat HIV (human immunodeficiency virus) infection. While not a cure for HIV infection, this drug may suppress the replication of the virus and delay the progression of the disease.

HOW THE DRUG WORKS
Stavudine (d4T) interferes with the activity of enzymes needed for the replication of DNA in viral cells, thus preventing the virus from reproducing.

DOSAGE
Adults and teenagers weighing 132 lbs or more: 40 mg, 2 times a day. Adults and teenagers weighing up to 132 lbs: 30 mg, 2 times a day. Doses of 20 mg, 2 times a day, are sometimes used in patients with advanced HIV disease or mild peripheral neuropathy. Stavudine is usually given in combination with other antiretroviral medications.

ONSET OF EFFECT
Unknown. With most antiretroviral drugs, an early response can be seen within the first few days of therapy, but the maximum effect may take 12 to 16 weeks.

DURATION OF ACTION
Unknown. Effects of the drug may be prolonged if stavudine is used in combination with other effective drugs and the virus is maximally suppressed.

DIETARY ADVICE
Drink plenty of fluids.

STORAGE
Store in a tightly sealed container away from heat and direct light.

IF YOU MISS A DOSE
Take it as soon as you remember. However, if it is near the time for the next dose, skip the missed dose and resume your regular dosage schedule. Do not double the next dose.

STOPPING THE DRUG
The decision to stop taking the drug should be made in consultation with your physician.

PROLONGED USE
See your doctor regularly for tests and examinations if you must take this medicine for a prolonged period.

PRECAUTIONS
Over 60: No special studies have been done on older patients. A lower dose may be warranted, especially if kidney function is impaired.

Driving and Hazardous Work: Do not drive or engage in hazardous work until you determine how the medicine affects you.

Alcohol: Avoid alcohol if liver function is impaired.

Pregnancy: Stavudine has been shown to cause birth defects in animals. Human studies have not been done. Nevertheless, stavudine is increasingly being used in combination with other antiretroviral drugs to treat pregnant HIV-infected women.

Breast Feeding: It is unknown whether stavudine passes into breast milk; however, women infected with HIV should not breast-feed, to avoid transmitting the virus to an uninfected child.

Infants and Children: It is not known whether stavudine causes different or more severe side effects in infants and children than it does in older persons.

Special Concerns: Use of stavudine does not reduce the risk of passing the AIDS virus to others. Take appropriate preventive measures.

OVERDOSE
Symptoms: No cases of overdose have been reported.

What to Do: An overdose of stavudine is unlikely to occur. Nonetheless, if you have any reason to suspect an overdose, call your doctor, emergency medical services (EMS), or the nearest poison control center.

DRUG INTERACTIONS
Consult your doctor for advice if you are taking any other prescription or over-the-counter medication, especially chloramphenicol, cisplatin, dapsone, didanosine, ethambutol, ethionamide, hydralazine, isoniazid, lithium, metronidazole, nitrofurantoin, phenytoin, vincristine, or zalcitabine.

FOOD INTERACTIONS
No known food interactions.

DISEASE INTERACTIONS
Caution is advised when taking stavudine. Consult your doctor if you have pancreatitis or peripheral neuropathy. Use of stavudine may cause complications in patients with kidney or liver disease, because these organs work to remove the drug from the body.

Sucralfate

Carafate 1 g
(HOECHST MARION ROUSSEL)

▶ Drug Class: Antiulcer/
antireflux agent

▶ Available in: Oral suspension,
tablets

▶ Available OTC? No

▶ As Generic? Yes

Side Effects

SERIOUS
Drowsiness, seizures. Call
your doctor immediately.

COMMON
Constipation.

LESS COMMON
Backache, diarrhea, dizziness or lightheadedness,
dry mouth, indigestion,
nausea, stomach pain or
cramps, skin rash, hives,
or itching.

PRINCIPAL USES
To treat and prevent ulcers
of the duodenum, the first
portion of the small intestine located just after the
stomach in the digestive
tract.

HOW THE DRUG WORKS
Sucralfate coats the surface
of an ulcer, protecting the
tissue from irritation by
stomach acids, digestive
enzymes, bile salts, and
other substances that are
present in the stomach
and duodenum.

DOSAGE
Suspension— 1 g, 4 times
a day, 1 hour before each
meal and at bedtime, or 2 g,
2 times a day, upon waking
and at bedtime. Tablets—
To treat ulcer: 1 g, 4 times
a day, 1 hour before each
meal and at bedtime. To
prevent the recurrence
of duodenal ulcers: 1 g, 2
times a day on an empty
stomach.

ONSET OF EFFECT
Unknown.

DURATION OF ACTION
Up to 6 hours.

DIETARY ADVICE
This medication should be
taken without food and with
an 8 oz glass of water.

STORAGE
Store in a tightly sealed container away from heat and
direct light. Do not refrigerate the liquid form; also
keep it from freezing.

IF YOU MISS A DOSE
Take it as soon as you
remember. If it is near
the time for the next dose,
skip the missed dose and
resume your regular dosage
schedule. Do not double the
next dose.

STOPPING THE DRUG
Take the drug as prescribed
for the full treatment period,
even if you begin to feel better before the scheduled
end of therapy.

PROLONGED USE
You should see your doctor
regularly for tests and
examinations if you take
this drug for a prolonged
period.

PRECAUTIONS
Over 60: There is no specific information about the
use of sucralfate in older
persons. It is not expected
to produce side effects
different from those in
younger persons.

**Driving and Hazardous
Work:** Do not drive or
engage in hazardous work
until you determine how
the medicine affects you.

Alcohol: Avoid alcohol
while using this drug.

Pregnancy: Sucralfate has
not caused birth defects in
animals. Human studies
have not been done. Before
you use sucralfate, tell your
doctor if you are pregnant
or plan to become pregnant.

Breast Feeding: Sucralfate
may pass into breast milk
but has not been shown to
cause problems in nursing
babies. Consult your doctor
for specific advice.

Infants and Children: In
limited trials sucralfate has
not been shown to cause
problems in children. The
dose must be determined
by your pediatrician.

Special Concerns: Take
other medications at least 2
hours before or after taking
sucralfate. Do not take
antacids within 30 minutes
of taking sucralfate. Regular
exercise and intake of

dietary fiber along with
plenty of fluid can help
to prevent drug-induced
constipation.

OVERDOSE
Symptoms: No specific
ones have been reported.

What to Do: An overdose
of sucralfate is unlikely to
be life-threatening. How-
ever, if someone takes a
much larger dose than prescribed, call your doctor,
emergency medical services
(EMS), or the nearest poison control center.

DRUG INTERACTIONS
Consult your doctor for specific advice if you are taking
ciprofloxacin, digoxin, norfloxacin, ofloxacin, phenytoin, theophylline, or any
antacid or other drug that
contains aluminum. Consult
your doctor or pharmacist
for advice if you are taking
any over-the-counter drug.

FOOD INTERACTIONS
No known food interactions.

DISEASE INTERACTIONS
Caution is advised when
taking sucralfate. Consult
your doctor if you have a
history of gastrointestinal
tract obstruction or kidney
failure.

Sulfacetamide

BRAND NAMES
Ak-Sulf, Bleph-10,
Cetamide, I-Sulfaset,
Isopto-Cetamide, Ocu-Sul,
Ocusulf-10, Ophthacet,
Sodium Sulamyd,
Spectro-Sulf, Steri-Units
Sulfacetamide, Sulf-10,
Sulfair, Sulfamide,
Sulten-10

▶ Drug Class: Anti-infective

▶ Available in: Ophthalmic
   solution, ointment

▶ Available OTC? No

▶ As Generic? Yes

Side Effects

SERIOUS
No serious side effects
have been reported.

COMMON
Eye itching, redness,
swelling, and other signs
of irritation not present
before use of the medi-
cine. Stop using the
medication and call
your doctor.

LESS COMMON
No less-common side
effects have been
reported.

PRINCIPAL USES
To treat bacterial conjunctivitis (inflammation of the
mucous membranes that
line the inner surface of
the eyelids and whites of
the eyes) and other eye
infections.

HOW THE DRUG WORKS
Sulfacetamide inhibits the
spread of bacteria by preventing the synthesis of
folic acid, which is necessary for bacterial growth
and multiplication.

DOSAGE
Adults and teenagers—
Solution: 1 drop, 4 to 6
times per day. Ointment:
Apply 3 to 4 times per day.
Infants and children— Both
the use and dosage must be
determined by your doctor.

ONSET OF EFFECT
Unknown.

DURATION OF ACTION
Unknown.

DIETARY ADVICE
This medication can be
used without regard to diet.

STORAGE
Store in a tightly sealed container away from heat, moisture, and direct light. Do
not allow it to freeze.

IF YOU MISS A DOSE
Apply it as soon as you
remember. If it is near
the time for the next dose,
skip the missed dose and
resume your regular dosage
schedule. Do not double the
next dose.

STOPPING THE DRUG
Use this drug as prescribed
for the full treatment period,
even if you begin to feel better before the scheduled
end of therapy.

PROLONGED USE
You should see your doctor
regularly for tests and
examinations if you use this
drug for a prolonged period.

PRECAUTIONS
Over 60: No special problems are expected.

**Driving and Hazardous
Work:** The use of sulfacetamide should not impair
your ability to perform
such tasks safely.

Alcohol: No special precautions are necessary.

Pregnancy: Sulfacetamide
has not been shown to
cause problems during
pregnancy. Before you take
sulfacetamide, tell your doctor if you are pregnant or
plan to become pregnant.

Breast Feeding: Sulfacetamide has not been
reported to cause problems
in nursing babies. Consult
your doctor for advice.

Infants and Children:
This drug is not recom-
mended for use by infants
under the age of 2 months.

Special Concerns: To use
the eye drops or the ointment, first wash your hands.
Tilt your head back. Gently
apply pressure to the inside
corner of the eyelid and
with the index finger of the
same hand, pull downward
on the lower eyelid to make
a space. Drop the medicine
or put a short strip of ointment (about ⅓ inch long)
into this space and close
your eye. Apply pressure for
1 or 2 minutes while keeping the eye closed without
blinking. Then wash your
hands again. Make sure the
tip of the dropper or the
applicator does not touch
your eye, finger, or any
other surface. If your
symptoms do not improve
in a few days or if they
become worse, check
with your doctor.

OVERDOSE
Symptoms: No specific
ones have been reported.

What to Do: An overdose
of sulfacetamide is unlikely
to be life-threatening. If a
large volume enters the eye,
flush with water. If someone
accidentally ingests the
medicine, call your doctor,
emergency medical services
(EMS), or the nearest poison control center.

DRUG INTERACTIONS
Other drugs may interact
with sulfacetamide. Consult
your doctor for specific
advice if you are taking eye
preparations containing silver such as silver nitrate.

FOOD INTERACTIONS
No known food interactions.

DISEASE INTERACTIONS
Caution is advised when
taking sulfacetamide. Consult your doctor if you have
any other medical condition.

Sulfasalazine

BRAND NAMES
Azaline, Azulfidine,
Azulfidine EN-Tabs

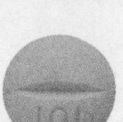

Azulfidine 500 mg
(Pharmacia)

▶ Drug Class: Anti-infective/
sulfa drug; anti-inflammatory
agent

▶ Available in: Tablets, enteric-
coated tablets

▶ Available OTC? No

▶ As Generic? Yes

Side Effects

SERIOUS
Aching joints and mus-
cles; pain in back, legs
or stomach; bloody diar-
rhea; blue fingernails,
lips, or skin; chest pain;
cough; breathing diffi-
culty; swallowing diffi-
culty; fever; sore throat;
general discomfort; loss
of appetite; paleness of
skin or redness, peeling,
blistering, or loosening of
skin; unusual bleeding or
bruising; unusual fatigue;
yellow discoloration of
eyes or skin; increased
sensitivity to sunlight.
Call your physician
immediately.

COMMON
Stomach or abdominal
discomfort and cramps,
diarrhea, loss of appetite,
nausea, vomiting. Call
your doctor; these symp-
toms may be alleviated
by lowering the dosage.

LESS COMMON
No less-common side
effects have been
reported.

PRINCIPAL USES
To prevent and treat inflammatory bowel disease
(ulcerative colitis, Crohn's
disease).

HOW THE DRUG WORKS
The exact mechanism of
action is unknown. One
explanation is that it acts as
an anti-inflammatory in the
bowel. It also has antibiotic
properties that may be
important in changing the
bacteria in the bowel.

DOSAGE
Adults and teenagers: To
start, 500 to 1,000 mg, 3 or
4 times a day. The dose may
be decreased to 500 mg, 4
times a day, to reduce the
incidence of gastrointestinal
side effects. Children age 6
and over: To start, 3 to 4.55
mg per lb of body weight.

ONSET OF EFFECT
Unknown.

DURATION OF ACTION
Unknown.

DIETARY ADVICE
Take it with or immediately
following meals. Take each
dose with a full glass of
water, and consume several
additional glasses of water
during the day to reduce
the chance of side effects.

STORAGE
Store in a tightly sealed container away from heat, moisture, and direct light.

IF YOU MISS A DOSE
Take it as soon as you
remember. If it is near
the time for the next dose,
skip the missed dose and
resume your regular dosage
schedule. Do not double the
next dose.

STOPPING THE DRUG
Take it as prescribed for the
full treatment period, even if
you feel better before the
scheduled end of therapy.

PROLONGED USE
Sulfasalazine can be used
for as long as it is needed;
see your doctor for periodic
evaluation if prolonged use
is necessary.

PRECAUTIONS
Over 60: No special problems are expected.

**Driving and Hazardous
Work:** Do not drive or
engage in hazardous work
until you determine how the
medicine affects you.

Alcohol: No special precautions are necessary.

Pregnancy: Adequate studies of use during pregnancy
have not been done,
although no problems have
been reported. Consult your
doctor for specific advice.

Breast Feeding: Small
amounts of sulfasalazine
pass into breast milk; use
of this drug is not recommended while nursing,
unless benefits clearly outweigh potential risks. Consult your doctor for advice.

Infants and Children:
Not recommended for use
by children under age 2.

Special Concerns: Since
some patients experience
sensitivity to sunlight, take
preventive measures when
starting therapy: use sunscreens, wear protective
clothing, and avoid expo-
sure to the sun. Be careful
when brushing or flossing
your teeth, because sul-
fasalazine can increase the
risk of mouth infections.
The drug may also turn
skin, urine, or contact
lenses yellow.

OVERDOSE
Symptoms: Nausea, vomiting, stomach upset, blood in
urine, decreased urine volume, low back pain; in more

serious cases, extreme
drowsiness or seizures.

What to Do: Call your
doctor, emergency medical
services (EMS), or the
nearest poison control
center immediately.

DRUG INTERACTIONS
Consult your doctor for specific advice if you are taking
acetaminophen, acetohy-
droxamic acid, alfentanil,
amiodarone, aminophylline,
anabolic steroids, andro-
gens, antithyroid drugs,
anticoagulants, oral antidiabetics, caffeine, carba-
mazepine, carmustine,
chloramphenicol, chloro-
quine, oral contraceptives,
dantrolene, dapsone,
daunorubicin, disulfiram,
divalproex, estrogens, etretinate, gold salts, hydroxychloroquine, methotrexate,
mercaptopurine, methyl-
dopa, naltrexone, oral contraceptives, phenothiazine,
phenytoin, plicamycin, primaquine, procainamide,
quinidine, quinine, sulfoxone, or vitamin K.

FOOD INTERACTIONS
No known food interactions.

DISEASE INTERACTIONS
Consult your doctor if you
have anemia, another blood
problem, G6PD deficiency,
kidney disease, liver disease, intestinal or urinary
obstruction, or porphyria.

Sulfinpyrazone

Anturane 100 mg
(NOVARTIS)

▶ Drug Class: Antigout drug

▶ Available in: Capsules, tablets

▶ Available OTC? No

▶ As Generic? Yes

Side Effects

SERIOUS
Shortness of breath, breathing difficulty, tightness in chest, sores, ulcers, or white spots on lips or in mouth, sore throat and fever with or without chills, swollen or painful glands, unusual bleeding or bruising. Call your doctor immediately.

COMMON
Pain in lower back or side, painful or bloody urination.

LESS COMMON
Skin rash, bloody or black stools, high blood pressure, tiny bright red spots on skin, sudden decrease in urine, swelling of face, fingers, feet, or lower legs, unusual fatigue, vomiting of blood or dark material, weight gain.

PRINCIPAL USES
To treat chronic (recurring) gout or gouty arthritis by preventing attacks. (It should not be used for treating acute gout attacks in progress.)

HOW THE DRUG WORKS
Gout occurs when too much uric acid builds up in the blood. This leads to the formation of uric-acid-based crystals that are deposited in the joints, causing inflammation and leading to the sharp, excruciating pain of a gout attack. Sulfinpyrazone promotes excretion of excess uric acid from the body and so eases or prevents gout attacks. It also slows the body's removal of antibiotics, thus increasing their levels in the blood and prolonging their duration of action.

DOSAGE
200 to 400 mg a day in 2 doses to start; can be increased to as much as 800 mg a day in 2 doses.

ONSET OF EFFECT
It may take months before this medicine begins to prevent gout attacks.

DURATION OF ACTION
6 to 8 hours.

DIETARY ADVICE
Sulfinpyrazone may be taken with meals or milk to reduce stomach upset.

STORAGE
Store in a tightly sealed container away from heat and direct light.

IF YOU MISS A DOSE
Take it as soon as you remember. However, if it is near the time for the next dose, skip the missed dose and resume your regular dosage schedule. Do not double the next dose.

STOPPING THE DRUG
The decision to stop taking the drug should be made by your doctor.

PROLONGED USE
You should see your doctor regularly for tests and examinations if you take this drug for a prolonged period.

PRECAUTIONS
Over 60: No special problems are expected.

Driving and Hazardous Work: The use of this drug should not impair your ability to perform such tasks safely.

Alcohol: Avoid alcohol.

Pregnancy: Sulfinpyrazone has not been reported to cause problems during pregnancy. Before you take sulfinpyrazone, tell your doctor if you are pregnant or plan to become pregnant.

Breast Feeding: Sulfinpyrazone may pass into breast milk; caution is advised. Consult your doctor for advice.

Infants and Children: There is no specific information on the use of sulfinpyrazone in children, since it is generally prescribed only for adults.

Special Concerns: Your doctor may advise you to drink 10 to 12 full glasses of fluid every day while you take sulfinpyrazone to help prevent the formation of uric acid kidney stones. Sulfinpyrazone will not relieve a gout attack that has already started. You may also be prescribed another medicine for gout while you take this drug.

OVERDOSE
Symptoms: Nausea, vomiting, diarrhea, stomach pain, clumsiness or unsteadiness, seizures, difficulty breathing, loss of consciousness.

What to Do: Call your doctor, emergency medical services (EMS), or the nearest poison control center immediately.

DRUG INTERACTIONS
Consult your physician for specific advice if you are taking anticoagulants, carbenicillin, cefamandole, cefoperazone, cefotetan, dipyridamole, divalproex, heparin, medicine for pain or inflammation, moxalactam, pentoxifylline, plicamycin, ticarcillin, valproic acid, any cancer medicine, aspirin or other salicylates, or nitrofurantoin.

FOOD INTERACTIONS
None are likely, but a low-purine diet is recommended to reduce the risk of gout attacks. Foods high in purines include anchovies, sardines, legumes, poultry, sweetbreads, liver, kidneys, and other organ meats.

DISEASE INTERACTIONS
Consult your physician if you have any of the following: blood disease, cancer being treated by drugs or radiation, kidney stones or any other kidney disease, stomach ulcer, or any other stomach or intestinal problem.

Sulfisoxazole Ophthalmic

BRAND NAME
Gantrisin Ophthalmic

▶ Drug Class: Anti-infective

▶ Available in: Ophthalmic solution, ointment

▶ Available OTC? No

▶ As Generic? No

Side Effects

SERIOUS
No serious side effects have been reported.

COMMON
Eye itching, redness, swelling, and other signs of irritation not present before use of the medicine. If this occurs, stop using the medication and call your doctor.

LESS COMMON
No less-common side effects have been reported.

PRINCIPAL USES
To treat bacterial conjunctivitis (inflammation of the mucous membranes that line the inner surface of the eyelids and whites of the eyes) and other eye infections.

HOW THE DRUG WORKS
Sulfisoxazole inhibits the spread of bacteria by preventing the synthesis of folic acid, which is necessary for bacterial growth and multiplication.

DOSAGE
Solution, adults and children 2 months of age and older: 1 drop 4 times a day. Ointment, adults and children: 3 times a day and at bedtime. All forms, infants up to 2 months of age: Use and dosage must be determined by your doctor.

ONSET OF EFFECT
Unknown.

DURATION OF ACTION
Unknown.

DIETARY ADVICE
This medication can be used without regard to diet.

STORAGE
Store in a tightly sealed container away from heat, moisture, and direct light. Do not allow it to freeze.

IF YOU MISS A DOSE
Apply it as soon as you remember. If it is near the time for the next dose, skip the missed dose and resume your regular dosage schedule. Do not double the next dose.

STOPPING THE DRUG
Use this drug as prescribed for the full treatment period, even if you begin to feel better before the scheduled end of therapy.

PROLONGED USE
You should see your doctor regularly for tests and examinations if you use this drug for a prolonged period.

PRECAUTIONS
Over 60: No special problems are expected.

Driving and Hazardous Work: The use of ophthalmic sulfisoxazole solution should not impair your ability to perform such tasks safely. The use of the ointment, however, may temporarily but significantly blur vision and may interfere with your ability to drive or perform other sight-dependent tasks.

Alcohol: No special precautions are necessary.

Pregnancy: Ophthalmic sulfisoxazole has not been shown to cause problems during pregnancy. Before you take it, tell your physician if you are pregnant or plan to become pregnant.

Breast Feeding: Ophthalmic sulfisoxazole has not been reported to cause problems in nursing babies. Consult your doctor for advice.

Infants and Children: Use and dosage for infants under the age of 2 months must be determined by your doctor.

Special Concerns: To use the eye drops or the ointment, first wash your hands. Tilt your head back. Gently apply pressure to the inside corner of the eyelid and with the index finger of the same hand, pull downward on the lower eyelid to make a space. Drop the medicine or put a short strip of ointment (about ⅓ inch long) into this space and close your eye. Apply gentle pressure for 1 or 2 minutes while keeping the eye closed without blinking. Then wash your hands again. Make sure the tip of the dropper or the applicator does not touch your eye, finger, or any other surface. If your symptoms do not improve in a few days or if they become worse, check with your doctor.

OVERDOSE
Symptoms: No specific ones have been reported.

What to Do: An overdose of ophthalmic sulfisoxazole is unlikely to be life-threatening. If a large volume enters the eye, flush with water. If someone accidentally ingests the medicine, call your doctor, emergency medical services (EMS), or the nearest poison control center immediately.

DRUG INTERACTIONS
Other drugs may interact with ophthalmic sulfisoxazole. Consult your doctor for specific advice if you are taking eye preparations containing silver such as silver nitrate.

FOOD INTERACTIONS
No known food interactions.

DISEASE INTERACTIONS
Caution is advised when taking ophthalmic sulfisoxazole. Consult your doctor if you have any other medical condition.

Sulfisoxazole Systemic

BRAND NAME
Gantrisin

▶ Drug Class: Anti-infective

▶ Available in: Oral suspension, syrup, tablets

▶ Available OTC? No

▶ As Generic? Yes

Side Effects

SERIOUS
Itching, skin rash, aching joints and muscles, difficulty swallowing, pale skin or reddened, blistered, and peeling skin, sore throat and fever, unusual bleeding or bruising, unusual fatigue, yellow discoloration of the eyes or skin, pain in stomach or abdomen, bloody urine, greatly increased or decreased urine output, pain or burning while urinating, unusual thirst, lower back pain, mood or mental changes, swelling in the neck, increased sensitivity to sunlight. Call your doctor right away.

COMMON
Dizziness, diarrhea, headache, loss of appetite, nausea, vomiting, fatigue. Call your doctor. These symptoms may be alleviated by lowering the dosage.

LESS COMMON
No less-common side effects have been reported.

PRINCIPAL USES
To treat bacterial infections. It is most commonly used to treat middle ear infections or urinary tract infections. It is also used, in combination with other medications, to treat malaria.

HOW THE DRUG WORKS
Sulfisoxazole kills bacterial cells by preventing them from utilizing folic acid, a vitamin essential to cell growth and reproduction.

DOSAGE
Adults and teenagers: To start, 2,000 to 4,000 mg for first dose. Then 750 to 1,500 mg, 6 times a day, or 1,000 to 2,000 mg, 4 times a day. Children over 2 months of age: To start, 34 mg per lb of body weight. Then 11.4 mg per lb, 6 times a day, or 37.5 mg per lb, 4 times a day.

ONSET OF EFFECT
Unknown.

DURATION OF ACTION
Unknown.

DIETARY ADVICE
Take it with or immediately after meals. Each dose should be taken with a full glass of water, and several additional glasses of water should be consumed daily to decrease the chance of side effects.

STORAGE
Store in a tightly sealed container away from heat, moisture, and direct light.

IF YOU MISS A DOSE
Take it as soon as you remember. If it is near the time for the next dose, skip the missed dose and resume your regular dosage schedule. Do not double the next dose.

STOPPING THE DRUG
Take it as prescribed for the full treatment period, even if you feel better before the scheduled end of therapy.

PROLONGED USE
See your doctor regularly for tests and examinations if you take it for a prolonged period.

PRECAUTIONS
Over 60: Adverse reactions may be more likely and more severe in older patients.

Driving and Hazardous Work: Do not drive or engage in hazardous work until you determine how the medicine affects you.

Alcohol: No special precautions are necessary.

Pregnancy: Adequate human studies have not been done. Before taking sulfisoxazole, tell your doctor if you are pregnant or plan to become pregnant.

Breast Feeding: Sulfisoxazole passes into breast milk; avoid or discontinue use while nursing.

Infants and Children: Not recommended for use by infants under the age of 2 months.

Special Concerns: Since some patients experience sensitivity to sunlight, take preventive measures when starting therapy: use sunscreens, wear protective clothing, and avoid exposure to the sun. Be careful when brushing or flossing your teeth, because sulfisoxazole can increase the risk of mouth infections. If your symptoms do not improve or become worse in a few days, consult your doctor.

OVERDOSE
Symptoms: Loss of appetite, nausea, vomiting, dizziness, headache, drowsiness, loss of consciousness, blood in the urine, decreased urination, low back pain, yellow discoloration of the eyes or skin.

What to Do: Call your doctor, emergency medical services (EMS), or the nearest poison control center immediately.

DRUG INTERACTIONS
Consult your doctor for specific advice if you are taking acetaminophen, acetohydroxamic acid, amiodarone, anabolic steroids, androgens, antithyroid drugs, anticoagulants, oral antidiabetics, carbamazepine, carmustine, chloroquine, oral contraceptives, dantrolene, dapsone, daunorubicin, disulfiram, divalproex, estrogens, etretinate, gold salts, hydroxychloroquine, methenamine, methotrexate, mercaptopurine, methyldopa, naltrexone, oral contraceptives, phenothiazines, phenytoin, plicamycin, primaquine, procainamide, quinidine, quinine, sulfoxone, or vitamin K.

FOOD INTERACTIONS
No known food interactions.

DISEASE INTERACTIONS
Consult your doctor if you have anemia, another blood problem, G6PD deficiency, kidney disease, liver disease, or porphyria.

Sulfur Topical

BRAND NAMES
Cuticura Ointment, Finac,
Fostex Regular Strength
Medicated Cover-Up,
Fostril Lotion, Lotio-
Asulfa, Sulpho-Lac

▶ Drug Class: Acne drug

▶ Available in: Cream, lotion,
ointment, bar soap

▶ Available OTC? Yes

▶ As Generic? Yes

Side Effects

SERIOUS
No serious side effects
have been reported.

COMMON
Mild redness and peeling
of skin.

LESS COMMON
Skin irritation or allergy
with redness, peeling,
burning, stinging, itching,
or rash. Contact your
doctor.

PRINCIPAL USES
To treat skin conditions
including acne, seborrheic
dermatitis, and scabies.

HOW THE DRUG WORKS
Topical sulfur is lethal to
various strains of bacteria
(which are a primary cause
of acne), fungus, parasites,
and other types of microorganisms. It also promotes
softening, dissolution, and
peeling of hard, scaly,
roughened, or irregular
surface skin.

DOSAGE
For acne, lotion, cream, or
bar soap: Use on skin as
needed. To use the soap,
work up a rich lather using
warm water. Wash the
affected area, rinse thoroughly, apply again and rub
in gently for a few minutes.
Remove excess lather with
a towel or tissue, without
rinsing. Lotion: Apply 2 or
3 times a day. Ointment:
Apply the 0.5% ointment as
needed. Wash the affected
area with soap and water
and dry thoroughly before
application. For seborrheic
dermatitis: Use 1 or 2 times
a day as directed on the
package instructions. For
scabies: Apply the 6% ointment every night for 3
nights. The ointment should
be applied to the entire
body from the neck down.
You may bathe before each
application and should
bathe 24 hours after the
last application.

ONSET OF EFFECT
Unknown.

DURATION OF ACTION
Unknown.

DIETARY ADVICE
Topical sulfur can be used
without regard to diet.

STORAGE
Store in a tightly sealed container away from heat and
direct light. Keep the
cream, lotion, and ointment
forms from freezing.

IF YOU MISS A DOSE
Resume your regular
dosage schedule with the
next application. Do not
double the next dose.

STOPPING THE DRUG
If you are using sulfur by
prescription, the decision to
stop taking the drug should
be made by your doctor. If
you are using it without prescription, you may stop taking the drug when your
skin has cleared; however, it
is likely that the condition
will recur.

PROLONGED USE
If prescribed, do not use
sulfur for longer than your
doctor recommends.

PRECAUTIONS
Over 60: No special precautions required.

**Driving and Hazardous
Work:** No special precautions are necessary.

Alcohol: No special precautions are necessary.

Pregnancy: Sulfur has not
been shown to cause birth
defects or other problems
during pregnancy. Before
you use sulfur, tell your doctor if you are pregnant or
plan to become pregnant.

Breast Feeding: Topical
sulfur has not been
reported to cause problems
in nursing infants. Consult
your doctor for specific
advice.

Infants and Children:
Use and dosage for children
must be determined by
your pediatrician.

Special Concerns: Anyone with a history of allergy
to sulfur and other ingredients in the medication
should not use this product.
Keep sulfur away from the
eyes. If you accidentally get
some of the medicine in
your eyes, flush them thoroughly with water.

OVERDOSE
Symptoms: Excessive
application of topical sulfur
may lead to more-severe
irritation of the skin.

What to Do: If topical sulfur is accidentally ingested,
call your doctor, emergency
medical services (EMS), or
the nearest poison control
center immediately.

DRUG INTERACTIONS
Consult your doctor for specific advice if you are using
abrasive soaps or cleansers,
alcohol-containing preparations, any other acne agent,
any preparation containing a
peeling agent such as benzoyl peroxide, salicylic acid,
alpha hydroxy acids, sulfur,
or vitamin A, or soaps, medicated cosmetics, or other
cosmetics that dry the skin.
Also tell your doctor if you
are using any other pre-
scription or over-the-counter
drug for a skin condition.

FOOD INTERACTIONS
No known food interactions.

DISEASE INTERACTIONS
You should not use sulfur if
you have had a prior allergic reaction to it.

Sulindac

BRAND NAMES
Apo-Sulin, Clinoril,
Novo-Sundac

Generic 150 mg
(MYLAN)

▶ Drug Class: Nonsteroidal
anti-inflammatory drug
(NSAID)

▶ Available in: Tablets

▶ Available OTC? No

▶ As Generic? Yes

Side Effects

SERIOUS
Shortness of breath or
wheezing, with or with-
out swelling of legs or
other signs of heart failure; chest pain; peptic
ulcer disease with vomit-
ing of blood; black, tarry
stools; decreasing kidney
function. Call your doctor
immediately.

COMMON
Nausea, vomiting, heart-
burn, diarrhea, constipa-
tion, headache, dizziness,
sleepiness.

LESS COMMON
Ulcers or sores in mouth,
depression, rashes or
blistering of skin, ringing
sound in the ears,
unusual tingling or
numbness of the hands
or feet, seizures, blurred
vision. Also elevated
potassium levels,
decreased blood counts;
such problems can be
detected by your doctor.

PRINCIPAL USES
To treat mild to moderate
pain and inflammation
caused by tendinitis, arthritis, bursitis, gout, soft tissue
injuries, migraine and other
vascular headaches, men-
strual cramps, and other
conditions. When patients
fail to respond to one
NSAID, another may be
tried. The greatest effectiveness often requires trial and
error of several different
NSAIDs.

HOW THE DRUG WORKS
NSAIDs work by interfering
with the formation of
prostaglandins, naturally
occurring substances in the
body that cause inflamma-
tion and make nerves more
sensitive to pain impulses.
NSAIDs also have other
modes of action that are
less well understood.

DOSAGE
Adults: 150 mg, 2 times a
day, up to a maximum dose
of 200 mg, 2 times a day.
For children's dose, consult
your pediatrician.

ONSET OF EFFECT
Initial effect occurs within
several hours; full effect
occurs in several days.

DURATION OF ACTION
Varies.

DIETARY ADVICE
Take with food; maintain
your usual food and fluid
intake.

STORAGE
Store in a tightly sealed container away from heat, moisture, and direct light.

IF YOU MISS A DOSE
Take it as soon as you
remember. If it is near
the time for the next dose,
skip the missed dose and
resume your regular dosage
schedule. Do not double the
next dose.

STOPPING THE DRUG
The decision to stop taking
the drug should be made
in consultation with your
physician.

PROLONGED USE
Prolonged use can cause
gastrointestinal problems,
including ulceration and
bleeding, kidney dysfunc-
tion, and liver inflammation.
Consult your doctor about
the need for medical examinations and laboratory tests.

PRECAUTIONS
Over 60: Because of the
potentially greater consequences of gastrointestinal
side effects, the dose of
NSAIDs for older patients,
especially those over age
70, is often cut in half.

**Driving and Hazardous
Work:** Avoid such activities
until you determine how the
medicine affects you.

Alcohol: Avoid alcohol
when using this medication
because it increases the risk
of stomach irritation.

Pregnancy: Avoid or discontinue this drug if you
are pregnant or are plan-
ning to become pregnant.

Breast Feeding: Sulindac
passes into breast milk;
avoid use while nursing.

Infants and Children:
May be used in exceptional
circumstances; consult your
doctor.

Special Concerns:
Because NSAIDs can inter-
fere with blood coagulation,
this drug should be stopped
at least 3 days prior to any
surgery.

OVERDOSE
Symptoms: Severe nausea,
vomiting, headache, confusion, seizures.

What to Do: Call your
doctor, emergency medical
services (EMS), or the
nearest poison control
center immediately.

DRUG INTERACTIONS
Do not take this drug with
aspirin or any other NSAIDs
without your doctor's
approval. In addition, consult your doctor if you are
taking antihypertensives,
steroids, anticoagulants,
antibiotics, itraconazole or
ketoconazole, plicamycin,
penicillamine, valproic acid,
phenytoin, cyclosporine,
digitalis drugs, lithium,
methotrexate, probenecid,
triamterene, or zidovudine.

FOOD INTERACTIONS
No known food interactions.

DISEASE INTERACTIONS
Caution is advised when
taking sulindac. Consult
your doctor if you have any
of the following: bleeding
problems, inflammation or
ulcers of the stomach and
intestines, diabetes mellitus,
systemic lupus erythematosus (SLE, lupus), anemia,
asthma, epilepsy, Parkin-
son's disease, kidney
stones, or a history of heart
disease or alcohol abuse.
Use of sulindac may cause
complications in patients
with liver or kidney disease,
since these organs work
together to remove the
medication from the body.

Sumatriptan Succinate

BRAND NAME
Imitrex

Imitrex 25 mg
(GLAXO WELLCOME)

▶ Drug Class: Antimigraine/
antiheadache drug

▶ Available in: Tablets,
injection, nasal spray

▶ Available OTC? No

▶ As Generic? No

Side Effects

SERIOUS
Chest pain (mild to
severe) or feeling of
heaviness or pressure in
the chest; wheezing or
shortness of breath, and
rapid, shallow, or irregular breathing; puffiness or
swelling of the eyelids,
face or, lips; hives;
intense itching. Seek
emergency medical
assistance immediately.

COMMON
Pain, burning, or redness
at injection site; a general
feeling of warmth or
heat; a feeling of numb-
ness, tightness, or tin-
gling; mild pain of the
jaw, mouth, tongue,
throat, nose, or sinuses;
dizziness; drowsiness;
feeling cold or weak;
feeling flushed or light-
headed; muscle aches,
cramps, or stiffness;
nausea or vomiting.

LESS COMMON
Mild chest pain; heavi-
ness or pressure in the
chest or neck; anxiety;
feeling tired or ill; vision
changes.

PRINCIPAL USES
To treat severe, acute
migraine headaches (suma-
triptan is not effective
against any other kinds of
pain or headache). Because
of the risk of side effects,
sumatriptan is generally
used only when other treatments prove ineffective.

HOW THE DRUG WORKS
It appears that sumatriptan
activates chemical messengers that cause blood
vessels in the brain to constrict, thus lessening the
effects of a migraine. The
drug not only relieves the
pain, but also nausea, vomiting, sensitivity to sound and
light, and other symptoms
associated with migraines.

DOSAGE
Tablets— A single dose of
25 to 100 mg taken with
fluid is generally effective. If
the headache returns or
there is only partial relief,
additional single doses of up
to 50 mg may be given at
intervals of least 2 hours,
but no more than 200 mg
should be taken in a 24-
hour period. Injection— Initial dose: 6 mg injection.
Additional doses: Another 6
mg injection separated by at
least one hour. Nasal
spray— A single dose of 5,
10, or 20 mg into one nostril. A 10-mg dose may be
achieved by administering
a 5-mg dose in each nostril.
If the headache returns or
there is only partial relief,
an additional single dose of
up to 20 mg may be given
at an interval of least 2
hours, but no more than
40 mg should be taken in
a 24-hour period.

ONSET OF EFFECT
Tablets: Within 30 minutes.
Injection: Within 10 to 20
minutes. Nasal spray:
Within 15 to 30 minutes.

DURATION OF ACTION
Unknown, but peak effect
occurs within 1 to 4 hours.

DIETARY ADVICE
The medication can be
taken with or without food.

STORAGE
Keep away from heat and
direct light; do not allow
solution to freeze.

IF YOU MISS A DOSE
Not applicable, since the
drug is taken only when
necessary.

STOPPING THE DRUG
Consult your doctor before
discontinuing sumatriptan.

PROLONGED USE
Consult your doctor if you
have used sumatriptan for
three migraine episodes and
have not had relief, there is
no improvement in symp-
toms after several weeks of
use, or migraines increase
in severity or frequency.

PRECAUTIONS
Over 60: Sumatriptan is
not recommended for use
in older patients.

**Driving and Hazardous
Work:** Sumatriptan may
cause drowsiness or dizziness. Do not drive or
engage in hazardous work
until you determine how the
medication affects you.

Alcohol: No special warnings, although alcohol may
trigger or exacerbate
migraine headaches.

Pregnancy: Do not use
this drug while pregnant.

Breast Feeding: Do not
use this drug while nursing.

Infants and Children:
Sumatriptan is not recom-
mended for children.

Special Concerns: Rare
but serious heart-related
problems may occur after
sumatriptan use. Anyone at
risk for unrecognized coronary artery disease—such
as post-menopausal women,
men over age 40, or those
with heart disease risk factors like high blood pressure, high cholesterol
levels, obesity, cigarette
smoking, diabetes, or a
family history of heart disease—should have the first
dose of sumatriptan administered in a doctor's office.
Sumatriptan should not be
used by anyone with any
symptoms of active heart
disease (chest pain or tightness, shortness of breath).

OVERDOSE
Symptoms: No overdoses
have been reported.

What to Do: Although
overdose is unlikely, if you
take a much larger dose
than prescribed, call your
doctor, emergency medical
services (EMS), or the
nearest poison control
center immediately.

DRUG INTERACTIONS
Do not take sumatriptan
within 24 hours of taking
any other migraine drug.
Consult your doctor for
advice if you are taking antidepressants, selective serotonin reuptake inhibitors
(SSRIs), or lithium.

FOOD INTERACTIONS
See Dietary Advice.

DISEASE INTERACTIONS
You should not take suma-
triptan if you have a history
of coronary artery disease,
especially angina, heart
attack, Prinzmetal's angina,
or uncontrolled high blood
pressure. Sumatriptan
should be used with caution
in patients with liver disease
or severely impaired kidney
function.

706

Tacrine

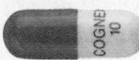

Cognex 10 mg
(**Parke-Davis**)

▶ Drug Class: Psychotherapeutic; antidementia agent

▶ Available in: Capsules

▶ Available OTC? No

▶ As Generic? No

Side Effects

SERIOUS
Clumsiness or unsteadiness, severe vomiting, rapid or pounding heartbeat, slow heartbeat, seizures, elevated liver function tests (detectable by your doctor). Call your doctor right away.

COMMON
Nausea and vomiting, stomach pain or cramps, indigestion, muscle aches or pains, headache, dizziness, loss of appetite, diarrhea.

LESS COMMON
Belching, general feeling of discomfort or illness, rapid breathing, flushed skin, increased urination, increased sweating, watering of the eyes and mouth, insomnia, runny nose, swelling of the feet or lower legs.

PRINCIPAL USES
To treat mild to moderate Alzheimer's disease.

HOW THE DRUG WORKS
Tacrine prevents the breakdown of acetylcholine, a brain chemical crucial to memory. Acetylcholine deficiency is thought to result in memory loss associated with Alzheimer's disease.

DOSAGE
To start, 10 mg, 4 times a day. The dose may be increased to 40 mg, 4 times a day.

ONSET OF EFFECT
Unknown.

DURATION OF ACTION
Unknown.

DIETARY ADVICE
Best taken on an empty stomach, at least 1 hour before or 2 hours after eating. Tacrine can be taken with food to minimize stomach upset, but this will decrease the absorption and effectiveness of the drug.

STORAGE
Store in a tightly sealed container away from heat, moisture, and direct light.

IF YOU MISS A DOSE
Take it as soon as you remember, unless the time for your next scheduled dose is within the next 2 hours. If so, do not take the missed dose. Take your next scheduled dose at the proper time and resume your regular dosage schedule. Do not double the next dose.

STOPPING THE DRUG
The decision to stop taking the drug should be made in consultation with your physician.

PROLONGED USE
You should see your doctor regularly for tests and examinations if you must take this drug for a prolonged period.

PRECAUTIONS
Over 60: No special problems are expected.

Driving and Hazardous Work: Do not drive or engage in hazardous work until you determine how the medicine affects you.

Alcohol: Avoid alcohol.

Pregnancy: Adequate studies on the use of tacrine during pregnancy have not been done. Consult your doctor for specific advice.

Breast Feeding: Tacrine may pass into breast milk and be harmful to the nursing infant; do not use the drug while nursing.

Infants and Children: Tacrine is not intended for use by infants and children.

Special Concerns: Have your blood tested every other week for at least 16 weeks when you start taking tacrine, to see if it is affecting your liver. Do not smoke tobacco products while taking tacrine. Smoking will decrease the effects of tacrine.

OVERDOSE
Symptoms: Sweating and watering of mouth, seizures, increased muscle weakness, low blood pressure, severe nausea or vomiting, fast and weak pulse, large pupils, irregular breathing, slow heartbeat.

What to Do: Call your doctor, emergency medical services (EMS), or the nearest poison control center immediately.

DRUG INTERACTIONS
The following drugs may interact with tacrine. Consult your doctor for specific advice if you are taking: cimetidine, medicine for inflammation or pain, or theophylline.

FOOD INTERACTIONS
No known food interactions.

DISEASE INTERACTIONS
Caution is advised when taking tacrine. Consult your doctor if you have any of the following: asthma, epilepsy or a history of seizures, heart problems, intestinal blockage, stomach or duodenal ulcer, liver disease, Parkinson's disease, urinary problems, brain disease, or history of a head injury that involved a loss of consciousness.

Tacrolimus (FK506)

Prograf 1 mg
(FUJISAWA)

▶ Drug Class: Immunosup-
pressant

▶ Available in: Capsules,
injection

▶ Available OTC? No

▶ As Generic? No

Side Effects

SERIOUS
Increased bleeding,
increased bruising, fluid
buildup in lungs causing
fever, chest pain, diffi-
culty breathing, and
cough. Call your doctor
immediately.

COMMON
Headache; fever; weak-
ness; tremor; high blood
pressure causing
headache and blurred
vision; diarrhea; nausea;
decreased urination; high
blood sugar levels caus-
ing increased thirst,
hunger, and urination.

LESS COMMON
Insomnia, swelling of feet
or lower legs, numbness
or tingling sensations,
constipation, loss of
appetite, abdominal pain,
abdominal swelling due
to fluid buildup, painful
urination, back pain, electrolyte imbalance causing
nausea, diarrhea, muscle
weakness, and fatigue.

PRINCIPAL USES
To slow down or reduce the
natural tendency of the
immune system to reject
liver or kidney transplants.

HOW THE DRUG WORKS
Tacrolimus suppresses the
immune system's reaction
against foreign tissue by
inhibiting the activity of
white blood cells, a major
component of the immune
system's arsenal.

DOSAGE
Adults— Capsules: 0.1 to
0.2 mg per 2.2 lbs (1 kg) of
body weight daily in 2
divided doses every 12
hours. Injection: Dosage to
be determined by your doctor. Children— 0.15 to 0.2
mg per 2.2 lbs of body
weight daily in capsules on
a schedule similar to that
of adults.

ONSET OF EFFECT
Unknown.

DURATION OF ACTION
Unknown.

DIETARY ADVICE
The oral medication is most
effective on an empty stomach; take it 30 minutes
before or 2 hours after a
meal. It can be taken with a
full glass of water to lessen
stomach upset. Do not take
tacrolimus with grapefruit
juice.

STORAGE
Capsules: Store in a tightly
sealed container away from
heat, moisture, and direct
light. Injection: Not applicable; administered only at a
health care facility.

IF YOU MISS A DOSE
Capsules: Take it as soon as
you remember. If it is near
the time for the next dose,
skip the missed dose and
resume your regular dosage
schedule. Do not double the
next dose. Injection: Not

applicable; administered by
health care professional.

STOPPING THE DRUG
The decision to stop taking
the drug should be made by
your doctor.

PROLONGED USE
See your doctor regularly
for tests and examinations if
you take this medication for
a prolonged period.

PRECAUTIONS
Over 60: Adverse reactions
may be more likely and
more severe in older
patients.

**Driving and Hazardous
Work:** Do not drive or
engage in hazardous work
until you determine how the
medicine affects you.

Alcohol: Avoid alcohol.

Pregnancy: Very high
doses of tacrolimus have
caused birth defects in animals. Human studies have
not been done. Before you
take tacrolimus, tell your
doctor if you are pregnant
or plan to become pregnant.

Breast Feeding:
Tacrolimus passes into
breast milk; discontinue
breast feeding while taking
the drug.

Infants and Children:
No special problems have
been observed, even though
children may actually
require higher doses
than adults.

Special Concerns: In
some cases, tacrolimus has
been shown to cause dia-
betes. Consult your doctor
right away if you develop
symptoms of increased
hunger, thirst, and urination
while taking this drug.

OVERDOSE
Symptoms: No acute
effects have been reported.

What to Do: Call your
doctor, emergency medical
services (EMS), or the
nearest poison control
center immediately.

DRUG INTERACTIONS
Tacrolimus should not be
taken within 24 hours of
receiving cyclosporine.
Avoid live vaccines. Consult
your doctor for specific
advice if you are taking
bromocriptine, cimetidine,
clarithromycin, danazol, erythromycin, antifungal drugs,
methylprednisolone, meto-
clopramide, calcium channel
blockers, carbamazepine,
phenobarbital, phenytoin,
rifabutin, rifampin, other
immunosuppressants, some
vaccinations, aminoglyco-
sides, amphotericin B, or
cisplatin.

FOOD INTERACTIONS
Do not take tacrolimus with
grapefruit juice.

DISEASE INTERACTIONS
Caution is advised when
taking tacrolimus. Consult
your doctor if you have a
history of high blood pressure, heart problems, kidney disease, or liver
disease.

Tamoxifen Citrate

Side Effects

SERIOUS
Endometrial cancer
(menstrual irregularities,
abnormal nonmenstrual
vaginal bleeding, changes
in vaginal discharge,
pelvic pain or pressure);
deep vein thrombosis
and pulmonary embolism
(pain or swelling in legs,
shortness of breath, sud-
den chest pain, coughing
up blood); cataracts
(blurred vision); new
breast lumps; confusion,
weakness, or drowsiness;
jaundice (yellowish tinge
to eyes or skin). Call your
doctor promptly.

COMMON
Hot flashes, weight gain.

LESS COMMON
Bone pain, headache,
nausea or vomiting, skin
dryness or rash, changes
in menstrual period, vaginal discharge, itching in
genital area of women,
depression, erectile dys-
function (impotence) or
decreased sexual interest
in men. Other less-com-
mon side effects include
high blood calcium levels
and liver dysfunction;
such problems can be
detected by your doctor.

PRINCIPAL USES
To treat breast cancer in
women and men; to help
reduce the incidence of
breast cancer in women
at high risk.

HOW THE DRUG WORKS
Tamoxifen blocks the
effects of the hormone
estrogen on certain organs
in the body. Because the
growth of some types of
breast cancer is stimulated
by estrogen, tamoxifen
interferes with the growth
of such tumors.

DOSAGE
For treatment and preven-
tion: 20 mg a day.

ONSET OF EFFECT
Several weeks.

DURATION OF ACTION
Several weeks.

DIETARY ADVICE
It is recommended that
tamoxifen be taken after
breakfast and after dinner.
Swallow the tablet whole
with a glass of water. Do
not crush or chew.

STORAGE
Store in a tightly sealed container away from heat, moisture, and direct light.

IF YOU MISS A DOSE
Take it as soon as you
remember and resume your
regular dosage schedule.

STOPPING THE DRUG
The decision to stop taking
the drug should be made by
your doctor.

PROLONGED USE
See your doctor regularly
for tests and examinations if
you take this medication for
a prolonged period. Tamoxifen does not prevent all
breast cancers, so women
taking the drug for prevention should continue to have
regular breast exams and
mammograms.

PRECAUTIONS
Over 60: No different side
effects or problems are
expected in older patients.

**Driving and Hazardous
Work:** Use of tamoxifen
should not impair your ability to perform such tasks
safely.

Alcohol: No special problems are expected, but you
should consult your doctor
about drinking alcohol while
taking tamoxifen.

Pregnancy: Tamoxifen
may cause miscarriage,
birth defects, fetal death,
and unexpected vaginal
bleeding, and so should not
be taken during pregnancy.
Avoid becoming pregnant
for at least two months after
stopping tamoxifen. A reliable birth control method
other than oral contraceptives is recommended while
undergoing tamoxifen therapy. Notify your physician
and stop taking tamoxifen
immediately if pregnancy
occurs.

Breast Feeding: Tamoxifen may pass into breast
milk; do not breast feed
while taking the drug.

Infants and Children:
Tamoxifen is not prescribed
for infants and children.

Special Concerns:
Women should have regular
gynecological examinations
while taking tamoxifen and
for months or years after
discontinuing it, since the
medication may increase
the long-term risk of uterine
cancer. Tamoxifen may
change or stop a woman's
normal menstrual cycle;
however, she may still be
fertile. A reliable birth control method other than oral
contraceptives (barrier
method) should therefore
be used while taking this
drug. Tamoxifen for breast
cancer risk reduction has
not been studied in women
under the age of 35. Risk
factors for breast cancer
include: early age at first
menstruation, late age at
first pregnancy, no pregnancies, breast cancer in a first-
degree relative, history of
previous breast biopsies, or
high-risk changes seen on
a biopsy.

OVERDOSE
Symptoms: Nausea, vomiting, irregular heartbeat,
tremor, dizziness, seizures,
exaggerated reflexes.

What to Do: Call your
doctor, emergency medical
services (EMS), or the
nearest poison control
center immediately.

DRUG INTERACTIONS
You should not take tamoxifen to prevent breast cancer if you are taking
anticoagulants (such as warfarin). Consult your doctor
for specific advice if you are
taking antacids, cimetidine,
famotidine, ranitidine, birth
control pills.

FOOD INTERACTIONS
No known food interactions.

DISEASE INTERACTIONS
Caution is advised when
taking tamoxifen. Consult
your doctor if you have a
medical history that
includes any of the following: cataracts or other vision
disturbances, high blood
levels of cholesterol or
triglycerides, blood clots,
low white blood cell and/or
platelet counts. Tamoxifen
should not be taken to prevent breast cancer by
women with a history of
deep vein thrombosis or
pulmonary embolism.

Tamsulosin Hydrochloride

BRAND NAME
Flomax

▶ Drug Class: BPH therapy agent

▶ Available in: Capsules

▶ Available OTC? No

▶ As Generic? No

Side Effects

SERIOUS
No serious side effects have been reported.

COMMON
Headache, increased susceptibility to infection, joint pain, back pain, muscle pain, dizziness, runny nose, diarrhea, abnormal ejaculation.

LESS COMMON
Mild chest pain, drowsiness, insomnia, decreased libido, sore throat, cough, sinus infection, nausea, mouth pain, vision problems. The drug may also promote orthostatic hypotension (episodes of low blood pressure most likely to occur when getting up quickly from a seated or lying position), which produces symptoms of lightheadedness, dizziness, confusion, or fainting.

PRINCIPAL USES
To treat symptoms of urinary difficulty that occur with benign prostatic hyperplasia (BPH)—a noncancerous enlargement of the prostate gland. BPH is extremely common among men over the age of 50.

HOW THE DRUG WORKS
By blocking a specific (alpha) receptor, tamsulosin relaxes muscle tissue in the prostate and the opening of the bladder. Note that tamsulosin will not shrink the prostate; symptoms may worsen and surgery may eventually be required. Unlike other alpha receptor blockers used to treat BPH, tamsulosin is not used to treat high blood pressure.

DOSAGE
0.4 mg once a day. It should be taken 30 minutes following the same meal each day. If patients fail to respond to the 0.4 mg dose after 2 to 4 weeks of therapy, they may increase the dose to 0.8 mg once a day.

ONSET OF EFFECT
Unknown.

DURATION OF ACTION
Unknown.

DIETARY ADVICE
There are no dietary restrictions. However, tamsulosin should be taken 30 minutes after the same meal every day. Do not chew, crush, or open the capsules.

STORAGE
Store in a tightly sealed container away from heat, moisture, and direct light.

IF YOU MISS A DOSE
If therapy is discontinued or interrupted for several days at either the 0.4 mg dose or the 0.8 mg dose, therapy should be started again with the 0.4 mg once daily dose.

STOPPING THE DRUG
Take tamsulosin as prescribed for the full treatment period.

PROLONGED USE
If you take this drug for a prolonged period, see your doctor regularly so that changes in prostate size can be monitored.

PRECAUTIONS
Over 60: No special problems are expected.

Driving and Hazardous Work: Tamsulosin may impair mental functioning, causing drowsiness, lightheadedness, or dizziness, especially when you take the medication for the first time. Caution is advised; for 24 hours after the initial dose, avoid driving or other activities requiring mental alertness. Effects should diminish after several doses.

Alcohol: May increase effects of dizziness or fainting; drink in moderation.

Pregnancy: Tamsulosin is not indicated for use by women.

Breast Feeding: Tamsulosin is not indicated for use by women.

Infants and Children: Tamsulosin is not indicated for use by children.

Special Concerns: The first dose is likely to cause dizziness or lightheadedness. Take the drug at night and get out of bed slowly the next day. Be cautious while exercising and during hot weather. Tell your primary care physician if you are planning to have surgery requiring general anesthesia, including dental surgery. Do not chew, crush, or open the capsules.

OVERDOSE
Symptoms: An overdose is unlikely to occur. Possible symptoms after an excessive dose may include severe headache or orthostatic hypotension (see Less Common Side Effects).

What to Do: If someone takes a much larger dose than prescribed, keep the patient lying down and call your doctor, emergency medical services (EMS), or the nearest poison control center immediately.

DRUG INTERACTIONS
Tamsulosin should not be used in conjunction with other BPH therapy agents. Consult your doctor if you are taking either cimetidine or warfarin, which may interact with tamsulosin.

FOOD INTERACTIONS
None reported.

DISEASE INTERACTIONS
None reported.

Tazarotene

BRAND NAME
Tazorac

▶ Drug Class: Retinoid

▶ Available in: Topical gel

▶ Available OTC? No

▶ As Generic? No

Side Effects

SERIOUS
No serious side effects are associated with the use of tazarotene.

COMMON
Common side effects are limited to the skin. When used for psoriasis: Itching, redness, burning, stinging, worsening of psoriasis, irritation, skin pain. When used for acne: Peeling, burning, stinging, dry skin, redness, itching.

LESS COMMON
When used for psoriasis: Skin rash, peeling or scaling, increased risk of dermatitis caused by external irritants, skin inflammation, cracking, bleeding, dry skin. When used for acne: Skin pain, irritation, cracking, swelling of treated area, skin discoloration.

PRINCIPAL USES
To treat psoriasis. Tazarotene is also used to treat mild to moderate acne.

HOW THE DRUG WORKS
The exact way in which tazarotene works is unknown. It appears to establish a more normal pattern of growth and shedding of skin cells.

DOSAGE
For psoriasis: Apply to the affected area once a day, in the evening, using enough to cover the lesion with a thin film. Be sure the area is clean and dry before applying. For acne: Apply once a day in the evening. First gently wash and dry your face, then spread a thin film on the area of skin where acne appears. Avoid applying tazarotene near the eyes, eyelids, and mouth.

ONSET OF EFFECT
1 to 4 weeks.

DURATION OF ACTION
Unknown.

DIETARY ADVICE
Tazarotene can be used without regard to diet.

STORAGE
Store in a tightly sealed container away from heat, moisture, and direct light.

IF YOU MISS A DOSE
If you fail to apply the medication on one day, return to your regular schedule the next day; do not apply an extra amount in an attempt to compensate for the missed dose.

STOPPING THE DRUG
In the treatment of psoriasis, you should apply it for the full treatment period as prescribed by your doctor. For acne, apply the drug for up to 12 weeks as directed by your doctor.

PROLONGED USE
Side effects are more likely with prolonged use.

PRECAUTIONS
Over 60: No special problems are expected.

Driving and Hazardous Work: The use of tazarotene should not impair your ability to perform such tasks safely.

Alcohol: No special precautions are necessary.

Pregnancy: Tazarotene should not be used if you are pregnant or plan to become pregnant. Adequate birth-control methods should be practiced when tazarotene is used in women of child-bearing age.

Breast Feeding: Tazarotene may pass into breast milk; caution is advised. Consult your doctor for specific advice.

Infants and Children: Not recommended for use by children under age 12.

Special Concerns: If tazarotene comes in contact with your eyes, flush your eyes with large amounts of cool water. If eye irritation persists, contact your doctor. Wash your hands after applying the medication. Do not cover the treated area with tight-fitting clothing or bandages. If the drug causes increased sensitivity to sunlight, wear protective clothing, use a sunblock, and try to avoid exposure to direct sunlight. Avoid sunlamps completely. Caution is advised for all patients with fair skin or who are particularly sensitive to sunlight. Weather extremes such as wind or cold may be more irritating to the skin while you use this drug. When tazarotene is used to treat psoriasis, avoid applying it to normal-appearing areas of skin.

OVERDOSE
Symptoms: Excessive use of tazarotene may lead to skin redness, peeling, or discomfort.

What to Do: An overdose is unlikely to occur. If someone accidentally ingests tazarotene, call your doctor.

DRUG INTERACTIONS
Consult your doctor for advice if you are taking any of the following drugs that may interact with tazarotene: vitamin A supplements; other skin medications, creams, or lotions; drugs that increase your sensitivity to sunlight (such as thiazide diuretics, tetracyclines, fluoroquinolone antibiotics, phenothiazines, or sulfonamides); or products such as astringents or medicated soaps that dry the skin.

FOOD INTERACTIONS
No known food interactions.

DISEASE INTERACTIONS
You should not use tazarotene if you have eczema or other chronic skin diseases, or a recent sunburn.

Telmisartan

▶ Drug Class: Antihypertensive/
angiotensin II antagonist

▶ Available in: Tablets

▶ Available OTC? No

▶ As Generic? No

Side Effects

SERIOUS
No serious side effects are associated with the use of telmisartan. (In clinical trials, the incidence of adverse effects was not significantly greater with the medication than with a placebo.)

COMMON
No common side effects are associated with the use of telmisartan.

LESS COMMON
Headache, dizziness, back pain, upper respiratory tract infection, sore throat, and nasal congestion.

PRINCIPAL USES
To control high blood pressure. This drug appears to have the same benefits as the class of antihypertensive drugs known as ACE inhibitors, without producing the common side effect (experienced by as many as 30% of patients) of a dry cough. Telmisartan may be used by itself or in conjunction with other antihypertensive medications.

HOW THE DRUG WORKS
Telmisartan blocks the effects of angiotensin II, a naturally occurring substance that causes blood vessels to narrow. Telmisartan causes the blood vessels to dilate, thereby lowering blood pressure and decreasing the workload of the heart.

DOSAGE
To start, 40 mg once a day when used as the only drug to treat hypertension. Usual maintenance dose is 20 to 80 mg daily.

ONSET OF EFFECT
Within 2 weeks.

DURATION OF ACTION
Up to 24 hours.

DIETARY ADVICE
No special restrictions, unless your doctor has advised a low-sodium diet or other dietary modifications to help you control your blood pressure.

STORAGE
Store in a tightly sealed container away from heat, moisture, and direct light.

IF YOU MISS A DOSE
Take it as soon as you remember. If it is near the time for the next dose, skip the missed dose and resume your regular dosage schedule. Do not double the next dose.

STOPPING THE DRUG
Take it as prescribed for the full treatment period. The decision to stop taking the drug should be made in consultation with your physician.

PROLONGED USE
Lifelong therapy may be necessary. However, if you do change certain health habits (for example, increasing exercise or losing weight), a reduced dose may be possible under a doctor's supervision.

PRECAUTIONS
Over 60: No special problems are expected.

Driving and Hazardous Work: Do not drive or engage in hazardous work until you determine how the medicine affects you.

Alcohol: No special precautions are necessary.

Pregnancy: Telmisartan should not be used by pregnant women. Discontinue taking the drug as soon as possible when pregnancy is detected and discuss treatment alternatives with your doctor.

Breast Feeding: Telmisartan may pass into breast milk; caution is advised. Consult your doctor for advice.

Infants and Children: The safety and effectiveness of use in children have not been established.

Special Concerns: Telmisartan may cause excessively low blood pressure with dizziness or lightheadedness, which is most noticeable when you change position. This may lead to fainting, falls, and injury. Sit or lie down immediately if you feel dizzy or light-headed. This side effect may be worsened by alcohol, hot weather, dehydration, salt depletion from diuretic use, fever, prolonged standing, prolonged sitting, or exercise.

OVERDOSE
Symptoms: Few cases of overdose have been reported. However, if you take a much larger dose than prescribed, you may experience fainting, dizziness, weak pulse that might be very slow or very fast.

What to Do: Call your doctor, emergency medical services (EMS), or the nearest poison control center immediately.

DRUG INTERACTIONS
No clinically significant drug interactions have yet been observed with telmisartan. Consult your doctor for specific advice if you are taking digoxin or any other medication, especially other drugs for high blood pressure. Telmisartan can be taken together with diuretics or other medications for high blood pressure, if your doctor approves.

FOOD INTERACTIONS
No known food interactions.

DISEASE INTERACTIONS
Patients with moderate to severe liver or kidney disease are advised to exercise caution when taking telmisartan.

Temazepam

Generic 15 mg
(PUREPAC)

▶ Drug Class: Benzodiazepine tranquilizer

▶ Available in: Capsules, tablets

▶ Available OTC? No

▶ As Generic? Yes

Side Effects

SERIOUS
Difficulty concentrating, outbursts of anger, other behavior problems, depression, convulsions, hallucinations, low blood pressure (causing faintness or confusion), memory impairment, muscle weakness, skin rash or itching, sore throat, fever and chills, sores or ulcers in throat or mouth, unusual bruising or bleeding, extreme fatigue, yellowish tinge to eyes or skin. Call your doctor immediately.

COMMON
Loss of coordination, unsteady gait, dizziness, lightheadedness, drowsiness, slurred speech.

LESS COMMON
Stomach cramps or pain, vision disturbances, change in sexual desire or ability, constipation or diarrhea, dry mouth or watering mouth, false sense of well-being, rapid or pounding heartbeat, headache, muscle spasms, nausea and vomiting, urinary problems, trembling.

PRINCIPAL USES
To treat insomnia.

HOW THE DRUG WORKS
In general, temazepam produces mild sedation by depressing activity in the central nervous system. In particular, temazepam appears to enhance the effect of gamma-aminobutyric acid (GABA), a natural chemical that inhibits the firing of neurons and dampens the transmission of nerve signals, thus decreasing nervous excitation.

DOSAGE
Adults: 15 mg, taken at bedtime. Older adults: To start, 7.5 mg, taken at bedtime. The dose may be increased. Use and dose for children under 18 must be determined by your doctor.

ONSET OF EFFECT
Unknown.

DURATION OF ACTION
Unknown. It may take more than 2 hours.

DIETARY ADVICE
Take it 30 minutes before bedtime with a full glass of water. Temazepam can be taken with food to prevent gastrointestinal upset.

STORAGE
Store in a tightly sealed container away from heat and direct light.

IF YOU MISS A DOSE
Take it as soon as you remember, unless it is late at night. Do not take the medicine unless your schedule allows a full night's sleep.

STOPPING THE DRUG
Discontinuing the drug abruptly may produce withdrawal symptoms (sleep disruption, nervousness, irritability, diarrhea, abdominal cramps, muscle aches, memory impairment). The dosage should be reduced gradually according to your doctor's instructions.

PROLONGED USE
This medication may slowly lose its effectiveness, and adverse reactions are more likely to occur with prolonged use. You should see your doctor for periodic evaluation if you must take it for an extended time.

PRECAUTIONS
Over 60: Adverse reactions may be more likely and more severe. A lower dose may be warranted.

Driving and Hazardous Work: Do not drive or engage in hazardous work until you determine how the medicine affects you.

Alcohol: Avoid alcohol.

Pregnancy: Use during pregnancy should be avoided if possible. Be sure to tell your doctor if you are pregnant or plan to become pregnant.

Breast Feeding: Temazepam passes into breast milk; do not take it while nursing.

Infants and Children: Safety and effectiveness have not been established for children under age 18.

Special Concerns: Temazepam use can lead to psychological or physical dependence if the drug is not taken in strict accordance with your doctor's instructions. Never take more than the prescribed daily dose.

OVERDOSE
Symptoms: Extreme drowsiness, confusion, slurred speech, slow reflexes, poor coordination, staggering gait, tremor, slowed breathing, loss of consciousness.

What to Do: Call your doctor, emergency medical services (EMS), or the nearest poison control center immediately.

DRUG INTERACTIONS
Consult your physician for advice if you are taking any drugs that depress the central nervous system; these include antihistamines, antidepressants or other psychiatric medications, barbiturates, sedatives, cough medicines, decongestants, and painkillers. Be sure your doctor knows about any over-the-counter medication you may take.

FOOD INTERACTIONS
None reported.

DISEASE INTERACTIONS
Consult your doctor if you have a history of alcohol or drug abuse, stroke or other brain disease, any chronic lung disease, glaucoma, hyperactivity, depression or other mental illness, myasthenia gravis, sleep apnea, epilepsy, porphyria, kidney disease, or liver disease.

Terazosin

Hytrin 1 mg
(ABBOTT)

▶ Drug Class: Antihypertensive;
BPH therapy agent

▶ Available in: Tablets,
capsules

▶ Available OTC? No

▶ As Generic? Yes

Side Effects

SERIOUS
No serious side effects
have been reported.

COMMON
Dizziness.

LESS COMMON
Chest pain; lightheaded-
ness or fainting, espe-
cially when getting up
quickly from a seated
or lying position. Such
symptoms are typically
more common when you
first take the medication,
and generally diminish
over time. These symp-
toms tend to recur when
the dosage is increased.
Take it at bedtime to minimize such problems.

PRINCIPAL USES
To lower and control high
blood pressure (hyperten-
sion). It is also used to treat
symptoms of urinary difficulty that occur with benign
prostatic hyperplasia (BPH).

HOW THE DRUG WORKS
Terazosin helps to control
hypertension by relaxing
blood vessels and permit-
ting them to expand,
decreasing blood pressure
in the process. When used
for BPH, it helps relax the
muscles in the prostate
gland and the opening of
the bladder, improving the
passage of urine.

DOSAGE
For high blood pressure:
Initially, 1 mg taken at bedtime, then 1 to 5 mg once
daily. For children, the dose
and frequency must be
determined by your pedia-
trician. For BPH: Initially,
1 mg taken at bedtime, then
5 to 10 mg once daily.

ONSET OF EFFECT
Within 15 minutes, with
peak blood pressure effect
within 2 to 3 hours. When
the drug is used to treat urinary difficulty associated
with BPH, the full effect
may not be seen for 4 to 6
weeks.

DURATION OF ACTION
24 hours.

DIETARY ADVICE
Terazosin can be taken
before, with, or after meals.

STORAGE
Store in a tightly sealed container away from heat, moisture, and direct light.

IF YOU MISS A DOSE
Take it as soon as possible
the same day. If it is the
next day, skip the missed
dose. Do not double the
dose. Resume your regular
dosage schedule.

STOPPING THE DRUG
Do not discontinue taking
the medication suddenly,
even if you start to experience unpleasant side
effects. Consult your physician. If terazosin is discontinued for several days, you
may need to start therapy
over, using the initial dosing
regimen.

PROLONGED USE
When taking the medication
for hypertension, blood
pressure measurement is
recommended at regular
intervals.

PRECAUTIONS

Over 60: Older persons
are generally more sensitive
to terazosin and more likely
to experience adverse side
effects, especially when getting up from a lying or
seated position. Rise slowly
to minimize symptoms.

**Driving and Hazardous
Work:** Terazosin may
impair mental ability, causing drowsiness, lightheadedness, or dizziness, especially
when you take the medica-
tion for the first time. Caution is advised; for 24 hours
after the initial dose, avoid
driving or other activities
requiring mental alertness.
Effects should diminish
after several doses.

Alcohol: May increase
effects of dizziness or fainting; drink in strict moderation, if at all.

Pregnancy: Well-controlled
studies have not been done.
Consult your physician if
you are pregnant or plan to
become pregnant.

Breast Feeding: It is not
known whether terazosin
passes into breast milk.
Consult your physician
for specific advice.

Infants and Children:
Adequate studies of tera-
zosin use in this age group
have not been performed.
Discuss the risks and benefits with your pediatrician.

Special Concerns: Be
sure to notify your doctor if
you are taking nonprescription medications for asthma,
colds, cough, allergy, or
appetite suppression. These
drugs can increase blood
pressure and cause other
complications if they are
taken with terazosin.

OVERDOSE
Symptoms: Extremely low
blood pressure (hypoten-
sion), with accompanying
fatigue, weakness, head-
ache, palpitations, fainting,
or dizziness.

What to Do: Call your
doctor, emergency medical
services (EMS), or the
nearest poison control
center immediately.

DRUG INTERACTIONS
Several drugs may interact
with terazosin, including
anti-inflammatory medica-
tions, especially indomethacin, which can cause fluid
and sodium retention, and
estrogen, which can reduce
the antihypertensive effects
of the drug. Consult your
doctor.

FOOD INTERACTIONS
None are expected.

DISEASE INTERACTIONS
Consult your physician if
you have kidney disease,
severe heart disease, or
chest pain caused by
angina. Terazosin may
aggravate these conditions.

Terbinafine Hydrochloride

BRAND NAME
Lamisil

▸ Drug Class: Antifungal

▸ Available in: Tablets, topical cream

▸ Available OTC? Yes

▸ As Generic? No

Side Effects

SERIOUS
Serious side effects with terbinafine are rare. However, terbinafine tablets may cause liver dysfunction; severe skin reactions such as Stevens-Johnson syndrome (a serious inflammatory disease affecting children and young adults, characterized by high fever, boils, ulceration of the mucous membranes, pneumonia, joint pain); severe blood disorders, potentially resulting in increased susceptibility to infection, uncontrolled bleeding or other problems; or severe allergic reactions. Seek emergency medical assistance immediately.

COMMON
Headache, diarrhea, rash, abdominal pain, indigestion, nausea.

LESS COMMON
Tablets may cause flatulence, itching, skin eruptions, loss of taste, weakness, fatigue, vomiting, joint and muscle pain, or hair loss. Terbinafine cream may cause redness, itching, burning, blistering, swelling, oozing, or other signs of skin irritation not present before using the drug.

PRINCIPAL USES
The tablets are used only to treat fungal infections of the fingernails and toenails (tinea unguium). The cream is used to treat fungal infections of the skin, such as tinea corporis (ringworm), tinea cruris (jock itch), and tinea pedis (athlete's foot).

HOW THE DRUG WORKS
Terbinafine inhibits an enzyme essential for the production of substances vital for the reproduction and survival of some types of fungal organisms.

DOSAGE
Tablets: 250 mg once a day for 6 weeks for fingernail fungus; 250 mg once a day for 12 weeks for toenail fungus. Cream: Apply a thin film of medicine to the affected area 1 to 2 times a day for ringworm or jock itch; 2 times a day for athlete's foot. Apply the cream for at least 1 week, but no longer than 4 weeks.

ONSET OF EFFECT
Tablets: The optimal effect is seen several months after the completion of treatment. Cream: Unknown.

DURATION OF ACTION
Unknown.

DIETARY ADVICE
Terbinafine can be taken or applied without regard to meals.

STORAGE
Store in a tightly sealed container away from heat, moisture, and direct light. Do not allow the cream to freeze.

IF YOU MISS A DOSE
It is important to not miss any doses. Take or apply as soon as you remember. If you do not remember until the next day, skip the missed dose and resume your regular dosage schedule. Do not double the next dose or use excessive amounts of the cream.

STOPPING THE DRUG
Take terbinafine tablets as prescribed for the full treatment period.

PROLONGED USE
Side effects are more likely to occur with prolonged use. Tests of liver function are recommended if the tablets are used for longer than 6 weeks.

PRECAUTIONS
Over 60: No special problems are expected.

Driving and Hazardous Work: This drug should not impair your ability to perform such tasks safely.

Alcohol: No special precautions are necessary.

Pregnancy: Adequate human studies have not been done. Terbinafine tablets are not recommended for pregnant women.

Breast Feeding: Terbinafine passes into breast milk; avoid or discontinue use of the tablets while nursing.

Infants and Children: Terbinafine is not recommended for children under the age of 18.

Special Concerns: Wash your hands before and after applying the cream. Avoid allowing topical terbinafine to come into contact with the eyes, nose, and mouth. If using terbinafine for ringworm, wear loose-fitting, well-ventilated clothing and avoid excess heat and humidity. It is also recommended to use a bland, absorbent powder like talcum once or twice a day after the cream has been applied and absorbed by the skin. If using the medication for jock itch, do not wear underwear that is tight or made from synthetic materials; wear loose-fitting cotton underwear. If using terbinafine for athlete's foot, dry your feet carefully after bathing and wear clean cotton socks with sandals or well-ventilated shoes. Before applying the medication, wash the affected area with soap and warm water and dry thoroughly.

OVERDOSE
Symptoms: Tablets: nausea, vomiting, abdominal pain, dizziness, rash, frequent urination, and headache.

What to Do: Call your doctor as soon as possible.

DRUG INTERACTIONS
Consult your doctor if you are taking the following drugs that may interact with terbinafine: rifampin, cimetidine, or any other prescription or over-the-counter preparation that is to be applied to the same area of skin as terbinafine cream.

FOOD INTERACTIONS
No known food interactions.

DISEASE INTERACTIONS
Use of terbinafine tablets may cause complications in patients with liver or kidney disease, since these organs work together to remove the medication from the body. Consult your doctor if you have a history of alcohol abuse (a potential cause of liver disease).

Terbutaline Sulfate

Brethine 5 mg
(NOVARTIS)

Additional photographs

▶ Drug Class: Bronchodilator/
sympathomimetic

▶ Available in: Inhalation
aerosol, tablets

▶ Available OTC? No

▶ As Generic? Yes

Side Effects

SERIOUS
Inhaled form: May
become ineffective if
used too often, resulting
in more-severe breathing
difficulty that does not
improve. Signs include
persistent wheezing,
coughing, or shortness of
breath; confusion; bluish
color to lips or finger-
nails; inability to speak.
Ingested form: Chest pain
or heaviness; irregular,
racing, fluttering, or
pounding heartbeat;
lightheadedness; fainting;
severe weakness; severe
headache.

COMMON
Insomnia, dry mouth,
sore throat, anxiety, nervousness, restlessness.

LESS COMMON
Trembling, sweating,
headache, nausea or
vomiting, flushing or redness to cheeks or other
skin surfaces, muscle
aches, cramps, or twitch-
ing, unpleasant or
unusual taste in the
mouth.

PRINCIPAL USES
Terbutaline is used to dilate
air passages in the lungs
that have become narrowed
as a result of disease or
inflammation. It is used in
the treatment of asthma and
chronic obstructive pul-
monary disease (COPD).

HOW THE DRUG WORKS
Terbutaline widens con-
stricted airways in the lungs
by relaxing the smooth
muscles that surround
bronchial passages.

DOSAGE
Use when needed to relieve
breathing difficulty. Inhalation aerosol— Adults and
children age 12 and older:
1 to 2 in-halations every 4
to 6 hours. Wait 1 minute
between first and second
inhalations. In-fants and
children under 12 years of
age: Not recommen-ded.
Tablets— Adults and chil-
dren age 12 and older: 2.5
to 5 mg taken 3 times a day,
ideally at 6-hour intervals.
Children under 12 years of
age: Consult a pediatrician.

ONSET OF EFFECT
Inhalation: Within 5 min-
utes. Oral: 1 to 2 hours.

DURATION OF ACTION
3 to 6 hours for the inhalation; up to 8 hours for
tablets.

DIETARY ADVICE
Maintain your usual food
and fluid intake.

STORAGE
Store in a tightly sealed container away from heat and
direct light. Do not refrigerate inhalation solutions.

IF YOU MISS A DOSE
Skip the missed dose and
resume your regular dosage
schedule. Do not double the
next dose.

STOPPING THE DRUG
It may not be necessary to
finish the recommended
course of therapy. Consult
your doctor.

PROLONGED USE
Therapy with this medica-
tion may require months or
years. Excessive use may
result in temporary loss of
the drug's effectiveness.

PRECAUTIONS
Over 60: Adverse reactions
may be more likely and
more severe.

**Driving and Hazardous
Work:** Avoid such activities
until you determine how the
medicine affects you.

Alcohol: No special precautions are necessary.

Pregnancy: Adequate studies have not been done; the
benefits must be weighed
against potential risks. Consult your doctor for advice.

Breast Feeding: It is not
known if terbutaline passes
into breast milk. Mothers
who wish to breast-feed
while taking this drug
should discuss the matter
with their doctor.

Infants and Children:
Use of the inhalation
aerosol is not recommended
in children younger than 12.

Special Concerns: Pay
heed to any asthma attack
or other breathing problem
that does not improve after
your usual nebulizer treatment or usual number of
puffs. Seek help immedi-
ately if you feel your lungs
are persistently constricted,
if you are using more than
the recommended number
of treatments or puffs per
day, or if you feel a recent
attack is somehow different
from others.

OVERDOSE
Symptoms: Chest pain or
heaviness; irregular, racing,
fluttering, or pounding
heartbeat; dizziness or lightheadedness; fainting; severe
weakness; severe headache.

What to Do: Call your
doctor, emergency medical
services (EMS), or the
nearest poison control
center immediately.

DRUG INTERACTIONS
Consult your doctor for specific advice if you are taking
a beta-blocker, ergotamine
or ergotamine-like medications, antidepressants, digitalis drugs, or an MAO
inhibitor.

FOOD INTERACTIONS
No known food interactions.

DISEASE INTERACTIONS
Consult your doctor if you
have a history of substance
abuse (especially cocaine),
seizures, brain damage,
heart disease, heartbeat
irregularities, high blood
pressure, anxiety disorders,
or a thyroid condition.

Terconazole

▶ Drug Class: Antifungal

▶ Available in: Cream, suppositories

▶ Available OTC? No

▶ As Generic? No

Side Effects

SERIOUS
Vaginal burning, itching, discharge, or irritation not present prior to treatment. Call your doctor immediately.

COMMON
No common side effects have been reported.

LESS COMMON
Headache, stomach cramps or pain, irritation or burning of sexual partner's penis.

PRINCIPAL USES
To treat candidiasis, a fungal infection of the vagina.

HOW THE DRUG WORKS
Terconazole prevents fungal organisms from producing vital substances required for growth and function. This drug is effective only for infections caused by fungal organisms. It will not work for bacterial or viral infections.

DOSAGE
Cream— 0.4% cream: 20 mg (1 applicator) inserted in the vagina at bedtime for 7 nights. 0.8% cream: 40 mg (1 applicator) inserted in the vagina at bedtime for 3 nights. Suppositories— 80 mg (1 suppository) inserted in the vagina at bedtime for 3 nights. Wash your hands before and after insertion or application.

ONSET OF EFFECT
Unknown.

DURATION OF ACTION
Unknown.

DIETARY ADVICE
Terconazole can be taken without regard to diet.

STORAGE
Store in a tightly sealed container away from heat, moisture, and direct light. Do not refrigerate or freeze.

IF YOU MISS A DOSE
Take it as soon as you remember. However, if it is near the time for the next dose, skip the missed dose and resume your regular dosage schedule. Do not double the next dose.

STOPPING THE DRUG
Take it as prescribed for the full treatment period, even if you begin to feel better before the scheduled end of therapy.

PROLONGED USE
If your symptoms do not improve after a few days, or if they become worse, consult your doctor.

PRECAUTIONS
Over 60: Adverse reactions may be more likely and more severe in older patients.

Driving and Hazardous Work: The use of terconazole should not impair your ability to perform such tasks safely.

Alcohol: No special precautions are necessary.

Pregnancy: Studies on the use of terconazole during the first 3 months (trimester) of pregnancy have not been done. No adverse effects from using terconazole during the second or third trimesters have been reported.

Breast Feeding: Terconazole may pass into breast milk; caution is advised. Consult your doctor for advice.

Infants and Children: Studies of the use of terconazole in infants and children have not been done.

Special Concerns: Sanitary napkins should be used to prevent staining of clothing. The affected area should be kept cool and dry. The patient should wear loose-fitting cotton clothing and freshly laundered cotton underwear or pantyhose with a cotton crotch. Avoid underwear made from nonventilating materials. Do not sit for a long time in a wet bathing suit. Avoid feminine hygiene sprays. Wash daily with unscented soap and dry thoroughly with a clean towel. Tampons should not be used during therapy. The patient's sexual partner should wear a condom during intercourse and should consult a doctor if penile redness, itching, or discomfort occur. Do not stop using this medicine during your menstrual period. After urination or a bowel movement, cleanse by wiping the area from front to back to prevent reinfection.

OVERDOSE
Symptoms: An overdose with terconazole is unlikely.

What to Do: Emergency instructions not applicable.

DRUG INTERACTIONS
Other drugs may interact with terconazole. Consult your doctor for specific advice if you are taking any other prescription or over-the-counter medication.

FOOD INTERACTIONS
No known food interactions.

DISEASE INTERACTIONS
Consult your doctor for advice if you have any other medical condition.

Testolactone

BRAND NAME
Teslac

Teslac 50 mg
(BRISTOL-MYERS SQUIBB)

▶ Drug Class: Antineoplastic (anticancer) agent

▶ Available in: Tablets

▶ Available OTC? No

▶ As Generic? No

Side Effects

SERIOUS
No serious side effects have been reported.

COMMON
No common side effects have been reported.

LESS COMMON
Skin rash; increased blood pressure; numbness or tingling of fingers, toes, or face; diarrhea; loss of appetite; nausea or vomiting; pain or swelling in feet or lower legs; swelling or redness of the tongue; hair loss; aching and swelling of arms and legs; high blood calcium levels causing confusion, increased thirst, and constipation.

PRINCIPAL USES
To treat some cases of advanced breast cancer in either postmenopausal women or premenopausal women in whom ovarian function has been terminated. It is not recommended for treatment of breast cancer in men.

HOW THE DRUG WORKS
Testolactone is chemically similar to the hormone testosterone. The mechanism by which testolactone inhibits breast cancer growth is unclear. The growth of some types of breast cancer is stimulated by the hormone estrogen; testolactone is thought to interfere with the synthesis of estrogen and thus slow the growth of such types of breast cancer.

DOSAGE
The dosage should be 250 mg, 4 times a day, for at least 3 months.

ONSET OF EFFECT
6 to 12 weeks.

DURATION OF ACTION
Unknown.

DIETARY ADVICE
Testolactone can be taken with or between meals. Be sure to get plenty of fluids.

STORAGE
Store in a tightly sealed container away from heat and direct light.

IF YOU MISS A DOSE
Take it as soon as you remember. If it is close to the next dose, skip the missed dose and resume your regular dosage schedule. Do not double the next dose. If you miss more than 1 dose, consult your doctor.

STOPPING THE DRUG
The decision to stop taking the drug should be made by your doctor.

PROLONGED USE
You should see your doctor regularly for tests and examinations if you must take this drug for a prolonged period.

PRECAUTIONS

Over 60: There is no specific information comparing the use of testolactone in the elderly with use in other age groups. However, no special problems or side effects are expected in older patients.

Driving and Hazardous Work: The use of testolactone should not impair your ability to perform such tasks safely.

Alcohol: Avoid alcohol.

Pregnancy: Large doses of testolactone have been shown to cause birth defects and other problems in animal studies. Human studies have not been done. Before you take testolactone, tell your doctor if you are pregnant or plan to become pregnant. If you become pregnant while taking testolactone, tell your doctor immediately.

Breast Feeding: Testolactone may pass into breast milk; caution is advised. Consult your doctor for advice.

Infants and Children: Safety and effectiveness of testolactone in infants and children have not been determined.

Special Concerns: If you vomit shortly after taking a dose of testolactone, check with your doctor to learn whether you should take the dose again or wait for the next dose. Testolactone may cause an excess buildup of calcium in the body, which can produce unwanted or even dangerous side effects. Therefore, drink large amounts of fluids while taking testolactone to rid your body of excess calcium. Your doctor may want to check blood calcium levels regularly while you take testolactone.

OVERDOSE
Symptoms: No specific ones have been reported.

What to Do: An overdose of testolactone is unlikely to be life-threatening. However, if someone takes a much larger dose than prescribed, call your doctor, emergency medical services (EMS), or the nearest poison control center.

DRUG INTERACTIONS
Consult your doctor for specific advice if you are taking anticoagulants such as warfarin. Testolactone may boost the anticlotting effect of such drugs, leading to uncontrolled internal or external bleeding.

FOOD INTERACTIONS
No known food interactions.

DISEASE INTERACTIONS
Caution is advised when taking testolactone. Consult your doctor if you have a medical history that includes heart or kidney disease.

Testosterone

BRAND NAMES
Andro L.A., Andro-Cyp, Androderm, Andronate, Andropository 100, Andryl 200, Delatest, Delatestryl, depAndro, Depotest, Durathate-200, Everone, T-Cypionate, Testoderm, Testoject, Virilon

▸ Drug Class: Male hormone (androgen)

▸ Available in: Injection, skin patch

▸ Available OTC? No

▸ As Generic? Yes

Side Effects

SERIOUS
In men: Prolonged, possibly painful erection (which may cause permanent damage to the tissues of the penis and result in the inability to achieve further erections), frequent head-ache, increased thirst, increased urination, nausea or vomiting, swollen feet or legs, unusual bleeding, unusual fatigue, rapid weight gain, hives, significant changes in emotions. Call your doctor immediately. In women: Enlarged clitoris, deepening of voice, male-pattern baldness. Such side effects are rare; call your doctor immediately if any occur.

COMMON
In men: Enlarged, sore breasts, frequent erections, acne, frequent urination. The skin patch may cause itching. In women: Acne, decreased breast size, excessive hair growth, irregular menstrual periods.

LESS COMMON
No less-common minor side effects are associated with testosterone.

PRINCIPAL USES
To replace the hormone when the body does not produce enough; to stimulate puberty in boys with delayed onset of puberty; to increase libido in women (prescribed in combination with estrogen; brand name: Estratest).

HOW THE DRUG WORKS
Testosterone supplementation replaces the natural testosterone normally produced by the body.

DOSAGE
For hormone replacement in men: 100 mg weekly intramuscular injection or 200 mg injection every 2 weeks. For delayed puberty in boys: Up to 100 mg injection once a month for 4 to 6 months. For all purposes—Scrotal patch: One new patch applied to scrotal skin in the morning. Nonscrotal patch: 2 to 3 patches a day applied to skin on the arm, back, or upper buttocks.

ONSET OF EFFECT
Blood levels of testosterone peak 5 to 12 hours with the skin patch and in 24 hours with intramuscular injection. Some long-term effects such as improved sexual function may occur after a few weeks of therapy. Other effects (such as those affecting body composition and maturation) may take months to years.

DURATION OF ACTION
Unknown.

DIETARY ADVICE
Testosterone can be taken without regard to diet.

STORAGE
Store skin patch in a tightly sealed container away from heat and direct light.

IF YOU MISS A DOSE
Take it as soon as you remember. If it is near the time for the next dose, skip the missed dose and resume your regular dosage schedule. Do not double the next dose.

STOPPING THE DRUG
The decision to stop taking the drug should be made by your doctor.

PROLONGED USE
You should see your doctor regularly if you are required to use this hormone for a prolonged period.

PRECAUTIONS
Over 60: Increased risk of causing dormant prostate cancer to grow in men. Repeated examinations should be done, using a blood test for prostate specific antigen (PSA) and a digital rectal examination by your doctor.

Driving and Hazardous Work: Do not drive or engage in hazardous work until you determine how the medicine affects you.

Alcohol: Moderate alcohol consumption is acceptable while taking this drug.

Pregnancy: Testosterone should not be taken during pregnancy.

Breast Feeding: Testosterone passes into breast milk and may be harmful; do not use it while breast feeding.

Infants and Children: Not recommended for use by children under the age of puberty.

Special Concerns: The scrotal skin patch should be applied to a shaved area of the scrotum. Men who have experienced skin irrita-tion using a nonscrotal patch can apply triamcinolone cream (0.1%) prior to placement.

OVERDOSE
Symptoms: No specific ones have been reported.

What to Do: An overdose of testosterone is unlikely to be life-threatening. However, if someone takes a much larger dose than prescribed, call your doctor.

DRUG INTERACTIONS
Consult your doctor if you are taking anabolic steroids, anticoagulants (blood thinners, such as warfarin), or an oral contraceptive.

FOOD INTERACTIONS
No known food interactions.

DISEASE INTERACTIONS
Consult your doctor if you have a history of breast cancer (men or women), prostate cancer, diabetes, edema (swelling due to fluid retention), kidney disease, liver disease, enlarged prostate, or cardiovascular disease.

Tetanus Toxoid

BRAND NAMES
Tetanus Toxoid Adsorbed,
Tetanus Toxoid Fluid

▶ Drug Class: Vaccine

▶ Available in: Injection

▶ Available OTC? No

▶ As Generic? No

Side Effects

SERIOUS
Serious allergic reaction involving difficulty swallowing or breathing; reddened skin, especially around the ears; itching, particularly of the hands or feet; hives; unusual and severe fatigue; and swollen face, eyes, or nasal passages. Call your doctor immediately.

COMMON
Hard lump or redness at site of injection.

LESS COMMON
Fever, chills, unusual fatigue, irritability. Also skin rash, pain, itching, swelling, or tenderness at site of injection.

PRINCIPAL USES
To prevent, but not to treat, tetanus (lockjaw).

HOW THE DRUG WORKS
Tetanus toxoid stimulates the body's immune system to produce protective antibodies against tetanus.

DOSAGE
Depending on the type of vaccine being administered, injections are given in the upper arm or midthigh, either into a muscle or under the skin. For adults, children, and infants 6 weeks of age and older: An initial dose at first visit, a second dose 8 weeks later. Depending on the vaccine being used, a third dose may be given 8 weeks after the second dose, and a fourth dose 6 to 12 months later (usually at 15 to 18 months of age in infants). Booster shots should be administered every 10 years. If you sustain a wound that is unclean or difficult to clean, you may need an emergency booster injection if more than 5 years have elapsed since your last booster shot.

ONSET OF EFFECT
Most patients develop immunity following the second dose.

DURATION OF ACTION
Up to 10 years.

DIETARY ADVICE
It may be administered without regard to diet.

STORAGE
Not applicable; the immunizations are administered only at a health care facility.

IF YOU MISS A DOSE
If you miss a scheduled vaccination, contact your doctor to reschedule it.

STOPPING THE DRUG
Follow the full immunization schedule unless a medical problem arises that rules out receiving a vaccination.

PROLONGED USE
No special problems are expected.

PRECAUTIONS
Over 60: Tetanus toxoid should not cause different or more severe side effects in older patients than in younger persons. Vaccine may be slightly less effective. Two-thirds of all tetanus cases in the past few years have been in people age 50 and older.

Driving and Hazardous Work: The administration of tetanus toxoid should not impair your ability to perform such tasks safely.

Alcohol: No special precautions are necessary.

Pregnancy: Adequate studies have not been done. However, if the mother is immune to tetanus, tetanus antibodies from the mother can protect the child from tetanus infection at birth.

Breast Feeding: Tetanus toxoid has not been shown to cause problems during breast feeding.

Infants and Children: Not recommended for use by children less than 6 weeks old.

Special Concerns: Regardless of immunization status, dirty wounds should always be properly cleaned and treated.

OVERDOSE
Symptoms: No specific ones have been reported.

What to Do: If any unexplained symptoms arise after receiving an immunization, call your doctor, emergency medical services (EMS), or the nearest poison control center.

DRUG INTERACTIONS
Other drugs may interact with tetanus toxoid. Consult your doctor for specific advice if you are taking any prescription or over-the-counter medication.

FOOD INTERACTIONS
No known food interactions.

DISEASE INTERACTIONS
Consult your doctor if you have had a severe reaction or a high fever following a previous injection; or if you have pneumonia, bronchitis, or another illness affecting the lungs; any severe illness that is causing fever; or neurological disorders or a history of seizures.

Tetracycline Hydrochloride

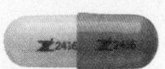

Generic 250 mg
(ZENITH)

▶ Drug Class: Tetracycline antibiotic

▶ Available in: Capsules, tablets, liquid, topical forms, ophthalmic forms, injection

▶ Available OTC? No

▶ As Generic? Yes

Side Effects

SERIOUS
Increased frequency of urination, increased thirst, unusual fatigue, discoloration of skin and mucous membranes. Call your doctor immediately.

COMMON
Stomach cramps and discomfort, diarrhea, nausea, vomiting, increased sensitivity of skin to sunlight, itching in genital or rectal area, sore mouth or tongue, dizziness, lightheadedness, or unsteadiness.

LESS COMMON
No less-common side effects have been reported.

PRINCIPAL USES
To treat infections caused by bacteria or protozoa (tiny single-celled organisms); also, to treat acne.

HOW THE DRUG WORKS
Tetracycline kills bacteria and protozoa by inhibiting the manufacture of specific proteins needed by the organisms to survive.

DOSAGE
Oral forms (capsules, tablets, liquid), for bacterial and protozoal infections: 500 to 2,000 mg,1 to 4 times a day, as determined by your doctor. Topical forms (cream, topical ointment, topical solution), for acne or skin infections: Apply 1 or 2 times a day to affected areas. Ophthalmic forms (ophthalmic ointment, oph-thalmic solution) for eye infections: Apply once every 2 to 12 hours as determined by your doctor.

ONSET OF EFFECT
Unknown.

DURATION OF ACTION
Unknown.

DIETARY ADVICE
Oral forms are best taken on an empty stomach with a full glass of water.

STORAGE
Store in a tightly sealed container away from heat and direct light. Refrigerate liquid forms but do not freeze.

IF YOU MISS A DOSE
Take it as soon as you remember. If it is near the time for the next dose, skip the missed dose and resume your regular dosage schedule. Do not double the next dose.

STOPPING THE DRUG
Take this antibiotic as prescribed for the full treatment period, even if you begin to feel better before the scheduled end of therapy.

PROLONGED USE
May increase susceptibility to infections by microorganisms resistant to antibiotics.

PRECAUTIONS
Over 60: It is not known whether tetracycline causes different or more severe adverse reactions in older patients than it does in younger persons.

Driving and Hazardous Work: Do not drive or engage in hazardous work until you determine how the medicine affects you.

Alcohol: It is advisable to abstain from alcohol when fighting an infection.

Pregnancy: Tetracycline should not be used during pregnancy.

Breast Feeding: Tetracycline passes into breast milk and may be harmful to the nursing infant. The patient must choose between using the drug or breast feeding.

Infants and Children: Tetracycline should be used by children younger than 8 years of age only if other antibiotics are unlikely to be effective, since it can cause permanent tooth staining.

Special Concerns: If tetracycline causes increased sensitivity of your skin to sunlight, wear protective clothing, use a sunscreen with an SPF (sun protection factor) of 15 or higher, and try to avoid direct exposure to sunlight, especially between 10 am and 3 pm. Before having surgery, tell the doctor or dentist in charge that you are taking tetracycline. If you use makeup, it is best to apply only water-based cosmetics and to keep the amount to a minimum during tetracycline therapy for the skin. Tetracycline can reduce the effectiveness of oral contraceptives. You should use a different method of birth control while taking this antibiotic. Absorption of tetracycline may be altered if you take antacids.

OVERDOSE
Symptoms: Severe nausea, vomiting, diarrhea, difficulty swallowing.

What to Do: An overdose is unlikely to be life-threatening. However, if someone takes a much larger dose than prescribed, call your doctor, emergency medical services (EMS), or the nearest poison control center immediately.

DRUG INTERACTIONS
Consult your physician for specific advice if you are taking antacids, calcium supplements, cholestyramine, choline and magnesium salicylates, medicines containing iron, laxatives containing magnesium, or oral contraceptives.

FOOD INTERACTIONS
Avoid dairy products while taking tetracycline.

DISEASE INTERACTIONS
Consult your doctor if you have a history of kidney disease or liver disease.

BRAND NAMES

Accurbron, Aerolate SR, Aquaphyllin, Asmalix, Bronkodyl, Chloledyl, Constant-T, Duraphyl, Elixophyllin, Hydro-Spec, Labid, Lanophyllin, Lixolin, Respbid, Slo-Bid, Slo-Phyllin, Somophyllin, Sustaire, T-Phyl, Theo-24, Theo-Dur, Theo-Time, Theobid, Theoclear-80, Theolair, Theovent, Truxophyllin, Uni-Dur, Uniphyl

Slo-Bid 50 mg
(RHONE-POULENC RORER)

Additional photographs

▶ Drug Class: Bronchodilator/ xanthine

▶ Available in: Tablets, capsules, extended release forms, elixir, syrup, oral solution

▶ Available OTC? No

▶ As Generic? Yes

Side Effects

SERIOUS
Vomiting, trembling, confusion, rapid, irregular, or pounding pulse, chest pain, dizziness, convulsions, skin rashes.

COMMON
Restlessness, insomnia, loss of appetite, nervousness, irritability, nausea.

LESS COMMON
Heartburn, diarrhea.

PRINCIPAL USES

Theophylline is used to reduce the frequency and severity of breathing problems in people with asthma, emphysema, bronchitis, and other lung disorders.

HOW THE DRUG WORKS

An asthma attack occurs when the smooth muscles in the bronchial passages of the lungs go into a spasm (bronchospasm). Theophylline relaxes these muscles, helping to widen the constricted airways and restore normal breathing.

DOSAGE

Adults not currently taking any theophylline medications: Your physician will prescribe a "loading dose," which is based on your weight and taken only once. This is followed by a daily maintenance dose, usually 300 to 600 mg per day, taken in 1 or 2 doses. Patients given extended-release capsules: After the loading dose, take one-half of the total daily dose at 12-hour intervals, unless otherwise directed by your doctor. Adults currently taking theophylline: Dose is determined by blood level of theophylline. Children: Consult a pediatrician.

ONSET OF EFFECT

Variable.

DURATION OF ACTION

Variable.

DIETARY ADVICE

Avoid large amounts of caffeine-containing foods or beverages, including colas. Otherwise, maintain your usual food and fluid intake.

STORAGE

Store in a tightly sealed container away from heat and direct light. Keep away from moisture and extremes in temperature.

IF YOU MISS A DOSE

Take it as soon as you remember. If it is near the time for the next dose, skip the missed dose and resume your regular dosage schedule. Do not double the next dose.

STOPPING THE DRUG

The decision to stop taking the drug should be made by your doctor.

PROLONGED USE

Therapy with this medication may require months or years.

PRECAUTIONS

Over 60: Adverse reactions may be more likely and more severe in older patients.

Driving and Hazardous Work: Do not drive or engage in hazardous work until you determine how the medicine affects you.

Alcohol: Avoid alcohol.

Pregnancy: Discuss the relative risks with your doctor. Generally, this drug should be used only if necessary and if a substitute cannot be prescribed.

Breast Feeding: Theophylline passes into breast milk and may be toxic to nursing infants; avoid or discontinue use while breast feeding.

Infants and Children: Theophylline has been used in children of all ages. Consult your pediatrician for specific dosages. Theophylline elixir contains alcohol and should not be used by children.

Special Concerns: You will need periodic blood tests to determine theophylline levels. Do not switch between different brands of theophylline, and especially do not switch between extended-release forms and other forms without notifying your doctor. Inform your doctor if you have stopped smoking; tobacco affects the level of theophylline in the blood.

OVERDOSE

Symptoms: Abdominal pain; disorientation, extreme anxiety, or unusual behavior; bloody vomiting; twitching, trembling, or shaking; seizures; rapid, pounding, or irregular heartbeat; lightheadedness, dizziness, or fainting.

What to Do: Call your doctor, emergency medical services (EMS), or the nearest poison control center immediately.

DRUG INTERACTIONS

Consult your doctor for specific advice if you are taking beta-blockers, cimetidine, ciprofloxacin, clarithromycin, enoxacin, erythromycin, fluvoxamine, mexiletine, pentoxifylline, propranolol, tacrine, thiabendazole, ticlopidine, troleandomycin; moricizine, phenytoin, or rifampin.

FOOD INTERACTIONS

Your doctor may suggest that you restrict caffeine intake.

DISEASE INTERACTIONS

Consult your doctor if you have a history of convulsions, heart failure, liver disease, or underactive thyroid.

Thiabendazole

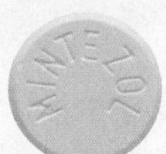

Mintezol 500 mg
(**MERCK**)

▶ Drug Class: Anthelmintic

▶ Available in: Oral suspension, chewable tablets

▶ Available OTC? No

▶ As Generic? No

Side Effects

SERIOUS
Severe nausea and vomiting, confusion, skin rash or itching, severe diarrhea, hallucinations, delirium, disorientation, loss of appetite, irritability, tingling or numbness of hands or feet, decreased pulse or blood pressure. Call your physician immediately.

COMMON
Dry eyes or mouth, dizziness, drowsiness, buzzing or ringing in ears, headache, asparagus-like odor from urine.

LESS COMMON
Elevated liver enzymes, temporary decrease in white blood cell count (these effects are detectable by your doctor); fever, flushing of the face, swelling.

PRINCIPAL USES
To treat infections caused by worms, primarily strongyloidiasis (threadworms). It may also be used to treat cutaneous larva migrans (creeping eruption), trichinosis, and visceral larva migrans, although less toxic drugs are available.

HOW THE DRUG WORKS
The exact way in which thiabendazole works is unknown. It appears to interfere with the metabolic or energy-producing processes of worms, including the uptake of glucose (sugar).

DOSAGE
Adults and children: 25 mg per 2.2 lbs (1 kg) of body weight twice a day (up to a maximum of 3,000 mg per day) for 2 to 5 days. Consult your doctor for specific dose. The oral suspension can be used topically for cutaneous larva migrans.

ONSET OF EFFECT
Unknown.

DURATION OF ACTION
Unknown.

DIETARY ADVICE
Take it after meals to reduce stomach upset and some of the common side effects.

STORAGE
Store in a tightly sealed container away from heat, moisture, and direct light. Keep the oral suspension from freezing.

IF YOU MISS A DOSE
Take it as soon as you remember. If it is near the time for the next dose, skip the missed dose and resume your regular dosage schedule. Do not double the next dose.

STOPPING THE DRUG
Take it as prescribed for the full treatment period, even if you feel better before the scheduled end of therapy.

PROLONGED USE
Thiabendazole is generally prescribed for short-term therapy (2 to 5 days). If your condition shows no signs of improvement or worsens within this time, consult your doctor. Another treatment regimen may be prescribed.

PRECAUTIONS
Over 60: Adverse reactions may be more likely and more severe in older patients.

Driving and Hazardous Work: Do not drive or engage in hazardous work while undergoing treatment.

Alcohol: No special precautions are necessary.

Pregnancy: Do not take thiabendazole while pregnant. Consult your doctor for advice if you are pregnant or plan to become pregnant.

Breast Feeding: Thiabendazole may pass into breast milk. Breast feeding may need to be discontinued while you take the drug. Consult your doctor for advice.

Infants and Children: Use and dosage for infants weighing less than 30 pounds should be determined by your doctor.

Special Concerns: To prevent reinfection with trichinosis, all pork, pork-containing products, and game meat should be cooked until the center is no longer pink. To prevent reinfection with cutaneous larva migrans or visceral larva migrans, keep your dogs or cats away from beaches and bathing areas, deworm them regularly, and keep children's sandboxes covered when not in use. Note that approximately half of all patients who take thiabendazole experience at least one side effect.

OVERDOSE
Symptoms: Sporadic vision disturbances, changes in mental state.

What to Do: An overdose of thiabendazole is unlikely to be life-threatening. However, if someone takes a much larger dose than prescribed, call your doctor, emergency medical services (EMS), or the nearest poison control center.

DRUG INTERACTIONS
Consult your doctor for specific advice if you are taking theophylline. Also tell your doctor if you are taking any other prescription or over-the-counter medicine. If you have trichinosis, your doctor may also prescribe a corticosteroid to help reduce inflammation from the pork worm larvae; it is important to take the corticosteroid and thiabendazole together.

FOOD INTERACTIONS
No known food interactions.

DISEASE INTERACTIONS
Use of thiabendazole may cause complications in patients with liver disease, since this organ removes the drug from the body.

Thioguanine

Generic 40 mg
(GLAXO WELLCOME)

▶ Drug Class: Antimetabolite; antineoplastic (anticancer) agent

▶ Available in: Tablets

▶ Available OTC? No

▶ As Generic? Yes

Side Effects

SERIOUS
Black, tarry, or bloody stools; blood-tinged (pink or maroon) urine; cough or hoarseness; fever and chills; lower back or flank pain; painful, difficult urination; tiny bright red spots on skin; bleeding from gums, nose, or other unusual places; easy bruising, shortness of breath. These side effects may mean that normal blood cells and special blood-clotting cells have been affected, or that normal immune cells have been affected and an infection is developing somewhere in your body. See your doctor immediately if any of these occur. Some of these side effects may occur after you stop taking thioguanine; notify your doctor if they do.

COMMON
No common side effects have been reported.

LESS COMMON
Diarrhea, loss of appetite, nausea and vomiting, skin rash or itching.

PRINCIPAL USES
To treat some forms of leukemia.

HOW THE DRUG WORKS
It kills cancer cells by interfering with the activity of their genetic material, which prevents the cells from reproducing. It may also affect the growth and development of other cells in the body, resulting in unpleasant side effects.

DOSAGE
2 mg per 2.2 lbs (1 kg) of body weight per day, usually in 1 dose. The dose can be increased to 3 mg per 2.2 lbs per day if there is no response after 3 weeks.

ONSET OF EFFECT
Unknown.

DURATION OF ACTION
Unknown.

DIETARY ADVICE
Maintain adequate food and fluid intake. Calorie, protein, and vitamin needs increase in patients with cancer. Good nutrition is essential to cope with chemotherapy.

STORAGE
Store in a tightly sealed container away from heat and direct light.

IF YOU MISS A DOSE
If you miss a dose, skip the missed dose and resume your regular dosage schedule. Do not double the next dose.

STOPPING THE DRUG
The decision to stop taking thioguanine should be made in consultation with your doctor.

PROLONGED USE
You should see your doctor regularly for tests and examinations if you take this drug for a prolonged period.

PRECAUTIONS
Over 60: No special problems are expected.

Driving and Hazardous Work: Do not drive or engage in hazardous work until you determine how the medicine affects you.

Alcohol: Consult your doctor about drinking alcohol while taking this drug.

Pregnancy: Thioguanine can cause birth defects if either the father or mother takes it. It is best to use some kind of birth control while taking thioguanine. Consult your doctor for specific advice if you are pregnant or plan to become pregnant.

Breast Feeding: Thioguanine may pass into breast milk; avoid or discontinue use while nursing.

Infants and Children: No special problems are expected.

Special Concerns: While taking thioguanine, do not receive any immunizations without consulting your doctor. Avoid people with infections and those who have recently had oral polio vaccine. Be careful when using a toothbrush, dental floss, or toothpick. Check with your doctor before having any dental work done. If you are going to have surgery, tell the doctor or dentist in charge that you are taking thioguanine. Do not touch your eyes or the inside of your nose unless you have just washed your hands. Be careful not to cut yourself when using sharp objects such as a razor. Avoid contact sports and other activities where bruising could occur. If you vomit shortly after taking a dose of thioguanine, consult your doctor about taking the dose again.

OVERDOSE
Symptoms: Nausea, vomiting, general malaise, high blood pressure.

What to Do: Call your doctor, emergency medical services (EMS), or the nearest poison control center immediately.

DRUG INTERACTIONS
Consult your doctor for specific advice if you are taking antithyroid agents, azathioprine, chloramphenicol, colchicine, flucytosine, interferon, plicamycin, zidovudine, probenecid, or sulfinpyrazone.

FOOD INTERACTIONS
No known food interactions.

DISEASE INTERACTIONS
Caution is advised when taking thioguanine. Consult your doctor if you have any of the following: chicken pox, shingles, gout, kidney stones, kidney disease, liver disease, or any infection.

Thioridazine Hydrochloride

Generic 100 mg
(CREIGHTON)

Additional photographs

▶ Drug Class: Neuroleptic;
antipsychotic

▶ Available in: Oral solution,
oral suspension, tablets

▶ Available OTC? No

▶ As Generic? Yes

Side Effects

SERIOUS
Rapid heartbeat, profuse sweating, seizures, difficulty breathing, neck stiffness, swelling of the tongue, difficulty swallowing. Also a rare condition can develop called neuroleptic malignant syndrome, characterized by stiffness or spasms of the muscles, high fever, and confusion or disorientation. Call your doctor immediately.

COMMON
Dizziness or faintness, drowsiness, constipation, decreased sweating, dry mouth, nasal congestion, shaking or trembling of the hands, stiffness, stooped posture.

LESS COMMON
Menstrual irregularities, sexual dysfunction, unusual milk secretion, breast pain or swelling, unexpected weight gain, difficult urination.

PRINCIPAL USES
To treat moderate to severe psychiatric conditions including schizophrenia, manic states, and drug-induced psychosis. It is also used to treat extreme behavior problems in children (including infantile autism), to ease the symptoms of Tourette's syndrome, and to reduce nausea and vomiting associated with chemotherapy for cancer.

HOW THE DRUG WORKS
Thioridazine blocks receptors of dopamine (a chemical that aids in the transmission of nerve impulses) in the central nervous system. Presumably, this produces a tranquilizing and antipsychotic effect.

DOSAGE
Adults: Initially, 25 to 100 mg, 3 times a day. Your doctor may increase the dose as needed and tolerated, not to exceed 800 mg a day.

ONSET OF EFFECT
Sedation may occur within minutes, but onset of antipsychotic effect may take hours to occur or may not occur until days or weeks after the beginning of therapy.

DURATION OF ACTION
12 to 24 hours, but effects may persist for several days.

DIETARY ADVICE
Should be taken with food and a full glass of water.

STORAGE
Store in a tightly sealed container away from heat and direct light. Do not allow liquid forms to freeze.

IF YOU MISS A DOSE
Take it as soon as you remember. If it is near the time for the next dose, skip the missed dose and resume your regular dosage schedule. Do not double the next dose.

STOPPING THE DRUG
The decision to stop taking the drug should be made in consultation with your doctor. Gradual reduction of doses may be required if you have taken this medication for an extended period.

PROLONGED USE
See your doctor regularly for tests and examinations if you must take this medicine for a prolonged period.

PRECAUTIONS
Over 60: Adverse reactions are more likely and more severe in older patients.

Driving and Hazardous Work: Do not drive or engage in hazardous work until you learn how this medication affects you.

Alcohol: Avoid alcohol.

Pregnancy: Avoid using thioridazine if you are pregnant or plan to become pregnant.

Breast Feeding: Either avoid taking the drug if possible or refrain from breast feeding.

Infants and Children: Adverse reactions may be more likely and more severe in children.

Special Concerns: Avoid prolonged exposure to high temperatures or hot climates. Drink plenty of fluids and stay cool in the summertime. Avoid overexposure to sunlight until you determine if the drug heightens your skin's sensitivity to ultraviolet light.

OVERDOSE
Symptoms: Extreme drowsiness or paradoxical restlessness or agitation, heart rhythm irregularities or palpitations, dry mouth, seizures, stiffness or impaired muscle control, loss of consciousness.

What to Do: Call your doctor, emergency medical services (EMS), or the nearest poison control center immediately.

DRUG INTERACTIONS
Thioridazine should not be used within 5 weeks of taking fluoxetine. Consult your doctor for specific advice if you are taking anticholinergics, anticonvulsants, antidepressants, antihistamines, antihypertensives, bupropion, central nervous system depressants such as barbiturates, clozapine, dronabinol, ethinamate, guanethidine, guanfacine, lithium, methyldopa, carbamazepine, rifampin, or trihexyphenidyl.

FOOD INTERACTIONS
No known food interactions.

DISEASE INTERACTIONS
Consult your doctor if you have Parkinson's disease or any movement disorder, glaucoma, epilepsy, liver disease, or kidney disease.

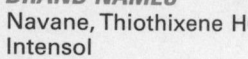

Generic 1 mg
(MYLAN)

807

Additional photographs

▶ Drug Class: Neuroleptic; antipsychotic

▶ Available in: Capsules, solution, injection

▶ Available OTC? No

▶ As Generic? Yes

Side Effects

SERIOUS
Rapid heartbeat, profuse sweating, seizures, difficulty breathing, neck stiffness, swelling of the tongue, difficulty swallowing. Also a rare condition can develop called neuroleptic malignant syndrome, characterized by stiffness or spasms of the muscles, high fever, and confusion or disorientation. Call your doctor immediately.

COMMON
Nausea, reduced perspiration, dry mouth, blurred vision, drowsiness, shaking of the hands, muscle stiffness, stooped posture.

LESS COMMON
Difficult urination, menstrual irregularities, breast pain or swelling, unexpected weight gain, uncontrolled movements of the tongue, fever, chills, sore throat, unusual bruising or bleeding, heart palpitations, skin rash, itching, increased sensitivity of the skin to sunlight.

PRINCIPAL USES
To treat psychotic conditions (severe mental disorders characterized by distorted thoughts, perceptions, and emotions), such as schizophrenia.

HOW THE DRUG WORKS
Thiothixene blocks receptors of dopamine (a chemical that allows the transmission of nerve impulses) in the central nervous system. Presumably, this produces a tranquilizing or antipsychotic effect.

DOSAGE
Oral forms: Initial dose is 2 mg, 3 times a day, or 5 mg, 2 times a day. The dose may be increased up to 60 mg a day. Injection: 4 mg injected into a muscle, 2 to 4 times a day. The dose may be increased up to 30 mg a day.

ONSET OF EFFECT
Sedation may occur within minutes, but onset of antipsychotic effect may take hours to occur or may not occur until days or weeks after the beginning of therapy.

DURATION OF ACTION
12 to 24 hours, but effects may persist for several days.

DIETARY ADVICE
This drug may be taken without regard to diet.

STORAGE
Store in a tightly sealed container away from heat and direct light. Do not allow liquid forms to freeze.

IF YOU MISS A DOSE
Take it as soon as you remember. However, if it is within 2 hours of the next dose, skip the missed dose and resume your regular dosage schedule. Do not double the next dose.

STOPPING THE DRUG
The decision to stop taking the drug should be made in consultation with your physician.

PROLONGED USE
Prolonged use may lead to tardive dyskinesia (involuntary movements of the jaw, lips, tongue, and, in rare cases, the arms, legs, hands, or body). Consult your doctor about the need for follow-up evaluations and tests if you must take this drug for an extended period.

PRECAUTIONS
Over 60: Adverse reactions are more likely and more severe in older patients.

Driving and Hazardous Work: Do not drive or engage in hazardous work until you determine how the medicine affects you.

Alcohol: Avoid alcohol.

Pregnancy: Adequate studies have not been done. Before you take thiothixene, tell your doctor if you are pregnant or plan to become pregnant.

Breast Feeding: It is unknown if thiothixene passes into breast milk; consult your doctor for advice.

Infants and Children: Thiothixene is not commonly prescribed for patients under age 12.

Special Concerns: Avoid prolonged exposure to high temperatures or hot climates. Drink plenty of fluids and stay cool in the summertime. Avoid overexposure to sunlight until you determine if the drug heightens your skin's sensitivity to ultraviolet light.

OVERDOSE
Symptoms: Severe breathing difficulty, severe dizziness, extreme fatigue or sedation, muscle spasms, stiffness, or twitching, constricted pupils, unusual excitability.

What to Do: Call your doctor, emergency medical services (EMS), or the nearest poison control center immediately.

DRUG INTERACTIONS
Other drugs may interact with thiothixene. Consult your doctor for specific advice if you are taking anticholinergics, anticonvulsants, antidepressants, antihistamines, antihypertensives, bupropion, central nervous system depressants such as barbiturates, clozapine, dronabinol, ethinamate, fluoxetine, guanethidine, guanfacine, lithium, methyldopa, carbamazepine, rifampin, or trihexyphenidyl.

FOOD INTERACTIONS
No known food interactions.

DISEASE INTERACTIONS
Consult your doctor if you have Parkinson's disease or any movement disorder, glaucoma, epilepsy, liver disease, or kidney disease.

Tiagabine Hydrochloride

BRAND NAME
Gabitril

▶ Drug Class: Anticonvulsant

▶ Available in: Tablets

▶ Available OTC? No

▶ As Generic? No

Side Effects

SERIOUS
No serious side effects are associated with the use of tiagabine.

COMMON
Dizziness, fatigue, lack of energy, drowsiness, nausea, nervousness, irritability, tremor.

LESS COMMON
Abdominal pain, diarrhea, vomiting, general pain, increased appetite, mouth sores, joint aches, insomnia, speech difficulties, clumsiness or incoordination, difficulty concentrating, amnesia, mental depression, emotional instability, hostility or agitation, confusion, abnormal eye movements, sore throat, numbness, prickling or tingling sensations, rash, flu-like symptoms.

PRINCIPAL USES
Used in combination with one or more anticonvulsant drugs to control partial seizures (those which begin with an abnormal burst of electrical activity in a small portion of the brain).

HOW THE DRUG WORKS
Although its precise mechanism of action is unknown, tiagabine is thought to increase the activity of an inhibiting neurotransmitter that depresses brain activity and suppresses the abnormal firing of neurons that causes seizures.

DOSAGE
Teenagers: For the first week, 4 mg once a day. At the beginning of the second week, the total daily dose may be increased by 4 mg. The total daily dose may be further adjusted by 4 to 8 mg on a weekly basis, up to 32 mg a day in 2 to 4 divided doses. Adults: For the first week, 4 mg once a day. The total daily dose may be further adjusted by 4 to 8 mg on a weekly basis, up to 56 mg a day in 2 to 4 divided doses.

ONSET OF EFFECT
Unknown.

DURATION OF ACTION
Unknown.

DIETARY ADVICE
Tiagabine should be taken with meals.

STORAGE
Store in a tightly sealed container away from heat, moisture, and direct light.

IF YOU MISS A DOSE
Take it as soon as you remember. If it is near the time for the next dose, skip the missed dose and resume your regular dosage schedule. Do not double the next dose.

STOPPING THE DRUG
The decision to stop taking the drug should be made by your doctor. Never stop this drug abruptly because this may cause seizures. The dose is typically tapered over a period of weeks.

PROLONGED USE
Side effects are more likely with prolonged use.

PRECAUTIONS
Over 60: Adverse reactions may be more likely and more severe.

Driving and Hazardous Work: Do not drive or engage in hazardous work until you determine how the medicine affects you.

Alcohol: May contribute to excessive drowsiness.

Pregnancy: Adequate human studies have not been done. Before taking tiagabine, tell your doctor if you are or are planning to become pregnant. Discuss with your doctor the relative risks and benefits of using this drug while pregnant.

Breast Feeding: Tiagabine may pass into breast milk; caution is advised. Consult your doctor for specific advice.

Infants and Children: Not recommended for use by children under age 12.

Special Concerns: Your doctor may want you to wear a medical alert bracelet or carry an identification card saying that you are taking this drug.

OVERDOSE
Symptoms: Few cases of overdose have been reported. In clinical trials, the most common symptoms following overdose have been drowsiness, agitation, confusion, speech problems, hostility, mental depression, weakness, and muscle spasms.

What to Do: Call your doctor, emergency medical services (EMS), or the nearest poison control center immediately.

DRUG INTERACTIONS
There are no significant drug interactions.

FOOD INTERACTIONS
No known food interactions.

DISEASE INTERACTIONS
A lower dose or longer dosing intervals may be warranted in patients with impaired liver function.

Ticlopidine Hydrochloride

BRAND NAME
Ticlid

Ticlid 250 mg
(ROCHE)

▶ Drug Class: Antiplatelet drug

▶ Available in: Tablets

▶ Available OTC? No

▶ As Generic? No

Side Effects

SERIOUS
Bleeding that is difficult to stop, bruising, increased susceptibility to infection, sores, ulcers or white spots in the mouth, severe abdominal or stomach pain, back pain, peeling or loosening of the skin or lips or mucous membranes, bloody or tarry stools, blood in urine, coughing up blood, dizziness, fever or chills, severe headache, loss of coordination, pinpoint red spots on skin, thickened or scaly skin, difficulty speaking, unusually heavy menstrual flow, vomiting of blood or dark material. Call your doctor immediately.

COMMON
Skin rash, mild stomach pain, diarrhea, indigestion, nausea.

LESS COMMON
Gas or bloating, dizziness, vomiting.

PRINCIPAL USES
To reduce the chance of stroke in patients who have had a stroke or have high risk factors for stroke. While beneficial in this regard, ticlopidine is potentially a very dangerous medication prescribed only when all other therapeutic measures have failed.

HOW THE DRUG WORKS
Blood clots are a primary cause of stroke and heart attack. Ticlopidine prevents platelets from clumping clumping together to form blood clots, thus reducing the risk of stroke.

DOSAGE
250 mg, 2 times a day.

ONSET OF EFFECT
Within 2 days.

DURATION OF ACTION
1 to 2 weeks.

DIETARY ADVICE
Should be taken with food.

STORAGE
Store in a tightly sealed container away from heat and direct light.

IF YOU MISS A DOSE
Take it as soon as you remember. If it is near the time for the next dose, skip the missed dose and resume your regular dosage schedule. Do not double the next dose.

STOPPING THE DRUG
The decision to stop taking the drug should be made by your doctor.

PROLONGED USE
You should see your doctor regularly for blood cell counts and physical examinations if you must take this medication for a prolonged period.

PRECAUTIONS
Over 60: No special problems are expected.

Driving and Hazardous Work: Do not drive or engage in hazardous work until you determine how the medicine affects you.

Alcohol: Avoid alcohol.

Pregnancy: In animal studies, ticlopidine has caused harmful effects; human studies have not been done. Before you take ticlopidine, be sure to tell your doctor if you are currently pregnant or plan to become pregnant.

Breast Feeding: It is not known whether ticlopidine passes into breast milk; caution is advised. Consult your doctor for specific advice.

Infants and Children: There are no studies of ticlopidine use in children.

Special Concerns: Be sure to tell all of your doctors, dentists, and pharmacists that you are taking ticlopidine. You may have to stop taking the drug 10 days to 2 weeks before an operation or dental work. Ticlopidine can cause serious bleeding, especially after an injury. Ask your doctor whether there are activities you should avoid while taking this drug. Frequent blood tests, every 1 or 2 weeks, should be done during the first 6 months of ticlopidine therapy.

OVERDOSE
Symptoms: Uncontrolled bleeding, fever, infection.

What to Do: Discontinue the medication and call your doctor, emergency medical services (EMS), or the nearest poison control center right away.

DRUG INTERACTIONS
Consult your doctor for specific advice if you are taking anticoagulants, carbenicillin, dipyridamole, divalproex, heparin, medicine for pain or inflammation, pentoxifylline, plicamycin, sulfinpyrazone, ticarcillin, or valproic acid.

FOOD INTERACTIONS
No known food interactions.

DISEASE INTERACTIONS
Caution is advised when taking ticlopidine. Consult your doctor if you have a history of any of the following: a blood clotting problem, severe liver disease, stomach ulcers, any blood disease, or severe kidney disease.

728

Tiludronate Disodium

BRAND NAME
Skelid

▶ Drug Class: Bisphosphonate inhibitor of bone resorption

▶ Available in: Tablets

▶ Available OTC? No

▶ As Generic? No

Side Effects

SERIOUS
No serious side effects are associated with the use of tiludronate.

COMMON
Diarrhea, nausea, stomach upset, indigestion.

LESS COMMON
Mild chest pain, swelling of the ankles, numbness, rash, vomiting, flatulence, increased susceptibility to infection, runny nose, sinus infection, cataract, conjunctivitis, glaucoma, dental problems.

PRINCIPAL USES
To treat Paget's disease, a disorder characterized by rapid breakdown and reformation of bone, which can lead to fragility and malformation of bones. Treatment is indicated if serum alkaline phosphatase (as measured in blood tests) is at least two times normal, or if the patient has symptoms or is at risk for complications.

HOW THE DRUG WORKS
Healthy bones are continuously remodeled (broken down and then reformed); the minerals and other components of bones are reabsorbed by one set of cells (osteoclasts) and replaced by another set of cells to form new bone. Tiludronate suppresses the activity of osteoclasts; consequently, the breakdown of bone tissue occurs more slowly than the laying down of new bone. As a result, bone density and strength are preserved.

DOSAGE
400 mg, once a day for 3 months.

ONSET OF EFFECT
Unknown.

DURATION OF ACTION
Unknown.

DIETARY ADVICE
Take it with a full glass of plain water. Taking tiludronate with food or beverages (including mineral water) other than plain water is likely to reduce the absorption of the drug from the intestine. Take the tablets at least 2 hours before or after eating. Maintain adequate vitamin D and calcium intake; however, vitamin or mineral supplements should also be taken at least 2 hours before or after taking the drug.

STORAGE
Store in a tightly sealed container away from heat, moisture, and direct light. Do not remove tablets from the foil strips until they are to be used.

IF YOU MISS A DOSE
If you miss a dose on one day, do not double the dose the next day. Resume your regular dosage schedule.

STOPPING THE DRUG
Take it as prescribed for the full treatment period. The decision to stop taking the drug should be made in consultation with your physician.

PROLONGED USE
Tiludronate is generally prescribed for a 3-month course of therapy. Adequate studies on the safety and effectiveness of tiludronate beyond this period of time have not been done.

PRECAUTIONS
Over 60: No special problems are expected.

Driving and Hazardous Work: The use of tiludronate should not impair your ability to perform such tasks safely.

Alcohol: No special precautions are necessary.

Pregnancy: Adequate human studies have not been done. Discuss with your doctor the relative risks and benefits of using this drug while pregnant.

Breast Feeding: Tiludronate may pass into breast milk; caution is advised. Consult your doctor for specific advice.

Infants and Children: Not recommended for use by children under age 18.

OVERDOSE
Symptoms: No cases of overdose have been reported.

What to Do: An overdose with tiludronate is unlikely. If someone takes a much larger dose than prescribed, call your doctor.

DRUG INTERACTIONS
Calcium supplements, aspirin, and indomethacin should not be taken within 2 hours before or after taking tiludronate. Aluminum- or magnesium-containing antacids, if needed, should be taken at least 2 hours after taking tiludronate.

FOOD INTERACTIONS
No known food interactions, although tiludronate works best when taken on an empty stomach.

DISEASE INTERACTIONS
Patients with severe kidney disease should not take tiludronate.

Timolol Maleate Ophthalmic

▶ Drug Class: Antiglaucoma drug; ophthalmic beta-blocker

▶ Available in: Ophthalmic solution

▶ Available OTC? No

▶ As Generic? No

Side Effects

SERIOUS
Palpitations; trouble breathing; dizziness and weakness caused by low blood pressure. Call your doctor right away.

COMMON
Stinging or irritation of the eye when drops are applied; tearing.

LESS COMMON
Decreased night vision; eyebrow pain; crusted eyelashes; dry eyes; increased sensitivity of eyes to light; redness, stinging, burning, watering, or other irritation of the eye; droopy eyelid; eye inflammation.

PRINCIPAL USES
To treat glaucoma.

HOW THE DRUG WORKS
Glaucoma, a sight-threatening disorder, occurs when aqueous humor (the fluid inside the eye) cannot drain properly, causing an increase in pressure within the eyeball (intraocular pressure). This can damage the optic nerve and lead to a gradually progressive loss of vision. Timolol decreases the production of aqueous humor, thereby reducing intraocular pressure.

DOSAGE
Adults and older children: 1 drop 1 or 2 times a day. Younger children and infants: Use and dosage must be determined by your doctor.

ONSET OF EFFECT
Within 30 minutes.

DURATION OF ACTION
12 to 24 hours.

DIETARY ADVICE
This medication can be used without regard to diet.

STORAGE
Store in a tightly sealed container away from heat, moisture, and direct light. Do not allow it to freeze.

IF YOU MISS A DOSE
Apply it as soon as you remember. If it is near the time for the next dose, skip the missed dose and resume your regular dosage schedule. Do not double the next dose.

STOPPING THE DRUG
The decision to stop using the drug should be made by your doctor.

PROLONGED USE
You should see your doctor regularly for tests and examinations as part of glaucoma follow up if you take this drug for a prolonged period.

PRECAUTIONS
Over 60: Adverse reactions may be more likely and more severe in older patients.

Driving and Hazardous Work: Do not drive or engage in hazardous work until you determine how the medicine affects your vision.

Alcohol: Use alcohol with caution.

Pregnancy: Timolol has not caused birth defects in animals. Human studies have not been completed. Before you take timolol, tell your doctor if you are pregnant or plan to become pregnant.

Breast Feeding: Timolol may pass into breast milk; caution is advised. Consult your doctor for advice.

Infants and Children: Adverse reactions may be more likely and more severe in infants.

Special Concerns: To use the eye drops, first wash your hands. Tilt your head back. Gently apply pressure to the inside corner of the eyelid and with the index finger of the same hand, pull downward on the lower eyelid to make a space. Drop the medicine into this space and close your eye. Apply pressure for 1 or 2 minutes while keeping the eye closed without blinking. Then wash your hands again. Make sure the tip of the dropper does not touch your eye, finger, or any other surface. Timolol may make your eyes more sensitive to bright light. If this occurs, wear sunglasses or avoid bright light as necessary. Before you have any surgery, dental treatment, or emergency treatment, tell the doctor or dentist in charge that you are using timolol.

OVERDOSE
Symptoms: Nervousness, chest pain, irregular or pounding heartbeat, hallucinations, wheezing, mental confusion.

What to Do: If a large volume enters the eye, flush with water. If someone accidentally ingests the medicine, call your doctor, emergency medical services (EMS), or the nearest poison control center.

DRUG INTERACTIONS
It is not recommended to use two ophthalmic beta-blockers at the same time. Special caution is warranted in people taking antidiabetic drugs, as timolol may mask symptoms of low blood sugar. Consult your doctor for specific advice if you are taking any other prescription or over-the-counter medication.

FOOD INTERACTIONS
No known food interactions.

DISEASE INTERACTIONS
Caution is advised when taking timolol. Consult your doctor if you have any of the following: asthma, emphysema or another lung disease, low blood sugar, heart disease, blood vessel disease, or an overactive thyroid. In diabetes, timolol can affect blood sugar levels or mask symptoms of low blood sugar.

Timolol Maleate Oral

Generic 5 mg
(GENEVA)

▶ Drug Class: Beta-blocker

▶ Available in: Tablets

▶ Available OTC? No

▶ As Generic? Yes

Side Effects

SERIOUS
Shortness of breath, wheezing; irregular or slow heartbeat (50 beats per minute or less); pain or feelings of tightness or pressure in the chest; swelling of the ankles, feet, and lower legs; mental depression. If you experience any such symptoms, stop taking timolol and contact your doctor right away.

COMMON
Dizziness or lightheadedness, especially when rising suddenly to a standing position; decreased sexual ability; unusual fatigue, weakness, or drowsiness; insomnia.

LESS COMMON
Anxiety, irritability, nervousness; constipation; diarrhea; dry, sore eyes; itching; nausea or vomiting; nightmares or intensely vivid dreams; numbness, tingling, or other unusual sensations in the fingers, toes, or scalp.

PRINCIPAL USES
To treat high blood pressure; to prevent recurrence of and lower mortality from heart attack; to prevent migraine headaches.

HOW THE DRUG WORKS
Beta-blockers such as timolol work by preventing—or blocking—nerve impulses from exerting an accelerating or intensifying effect on specific parts of the body, especially blood vessels and the heart. This slows the heart and widens the vessels, thus lowering blood pressure. By relaxing blood vessels in the brain, timolol also helps prevent migraines.

DOSAGE
For high blood pressure: 10 mg, 2 times a day; may be increased to a maximum of 60 mg per day. After heart attack: 10 mg, 2 times a day. Migraine headache prevention: 10 mg, 2 times a day; may be increased to 30 mg per day.

ONSET OF EFFECT
Within 15 to 30 minutes.

DURATION OF ACTION
Up to 12 hours.

DIETARY ADVICE
Timolol can be taken with meals to minimize the risk of stomach upset.

STORAGE
Store in a tightly sealed container away from heat and direct light.

IF YOU MISS A DOSE
Take it as soon as you remember. If it is near the time for the next dose, skip the missed dose and resume your regular dosage schedule. Do not double the next dose.

STOPPING THE DRUG
Do not discontinue the drug suddenly, as this may cause serious health problems. The dosage must be gradually tapered in accordance with your physician's instructions.

PROLONGED USE
Lifelong therapy with timolol may be necessary. Visit your doctor regularly if you take it for a prolonged period.

PRECAUTIONS
Over 60: Adverse reactions may be more likely and more severe. Resistance to cold temperatures may be decreased in older patients.

Driving and Hazardous Work: Do not drive or engage in hazardous work until you determine how the medicine affects you.

Alcohol: Avoid alcohol.

Pregnancy: Discuss with your doctor the relative risks and benefits of using this drug while pregnant.

Breast Feeding: Timolol passes into breast milk; consult your doctor about its use while nursing.

Infants and Children: The dosage must be determined by your pediatrician.

Special Concerns: Take extra care during exercise or hot weather to avoid dizziness and fainting. Check your pulse regularly while taking timolol. If it is slower than your usual rate or less than 50 beats a minute, check with your doctor.

OVERDOSE
Symptoms: Unusually slow or rapid heartbeat, severe dizziness or fainting, poor circulation in the hands (bluish skin), breathing difficulty, seizures.

What to Do: Call your doctor, emergency medical services (EMS), or the nearest poison control center immediately.

DRUG INTERACTIONS
Consult your doctor for specific advice if you are taking amphetamines, oral antidiabetic agents, asthma medication (such as aminophylline or theophylline), calcium channel blockers, clonidine, guanabenz, halothane, immunotherapy for allergies (allergy shots), insulin, MAO inhibitors, reserpine, other beta-blockers, or any over-the-counter medicine.

FOOD INTERACTIONS
No known food interactions.

DISEASE INTERACTIONS
Timolol should be used with caution in people with diabetes, especially insulin-dependent diabetes, since the drug may mask symptoms of hypoglycemia. People with the following conditions should consult their doctor before using timolol: allergies or asthma, heart or blood vessel disease (including congestive heart failure and peripheral vascular disease), hyperthyroidism, irregular (slow) heartbeat, myasthenia gravis, psoriasis, respiratory problems such as bronchitis or emphysema, kidney or liver disease, or a history of mental depression.

Tioconazole

▶ Drug Class: Antifungal

▶ Available in: Vaginal ointment

▶ Available OTC? Yes

▶ As Generic? No

Side Effects

SERIOUS
Vaginal itching, burning, discharge, or irritation not present prior to treatment. Call your doctor as soon as possible.

COMMON
No common side effects have been reported.

LESS COMMON
Headache, stomach cramps or pain, irritation or burning of sexual partner's penis.

PRINCIPAL USES
To treat fungal (yeast) infections of the vagina.

HOW THE DRUG WORKS
Tioconazole prevents the growth and function of some fungal organisms by interfering with the production of substances needed to preserve the cell membrane. This drug is effective only for infections caused by fungal organisms. It will not work for bacterial or viral infections.

DOSAGE
A single 300 mg (1 applicatorful) dose of ointment, inserted with an applicator into the vagina at bedtime.

ONSET OF EFFECT
Some relief may be felt within 1 day. Complete relief of symptoms generally occurs within 7 days.

DURATION OF ACTION
Unknown.

DIETARY ADVICE
Tioconazole may be used without regard to diet.

STORAGE
Store in a tightly sealed container away from heat, moisture, and direct light. Do not allow it to freeze.

IF YOU MISS A DOSE
Not applicable. Tioconazole is usually effective with a single, one-time use.

STOPPING THE DRUG
Tioconazole is generally used on a one-time basis. If needed, a second dose may be applied 1 to 2 weeks following the first dose.

PROLONGED USE
Tioconazole is for short-term use only.

PRECAUTIONS
Over 60: No special problems are expected.

Driving and Hazardous Work: This drug should not impair your ability to perform such tasks safely.

Alcohol: No special precautions are necessary.

Pregnancy: Adequate studies on the use of tioconazole during pregnancy have not been done; however, there are no reports of adverse effects while using it. Consult your doctor.

Breast Feeding: No problems are expected. Consult your doctor before using this medicine while nursing.

Infants and Children: No studies have been done on the use of tioconazole in children. Consult your pediatrician for specific advice.

Special Concerns: Tioconazole may be used with oral contraceptives and antibiotic therapy. Sanitary napkins should be used to prevent staining of clothing. The affected area should be kept cool and dry. The patient should wear loose-fitting cotton clothing and freshly laundered cotton underwear or pantyhose with a cotton crotch. Avoid underwear made from non-ventilating materials. Do not sit for a long time in a wet bathing suit. Avoid feminine hygiene sprays. Wash daily with unscented soap and dry thoroughly with a clean towel. Tampons should not be used during therapy. Do not have sex for 3 days after treatment and wait an additional 3 days before relying upon a condom or diaphragm, since the medication may weaken latex. After this time, the patient's sexual partner should wear a condom during intercourse and should consult a doctor if penile redness, itching, or discomfort occurs. You may use this medicine during your menstrual period. After urination or a bowel movement, cleanse by wiping the area from front to back to prevent reinfection.

OVERDOSE
Symptoms: An overdose with tioconazole is unlikely.

What to Do: If someone should swallow a large amount of the medicine, call your doctor.

DRUG INTERACTIONS
Tell your doctor if you are using any other vaginal prescription or over-the-counter medication.

FOOD INTERACTIONS
No food interactions have been reported.

DISEASE INTERACTIONS
No disease interactions have been reported.

Tizanidine Hydrochloride

▶ Drug Class: Muscle relaxant

▶ Available in: Tablets

▶ Available OTC? No

▶ As Generic? No

Side Effects

SERIOUS
Liver damage causing nausea, vomiting, loss of appetite, and yellowish tinge to eyes and skin (jaundice). Call your doctor immediately.

COMMON
Drowsiness, dry mouth, dizziness, slowed heartbeat, very low blood pressure causing light-headedness when arising from a sitting or lying position.

LESS COMMON
Infection, constipation, rapid heartbeat, vomiting, speech problems, blurred vision, frequent urination, flu syndrome, nervousness, movement difficulties, inflamed mucous membranes, nasal inflammation.

PRINCIPAL USES
To relieve the muscle spasticity and cramping associated with multiple sclerosis and spinal cord injury.

HOW THE DRUG WORKS
Tizanidine is a short-acting drug that temporarily inhibits nerve activity that causes spasticity. Because of the risk of side effects, it should be taken only at times of the day when reduced spasticity is most important.

DOSAGE
Initial dose is 4 mg, every 6 to 8 hours. This may be increased as needed in 2 to 4 mg increments to 8 mg every 6 to 8 hours (not exceeding 3 doses in 24 hours), until a satisfactory therapeutic effect is achieved. Maximum dose is 36 mg a day.

ONSET OF EFFECT
Within 1 hour.

DURATION OF ACTION
Up to 6 hours.

DIETARY ADVICE
It can be taken with or between meals. Dry mouth is a common complaint with such drugs; maintain adequate fluid intake and suck on ice chips if desired.

STORAGE
Store in a tightly sealed container away from heat and direct light.

IF YOU MISS A DOSE
Take it as soon as you remember. If it is near the time for the next dose, skip the missed dose and resume your regular dosage schedule. Do not double the next dose.

STOPPING THE DRUG
The decision to stop taking the drug should be made by your doctor.

PROLONGED USE
You should see your doctor regularly for tests and examinations if you must take this drug for a prolonged period.

PRECAUTIONS
Over 60: Adverse reactions may be more likely and more severe in older patients.

Driving and Hazardous Work: Do not drive or engage in hazardous work until you determine how the medicine affects you.

Alcohol: Avoid alcohol.

Pregnancy: In some animal studies, large doses of tizanidine have been shown to cause problems. Human studies have not been done. This drug should be used during pregnancy only if clearly needed. Consult your doctor for advice.

Breast Feeding: Tizanidine may pass into breast milk; caution is advised. Consult your doctor for advice.

Infants and Children: There is no specific information about the use of tizanidine in infants and children.

Special Concerns: Tizanidine is a newly introduced medication, and it is possible that side effects not found in early studies may occur with widespread use. Patients should be alert for the signs of significantly lowered blood pressure (dizziness, faintness, disorientation). In clinical trials of tizanidine, a small number of patients experienced hallucinations that continued after treatment was stopped. Dose-related eye damage (retinal degeneration and corneal opacities) was detected in some animal studies but has not been seen in human clinical trials.

OVERDOSE
Symptoms: Loss of consciousness and respiratory depression have been noted thus far in limited experience with the drug. Other symptoms may occur.

What to Do: If apparent overdose occurs, call your doctor, emergency medical services (EMS), or the nearest poison control center immediately.

DRUG INTERACTIONS
Consult your doctor for specific advice if you are taking oral contraceptives or any other prescription or over-the-counter medication, especially those that produce sedation as a side effect, such as benzodiazepine tranquilizers and baclofen, or medications that are used for lowering high blood pressure.

FOOD INTERACTIONS
No known food interactions.

DISEASE INTERACTIONS
Caution is advised when taking tizanidine. Consult your doctor if you have any other medical condition. Tizanidine may cause complications in patients with kidney disease, since the kidneys are involved in the removal of the drug from the body.

Tobramycin

▶ Drug Class: Aminoglycoside antibiotic

▶ Available in: Injection, ophthalmic solution and ointment, inhalation

▶ Available OTC? No

▶ As Generic? Yes

Side Effects

SERIOUS
Loss of balance, dizziness; ringing, buzzing, or feeling of fullness in the ears, any loss of hearing; increased thirst, greatly decreased or increased amount of urine or frequency of urination, loss of appetite, nausea or vomiting; muscle twitching or seizures; skin rash, itching, redness, or swelling (especially around the eye or eyelid) not present prior to treatment. Call your doctor immediately.

COMMON
Ophthalmic ointment: Temporary blurred vision immediately following administration.

LESS COMMON
Ophthalmic forms: Stinging or burning of the eyes.

PRINCIPAL USES
To treat a variety of bacterial infections including those of the bones and joints, central nervous system, the abdominal cavity, eyes, lungs, skin and soft tissue, urinary tract, and the blood. Tobramycin is also used in the management of lung infections in patients with cystic fibrosis.

HOW THE DRUG WORKS
Tobramycin interferes with bacteria's genetic material—specifically its RNA, which is necessary in the manufacture of proteins. Without the ability to manufacture protein, the bacteria cannot survive.

DOSAGE
Standard dose for most infections— Injection: Dosage depends on the weight of the patient and the infection being treated. Mild eye infections— Adults and teenagers: 1 drop of solution in the affected eye every 4 hours or a thin strip of ointment applied every 8 to 12 hours. Severe eye infections— Apply the solution or ointment every 3 to 4 hours until improvement occurs, then adjust the frequency of doses as directed by your doctor. Lung infections in those with cystic fibrosis— Injection: Initially, 10 mg per 2.2 lbs (1 kg) of body weight a day in 4 divided doses. Inhalation: 300 mg (1 single-use ampule) 2 times a day for 28 days. Stop therapy for 28 days, and then resume therapy for the next 28 days. Inhalations should be taken as close to 12 hours apart as possible and not less than 6 hours apart.

ONSET OF EFFECT
Variable.

DURATION OF ACTION
Variable.

DIETARY ADVICE
Drink plenty of fluids.

STORAGE
Store in a tightly sealed container away from heat and direct light. Refrigerate the inhalation form.

IF YOU MISS A DOSE
Take it as soon as you remember. If it is near the time (within 6 hours for the inhalation) for the next dose, skip the missed dose and resume your regular dosage schedule. Do not double the next dose.

STOPPING THE DRUG
Take as prescribed for the full treatment period, even if your symptoms subside.

PROLONGED USE
Periodic kidney function tests may be needed. Consult your doctor if your condition does not improve after 7 days, or 1 to 3 days for eye infections.

PRECAUTIONS
Over 60: Adverse reactions may be more likely and more severe.

Driving and Hazardous Work: Avoid such activities until you determine how the medicine affects you.

Alcohol: Avoid alcohol.

Pregnancy: Discuss with your doctor the relative risks and benefits of using this drug while pregnant. Some studies show that injectable tobramycin may cause damage to the infant's hearing, sense of balance, and kidneys. However, this medication may be necessary for the mother.

Breast Feeding: Tobramycin may pass into breast milk; caution is advised. Consult your doctor for advice.

Infants and Children: Tobramycin may be used by infants and children with proper doses.

Special Concerns: To use the eye drops or the ointment, first wash your hands. Tilt your head back. Gently apply pressure to the inside corner of the eyelid and with the index finger of the same hand, pull downward on the lower eyelid to make a space. Drop the medicine or put a short strip of ointment (about ⅓ inch long) into this space and close your eye. Apply pressure for 1 or 2 minutes while keeping the eye closed. Wash hands again. Make sure the tip of the dropper or applicator does not touch your eye, finger, or any other surface.

OVERDOSE
Symptoms: Injection: Decreased urine output, blood in the urine, swelling of the ankles or other body parts, impaired muscle control, severe breathing difficulty. Ophthalmic forms: Eye pain and redness, increased tear production, swelling and itching of the eyes or eyelids. Inhalation: None reported.

What to Do: Seek medical attention immediately.

DRUG INTERACTIONS
Consult your doctor for specific advice if you are taking any other aminoglycoside, capreomycin, methoxyflurane, polymyxins, cyclosporine, dornase alfa, or vancomycin.

FOOD INTERACTIONS
No known food interactions.

DISEASE INTERACTIONS
Consult your doctor for specific advice if you have loss of hearing or balance, kidney disease, Parkinson's disease, or myasthenia gravis.

Tocainide Hydrochloride

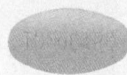

Tonocard 400 mg
(ASTRA MERCK)

▶ Drug Class: Antiarrhythmic

▶ Available in: Tablets

▶ Available OTC? No

▶ As Generic? No

Side Effects

SERIOUS
Fainting; rapid or irregular heartbeats (palpitations); trembling or shaking; severe rash, blisters, peeling or scaling of skin; cough or shortness of breath; fever or chills; unusually slow heartbeat; mouth sores; unusual bleeding or bruising, loss of appetite, unusual anxiety; jaundice (yellowish tinge to skin or whites of eyes); profuse sweating. Call your doctor immediately.

COMMON
Dizziness or lightheadedness, loss of appetite, nausea.

LESS COMMON
Mental confusion, blurred vision, headache, anxiety or irritability, skin rash, sweating, vomiting, numbness or tingling of fingers and toes.

PRINCIPAL USES
To correct irregular heartbeats (cardiac arrhythmias). This drug is used only to treat severe, life-threatening heart rhythm disorders, since it has been shown to cause serious adverse side effects in some patients.

HOW THE DRUG WORKS
Tocainide slows nerve impulses in the heart and reduces the sensitivity of heart tissue to certain nerve impulses, thus stabilizing heartbeat.

DOSAGE
To start, 400 mg every 8 hours. The dose may be increased to 600 mg, 3 times a day. It is best to take doses at equally spaced intervals. Early adverse effects may be decreased by administering the medication in smaller, more frequent doses.

ONSET OF EFFECT
Within 2 hours.

DURATION OF ACTION
Approximately 8 to 11 hours.

DIETARY ADVICE
Tocainide can be taken with food or milk to avoid gastrointestinal upset.

STORAGE
Store in a tightly sealed container in a dry place away from heat and direct light.

IF YOU MISS A DOSE
Take it as soon as you remember. However, if it is near the time for the next dose, skip the missed dose and resume your regular dosage schedule. Do not double the next dose.

STOPPING THE DRUG
Take tocainide as prescribed for the full treatment period, even if you begin to feel better before the scheduled end of therapy. The decision to stop taking the drug should be made by your doctor.

PROLONGED USE
Lifelong therapy may be necessary. See your doctor regularly for examinations and diagnostic tests if you must take this medicine for a prolonged period.

PRECAUTIONS
Over 60: Adverse reactions may be more likely and more severe in older patients.

Driving and Hazardous Work: Avoid such activities until you determine how the medicine affects you.

Alcohol: Avoid alcohol.

Pregnancy: Animal studies have shown that high doses of tocainide can cause fetal deaths. No defects or other problems have been found in humans. Before you take tocainide, tell your doctor if you are pregnant or plan to become pregnant.

Breast Feeding: Tocainide may pass into breast milk; caution is advised. Consult your doctor for advice.

Infants and Children: Studies of tocainide in infants and children have not been done. Use and dose must be determined by your pediatrician.

Special Concerns: Before having any kind of surgery, tell the doctor or dentist in charge that you are taking tocainide. Your doctor may require weekly blood tests for the first 3 weeks of treatment and frequently after that. Tell your doctor if you have any unusual allergic reaction to tocainide or to an anesthetic.

OVERDOSE
Symptoms: Tremors, seizures, heartbeat irregularities, nausea, vomiting, weakness, cardiac arrest.

What to Do: Call your doctor, emergency medical services (EMS), or the nearest poison control center immediately.

DRUG INTERACTIONS
Consult your doctor for specific advice if you are taking rifampin, beta-blockers, or any other prescription or over-the-counter medication.

FOOD INTERACTIONS
No known food interactions.

DISEASE INTERACTIONS
Caution is advised when taking tocainide. Avoid this medication if you have congestive heart failure. Use of tocainide may cause complications in patients with liver or kidney disease, since these organs work together to remove the medication from the body.

Tolazamide

BRAND NAME
Tolinase

Generic 100 mg
(ZENITH)

▶ Drug Class: Antidiabetic
agent/sulfonylurea

▶ Available in: Tablets

▶ Available OTC? No

▶ As Generic? Yes

Side Effects

SERIOUS
Convulsions, fainting, low blood sugar causing anxious feeling, blurred vision, cold sweats, confusion, drowsiness, excessive hunger, rapid heartbeat, headache, nausea, nervousness, restless sleep, shortness of breath, unusual weight gain, unusual bleeding or bruising. Call your doctor at once. Other serious but less common side effects include bone marrow suppression, hemolytic anemia, and elevation of liver-associated enzymes; these problems can be detected by your doctor.

COMMON
Changes in taste, constipation or diarrhea, more frequent urination, headache, heartburn, increased or decreased appetite, nausea, stomach pain or fullness, vomiting.

LESS COMMON
Increased sensitivity of skin to the sun.

PRINCIPAL USES
To help control blood sugar in patients with non-insulin-dependent (type 2) diabetes.

HOW THE DRUG WORKS
Tolazamide stimulates insulin release from the pancreas and reduces glucose output by the liver.

DOSAGE
Adults: 100 to 250 mg once a day to start. It can be increased to 1,000 mg per day. If more than 500 mg per day, tablets are usually taken in 2 doses. Children: The dose must be determined by your doctor.

ONSET OF EFFECT
Within 4 to 6 hours.

DURATION OF ACTION
12 to 24 hours.

DIETARY ADVICE
If 1 dose daily, take it before breakfast. If 2 doses, take one before breakfast and one before dinner.

STORAGE
Store in a tightly sealed container away from heat and direct light.

IF YOU MISS A DOSE
Take it as soon as you remember. If it is near the time for the next dose, skip the missed dose and resume your regular dosage schedule. Do not double the next dose.

STOPPING THE DRUG
The decision to stop taking the drug should be made by your doctor.

PROLONGED USE
At some point, tolazamide may stop working effectively and your blood sugar may go up. Consult your doctor about the need for periodic examinations and blood tests.

PRECAUTIONS
Over 60: Adverse reactions may be more likely and more severe in older patients.

Driving and Hazardous Work: Do not drive or engage in hazardous work until you determine how the medicine affects you.

Alcohol: Alcohol should be avoided while taking this medication.

Pregnancy: Before you take tolazamide, tell your doctor if you are pregnant or plan to become pregnant. This medicine is rarely used during pregnancy (insulin is the treatment of choice for pregnant diabetic women).

Breast Feeding: Tolbutamide may pass into breast milk; caution is advised. Consult your doctor for advice.

Infants and Children: Non-insulin-dependent (type 2) diabetes is rare in infants and children.

Special Concerns: Be sure to carry a card or medical ID bracelet saying that you have this type of diabetes. Follow your prescribed diet closely. Consult your doctor about exercises you should do. Be sure you take your daily dose of tolazamide even when you become ill. You may have to be switched temporarily to insulin. Test your blood sugar level at least every 4 hours when you are ill. Keep some source of quick-acting sugar readily available to handle episodes of low blood sugar.

OVERDOSE
Symptoms: Tingling of lips and tongue, lethargy, confusion, nausea, nervousness, sweating, tremors, hunger, convulsions, loss of consciousness. (Most symptoms of overdose are due to serious hypoglycemia.)

What to Do: Call your doctor, emergency medical services (EMS), or the nearest poison control center immediately.

DRUG INTERACTIONS
Consult your doctor if you are taking anticoagulants, antifungal agents, aspirin, chloramphenicol, cimetidine, ciprofloxacin, quinidine, ranitidine, asparaginase, corticosteroids, lithium, asthma medicine, allergy medicine, beta-blockers, cyclosporine, guanethidine, MAO inhibitors, octreotide, pentamidine, or anticonvulsants.

FOOD INTERACTIONS
Be careful to follow the low-sugar diet prescribed for you by your doctor.

DISEASE INTERACTIONS
Consult your physician if you have any of the following: diarrhea, heart disease, hyperthyroidism, or underactive adrenal or pituitary gland. Use of tolazamide may cause complications in patients with liver or kidney disease, since these organs work together to remove the medication from the body.

Tolbutamide

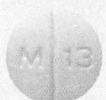

Generic 500 mg
(MYLAN)

▶ Drug Class: Antidiabetic
agent/sulfonylurea

▶ Available in: Tablets

▶ Available OTC? No

▶ As Generic? Yes

Side Effects

SERIOUS
Seizures, fainting, low blood sugar causing anxious feeling, blurred vision, cold sweats, confusion, drowsiness, excessive hunger, fast heartbeat, headache, nausea, nervousness, restless sleep, shortness of breath, unusual weight gain, unusual bleeding or bruising. Call your doctor at once. Other serious but less common side effects include bone marrow suppression, hemolytic anemia, and elevation of liver-associated enzymes; these problems can be detected by your doctor.

COMMON
Changes in taste, constipation or diarrhea, more frequent urination, headache, heartburn, increased or decreased appetite, nausea, stomach pain or fullness, vomiting.

LESS COMMON
Increased sensitivity of skin to the sun.

PRINCIPAL USES
To help control blood sugar in patients with non-insulin-dependent (type 2) diabetes.

HOW THE DRUG WORKS
Tolbutamide stimulates insulin release from the pancreas and reduces glucose output by the liver.

DOSAGE
Adults: 1,000 to 2,000 mg per day to start, in 2 divided doses. It can be increased to 3,000 mg (3 g) a day, although little additional benefit is derived from more than 2 g a day. Children: The dose must be set by a pediatrician.

ONSET OF EFFECT
Within 1 hour.

DURATION OF ACTION
6 to 12 hours.

DIETARY ADVICE
Tolbutamide should be taken 30 minutes before the morning and evening meals.

STORAGE
Store in a tightly sealed container away from heat and direct light.

IF YOU MISS A DOSE
Take it as soon as you remember. If it is near the time for the next dose, skip the missed dose and resume your regular dosage schedule. Do not double the next dose.

STOPPING THE DRUG
The decision to stop taking the drug should be made by your doctor.

PROLONGED USE
At some point, tolbutamide may stop working effectively and your blood sugar may rise unexpectedly. Consult your doctor about the need for periodic examinations and blood tests.

PRECAUTIONS
Over 60: Adverse reactions may be more likely and more severe in older patients.

Driving and Hazardous Work: Do not drive or engage in hazardous work until you determine how the medicine affects you.

Alcohol: Avoid alcohol.

Pregnancy: Before you take tolbutamide, tell your doctor if you are pregnant or plan to become pregnant. This medicine is rarely used during pregnancy.

Breast Feeding: Tolbutamide may pass into breast milk; caution is advised. Consult your doctor for specific advice.

Infants and Children: The safety and effectiveness have not been established for young patients.

Special Concerns: Be sure to carry a card or medical ID bracelet saying that you have this type of diabetes. Follow your prescribed diet closely. Consult your doctor about exercises you should do. Be sure you take your daily dose of tolbutamide even when you become ill. You may have to be switched temporarily to insulin. Test your blood sugar level at least every 4 hours when you are ill.

OVERDOSE
Symptoms: Tingling of lips and tongue, lethargy, confusion, nausea, nervousness, sweating, tremors, hunger, convulsions, loss of consciousness. (Most symptoms of overdose are due to serious hypoglycemia.)

What to Do: Call your doctor, emergency medical services (EMS), or the nearest poison control center immediately.

DRUG INTERACTIONS
Consult your doctor if you are taking anticoagulants, antifungal agents, aspirin, chloramphenicol, cimetidine, ciprofloxacin, quinidine, ranitidine, antiseizure medication, asparaginase, corticosteroids, lithium, asthma medicine, allergy medicine, beta-blockers, cyclosporine, guanethidine, MAO inhibitors, octreotide, or pentamidine.

FOOD INTERACTIONS
Be careful to follow the low-sugar diet as prescribed.

DISEASE INTERACTIONS
Caution is advised when taking tolbutamide. Consult your doctor if you have any of the following: diarrhea, heart disease, overactive thyroid, or underactive adrenal or pituitary gland. Use of tolbutamide may cause complications in patients who have liver or kidney disease, since these organs work together to remove the medication from the body.

Tolcapone

Side Effects

SERIOUS
Liver damage is a significant serious side effect. Symptoms include persistent nausea, fatigue, lethargy, loss of appetite, yellow discoloration of the skin and eyes (jaundice), dark urine, itchiness, and abdominal pain on the right side. Call your doctor immediately. Dizziness, lightheadedness, or fainting, especially when rising from a sitting or lying position, owing to a sudden drop in blood pressure (orthostatic hypotension). Such symptoms, in addition to nausea, are more common at the beginning of therapy.

COMMON
Impaired ability to execute voluntary movements, nausea, sleep difficulties, quirky involuntary muscle movements that contort the body, excessive dreaming, loss of appetite, muscle cramps, drowsiness, diarrhea, confusion, headaches, hallucinations, vomiting.

LESS COMMON
Constipation, increased susceptibility to upper respiratory tract infection, increased incidence of falling, increased sweating, dry mouth, abdominal pain, discolored urine.

PRINCIPAL USES
To treat Parkinson's disease in conjunction with standard levodopa/carbidopa therapy. It should only be used by patients who are experiencing symptom fluctuations and are not responding satisfactorily or those who are inappropriate candidates for other adjunctive therapies.

HOW THE DRUG WORKS
When used with levodopa/carbidopa, tolcapone sustains higher levels of levodopa in the blood. Tolcapone is believed to increase blood levels of levodopa by blocking the action of catechol-O-methyltransferase (COMT), one of the enzymes responsible for breaking down levodopa, before it reaches its receptors in the brain. Levodopa raises the amount of dopamine available in the brain; dopamine plays an essential role in smooth movement of muscles and is deficient in patients with Parkinson's disease.

DOSAGE
Initial dose: 100 mg, 3 times a day in conjunction with levodopa/carbidopa. The first dose of the day should be taken together with levodopa/carbidopa and the remaining doses should be taken 6 and 12 hours later. The dose can be increased to 200 mg 3 times a day if the anticipated increase in benefit is justified. Tolcapone may be taken with either the immediate or the sustained-release forms of levodopa/carbidopa. Many patients may need to reduce their daily dose of levodopa.

ONSET OF EFFECT
Unknown.

DURATION OF ACTION
Unknown.

DIETARY ADVICE
Tolcapone can be taken without regard to meals.

STORAGE
Store in a tightly sealed container away from heat, moisture, and direct light.

IF YOU MISS A DOSE
Take it as soon as you remember. If it is near the time for the next dose, skip the missed dose and resume your regular dosage schedule. Do not double the next dose.

STOPPING THE DRUG
Take it as prescribed for the full treatment period. The decision to stop taking the drug should be made in consultation with your physician.

PROLONGED USE
Liver function tests are strongly recommended just prior to treatment, every 2 weeks for the first year of therapy, every 4 weeks for the next 6 months, and then every 8 weeks thereafter if you must take this medicine for a prolonged period.

PRECAUTIONS
Over 60: Adverse reactions may be more likely and more severe in older patients.

Driving and Hazardous Work: Do not drive or engage in hazardous work until you determine how the medicine affects you.

Alcohol: Avoid alcohol.

Pregnancy: Adequate human studies have not been done. Before taking tolcapone, tell your doctor if you are or are planning to become pregnant. Discuss with your doctor the relative risks and benefits of using this drug while pregnant.

Breast Feeding: Tolcapone may pass into breast milk; caution is advised. Consult your doctor for specific advice.

Infants and Children: Not applicable. No potential use for tolcapone has been identified in children.

Special Concerns: If tolcapone does does not provide significant benefit within three weeks of the initiation of treatment, therapy should be discontinued. Your doctor should be thoroughly familiar with tolcapone and should ask you to sign a patient consent form that helps spell out the risks of taking this medication.

OVERDOSE
Symptoms: An overdose with tolcapone is unlikely. However, nausea, vomiting, and dizziness or fainting may occur with an excessive dose.

What to Do: If someone takes a much larger dose than prescribed, seek medical attention immediately.

DRUG INTERACTIONS
Consult your doctor for specific advice if you are taking any of the following drugs, which may interact with tolcapone: desipramine, MAO inhibitor antidepressants (such as phenelzine sulfate or tranylcypromine sulfate, but not selegiline), or antihypertensive drugs.

FOOD INTERACTIONS
No known food interactions.

DISEASE INTERACTIONS
Do not use tolcapone if you have liver disease or have had a prior reaction to tolcapone. Caution is advised for patients with low blood pressure or severe kidney dysfunction.

Tolmetin Sodium

BRAND NAMES
Tolectin, Tolectin DS

Generic 600 mg
(PUREPAC)

▶ Drug Class: Nonsteroidal anti-inflammatory drug (NSAID)

▶ Available in: Tablets, capsules

▶ Available OTC? No

▶ As Generic? Yes

Side Effects

SERIOUS
Shortness of breath or wheezing, with or without swelling of legs or other signs of heart failure; chest pain; peptic ulcer disease with vomiting of blood; black, tarry stools; decreasing kidney function. Call your doctor immediately.

COMMON
Nausea, vomiting, heartburn, diarrhea, constipation, headache, dizziness, sleepiness.

LESS COMMON
Ulcers or sores in mouth, depression, rashes or blistering of skin, ringing sound in the ears, unusual tingling or numbness of the hands or feet, seizures, blurred vision. Also elevated potassium levels, decreased blood counts; such problems can be detected by your doctor.

PRINCIPAL USES
To treat mild to moderate pain and inflammation caused by tendinitis, arthritis, bursitis, gout, soft tissue injuries, migraine and other vascular headaches, menstrual cramps, and other conditions. When patients fail to respond to one NSAID, another may be tried. The greatest effectiveness often requires trial and error of several different NSAIDs.

HOW THE DRUG WORKS
NSAIDs work by interfering with the formation of prostaglandins, naturally occurring substances in the body that cause inflammation and make nerves more sensitive to pain impulses. NSAIDs also have other modes of action that are less well understood.

DOSAGE
Adults: 400 mg, 3 times a day. Maximum dose is 1,800 mg a day. Children: Consult your pediatrician.

ONSET OF EFFECT
From 30 minutes to several hours or longer.

DURATION OF ACTION
Varies.

DIETARY ADVICE
Take with food; maintain your usual food and fluid intake.

STORAGE
Store in a tightly sealed container away from heat, moisture, and direct light.

IF YOU MISS A DOSE
Take it as soon as you remember. If it is near the time for the next dose, skip the missed dose and resume your regular dosage schedule. Do not double the next dose.

STOPPING THE DRUG
The decision to stop taking the drug should be made in consultation with your physician.

PROLONGED USE
Prolonged use can cause gastrointestinal problems, including ulceration and bleeding, kidney dysfunction, and liver inflammation. Consult your doctor about the need for medical examinations and laboratory tests.

PRECAUTIONS
Over 60: Because of the potentially greater consequences of gastrointestinal side effects, the dose of NSAIDs for older patients, especially those over age 70, is often cut in half.

Driving and Hazardous Work: Avoid such activities until you determine how the medicine affects you.

Alcohol: Avoid alcohol when using this medication because it increases the risk of stomach irritation.

Pregnancy: Avoid or discontinue this drug if you are pregnant or are planning to become pregnant.

Breast Feeding: Tolmetin passes into breast milk; avoid use while nursing.

Infants and Children: May be used in exceptional circumstances; consult your doctor.

Special Concerns: Because NSAIDs can interfere with blood coagulation, this drug should be stopped at least 3 days prior to any surgery.

OVERDOSE
Symptoms: Severe nausea, vomiting, headache, confusion, seizures.

What to Do: Call your doctor, emergency medical services (EMS), or the nearest poison control center immediately.

DRUG INTERACTIONS
Do not take this drug with aspirin or any other NSAIDs without your doctor's approval. In addition, consult your doctor if you are taking antihypertensives, steroids, anticoagulants, antibiotics, itraconazole or ketoconazole, plicamycin, penicillamine, valproic acid, phenytoin, cyclosporine, digitalis drugs, lithium, methotrexate, probenecid, triamterene, or zidovudine.

FOOD INTERACTIONS
No known food interactions.

DISEASE INTERACTIONS
Consult your doctor if you have any of the following: bleeding problems, inflammation or ulcers of the stomach and intestines, diabetes mellitus, systemic lupus erythematosus (SLE, lupus), anemia, asthma, epilepsy, Parkinson's disease, kidney stones, or a history of heart disease or alcohol abuse. Use of tolmetin may cause complications in patients with liver or kidney disease, since these organs work together to remove the medication from the body.

Tolnaftate

BRAND NAMES
Aftate, Genaspore, NP-27,
Tinactin, Ting, Zeasorb-AF

▶ Drug Class: Topical antifungal

▶ Available in: Cream, gel, powder, solution

▶ Available OTC? Yes

▶ As Generic? Yes

Side Effects

SERIOUS
Skin irritation that was not present before use of tolnaftate. Call your doctor immediately.

COMMON
No common side effects have been reported.

LESS COMMON
No less-common side effects have been reported.

PRINCIPAL USES
To treat a variety of fungal infections of the skin, including tinea corporis (ringworm), tinea cruris (jock itch), and tinea pedis (athlete's foot).

HOW THE DRUG WORKS
Tolnaftate prevents fungi from manufacturing vital substances required for growth and function. This medication is effective only for infections caused by ringworm fungal organisms. It will not work for bacterial or viral infections.

DOSAGE
Apply to the affected area 2 times a day. All forms should be used immediately after the affected area is washed and dried. Wash your hands before and after application.

ONSET OF EFFECT
Unknown.

DURATION OF ACTION
Unknown.

DIETARY ADVICE
No special restrictions.

STORAGE
Store in a tightly sealed container away from heat, moisture, and direct light.

IF YOU MISS A DOSE
Apply it as soon as you remember. If it is near the time for the next dose, skip the missed dose and resume your regular dosage schedule. Do not double the next dose.

STOPPING THE DRUG
Use of tolnaftate should continue for 2 weeks beyond the time that symptoms disappear. This helps to ensure eradication of the fungus.

PROLONGED USE
You should consult your doctor if symptoms do not improve within 10 days of beginning therapy.

PRECAUTIONS
Over 60: No special problems are expected.

Driving and Hazardous Work: The use of tolnaftate should not impair your ability to perform such tasks safely.

Alcohol: No special precautions are necessary.

Pregnancy: Tolnaftate has not been shown in studies to cause problems when used during pregnancy.

Breast Feeding: Tolnaftate may pass into breast milk, but no problems have been reported. Consult your doctor for specific advice.

Infants and Children: Tolnaftate should be used by children under the age of 2 years only under a doctor's close supervision.

Special Concerns: Do not allow tolnaftate to come into contact with your eyes. If your skin condition does not improve or instead gets worse after 10 days of treatment, consult your doctor. Tolnaftate should not be used alone to treat fungal infections of the hair or nails; your doctor will prescribe an additional medication. If you are using tolnaftate for an infection of the feet, be sure to wear well-fitting and well-ventilated shoes and to change your shoes and socks every day. Do not cover the treated area of skin with bandages unless your doctor instructs you to do so.

OVERDOSE
Symptoms: None are known; no cases of overdose have been reported.

What to Do: An overdose of tolnaftate is unlikely to occur. However, if someone accidentally ingests some of the medication, call your doctor, emergency medical services (EMS), or the nearest poison control center immediately.

DRUG INTERACTIONS
Some drugs may interact adversely with tolnaftate. Consult your doctor for specific advice if you are taking any other prescription or over-the-counter medication that is applied to the same area of skin being treated by tolnaftate.

FOOD INTERACTIONS
No known food interactions.

DISEASE INTERACTIONS
Caution is advised when taking tolnaftate. Consult your doctor for specific advice if you have a history of any other skin condition.

Tolterodine Tartrate

BRAND NAME
Detrol

▶ Drug Class: Anticholinergic

▶ Available in: Tablets

▶ Available OTC? No

▶ As Generic? No

Side Effects

SERIOUS
Chest pain. Consult your doctor immediately.

COMMON
Headache, constipation, indigestion, dry eye, dry mouth.

LESS COMMON
Numbness, tingling or prickling sensation, abdominal pain, flatulence, nausea or vomiting, bronchitis, cough, dry skin, nervousness, drowsiness, blurred vision.

PRINCIPAL USES
To treat overactive bladder with symptoms of urinary frequency, urgency, or urge incontinence.

HOW THE DRUG WORKS
Tolterodine decreases the urge to urinate by blocking nerve receptors that trigger contractions of the bladder.

DOSAGE
Adults: 2 mg, twice a day. Dose may be lowered by your doctor to 1 mg, twice a day, depending upon response to the medication. Adults with impaired liver function: no more than 1 mg, twice a day.

ONSET OF EFFECT
Unknown.

DURATION OF ACTION
Unknown.

DIETARY ADVICE
Tolterodine can be taken without regard to diet.

STORAGE
Store in a tightly sealed container away from heat, moisture, and direct light.

IF YOU MISS A DOSE
Take it as soon as you remember. If it is near the time for the next dose, skip the missed dose and resume your regular dosage schedule. Do not double the next dose.

STOPPING THE DRUG
The decision to stop taking the drug should be made in consultation with your physician.

PROLONGED USE
See your doctor periodically if you must take this drug for a prolonged period.

PRECAUTIONS
Over 60: No special problems are expected.

Driving and Hazardous Work: The use of tolterodine should not impair your ability to perform such tasks safely.

Alcohol: No special problems are expected.

Pregnancy: No human studies have been done. Before taking tolterodine, tell your doctor if you are pregnant or plan to become pregnant.

Breast Feeding: Tolterodine may pass into breast milk; avoid use while nursing. Consult your doctor for specific advice.

Infants and Children: Not recommended for use by children under the age of 18.

OVERDOSE
Symptoms: Drowsiness, mental confusion, dizziness, loss of coordination, dry mouth.

What to Do: Few cases of overdose have been reported. However, if someone takes a much larger dose than prescribed, call your doctor, emergency medical services (EMS), or the nearest poison control center immediately.

DRUG INTERACTIONS
The following drugs may interact with tolterodine. Consult your doctor for specific advice if you are taking fluoxetine, macrolide antibiotics, or antifungal drugs.

FOOD INTERACTIONS
No known food interactions.

DISEASE INTERACTIONS
You should not take tolterodine if you have: urinary retention, gastric retention, or uncontrolled narrow-angle glaucoma. Tolterodine should be used with caution in patients with liver or kidney disease, since these organs work together to remove the medication from the body.

Topiramate

Side Effects

SERIOUS
Intense pain in the kidney area (the lower back or flanks) may be a sign of kidney stones, which occur with greater frequency in those taking topiramate.

COMMON
Drowsiness, fatigue, dizziness, anxiety, loss of coordination, unusual eye movements, tingling sensations, confusion, speech problems, depression, poor concentration or attention, mood changes, memory impairment, poor appetite, weight loss, tremor.

LESS COMMON
Back pain, nausea and vomiting, indigestion, dry mouth, abdominal pain, constipation, muscle aches, hearing difficulty, menstrual irregularities, sinus infections, double vision. Many additional side effects can occur; consult your doctor if you are concerned about any adverse or unusual reactions you experience while taking this drug.

PRINCIPAL USES
To help control certain types of seizures in the treatment of epilepsy and other disorders. It is often used in conjunction with other anticonvulsant drugs after they have failed to be effective on their own.

HOW THE DRUG WORKS
Topiramate appears to block the uncontrolled firing of neurons that causes seizures, but its precise mechanism of action is unknown.

DOSAGE
Adults: 100 to 400 mg a day, in 2 divided doses. Some patients require higher doses. Initially, a low dose is prescribed; it may then be gradually increased by your doctor. Children ages 2 to 16: 5 to 9 mg per 2.2 lbs (1 kg) a day, in 2 divided doses. As with adults, dosage may be adjusted by a doctor on an individual basis.

ONSET OF EFFECT
Several hours.

DURATION OF ACTION
Maximum effectiveness lasts 24 hours or longer; effectiveness then gradually decreases.

DIETARY ADVICE
Take it with food or milk to minimize stomach upset. Because of their bitter taste, tablets should be swallowed whole, without breaking, crushing, or chewing. Capsules may be swallowed whole or opened and the contents sprinkled on a small amount (one teaspoon) of soft food to make the drug more palatable. It should be swallowed immediately, without chewing.

STORAGE
Store in a tightly sealed container away from heat, moisture, and direct light.

IF YOU MISS A DOSE
Take it as soon as you remember. If it is near the time for the next dose, skip the missed dose and resume your regular dosage schedule. Do not double the next dose unless so advised by your doctor.

STOPPING THE DRUG
Never stop this drug abruptly, because seizures may ensue. The dose is typically tapered over a period of weeks to months under your doctor's supervision.

PROLONGED USE
This drug may be taken on a long-term basis. See your doctor regularly for tests.

PRECAUTIONS
Over 60: Older patients may require lower doses to minimize side effects.

Driving and Hazardous Work: Avoid such activities until you determine how this medication affects you.

Alcohol: May contribute to excessive drowsiness.

Pregnancy: Topiramate has caused birth defects in animal studies. Human studies with this drug have not been done, but other anticonvulsants are known to increase the risk of birth defects. However, seizures during pregnancy can also increase the risks to the fetus. Discuss with your doctor the potential risks and benefits of using this drug during pregnancy. Folate supplementation is advised starting 1 to 2 months before conception and throughout pregnancy.

Breast Feeding: Topiramate may pass into breast milk, although at low levels. Consult your doctor for advice.

Infants and Children: Special caution is advised in children. Use of the drug in children has been limited.

Special Concerns: Because this drug may predispose to the formation of kidney stones, you should drink plenty of fluids while taking it. Your doctor may suggest that you carry an ID card or bracelet saying that you are taking this medication.

OVERDOSE
Symptoms: No specific symptoms of overdose have been reported.

What to Do: Call your doctor, emergency medical services (EMS), or the nearest poison control center immediately.

DRUG INTERACTIONS
Topiramate interacts with a number of other drugs, including other anticonvulsants (carbamazepine, phenytoin, valproic acid); carbonic anhydrase inhibitors, such as acetazolamide or dichlorphenamide; and digoxin. This drug can interfere with oral contraceptives, leading to contraceptive failure.

FOOD INTERACTIONS
No known food interactions.

DISEASE INTERACTIONS
Special caution is advised if you have liver disease or kidney disease, including a history of kidney stones or hemodialysis.

Toremifene Citrate

BRAND NAME
Fareston

▶ Drug Class: Antiestrogen; antineoplastic (anticancer) agent

▶ Available in: Tablets

▶ Available OTC? No

▶ As Generic? No

Side Effects

SERIOUS
Vaginal bleeding, cataracts or other eye problems.

COMMON
Hot flashes, sweating, nausea, vaginal discharge, dizziness.

LESS COMMON
Swelling in the extremities, vomiting.

PRINCIPAL USES
To treat metastatic breast cancer in postmenopausal women.

HOW THE DRUG WORKS
Toremifene blocks the effects of the hormone estrogen by interfering with the binding of estrogen to its receptors on estrogen-sensitive cells. The growth of some breast tumors is stimulated by estrogens; toremifene may therefore slow the growth of such tumors.

DOSAGE
60 mg once a day.

ONSET OF EFFECT
Unknown.

DURATION OF ACTION
Unknown.

DIETARY ADVICE
Toremifene can be taken without regard to meals. Maintain adequate food and fluid intake, since calorie, protein, and vitamin needs increase in patients with cancer.

STORAGE
Store in a tightly sealed container away from heat, moisture, and direct light.

IF YOU MISS A DOSE
Toremifene is prescribed for once-daily use only. If you are unable to take the medication on a particular day, simply resume your regular dosage schedule the following day. Do not double the next dose.

STOPPING THE DRUG
You may need to remain on this medication for an extended period, and you should take toremifene exactly as prescribed throughout the course of treatment. The decision to stop taking the drug should be made in consultation with your physician. Do not stop taking toremifene on your own.

PROLONGED USE
There is no standard duration of therapy with toremifene, although you can expect to remain on it for at least several weeks in order to determine if it is effective. Your doctor will decide whether your response to the drug is satisfactory or not, and will recommend continuation or discontinuation of therapy.

PRECAUTIONS
Over 60: No special problems are expected.

Driving and Hazardous Work: The use of toremifene should not impair your ability to perform such tasks safely.

Alcohol: No special precautions are necessary.

Pregnancy: Toremifene must not be used in pregnant women. Although toremifene is not generally prescribed for premenopausal women, it is important that patients be sure they are not pregnant before starting treatment with this drug.

Breast Feeding: Use of this drug is not recommended while nursing; the benefits must clearly outweigh potential risks. Consult your doctor for advice.

Infants and Children: Use of toremifene is not approved for infants and children.

Special Concerns: Patients with cancer are very often weakened by their illness, by poor nutrition, and by the effects of chemotherapy, radiation, and surgery. Such patients are more likely to experience undesirable side effects of a medication. In addition, these side effects may be more pronounced. Follow all medication directions carefully. Some women with metastases to bone may develop musculoskeletal pain and elevated levels of blood calcium during the first week of treatment.

OVERDOSE
Symptoms: No cases of overdose have been reported.

What to Do: An overdose is unlikely; however, if you have any reason to suspect that one has occurred, call emergency medical services (EMS) to receive evaluation and treatment in the closest emergency facility.

DRUG INTERACTIONS
Consult your doctor for specific advice if you are taking thiazide diuretics or warfarin, which may interact with toremifene.

FOOD INTERACTIONS
No known food interactions.

DISEASE INTERACTIONS
Toremifene should not be used in women with a history of thromboembolic disease. Long-term treatment is not generally advised in women with preexisting endometrial hyperplasia.

Torsemide

Demadex 10 mg
(BOEHRINGER MANNHEIM)

807

Additional photographs

▶ Drug Class: Loop diuretic

▶ Available in: Tablets, injection

▶ Available OTC? No

▶ As Generic? No

Side Effects

SERIOUS
Skin rash, hives, intense itching, swelling of the mouth and throat, breathing difficulty, heart rhythm irregularities, lightheadedness, unusual bleeding or bruising, black or tarry stools. Call your doctor immediately.

COMMON
Muscle cramps or pain. Potassium depletion may lead to heart palpitations and weakness. Fluid depletion may lead to dizziness, especially upon arising from a sitting or lying position, as well as thirst, dry mouth, and constipation.

LESS COMMON
Buzzing or ringing in ears, loss of hearing (particularly after intravenous treatment or with very high doses), diarrhea, loss of appetite, gout, increased blood sugar (a problem for diabetic patients).

PRINCIPAL USES
To reduce fluid (salt and water) accumulation that leads to edema (swelling of body tissues) and breathlessness in patients with heart disease, liver disease, and kidney disease. Torsemide is also sometimes prescribed to help control high blood pressure.

HOW THE DRUG WORKS
Loop diuretics work on a specific portion of the kidney (the loop of Henle) to increase the excretion of water and sodium (and other salts) in the urine.

DOSAGE
For high blood pressure—Tablets: 5 to 10 mg once a day. The dose may be increased as determined by your doctor. For eliminating excess body water (edema)— Tablets: 5 to 60 mg once a day. Injection: 5 to 20 mg, injected once a day. The dose may be increased.

ONSET OF EFFECT
For injection, 10 minutes; for tablets, 1 hour.

DURATION OF ACTION
6 to 8 hours.

DIETARY ADVICE
Take it with or after meals to reduce stomach irritation.

STORAGE
Store in a tightly sealed container away from heat and direct light.

IF YOU MISS A DOSE
Take it as soon as you remember. If it is near the time for the next dose, skip the missed dose and resume your regular dosage schedule. Do not double the next dose.

STOPPING THE DRUG
The decision to stop taking the drug should be made by your doctor.

PROLONGED USE
See your doctor regularly if you must take this medicine for a prolonged period.

PRECAUTIONS
Over 60: No special precautions are warranted.

Driving and Hazardous Work: The use of this drug should not impair your ability to perform such tasks safely.

Alcohol: No special precautions are necessary.

Pregnancy: Human studies have not been done. Consult your doctor about taking torsemide during pregnancy.

Breast Feeding: Torsemide may pass into breast milk; caution is advised. Consult your doctor for advice.

Infants and Children: There is no specific information on the use of torsemide in infants and children. Use and dose must be determined by a pediatrician.

Special Concerns: If you take torsemide for high blood pressure, follow your doctor's advice on diet and weight control. This medicine may cause your body to lose potassium. Consult your doctor about eating potassium-rich foods or taking a supplement.

OVERDOSE
Symptoms: Dehydration, palpitations or heartbeat irregularities, weakness, dizziness, confusion, vomiting, cramps, loss of consciousness.

What to Do: Call your doctor, emergency medical services (EMS), or the nearest poison control center immediately.

DRUG INTERACTIONS
Consult your doctor for specific advice if you are taking any ACE inhibitor, antibiotics, amphotericin B, carmustine, cisplatin, corticosteroids, corticotropin, cyclosporine, deferoxamine, dichlorphenamide, digitalis drugs, lithium, methazolamide, methotrexate, penicillamine, gold salts, pentamidine, streptozocin, tiopronin, or vitamin B12.

FOOD INTERACTIONS
No known food interactions.

DISEASE INTERACTIONS
Caution is advised when taking torsemide. Consult your doctor for advice if you have diabetes, gout, or a hearing problem, or have had a recent heart attack.

Tramadol Hydrochloride

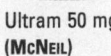

Ultram 50 mg
(McNEIL)

▶ Drug Class: Analgesic

▶ Available in: Tablets

▶ Available OTC? No

▶ As Generic? No

Side Effects

SERIOUS
Blurred vision, difficulty urinating, frequent urge to urinate, blisters under the skin, change in walking balance, dizziness or lightheadedness when getting up, fainting, fast heartbeat, memory loss, hallucinations, shortness of breath. Also numbness, tingling, pain, or weakness in hands or feet; redness, swelling, and itching of skin; trembling and shaking of hands or feet; trouble performing routine tasks. Call your doctor immediately.

COMMON
Dizziness, vertigo, headache, drowsiness, nausea, vomiting, constipation.

LESS COMMON
Weakness, lack of energy, anxiety, confusion, euphoria, nervousness, insomnia, visual disturbances, stomach upset, dry mouth, diarrhea, abdominal pain, loss of appetite, gas, menopausal symptoms, sweating, muscle spasm, rash.

PRINCIPAL USES
To help manage moderate to somewhat severe pain, such as that which occurs following joint surgery and certain gynecological procedures (for example, cesarean section).

HOW THE DRUG WORKS
Tramadol acts on the central nervous system to block the transmission of pain signals. It works similarly to narcotic analgesics, and while not a narcotic, it can be habit-forming, leading to mental and physical drug dependence.

DOSAGE
1 or 2 tablets (50 mg each) every 6 hours as needed. For severe pain, your doctor may prescribe 2 tablets for the first dose.

ONSET OF EFFECT
Usually within 1 hour, with a peak effect at 2 hours.

DURATION OF ACTION
6 to 7 hours.

DIETARY ADVICE
Tramadol can be taken with or without food.

STORAGE
Store in a tightly sealed container away from heat and direct light.

IF YOU MISS A DOSE
Take it as soon as you remember. However, if it is near the time for the next dose, skip the missed dose and resume your regular dosage schedule. Do not double the next dose.

STOPPING THE DRUG
The decision to stop taking the drug should be made by your doctor.

PROLONGED USE
You should see your doctor regularly for tests and examinations if you must take this drug for a prolonged period of time.

PRECAUTIONS
Over 60: Tramadol stays longer in the body of older patients than younger ones; your doctor may adjust the dose accordingly.

Driving and Hazardous Work: Do not drive or engage in hazardous work until you determine how the medicine affects you.

Alcohol: Do not consume alcohol while taking this medication since it may compound the drug's sedative effect on the central nervous system.

Pregnancy: Tramadol has caused birth defects and other problems in animals. Human studies have not been done. Before you take tramadol, tell your doctor if you are pregnant or are planning to become pregnant.

Breast Feeding: Tramadol passes into breast milk; avoid or discontinue use while nursing.

Infants and Children: Safety and effectiveness have not been established for the use of tramadol in children under 16 years old.

Special Concerns: Before undergoing any kind of surgery, including dental surgery, be sure your doctor or dentist knows that you are taking tramadol.

OVERDOSE
Symptoms: Breathing difficulty, seizures, vomiting.

What to Do: Call your doctor, emergency medical services (EMS), or the nearest poison control center immediately.

DRUG INTERACTIONS
Consult your doctor for specific advice if you are taking carbamazepine, anesthetics, MAO inhibitors, or any drugs known to depress the central nervous system, including antihistamines, sedatives, tranquilizers, sleeping pills, other prescription pain medicines, barbiturates, medications for seizures, or muscle relaxants.

FOOD INTERACTIONS
No known food interactions.

DISEASE INTERACTIONS
Caution is advised when taking tramadol. Consult your doctor if you have severe abdominal or stomach conditions, or a history of alcohol abuse, drug abuse, head injury, or seizure disorders. Use of tramadol may cause complications in patients with liver or kidney disease, since these organs work together to remove the medication from the body.

Trandolapril

Mavic 1 mg
(KNOLL)

▶ Drug Class: Angiotensin-converting enzyme (ACE) inhibitor

▶ Available in: Tablet

▶ Available OTC? No

▶ As Generic? No

Side Effects

SERIOUS
Fever and chills, sore throat and hoarseness, sudden difficulty breathing or swallowing, swelling of the face, mouth, or extremities, impaired kidney function (ankle swelling, decreased urination), confusion, yellow discoloration of the eyes or skin (indicating liver disorder), intense itching, chest pain or palpitations, abdominal pain. Serious side effects are very rare; contact your doctor immediately.

COMMON
Dry, persistent cough.

LESS COMMON
Dizziness or fainting, skin rash, numbness or tingling in the hands, feet, or lips, unusual fatigue or muscle weakness, nausea, drowsiness, loss of taste, headache.

PRINCIPAL USES
To control high blood pressure; to treat congestive heart failure; to treat patients with left ventricular dysfunction (damage to the pumping chamber of the heart); and to minimize further kidney damage in diabetics with mild kidney disease.

HOW THE DRUG WORKS
Angiotensin-converting enzyme (ACE) inhibitors block an enzyme that produces angiotensin, a naturally occurring substance that causes blood vessels to constrict and stimulates production of the adrenal hormone, aldosterone, which promotes sodium retention in the body. As a result, ACE inhibitors relax blood vessels (causing them to widen) and reduces sodium retention, which lowers blood pressure and so decreases the workload of the heart.

DOSAGE
To start, 1 mg once a day, except black patients, who should start with 2 mg once a day. Doses may be increased to a maximum of 8 mg a day in 1 or 2 doses.

ONSET OF EFFECT
Within 4 hours.

DURATION OF ACTION
Up to 24 hours.

DIETARY ADVICE
Take it on an empty stomach, about 1 hour before mealtime. Follow your doctor's dietary advice (such as low-salt or low-cholesterol restrictions) to improve control over high blood pressure and heart disease. Avoid high-potassium foods like bananas and citrus fruits and juices, unless you are also taking medications, such as diuretics, that lower potassium levels.

STORAGE
Store in a tightly sealed container away from heat, moisture, and direct light.

IF YOU MISS A DOSE
Take it as soon as you remember. If it is near the time for the next dose, skip the missed dose and resume your regular dosage schedule. Do not double the next dose.

STOPPING THE DRUG
Do not stop taking this drug abruptly, as this may cause potentially serious health problems. Dosage should be reduced gradually, according to your doctor's instructions.

PROLONGED USE
See your doctor regularly for examinations and tests if you must take this medicine for a prolonged period. Remember that trandolapril helps control high blood pressure but does not cure it. Lifelong therapy may be necessary.

PRECAUTIONS
Over 60: Some elderly patients may be more sensitive to the effects of this drug; smaller doses may be warranted.

Driving and Hazardous Work: Exercise caution until you determine how the medicine affects you.

Alcohol: Consume alcohol only in moderation since it may increase the effect of the drug and cause an excessive drop in blood pressure. Consult your doctor for advice.

Pregnancy: Not recommended, especially during the last 2 trimesters (final 6 months) of pregnancy. If you become pregnant, notify your doctor as soon as possible.

Breast Feeding: Trace amounts of trandolapril can be found in breast milk; however, adverse effects in infants have not been documented. Consult your doctor for advice.

Infants and Children: The safety and effectiveness of trandolapril in children 18 and under have not been established.

OVERDOSE
Symptoms: No specific ones have been reported.

What to Do: While overdose is unlikely, call your doctor, emergency medical services (EMS), or the nearest poison control center immediately if you suspect that someone has taken a much larger dose than prescribed.

DRUG INTERACTIONS
Consult your doctor if you are taking diuretics (especially potassium-sparing diuretics), potassium supplements or drugs containing potassium, lithium, anticoagulants, anti-inflammatory drugs, any over-the-counter drugs (especially cold remedies and diet pills).

FOOD INTERACTIONS
Avoid low-salt milk and salt substitutes. Many of these products contain potassium.

DISEASE INTERACTIONS
Consult your doctor if you have systemic lupus erythematosus (SLE) or if you have had a prior allergic reaction to ACE inhibitors. Trandolapril should be used with caution by patients with severe kidney disease or renal artery stenosis (narrowing of one or both of the arteries that supply blood to the kidneys).

Trandolapril/Verapamil Hydrochloride

BRAND NAME
Tarka

▶ Drug Class: ACE inhibitor/
calcium channel blocker
combination

▶ Available in: Tablets

▶ Available OTC? No

▶ As Generic? No

Side Effects

SERIOUS
Serious side effects are very rare; they include fever and chills, sore throat and hoarseness, sudden difficulty breathing or swallowing, swelling of the face, mouth, or extremities, worsening kidney function (ankle swelling, decreased urination), confusion, jaundice (yellowish tinge to eyes or skin, indicating liver problems), intense itching, chest pain or heart palpitations, abdominal pain, irregular or slow heartbeats, low blood pressure (causing dizziness or faintness). Call your doctor immediately.

COMMON
Mild swelling of arms and legs (edema), fatigue, mild headache, dizziness, constipation, cough, flushed skin.

LESS COMMON
Fainting, dry mouth, diarrhea, gas, nausea, vomiting, rectal pain, gout, neck pain, joint swelling, nervousness, insomnia, drowsiness, skin rash, increased eye pressure, impotence, hot flashes.

PRINCIPAL USES
To control high blood pressure (hypertension).

HOW THE DRUG WORKS
Angiotensin-converting enzyme (ACE) inhibitors such as trandolapril block an enzyme that produces angiotensin, a naturally occurring substance that causes blood vessels to constrict and stimulates production of the adrenal hormone, aldosterone, which promotes sodium retention in the body. As a result, ACE inhibitors relax blood vessels (causing them to widen) and reduces sodium retention. Verapamil, a calcium channel blocker, interferes with the movement of calcium into heart muscle cells and the smooth muscle cells in the walls of the arteries. As a result of the combined action of trandolapril and verapamil, blood vessels relax (causing them to widen), which lowers blood pressure and thereby decreases the workload of the heart.

DOSAGE
From 1 to 4 mg of trandolapril and 120 to 480 micrograms (mcg) of verapamil per day. Tablets containing both active ingredients are taken either once a day or in 2 divided doses.

ONSET OF EFFECT
Within 15 hours.

DURATION OF ACTION
Unknown.

DIETARY ADVICE
Best taken without food. Can be taken with grapefruit juice.

STORAGE
Store in a tightly sealed container away from heat, moisture, and direct light.

IF YOU MISS A DOSE
Take it as soon as you remember. If it is near the time for the next dose, skip the missed dose and resume your regular dosage schedule. Do not double the next dose.

STOPPING THE DRUG
The decision to stop taking the drug should be made by your doctor.

PROLONGED USE
See your doctor periodically for tests and examinations if you must take this medication for a prolonged period.

PRECAUTIONS
Over 60: No special problems are expected.

Driving and Hazardous Work: Avoid such activities until you determine how the medicine affects you.

Alcohol: Consume alcohol only in moderation since it may increase the effect of the drug and cause an excessive drop in blood pressure.

Pregnancy: This drug should not be used during pregnancy and is especially dangerous to the unborn child during the final 6 months (second and third trimesters). Consult your doctor if you are pregnant or plan to become pregnant.

Breast Feeding: Trandolapril with verapamil passes into breast milk; avoid use while nursing or discontinue breast feeding.

Infants and Children: The safety and effectiveness of trandolapril with verapamil use by children have not been established.

Special Concerns: Trandolapril with verapamil is not recommended as the first line of therapy when high blood pressure is diagnosed. It may be prescribed after other medications have proved unsatisfactory. Before you undergo surgery, tell the doctor or dentist in charge that you are taking this drug.

OVERDOSE
Symptoms: No cases of overdose have been reported. Symptoms might include extreme dizziness, fainting, or confusion.

What to Do: If someone takes a much larger dose than prescribed, seek medical assistance right away.

DRUG INTERACTIONS
Consult your physician for specific advice if you are taking digitalis drugs, lithium, cimetidine, beta-blockers, antiarrhythmic drugs (such as disopyramide, flecainide, and quinidine), anticonvulsants, cyclosporine, or theophylline.

FOOD INTERACTIONS
No known food interactions.

DISEASE INTERACTIONS
Consult your doctor if you have congestive heart failure (CHF), heart rhythm irregularities (cardiac arrhythmia), or any other medical condition. This drug should be used with caution by patients with severe kidney disease or renal artery stenosis (narrowing of one or both of the arteries that supply blood to the kidneys).

Tranylcypromine Sulfate

Parnate 10 mg
(SMITHKLINE BEECHAM)

▶ Drug Class: Monoamine oxidase (MAO) inhibitor antidepressant

▶ Available in: Tablets

▶ Available OTC? No

▶ As Generic? No

Side Effects

SERIOUS
Severe chest pain, dilated pupils, irregular heartbeat, sensitivity of eyes to light, sweating or fever, nausea and vomiting, stiff neck, extreme dizziness. Call your doctor immediately.

COMMON
Blurring of vision, decreased urination, sexual dysfunction, mild dizziness or lightheadedness, mild headache, appetite changes including cravings for sweets, weight gain, increase in sweating, muscle twitching during sleep, restlessness, shakiness, fatigue, insomnia.

LESS COMMON
Chills, constipation, decrease in appetite, dry mouth.

PRINCIPAL USES
To treat symptoms of major mental depression.

HOW THE DRUG WORKS
Tranylcypromine inhibits the activity of monoamine oxidase, an enzyme that renders certain brain chemicals (epinephrine, norepinephrine, and dopamine) inactive. Consequently, this drug increases the availability of these chemicals in the nervous system; this is thought to have an antidepressant effect.

DOSAGE
Adults: To start, 10 mg, 3 times a day; this may be increased to 60 mg a day. Older adults: To start, 10 mg, 2 times a day; this may be increased to 40 mg a day.

ONSET OF EFFECT
48 hours; it may take up to 3 weeks for full effect.

DURATION OF ACTION
Up to 10 days after stopping treatment.

DIETARY ADVICE
See Food Interactions.

STORAGE
Store in a tightly sealed container away from heat, moisture, and direct light.

IF YOU MISS A DOSE
Take it as soon as you remember. However, if it is near the time for the next dose, skip the missed dose and resume your regular dosage schedule. Do not double the next dose.

STOPPING THE DRUG
Take it as prescribed for the full treatment period. The decision to stop taking the drug should be made in consultation with your physician.

PROLONGED USE
The usual course of therapy lasts 6 months to 1 year; some patients benefit from additional therapy.

PRECAUTIONS
Over 60: Adverse reactions may be more likely and more severe in older patients. A lower dose may be warranted.

Driving and Hazardous Work: Use caution until you determine how the medicine affects you.

Alcohol: Avoid alcohol.

Pregnancy: Use during pregnancy may increase the risk of birth defects.

Breast Feeding: Tranylcypromine may pass into breast milk; caution is advised. Consult your doctor for specific advice.

Infants and Children: This drug is not recommended for children age 16 and under.

Special Concerns: Before having any surgery, emergency treatment, or dental treatment, tell the doctor or dentist in charge that you are taking tranylcypromine. Your doctor may advise you to carry a card saying that you use tranylcypromine.

OVERDOSE
Symptoms: Profound anxiety, confusion, seizures, cold, clammy skin, severe drowsiness, irregular pulse, hallucinations, severe headache, fainting, stiff muscles, sweating, breathing difficulty.

What to Do: Call your doctor, emergency medical services (EMS), or the nearest poison control center immediately.

DRUG INTERACTIONS
Consult your doctor for specific advice if you are taking or have recently taken amphetamines, blood pressure medications, diet pills, cyclobenzaprine, fluoxetine, levodopa, maprotiline, asthma medication, cold or allergy medication, meperidine, methylphenidate, another MAO inhibitor, paroxetine, sertraline, a tricyclic antidepressant, an oral diabetes drug, insulin, bupropion, buspirone, carbamazepine, a central nervous system depressant, dextromethorphan, trazodone, or tryptophan.

FOOD INTERACTIONS
Do not eat foods with a high tyramine content, such as cheeses; yeast or meat extracts; pickled or smoked meat, poultry, or fish; processed meats like bologna, salami, and pepperoni; and sauerkraut. Do not drink alcohol-free or reduced-alcohol beer and wine. Do not drink beverages or eat food with a high caffeine content, such as coffee and chocolate.

DISEASE INTERACTIONS
Consult your physician if you have any of the following: a history of alcohol abuse, angina, frequent headaches, asthma, bronchitis, diabetes mellitus, epilepsy, heart disease or a recent heart attack, blood vessel disease, liver disease, Parkinson's disease, a recent stroke, kidney disease, an overactive thyroid, or pheochromocytoma.

Trazodone

BRAND NAMES
Desyrel, Trazon, Trialodine

Generic 50 mg
(PUREPAC)

▶ Drug Class: Antidepressant

▶ Available in: Tablets

▶ Available OTC? No

▶ As Generic? Yes

Side Effects

SERIOUS
Muscle twitching, confusion. Call your doctor immediately.

COMMON
Drowsiness, dry mouth, dizziness, lightheadedness, unpleasant taste in mouth, nausea and vomiting, headache.

LESS COMMON
Blurred vision, muscle pains, diarrhea, constipation, unusual fatigue.

PRINCIPAL USES
To treat symptoms of major depression. It may be taken with selective serotonin reuptake inhibitor (SSRI) antidepressants such as fluoxetine, sertraline, and paroxetine when these drugs cause insomnia.

HOW THE DRUG WORKS
Trazodone helps to balance levels of serotonin, a brain chemical that is profoundly linked to mood, emotions, and mental state.

DOSAGE
Adults: To start, 50 mg, 3 times a day, or 75 mg, 2 times a day, or 100 mg at bedtime. The dose may be gradually increased by your doctor to 400 mg a day. Older adults: To start, 25 mg, 3 times a day, or 50 mg at bedtime. The dose may be increased by your doctor.

ONSET OF EFFECT
1 to 4 weeks.

DURATION OF ACTION
Unknown.

DIETARY ADVICE
It can be taken with a meal or light snack to reduce the chance of dizziness and to increase the absorption of the drug by the body.

STORAGE
Store in a tightly sealed container away from heat, moisture, and direct light.

IF YOU MISS A DOSE
Take it as soon as you remember, unless the time for your next scheduled dose is within the next 4 hours. If so, do not take the missed dose. Take your next scheduled dose at the proper time and resume your regular dosage schedule. Do not double the next dose.

STOPPING THE DRUG
Take as prescribed for the full treatment period, even if you begin to feel better before the scheduled end of therapy. The decision to stop taking the drug should be made in consultation with your doctor.

PROLONGED USE
The usual course of therapy lasts for 6 months to 1 year; some patients benefit from additional therapy beyond that period.

PRECAUTIONS
Over 60: Adverse reactions may be more likely and more severe in older patients. Lower doses may be needed.

Driving and Hazardous Work: Use caution when driving or engaging in hazardous work until you determine how the medicine affects you. Drowsiness may occur.

Alcohol: Avoid alcohol.

Pregnancy: Adequate studies of trazodone use during pregnancy have not been done. Before you take trazodone, tell your doctor if you are pregnant or plan to become pregnant.

Breast Feeding: Trazodone passes into breast milk; caution is advised. Consult your doctor for specific advice.

Infants and Children: The safety and effectiveness of trazodone use by infants and children have not been established.

OVERDOSE
Symptoms: Severe nausea and vomiting, loss of coordination, drowsiness.

What to Do: Call your doctor, emergency medical services (EMS), or the nearest poison control center immediately.

DRUG INTERACTIONS
The following drugs may interact with trazodone. Consult your doctor for specific advice if you are taking high blood pressure medication, central nervous system depressants (including cold and allergy drugs, narcotic pain relievers, and muscle relaxants), fluoxetine, or tricyclic antidepressants.

FOOD INTERACTIONS
No known food interactions.

DISEASE INTERACTIONS
Caution is advised when taking trazodone. Consult your doctor if you have a history of alcohol abuse or any heart condition. Use of trazodone may cause complications in patients with liver or kidney disease, since these organs work together to remove the medication from the body.

Tretinoin

▶ Drug Class: Acne drug

▶ Available in: Cream, gel,
liquid

▶ Available OTC? No

▶ As Generic? Yes

Side Effects

SERIOUS
No serious side effects
are associated with
regular applications of
tretinoin when used as
directed.

COMMON
Mild redness and peel-
ing, or excessive dryness,
at the site of application.

LESS COMMON
Irritation or allergy with
severe redness, swelling,
blistering, pain, rash, or
crusting at sites of application; changes in pig-
ment (either lightening or
darkening of skin color).
These problems generally
improve when the med-
ication is stopped or
reduced in dosage or fre-
quency of application.
Consult your doctor.

PRINCIPAL USES
Tretinoin is used to treat
mild to moderate acne.

HOW THE DRUG WORKS
Although the exact mecha-
nism of action is unknown,
tretinoin appears to affect
skin cells so that they are
shed in a more normal fashion, therefore "unplugging"
blackheads and whiteheads
(comedones), the initial
changes in acne formation.

DOSAGE
Adults: Apply once daily at
bedtime.

ONSET OF EFFECT
Variable, usually within 2 to
6 weeks after starting therapy.

DURATION OF ACTION
The effect of tretinoin typically persists for as long as
the drug is being used.

DIETARY ADVICE
No special restrictions.

STORAGE
Store in a tightly sealed container away from heat and
direct light. Keep away from
moisture and extremes in
temperature. The gel form
of this medication is flammable; keep away from heat
and open flame.

IF YOU MISS A DOSE
This drug is applied once
every 24 hours, at night.
If you miss a day, resume
your regular dosage schedule the next day. There is
no need to apply extra
medication with the next
dose to compensate for the
missed dose.

STOPPING THE DRUG
Use as prescribed for the
full treatment period, even if
you show signs of improvement before the scheduled
end of therapy.

PROLONGED USE
Therapy with this medica-
tion is frequently prolonged.

PRECAUTIONS
Over 60: No special problems are expected.

**Driving and Hazardous
Work:** No special precautions are necessary.

Alcohol: No special precautions are necessary.

Pregnancy: Avoid or discontinue tretinoin if you are
pregnant or trying to
become pregnant.

Breast Feeding: Tretinoin
may pass into breast milk;
caution is advised. Consult
your doctor for advice.

Infants and Children:
Not recommended for use
on children.

Special Concerns: Persons with a history of
allergy to tretinoin or any
other ingredients in the
medication should not use
the product. Do not apply
large amounts of tretinoin
to your skin in expectation
of better or faster results.
This will only lead to unnecessary irritation of affected
skin and surrounding areas.
Sunburned skin is more
susceptible to irritation
from tretinoin, and application should be avoided.
Avoid excessive exposure to
sunlight or use of sunlamps.
Keep this medication away
from your eyes, mouth, and
nostrils. Severe irritation
and redness may result.
Do not apply tretinoin to
inflamed skin. If your skin
becomes reddened and
painful while using tretinoin, discontinue use of the
medication and call your
doctor. If you are using cosmetics, gently cleanse skin
to be treated before applying the medication.

OVERDOSE
Symptoms: Excessive
application of tretinoin may
lead to severe irritation of
the skin.

What to Do: If tretinoin is
ingested, call your doctor,
emergency medical services
(EMS), or the nearest poison control center.

DRUG INTERACTIONS
Consult your doctor for specific advice if you are taking
other acne medications that
are applied to the same area
of skin, including prescription and nonprescription
treatments containing
sulfur, resorcinol, alpha
hydroxy acids, or salicylic
acid; medicated soaps, abra-
sives, cleansers, or cosmetics; topical preparations
with a high concentration of
alcohol, astringents, extract
of lime, or spices; and medications used for a drying
effect.

FOOD INTERACTIONS
No known food interactions.

DISEASE INTERACTIONS
Caution is advised when
using tretinoin. Consult
your doctor if you have
eczema.

▶ Drug Class: Respiratory corticosteroid

▶ Available in: Nasal spray, oral inhalation

▶ Available OTC? No

▶ As Generic? No

Side Effects

SERIOUS
No serious side effects have been reported.

COMMON
Oral inhalation: Sore throat, white patches in mouth or throat, hoarseness. Nasal spray: Nosebleeds or bloody nasal secretions, nasal burning or irritation, sore throat.

LESS COMMON
Eye pain, watering eyes, gradual decrease of vision, stomach pain and digestive disturbances.

PRINCIPAL USES
Oral inhalation: To treat bronchial asthma. Nasal spray: To treat allergic rhinitis (seasonal or perennial allergies such as hay fever), and to prevent recurrence of nasal polyps after surgical removal.

HOW THE DRUG WORKS
Respiratory corticosteroids such as triamcinolone primarily reduce or prevent inflammation of the lining of the airways (the underlying cause of asthma), reduce the allergic response to inhaled allergens, and inhibit the secretion of mucus within the airways.

DOSAGE
Adults and children ages 12 and older— Oral inhalation: 2 inhalations of 100 mcg each, 3 or 4 times a day. Maximum dose is 16 inhalations a day. In some patients maintenance can be achieved when the total daily dose is given 2 times a day. Nasal spray: 2 sprays (55 micrograms [mcg] each) in each nostril once a day. It can be increased to 440 mcg per day in 1 or up to 4 doses. After relief is achieved, it can be decreased to as little as 1 spray (55 mcg) in each nostril once a day.

ONSET OF EFFECT
Usually within 1 week; it may take 3 weeks for the full effect to occur.

DURATION OF ACTION
Several days.

DIETARY ADVICE
No special restrictions.

STORAGE
Store in a tightly sealed container away from heat and direct light.

IF YOU MISS A DOSE
Take it as soon as you remember. However, if it is near the time for the next dose, skip the missed dose and resume your regular dosage schedule. Do not double the next dose.

STOPPING THE DRUG
The decision to stop taking the drug should be made in consultation with your physician.

PROLONGED USE
Consult your doctor about the need for regular periodic medical tests and examinations if you must take this drug for a prolonged period.

PRECAUTIONS
Over 60: No special problems are expected with older patients.

Driving and Hazardous Work: The use of triamcinolone should not impair your ability to perform such tasks safely.

Alcohol: No special precautions are necessary.

Pregnancy: Inhaled or nasal steroids have not been reported to cause birth defects if taken during pregnancy. Before using such drugs, tell your doctor if you are or are planning to become pregnant.

Breast Feeding: Triamcinolone may pass into breast milk; caution is advised. Consult your doctor for advice.

Infants and Children: No special problems are expected in children, but the lowest possible dose should be used.

Special Concerns: Inhaled steroids will not help an asthma attack in progress. Inhaled steroids can lower resistance to yeast infections of the mouth, throat, or voice box. To prevent yeast infections, gargle or rinse your mouth with water after each use; do not swallow the water. Know how to use the spray properly; read and follow the directions that come with the device. Before you have surgery, tell the doctor or dentist that you are using a steroid.

OVERDOSE
Symptoms: No specific ones have been reported.

What to Do: Call your doctor, emergency medical services (EMS), or the nearest poison control center if you have any reason to suspect an overdose.

DRUG INTERACTIONS
Consult your physician for advice if you are taking systemic corticosteroids, other inhaled corticosteroids, or any drugs that suppress the immune system.

FOOD INTERACTIONS
No known food interactions.

DISEASE INTERACTIONS
Consult your physician if you have any of the following: nasal septal ulcers, ocular herpes simplex, or any fungal, bacterial, or systemic viral infection. If you are exposed to chicken pox or measles, tell your doctor at once.

Triamcinolone Systemic

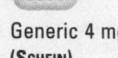

Generic 4 mg
(Schein)

▶ Drug Class: Corticosteroid

▶ Available in: Syrup, tablets, injection

▶ Available OTC? No

▶ As Generic? Yes

Side Effects

SERIOUS
Vision problems, frequent urination, increased thirst, rectal bleeding, blistering skin, confusion, hallucinations, paranoia, euphoria, depression, mood swings, redness and swelling at injection site. Call your doctor immediately.

COMMON
Increased appetite, indigestion, nervousness, insomnia, greater susceptibility to infections, increased blood pressure, slowed wound healing, weight gain, easy bruising, fluid retention.

LESS COMMON
Change in skin color, dizziness, headache, increased sweating, unusual growth of body or facial hair, increased blood sugar, peptic ulcers, adrenal insufficiency, muscle weakness, cataracts, glaucoma, osteoporosis.

PRINCIPAL USES
To treat numerous conditions that involve inflammation (a response by body tissues, producing redness, warmth, swelling, and pain). Such conditions include arthritis, allergic reactions, asthma, some skin diseases, multiple sclerosis flare-ups, and other autoimmune diseases. Also prescribed to treat deficiency of natural steroid hormones.

HOW THE DRUG WORKS
This hormone mimics the effects of the body's natural corticosteroids. It depresses the synthesis, release, and activity of inflammation-producing body chemicals. It also suppresses the activity of the immune system.

DOSAGE
Adults and teenagers: 4 to 60 mg a day in 1 or several doses. Children's doses depend on size and body weight and should be determined by your doctor.

ONSET OF EFFECT
Variable.

DURATION OF ACTION
Variable.

DIETARY ADVICE
It can be taken with food or milk to minimize stomach upset. Your doctor may recommend a special diet.

STORAGE
Store in a tightly sealed container away from heat, moisture, and direct light. Do not freeze the liquid form.

IF YOU MISS A DOSE
If you take several doses a day and it is close to the next dose, double the next dose. If you take 1 dose a day and you do not remember until the next day, skip the missed dose and do not double the next dose.

STOPPING THE DRUG
The decision to stop taking the drug should be made by your doctor.

PROLONGED USE
Long-term use may lead to cataracts, diabetes, hypertension, or osteoporosis; see your physician for regular visits.

PRECAUTIONS
Over 60: Adverse reactions may be more likely and more severe in older patients.

Driving and Hazardous Work: Avoid such activities until you determine how the medicine affects you.

Alcohol: May cause stomach problems; avoid it unless your physician approves occasional moderate drinking.

Pregnancy: Overuse during pregnancy can impair growth and development of the child.

Breast Feeding: Do not use this drug while nursing.

Infants and Children: Triamcinolone may retard the development of bone and other tissues.

Special Concerns: This drug can lower your resistance to infection. Avoid immunizations with live vaccines. Patients undergoing long-term therapy should wear a medical-alert bracelet. Call your doctor right away if you develop a fever.

OVERDOSE
Symptoms: Fever, muscle or joint pain, nausea, dizziness, fainting, difficulty breathing. Prolonged overuse: Moonface, obesity, unusual hair growth, acne, loss of sexual function, muscle wasting.

What to Do: Call your doctor, emergency medical services (EMS), or the nearest poison control center immediately.

DRUG INTERACTIONS
Consult your doctor for specific advice if you are taking aminoglutethimide, antacids, barbiturates, carbamazepine, griseofulvin, mitotane, phenylbutazone, phenytoin, primidone, rifampin, injectable amphotericin B, oral antidiabetes agents, insulin, digitalis drugs, diuretics, or medications containing potassium or sodium.

FOOD INTERACTIONS
Avoid excess sodium.

DISEASE INTERACTIONS
Consult your doctor if you have a history of bone disease, chicken pox, measles, gastrointestinal disorders, diabetes, recent serious infection, glaucoma, heart disease, hypertension, liver or kidney disorders, high blood cholesterol, thyroid problems, myasthenia gravis, or lupus.

Triamcinolone Topical

▶ Drug Class: Topical corticosteroid

▶ Available in: Cream, lotion, ointment, aerosol, dental paste

▶ Available OTC? No

▶ As Generic? Yes

Side Effects

SERIOUS
Serious side effects from the use of topical triamcinolone are very rare.

COMMON
Burning, itching, irritation, redness, dryness, acne, stinging and cracking of skin, and numbness or tingling in the extremities have been reported in 0.5% to 1% of patients, although the risk is increased when the medication is used with bandages or other occlusive dressings.

LESS COMMON
Blistering and pus near hair follicles, unusual bleeding or easy bruising, darkening or prominence of small surface veins, increased susceptibility to infection.

PRINCIPAL USES
To treat rashes and inflammation of the skin. It is also used for treatment of inflammatory conditions within the mouth.

HOW THE DRUG WORKS
Topical triamcinolone appears to interfere with the formation of natural substances within the body that are directly responsible for the process of inflammation, which produces swelling, redness, and pain.

DOSAGE
Cream (0.025%, 0.1%, and 0.5% strength)— Adults: Apply 2 to 3 times daily. Children: 1 to 2 times daily (0.025%); once daily for all others (0.1% and 0.5%). Lotion (0.025% and 0.1% strength)— Adults: Apply 2 to 4 times daily. Children: 1 to 2 times daily (0.025%); once daily for all others (0.1%). Ointment (0.025%, 0.1%, and 0.5% strength)— Adults: Apply 2 to 4 times daily. Children: 1 to 2 times daily (0.025%); once daily for all others (0.1% and 0.5%). Aerosol (0.015% strength)— Adults: Apply 3 or 4 times daily. Children: 1 or 2 times daily. Dental paste (0.1% strength)— Adults: Apply to affected areas of the mouth 2 to 3 times daily after meals and at bedtime. Children: Consult a pediatrician.

ONSET OF EFFECT
Soon after application. However, recognizable changes in your condition may take several days or more to develop.

DURATION OF ACTION
Unknown.

DIETARY ADVICE
No special restrictions.

STORAGE
Store in a tightly sealed container away from heat and direct light.

IF YOU MISS A DOSE
Apply it as soon as you remember. If it is near the time for the next dose, skip the missed dose and resume your regular dosage schedule.

STOPPING THE DRUG
Take as prescribed for the full treatment period, even if you begin to feel better before the scheduled end of therapy.

PROLONGED USE
Avoid prolonged use, particularly near the eyes, on the face, genital, or rectal areas, or in the folds of the skin.

PRECAUTIONS
Over 60: Side effects may be more likely and more severe in elderly patients.

Driving and Hazardous Work: No special precautions are necessary.

Alcohol: No special precautions are necessary.

Pregnancy: This drug should not be used for prolonged periods by pregnant women or by women trying to become pregnant.

Breast Feeding: Although problems have not been documented, caution is advised. Do not apply to breasts prior to nursing. Consult your doctor for specific advice.

Infants and Children: This medication should not be used for more than 2 weeks in children and adolescents, unless otherwise directed by your doctor. Do not use tight-fitting diapers or plastic pants on children when treating skin irritation in the diaper area.

Special Concerns: Wash your hands thoroughly after application. Do not wrap the treated area with bandages or tight-fitting clothing unless otherwise instructed by your doctor.

OVERDOSE
Symptoms: None known.

What to Do: An overdose of a topical corticosteroid is unlikely to be life-threatening. However, in case of accidental ingestion or an apparent overdose, call your doctor, emergency medical services (EMS), or the nearest poison control center right away.

DRUG INTERACTIONS
Do not mix topical triamcinolone with other products, especially alcohol-containing preparations (which include colognes, aftershave, and many moisturizer lotions), since this may cause dryness and irritation, or increase the risk of an allergic reaction.

FOOD INTERACTIONS
Potassium supplements may decrease this drug's effects. Avoid foods high in sodium.

DISEASE INTERACTIONS
Caution is advised when taking this drug. Consult your doctor if you have any of the following: cataracts; diabetes mellitus; glaucoma; infection, sores, or ulcerations of the skin; infection at another site in your body; tuberculosis.

Triamterene

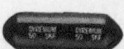

Dyrenium 50 mg
(SmithKline Beecham)

▶ Drug Class: Potassium-sparing diuretic

▶ Available in: Capsules

▶ Available OTC? No

▶ As Generic? No

Side Effects

SERIOUS
Skin rash, hives, light-headedness, unusual bleeding. Call your doctor immediately.

COMMON
No common side effects have been reported.

LESS COMMON
Dizziness, nausea, vomiting, stomach cramps, diarrhea, headache, increased sensitivity of skin to sunlight.

PRINCIPAL USES
Used as an adjunctive, supplementary treatment with other diuretics to conserve potassium while promoting the excretion of sodium and water. In conjunction with thiazide or loop diuretics, triamterene reduces the overall fluid volume in the body and so helps to control symptoms of heart disease, kidney disease, and liver disease.

HOW THE DRUG WORKS
Triamterene promotes the excretion of sodium and excess water by altering kidney enzymes that control urine production. Unlike most other types of diuretics, triamterene promotes fluid and salt loss but does not deplete normal levels of potassium.

DOSAGE
Adults: 25 to 100 mg a day. Dose may be increased to no more than 300 mg a day. Children: 0.9 to 1.82 mg per lb of body weight, once a day or once every other day. Dose may be increased.

ONSET OF EFFECT
Within 2 to 4 hours.

DURATION OF ACTION
From 7 to 9 hours.

DIETARY ADVICE
Triamterene should be taken after meals, though it can be taken with food or a full glass of milk to minimize the risk of stomach upset.

STORAGE
Store in a tightly sealed container away from heat, moisture, and direct light.

IF YOU MISS A DOSE
Take it as soon as you remember. However, if it is near the time for the next dose, skip the missed dose and resume your regular dosage schedule. Do not double the next dose.

STOPPING THE DRUG
The decision to stop taking the drug should be made by your doctor.

PROLONGED USE
See your doctor regularly for tests and examinations if you must take this drug for a prolonged period.

PRECAUTIONS
Over 60: Adverse reactions may be more likely and more severe in older patients. In particular, signs of excess potassium levels are more likely to occur in older patients.

Driving and Hazardous Work: The use of triamterene should not impair your ability to perform such tasks safely.

Alcohol: No special precautions are necessary.

Pregnancy: Adequate human studies have not been done. Before taking triamterene, tell your doctor if you are pregnant or plan to become pregnant.

Breast Feeding: Triamterene passes into breast milk; caution is advised. Consult your doctor for specific advice.

Infants and Children: No special problems are expected.

Special Concerns: Avoid exposure to the sun until you determine how the medicine affects you. Before having any kind of surgery, tell the doctor or dentist in charge that you are taking triamterene.

OVERDOSE
Symptoms: Dizziness or faintness, nausea, vomiting, confusion, heartbeat irregularities, nervousness, numbness or tingling in hands, feet, or lips, weak or heavy legs, unusual fatigue or tiredness.

What to Do: Call your doctor, emergency medical services (EMS), or the nearest poison control center immediately.

DRUG INTERACTIONS
Other drugs may interact with triamterene. Consult your doctor for specific advice if you are taking ACE inhibitors, cyclosporine, potassium-containing medicines or supplements, digoxin, or lithium.

FOOD INTERACTIONS
Avoid foods and beverages high in potassium, such as some salt substitutes, bananas, and citrus juices.

DISEASE INTERACTIONS
Consult your doctor if you have a history of gout or kidney stones. Use of triamterene may cause complications in patients with liver or kidney disease, since these organs work together to remove the medication from the body.

Triazolam

BRAND NAME
Halcion

Generic 0.125 mg
(GENEVA)

▶ Drug Class: Benzodiazepine tranquilizer

▶ Available in: Tablets

▶ Available OTC? No

▶ As Generic? Yes

Side Effects

SERIOUS
Difficulty concentrating, outbursts of anger, other behavior problems, depression, convulsions, hallucinations, low blood pressure (causing faintness or confusion), memory impairment, muscle weakness, skin rash or itching, sore throat, fever and chills, sores or ulcers in throat or mouth, unusual bruising or bleeding, extreme fatigue, yellowish tinge to eyes or skin. Call your doctor immediately.

COMMON
Loss of coordination, unsteady gait, dizziness, lightheadedness, drowsiness, slurred speech.

LESS COMMON
Stomach cramps or pain, vision disturbances, change in sexual desire or ability, constipation or diarrhea, dry mouth or watering mouth, false sense of well-being, rapid or pounding heartbeat, headache, muscle spasms, nausea and vomiting, urinary problems, trembling, unusual fatigue.

PRINCIPAL USES
To treat insomnia.

HOW THE DRUG WORKS
In general, triazolam produces mild sedation by depressing activity in the central nervous system (brain and spinal cord). In particular, triazolam appears to enhance the effect of gamma-aminobutyric acid (GABA), a natural chemical that inhibits the firing of neurons and dampens the transmission of nerve signals, thus decreasing nervous excitation.

DOSAGE
Adults: 0.125 to 0.250 mg at bedtime. Use and dose for children under 18 must be determined by your doctor.

ONSET OF EFFECT
Unknown.

DURATION OF ACTION
Unknown.

DIETARY ADVICE
Take with a full glass of water. Can be taken with food to lessen stomach upset.

STORAGE
Store in a tightly sealed container away from heat and direct light.

IF YOU MISS A DOSE
Take it as soon as you remember, unless it is late at night. Do not take the medicine unless your schedule allows a full night's sleep.

STOPPING THE DRUG
Stopping the drug abruptly may produce withdrawal symptoms (sleep disruption, nervousness, irritability, diarrhea, abdominal cramps, muscle aches, memory impairment). Dose should be reduced gradually according to your doctor's instructions.

PROLONGED USE
Triazolam may slowly lose its effectiveness, and adverse reactions are more likely to occur with prolonged use. You should see your doctor for periodic evaluation if you must take it for an extended time.

PRECAUTIONS
Over 60: Adverse reactions may be more likely and more severe. A lower dose may be warranted.

Driving and Hazardous Work: Triazolam can impair mental alertness and physical coordination. Adjust your activities accordingly.

Alcohol: Avoid alcohol.

Pregnancy: Use during pregnancy should be avoided if possible. Be sure to tell your doctor if you are pregnant or plan to become pregnant.

Breast Feeding: Triazolam passes into breast milk; do not take it while nursing.

Infants and Children: Safety and effectiveness have not been established for children under age 18.

Special Concerns: Triazolam use can lead to psychological or physical dependence if it is not taken in strict accordance with your doctor's instructions. Never take more than the prescribed daily dose.

OVERDOSE
Symptoms: Extreme drowsiness, confusion, slurred speech, slow reflexes, poor coordination, staggering gait, tremor, slowed breathing, loss of consciousness.

What to Do: Call your doctor, emergency medical services (EMS), or the nearest poison control center immediately.

DRUG INTERACTIONS
Other drugs may interact with triazolam. Consult your doctor for specific advice if you are taking any drugs that depress the central nervous system; these include antihistamines, antidepressants or other psychiatric medications, barbiturates, sedatives, cough medicines, decongestants, and painkillers. Be sure your physician knows about any over-the-counter medication you may take.

FOOD INTERACTIONS
None reported.

DISEASE INTERACTIONS
Caution is advised when taking triazolam. Consult your doctor if you have a history of alcohol or drug abuse, stroke or other brain disease, any chronic lung disease, glaucoma, hyperactivity, depression or other mental illness, myasthenia gravis, sleep apnea, epilepsy, porphyria, kidney disease, or liver disease.

Trifluoperazine Hydrochloride

Generic 10 mg
(GENEVA)

Additional photographs

▶ Drug Class: Neuroleptic;
antipsychotic

▶ Available in: Oral solution,
tablets, injection

▶ Available OTC? No

▶ As Generic? Yes

Side Effects

SERIOUS
Rapid heartbeat, profuse sweating, seizures, difficulty breathing, neck stiffness, swelling of the tongue, difficulty swallowing. Also a rare condition can develop called neuroleptic malignant syndrome, characterized by stiffness or spasms of the muscles, high fever, and confusion or disorientation. Call your doctor immediately.

COMMON
Nausea, reduced perspiration, dry mouth, blurred vision, drowsiness, shaking of the hands, muscle stiffness, stooped posture.

LESS COMMON
Difficult urination, menstrual irregularities, breast pain or swelling, unexpected weight gain, uncontrolled movements of the tongue, fever, chills, sore throat, unusual bruising or bleeding, heart palpitations, skin rash, itching, increased sensitivity of the skin to sunlight.

PRINCIPAL USES
To treat psychotic conditions (severe mental disorders characterized by distorted thoughts, perceptions, and emotions), such as schizophrenia.

HOW THE DRUG WORKS
Trifluoperazine appears to block receptors of dopamine (a chemical that aids in the transmission of nerve impulses) in the central nervous system. Presumably, this produces a tranquilizing and antipsychotic effect.

DOSAGE
Usual adult dose: Initially, 2 to 5 mg, 2 times a day. Your doctor may increase the dose if necessary (and if side effects are tolerated) up to a maximum of 40 mg a day.

ONSET OF EFFECT
Sedation may occur within minutes, but onset of antipsychotic effect may take hours to occur or may not occur until days or weeks after the beginning of therapy.

DURATION OF ACTION
12 to 24 hours, but effects may persist for several days.

DIETARY ADVICE
Can be taken with food or a full glass of milk or water.

STORAGE
Store in a tightly sealed container away from heat and direct light.

IF YOU MISS A DOSE
Take it as soon as you remember. However, if it is near the time for the next dose, skip the missed dose and resume your regular dosage schedule. Do not double the next dose.

STOPPING THE DRUG
The decision to stop taking the drug should be made in consultation with your doctor. Gradual reduction of doses may be required if you have taken this medication for an extended period.

PROLONGED USE
Prolonged use may lead to tardive dyskinesia (involuntary movements of the jaw, lips, tongue, and, in rare cases, the arms, legs, hands, or body). Consult your doctor about the need for follow-up evaluations and tests if you must take this drug for an extended period.

PRECAUTIONS
Over 60: Adverse reactions are more common in elderly patients. A lower dose may be warranted.

Driving and Hazardous Work: Do not drive or engage in hazardous work until you determine how the medicine affects you.

Alcohol: Avoid alcohol.

Pregnancy: Avoid using this drug during pregnancy.

Breast Feeding: Either avoid taking the drug if possible or refrain from breast feeding.

Infants and Children: Adverse reactions may be more likely and more severe in children.

Special Concerns: Avoid prolonged exposure to high temperatures or hot climates. Drink plenty of fluids and stay cool in the summertime. Also, avoid overexposure to sunlight until you determine if the drug heightens your skin's sensitivity to ultraviolet light.

OVERDOSE
Symptoms: Extreme drowsiness or paradoxical restlessness or agitation, heart rhythm irregularities or palpitations, dry mouth, seizures, stiffness or impaired mental control, loss of consciousness.

What to Do: Call your doctor, emergency medical services (EMS), or the nearest poison control center immediately.

DRUG INTERACTIONS
Consult your physician for specific advice if you are taking amantadine, high blood pressure medication, bromocriptine, deferoxamine, diuretics, levobunolol, heart medication, metipranolol, nabilone, other psychiatric drugs, pentamidine, pimozide, promethazine, trimeprazine, a thyroid agent, central nervous system depressants, epinephrine, lithium, levodopa, methyldopa, metoclopramide, metyrosine, pemoline, a rauwolfia alkaloid, or metrizamide.

FOOD INTERACTIONS
No known food interactions.

DISEASE INTERACTIONS
Consult your doctor if you have Parkinson's disease or any movement disorder, glaucoma, epilepsy, liver disease, or kidney disease.

Trihexyphenidyl Hydrochloride

Generic 5 mg
(LEDERLE)

▶ Drug Class: Antiparkinsonism drug

▶ Available in: Tablets, sustained-release capsules, elixir

▶ Available OTC? No

▶ As Generic? Yes

Side Effects

SERIOUS
Confusion, hallucinations, blurred vision, glaucoma. Call your doctor at once.

COMMON
Dry mouth, nausea.

LESS COMMON
Difficult urination.

PRINCIPAL USES
To treat Parkinson's disease and the Parkinson-like symptoms induced by certain central nervous system drugs. Such symptoms include slowed movement, stiffness and muscle rigidity, tremor, and loss of balance. Trihexyphenidyl is also used to treat Parkinson-like syndromes that can occur as a result of injury to or infection of the central nervous system, damage to blood vessels in the brain, or exposure to certain toxins.

HOW THE DRUG WORKS
The exact mechanism of action of trihexyphenidyl is unknown, although it is thought to increase the availability of dopamine, a brain chemical that is critical in the initiation and smooth control of voluntary muscle movement.

DOSAGE
Adults: To start, 2 mg, 3 times a day. The dose is gradually increased until the desired therapeutic response is achieved. The usual maximum maintenance dose is 5 mg, 3 times a day. Once a maintenance dosage is established, your physician may switch you to sustained-release capsules (sequels), which can be taken less frequently (once or twice a day). Children: The dosage for children has not been established; consult your pediatrician for advice.

ONSET OF EFFECT
Usually within 1 hour.

DURATION OF ACTION
The effect may last for at least 24 hours.

DIETARY ADVICE
No special restrictions.

STORAGE
Store in a tightly sealed container away from heat, moisture, and direct light.

IF YOU MISS A DOSE
Take it as soon as you remember, unless the time for your next scheduled dose is within the next 2 hours. If so, skip the missed dose and resume your regular dosage schedule. Do not double the next dose.

STOPPING THE DRUG
The decision to stop taking the drug should be made in consultation with your doctor. The dosage is typically tapered gradually over the course of 7 days.

PROLONGED USE
The prolonged use of trihexyphenidyl may cause glaucoma (elevated pressure within the eye, and a leading cause of blindness) or increase its severity. Arrange for regular checkups with your eye doctor to have your eye pressure monitored.

PRECAUTIONS
Over 60: Adverse reactions may be more likely and more severe in older patients. Lower doses may be needed.

Driving and Hazardous Work: Do not drive or engage in hazardous work until you determine how the medicine affects you.

Alcohol: Avoid alcohol.

Pregnancy: This drug should not be used by pregnant women.

Breast Feeding: Trihexyphenidyl passes into breast milk; this drug should not be used by nursing mothers.

Infants and Children: Very low doses may be used by children; consult your pediatrician. The drug is not recommended for use by children under age 10.

Special Concerns: Your eye doctor should regularly monitor your intraocular pressure to check for glaucoma. Consult your doctor to determine the best schedule for regular physical examinations.

OVERDOSE
Symptoms: Clumsiness, confusion, delirium, inability to urinate, seizures.

What to Do: Call your doctor, emergency medical services (EMS), or the nearest poison control center immediately.

DRUG INTERACTIONS
Consult your doctor for specific advice if you are taking any of the following: other drugs for Parkinson's disease (such as levodopa), medications that depress the central nervous system (such as alcohol, barbiturates, or other sleep-inducing drugs), or MAO inhibitor antidepressants (such as phenelzine sulfate or tranylcypromine sulfate).

FOOD INTERACTIONS
No known food interactions.

DISEASE INTERACTIONS
Caution is advised when taking trihexyphenidyl. Consult your doctor for specific advice if you have glaucoma, prostate disease, or enlarged prostate (benign prostatic hyperplasia).

Trimethobenzamide Hydrochloride

▶ Drug Class: Antiemetic

▶ Available in: Capsules, injection, suppositories

▶ Available OTC? No

▶ As Generic? Yes

Side Effects

SERIOUS
Seizures, yellow discoloration of the eyes and skin, skin rash, body spasms, convulsions, mental depression, shakiness or tremors, sore throat and fever, unusual fatigue, severe or continuing vomiting. Call your doctor immediately.

COMMON
Drowsiness.

LESS COMMON
Dizziness, lightheadedness, muscle cramps, fainting, blurred vision, diarrhea, headache.

PRINCIPAL USES
To treat nausea, vomiting, and motion sickness.

HOW THE DRUG WORKS
Trimethobenzamide acts on the brain center that controls vomiting.

DOSAGE
Capsules— Adults and children 12 years and older: 250 mg, 3 or 4 times a day, as needed. Children weighing 30 to 90 lbs: 6.8 mg per lb of body weight, not to exceed 200 mg, 3 or 4 times a day. Injection— Adults and children 12 years and older: 200 mg into a muscle, 3 or 4 times a day. Suppositories— Adults and children 12 years and older: 200 mg, 3 or 4 times a day. Children 30 to 90 lbs: 1/2 to 1 suppository (100 to 200 mg), 3 or 4 times a day. Children under 30 lbs: 1/2 suppository (100 mg), 3 or 4 times a day.

ONSET OF EFFECT
Capsules: 10 to 20 minutes. Injection: 15 to 35 minutes. Suppositories: Variable.

DURATION OF ACTION
Capsules: 3 to 4 hours. Injection: 2 to 3 hours. Suppositories: Variable.

DIETARY ADVICE
Capsules can be opened and the contents mixed with food if so desired.

STORAGE
Store in a tightly sealed container away from heat, moisture, and direct light. Suppositories should be refrigerated.

IF YOU MISS A DOSE
Take it as soon as you remember. If it is near the time for the next dose, skip the missed dose and resume your regular dosage schedule. Do not double the next dose.

STOPPING THE DRUG
The decision to stop taking the drug should be made by your doctor.

PROLONGED USE
See your doctor regularly for tests and examinations if you take trimethobenzamide for a prolonged period. Using more than the recommended dosage or taking it more often than directed can increase the possibility of side effects.

PRECAUTIONS
Over 60: No special problems are expected.

Driving and Hazardous Work: Do not drive or engage in hazardous work until you determine how the medicine affects you.

Alcohol: Avoid alcohol.

Pregnancy: Adequate human studies have not been completed. Before taking trimethobenzamide, tell your doctor if you are pregnant or plan to become pregnant.

Breast Feeding: Trimethobenzamide may pass into breast milk; caution is advised. Consult your doctor for advice.

Infants and Children: Trimethobenzamide should be used in infants and children only under the direction of your doctor. Some side effects may be more severe in children. Do not use the injectable form in children. Do not use the suppository form in either premature or newborn infants.

Special Concerns: When used for motion sickness, trimethobenzamide should be taken 30 minutes before exposure to motion. If the suppository is too soft to insert, chill it with running water or refrigerate it for 30 minutes. To reduce irritation and pain around the area of the injection, inject the medicine deeply into the outer area of the buttocks.

OVERDOSE
Symptoms: Seizures, unconsciousness.

What to Do: Call your doctor, emergency medical services (EMS), or the nearest poison control center immediately.

DRUG INTERACTIONS
Consult your doctor for specific advice if you are taking aspirin, phenobarbital, tricyclic antidepressants, or other central nervous system depressants such as tranquilizers, sleeping pills, or cold and allergy drugs.

FOOD INTERACTIONS
No known food interactions.

DISEASE INTERACTIONS
Caution is advised when taking trimethobenzamide. Consult your doctor if you have a high fever, severe vomiting, dehydration, or an intestinal infection, or if a child has Reye's syndrome.

BRAND NAMES
Bactrim, Cotrim, Septra, Sulfamethoprim, Uro-D/S, Uroplus

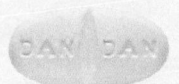

Generic 160/800 mg
(SCHEIN/DANBURY)

▶ Drug Class: Anti-infective

▶ Available in: Tablets, injection

▶ Available OTC? No

▶ As Generic? Yes

Side Effects

SERIOUS
Skin rash, sore throat, fever, joint pain, shortness of breath, pale skin, reddish spots on skin, unusual bleeding or bruising. Call your doctor immediately.

COMMON
Nausea, vomiting, loss of appetite, allergic skin reactions, itching, hives.

LESS COMMON
Abdominal pain, diarrhea, seizures, dizziness, ringing in ears, headache, hallucinations, depression, unusual sensitivity to sunlight.

PRINCIPAL USES
To treat urinary tract infections, ear infections, chronic bronchitis, Pneumocystis carinii pneumonia (a lung infection commonly seen in patients with compromised immune systems), traveler's diarrhea, and other types of diarrheal disease.

HOW THE DRUG WORKS
This medication is a combination of two active ingredients. Both trimethoprim and sulfamethoxazole kill or inhibit growth of bacteria by disrupting their ability to make necessary proteins.

DOSAGE
For common bacterial infections— Adults: The usual dose is 1 double strength (DS) tablet 2 times a day. Duration of therapy depends on the type of infection and will be determined by your doctor. For alternative dosages and for treatment of children, consult your pediatrician, as dosages can vary considerably depending on age, weight, and kidney function.

ONSET OF EFFECT
Unknown.

DURATION OF ACTION
Unknown.

DIETARY ADVICE
Tablets should be taken with a full glass of water and can be taken with food to lessen stomach upset.

STORAGE
Store in a tightly sealed container away from heat and direct light.

IF YOU MISS A DOSE
Take it as soon as you remember. However, if it is near the time for the next dose, skip the missed dose and resume your regular dosage schedule. Do not double the next dose.

STOPPING THE DRUG
Take the drug as prescribed for the full treatment period, even if you begin to feel better before the scheduled end of therapy.

PROLONGED USE
See your doctor regularly for tests and examinations if you must take this medicine for a prolonged period.

PRECAUTIONS
Over 60: Adverse reactions may be more likely and more severe in older patients.

Driving and Hazardous Work: Do not drive or engage in hazardous work until you determine how the medicine affects you.

Alcohol: No special problems are expected, although it is generally advisable to abstain from alcohol when fighting an infection.

Pregnancy: Trimethoprim with sulfamethoxazole has caused birth defects in animals. Human studies have not been done. It should be used during pregnancy only if the benefits clearly outweigh the possible risks. Before you take this medication, tell your doctor if you are pregnant or plan to become pregnant.

Breast Feeding: Trimethoprim with sulfamethoxazole passes into breast milk; avoid or discontinue use while nursing.

Infants and Children: This medication is not recommended for use by children under the age of 2 months.

Special Concerns: Since some patients experience increased sensitivity to sunlight, take preventive measures: use sunscreens, wear protective clothing, and avoid exposure to the sun. Patients with acquired immunodeficiency syndrome (AIDS) may have a higher incidence of side effects, especially rash. Nonetheless, trimethoprim with sulfamethoxazole remains valuable for treating a number of problems associated with this disease.

OVERDOSE
Symptoms: Loss of appetite, nausea, vomiting, dizziness, headache, drowsiness, depression, confusion, altered mental status, fever, blood in urine, yellow skin or eyes.

What to Do: Call your doctor, emergency medical services (EMS), or the nearest poison control center immediately.

DRUG INTERACTIONS
The following drugs may interact with trimethoprim with sulfamethoxazole. Consult your doctor for specific advice if you are taking cyclosporine, methotrexate, phenytoin, procainamide, sulfonylureas, or warfarin.

FOOD INTERACTIONS
No known food interactions.

DISEASE INTERACTIONS
Use of sulfamethoxazole may cause complications in patients with liver or kidney disease, since these organs work together to remove the medication from the body. This drug can also cause complications in patients with certain types of anemia. Consult your doctor for specific advice if you have any other medical condition.

Triprolidine Hydrochloride

▶ Drug Class: Antihistamine

▶ Available in: Syrup

▶ Available OTC? Yes

▶ As Generic? Yes

Side Effects

SERIOUS
Sore throat and fever, unusual tiredness or weakness, unusual bleeding or bruising. Call your doctor immediately.

COMMON
Drowsiness, thickening of mucus.

LESS COMMON
Blurred vision; rapid heartbeat; skin rash; stomach upset; nervousness; increased sensitivity of skin to sunlight; confusion; difficult or painful urination; dizziness; dry mouth, nose, or throat; loss of appetite; nightmares; ringing or buzzing in ears; restlessness; irritability.

PRINCIPAL USES
To relieve symptoms of hay fever and other allergies.

HOW THE DRUG WORKS
Triprolidine blocks the effects of histamine, a naturally occurring substance that causes swelling, itching, sneezing, watery eyes, hives, and other symptoms of allergic reaction.

DOSAGE
Adults and children age 12 and over: 2.5 mg every 4 to 6 hours. The maximum dose is 10 mg per day. Children ages 6 to 12: 1.25 mg (1 teaspoon) every 4 to 6 hours. The maximum dose is 5 mg per day. Children ages 4 to 6: 0.938 mg (¾ teaspoon) every 4 to 6 hours. The maximum dose is 3.744 mg per day. Children ages 2 to 4: 0.625 mg (½ teaspoon) every 4 to 6 hours. The maximum dose is 2.5 mg per day. Children ages 4 months to 2 years: 0.313 mg (¼ teaspoon) every 4 to 6 hours. The maximum dose is 1.25 mg per day.

ONSET OF EFFECT
15 to 60 minutes.

DURATION OF ACTION
4 to 6 hours.

DIETARY ADVICE
This drug should be taken with food or milk to reduce stomach upset.

STORAGE
Store in a tightly sealed container away from heat and direct light. Do not allow the drug to freeze.

IF YOU MISS A DOSE
Take it as soon as you remember. If it is near the time for the next dose, skip the missed dose and resume your regular dosage schedule. Do not double the next dose.

STOPPING THE DRUG
The decision to stop taking the drug should be made by your doctor.

PROLONGED USE
Tolerance, or decreased responsiveness to the drug, usually does not develop with prolonged use. If it does, consult your doctor.

PRECAUTIONS
Over 60: Adverse reactions may be more likely and more severe in older patients.

Driving and Hazardous Work: Do not drive or engage in hazardous work until you determine how the medicine affects you.

Alcohol: Avoid alcohol.

Pregnancy: Before you take triprolidine, tell your doctor if you are pregnant or plan to become pregnant.

Breast Feeding: Triprolidine passes into breast milk; avoid or discontinue use while nursing. Flow of breast milk may be reduced.

Infants and Children: Adverse effects may be more likely and more severe in children.

Special Concerns: Stop taking triprolidine 4 days before you have an allergy skin test. Drink water frequently or use ice chips, sugarless candy, or sugarless gum if dry mouth occurs. Coffee or tea may reduce the common side effect of drowsiness.

OVERDOSE
Symptoms: Central nervous system depression or, paradoxically, nervous system stimulation; very low blood pressure; breathing difficulty; seizures; loss of consciousness; severe dryness of the mouth, nose, or throat.

What to Do: Call your doctor, emergency medical services (EMS), or the nearest poison control center immediately.

DRUG INTERACTIONS
Consult your doctor for specific advice if you are taking anticholinergics, clarithromycin, erythromycin, itraconazole, ketoconazole, bepridil, disopyramide, maprotiline, phenothiazines, pimozide, procainamide, quinidine, tricyclic antidepressants, central nervous system depressants, MAO inhibitors, or quinine.

FOOD INTERACTIONS
No known food interactions.

DISEASE INTERACTIONS
Caution is advised when taking triprolidine. Consult your doctor if you have an enlarged prostate, urinary tract blockage, difficult urination, or glaucoma. Use of triprolidine may cause complications in patients with liver disease, since this organ works to remove the medication from the body.

Trovafloxacin

BRAND NAME
Trovan

▶ Drug Class: Antibiotic

▶ Available in: Tablets, injection

▶ Available OTC? No

▶ As Generic? No

Side Effects

SERIOUS
Serious reactions are rare. The most serious potential side effect is liver toxicity, which can cause jaundice (characterized by yellowish discoloration of the skin and eyes), nausea, vomiting, abdominal pain, fatigue, loss of appetite, and dark urine. Liver failure has led to a small number of deaths and liver transplants. Other serious side effects may include chest pain, heart rhythm irregularities, diarrhea, anaphylaxis (a severe allergic reaction marked by sudden swelling of the lips, tongue, face, or throat; breathing difficulty; skin rash, itching, or hives), seizures, and confusion or other mental disturbances such as restlessness, nightmares, and insomnia. Call your doctor immediately.

COMMON
Dizziness, lightheadedness, nausea, headache.

LESS COMMON
Vomiting, abdominal pain, yeast infection (females), itching, increased sensitivity to sunlight.

PRINCIPAL USES
To treat a number of serious bacterial infections such as pneumonia, gynecological infections, and complicated skin infections, especially when acquired in a hospital or nursing home. Your doctor will determine if this drug is appropriate for your condition.

HOW THE DRUG WORKS
Trovafloxacin inhibits the activity of two bacterial enzymes, including DNA gyrase, that are necessary for proper DNA formation and replication. This fights infection by preventing bacteria cells from reproducing.

DOSAGE
The dosage varies, depending on the site and type of infection. Daily doses of the tablets range from 100 to 200 mg for periods of 3 to 14 days. Your doctor will determine the correct dosage for your specific condition. Intravenous doses, when necessary, are administered by a health care professional.

ONSET OF EFFECT
Unknown.

DURATION OF ACTION
Unknown.

DIETARY ADVICE
Trovafloxacin can be taken without regard to meals.

STORAGE
Tablets: Store in a tightly sealed container away from heat, moisture, and direct light. Injection: Not applicable; injectable dose is administered only at a health care facility.

IF YOU MISS A DOSE
Tablet: Take it as soon as you remember. If you miss the dose one day, resume your regular dosage schedule. Do not double the next dose. Injection: Consult your doctor.

STOPPING THE DRUG
Take it as prescribed for the full treatment period, even if you begin to feel better before the scheduled end of therapy. The decision to stop taking the drug should be made by your doctor.

PROLONGED USE
Trovafloxacin is generally prescribed only for short-term use and should not be used for more than 14 days.

PRECAUTIONS

Over 60: No special problems are expected.

Driving and Hazardous Work: Do not drive or engage in hazardous work until you determine how the medicine affects you.

Alcohol: It is advisable to abstain from alcohol when fighting an infection.

Pregnancy: Adequate human studies have not been done. Before taking trovafloxacin, discuss with your doctor the relative risks and benefits of using this drug while pregnant.

Breast Feeding: Trovafloxacin passes into breast milk; extreme caution is advised. Consult your doctor for specific advice.

Infants and Children: Not recommended for use by children under the age of 18 years.

Special Concerns: Take trovafloxacin with food or at bedtime to reduce the likelihood of dizziness. If trovafloxacin causes heightened sensitivity to sunlight, stop taking the drug and try to avoid exposure to sunlight for the next 5 days; also wear protective clothing and use a sunblock.

OVERDOSE

Symptoms: An overdose with trovafloxacin is unlikely to occur.

What to Do: If someone takes a much larger dose than prescribed, call your doctor, emergency medical services (EMS), or the nearest poison control center immediately.

DRUG INTERACTIONS
Trovafloxacin should be taken at least 2 hours before or after taking certain antacids, sucralfate, citric acid buffered with sodium citrate, or vitamin or mineral supplements containing iron.

FOOD INTERACTIONS
No known food interactions.

DISEASE INTERACTIONS
Trovafloxacin should not be used at all in patients with liver disease or those who have had an allergic reaction to quinolone antibiotics in the past. The drug should be used with caution in those with a history of seizures or any nervous system disorders that may increase the risk of seizures. Be sure to inform your doctor if you have any other medical condition.

Undecylenic Acid

▶ Drug Class: Topical antifungal

▶ Available in: Aerosol foam, aerosol powder, cream, ointment, powder, solution

▶ Available OTC? Yes

▶ As Generic? Yes

Side Effects

SERIOUS
No serious side effects have been reported.

COMMON
No common side effects have been reported.

LESS COMMON
Skin irritation that was not present before use of this medicine. Call your doctor promptly.

PRINCIPAL USES
To treat fungal infections of the skin. (Note: Undecylenic acid has generally been replaced by newer and more effective topical antifungal medications; however, your physician may find it worthwhile to prescribe undecylenic acid under certain circumstances—for example, if you have a history of allergic reaction to other antifungal preparations.)

HOW THE DRUG WORKS
Undecylenic acid prevents the growth and reproduction of fungus cells.

DOSAGE
Aerosol foam, aerosol powder, ointment, powder, or solution: Apply to the affected area of the skin 2 times a day. The aerosol powder and aerosol spray form of the medicine should be sprayed on the affected area from a distance of 4 to 6 inches. The powder may also be sprayed in socks and shoes. If the powder is used on the feet, sprinkle it between the toes, on the feet, and in shoes and socks. Cream: Apply to the affected area of the skin as often as necessary.

ONSET OF EFFECT
Unknown.

DURATION OF ACTION
Unknown.

DIETARY ADVICE
No special restrictions.

STORAGE
Store in a tightly sealed container away from heat and direct light. Keep aerosol, cream, ointment, and liquid solution forms of undecylenic acid from freezing. Do not puncture, rupture, or incinerate the aerosol container.

IF YOU MISS A DOSE
Apply a missed dose as soon as you remember. If it is close to the next dose, skip the missed dose and resume your regular dosage schedule. Do not apply a double dose.

STOPPING THE DRUG
Take as prescribed for the full treatment period, even if you begin to feel better before the scheduled end of therapy. Discontinuing the drug prematurely may result in an even worse fungal infection later (known as rebound infection). In general, keep using this medication for two weeks after burning, itching, and other symptoms have cleared up.

PROLONGED USE
If your skin problem does not improve or becomes worse after 4 weeks of treatment, consult your doctor.

PRECAUTIONS
Over 60: There is no specific information comparing use of undecylenic acid in older persons with use in other age groups.

Driving and Hazardous Work: No special precautions are necessary.

Alcohol: No special precautions are necessary.

Pregnancy: Undecylenic acid has not been shown to cause birth defects or other problems in humans.

Breast Feeding: Undecylenic acid may pass into breast milk; caution is advised. Consult your doctor for advice.

Infants and Children: Not recommended for use on children under age 2.

Special Concerns: Keep this medicine away from the eyes, nose, and mouth. To help prevent reinfection, the powder or spray form of undecylenic acid may be used every day after bathing and careful drying. Do not use on pus-producing sores or on badly broken skin.

OVERDOSE
Symptoms: No specific ones have been reported.

What to Do: An overdose of undecylenic acid is unlikely. However, if someone accidentally ingests the drug, call your doctor, emergency medical services (EMS), or the nearest poison control center.

DRUG INTERACTIONS
Consult your doctor for specific advice if you are taking any other topical prescription or over-the-counter medication that is to be applied to the same area of the skin.

FOOD INTERACTIONS
No known food interactions.

DISEASE INTERACTIONS
Caution is advised when taking undecylenic acid. Consult your doctor if you have any other medical condition that affects the skin.

Uracil Mustard

▶ Drug Class: Alkylating agent

▶ Available in: Capsules

▶ Available OTC? No

▶ As Generic? Yes

Side Effects

SERIOUS
Black, tarry, or bloody stools; blood in urine; fever and chills; cough or hoarseness; pain in lower back or side; difficult or painful urination; red spots on skin; unusual bleeding or bruising; joint pain; sores on lips or in mouth; swollen feet or lower legs; yellow tinge to eyes or skin (jaundice). Call your doctor immediately. Some of these side effects may recur after you stop taking uracil mustard. Consult your doctor if they do.

COMMON
Diarrhea; nausea or vomiting; temporary hair loss.

LESS COMMON
Darkening of the skin, irritability, depression, nervousness, skin rash and itching.

PRINCIPAL USES
To treat leukemia, Hodgkin's disease and other lymphomas (a type of cancer affecting the lymphatic system), polycythemia vera (a blood disease characterized by the overproduction of some types of blood cells), and mycosis fungoides (a rare type of skin cancer that affects the lymphatic system).

HOW THE DRUG WORKS
Uracil mustard kills cancer cells by interfering with the activity of their genetic material, thus preventing the cells from reproducing. The drug may also affect the growth and development of healthy cells in the body, resulting in unpleasant side effects.

DOSAGE
Initial weekly dose of 0.15 mg per 2.2 lbs (1 kg) of body weight for at least 4 weeks to provide an adequate trial period. Dosage and duration of treatment can then be altered to meet the needs of individual patients.

ONSET OF EFFECT
Unknown.

DURATION OF ACTION
Unknown.

DIETARY ADVICE
Best taken at bedtime to minimize stomach upset.

STORAGE
Store in a tightly sealed container away from heat and direct light.

IF YOU MISS A DOSE
Take it as soon as you remember. If it is near the time for the next dose, skip the missed dose and resume your regular dosage schedule. Do not double the next dose.

STOPPING THE DRUG
The decision to stop taking the drug should be made by your doctor.

PROLONGED USE
You should see your doctor regularly for tests and examinations if you must take this medication for a prolonged period of time.

PRECAUTIONS
Over 60: No special problems are expected.

Driving and Hazardous Work: The use of this medication should not impair your ability to perform such tasks safely.

Alcohol: Avoid alcohol.

Pregnancy: Uracil mustard can cause birth defects if taken by either the father or the mother. Persons of childbearing years should take steps to prevent pregnancy when taking it.

Breast Feeding: Not recommended during therapy.

Infants and Children: Although there is no specific information about the use of uracil mustard in infants and children, it is not expected to cause different side effects than it does in adults.

Special Concerns: Do not receive any immunizations without your doctor's approval while taking uracil mustard. Avoid persons who have recently had oral polio vaccine and those with any infection. Check with your doctor before having any dental work done. Consult your doctor or dentist about appropriate ways to clean your teeth to avoid injury. Be careful not to cut yourself when using sharp objects such as a safety razor or nail cutters. Avoid activities and contact sports where bruising or injury could occur. If you vomit shortly after taking a dose of uracil mustard, check with your doctor. You may be told to take the dose again. After completing a different regimen of chemotherapy or radiation, a period of 2 to 3 weeks is recommended before starting uracil mustard because of the risk of bone marrow damage.

OVERDOSE
Symptoms: Vomiting, severe nausea, severe diarrhea, unusual weakness, hemorrhaging.

What to Do: Call your doctor, emergency medical services (EMS), or the nearest poison control center immediately.

DRUG INTERACTIONS
Consult your doctor for advice if you are taking amphotericin B, antithyroid agents, azathioprine, chloramphenicol, colchicine, flucytosine, interferon, plicamycin, probenecid, sulfinpyrazone, or zidovudine. Also consult your doctor if you are taking any over-the-counter drugs.

FOOD INTERACTIONS
None are known.

DISEASE INTERACTIONS
Caution is advised when taking uracil mustard. Consult your doctor if you have any of the following: chicken pox, shingles, any infection, gout, kidney disease, or liver disease.

Ursodiol

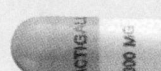

Actigall 300 mg
(Summit)

▶ Drug Class: Antigallstone agent

▶ Available in: Capsules, tablets

▶ Available OTC? No

▶ As Generic? Yes

Side Effects

SERIOUS
No serious side effects have been reported.

COMMON
No common side effects have been reported.

LESS COMMON
Diarrhea.

PRINCIPAL USES
To treat gallstones as an alternative to surgical removal of the gallbladder (cholecystectomy). Ursodiol works only when gallstones are composed entirely of cholesterol, and works best when the gallstones are small.

HOW THE DRUG WORKS
Ursodiol is a natural bile acid that safely dissolves cholesterol gallstones over a period of months or years. The time required to dissolve a stone is proportional to the stone's size. Multiple stones usually dissolve more easily than a single large stone.

DOSAGE
Adults and teenagers: 3.6 to 4.5 mg per lb of body weight a day, divided into 2 or 3 equal doses.

ONSET OF EFFECT
Variable. It may take 6 months to 2 years for gallstones to dissolve.

DURATION OF ACTION
For as long as the medication is taken.

DIETARY ADVICE
Ursodiol should be taken with or immediately after meals.

STORAGE
Store in a tightly sealed container away from heat, moisture, and direct light.

IF YOU MISS A DOSE
Take as soon as you remember or double the next dose.

STOPPING THE DRUG
Take it as prescribed for the full treatment period.

PROLONGED USE
You should see your doctor regularly for tests and examinations if you take this medicine for a prolonged period. Liver function tests (AST and ALT) should be done periodically. Ultrasound imaging should be done every 6 months for the first year of therapy to monitor the response to ursodiol. It may take 6 months to 2 years to dissolve gallstones, depending on their size and composition. Ursodiol treatment is not likely to be effective if gallstones are not partially dissolved after 12 months of therapy. Ursodiol should be continued for at least 3 months after the gallstones have dissolved.

PRECAUTIONS
Over 60: No special precautions are needed.

Driving and Hazardous Work: The use of ursodiol should not impair your ability to perform such tasks safely.

Alcohol: No special precautions are necessary.

Pregnancy: Adequate human studies have not been done. Before taking ursodiol, tell your doctor if you are or are planning to become pregnant.

Breast Feeding: It is not known whether ursodiol passes into breast milk; caution is advised. Consult your doctor for specific advice.

Infants and Children: Ursodiol is not expected to cause different or more severe side effects in children than it does in older persons.

Special Concerns: If you experience severe pain in the abdomen or stomach, particularly on the upper right side, or nausea and vomiting, call your doctor immediately. These symptoms may indicate the presence of other medical problems or that your gallbladder condition requires immediate care. Gallstones recur after 5 years in about half of those patients whose stones were successfully dissolved by ursodiol.

OVERDOSE
Symptoms: An overdose with ursodiol is unlikely.

What to Do: If someone takes a much larger dose than prescribed, call your doctor, emergency medical services (EMS), or the nearest poison control center right away.

DRUG INTERACTIONS
Other drugs may interact with ursodiol. Cholestyramine, colestipol, and antacids that contain aluminum can prevent the absorption of ursodiol from the intestine. Estrogen and oral contraceptives may interfere with the action of this medication.

FOOD INTERACTIONS
No known food interactions.

DISEASE INTERACTIONS
Ursodiol treatment is usually inappropriate when complications of gallstone disease, such as obstruction of the bile duct, cholecystitis (inflammation of the gallbladder) or pancreatitis (inflammation of the pancreas) are present. These conditions may require gallbladder surgery, because benefits from ursodiol would take too long to achieve.

Valacyclovir Hydrochloride

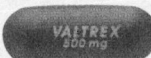

Valtrex 500 mg
(GLAXO WELLCOME)

▶ Drug Class: Antiviral

▶ Available in: Tablets

▶ Available OTC? No

▶ As Generic? No

Side Effects

SERIOUS
A rare but serious bleeding disorder marked by symptoms such as bruising, pinpoint red spots on the skin, and blood in the urine has been reported in a few patients with severely weakened immune systems.

COMMON
Headache, nausea.

LESS COMMON
Constipation or diarrhea, loss of appetite, dizziness, stomach pain, vomiting, unusual fatigue.

PRINCIPAL USES
To treat the symptoms of shingles (herpes zoster). Also used for the treatment and suppression of genital herpes.

HOW THE DRUG WORKS
Valacyclovir is converted in the body to acyclovir, which interferes with the activity of enzymes needed for the replication of viral DNA in cells, thus preventing the virus from multiplying. Although it cannot cure herpes infections, it can relieve symptoms and speed the healing of herpes lesions. It may also reduce the duration of any lingering pain (postherpetic neuralgia).

DOSAGE
For shingles: Adults: 1 gram (g), 3 times a day for 7 days. To treat initial episodes of genital herpes: 1 g, 2 times a day for 10 days. To treat recurrent genital herpes: 500 mg, 2 times a day for 5 days. For suppression of chronic recurrent genital herpes: 1 g, once a day. In patients with a history of 9 or fewer recurrences per year: 500 mg, once a day.

ONSET OF EFFECT
Within 30 minutes.

DURATION OF ACTION
Unknown.

DIETARY ADVICE
No special restrictions.

STORAGE
Store in a tightly sealed container away from heat, moisture, and direct light.

IF YOU MISS A DOSE
Take it as soon as you remember. If it is near the time for the next dose, skip the missed dose and resume your regular dosage schedule. Do not double the next dose.

STOPPING THE DRUG
The decision to stop taking the drug should be made with your doctor.

PROLONGED USE
Usual course of therapy lasts 7 to 10 days. If for any reason you must take the drug for a longer period, see your doctor for regular tests and examinations.

PRECAUTIONS
Over 60: No special problems are expected, although a smaller dose may be warranted for those with a history of impaired renal (kidney) function.

Driving and Hazardous Work: Exercise caution until you determine how the medication affects you.

Alcohol: No special precautions are necessary.

Pregnancy: Human studies of valacyclovir in pregnancy have not been done, but birth defects or other problems have not been reported. Before you take valacyclovir, tell your doctor if you are pregnant or plan to become pregnant.

Breast Feeding: Valacyclovir may pass into breast milk, although it is unknown if this poses any risks to the nursing infant; no problems have been reported. Consult your doctor for specific advice.

Infants and Children: The safety and effectiveness of this drug in children have not been established.

Special Concerns: Keep the body areas affected by shingles or herpes clean and dry, and wear comfortable, loose-fitting clothes to avoid irritation. Start taking valacyclovir as soon as possible after the symptoms

appear, ideally within 72 hours. Do not take valacyclovir if you have ever had an allergic reaction to antiviral drugs.

OVERDOSE
Symptoms: No cases of overdose of valacyclovir have been reported. If an overdose were to occur, symptoms would likely be those of acute kidney failure, which include blood in the urine, passing only small amounts of urine, swelling of the ankles, hands, face, or other areas, shortness of breath, itching, fever, and flank pain.

What to Do: Seek medical assistance right away.

DRUG INTERACTIONS
Consult your doctor for specific advice if you are taking any other prescription or over-the-counter medication, especially cimetidine or probenecid. These drugs slow the kidney's removal of valacyclovir, increasing the possibility of adverse side effects.

FOOD INTERACTIONS
No known food interactions.

DISEASE INTERACTIONS
Caution is advised when taking valacyclovir. Use of valacyclovir may cause complications in patients with kidney disease, since this organ works to remove the medication from the body. Consult your doctor if you have a weakened immune system; for example, if you are infected with the human immunodeficiency virus (HIV), or are taking immunosuppressant drugs to prevent organ rejection following a kidney or bone marrow transplant. Use of valacyclovir by patients with weakened immune systems can cause extreme side effects that may be fatal.

Depakote 500 mg
(ABBOTT)

Additional photographs

▶ Drug Class: Anticonvulsant

▶ Available in: Capsules, syrup

▶ Available OTC? No

▶ As Generic? Yes

Side Effects

SERIOUS
Severe abdominal pain and vomiting, muscle weakness and lethargy, yellow discoloration of the skin or eyes, facial swelling, abnormal bleeding or bruising, or seizures may be a sign of liver failure or other potentially fatal complications. Call your doctor immediately.

COMMON
Nausea and vomiting, heartburn, diarrhea, cramps, loss of appetite and weight loss, increased appetite and weight gain, hair loss, tremor, dizziness, clumsiness or unsteadiness, confusion, sedation.

LESS COMMON
Drowsiness, restlessness, constipation, unusual excitability, skin rash, headache, blurred or double vision, irritability or other changes in mental state. There are numerous additional side effects; consult your doctor if you are concerned about any adverse or unusual reactions.

Valproic Acid (Valproate; Divalproex Sodium)

PRINCIPAL USES
To control certain types of seizures in the treatment of epilepsy and other disorders. Also used to treat acute mania in the treatment of bipolar disorder.

HOW THE DRUG WORKS
Valproic acid is thought to depress the activity of certain parts of the brain and suppress the abnormal firing of neurons that causes seizures.

DOSAGE
Adults and children: 7 to 27 mg per lb of body weight, in 3 or 4 divided doses. Higher doses may be required. A low dose is used to start; it may be gradually increased by your doctor to achieve maximum therapeutic benefit with a minimum of side effects.

ONSET OF EFFECT
Within several hours.

DURATION OF ACTION
Maximum effect lasts for 12 hours or longer. Effectiveness then gradually decreases.

DIETARY ADVICE
Take it with food to minimize stomach upset. The syrup can be taken with liquids, but avoid carbonated beverages because the combination can irritate the mouth and throat.

STORAGE
Store in a tightly sealed container away from heat, moisture, and direct light. Do not allow the syrup to freeze.

IF YOU MISS A DOSE
Take it as soon as you remember. If it is almost time for the next dose, skip the missed dose and resume your regular dosage schedule. Do not double the

next dose without doctor's approval.

STOPPING THE DRUG
Abruptly stopping this drug may cause seizures. Your doctor will taper the dose over a period of weeks.

PROLONGED USE
See your doctor regularly for tests if you must take this drug for a prolonged period.

PRECAUTIONS
Over 60: Older patients may require lower doses to minimize side effects.

Driving and Hazardous Work: This drug may cause drowsiness or dizziness. Do not drive or engage in hazardous work until you determine how it affects you.

Alcohol: May contribute to excessive drowsiness.

Pregnancy: Valproic acid is associated with an increased risk of birth defects when taken during pregnancy. However, seizures during pregnancy can also increase the risks to the fetus. Discuss with your doctor the potential risks and benefits of using this drug during pregnancy. Folate supplementation is recommended starting 1 to 2 months before conception and throughout pregnancy.

Breast Feeding: Valproic acid passes into breast milk, although at low levels. Consult your doctor for specific advice before nursing.

Infants and Children: Adverse reactions may be more likely and more severe in children.

Special Concerns: The generic version of this drug is not recommended. Your

doctor may advise you to wear a medical bracelet or carry an identification card saying that you are taking this drug.

OVERDOSE
Symptoms: Restlessness, sleepiness, hallucinations, trembling arms and hands, loss of consciousness.

What to Do: Call your doctor, emergency medical services (EMS), or the nearest poison control center immediately.

DRUG INTERACTIONS
Valproic acid can interact with many drugs, including other anticonvulsants (carbamazepine, clonazepam, ethosuximide, felbamate, lamotrigine, phenobarbital, phenytoin, primidone), antacids, aspirin and other NSAIDs, barbiturates, cholestyramine, haloperidol, heparin, isoniazid, loxapine, MAO inhibitors, maprotiline, phenobarbital, tricyclic antidepressants, and warfarin.

FOOD INTERACTIONS
No known food interactions.

DISEASE INTERACTIONS
Special caution is advised if you have a history of blood disease, brain disease, or kidney or liver disease.

Valsartan

▶ Drug Class: Antihypertensive/
angiotensin II antagonist

▶ Available in: Capsules

▶ Available OTC? No

▶ As Generic? No

Side Effects

SERIOUS
No serious side effects
have been reported.

COMMON
No common side effects
have been reported.

LESS COMMON
Headache, dizziness,
upper respiratory infec-
tion, cough, diarrhea,
rhinitis, sinusitis, nausea,
viral infection, abdominal
pain, fatigue, edema,
joint pains, heart palpitations, skin rash, constipation, dry mouth, gas,
anxiety, insomnia, erec-
tile dysfunction (impo-
tence) in men.

PRINCIPAL USES
To control high blood pressure. This drug appears to
have the same benefits as
the class of antihypertensive
drugs known as ACE
inhibitors, without producing the common side effect
(experienced by as many as
30% of patients) of a dry
cough. Valsartan may be
used by itself or in conjunction with other antihypertensive medications.

HOW THE DRUG WORKS
Valsartan blocks the effects
of angiotensin II, a naturally
occurring substance that
causes blood vessels to narrow. Valsartan causes the
blood vessels to dilate,
thereby lowering blood
pressure and decreasing
the workload of the heart.

DOSAGE
To start, 80 mg once a day.
It may be increased by your
doctor to a maximum dose
of 320 mg per day.

ONSET OF EFFECT
Within 2 to 4 weeks.

DURATION OF ACTION
Unknown.

DIETARY ADVICE
Follow a healthy diet (low-
salt, low-fat, low-cholesterol)
as advised by your doctor to
help control blood pressure
and prevent heart disease.

STORAGE
Store in a tightly sealed container away from heat, moisture, and direct light.

IF YOU MISS A DOSE
Take it as soon as you
remember. If it is near the
time for the next dose, skip
the missed dose and
resume your regular dosage
schedule. Do not double the
next dose.

STOPPING THE DRUG
Take it as prescribed for the
full treatment period. The
decision to stop taking the
drug should be made in
consultation with your
physician.

PROLONGED USE
Lifelong therapy may be
necessary. However, if you
do change certain health
habits (for example, increasing exercise or losing
weight), a reduced dose
may be possible under a
doctor's supervision.

PRECAUTIONS
Over 60: No special problems are expected.

**Driving and Hazardous
Work:** Do not drive or
engage in hazardous work
until you determine how the
medicine affects you.

Alcohol: No special precautions are necessary.

Pregnancy: In certain
ways valsartan is similar to
a class of drugs that have
caused damage to the
unborn child when taken
in the second or third
trimester of pregnancy.
Because safer, more effective medications can lower
blood pressure during pregnancy, and because ade-
quate studies on the use of
valsartan during pregnancy
have not been done, women
who are pregnant or plan-
ning to become pregnant
should not take it.

Breast Feeding: Valsartan
may pass into breast milk;
caution is advised. Consult
your doctor for advice.

Infants and Children:
The safety and effectiveness
of use in children have not
been established.

Special Concerns: Valsartan may cause dizziness or

lightheadedness, which is
most noticeable when you
change position. This may
lead to fainting, falls, and
injury. Sit or lie down immediately if you feel dizzy or
lightheaded. This side effect
may be worsened by alco-
hol, hot weather, dehydration, fever, prolonged
standing, prolonged sitting,
or exercise.

OVERDOSE
Symptoms: Fainting, dizziness, weak pulse that might
be very slow or very fast,
nausea, vomiting, confusion,
chest pain.

What to Do: An overdose
of valsartan is unlikely to be
life-threatening. However,
if someone takes a much
larger dose than prescribed,
call your doctor, emergency
medical services (EMS), or
the nearest poison control
center immediately.

DRUG INTERACTIONS
No drug interactions have
yet been observed with valsartan. Consult your doctor
for specific advice if you are
taking any other medica-
tion, including other drugs
for high blood pressure.
Valsartan can be taken
together with diuretics or
other medications for high
blood pressure, if your doctor approves.

FOOD INTERACTIONS
No known food interactions.

DISEASE INTERACTIONS
Caution is advised when
taking valsartan. Use of valsartan may cause complications in patients with liver
or kidney disease, since
these organs work together
to remove the medication
from the body.

Valsartan/Hydrochlorothiazide

▶ Drug Class: Antihypertensive/ angiotensin II antagonist; thiazide diuretic

▶ Available in: Tablets

▶ Available OTC? No

▶ As Generic? No

Side Effects

SERIOUS
No serious side effects have been reported.

COMMON
Dizziness, fatigue.

LESS COMMON
Viral infection, sore throat, coughing, diarrhea.

PRINCIPAL USES
To control high blood pressure (hypertension). Valsartan appears to have the same benefits as the class of antihypertensive drugs known as ACE inhibitors, without producing the common side effect (experienced by as many as 30% of patients) of a dry cough. This drug combination is not used as initial treatment for hypertension.

HOW THE DRUG WORKS
This drug combines an angiotensin II antagonist (valsartan) and a thiazide diuretic (hydrochlorothiazide). Valsartan blocks the effects of angiotensin II, a naturally occurring substance that causes blood vessels to narrow. Valsartan causes the blood vessels to dilate, thereby lowering blood pressure and decreasing the workload of the heart. Hydrochlorothiazide (HCTZ) increases the excretion of salt and water in the urine. By reducing the overall fluid volume in the body, it decreases blood volume and so reduces pressure within the blood vessels.

DOSAGE
To start, 1 tablet containing 80 mg valsartan and 12.5 mg HCTZ once a day. The dose may be increased by your doctor to a maximum of 4 of these tablets or 2 tablets containing 160 mg valsartan and 12.5 mg HCTZ once a day.

ONSET OF EFFECT
Valsartan component: 2 to 4 weeks. HCTZ component: 2 to 4 hours.

DURATION OF ACTION
Valsartan component: Unknown. HCTZ component: 6 to 12 hours.

DIETARY ADVICE
It can be be taken with food to avoid stomach upset.

STORAGE
Store in a tightly sealed container away from heat, moisture, and direct light.

IF YOU MISS A DOSE
If you miss a dose on one day, do not double the dose the next day.

STOPPING THE DRUG
The decision to stop taking it should be made in consultation with your doctor.

PROLONGED USE
Lifelong therapy may be necessary.

PRECAUTIONS
Over 60: No special problems are expected.

Driving and Hazardous Work: Exercise caution until you determine how the medicine affects you.

Alcohol: No special precautions are necessary.

Pregnancy: Because safer, more effective medications can lower blood pressure during pregnancy, and because adequate studies have not been done on the use of this drug during pregnancy, women who are pregnant or planning to become pregnant should not take this medication unless recommended by your doctor.

Breast Feeding: Because of the potential for side effects on the infant, discuss with your doctor the relative risks and benefits of using this drug while nursing.

Infants and Children: The safety and effectiveness of use in children have not been established.

Special Concerns: The drug may cause dizziness or lightheadedness, which is most noticeable when you change position. This may lead to fainting, falls, and injury. Sit or lie down immediately if you feel dizzy or lightheaded. This side effect may be worsened by alcohol, hot weather, dehydration, fever, prolonged standing or sitting, or exercise. This medicine may cause your body to lose potassium. However, do not eat potassium-rich foods, salt substitutes, or take a potassium supplement without consulting your doctor.

OVERDOSE
Symptoms: Few cases of overdose have been reported. Symptoms may include: fainting, lethargy, dizziness, drowsiness, weak pulse that might be very slow or very fast, nausea, vomiting, confusion, chest pain.

What to Do: Call your doctor, emergency medical services (EMS), or the nearest poison control center immediately.

DRUG INTERACTIONS
Consult your doctor for specific advice if you are taking anticoagulants, cholestyramine, colestipol, drugs for diabetes, nonsteroidal anti-inflammatory drugs, digitalis drugs, or lithium.

FOOD INTERACTIONS
No known food interactions.

DISEASE INTERACTIONS
Consult your doctor if you have any of the following: diabetes, gout, systemic lupus erythematosus (SLE), pancreatitis, heart disease, blood vessel disease. This medication should be used with caution in patients with moderate to severe liver or kidney disease.

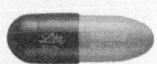

Vancocin 125 mg
(LILLY)

▶ Drug Class: Antibiotic

▶ Available in: Capsules, oral solution, injection

▶ Available OTC? No

▶ As Generic? Yes

Side Effects

SERIOUS
Skin rash (with oral forms), change in the frequency or amount of urination, breathing difficulty, drowsiness, unusual thirst, loss of appetite, weakness, hearing loss, ringing or buzzing in ears, chills or fever, fast heartbeat, fainting, nausea or vomiting, itching, redness of face, neck, upper back, and arms, tingling, unpleasant taste. Call your doctor immediately.

COMMON
Bitter or unpleasant taste, mouth irritation.

LESS COMMON
There are no less-common side effects associated with the use of vancomycin.

PRINCIPAL USES
To treat severe bacterial infections such as colitis (infection and inflammation of the colon); also used prior to surgical or dental procedures to prevent heart valve infection in susceptible patients (for example, those with a history of rheumatic fever or heart valve replacement) who are allergic to penicillin.

HOW THE DRUG WORKS
Vancomycin kills and inhibits the growth of bacteria by interrupting their formation of cell walls.

DOSAGE
To treat bacterial infections— Oral forms: Adults and teenagers: 125 to 500 mg, 4 times a day for 5 to 10 days. Children: 4.5 mg per lb of body weight (up to 125 mg), 4 times a day for 5 to 10 days. Injection: Adults and teenagers: 1,000 mg twice a day or 500 mg, 4 times a day. Children: 4.5 mg per lb, 4 times a day or 9.1 mg per lb, 2 times a day. Infants over 1 week: 6.8 mg per lb to start, then 4.5 mg per lb, 3 times a day. Newborns up to 1 week: 6.8 mg per lb to start, then 4.5 mg per lb, 2 times a day. To prevent heart valve infection— Injection: Adults and teenagers: 1,000 mg 1 hour before surgery or dental work, then 1,000 mg, 8 hours later. Children: 9.1 mg per lb of body weight 1 hour before surgery or dental work, then 9.1 mg per lb, 8 hours later.

ONSET OF EFFECT
Unknown.

DURATION OF ACTION
Unknown.

DIETARY ADVICE
No special restrictions.

STORAGE
Store the medicine in a tightly sealed container away from heat, moisture, and direct light. Refrigerate any liquid form but do not allow it to freeze.

IF YOU MISS A DOSE
Take it as soon as you remember. If it is near the time for the next dose, skip the missed dose and resume your regular dosage schedule. Do not double the next dose.

STOPPING THE DRUG
Take it as prescribed for the full treatment period, even if you feel better before the scheduled end of therapy.

PROLONGED USE
If your symptoms do not improve or instead become worse after a few days, consult your doctor.

PRECAUTIONS
Over 60: Adverse reactions may be more likely and more severe in older patients.

Driving and Hazardous Work: No special precautions are necessary.

Alcohol: No special problems are expected, although it is generally advisable to avoid alcohol when recovering from an infection.

Pregnancy: Adequate studies of the use of vancomycin during pregnancy have not been done, although no problems are expected. Before using vancomycin, consult your doctor if you are pregnant or plan to become pregnant.

Breast Feeding: Vancomycin passes into breast milk; caution is advised. Consult your doctor for specific advice.

Infants and Children: Consult your pediatrician about the relative risks and benefits of using vancomycin for children.

Special Concerns: If you take vancomycin for diarrhea caused by other antibiotics, do not take any other diarrhea medicine without consulting your doctor.

OVERDOSE
Symptoms: Hearing loss, ringing in ears, dizziness.

What to Do: Call your doctor, emergency medical services (EMS), or the nearest poison control center immediately.

DRUG INTERACTIONS
Other drugs may interact with vancomycin. Consult your doctor for specific advice if you are taking cholestyramine, colestipol (with oral forms of vancomycin), aminoglycosides, amphotericin B, bacitracin, bumetanide, capreomycin, cisplatin, cyclosporine, ethacrynic acid, furosemide, paromomycin, polymixins, or streptozocin.

FOOD INTERACTIONS
No known food interactions.

DISEASE INTERACTIONS
Consult your doctor if you have a history of kidney disease, inflammatory bowel disease, or hearing loss.

▶ Drug Class: Antidiuretic hormone

▶ Available in: Injection, nasal spray

▶ Available OTC? No

▶ As Generic? No

Side Effects

SERIOUS
Allergic response characterized by wheezing, rash, hives, itching, swelling of face, lips, hands, or feet, closing of throat, breathing difficulty, and slow or irregular pulse; drowsiness; water intoxication causing listlessness, headache, confusion, weight gain, seizures, loss of consciousness. Call your doctor immediately.

COMMON
No common side effects have been reported.

LESS COMMON
Tremor, dizziness, chest pain, abdominal cramps, nausea, vomiting, diarrhea, inability to urinate, pale skin around mouth, profuse or unusual sweating, uterine cramps. Such symptoms are generally associated only with excessively large doses.

PRINCIPAL USES
To treat diabetes insipidus, a relatively rare disorder characterized by excessive loss of water in the urine, potentially leading to dehydration. Vasopressin is generally prescribed for short-term use only and has largely been replaced by a long-lasting analog known as DDAVP (desmopressin acetate).

HOW THE DRUG WORKS
Vasopressin is a hormone involved in kidney function. It helps the kidneys to reabsorb water from urine before it is excreted, thereby maintaining proper fluid and electrolyte balance in the body.

DOSAGE
Subcutaneous (under the skin) injection— Adults: 5 to 10 units, 2 or 3 times a day. Children: 2.5 to 10 units, 3 or 4 times a day. Nasal spray— Adults or children: Spray into nostril as directed by your doctor.

ONSET OF EFFECT
Within 1 hour.

DURATION OF ACTION
From 6 to 8 hours.

DIETARY ADVICE
It can be taken with or between meals. Take it with 1 or 2 glasses of water to prevent nausea, skin whitening, and abdominal cramps.

STORAGE
Store in a tightly sealed container away from heat and direct light.

IF YOU MISS A DOSE
Take it as soon as you remember. If it is near the time for the next dose, skip the missed dose and resume your regular dosage schedule. Do not double the next dose.

STOPPING THE DRUG
The decision to stop taking the drug should be made by your doctor.

PROLONGED USE
No apparent problems are associated with prolonged use of vasopressin.

PRECAUTIONS
Over 60: Adverse reactions may be more likely and more severe in older patients.

Driving and Hazardous Work: Do not drive or engage in hazardous work until you determine how the medicine affects you.

Alcohol: Drink alcohol only in moderation.

Pregnancy: Vasopressin has not been shown to cause birth defects or other problems in humans. Animal and human studies have not been done. Before you take the drug, tell your doctor if you are pregnant or are planning to become pregnant.

Breast Feeding: Vasopressin has not been shown to cause problems in nursing babies. Consult your doctor about its use if you are breast feeding.

Infants and Children: Adverse reactions may be more likely and more severe in children under the age of 18.

Special Concerns: Electrocardiograms and laboratory tests of fluid status should be done periodically while you take vasopressin. Tell your doctor if you are allergic to any preservative or dye. Vasopressin may worsen the effect of migraine headaches.

OVERDOSE
Symptoms: Drowsiness, listlessness, headache, confusion, inability to urinate, unexpected weight gain or fluid retention.

What to Do: An overdose of vasopressin is unlikely to be life-threatening, but it can cause excessive retention of water (water intoxication) and spasm of the blood vessels. If someone takes a much larger dose than prescribed, call your doctor, emergency medical services (EMS), or poison control center immediately.

DRUG INTERACTIONS
Consult your physician for specific advice if you are taking carbamazepine, chlorpropamide, demeclocycline, ethanol, fludrocortisone, heparin, lithium, norepinephrine, or tricyclic antidepressants.

FOOD INTERACTIONS
No known food interactions.

DISEASE INTERACTIONS
Consult your doctor if you have a history of any of the following: seizures, migraine headaches, asthma, heart disease, blood vessel disease, heart failure, or kidney disease.

Venlafaxine

BRAND NAMES
Effexor, Effexor XR

Effexor 37.5 mg
(WYETH-AYERST)

▶ Drug Class: Antidepressant

▶ Available in: Tablets, extended-release capsules

▶ Available OTC? No

▶ As Generic? No

Side Effects

SERIOUS
Headache, changes in or blurred vision, decreased sexual ability or desire, difficulty urinating, itching, skin rash, chest pain, heartbeat irregularities, changes in moods or mental state, extreme drowsiness or fatigue. Call your physician immediately.

COMMON
Fatigue, dizziness or drowsiness, anxiety, dry mouth, changed sense of taste, loss of appetite, nausea, vomiting, chills, diarrhea, constipation, prickly sensation of skin, heartburn, increased sweating, runny nose, stomach gas or pain, insomnia, unusual dreams, weight loss.

LESS COMMON
Frequent yawning, twitching.

PRINCIPAL USES
To treat symptoms of major depression and generalized anxiety disorder (GAD).

HOW THE DRUG WORKS
Venlafaxine helps to balance levels of serotonin and norepinephrine, brain chemicals that are profoundly linked to mood, emotions, and mental state.

DOSAGE
Tablets: Adults: To start, 75 mg a day in 2 or 3 divided doses. The dose may be gradually increased by your doctor to 375 mg a day. Extended-release capsules: To start, 75 mg, once a day. The dose may be increased by up to 75 mg at a time at intervals of not less than 4 days, up to a maximum dose of 225 mg a day.

ONSET OF EFFECT
2 weeks or more.

DURATION OF ACTION
Unknown.

DIETARY ADVICE
Venlafaxine should be taken with meals.

STORAGE
Store in a tightly sealed container away from heat, moisture, and direct light.

IF YOU MISS A DOSE
Tablets: Take it as soon as you remember, unless the time for your next scheduled dose is within the next 2 hours. If so, skip the missed dose, take the next scheduled dose, and resume your regular schedule. Do not double the next dose. Extended-release capsules: If you miss a dose on one day, do not double the dose the next day.

STOPPING THE DRUG
Take this medication as prescribed for the full treatment period, even if you begin to feel better before the scheduled end of therapy.

PROLONGED USE
See your doctor regularly for tests and examinations if you must take this medicine for a prolonged period.

PRECAUTIONS
Over 60: No special problems are expected.

Driving and Hazardous Work: Do not drive or engage in hazardous work until you determine how the medicine affects you.

Alcohol: Avoid alcohol.

Pregnancy: Adequate studies of venlafaxine use during pregnancy have not been done. Before you take venlafaxine, tell your doctor if you are pregnant or plan to become pregnant.

Breast Feeding: It is not known whether venlafaxine passes into breast milk; caution is advised. Consult your doctor for specific advice.

Infants and Children: The safety and effectiveness of venlafaxine use by infants and children have not been established.

Special Concerns: Venlafaxine can cause an elevation in blood pressure. Therefore, blood pressure should be monitored regularly, especially in the first several months of therapy.

OVERDOSE
Symptoms: Extreme drowsiness or fatigue.

What to Do: Call your doctor, emergency medical services (EMS), or the nearest poison control center immediately.

DRUG INTERACTIONS
Venlafaxine and MAO inhibitors should not be used within 14 days of each other. Serious side effects such as myoclonus (uncontrolled muscle spasms), hyperthermia (excessive rise in body temperature), and extreme stiffness may result. Consult your doctor for specific advice if you are taking any other prescription or over-the-counter medication.

FOOD INTERACTIONS
No known food interactions.

DISEASE INTERACTIONS
Consult your physician if you have a history of any of the following: high or low blood pressure, alcohol or drug abuse, heart disease, or seizures. Use of venlafaxine may cause complications in patients with liver or kidney disease, since these organs work together to remove the medication from the body.

Isoptin SR 120 mg
(KNOLL)

808

Additional photographs

▶ Drug Class: Calcium channel blocker

▶ Available in: Extended-release capsules, tablets, injection

▶ Available OTC? No

▶ As Generic? Yes

Side Effects

SERIOUS
Breathing difficulty, coughing, or wheezing; irregular or pounding heartbeat; chest pain; extreme dizziness; fainting. Call your doctor immediately.

COMMON
Headache, dizziness, constipation, flushing and a feeling of warmth, swelling in the feet, ankles, or calves, heart palpitations.

LESS COMMON
Diarrhea, nausea, unusual fatigue and weakness, skin rash, increased urination, ringing in the ears.

PRINCIPAL USES
To treat high blood pressure, angina pectoris (chest pain associated with heart disease), and heartbeat irregularities (cardiac arrhythmias).

HOW THE DRUG WORKS
Verapamil interferes with the movement of calcium into heart muscle cells and the smooth muscle cells in the walls of the arteries. This action relaxes blood vessels (causing them to widen), which lowers blood pressure, increases the blood supply to the heart, and decreases the heart's overall workload.

DOSAGE
Adults: 40 to 160 mg, 3 times a day. Your doctor may increase dose as necessary, up to a maximum of 480 mg per day. Extended-release capsules: 200 to 480 mg once a day. Extended-release tablets: 120 mg once a day to 240 mg every 12 hours. Children: Dose is determined by a pediatrician.

ONSET OF EFFECT
Oral forms: 1 to 2 hours. Injection: 1 to 5 minutes.

DURATION OF ACTION
Extended-release capsules: 24 hours. Tablets: 8 to 10 hours. Injection: 1 to 6 hours.

DIETARY ADVICE
Take oral forms with food.

STORAGE
Store in a tightly sealed container away from heat and direct light.

IF YOU MISS A DOSE
Take it as soon as you remember. If it is near the time for the next dose, skip the missed dose and resume your regular dosage schedule. Do not double the next dose.

STOPPING THE DRUG
Do not stop taking this drug suddenly, as this may cause potentially serious health problems. If therapy is to be discontinued, dosage should be reduced gradually, according to doctor's instructions.

PROLONGED USE
Lifetime therapy with verapamil may be necessary; regular medical exams and tests are important in such cases.

PRECAUTIONS
Over 60: Adverse reactions may be more likely and more severe in older patients.

Driving and Hazardous Work: Do not drive or engage in hazardous work until you determine how the medicine affects you.

Alcohol: Avoid alcohol.

Pregnancy: Large doses of verapamil have been shown to cause birth defects in animals; human studies have not been done. Before you take verapamil, tell your doctor if you are pregnant or plan to become pregnant.

Breast Feeding: Verapamil passes into breast milk but has not been reported to cause problems; caution is advised. Consult your doctor for advice.

Infants and Children: Oral doses for children 1 to 15 years old must be determined by your pediatrician.

Special Concerns: In addition to taking verapamil, be sure to follow all special instructions on weight control and diet. Your doctor will tell you which specific factors are most important for you. Check with your doctor before making changes in your diet. Extended-release forms should not be crushed or chewed.

OVERDOSE
Symptoms: Extremely slow heartbeat and heart palpitations; dizziness or fainting (due to excessively low blood pressure).

What to Do: Call your doctor, emergency medical services (EMS), or the nearest poison control center immediately.

DRUG INTERACTIONS
Consult your physician for specific advice if you are taking acetazolamide, amphotericin B, corticosteroids, dichlorphenamide, diuretics, methazolamide, beta-blockers, carbamazepine, cyclosporine, lithium, procainamide, quinidine, digitalis, disopyramide or the following eye medicines: betaxolol, levobunolol, metipranolol, or timolol.

FOOD INTERACTIONS
Avoid foods high in sodium.

DISEASE INTERACTIONS
Caution is advised when taking verapamil. Consult your doctor if you have any of the following: abnormal heart rhythm or other disorders of the heart and blood vessels, mental depression, or Parkinson's disease. Verapamil may cause complications in patients with liver or kidney disease, since these organs work together to remove the medication from the body.

Vitamin A (Retinol)

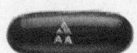

Aquasol A 25,000 IU
(ASTRA)

▶ Drug Class: Vitamin

▶ Available in: Capsules, oral solution, tablets

▶ Available OTC? Yes

▶ As Generic? Yes

Side Effects

SERIOUS
No serious side effects occur with recommended doses of vitamin A (see Overdose).

COMMON
No common side effects occur with recommended doses of vitamin A.

LESS COMMON
No less-common side effects occur with recommended doses of vitamin A.

PRINCIPAL USES
To treat vitamin A deficiency. Most Americans get sufficient amounts of vitamin A from their diet. Most vitamin A is obtained from the conversion of dietary beta-carotene to vitamin A in the intestine. Foods rich in beta-carotene include yellow-orange fruits and vegetables; dark-green leafy vegetables such as spinach and lettuce; liver; and fortified milk and margarine. Supplementation may be necessary with certain medical conditions such as long-term chronic illness, liver disorders, intestinal malabsorption associated with chronic diarrhea or pancreatic disease, and surgical removal of the stomach. Vitamin A deficiency can cause night blindness, dry eyes, eye infections, and skin problems.

HOW THE DRUG WORKS
Vitamin A plays an essential role in night vision and proper growth and maintenance of the skin, bones, and reproductive organs.

DOSAGE
For severe vitamin A deficiency: 100,000 International Units (IU) daily for 3 days, followed by 25,000 to 50,000 IU daily for 2 weeks, then 10,000 to 20,000 IU daily for 2 months. To prevent vitamin deficiency, recommended dietary allowances (RDAs)— Adults: 3,330 IU daily for men, 2,665 IU daily for women. Children ages 7 to 10: 2,330 IU daily. Children ages 4 to 6: 1,665 IU daily. Children ages 1 to 3: 1,330 IU daily. Infants: 1,250 IU daily.

ONSET OF EFFECT
Unknown.

DURATION OF ACTION
Unknown.

DIETARY ADVICE
Absorption of vitamin A requires some fat in the diet.

STORAGE
Store in a tightly sealed container away from heat, moisture, and direct light.

IF YOU MISS A DOSE
Take it as soon as you remember.

STOPPING THE DRUG
If you are taking vitamin A because of a deficiency, take it as prescribed for the full treatment period.

PROLONGED USE
Prolonged use of high doses may cause serious toxicity (see Overdose).

PRECAUTIONS
Over 60: Adverse reactions associated with high-dose, long-term use may be more likely and more severe in older patients.

Driving and Hazardous Work: The use of recommended doses of vitamin A should not impair your ability to perform such tasks safely.

Alcohol: No special precautions are necessary.

Pregnancy: Adequate vitamin A intake is essential during pregnancy. However, vitamin A overdose (more than 6,000 IU daily) can cause birth defects or slow or reduce growth in the fetus.

Breast Feeding: Vitamin A passes into breast milk; caution is advised. Ingesting too much vitamin A during breast feeding can be harmful to the nursing infant.

Infants and Children: Children are more sensitive to side effects from high doses of vitamin A.

Special Concerns: Vitamin A can be highly toxic (see Overdose) when taken in high doses. Take only as directed.

OVERDOSE
Symptoms: Acute overdose: Bleeding from gums, sore mouth, confusion or unusual excitement, diarrhea, drowsiness or dizziness, double vision, severe headache, irritability, peeling skin, especially on lips and palms, severe vomiting. Chronic overdose (with prolonged overuse): Drying or cracking of skin or lips, bone or joint pain, fever, general feeling of discomfort, increased sensitivity of skin to sunlight, increased urination, loss of appetite, hair loss, stomach pain, unusual fatigue, yellow-orange patches on soles of feet, palms of hands, or skin around the nose and lips.

What to Do: For an acute overdose, call your doctor, emergency medical services (EMS), or the nearest poison control center immediately. For symptoms of chronic overdose, contact your doctor.

DRUG INTERACTIONS
Consult your doctor for specific advice if you are taking etretinate or isotretinoin.

FOOD INTERACTIONS
No known food interactions.

DISEASE INTERACTIONS
Consult your doctor if you have a history of alcohol abuse, liver disease, or kidney disease.

Vitamin B₁ (Thiamine)

Generic 50 mg
(NUTRO)

▶ Drug Class: Vitamin

▶ Available in: Tablets, injection

▶ Available OTC? Yes

▶ As Generic? Yes

Side Effects

SERIOUS
There are no serious side effects associated with the use of thiamine (except in very rare cases pertaining to high doses administered by injection, which occur exclusively in a hospital setting).

COMMON
No common side effects have been reported.

LESS COMMON
No less-common side effects have been reported.

PRINCIPAL USES
To prevent and treat a vitamin B₁ deficiency. Vitamin B₁ deficiency can lead to either beriberi, which affects many body tissues, including the heart and nervous system (symptoms include constipation, loss of appetite, pain or tingling in arms and legs, emaciation, paralysis, heart failure, and mental deficits), or a severe brain disorder known as Wernicke's encephalopathy.

HOW THE DRUG WORKS
Thiamine is one of the B-complex vitamins, which are essential for normal metabolism and for the health and proper functioning of the cardiovascular and nervous systems. Thiamine is required for the formation of a factor needed for the function of enzymes involved in the metabolism of carbohydrates.

DOSAGE
Recommended dietary allowance (RDAs)— Infants, birth to 3 years: 0.2 to 0.5 mg per day. Children ages 4 to 8: 0.6 mg. Children ages 9 to 13: 0.9 mg. Adolescent and adult males: 1.2 mg. Males ages 51 and over: 1.0 mg. Adolescent and adult women: 1.0 to 1.1 mg. Women ages 51 and over: 0.9 mg. Pregnant women: 1.4 mg. Breast-feeding women: 1.5 mg.

ONSET OF EFFECT
Unknown.

DURATION OF ACTION
Unknown.

DIETARY ADVICE
Take it with or between meals.

STORAGE
Store in a tightly sealed container away from heat, moisture, and direct light.

IF YOU MISS A DOSE
Take it as soon as you remember.

STOPPING THE DRUG
If thiamine is being taken to treat beriberi, the decision to stop taking the drug should be made by your doctor.

PROLONGED USE
No problems are expected.

PRECAUTIONS
Over 60: No problems have been reported in older persons, who are more likely to have low blood levels of thiamine and thus require a supplement.

Driving and Hazardous Work: No special precautions are necessary.

Alcohol: No special precautions are necessary.

Pregnancy: A thiamine-containing vitamin supplement may be recommended, but taking large amounts of a supplement during pregnancy may be harmful to the mother or fetus. Consult your doctor for advice.

Breast Feeding: Taking large amounts of a dietary supplement while breast feeding may be harmful to the infant. Consult your doctor for specific advice. If thiamine deficiency occurs during breast feeding, both the mother and the nursing infant should be treated.

Infants and Children: No problems reported in infants and children with the intake of recommended daily allowances.

Special Concerns: Good nutritional habits are necessary to avoid vitamin deficiency. Thiamine-rich foods include pork, organ meats, green leafy vegetables, legumes, sweet corn, corn meal, egg yolks, brown rice, yeast, whole grains, berries, and nuts. Supplements of more than 15 mg taken 3 times a day are poorly absorbed from the intestine.

OVERDOSE
Symptoms: No cases of thiamine overdose have been reported.

What to Do: Emergency instructions not applicable.

DRUG INTERACTIONS
Consult your doctor for specific advice if you are taking any prescription or over-the-counter medication.

FOOD INTERACTIONS
No known food interactions.

DISEASE INTERACTIONS
Thiamine deficiency is most likely to occur in people on extremely low-calorie diets or those suffering from gastrointestinal disease (leading to chronic malabsorption), cirrhosis, or alcoholism. A clinically significant deficiency can occur after a few weeks of a diet with little or no thiamine.

Vitamin B₂ (Riboflavin)

Side Effects

SERIOUS
No serious side effects have been reported.

COMMON
Urine may appear bright yellow when riboflavin is taken in high doses.

LESS COMMON
No less-common side effects have been reported.

PRINCIPAL USES

To treat vitamin B₂ deficiency. Riboflavin must be included in the nutrients administered to patients receiving all their nutrition intravenously. A riboflavin deficiency may have symptoms that include sensitivity of eyes to light; itching and burning eyes; itching and peeling skin on the nose and scrotum; and sores at the corners of the mouth and on the tongue. Riboflavin requirements may be increased in people suffering from severe burns, chronic diarrhea, cirrhosis of the liver, alcoholism, cancer, or in those who have undergone surgical removal of the stomach.

HOW THE DRUG WORKS

Riboflavin is one of the B-complex vitamins, which are essential for normal metabolism and for the health and proper functioning of the cardiovascular and nervous systems. Specifically, body cells convert riboflavin into two products essential to the activity of enzymes that break down carbohydrates, proteins, and fats, and that enable oxygen to be used by the body's cells.

DOSAGE

Recommended dietary allowances (RDAs)— Adult and teenage males: 1.3 mg daily. Adult and teenage females: 1.0 to 1.1 mg daily. Children ages 9 to 13: 0.9 mg daily. Children ages 4 to 8: 0.6 mg daily. Infants from birth to 3: 0.3 to 0.5 mg daily. Pregnant women: 1.4 mg daily. Breast-feeding women: 1.6 mg daily. Sufficient vitamin B₂ is usually provided by adequate diets.

ONSET OF EFFECT

Unknown.

DURATION OF ACTION

Unknown.

DIETARY ADVICE

Avoid alcohol; it reduces the absorption of riboflavin from the intestine.

STORAGE

Store in a tightly sealed container away from heat, moisture, and direct light.

IF YOU MISS A DOSE

Take it as soon as you remember. No problems are expected as a result of missing a dose.

STOPPING THE DRUG

If riboflavin is prescribed for a vitamin deficiency, take it as prescribed for the full treatment period.

PROLONGED USE

No special problems are expected.

PRECAUTIONS

Over 60: No special problems are expected.

Driving and Hazardous Work: No special precautions are necessary.

Alcohol: Alcohol may reduce the absorption of vitamin B₂ from the intestine.

Pregnancy: No known problems. Riboflavin requirements are increased slightly during pregnancy.

Breast Feeding: Recommended intake of riboflavin and other vitamins is increased during breast feeding. Taking excessive amounts while breast feeding may be harmful to the nursing baby. Consult your doctor for specific advice.

Infants and Children: No problems are expected.

Special Concerns: Riboflavin supplements may cause a harmless yellow discoloration of the urine. Severe weight reducing diets may reduce riboflavin intake below recommended amounts, and require supplementation or increased intake of riboflavin-rich foods like eggs, organ meats, whole-grain cereals and breads, green leafy vegetables, mushrooms, avocados, legumes (such as kidney beans), cashews, chestnuts, milk, and cheeses.

OVERDOSE

Symptoms: No specific ones have been reported.

What to Do: Emergency instructions not applicable.

DRUG INTERACTIONS

Consult your doctor for specific advice if you are taking propantheline, phenothiazines, tricyclic antidepressants, or probenecid.

FOOD INTERACTIONS

None expected.

DISEASE INTERACTIONS

None expected.

Vitamin B₃ (Niacin)

Generic 50 mg
(NUTRO)

▶ Drug Class: Dietary supplement; antilipidemic (lipid-lowering) agent

▶ Available in: Tablets, extended-release tablets

▶ Available OTC? Yes

▶ As Generic? Yes

Side Effects

SERIOUS
Liver toxicity leading to jaundice (yellow discoloration of skin and eyes) and fatigue (more common with slow-release forms of niacin); gastrointestinal irritation causing nausea, vomiting, and abdominal pain; peptic ulcer; increased uric acid levels leading to gout attacks; elevated blood glucose levels.

COMMON
Itching, flushing, sweating, and dizziness, often within 20 to 40 minutes after taking niacin. These symptoms can usually be reduced or eliminated by taking an aspirin 30 minutes before the niacin. They tend to diminish or disappear with prolonged use. Slow-release forms reduce these side effects. Nausea and vomiting may also occur.

LESS COMMON
Dry skin, headaches, eye problems.

PRINCIPAL USES

As a dietary supplement: To prevent or treat niacin deficiency (pellagra). Symptoms include dermatitis, diarrhea, and dementia. (Healthy people eating a well-rounded diet do not develop niacin deficiency.) As an antilipidemic: Large doses of niacin are used to lower total and LDL cholesterol and triglyceride levels. It is the most effective drug currently available to increase HDL cholesterol levels.

HOW THE DRUG WORKS

Niacin is required for the proper action of enzymes involved in energy metabolism. It lowers blood lipids by partially blocking the release of fatty acids from adipose (fat) tissue and reducing the liver's production of the triglyceride-carrying lipoprotein, very-low-density lipoprotein (VLDL).

DOSAGE

Recommended dietary allowances (RDAs) for niacin are 6 to 12 mg a day for children; 16 mg a day for adolescent and adult men; and 14 mg a day for adolescent and adult women. As an antilipidemic: 500 to 4,500 mg a day in divided doses with meals. Initial dose is usually low and gradually increased to minimize side effects. Extended-release tablets— As an antilipidemic: All doses are taken once a day at bedtime following a low-fat snack. Week 1: 375 mg. Week 2: 500 mg. Week 3: 750 mg. Weeks 4 to 7: 1,000 mg. After week 7, your doctor will evaluate your response to your dose. The daily dose should not be increased more than 500 mg in a 4-week period, and doses above 2,000 mg daily are not recommended.

ONSET OF EFFECT

2 to 4 weeks.

DURATION OF ACTION

As long as it is taken.

DIETARY ADVICE

A well-balanced diet will prevent niacin deficiency. Persons with elevated blood lipids should follow a diet containing no more than 30% calories from fat, with only 10% calories from saturated fat, and less than 300 mg a day of cholesterol.

STORAGE

Avoid heat and direct light.

IF YOU MISS A DOSE

Skip the missed dose and resume you regular dosage schedule. Do not double the next dose.

STOPPING THE DRUG

If you take this vitamin as an antilipidemic, do not stop unless so instructed by your doctor. Once niacin is stopped, lipids will increase to pretreatment levels.

PROLONGED USE

Side effects are more likely with prolonged use.

PRECAUTIONS

Over 60: Possible increase in side effects and risk of developing diabetes.

Driving and Hazardous Work: No special precautions are necessary.

Alcohol: Niacin deficiency is more common in alcoholics because of their poor diets. Alcohol can increase blood triglycerides in people with blood lipid abnormalities. Alcohol also increases the likelihood of flushing reactions.

Pregnancy: Pregnancy increases dietary niacin needs to 18 mg a day. If taken as an antilipidemic, niacin therapy should be discontinued unless the doctor believes benefits clearly outweigh possible risks.

Breast Feeding: Breast feeding increases dietary niacin needs to 17 mg a day. There is no evidence of danger to the infant from niacin as an antilipidemic, but your doctor should reconsider whether continued therapy is absolutely necessary.

Infants and Children: Safety has not been established for treatment of lipid problems.

Special Concerns: Periodic tests to assess liver function, blood glucose, and uric acid levels are needed.

OVERDOSE

Symptoms: Flushing, abdominal pain, nausea, vomiting.

What to Do: Call your doctor.

DRUG INTERACTIONS

Niacin combined with HMG-CoA reductase inhibitors (lipid-lowering drugs known as statins) can cause myositis (muscle inflammation) with muscle pain and tenderness. Severe myositis can damage kidneys and lead to kidney failure. The drugs must be stopped immediately if symptoms of myositis occur.

FOOD INTERACTIONS

Flushing may be worse when niacin is taken with hot foods or drinks.

DISEASE INTERACTIONS

Niacin should not be used by those with a history of gout or peptic ulcer. It should be used with caution by people with diabetes, borderline high glucose levels, or any evidence of liver abnormalities.

BRAND NAMES
Beesix, Doxine, Nestrex, Pyri, Rodex, Vitabee 6

▶ Drug Class: Dietary supplement

▶ Available in: Tablets

▶ Available OTC? Yes

▶ As Generic? Yes

Side Effects

SERIOUS
When taken for several months, high doses of vitamin B6 (2 to 6 grams daily) may cause reversible nerve damage; symptoms include numbness, tingling, or prickling in the feet, loss of manual dexterity, and unsteady gait.

COMMON
No common side effects are associated with recommended doses.

LESS COMMON
No less-common side effects are associated with recommended doses.

PRINCIPAL USES
To treat or prevent vitamin B₆ deficiency, which can cause anemia, dermatitis, nervous system problems, and painful cracking at the outer sides of the mouth. Deficiency does not occur in healthy people eating a well-balanced diet. However, several genetic abnormalities may lead to a requirement for higher doses of vitamin B₆ than can be obtained from the diet. Supplements may also be necessary in people with alcoholism, an overactive thyroid, or intestinal diseases associated with nutritional malabsorption.

HOW THE DRUG WORKS
Vitamin B₆ is used to manufacture a substance required for the proper action of enzymes involved in the metabolism of carbohydrates, fats, and proteins.

DOSAGE
Recommended dietary allowances (RDAs) for vitamin B₆ are 0.1 to 0.5 mg from birth to age 3; 0.6 mg from age 4 to 8; 1.0 mg from age 9 to 13; 1.3 mg in adolescent and adult males; and 1.2 to 1.3 mg in adolescent and adult females. For men over 51: 1.7 mg; For women over 51: 1.5 mg. For vitamin B6 deficiency or an inherited abnormality causing increased vitamin B₆ requirements, consult your doctor.

ONSET OF EFFECT
Unknown.

DURATION OF ACTION
As long as the vitamin is taken.

DIETARY ADVICE
Eat a well-balanced diet. Foods rich in vitamin B₆ include egg yolks, meats, bananas, and whole grain cereals.

STORAGE
Store in a cool, dry place.

IF YOU MISS A DOSE
Take the next regularly scheduled dose.

STOPPING THE DRUG
If the vitamin was prescribed for a deficiency, consult your doctor before stopping.

PROLONGED USE
No problems are expected with recommended doses of vitamin B₆.

PRECAUTIONS
Over 60: No special problems are expected with recommended doses.

Driving and Hazardous Work: No special precautions are necessary.

Alcohol: Alcoholism can lead to a vitamin B₆ deficiency. Conversely, those who are being treated for vitamin B₆ deficiency should abstain from alcohol.

Pregnancy: Vitamin B₆ requirements increase during pregnancy to 1.9 mg per day. Very large doses may cause vitamin B₆ dependency in the newborn child.

Breast Feeding: Vitamin B₆ requirements increase during breast feeding to 2.0 mg per day.

Infants and Children: No problems are expected with recommended doses.

OVERDOSE
Symptoms: Overdose is extremely rare. Two cases that caused central nervous system toxicity (see Serious Side Effects) have been reported.

What to Do: Although an overdose is highly unlikely to occur, call your doctor right away if you have any reason to suspect that one has occurred.

DRUG INTERACTIONS
Vitamin B₆ is used in the treatment of toxicity associated with the drugs cycloserine and isoniazid. Other drugs that may increase the daily requirement for vitamin B₆ include ethionamide, hydralazine, penicillamine, immunosuppressants, and estrogen.

FOOD INTERACTIONS
No food interactions have been reported.

DISEASE INTERACTIONS
No disease interactions have been reported.

Vitamin B$_{12}$ (Cyanocobalamin)

▶ Drug Class: Dietary supplement

▶ Available in: Tablets, extended-release tablets, injection, nasal gel

▶ Available OTC? Yes

▶ As Generic? Yes

Side Effects

SERIOUS
Breathing difficulty, fever, hives, rash, swelling of face, mouth, lips, throat, or tongue. These may be signs of a rare but potentially serious allergic reaction. Seek medical assistance immediately.

COMMON
No common side effects have been reported with recommended doses.

LESS COMMON
Mild allergic reaction, diarrhea, itching.

PRINCIPAL USES
Cyanocobalamin is a synthetic form of vitamin B$_{12}$, prescribed to correct vitamin B$_{12}$ deficiency and to remedy the associated medical conditions (anemia and nerve damage) that may result from such a deficiency. B$_{12}$ deficiency can occur for a number of reasons, including a diet lacking in animal protein, pernicious anemia, intestinal malabsorption, surgical removal of portions of the stomach or small intestine, the effects of certain drugs (including colchicine, neomycin, and PAS), or because an individual is unable to keep up with an increase in the daily requirements of the vitamin (as occurs during pregnancy or during periods of great physical stress).

HOW THE DRUG WORKS
Vitamin B$_{12}$ is essential for the proper production of blood platelets and red and white blood cells, the manufacture of vital substances needed for cell function, and the metabolism of nutrients necessary for cell growth.

DOSAGE
Recommended dietary allowances (RDAs)— Adults and teenagers: 2.4 micrograms (mcg). Pregnant or breast-feeding women: 2.6 to 2.8 mcg. Children ages 9 to 13: 1.8 mcg. Children ages 4 to 8: 1.2 mcg. From birth to 3 years of age: 0.4 to 0.9 mcg. (Extended-release tablets are not recommended for children.) To treat severe vitamin B$_{12}$ deficiency— The dose will be determined by your doctor based on individual criteria. Patients with pernicious anemia or loss of intestinal function require the injection form of vitamin B$_{12}$. As an alternative to the injection, patients may use the nasal gel with a dose of 500 mcg, once a week.

ONSET OF EFFECT
Immediate.

DURATION OF ACTION
For as long as the supplement is taken.

DIETARY ADVICE
Eat a healthy, well-balanced diet. Foods rich in vitamin B$_{12}$ include animal protein (such as beef, lamb, and veal), clams and oysters, liver, fish, milk, and egg yolks.

STORAGE
Store in a tightly sealed container away from heat, moisture, and direct light.

IF YOU MISS A DOSE
Take the next regularly scheduled dose.

STOPPING THE DRUG
If the vitamin was prescribed for a deficiency, consult your doctor before stopping.

PROLONGED USE
Therapy may require weeks or months. Lifelong therapy is necessary for pernicious anemia or following certain types of gastrointestinal surgery. No problems are expected with prolonged use when the vitamin is taken as directed.

PRECAUTIONS
Over 60: No special problems are expected with recommended doses.

Driving and Hazardous Work: No special precautions are necessary.

Alcohol: Alcoholism can lead to pancreatic insufficiency and vitamin B$_{12}$ malabsorption.

Pregnancy: Vitamin B$_{12}$ requirements increase during pregnancy to 2.6 mcg daily.

Breast Feeding: Vitamin B$_{12}$ requirements increase during breast feeding to 2.8 mcg per day.

Infants and Children: No problems are expected with recommended doses.

Special Concerns: Vitamin B$_{12}$ deficiency is unlikely to occur in healthy people who are able to consume a normal, balanced diet. However, nutritional supplements should be considered for those who are ill or weakened by radiation therapy, chemotherapy, or any other condition that interferes with normal food and fluid intake. Also, healthy adults over age 51 should aim to meet their vitamin B$_{12}$ requirements with the use of B$_{12}$-fortified foods (such as fortified ready-to-eat cereal) or supplements.

OVERDOSE
Symptoms: Overdose is extremely rare.

What to Do: Although an overdose is highly unlikely, call your doctor right away if you have any reason to suspect that one has occurred.

DRUG INTERACTIONS
Consult your doctor for specific advice if you are taking analgesics, antibiotics, colchicine, folic acid, or other vitamin supplements.

FOOD INTERACTIONS
No known food interactions.

DISEASE INTERACTIONS
Consult your doctor if you have Leber's disease (a very rare eye disease).

Vitamin C (Ascorbic Acid)

Generic 500 mg
(NUTRO)

Additional photographs

► Drug Class: Dietary supplement

► Available in: Tablets, capsules

► Available OTC? Yes

► As Generic? Yes

Side Effects

SERIOUS
Occasionally, kidney stones may develop (especially with doses greater than 1 g per day over a prolonged period of time), causing back, side, or flank pain.

COMMON
No common side effects are associated with recommended doses.

LESS COMMON
High doses may cause diarrhea, flushing and redness of the skin, nausea and vomiting, or headache.

PRINCIPAL USES
To prevent or treat vitamin C deficiency, which causes scurvy, a disorder characterized by bleeding into the skin, swollen and bleeding gums, poor wound healing, muscle weakness, and fatigue. Deficiency does not occur in healthy people eating a well-balanced diet. Vitamin C requirements may be increased in those with AIDS, alcoholism, overactive thyroid, chronic infection, and intestinal diseases associated with nutritional malabsorption.

HOW THE DRUG WORKS
Vitamin C is required for the body's synthesis of collagen (tissue that constitutes the tendons, ligaments, and other inelastic fibers), for the metabolism of a variety of body substances, and to maintain structural and functional integrity of cell walls and small blood vessels.

DOSAGE
Recommended dietary allowances (RDAs) for vitamin C are as follows: 40 to 50 mg from birth to 1 year of age; 15 to 25 mg from age 1 to 8; 45 to 75 mg for boys from age 9 to 18; 45 to 65 mg for girls from age 9 to 18; 90 mg for adult men; 75 mg for adult women; smokers require an additional 35 mg daily.

ONSET OF EFFECT
Unknown.

DURATION OF ACTION
As long as it is taken.

DIETARY ADVICE
Eat a well-balanced diet to avoid vitamin C deficiency. Foods rich in vitamin C include citrus fruits and juices, green vegetables, and tomatoes.

STORAGE
Store in tightly sealed container away from heat, moisture, and direct light.

IF YOU MISS A DOSE
No problems are expected. Take the next dose at the regularly scheduled time and do not double the next dose.

STOPPING THE DRUG
If vitamin C is taken for a deficiency or because of a disorder associated with a need for a higher intake of the vitamin, consult your doctor before stopping.

PROLONGED USE
No problems are expected with prolonged use.

PRECAUTIONS
Over 60: No special problems are expected.

Driving and Hazardous Work: No special precautions are necessary.

Alcohol: Alcoholism may lead to vitamin C deficiency.

Pregnancy: Vitamin C requirements increase during pregnancy to 85 mg per day. Very large doses during pregnancy may harm the fetus.

Breast Feeding: Vitamin C requirements increase during breast feeding to 120 mg per day. Vitamin C does enter breast milk, but so far no problems have been reported from taking the recommended amounts of the vitamin.

Infants and Children: No problems are associated with recommended doses.

Special Concerns: Use of large doses of vitamin C is commonplace for the prevention of colds, cancer, and other disorders. However,

studies have shown that blood levels of the vitamin do not increase further when vitamin C doses exceed 250 to 500 mg per day. High doses of vitamin C may cause kidney stones in people with a prior history of the disorder or those with kidney disease treated with hemodialysis.

OVERDOSE
Symptoms: No specific ones have been reported.

What to Do: Emergency instructions not applicable.

DRUG INTERACTIONS
None reported with recommended doses.

FOOD INTERACTIONS
No known food interactions. However, it is worth noting that vitamin C can improve the body's absorption of iron, specifically nonheme iron (the type of iron found in foods derived from plant sources).

DISEASE INTERACTIONS
None reported.

Vitamin D

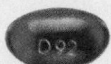

Drisdol 50,000 IU
(SANOFI WINTHROP)

▶ Drug Class: Dietary supplement

▶ Available in: Capsules, oral solution, tablets

▶ Available OTC? Yes

▶ As Generic? Yes

Side Effects

SERIOUS
Serious side effects are associated with excessively high doses (see Overdose).

COMMON
No common side effects are expected with recommended doses.

LESS COMMON
No less-common side effects are expected with recommended doses.

PRINCIPAL USES

Vitamin D is necessary for good health, and especially to maintain strong, healthy bones. It is derived from dietary sources, plus the body manufactures its own vitamin D upon exposure to sunlight. Vitamin D deficiency is thus rare among Americans, but some people—notably, those who are bedridden, have poor or highly restricted (vegan or macrobiotic) diets, or who cannot get adequate nutrition due to intestinal malabsorption—require supplementation. Supplements may also be prescribed for people with chronically low blood levels of calcium, and for alcoholics, dark-skinned people (who manufacture smaller amounts of vitamin D on their own), pregnant women, and nursing infants who get inadequate exposure to sunlight. Vitamin D supplements are also often recommended to increase calcium absorption and prevent osteoporosis in postmenopausal women.

HOW THE DRUG WORKS

Vitamin D promotes the absorption of calcium from the intestine and the utilization of calcium and phosphorus in the body. This ensures that levels of these minerals are high enough to support the constant breakdown and rebuilding of bone tissue, and to supply cells with the calcium needed to perform essential functions.

DOSAGE

Adequate intakes—
Teenagers and adults up to age 50: 200 international units (IU). Adults age 51 to 70: 400 IU. Adults over age 70: 600 IU. Infants and children up to age 12: 200 IU. Pregnant or breast-feeding women: 200 IU. Vitamin D supplementation for defi-

ciency or other medical condition— Same as above or higher, as determined by your doctor.

ONSET OF EFFECT

Within 12 to 24 hours; maximum effect: 10 to 14 days.

DURATION OF ACTION

As long as vitamin is taken.

DIETARY ADVICE

The best sources of vitamin D are fish and vitamin D fortified milk.

STORAGE

Store in a tightly sealed container away from heat and direct light.

IF YOU MISS A DOSE

When vitamin D is used as a dietary supplement, no problems are expected if you miss a dose. When it is prescribed to treat a specific medical condition, take the missed dose as soon as you remember. If it is near the time for the next dose, skip the missed dose and resume your regular dosage schedule. Do not double the next dose.

STOPPING THE DRUG

Do not stop taking the supplement without first consulting your doctor.

PROLONGED USE

Your doctor will take periodic blood tests to check levels of calcium and phosphorus if you are taking vitamin D for the treatment of low blood calcium levels.

PRECAUTIONS

Over 60: No special problems are expected.

Driving and Hazardous Work: No special precautions are necessary.

Alcohol: No special precautions are necessary.

Pregnancy: No problems are expected with recommended dose.

Breast Feeding: Trace amounts pass into breast milk; however, no problems have been reported.

Infants and Children: Infants who get little exposure to the sun and are totally breast-fed, especially those with dark-skinned mothers, may require vitamin D supplementation. Problems have not been reported with recommended amounts; however, prolonged excess doses may stunt a child's growth.

OVERDOSE

Symptoms: Early symptoms: Constipation (especially in children), diarrhea, dry mouth, increased thirst and frequency of urination, persistent headache, loss of appetite, metallic taste, nausea and vomiting, unusual fatigue. Advanced symptoms: Bone and muscle pain, irregular heartbeat, persistent itching, extreme drowsiness, mental changes. Severe vitamin D toxicity may be fatal.

What to Do: See your doctor at once.

DRUG INTERACTIONS

Consult your doctor if you are taking calcium-containing preparations, magnesium-containing antacids, or thiazide diuretics.

FOOD INTERACTIONS

No known food interactions.

DISEASE INTERACTIONS

Consult your doctor if you have high blood levels of calcium (hypercalcemia), a history of heart or blood vessel disease, pancreatitis, or impaired kidney function.

Vitamin E (Tocopherol)

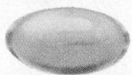

Generic 400 IU
(GOLD CAPS)

▶ Drug Class: Dietary supplement

▶ Available in: Capsules

▶ Available OTC? Yes

▶ As Generic? Yes

Side Effects

SERIOUS
No serious side effects are associated with recommended doses.

COMMON
No common side effects are associated with recommended doses.

LESS COMMON
Large doses (greater than 400 IU per day) have been associated with diarrhea, nausea, headache, blurred vision, dizziness, and fatigue. Doses greater than 800 IU per day have been reported to increase the danger of bleeding, especially in people deficient in vitamin K.

PRINCIPAL USES
For the prevention and treatment of vitamin E deficiency. Vitamin E deficiency is extremely rare and does not occur in healthy individuals eating a well-balanced diet. However, a deficiency of vitamin E can result from any disorder that causes poor absorption of fat from the intestine. Vitamin E is an antioxidant that is often prescribed to prevent the oxidation of low-density lipoprotein in an effort to prevent atherosclerosis (buildup of fatty plaques within the arteries), the underlying cause of coronary heart disease. The value of vitamin E supplements for this purpose is unproven.

HOW THE DRUG WORKS
Although considered an essential vitamin, the exact function of vitamin E remains unknown. It does help to prevent oxidation of the fatty acids present in the membranes of all cells (that is, it has antioxidant properties).

DOSAGE
Vitamin E requirements are small, ranging from 6 international units (IU) at birth to 28 IU in breast-feeding women. Recommended dietary allowance (RDA) for adults is 22 IU. Large doses (100 IU) are given when deficiency results from intestinal malabsorption. The usual doses prescribed for protection against coronary heart disease range from 400 to 800 IU per day.

ONSET OF EFFECT
Unknown.

DURATION OF ACTION
Unknown.

DIETARY ADVICE
Eat a well-balanced diet. Foods rich in vitamin E include vegetable oils, whole grains, and leafy green vegetables. Cooking and storage may cause significant losses of vitamin E.

STORAGE
Store in a tightly sealed container away from heat, moisture, and direct light.

IF YOU MISS A DOSE
No problems are expected. Take the next dose at the regularly scheduled time and do not double the next dose.

STOPPING THE DRUG
If prescribed for a deficiency, do not stop taking vitamin E without consulting your doctor first. There is no evidence that stopping vitamin E when it is taken to prevent coronary heart disease is harmful.

PROLONGED USE
No problems are associated with prolonged use.

PRECAUTIONS
Over 60: No problems are expected at recommended doses.

Driving and Hazardous Work: No special precautions are necessary.

Alcohol: No special precautions are necessary.

Pregnancy: No problems are expected with recommended doses.

Breast Feeding: Vitamin E enters breast milk, but no problems have been reported with recommended doses.

Infants and Children: No problems have been documented at recommended doses.

OVERDOSE
Symptoms: No cases of vitamin E overdose have been reported.

What to Do: Emergency instructions not applicable.

DRUG INTERACTIONS
Consumption of large doses of vitamin E in combination with anticoagulants (such as warfarin) might lead to uncontrolled bleeding.

FOOD INTERACTIONS
Absorption of vitamin E from the intestine requires the consumption of some dietary fat.

DISEASE INTERACTIONS
No disease interactions have been reported.

Vitamin K (Phytonadione; Menadiol)

BRAND NAMES
Aquamephyton (phytonadione), Konakion (phytonadione), Mephyton (phytonadione), Synkayvite (menadiol)

Mephyton 5 mg
(MERCK)

▸ Drug Class: Dietary supplement

▸ Available in: Tablets, injection

▸ Available OTC? No

▸ As Generic? No

Side Effects

SERIOUS
Menadiol has been associated with anemia and jaundice (yellow discoloration of the eyes and skin) in some newborns because their liver function is still poorly developed. Unless high doses are used, the risk is less with phytonadione.

COMMON
No common side effects are associated with recommended doses.

LESS COMMON
Flushing of the face, reactions at injection site.

PRINCIPAL USES
Vitamin K is used to prevent or treat bleeding disorders resulting from reduced formation of proteins needed for blood coagulation. The need may be due either to vitamin K deficiency or impairment of its function by anticoagulant drugs such as warfarin, salicylates, and some antibiotics. Vitamin K does not overcome the anticoagulant effects of heparin. Because vitamin K is normally made by bacteria in the intestine, dietary deficiency is rare. Bile salts are needed for absorption of vitamin K from the intestine, so absorption may be poor when obstruction of the bile ducts prevents entry of bile salts into the intestine. In newborns, the American Academy of Pediatrics recommends administration of phytonadione at birth to prevent bleeding disorders that can occur because adequate amounts of vitamin K may fail to cross the placenta from the mother to the fetus, and newborns have no bacteria in their intestines at birth. In people receiving all nutrition by injection for long periods, intramuscular injections of vitamin K are needed.

HOW THE DRUG WORKS
Vitamin K is necessary before a number of blood coagulation factors can become active in preventing or stopping bleeding.

DOSAGE
Oral doses— Menadiol sodium phosphate: Adults: For obstruction of bile duct: 5 mg a day. For problems related to use of antibacterials or salicylates: 5 to 10 mg a day. Children: 5 mg a day. Phytonadione: Adults: 2.5 to 10 mg (but up to 25 mg) if needed; can be repeated after 12 to 48 hours. Injections— Menadiol sodium phosphate: Adults: 5 to 15 mg once or twice a day. Children: 5 to 10 mg once or twice a day. Phytonadione: Adolescents and adults: 2.5 to 25 mg; can be repeated if necessary. Children: 5 to 10 mg. Infants: 1 to 2 mg. During long-term total parenteral (intravenous) nutrition: Adults: 5 to 10 mg a week. Children: 2 to 5 mg a week.

ONSET OF EFFECT
Oral phytonadione: 6 to 12 hours. Injected phytonadione: 1 to 2 hours. Injected menadiol sodium phosphate: 8 to 24 hours.

DURATION OF ACTION
12 to 24 hours.

DIETARY ADVICE
No interactions. The best dietary sources of vitamin K are leafy green vegetables, meats, and dairy products.

STORAGE
Store in a cool dry place away from light. Avoid allowing injectable forms to freeze.

IF YOU MISS A DOSE
Take as soon as remembered unless close to next dose. Do not double the next dose.

STOPPING THE DRUG
Do not stop taking vitamin K unless instructed to do so by your doctor.

PROLONGED USE
Prolonged use is uncommon; no problems are expected at recommended doses.

PRECAUTIONS
Over 60: No information is available on the effects of age on vitamin K doses.

Driving and Hazardous Work: No special precautions are necessary.

Alcohol: No special precautions are necessary.

Pregnancy: No information is available.

Breast Feeding: No problems have been reported.

Infants and Children: Caution is required with vitamin K injections in newborns because of the risk of anemia and liver toxicity.

Special Concerns: The smallest effective dose should be given to overcome bleeding due to an overdose of anticoagulant. Too large a dose may delay the subsequent action of the anticoagulant. Laboratory tests of clotting function (prothrombin time) are needed to determine the proper dose of vitamin K.

OVERDOSE
Symptoms: No specific ones have been reported.

What to Do: Emergency instructions not applicable.

DRUG INTERACTIONS
Antacids, antibiotics, and sucralfate can decrease vitamin K absorption. Vitamin K can interfere with the action of drugs like salicylates and anticoagulants. Other drugs may interact with vitamin K; consult your doctor if you are taking any prescription or over-the-counter drug.

FOOD INTERACTIONS
None reported.

DISEASE INTERACTIONS
Caution is advised in people with liver disease.

Warfarin

Coumadin 2 mg
(DUPONT)

Additional photographs

▸ Drug Class: Anticoagulant

▸ Available in: Tablets, injection

▸ Available OTC? No

▸ As Generic? Yes

Side Effects

SERIOUS
Allergic reaction (marked by wheezing, breathing difficulty, hives, or swelling of lips, tongue, and throat); bleeding into skin and soft tissue; abnormal bleeding from nose, gastrointestinal tract, urinary tract, or uterus; severe infection; excessive or unexpected menstrual bleeding; black vomit; bruises or purple marks on skin. Consult your doctor immediately.

COMMON
No common side effects have been reported.

LESS COMMON
Loss of appetite, unusual weight loss, nausea, vomiting, skin rash, diarrhea, cramping.

PRINCIPAL USES
To prevent blood clot formation in patients suffering from heart, lung, and blood vessel disorders that could lead to heart attack, stroke, or other problems.

HOW THE DRUG WORKS
Warfarin blocks the action of vitamin K, a compound necessary for blood clotting.

DOSAGE
Adults: To start, 10 to 15 mg daily, taken once a day. Long-term, usually 2 to 10 mg per day, taken once a day. Children: The dose must be determined by a pediatrician. It should be taken at the same time every day.

ONSET OF EFFECT
36 to 48 hours.

DURATION OF ACTION
24 to 96 hours.

DIETARY ADVICE
Warfarin can be taken with liquid or food.

STORAGE
Store in a tightly sealed container away from heat and direct light.

IF YOU MISS A DOSE
If you miss a dose, take it as soon as you remember, unless it is almost time for the next dose. In that case, skip the missed dose and go back to your regular schedule. Do not double the next dose.

STOPPING THE DRUG
Take it as prescribed for the full treatment period, even if you begin to feel better before the scheduled end of therapy. The decision to stop taking the drug should be made by your doctor.

PROLONGED USE
Regular tests of prothrombin time (a simple test that measures the time it takes for one stage of blood coagulation to occur) are needed when taking this drug. Your doctor may also take stool and urine samples periodically to check for the presence of blood.

PRECAUTIONS
Over 60: Adverse reactions may be more likely and more severe in older patients.

Driving and Hazardous Work: Avoid if you have blurred vision or feel dizzy. Avoid activities that could cause injury.

Alcohol: Use with caution. Alcohol can increase or decrease the effect of warfarin. Usually, consume no more than one drink a day.

Pregnancy: Warfarin may cause birth defects. Do not use during pregnancy.

Breast Feeding: Warfarin passes into breast milk. Do not use while nursing.

Infants and Children: Not recommended for children under 18.

OVERDOSE
Symptoms: Bleeding gums, uncontrolled nosebleeds, blood in the urine or stools.

What to Do: Discontinue the medication and call your doctor, emergency medical services (EMS), or the nearest poison control center right away.

DRUG INTERACTIONS
Consult your doctor for specific advice if you are taking steroid drugs, acetaminophen, allopurinol, aminogluthemide, antibiotics, antiarrhythmic heart drugs, androgens, antacids, antifungal drugs, antihistamines, aspirin, antidiabetic drugs, disulfiram, a nonsteroidal anti-inflammatory drug (NSAID), barbiturates, benzodiazepine tranquilizers, calcium supplements, chloramphenicol, or any cholesterol-lowering drugs.

FOOD INTERACTIONS
Avoid green, leafy vegetables and other foods that are rich in vitamin K (liver, broccoli, cauliflower, kale, spinach, and cabbage). Intake of too much vitamin K can override the anticlotting effect of warfarin and render the drug useless. Conversely, certain substances can interfere with the absorption of vitamin K so much that normal, healthy clotting (necessary for wounds to heal) is impaired. Megadoses of vitamin E can do this, as can fish oil supplements and foods high in omega-3 fatty acids. These substances can enhance the effect of anticlotting drugs so much that a tendency to hemorrhage may result.

DISEASE INTERACTIONS
Consult your doctor about taking warfarin if you have high blood pressure, diabetes, serious liver or kidney disease, or a severe allergy.

Yohimbine

Generic 5.4 mg
(MIKART)

▶ Drug Class: Alpha-adrenergic blocking agent

▶ Available in: Tablets

▶ Available OTC? Yes

▶ As Generic? Yes

Side Effects

SERIOUS
Rapid heartbeat; increased blood pressure, possibly causing symptoms such as persistent headaches or ringing in the ears. Call your doctor immediately.

COMMON
No common side effects have been reported.

LESS COMMON
Headache, dizziness, irritability, nervousness, restlessness, flushing of skin, shakiness, increased sweating.

PRINCIPAL USES
To aid in the treatment of male erectile dysfunction (impotence).

HOW THE DRUG WORKS
The exact way in which yohimbine works has not been determined. It is believed to block certain chemical receptors that cause constriction of blood vessels. In doing so, yohimbine theoretically improves blood flow into (and inhibits blood flow out of) the spongy columns of tissue in the penis involved in the mechanics of erection. Yohimbine may also have a mild stimulant effect and may promote the release of brain chemicals that control mood, relaxation, and sex drive, among other functions.

DOSAGE
Adult males: 5.4 mg, 3 times a day.

ONSET OF EFFECT
Within 2 to 3 weeks in most cases.

DURATION OF ACTION
Unknown.

DIETARY ADVICE
No special restrictions.

STORAGE
Store in a tightly sealed container away from heat, moisture, and direct light. Do not refrigerate medication or allow it to freeze.

IF YOU MISS A DOSE
Take it as soon as you remember. If it is near the time for the next dose, skip the missed dose and resume your regular dosage schedule. Do not double the next dose.

STOPPING THE DRUG
The decision to stop taking the drug should be made in consultation with your physician.

PROLONGED USE
See your doctor regularly for tests and examinations if you take this drug for a prolonged period of time.

PRECAUTIONS
Over 60: No special problems are expected.

Driving and Hazardous Work: Do not drive or engage in hazardous work until you determine how the medicine affects you.

Alcohol: No special restrictions; however, excess alcohol consumption may impair sexual function.

Pregnancy: Yohimbine is generally not prescribed for women and should not be used during pregnancy.

Breast Feeding: Not applicable to female patients.

Infants and Children: Not applicable to children.

Special Concerns: This drug should be used only by men who have been diagnosed with and are being medically treated for erectile dysfunction.

OVERDOSE
Symptoms: Agitation, restlessness, dizziness, heart palpitations.

What to Do: An overdose with yohimbine is unlikely. However, if someone takes a much larger dose than prescribed, call your doctor, emergency medical services (EMS), or the nearest poison control center.

DRUG INTERACTIONS
Consult your doctor for specific advice if you are taking antidepressants (especially MAO inhibitors) or any other mood-modifying medications, including selective serotonin reuptake inhibitors (SSRIs), such as fluoxetine. Before you take yohimbine, tell your doctor if you are taking any other prescription or over-the-counter drugs, especially cold remedies or weight-loss aids.

FOOD INTERACTIONS
Since yohimbine is a mild MAO inhibitor, it should not be taken with any food or drink containing tyramines, including cheese, chocolate, beer, aged meats, and nuts, and particularly not with the amino acids tyrosine or phenylalanine. A dangerous rise in blood pressure may result.

DISEASE INTERACTIONS
Caution is advised when taking yohimbine. Consult your doctor if you have a history of angina pectoris, mental depression or any other psychiatric illness, heart disease, high blood pressure, or impaired kidney function. Use of yohimbine may cause complications in patients with liver disease, since this organ works to remove the medication from the body.

Zafirlukast

BRAND NAME
Accolate

Accolate 20 mg
(ZENECA)

▶ Drug Class: Leukotriene receptor antagonist

▶ Available in: Tablets

▶ Available OTC? No

▶ As Generic? No

Side Effects

SERIOUS
Burning or prickling sensation, skin rash. A rare side effect with high doses is liver dysfunction (symptoms include: abdominal pain, nausea, fatigue, lethargy, itching, yellow discoloration of the eyes or skin, and flu-like symptoms). Call your doctor immediately.

COMMON
Headache.

LESS COMMON
Weakness, abdominal pain, back pain, diarrhea, dizziness, mouth ulcers, nausea, vomiting.

PRINCIPAL USES
To prevent the symptoms of asthma on a maintenance basis and to prevent bronchospasm (contraction of the smooth muscle tissue surrounding the airways, which results in narrowing and obstruction of the air passages). Zafirlukast may be used in conjunction with other asthma treatments, such as bronchodilators.

HOW THE DRUG WORKS
Zafirlukast blocks cell receptors for leukotrienes, chemicals that cause inflammation and constriction of the bronchial airways. Unlike bronchodilators, which relieve the acute symptoms of an asthma attack, zafirlukast is prescribed to be taken regularly when no symptoms are present, to reduce the chronic inflammation of the airways that underlies asthma. This prevents symptomatic asthma attacks.

DOSAGE
Adults and teenagers: 20 mg twice a day. Children ages 7 to 11: 10 mg twice a day. Doses are usually taken in the morning and evening, on an empty stomach (at least 1 hour before or 2 hours after eating).

ONSET OF EFFECT
Within 1 week.

DURATION OF ACTION
Unknown.

DIETARY ADVICE
Zafirlukast should be taken 1 hour before or 2 hours after meals. Taking it with a high-fat or high-protein meal reduces its availability in the body by 40%.

STORAGE
Store in a tightly sealed container away from heat and direct light.

IF YOU MISS A DOSE
Take it as soon as you remember. If it is near the time for the next dose, skip the missed dose and resume your regular dosage schedule. Do not double the next dose.

STOPPING THE DRUG
The decision to stop taking the drug should be made by your doctor.

PROLONGED USE
No problems are expected. It is important to take zafirlukast every day, even during symptom-free periods.

PRECAUTIONS
Over 60: In clinical trials, mild or moderate infections, primarily of the respiratory tract, occurred more often than expected in older patients. The rate of infection was proportional to the dose of zafirlukast taken. Other adverse reactions were no more likely or more severe in older patients than in younger persons.

Driving and Hazardous Work: Do not drive or engage in hazardous work until you determine how the medication affects you.

Alcohol: No special precautions are necessary.

Pregnancy: In some animal studies, zafirlukast caused birth defects and other problems. Human studies have not been done. Before you take zafirlukast, tell your doctor if you are pregnant or plan to become pregnant.

Breast Feeding: Zafirlukast passes into breast milk; do not use it while nursing.

Infants and Children: The safety and effectiveness of zafirlukast in children under the age of 7 have not been established.

Special Concerns: Zafirlukast has no effect on an asthma attack already in progress. In very rare cases, the drug may cause Churg-Strauss syndrome, a tissue disorder that strikes adult asthma patients and, if untreated, can destroy organs. Early symptoms include fever, muscle aches, and weight loss.

OVERDOSE
Symptoms: None.

What to Do: Call your doctor if you suspect an overdose.

DRUG INTERACTIONS
Consult your doctor for specific advice if you are taking aspirin, carbamazepine, cyclosporine, felodipine, isradipine, nicardipine, nifedipine, nimodipine, phenytoin, tolbutamide, erythromycin, terfenadine, theophylline, or warfarin. Patients who are taking warfarin or any other anticoagulant should have their prothrombin time monitored closely, and appropriate changes made in the anticoagulant dosage, when they start taking zafirlukast. Before you take zafirlukast, tell your doctor if you are allergic to any prescription or over-the-counter medicine.

FOOD INTERACTIONS
No known food interactions.

DISEASE INTERACTIONS
Consult your doctor if you have any other medical condition. Use of zafirlukast can cause complications in patients with liver disease, since this organ works to remove the medication from the body.

Zalcitabine (Dideoxycytidine; ddC)

HIVID 0.375 mg
(ROCHE)

▶ Drug Class: Antiviral

▶ Available in: Tablets

▶ Available OTC? No

▶ As Generic? No

Side Effects

SERIOUS
Burning, tingling, pain, or numbness in hands or feet, fever, muscle pain, joint pain, skin rash, ulcers in mouth and throat, nausea, vomiting, fever, sore throat, yellow discoloration of eyes or skin. Call your doctor immediately.

COMMON
No common side effects are associated with the use of zalcitabine.

LESS COMMON
Diarrhea, headache.

PRINCIPAL USES
To treat HIV (human immunodeficiency virus) infection, usually in combination with other antiretroviral drugs. While not a cure for HIV, such medications may suppress the replication of the virus and delay the progression of the disease.

HOW THE DRUG WORKS
Zalcitabine (ddC) interferes with the activity of enzymes needed for the replication of DNA in viral cells, thus preventing the virus from reproducing.

DOSAGE
Adults and teenagers: 0.75 mg, 3 times a day in combination with other antiretroviral drugs. Children: Dose must be determined by your pediatrician.

ONSET OF EFFECT
Unknown. With most antiretroviral drugs, an early response can be seen within the first few days of therapy, but the maximum effect may take 12 to 16 weeks.

DURATION OF ACTION
Unknown. Effects of the drug may be prolonged if zalcitabine is used in combination with other effective drugs and the virus is maximally suppressed.

DIETARY ADVICE
No special restrictions.

STORAGE
Store in a tightly sealed container away from heat and direct light.

IF YOU MISS A DOSE
Take it as soon as you remember. If it is near the time for the next dose, skip the missed dose and resume your regular dosage schedule. Do not double the next dose.

STOPPING THE DRUG
The decision to stop taking the drug should be made in consultation with your physician.

PROLONGED USE
See your doctor regularly for tests and examinations if you must take this medicine for a prolonged period.

PRECAUTIONS
Over 60: No special studies have been done on older patients. A lower dose may be warranted, especially if kidney function is impaired.

Driving and Hazardous Work: Do not drive or engage in hazardous work until you determine how the medicine affects you.

Alcohol: Avoid alcohol if liver function is impaired.

Pregnancy: Zalcitabine has been shown to cause birth defects in animals. Human studies have not been done. Nevertheless, zalcitabine is increasingly being used in combination with other antiretroviral drugs to treat pregnant HIV-infected women.

Breast Feeding: It is unknown whether zalcitabine passes into breast milk; however, women infected with HIV should not breast feed, to avoid transmitting the virus to an uninfected child.

Infants and Children: It is not known whether zalcitabine causes different or more severe side effects in children than it does in older persons. Use it for young patients only under close medical supervision.

Special Concerns: Use of zalcitabine does not reduce the risk of passing HIV to other persons. Take appropriate preventive measures.

OVERDOSE
Symptoms: Rash; fever; numbness, tingling, or prickling sensation in the arms and legs.

What to Do: An overdose of zalcitabine is unlikely to occur. Nonetheless, if you have any reason to suspect an overdose, call your doctor, emergency medical services (EMS), or the nearest poison control center.

DRUG INTERACTIONS
Consult your doctor for specific advice if you are taking asparaginase, azathioprine, estrogens, furosemide, methyldopa, pentamidine, sulfonamides, sulindac, tetracyclines, thiazide diuretics, valproic acid, injected aminoglycosides, amphotericin B, foscarnet, antacids, chloramphenicol, cisplatin, dapsone, didanosine, ethambutol, ethionamide, hydralazine, isoniazid, lithium, metronidazole, nitrous oxide, phenytoin, stavudine, vincristine, cimetidine, probenecid, or nitrofurantoin.

FOOD INTERACTIONS
No known food interactions.

DISEASE INTERACTIONS
Consult your doctor if you have a history of pancreatitis, peripheral neuropathy, or high levels of cholesterol or triglycerides in the blood. Use of zalcitabine may cause complications in patients who have kidney or liver disease, because these organs work to remove the medication from the body.

BRAND NAME
Sonata

▶ Drug Class: Sedative/hypnotic

▶ Available in: Capsules

▶ Available OTC? No

▶ As Generic? No

Side Effects

SERIOUS
Hallucinations, abnormal thoughts or behavior, confusion or disorientation, unsteadiness, dizziness, lightheadedness, unusual nervousness, agitation, difficulty breathing. Call your doctor immediately.

COMMON
Daytime drowsiness, general pain or discomfort, memory problems, headache.

LESS COMMON
Abdominal pain, weakness, fever.

PRINCIPAL USES
For the short-term treatment of insomnia.

HOW THE DRUG WORKS
By depressing activity in the central nervous system (the brain and spinal cord), zaleplon causes drowsiness and mild sedation. Because the drug is metabolized quickly compared with similar medications, zaleplon is associated with a lower incidence of side effects such as daytime drowsiness.

DOSAGE
The appropriate dosage will be determined by your doctor. The recommended dosage for adults: 10 mg. Debilitated patients and people over 60: 5 mg. Zaleplon should only be taken at bedtime or after the patient has gone to bed and has difficulty falling asleep.

ONSET OF EFFECT
Within 1 hour.

DURATION OF ACTION
About 4 hours.

DIETARY ADVICE
Do not take following a high-fat, heavy meal. The absorption of zaleplon may be slowed and reduce the drug's effectiveness.

STORAGE
Store in a tightly sealed container away from heat, moisture, and direct light.

IF YOU MISS A DOSE
If the medication was not taken at bedtime and you are unable to fall asleep, the drug may be used unless it is within 4 hours of when you need to be awake.

STOPPING THE DRUG
The decision to stop taking the drug should be made in consultation with your doctor.

PROLONGED USE
Zaleplon is usually prescribed only for short-term therapy (lasting several days or up to 4 weeks). See your doctor for periodic evaluation if you must take this drug for a longer time. Persistent insomnia may be a sign of an underlying medical problem.

PRECAUTIONS
Over 60: Adverse reactions may be more likely in older patients. Smaller doses usually are prescribed.

Driving and Hazardous Work: Avoid such activities until you determine how this medication affects you.

Alcohol: Avoid alcohol.

Pregnancy: In large doses zaleplon has been shown to slow the progress of fetal development in animals. Human studies have not been done. Zaleplon is not recommended for use by pregnant women. Before you take zaleplon, be sure to tell your doctor if you are pregnant or plan to become pregnant.

Breast Feeding: Zaleplon passes into breast milk, but its effect on the nursing infant is unknown. Women who are nursing should not take this medication.

Infants and Children: Safety and effectiveness have not been established for patients under age 18.

Special Concerns: When you stop taking zaleplon, you may have trouble falling asleep for the first few nights.

OVERDOSE
Symptoms: Severe drowsiness, breathing difficulty, severe clumsiness or unsteadiness, severe dizziness, severe nausea and vomiting, slow heartbeat, vision problems.

What to Do: Call your doctor, emergency medical services (EMS), or the nearest poison control center immediately.

DRUG INTERACTIONS
Other drugs may interact with zaleplon. Consult your doctor for specific advice if you are taking rifampin, phenytoin, carbamazepine, phenobarbital or other drugs that depress the central nervous system; these include antihistamines, other psychiatric medications, barbiturates, sedatives, cough medicines, decongestants, and painkillers. Be sure your doctor knows about any over-the-counter medication you may take.

FOOD INTERACTIONS
No known food interactions.

DISEASE INTERACTIONS
Caution is advised when taking zaleplon. Consult your doctor if you have a history of alcohol abuse or drug dependence, chronic respiratory disease (including asthma, bronchitis, or emphysema), mental depression, or sleep apnea. Use of zaleplon may cause complications in patients with liver disease, since this organ works to remove the medication from the body.

Zanamivir

▶ Drug Class: Antiviral

▶ Available in: Inhalant

▶ Available OTC? No

▶ As Generic? No

Side Effects

SERIOUS
No serious side effects are associated with zanamivir.

COMMON
There are no common side effects associated with zanamivir.

LESS COMMON
Dizziness.

PRINCIPAL USES
To treat influenza type A or B. Zanamivir can reduce the severity of symptoms and shorten the duration of flu episodes.

HOW THE DRUG WORKS
Zanamivir is believed to interfere with the synthesis of the viral enzyme neuraminidase, which is needed in order for the virus to infect cells in the respiratory tract and elsewhere in the body. The drug affects only certain susceptible strains of the influenza type A or B viruses.

DOSAGE
Adults and teenagers: 2 inhalations (one 5-mg blister per inhalation) every 12 hours for 5 days. On the first day of treatment, however, 2 doses should be taken whenever possible provided there is at least 2 hours between doses. On subsequent days, follow the above dosage schedule. Treatment should be initiated within 2 days after the onset of signs or symptoms of the flu.

ONSET OF EFFECT
Unknown.

DURATION OF ACTION
Unknown.

DIETARY ADVICE
No special restrictions.

STORAGE
Store in a tightly sealed container away from heat and direct light.

IF YOU MISS A DOSE
Take it as soon as you remember. If it is near the time for the next dose, skip the missed dose and resume your regular dosage schedule. Do not double the next dose.

STOPPING THE DRUG
It is important to take zanamivir for the full treatment period as prescribed. Do not stop taking the drug before the scheduled end of therapy even if you begin to feel better, as this may lead to a relapse.

PROLONGED USE
If your symptoms do not improve or if they become worse in a few days, you should consult your doctor.

PRECAUTIONS
Over 60: No special problems are expected.

Driving and Hazardous Work: Do not drive or engage in hazardous work until you determine how the medicine affects you.

Alcohol: No special precautions are necessary.

Pregnancy: Adequate studies have not been completed. Discuss with your doctor the relative risks and benefits of using this drug while pregnant.

Breast Feeding: Zanamivir may pass into breast milk, although it is unknown if this poses any risks to the nursing infant. Consult your doctor for specific advice.

Infants and Children: Zanamivir is not recommended for children under the age of 12.

Special Concerns: Zanamivir should be administered using the Diskhaler device. See your doctor for instructions and a demonstration of the proper use of this device.

OVERDOSE
Symptoms: No specific ones have been reported.

What to Do: If you have any reason to suspect an overdose, call your doctor, emergency medical services (EMS), or the nearest poison control center.

DRUG INTERACTIONS
No known drug interactions.

FOOD INTERACTIONS
No known food interactions.

DISEASE INTERACTIONS
Consult your doctor if you have any respiratory illness, such as chronic obstructive pulmonary disease or asthma.

Zidovudine (AZT)

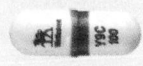

Retrovir 100 mg
(**GLAXO WELLCOME**)

▶ Drug Class: Antiviral

▶ Available in: Capsules, syrup, injection

▶ Available OTC? No

▶ As Generic? No

Side Effects

SERIOUS
Anemia (low red blood cell count) causing paleness, fatigue, or shortness of breath; fever. If such symptoms occur, call your doctor right away.

COMMON
Headaches, nausea, muscle aches, insomnia, mood swings, stomach upset, loss of appetite.

LESS COMMON
Bands of discoloration on the fingernails; hepatitis (liver inflammation, which may cause yellowish discoloration of skin and eyes).

PRINCIPAL USES
To treat HIV infection in combination with other drugs and to prevent passage of the virus from pregnant women to their babies. While not a cure for HIV, this drug may suppress the replication of the virus and delay the progression of the disease. Also used to treat HIV-related dementia and HIV-related thrombocytopenia (low platelet count).

HOW THE DRUG WORKS
Zidovudine (AZT) interferes with the activity of enzymes needed for the replication of DNA in viral cells, thus preventing the human immunodeficiency virus (HIV) from reproducing.

DOSAGE
For HIV infection— Adults and teenagers: Capsules: 200 mg, 3 times a day, or 300 mg, 2 times a day. Injection (given until oral dose can be taken): Adults and teenagers: 0.9 mg per lb of body weight injected slowly into a vein every 4 hours (6 times a day). To prevent the transmission of HIV to newborns— For pregnant women: Capsules: 100 mg, 5 times a day from 14th week of pregnancy to delivery. Injection: 0.9 mg per lb of body weight for first hour of delivery, followed by 0.45 mg per lb until baby is delivered. For newborns: Syrup: 0.9 mg per lb of body weight starting within 12 hours of birth and continuing for 6 weeks. Higher doses (up to 1,200 mg per day) are sometimes use to treat HIV-related dementia or thrombocytopenia.

ONSET OF EFFECT
Unknown. With most antiretroviral drugs, an early response can be seen within the first few days of therapy, but the maximum effect may take 12 to 16 weeks.

DURATION OF ACTION
Unknown. Effects of the drug may be prolonged if zidovudine is used in combination with other effective drugs and the virus is maximally suppressed.

DIETARY ADVICE
Take with food to minimize side effects.

STORAGE
Store in a tightly sealed container away from heat and direct light.

IF YOU MISS A DOSE
Take it as soon as you remember. If it is near the time for the next dose, skip the missed dose and resume your regular dosage schedule. Do not double the next dose.

STOPPING THE DRUG
The decision to stop taking the drug should be made in consultation with your physician.

PROLONGED USE
See your doctor regularly for tests and examinations as long as you take this medication.

PRECAUTIONS
Over 60: No special studies have been done on older patients. A lower dose may be warranted, especially if kidney function is impaired.

Driving and Hazardous Work: Do not drive or engage in hazardous work until you determine how the medicine affects you.

Alcohol: Avoid alcohol if liver function is impaired.

Pregnancy: Zidovudine can decrease the risk of passing the AIDS virus to the unborn child; in animal studies it has not caused birth defects.

Breast Feeding: Women who are infected with HIV should not breast feed, to avoid transmitting the virus to an uninfected child.

Infants and Children: Use and dose in infants and children must be established by your doctor.

Special Concerns: Use of zidovudine does not eliminate the risk of passing HIV to other persons. You should take appropriate preventive measures.

OVERDOSE
Symptoms: Sudden nausea and vomiting; headache, dizziness, or drowsiness.

What to Do: Seek medical assistance right away.

DRUG INTERACTIONS
Consult your doctor for specific advice if you are taking amphotericin B (by injection), anticancer agents, thyroid drugs, azathioprine, chloramphenicol, colchicine, cyclophosphamide, flucytosine, ganciclovir, interferon, mercaptopurine, methotrexate, plicamycin, clarithromycin, or probenecid. Also consult your doctor for specific advice if you are taking any other prescription or over-the-counter medication.

FOOD INTERACTIONS
Zidovudine may be better tolerated if taken with food.

DISEASE INTERACTIONS
Caution is advised when taking zidovudine. Consult your doctor if you have anemia or another blood problem or liver disease.

Zileuton

BRAND NAME
Zyflo

▶ Drug Class: Selective
5-lipoxygenase inhibitor

▶ Available in: Tablets

▶ Available OTC? No

▶ As Generic? No

Side Effects

SERIOUS
Liver problems causing nausea, fatigue, lethargy, skin rash or itching, yellow discoloration of the eyes or skin, flu-like symptoms, urine that is darker than normal. Call your doctor immediately.

COMMON
Headache, general pain, abdominal pain, nausea, indigestion, muscle soreness, weakness.

LESS COMMON
Joint pain, chest pain, inflammation of the tissues surrounding the eye (conjunctivitis), constipation, dizziness, fever, gas, insomnia or sleepiness, neck pain, nervousness, urinary tract infection, vomiting.

PRINCIPAL USES
To prevent and treat chronic asthma. Zileuton will not relieve a chronic asthma attack once it has started.

HOW THE DRUG WORKS
Zileuton blocks the activity of a specific enzyme needed in the manufacture of certain substances known as leukotrienes, which are known to contribute to allergic and inflammatory reactions, and appear to play a role in the development of inflammatory diseases including asthma and rheumatoid arthritis.

DOSAGE
Adults and teenagers: 600 mg, 4 times a day.

ONSET OF EFFECT
Within 1 to 2 hours. Several days or weeks may be required for the full effect in preventing asthma attacks.

DURATION OF ACTION
Unknown.

DIETARY ADVICE
Zileuton can be taken with meals and at bedtime, without regard to diet.

STORAGE
Store in a tightly sealed container away from heat, moisture, and direct light.

IF YOU MISS A DOSE
Take it as soon as you remember. If it is near the time for the next dose, skip the missed dose and resume your regular dosage schedule. Do not double the next dose.

STOPPING THE DRUG
Take it as prescribed for the full treatment period, even if you feel better before the scheduled end of therapy.

PROLONGED USE
See your doctor regularly for examinations and tests, especially of liver function, if you must take zileuton for a prolonged period.

PRECAUTIONS
Over 60: No special problems are expected.

Driving and Hazardous Work: Do not drive or engage in hazardous work until you determine how the medicine affects you.

Alcohol: Avoid alcohol.

Pregnancy: Adequate studies have not been done. Before taking zileuton, tell your doctor if you are pregnant or plan to become pregnant, and discuss the relative risks and benefits of using this drug.

Breast Feeding: Zileuton may pass into breast milk and be harmful to the nursing infant; avoid or discontinue using the drug while nursing or discontinue breast feeding.

Infants and Children: The safety and effectiveness of zileuton for children under the age of 12 have not been determined.

Special Concerns: Liver function should be tested before you start taking zileuton. While taking the drug, you should continue to take any other asthma medications that your doctor has prescribed. Tell your doctor if your use of short-acting bronchodilators increases when you start taking zileuton. It may indicate a worsening of your asthma that may require a change in dosage.

OVERDOSE
Symptoms: None are known; no cases of overdose have been reported.

What to Do: An overdose is unlikely to occur. However, if someone takes a much larger dose than prescribed, call your doctor, emergency medical services (EMS), or the nearest poison control center.

DRUG INTERACTIONS
Other drugs may interact with zileuton. Consult your doctor for specific advice if you are taking warfarin, propranolol, terfenadine, theophylline, calcium channel blockers, cyclosporine, and astemizole. Before you start taking zileuton, tell your doctor if you regularly take any other prescription or over-the-counter medication.

FOOD INTERACTIONS
No known food interactions.

DISEASE INTERACTIONS
Caution is advised when taking zileuton. Consult your doctor if you have hepatitis or jaundice. Use of zileuton may cause complications in patients with liver disease, since this organ works to remove the medication from the body.

Zinc Oxide

BRAND NAME
Ken Tox

▸ Drug Class: Sunscreen

▸ Available in: Cream, ointment

▸ Available OTC? Yes

▸ As Generic? Yes

Side Effects

SERIOUS
Acne, folliculitis (burning, pain, inflammation, and itching in hairy regions of the skin; pus in hair follicles), and skin rash may occur with zinc oxide and other physical sunscreens that block the pores. Notify your doctor if you experience such side effects.

COMMON
No common side effects have been reported.

LESS COMMON
No less-common side effects have been reported.

PRINCIPAL USES
To prevent sunburn.

HOW THE DRUG WORKS
Zinc oxide blocks ultraviolet radiation in sunlight from reaching the skin.

DOSAGE
Apply as needed before exposure to sunlight. A sunscreen should be applied uniformly to all exposed skin surfaces, including the lips.

ONSET OF EFFECT
Immediate.

DURATION OF ACTION
Keeps working until removed or worn off from perspiration or swimming.

DIETARY ADVICE
Zinc oxide can be used without regard to diet.

STORAGE
Store in a tightly sealed container away from heat and direct light.

IF YOU MISS A DOSE
If you forget to apply zinc oxide before exposure to sunlight, apply as soon as you remember.

STOPPING THE DRUG
No special warnings.

PROLONGED USE
No problems are expected.

PRECAUTIONS
Over 60: Studies suggest that frequent use of sunscreens like zinc oxide may increase the risk of vitamin D deficiency, which may promote osteoporosis or bone fractures later in life. Oral vitamin D supplements and consumption of foods rich in vitamin D may be recommended.

Driving and Hazardous Work: The use of zinc oxide should not impair your ability to perform such tasks safely.

Alcohol: No special precautions are necessary.

Pregnancy: No problems have been reported.

Breast Feeding: No problems have been reported.

Infants and Children: Zinc oxide should not be used on children (especially infants under 6 months of age) who have shown signs of allergic skin reaction (hypersensitivity). Otherwise, it is safe for use in children. To prevent accidental ingestion, do not allow small children to apply sunscreens themselves. In general, children should be kept out of the sun during peak daylight hours (from 10 am to 2 pm) and physically protected from direct sun exposure with clothing and other physical barriers (such as a beach umbrella). Infants over 6 months of age should be protected by a sunscreen with an SPF (sun protection factor) of 15 or higher. Older children should regularly use a sunscreen with an SPF of 15 or higher to protect against excess and repeated exposure to solar ultraviolet radiation, which can lead to skin cancer and other skin damage later in life.

Special Concerns: Zinc oxide sunscreen should be applied liberally before exposure to sunlight and reapplied every 1 to 2 hours, especially after swimming or heavy perspiration and after eating and drinking. Contact of zinc oxide with the eyes should be avoided. If skin rash or irritation develops, consult your doctor. Keep sun exposure to a minimum during peak daylight hours (10 am to 2 pm), when the sun's rays are strongest. Extra precautions should be taken around reflective surfaces such as sand, water, and concrete.

OVERDOSE
Symptoms: No specific ones have been reported.

What to Do: Not applicable. However, if someone accidentally ingests zinc oxide, call a doctor, emergency medical services (EMS), or the nearest poison control center.

DRUG INTERACTIONS
Consult your doctor for specific advice if you are using any other topical medications or skin preparations.

FOOD INTERACTIONS
No known food interactions.

DISEASE INTERACTIONS
Consult your doctor for advice if you have a history of any of the following: dermatitis (skin inflammation), herpes labialis (herpes simplex of the mouth and face), lichen planus (a rare non-malignant skin condition causing chronic itching and a distinctive skin eruption), systemic lupus erythematosus (lupus), photosensitivity (heightened sensitivity to sunlight), phytophotodermatitis (dermatitis caused by contact with certain plants followed by exposure to sunlight), polymorphous light eruption (skin lesions occurring after exposure to sunlight), or xeroderma pigmentosum (a rare genetic disorder causing extreme sensitivity to ultraviolet light, skin lesions including malignancies, and serious eye problems).

Zinc Sulfate Ophthalmic

BRAND NAMES
Clear Eyes ACR, Eye-Sed, VasoClear A, Visine Maximum Strength Allergy Relief, Zincfrin

▶ Drug Class: Ophthalmic astringent/analgesic

▶ Available in: Ophthalmic solution

▶ Available OTC? Yes

▶ As Generic? Yes

Side Effects

SERIOUS
No serious side effects have been reported.

COMMON
Overuse of this drug may cause increased eye irritation and redness.

LESS COMMON
No less-common side effects have been reported.

PRINCIPAL USES
For the temporary relief of discomfort and redness from minor eye irritation. It is prescribed in combination with other drugs such as phenylephrine, naphazoline, and tetrahydrozoline.

HOW THE DRUG WORKS
The mineral zinc is an integral component in the proper functioning of several important enzymes involved in wound healing and the general maintenance and proper hydration of certain body tissues. Zinc sulfate ophthalmic solution has a mild astringent effect (that is, it causes tissues to contract when applied topically), which can help to shrink the tiny blood vessels in the whites of the eye (sclera) and so relieve redness and irritation.

DOSAGE
Instill 1 to 2 drops in the affected eye(s) up to 4 times a day.

ONSET OF EFFECT
Rapid.

DURATION OF ACTION
Up to several hours.

DIETARY ADVICE
No special restrictions.

STORAGE
Store in a tightly sealed container away from heat and direct light. Do not allow the solution to freeze.

IF YOU MISS A DOSE
Instill the missed dose as soon as possible unless it is near the time for the next dose. In that case, skip the missed dose and go back to your regular schedule. Do not double the next dose.

STOPPING THE DRUG
You may stop applying this drug, or resume using it after discontinuing, as comfort dictates. No complications are expected.

PROLONGED USE
Eye drops containing zinc sulfate should generally not be used for self-medication for more than 3 days. If relief is not achieved in this time, or if redness and irritation persist or worsen, discontinue using it and contact your doctor or ophthalmologist right away.

PRECAUTIONS
Over 60: No special problems are expected.

Driving and Hazardous Work: The use of this medication should not affect your ability to perform such tasks safely.

Alcohol: No special precautions are necessary.

Pregnancy: No problems are expected; however, if you are pregnant or plan to become pregnant and you have any concerns about the safe use of this or any other medication, consult your doctor.

Breast Feeding: Adequate studies on the use of ophthalmic zinc sulfate during breast feeding have not been done; however, no adverse consequences have been reported. Consult your doctor for specific advice.

Infants and Children: No specific information is available on the use of this medication by children.

Special Concerns: Contact your ophthalmologist or general practitioner right away if you experience eye pain, changes in vision, or if eye irritation persists for more than 72 hours. To use the eye drops, first wash your hands. Tilt your head back. Gently apply pressure to the inside corner of the lower eyelid and with the index finger of the same hand, pull downward on the eyelid to make a space. Drop the medicine into this space and close your eye. Apply pressure for 1 or 2 minutes while keeping the eye closed without blinking. Then wash your hands again. Make sure that the tip of the dropper does not touch your eye, finger, or any other surface.

OVERDOSE
Symptoms: No cases of overdose have been reported.

What to Do: An overdose is unlikely to occur; in case of accidental ingestion, call your doctor, emergency medical services (EMS), or the nearest poison control center right away.

DRUG INTERACTIONS
No drug interactions have been reported, although phenylephrine, naphazoline, and tetrahydrozoline (other medications prescribed in combination with zinc sulfate ophthalmic solution) may adversely affect the action of certain glaucoma drops. Consult your doctor first before taking any other prescription or over-the-counter eye medications.

FOOD INTERACTIONS
No known food interactions.

DISEASE INTERACTIONS
If you have glaucoma, do not use this medication without consulting your doctor first. It is not an over-the-counter substitute for antibiotic or anti-inflammatory drops. Consult your doctor for specific advice if you have any other eye disorders or a history of allergic reaction to any other ophthalmic preparations.

Zinc Sulfate Systemic

BRAND NAMES
Orazinc, Verazinc, Zinc 15,
Zinc-220, Zincate,
Zinka-Pac

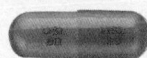

Generic 220 mg
(UPSHER-SMITH)

▶ Drug Class: Dietary
supplement

▶ Available in: Capsules,
tablets, extended-release
tablets, injection

▶ Available OTC? Yes

▶ As Generic? Yes

Side Effects

SERIOUS
Side effects are rare and occur only with large doses. Zinc itself may cause indigestion, heartburn, and nausea from irritation of the stomach. By interfering with the absorption of copper, zinc may interfere with the production of white and red blood cells, leading to infections, sores, or ulcers in the mouth or throat, and weakness due to anemia. Call your doctor if such symptoms occur.

COMMON
No common side effects have been reported.

LESS COMMON
No less-common side effects have been reported.

PRINCIPAL USES
To prevent or treat zinc deficiency. Zinc deficiency does not occur in healthy people who eat a proper, balanced diet. Conditions associated with zinc deficiency include alcoholism, eating disorders, and intestinal problems that result from malabsorption.

HOW THE DRUG WORKS
Zinc is essential to numerous physiological processes, including the function of many enzymes in the body. Deficiency may lead to poor night vision, slow healing of wounds, poor sexual development and function in males, poor appetite (perhaps owing to a decrease in the sense of taste and smell), a reduced ability to ward off infections, diarrhea, dermatitis, and, in children, retarded growth.

DOSAGE
Recommended daily allowances are as follows: 5 to 10 mg a day for children from birth to age 3; 10 mg a day for children ages 4 to 10; 15 mg a day for adolescent and adult males; 12 mg a day for adolescent and adult females; 15 mg a day for pregnant women; and 16 to 19 mg a day for breast-feeding women.

ONSET OF EFFECT
Unknown.

DURATION OF ACTION
Unknown.

DIETARY ADVICE
Most effective if taken 1 hour before or 2 hours after meals. It can be taken with food if stomach upset occurs.

STORAGE
Store in a tightly sealed container away from heat, moisture, and direct light.

IF YOU MISS A DOSE
No cause for concern.

STOPPING THE DRUG
If you are taking zinc sulfate by prescription, the decision to stop should be made by your doctor.

PROLONGED USE
You should see your doctor regularly for tests and examinations if you take zinc sulfate for a prolonged period.

PRECAUTIONS
Over 60: Zinc deficiency is more likely to occur in older persons; no special problems are expected from zinc supplementation.

Driving and Hazardous Work: The use of zinc sulfate should not impair your ability to perform such tasks safely.

Alcohol: Excessive alcohol intake can increase the likelihood of zinc deficiency.

Pregnancy: There are no known problems with recommended doses, but taking large amounts of zinc during pregnancy may be harmful to the fetus.

Breast Feeding: No problems have been reported with recommended doses.

Infants and Children: Problems have not been reported in infants and children receiving the recommended daily intake of zinc sulfate.

Special Concerns: Injectable zinc sulfate should be given under the supervision of a health care professional. Zinc is found in peas, beans, seafood such as oysters and herring, and in lean red meats. It is also found in whole grains, but consuming large amounts of whole grains can decrease the amount of zinc absorbed from the intestine. Be aware that food stored in uncoated tin cans may have less zinc available for absorption.

OVERDOSE
Symptoms: Chest pain, vomiting, yellowish tinge to eyes or skin, dehydration, shortness of breath, restlessness, profuse sweating, dizziness.

What to Do: Call your doctor, emergency medical services (EMS), or the nearest poison control center immediately.

DRUG INTERACTIONS
Consult your doctor for specific advice if you are taking copper supplements or oral tetracyclines.

FOOD INTERACTIONS
Some foods can interfere with absorption of zinc sulfate into your body. Avoid taking zinc sulfate within 2 hours of eating bran, whole-wheat breads and cereals, and other fiber-rich foods, or phosphorus-containing foods such as milk and poultry.

DISEASE INTERACTIONS
Consult your doctor if you have a copper deficiency or any other medical condition. Zinc supplements make a copper deficiency worse.

Zolmitriptan

Side Effects

SERIOUS
Serious side effects with zolmitriptan are rare. However, zolmitriptan may cause a heart attack, chest pain or tightness, sudden or severe abdominal pain, shortness of breath, wheezing, heartbeat irregularities, swelling of eyelids, face, or lips, skin rash, or hives. Seek emergency medical assistance immediately.

COMMON
Hot flashes or chills, numbness, prickling or tingling sensations, dry mouth, dizziness, drowsiness, weakness.

LESS COMMON
Indigestion, nausea, muscle ache.

PRINCIPAL USES
To treat severe, acute migraine headaches. Zolmitriptan is not intended as a migraine preventive or for use against any other kinds of pain or headache, including basilar and hemiplegic migraines. Your doctor will determine whether this medication is appropriate in your particular case.

HOW THE DRUG WORKS
The exact mechanism of zolmitriptan's action is unknown.

DOSAGE
A single dose ranging from half of a 2.5 mg tablet to one 5 mg tablet is generally effective. If the migraine returns or there is only partial relief, the dose may be repeated once after 2 hours, but no more than 10 mg should be taken in a 24-hour period. Since individual response to zolmitriptan may vary, your doctor will determine the appropriate dosage. A general recommendation is to take one 2.5 mg tablet as the initial dose.

ONSET OF EFFECT
Within 2 hours.

DURATION OF ACTION
Up to 24 hours.

DIETARY ADVICE
The medication can be taken with or without food.

STORAGE
Store in a tightly sealed container away from heat, moisture, and direct light.

IF YOU MISS A DOSE
Not applicable, since the drug is taken only when necessary.

STOPPING THE DRUG
Consult your doctor before discontinuing zolmitriptan.

PROLONGED USE
No special problems are expected. Patients at risk for heart disease should undergo periodic medical tests and evaluation.

PRECAUTIONS
Over 60: Zolmitriptan is not recommended for use in older patients.

Driving and Hazardous Work: Do not drive or engage in dangerous work until you determine how the medication affects you.

Alcohol: No special warnings, although alcohol may trigger or exacerbate migraine headaches.

Pregnancy: Do not use zolmitriptan without first consulting your doctor if you are pregnant or suspect you might be pregnant.

Breast Feeding: Zolmitriptan may pass into breast milk; consult your doctor for specific advice.

Infants and Children: The safety and effectiveness of zolmitriptan in patients under age 18 have not been established.

Special Concerns: Serious, but rare, heart-related problems may occur after using zolmitriptan. Anyone at risk for unrecognized coronary artery disease—such as postmenopausal women, men over the age of 40, or those with known risk factors for heart disease (hypertension, high blood cholesterol levels, obesity, diabetes, strong family history of heart disease, or cigarette smoking)—should have the first dose of zolmitriptan administered in a doctor's office. Zolmitriptan should not be used by anyone with any symptoms of active heart disease (chest pain or tightness, shortness of breath).

OVERDOSE
Symptoms: Increase in blood pressure resulting in lightheadedness, tension in the neck, fatigue, and loss of coordination.

What to Do: An overdose with zolmitriptan is unlikely. If someone takes a much larger dose than prescribed, call your doctor, emergency medical services (EMS), or the nearest poison control center immediately.

DRUG INTERACTIONS
Do not take zolmitriptan within 24 hours of taking almotriptan, naratriptan, sumatriptan, rizatriptan, ergotamine-containing medication, dihydroergotamine mesylate, or methysergide mesylate. Zolmitriptan and MAO inhibitors such as phenelzine, tranylcypromine, procarbazine, and selegiline should not be used within 14 days of each other. Zolmitriptan should be used with caution in patients taking SSRIs (selective serotonin reuptake inhibitors), which include fluoxetine, fluvoxamine, paroxetine, and sertraline.

FOOD INTERACTIONS
See Dietary Advice.

DISEASE INTERACTIONS
You should not take zolmitriptan if you have a history of angina, heart disease, stroke, uncontrolled hypertension, heartbeat irregularities, or peripheral vascular disease. Zolmitriptan should be used with caution in patients with liver disease or severely impaired kidney function.

Zolpidem Tartrate

Ambien 5 mg
(SEARLE)

▶ Drug Class: Sedative/hypnotic

▶ Available in: Tablets

▶ Available OTC? No

▶ As Generic? No

Side Effects

SERIOUS
Hallucinations, abnormal thoughts or behavior, confusion or disorientation, unsteadiness, dizziness, lightheadedness, unusual nervousness, agitation, difficulty breathing. Call your doctor immediately.

COMMON
Daytime drowsiness, diarrhea, general pain or discomfort, memory problems, nausea, bizarre or unusually vivid dreams, vomiting.

LESS COMMON
Stomach discomfort, agitation, feelings of panic, convulsions, muscle cramps, nausea, vomiting, unusual fatigue, uncontrolled weeping, worsening of emotional problems, vision problems, dry mouth.

PRINCIPAL USES
For the short-term treatment of insomnia.

HOW THE DRUG WORKS
Zolpidem depresses activity in the central nervous system (the brain and spinal cord), which causes drowsiness and mild sedation.

DOSAGE
Adults: 10 mg at bedtime. Patients over 60: 5 mg at bedtime.

ONSET OF EFFECT
Within minutes.

DURATION OF ACTION
2 to 4 hours.

DIETARY ADVICE
Zolpidem may be taken without regard to diet, although it generally works faster on an empty stomach.

STORAGE
Store in a tightly sealed container away from heat and direct light.

IF YOU MISS A DOSE
Take it as soon as you remember unless it is late at night. Do not take the drug unless your schedule permits 7 or 8 hours of sleep.

STOPPING THE DRUG
The decision to stop taking the drug should be made in consultation with your doctor. Discontinuing the drug abruptly may produce withdrawal symptoms (sleep disruption, nervousness, irritability, diarrhea, abdominal cramps, muscle aches, memory impairment). The dosage should be reduced gradually according to your doctor's instructions.

PROLONGED USE
Zolpidem is usually prescribed only for short-term therapy (lasting several days or up to 2 weeks). See your doctor for periodic evaluation if you must take this drug for a longer time. Persistent insomnia may be a sign of an underlying medical problem.

PRECAUTIONS
Over 60: Adverse reactions may be more likely and more severe in older patients. Smaller doses usually are prescribed.

Driving and Hazardous Work: Zolpidem may impair mental alertness and physical coordination. Adjust your activities accordingly.

Alcohol: Avoid alcohol.

Pregnancy: In large doses zolpidem has been shown to slow the progress of fetal development in animals. Human studies have not been done. Before you take zolpidem, be sure to tell your doctor if you are pregnant or plan to become pregnant.

Breast Feeding: Zolpidem passes into breast milk, but its effect on the nursing infant is unknown. Consult your doctor for advice.

Infants and Children: Safety and effectiveness have not been established for patients under age 18.

Special Concerns: When you stop taking zolpidem, you may have trouble falling asleep for the first few nights.

OVERDOSE
Symptoms: Severe drowsiness, breathing difficulty, severe clumsiness or unsteadiness, severe dizziness, severe nausea and vomiting, slow heartbeat, vision problems.

What to Do: Call your doctor, emergency medical services (EMS), or the nearest poison control center immediately.

DRUG INTERACTIONS
Other drugs may interact with zolpidem. Consult your doctor for specific advice if you are taking tricyclic antidepressants (such as amitriptyline, clomipramine, doxepin, or nortriptyline) or other drugs that depress the central nervous system; these include antihistamines, other psychiatric medications, barbiturates, sedatives, cough medicines, decongestants, and painkillers. Be sure your doctor knows about any over-the-counter medication you may take.

FOOD INTERACTIONS
No known food interactions.

DISEASE INTERACTIONS
Caution is advised when taking zolpidem. Consult your doctor if you have a history of alcohol abuse or drug dependence, chronic respiratory disease (including asthma, bronchitis, or emphysema), mental depression, or sleep apnea. Use of zolpidem may cause complications in patients with liver or kidney disease, since these organs work together to remove the medication from the body.

The following pages contain additional examples of many of the pills described in the individual drug profiles throughout the book. They are organized alphabetically by generic name (consult index for brand names).

Please note that the physical appearance of a particular drug may vary considerably from one manufacturer to another, or from one dosage strength to another even when made by the same manufacturer. Each picture that appears here (and elsewhere in the book) represents but one dosage strength of one brand of a drug made by one manufacturer. If the pill you take looks different from the one you see in the photograph, do not be alarmed. However, if you have any doubts, concerns, or questions whatsoever about the medication you take, consult your doctor or pharmacist.

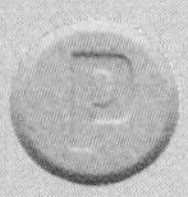

Acetaminophen
80 mg
Panadol Children's
SMITHKLINE BEECHAM

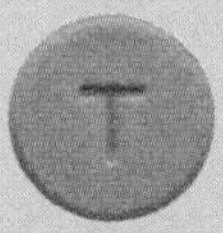

Acetaminophen
160 mg
Tempra Quicklets Junior Strength
BRISTOL-MYERS SQUIBB

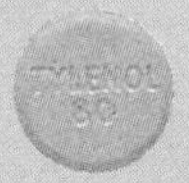

Acetaminophen
80 mg
Tylenol Children's
MCNEIL

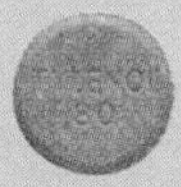

Acetaminophen
80 mg
Tylenol Children's
MCNEIL

Acetaminophen
650 mg
Tylenol Extended Relief
MCNEIL

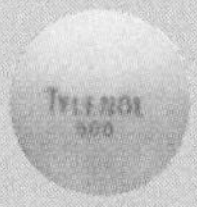

Acetaminophen
500 mg
Tylenol Extra Strength
MCNEIL

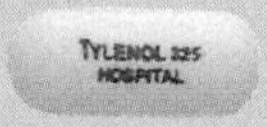

Acetaminophen
325 mg
Tylenol Hospital
MCNEIL

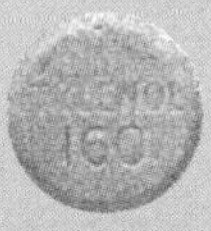

Acetaminophen
160 mg
Tylenol Junior Strength
MCNEIL

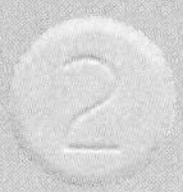

Acetaminophen/Codeine
300/15 mg
Generic
GOLDLINE

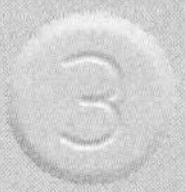

Acetaminophen/Codeine
300/30 mg
Generic
GOLDLINE

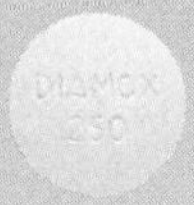

Acetazolamide
250 mg
Diamox
STORZ

Allopurinol
100 mg
Generic
SCHEIN/DANBURY

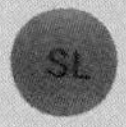

Amitriptyline Hydrochloride
10 mg
Generic
SIDMAK

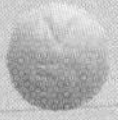

Amitriptyline Hydrochloride
25 mg
Generic
MYLAN

Amlodipine
5 mg
Norvasc
PFIZER

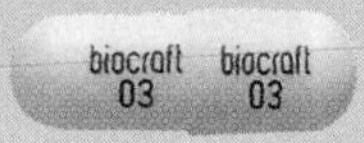

Amoxicillin
500 mg
Generic
BIOCRAFT

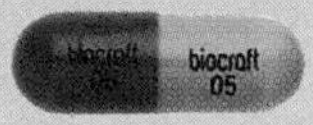

Ampicillin
250 mg
Generic
BIOCRAFT

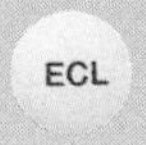

Aspirin
81 mg
Ascriptin Adult Low Strength
NOVARTIS

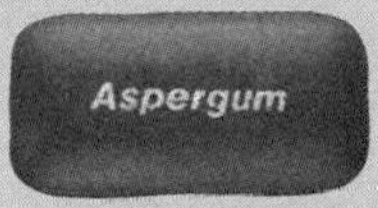

Aspirin
227 mg
Aspergum
SCHERING-PLOUGH

Aspirin
325 mg
Bayer
BAYER

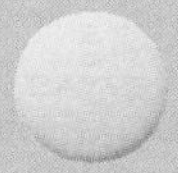

Aspirin
325 mg
Bayer
BAYER

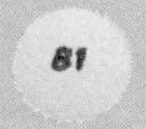

Aspirin
81 mg
Bayer Adult Low Strength
BAYER

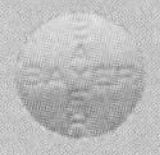

Aspirin
81 mg
Bayer Children's
BAYER

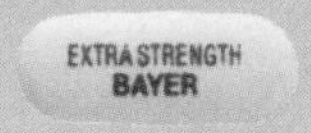

Aspirin
500 mg
Bayer Extra Strength
BAYER

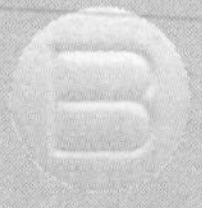

Aspirin
325 mg
Bufferin
BRISTOL-MYERS SQUIBB

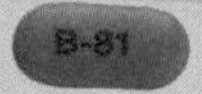

Aspirin
81 mg
Bufferin Low Dose
BRISTOL-MYERS SQUIBB

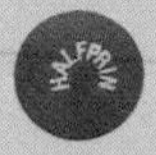

Aspirin
162 mg
Halfprin
KRAMER

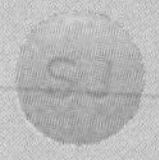

Aspirin
81 mg
St. Joseph Adult Chewable
SCHERING-PLOUGH

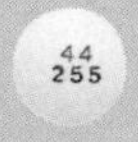

Aspirin
81 mg
Generic
LNK

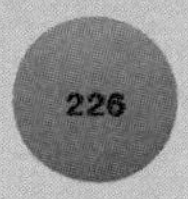

Aspirin
325 mg
Generic
TIME-CAP

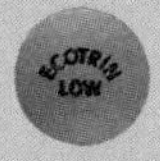

Aspirin (Enteric Coated)
81 mg
Ecotrin
SMITHKLINE BEECHAM

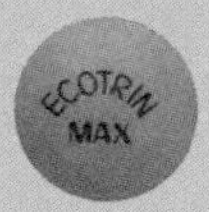

Aspirin (Enteric Coated)
500 mg
Ecotrin Maximum Strength
SMITHKLINE BEECHAM

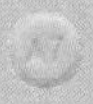

Atenolol
25 mg
Generic
LEDERLE

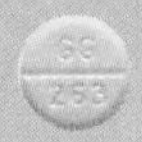

Atenolol
50 mg
Generic
GENEVA

Benztropine Mesylate
0.5 mg
Generic
PAR

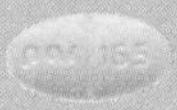

Benztropine Mesylate
1 mg
Generic
PAR

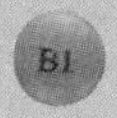

Bisacodyl
5 mg
Dulcolax
BOEHRINGER INGELHEIM

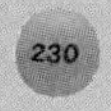

Bisacodyl
5 mg
Generic
PADDOCK

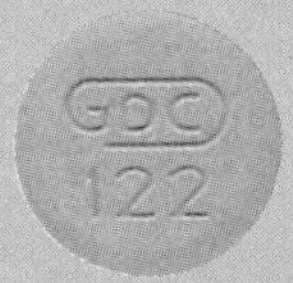

Bismuth Subsalicylate
262 mg
Pepto-Bismol
PROCTER & GAMBLE

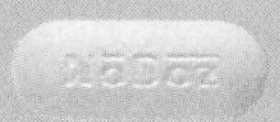

Caffeine
200 mg
Nōdōz
BRISTOL-MYERS SQUIBB

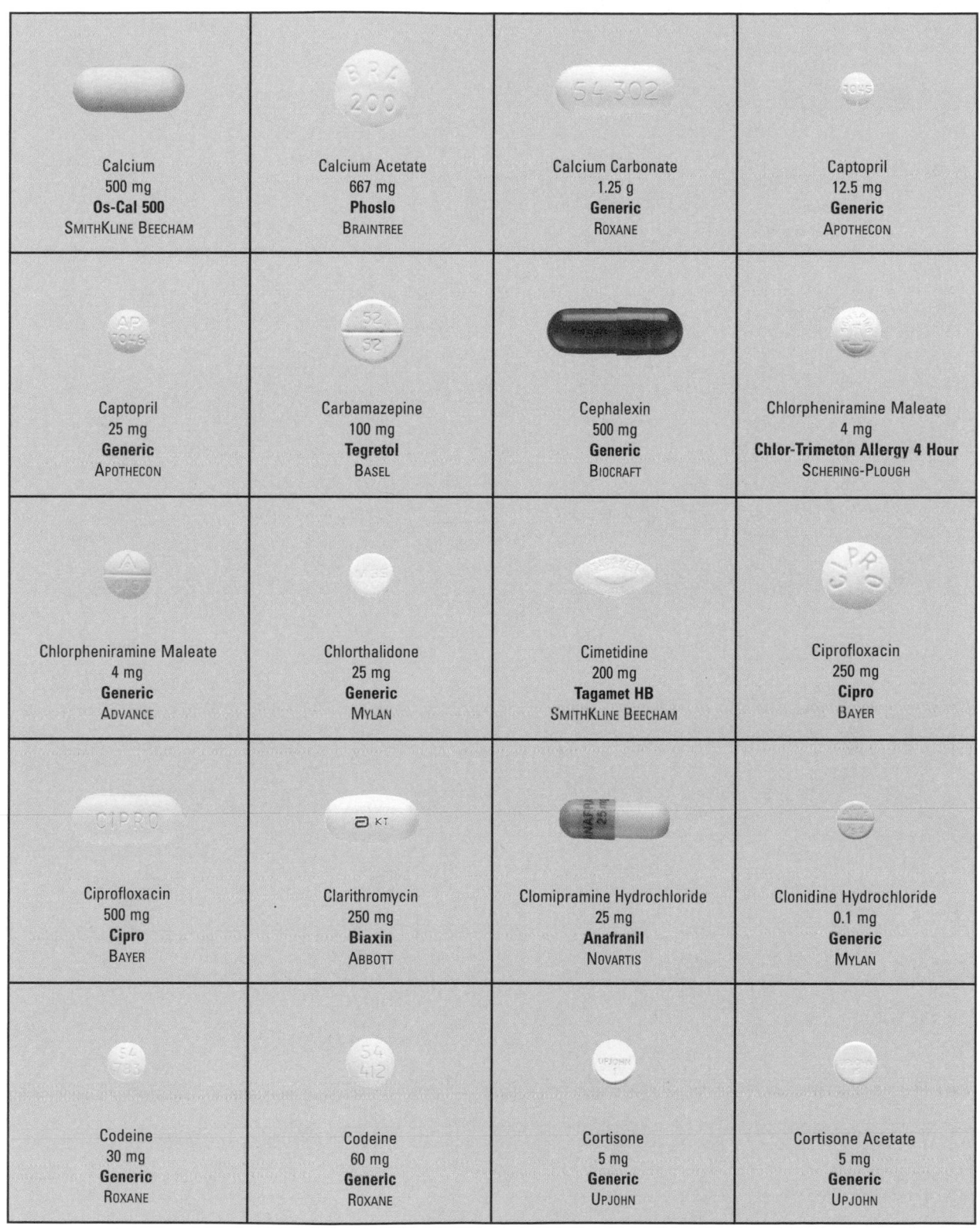

Calcium
500 mg
Os-Cal 500
SMITHKLINE BEECHAM

Calcium Acetate
667 mg
Phoslo
BRAINTREE

Calcium Carbonate
1.25 g
Generic
ROXANE

Captopril
12.5 mg
Generic
APOTHECON

Captopril
25 mg
Generic
APOTHECON

Carbamazepine
100 mg
Tegretol
BASEL

Cephalexin
500 mg
Generic
BIOCRAFT

Chlorpheniramine Maleate
4 mg
Chlor-Trimeton Allergy 4 Hour
SCHERING-PLOUGH

Chlorpheniramine Maleate
4 mg
Generic
ADVANCE

Chlorthalidone
25 mg
Generic
MYLAN

Cimetidine
200 mg
Tagamet HB
SMITHKLINE BEECHAM

Ciprofloxacin
250 mg
Cipro
BAYER

Ciprofloxacin
500 mg
Cipro
BAYER

Clarithromycin
250 mg
Biaxin
ABBOTT

Clomipramine Hydrochloride
25 mg
Anafranil
NOVARTIS

Clonidine Hydrochloride
0.1 mg
Generic
MYLAN

Codeine
30 mg
Generic
ROXANE

Codeine
60 mg
Generic
ROXANE

Cortisone
5 mg
Generic
UPJOHN

Cortisone Acetate
5 mg
Generic
UPJOHN

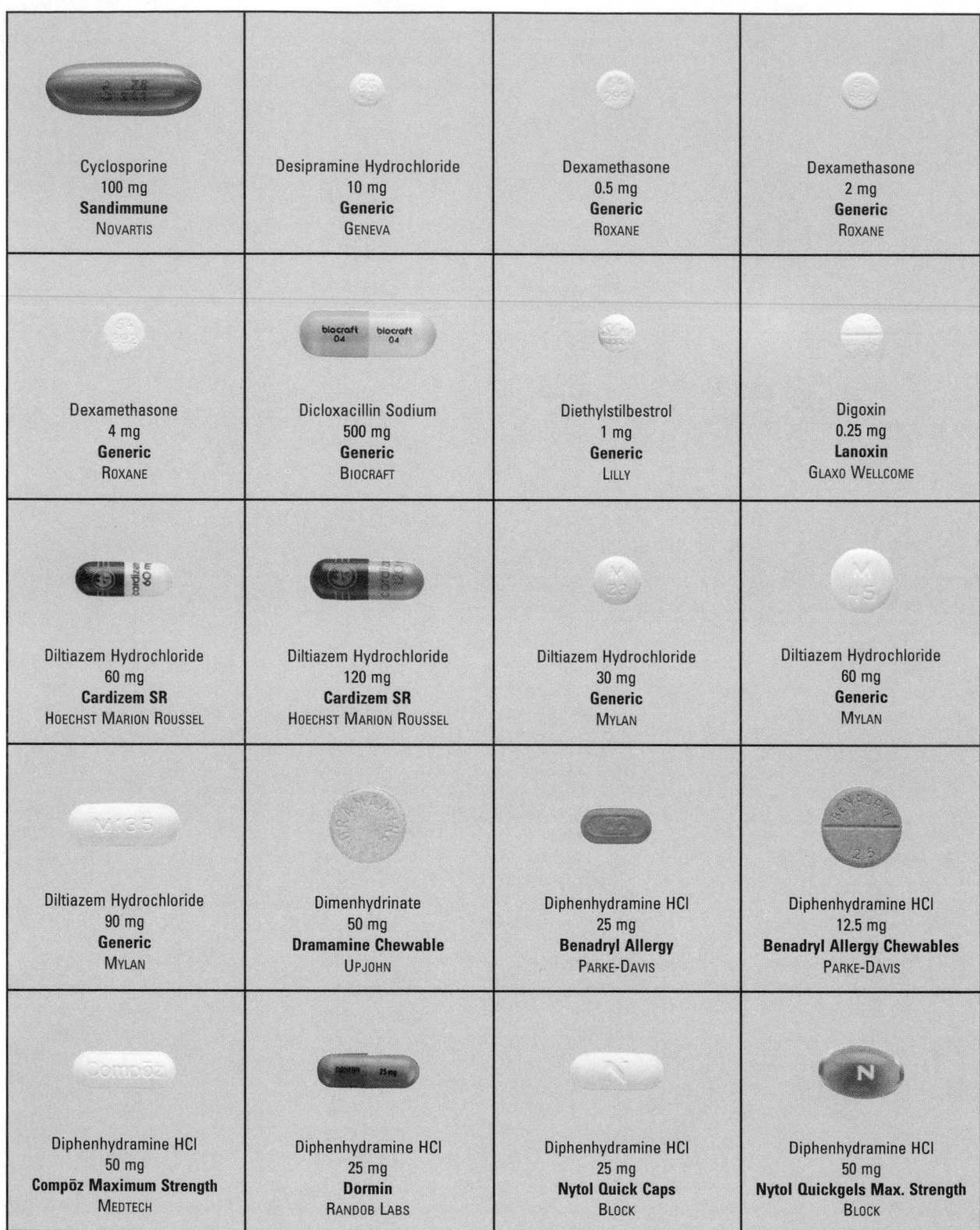

Cyclosporine
100 mg
Sandimmune
NOVARTIS

Desipramine Hydrochloride
10 mg
Generic
GENEVA

Dexamethasone
0.5 mg
Generic
ROXANE

Dexamethasone
2 mg
Generic
ROXANE

Dexamethasone
4 mg
Generic
ROXANE

Dicloxacillin Sodium
500 mg
Generic
BIOCRAFT

Diethylstilbestrol
1 mg
Generic
LILLY

Digoxin
0.25 mg
Lanoxin
GLAXO WELLCOME

Diltiazem Hydrochloride
60 mg
Cardizem SR
HOECHST MARION ROUSSEL

Diltiazem Hydrochloride
120 mg
Cardizem SR
HOECHST MARION ROUSSEL

Diltiazem Hydrochloride
30 mg
Generic
MYLAN

Diltiazem Hydrochloride
60 mg
Generic
MYLAN

Diltiazem Hydrochloride
90 mg
Generic
MYLAN

Dimenhydrinate
50 mg
Dramamine Chewable
UPJOHN

Diphenhydramine HCl
25 mg
Benadryl Allergy
PARKE-DAVIS

Diphenhydramine HCl
12.5 mg
Benadryl Allergy Chewables
PARKE-DAVIS

Diphenhydramine HCl
50 mg
Compōz Maximum Strength
MEDTECH

Diphenhydramine HCl
25 mg
Dormin
RANDOB LABS

Diphenhydramine HCl
25 mg
Nytol Quick Caps
BLOCK

Diphenhydramine HCl
50 mg
Nytol Quickgels Max. Strength
BLOCK

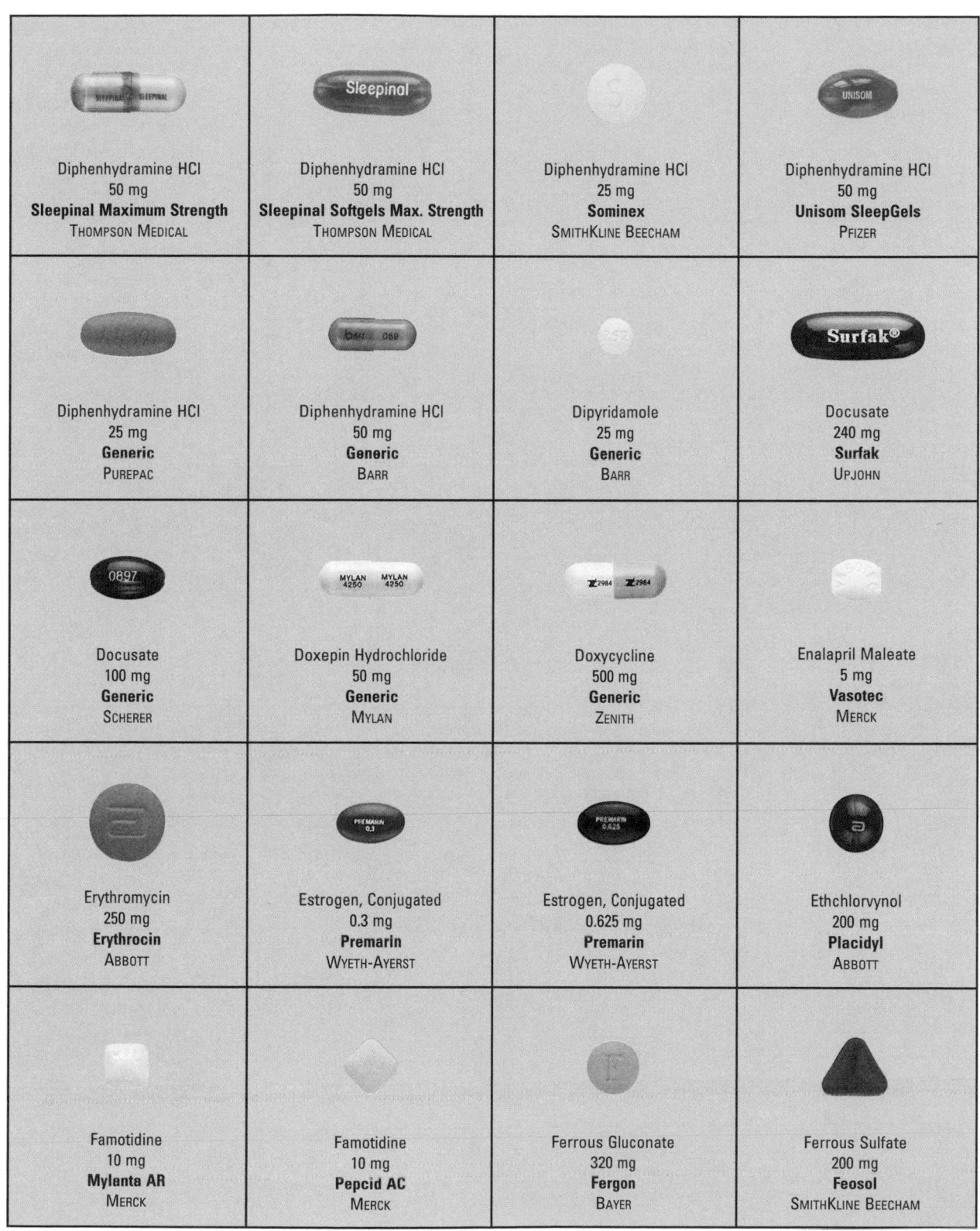

Diphenhydramine HCl 50 mg **Sleepinal Maximum Strength** THOMPSON MEDICAL	Diphenhydramine HCl 50 mg **Sleepinal Softgels Max. Strength** THOMPSON MEDICAL	Diphenhydramine HCl 25 mg **Sominex** SMITHKLINE BEECHAM	Diphenhydramine HCl 50 mg **Unisom SleepGels** PFIZER
Diphenhydramine HCl 25 mg **Generic** PUREPAC	Diphenhydramine HCl 50 mg **Generic** BARR	Dipyridamole 25 mg **Generic** BARR	Docusate 240 mg **Surfak** UPJOHN
Docusate 100 mg **Generic** SCHERER	Doxepin Hydrochloride 50 mg **Generic** MYLAN	Doxycycline 500 mg **Generic** ZENITH	Enalapril Maleate 5 mg **Vasotec** MERCK
Erythromycin 250 mg **Erythrocin** ABBOTT	Estrogen, Conjugated 0.3 mg **Premarin** WYETH-AYERST	Estrogen, Conjugated 0.625 mg **Premarin** WYETH-AYERST	Ethchlorvynol 200 mg **Placidyl** ABBOTT
Famotidine 10 mg **Mylanta AR** MERCK	Famotidine 10 mg **Pepcid AC** MERCK	Ferrous Gluconate 320 mg **Fergon** BAYER	Ferrous Sulfate 200 mg **Feosol** SMITHKLINE BEECHAM

ADDITIONAL PILL PHOTOGRAPHS

Ferrous Sulfate
324 mg
Generic
CHASE

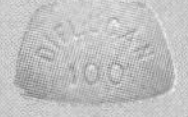

Fluconazole
100 mg
Diflucan
ROERIG

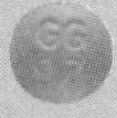

Fluphenazine
1 mg
Generic
GENEVA

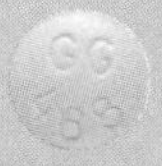

Fluphenazine
2.5 mg
Generic
GENEVA

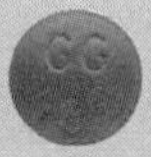

Fluphenazine
5 mg
Generic
GENEVA

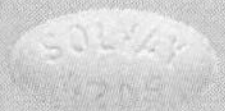

Fluvoxamine Maleate
50 mg
Luvox
SOLVAY

Fosinopril
20 mg
Monopril
BRISTOL-MYERS SQUIBB

Furosemide
40 mg
Generic
ROXANE

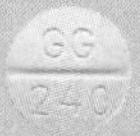

Glyburide
5 mg
Generic
GENEVA

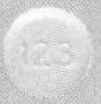

Haloperidol
1 mg
Generic
GENEVA

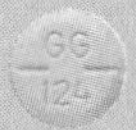

Haloperidol
2 mg
Generic
GENEVA

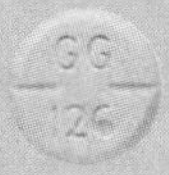

Haloperidol
10 mg
Generic
GENEVA

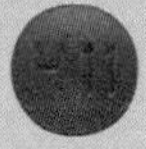

Hydralazine Hydrochloride
25 mg
Generic
LEDERLE

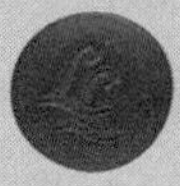

Hydralazine Hydrochloride
50 mg
Generic
LEDERLE

Hydroxyzine Hydrochloride
10 mg
Generic
SCHEIN/DANBURY

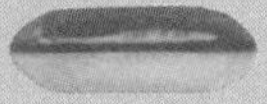

Ibuprofen
200 mg
Advil Gel Caplets
WHITEHALL

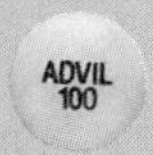

Ibuprofen
100 mg
Advil Junior Strength
WHITEHALL-ROBINS

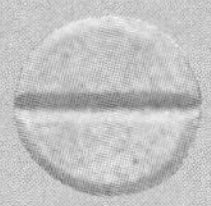

Ibuprofen
50 mg
Motrin Children's
MCNEIL

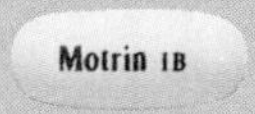

Ibuprofen
200 mg
Motrin IB
PHARMACIA & UPJOHN

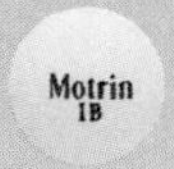

Ibuprofen
200 mg
Motrin IB
PHARMACIA & UPJOHN

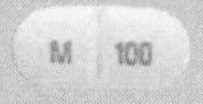

Ibuprofen
100 mg
Motrin Junior Strength
MCNEIL

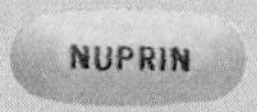

Ibuprofen
200 mg
Nuprin
BRISTOL-MYERS SQUIBB

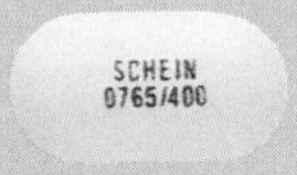

Ibuprofen
400 mg
Generic
SCHEIN

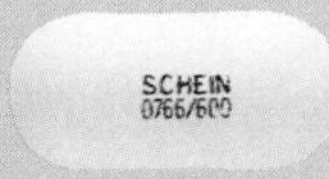

Ibuprofen
600 mg
Generic
SCHEIN

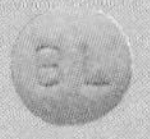

Imipramine
10 mg
Generic
BIOCRAFT

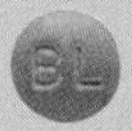

Imipramine
50 mg
Generic
BIOCRAFT

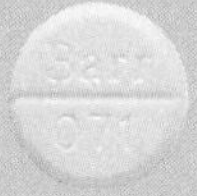

Isoniazid
300 mg
Generic
BARR

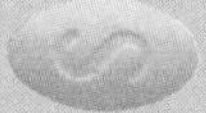

Isosorbide Dinitrate
40 mg
Sorbitrate
ZENECA

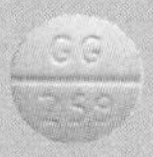

Isosorbide Dinitrate
5 mg
Generic
GENEVA

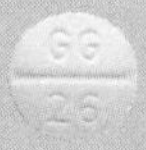

Isosorbide Dinitrate
10 mg
Generic
GENEVA

Ketoprofen
12.5 mg
Actron
BAYER

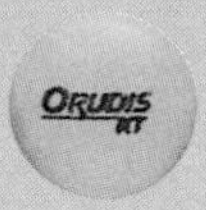

Ketoprofen
12.5 mg
Orudis KT
WHITEHALL-ROBINS

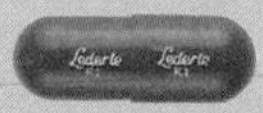

Ketoprofen
25 mg
Generic
LEDERLE

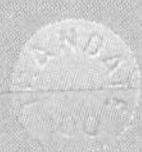

Labetalol Hydrochloride
100 mg
Trandate
GLAXO WELLCOME

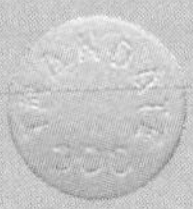

Labetalol Hydrochloride
300 mg
Trandate
GLAXO WELLCOME

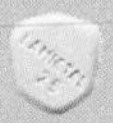

Lamotrigine
25 mg
Lamictal
GLAXO WELLCOME

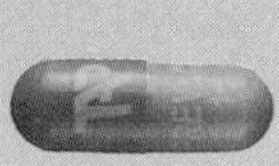

Lansoprazole
15 mg
Prevacid
TAP

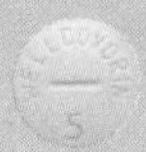

Leucovorin Calcium
5 mg
Wellcovorin
GLAXO WELLCOME

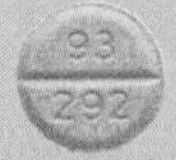

Levodopa/Carbidopa
100/10 mg
Generic
LEMMON

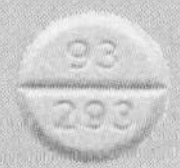

Levodopa/Carbidopa
100/25 mg
Generic
LEMMON

ADDITIONAL PILL PHOTOGRAPHS

Levodopa/Carbidopa 250/25 mg **Generic** LEMMON	Levothyroxine Sodium 0.3 mg **Levothroid** FOREST	Levothyroxine Sodium 0.025 mg **Levoxyl** DANIELS	Levothyroxine Sodium 0.05 mg **Levoxyl** DANIELS
Levothyroxine Sodium 0.15 mg **Levoxyl** DANIELS	Levothyroxine Sodium 0.2 mg **Levoxyl** DANIELS	Lisinopril 10 mg **Zestril** ZENECA	Lisinopril 20 mg **Zestril** ZENECA
Loperamide Hydrochloride 2 mg **Imodium A-D** MCNEIL	Loxapine 5 mg **Generic** WATSON	Meclizine 25 mg **Bonine** PFIZER	Medroxyprogesterone 2.5 mg **Cycrin** ESI
Megestrol Acetate 40 mg **Generic** PAR	Methyldopa 500 mg **Generic** LEDERLE	Methylphenidate 10 mg **Generic** MD PHARM	Methylprednisolone 4 mg **Medrol** UPJOHN
Metolazone 2.5 mg **Zaroxolyn** FISONS	Mexiletine Hydrochloride 150 mg **Mexitil** BOEHRINGER INGELHEIM	Molindone 25 mg **Moban** GATE	Morphine 30 mg **M S Contin** PURDUE FREDERICK

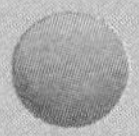

Morphine
60 mg
M S Contin
PURDUE FREDERICK

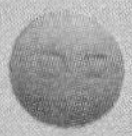

Morphine
100 mg
M S Contin
PURDUE FREDERICK

Nadolol
40 mg
Generic
MYLAN

Naproxen
250 mg
Generic
MYLAN

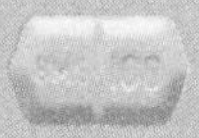

Nefazodone Hydrochloride
100 mg
Serzone
BRISTOL-MYERS SQUIBB

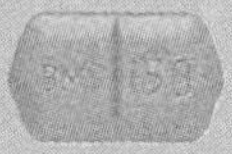

Nefazodone Hydrochloride
150 mg
Serzone
BRISTOL-MYERS SQUIBB

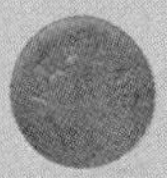

Nifedipine
60 mg
Adalat CC
BAYER

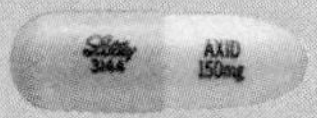

Nizatidine
150 mg
Axid
LILLY

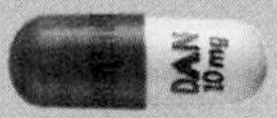

Nortriptyline Hydrochloride
10 mg
Generic
SCHEIN/DANBURY

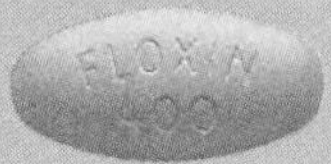

Ofloxacin
400 mg
Floxin
ORTHO

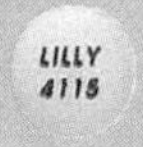

Olanzapine
5 mg
Zyprexa
LILLY

Oxycodone Hydrochloride
10 mg
Oxycontin
PURDUE

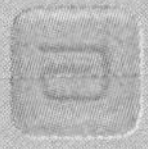

Pemoline
37.5 mg
Cylert
ABBOTT

Penicillin V
250 mg
Generic
BIOCRAFT

Perphenazine
4 mg
Generic
GENEVA

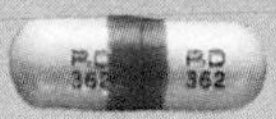

Phenytoin
100 mg
Dilantin
PARKE-DAVIS

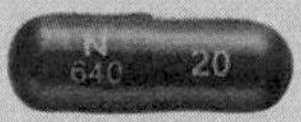

Piroxicam
20 mg
Generic
NOVOPHARM

Potassium Chloride
1,500 mg
K-Dur 20
KEY

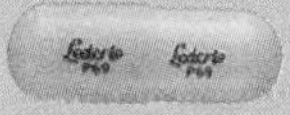

Prazosin
1 mg
Generic
LEDERLE

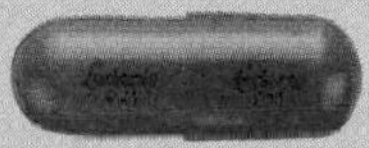

Prazosin
5 mg
Generic
LEDERLE

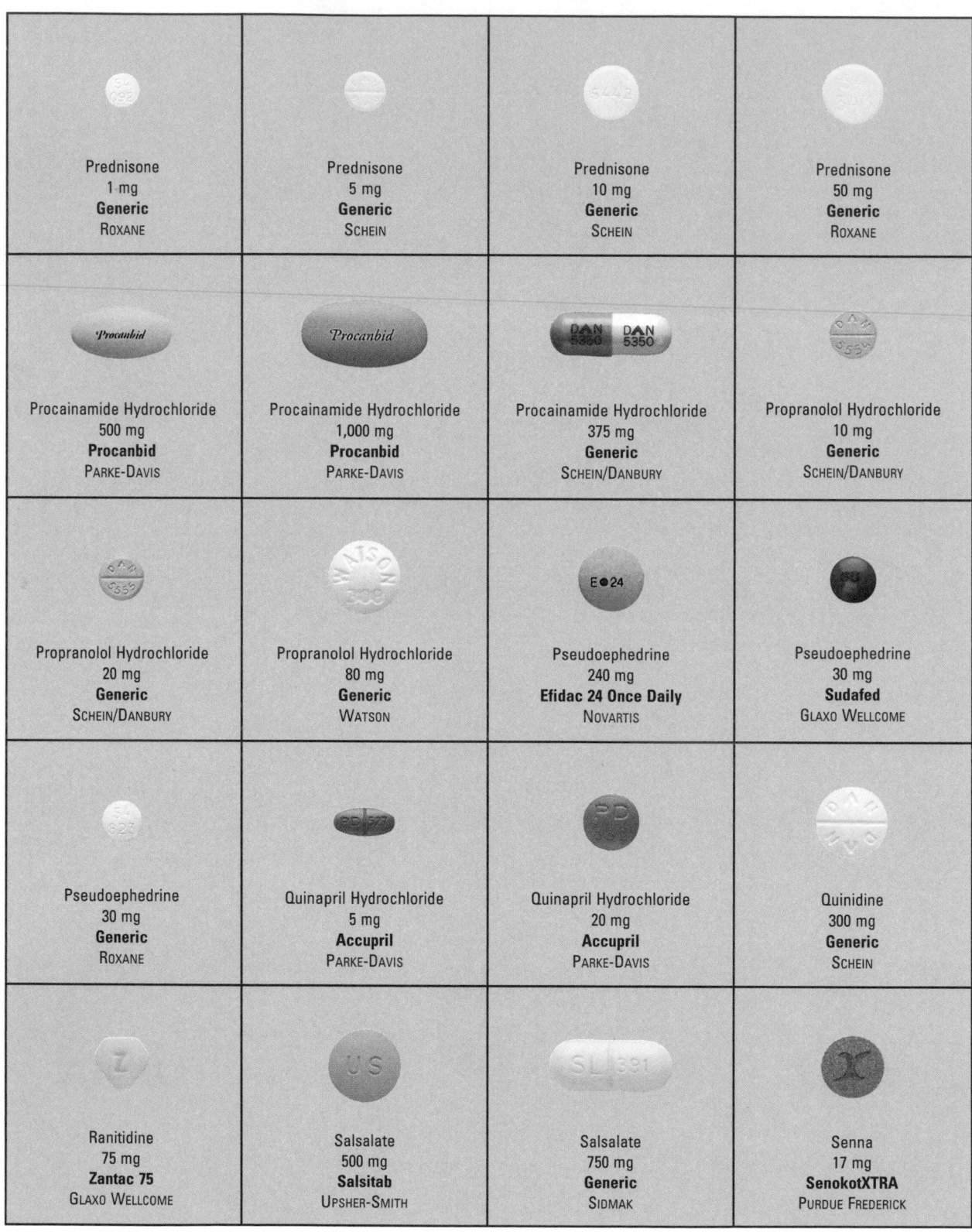

Prednisone
1 mg
Generic
ROXANE

Prednisone
5 mg
Generic
SCHEIN

Prednisone
10 mg
Generic
SCHEIN

Prednisone
50 mg
Generic
ROXANE

Procainamide Hydrochloride
500 mg
Procanbid
PARKE-DAVIS

Procainamide Hydrochloride
1,000 mg
Procanbid
PARKE-DAVIS

Procainamide Hydrochloride
375 mg
Generic
SCHEIN/DANBURY

Propranolol Hydrochloride
10 mg
Generic
SCHEIN/DANBURY

Propranolol Hydrochloride
20 mg
Generic
SCHEIN/DANBURY

Propranolol Hydrochloride
80 mg
Generic
WATSON

Pseudoephedrine
240 mg
Efidac 24 Once Daily
NOVARTIS

Pseudoephedrine
30 mg
Sudafed
GLAXO WELLCOME

Pseudoephedrine
30 mg
Generic
ROXANE

Quinapril Hydrochloride
5 mg
Accupril
PARKE-DAVIS

Quinapril Hydrochloride
20 mg
Accupril
PARKE-DAVIS

Quinidine
300 mg
Generic
SCHEIN

Ranitidine
75 mg
Zantac 75
GLAXO WELLCOME

Salsalate
500 mg
Salsitab
UPSHER-SMITH

Salsalate
750 mg
Generic
SIDMAK

Senna
17 mg
SenokotXTRA
PURDUE FREDERICK

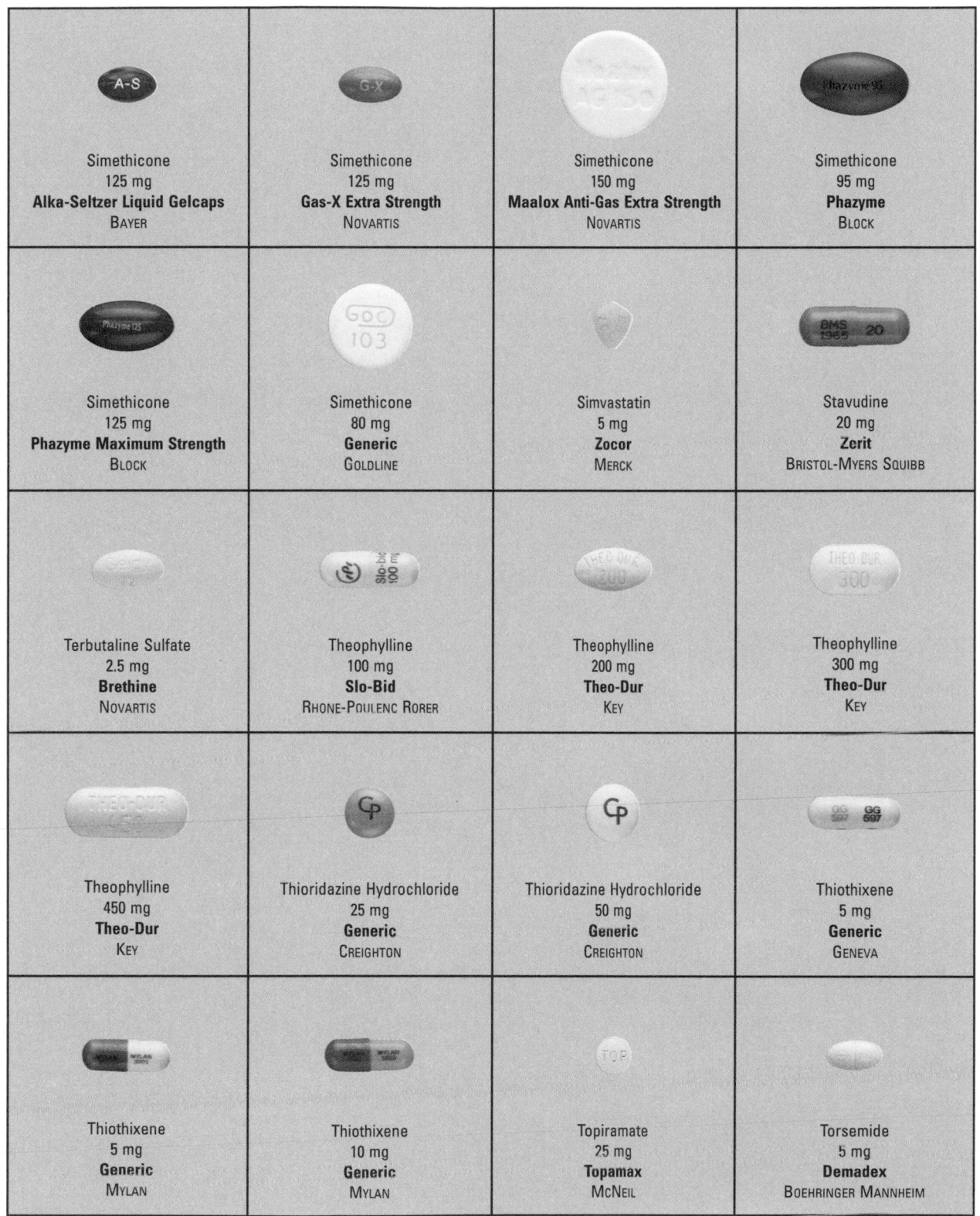

Simethicone 125 mg **Alka-Seltzer Liquid Gelcaps** BAYER	Simethicone 125 mg **Gas-X Extra Strength** NOVARTIS	Simethicone 150 mg **Maalox Anti-Gas Extra Strength** NOVARTIS	Simethicone 95 mg **Phazyme** BLOCK
Simethicone 125 mg **Phazyme Maximum Strength** BLOCK	Simethicone 80 mg **Generic** GOLDLINE	Simvastatin 5 mg **Zocor** MERCK	Stavudine 20 mg **Zerit** BRISTOL-MYERS SQUIBB
Terbutaline Sulfate 2.5 mg **Brethine** NOVARTIS	Theophylline 100 mg **Slo-Bid** RHONE-POULENC RORER	Theophylline 200 mg **Theo-Dur** KEY	Theophylline 300 mg **Theo-Dur** KEY
Theophylline 450 mg **Theo-Dur** KEY	Thioridazine Hydrochloride 25 mg **Generic** CREIGHTON	Thioridazine Hydrochloride 50 mg **Generic** CREIGHTON	Thiothixene 5 mg **Generic** GENEVA
Thiothixene 5 mg **Generic** MYLAN	Thiothixene 10 mg **Generic** MYLAN	Topiramate 25 mg **Topamax** McNEIL	Torsemide 5 mg **Demadex** BOEHRINGER MANNHEIM

Trifluoperazine Hydrochloride 1 mg **Generic** GENEVA	Trifluoperazine Hydrochloride 2 mg **Generic** GENEVA	Trifluoperazine Hydrochloride 5 mg **Generic** GENEVA	Valproic Acid 250 mg **Depakene** ABBOTT
Valproic Acid 250 mg **Depakote** ABBOTT	Verapamil Hydrochloride 180 mg **Isoptin SR** KNOLL	Verapamil Hydrochloride 240 mg **Isoptin SR** KNOLL	Verapamil Hydrochloride 80 mg **Generic** GENEVA
Verapamil Hydrochloride 120 mg **Generic** SCHEIN/DANBURY	Vitamin B1 100 mg **Generic** NUTRO	Vitamin B6 (Pyridoxine) 50 mg **Generic** NUTRO	Vitamin C 250 mg **Generic** NUTRO
Warfarin 2.5 mg **Coumadin** DUPONT	Warfarin 5 mg **Coumadin** DUPONT	Warfarin 10 mg **Coumadin** DUPONT	

A GUIDE TO
Dietary Supplements

A GUIDE TO
Dietary Supplements

DIETARY SUPPLEMENTS: AN OVERVIEW

As the use of medications increases, more people than ever are also using a constantly expanding variety of "dietary supplements," as they are officially called, to prevent, treat, or manage a range of health problems.

As defined by the Food and Drug Administration (FDA), dietary supplements encompass not only vitamins and minerals, but also herbs and other plant-derived substances ("botanicals"), various enzymes, amino acids, and even some human hormones.

Available without a prescription, these products are now sold in supermarkets, drug stores, and specialty stores, through whole-sale catalogs, and on the Internet. They have become enormously popular, with users numbering in the millions. In one national telephone survey done recently, 49 percent of interviewees had used an herbal supplement within the past year, and 24 percent reported using them regularly. Supplements are also big business. Though growth has slowed somewhat since the mid-1990s, the supplements industry sold an estimated $16 billion worth of products in 2000, of which more than $4 billion was spent on herbal supplements.

Supplements, and particularly herbs, are among the therapies considered part of alternative and complementary medicine, or CAM. Like other CAM practices, such as acupuncture or massage therapy, supplements may be used alone or in addition to conventional mainstream medicine. The following overview explains the key differences between dietary supplements and conventional medications, and sorts through the dilemmas and confusions facing the consumer interested in using supplements. As a further guide, starting on page 816, there are individual profiles of 10 of the most popular supplements marketed in the United States. The profiles summarize and assess the principal claims made for each supplement and offer precautions and guidelines concerning their use.

THE BASIC PROBLEM: A LACK OF RELIABLE EVIDENCE

Despite the widespread use of dietary supplements, there are surprisingly few places a consumer can find reliable, authoritative information on their effectiveness and safety. The use of supplements of vitamins and certain minerals to help prevent or treat diseases resulting from nutritional deficiencies is well established. Those uses—for which doses are based on the government's Recommended Dietary Allowances (RDAs)—are covered in the main section of this book. But most other benefits claimed for dietary supplements—benefits that range from curing colds to preventing heart disease—are largely unproven.

As interest in supplements has increased, so has scientific scrutiny of their therapeutic potential and safety. Some supplements, perhaps many of them, may prove to have real therapeutic value. However, most of the research on supplements, especially on herbs, has had limitations. Much "evidence" is anecdotal; clinical studies are often small, short-term, and poorly designed; negative results may be underreported; and effects of long-term use of supplements are lacking.

Even in Germany, where a government-approved body of experts known as Commission E has systematically reviewed the evidence on some 300 herbs over the past three decades, the scientific basis for the Commission E recommendations has not been made public. Only recently have researchers begun to undertake the kind of well-designed clinical trials that are routinely used to assess the safety and efficacy of conventional medications. Some supplements show promise. To date, however, there is simply a lack of definitive evidence for or against the effectiveness of most products that are within easy reach of the consumer.

Perhaps the greatest misconception many people have about dietary supplements, and herbal preparations in particular, is that they are safe because they are derived from a natural source. This is not necessarily true. Many herbs do have physiological effects; some are mild, but some are severe and dangerous, just like the effects from certain drugs. In fact, many drugs are "natural" in the sense that they originally came from plants. And just as drugs do, different herbs can interact with one another, or with conventional medications, in ways that can have serious consequences.

The difference is that a drug, in order to be marketed, must undergo clinical studies to determine its effectiveness, safety, possible interactions with other substances, and appropriate dosages; then the FDA must review these data and authorize the drug's use before it can be put on the market. Supplements do not have to undergo testing or authorization by the FDA. No authoritative body oversees the effectiveness and safety of supplements or their manufacture.

In addition, American physicians generally receive little or no training concerning the use of herbal medicines or other types of dietary supplements. In a number of Western European countries, medical students are routinely taught about medicinal herbs, and physicians commonly prescribe herbal preparations for a wide range of ailments. For example, the herb St. John's wort is widely prescribed for treating depression by doctors in Germany, where it outsells Prozac, the world's best-selling antidepressant medication, by a substantial margin. Herbal products in Europe must also conform to manufacturing standards, and studies examining supplements in European countries typically use standardized products containing consistent amounts of active ingredients—products that you can't be assured of purchasing in the United States.

WHY CLAIMS CAN'T BE TRUSTED

In many ways, American consumers are on their own when it comes to using supplements—and the primary reason for this is government legislation. With the Dietary Supplement Health and Education Act (DSHEA) of 1994, Congress essentially removed dietary supplements from regulatory control by the FDA. Provided the label for a supplement makes no claims about the product's effectiveness against specific diseases, it is exempt from the normally rigor-

ous testing the FDA requires to establish the safety and efficacy of drugs and food additives. So although labels can state dosages and make health-related claims that give them an air of authority, such information is not based on the kind of data that drug manufacturers must submit to the FDA in order to get a medication approved. Indeed, supplement manufacturers can make claims about a product without any scientific evidence to support the claims.

In 2000 the FDA published a ruling that defines the types of claims supplement manufacturers can make on product labels. This ruling continues to prohibit statements claiming that a supplement can prevent, treat, or cure a specific disease—unless such a claim has passed an FDA review for efficacy. A few dietary supplements have met this condition: calcium supplements, for example, can carry the claim that they help prevent osteoporosis; likewise, labels for folic acid supplements can claim that they help prevent birth defects. But these are exceptions. In practical terms, supplements cannot state, for example, that they prevent cardiovascular disease or treat depression.

However, manufacturers are permitted to make claims about how their supplements affect the "structure or function" of the body. This is where language can become misleading, since such claims may imply that a product can help treat a health problem. The label on a bottle of St. John's wort, for example, cannot claim to "treat depression." But it can state that the supplement "helps improve mood"—leaving open the question as to whether it can actually help someone who is depressed.

The FDA had initially hoped to limit such claims, but some consumer groups and virtually all supplement manufacturers expressed concern that government interference might take popular supplements off the market. Under considerable pressure, the agency reconsidered and ultimately relaxed the proposed restrictions. Products that carry structure/function claims must also display a disclaimer stating that the claim has not been approved by the FDA, nor is it intended to "diagnose, treat, cure, or prevent any disease." But the disclaimer can appear in small type and may be overlooked by—or fail to impress—many consumers.

The result is that it's often impossible for consumers to distinguish between claims that may be reasonable and ones that have little if any validity.

Consumers are often left with no more knowledge about the judicious use of supplements than their marketers deign to offer. To complicate matters, many supplements contain two or more ingredients whose individual and combined effects are anybody's guess.

As if all this wasn't sufficiently confusing to consumers, the limited restrictions imposed on the labeling of supplements don't apply to their marketing. As a result, ads for supplements in magazines, catalogs, or on the Internet can claim almost any benefit. To date, the Federal Trade Commission (FTC), which regulates claims made in advertising, has taken enforcement actions against a number of manufacturers making demonstrably false or misleading claims. For example, the FTC recently brought charges against several companies that had been promoting St. John's wort as a safe and effective treatment for HIV/AIDS. Not only is the herb unproven as a treatment, but it poses a risk of adverse interactions with prescription medications commonly used for treating the disease. Unfortunately, given its resources, the FTC can only monitor and challenge a fraction of the dizzying number of claims made in the promotional materials used to sell supplements.

NO GUARANTEES OF PURITY

The deregulation of supplements also means that the government does nothing to ensure that supplements meet quality control standards. Because the purity and consistency of products is left up to the manufacturers, consumers can't be sure that a product contains precisely what the label states. This is less of an issue with vitamin and mineral supplements, which are relatively simple to standardize. Herbal supplements are another matter. The amount of active chemical ingredients can vary considerably among different batches of the same plant. In addition, manufacturers usually do not isolate the active ingredients. Instead, many products contain all the compounds extracted from a plant—either because separating out the active ingredients is too expensive or, in many cases, because it's not known which components of an herb are most important.

Tests conducted by independent laboratories in recent years have shown that the ingredients contained in different brands of an herbal supplement, such as St. John's wort or saw palmetto, can vary widely. In one study assessing the content of 24 ginseng products, a third of the products contained no ginseng components at all. And because many herbal products are formulated using the entire plant, they may contain not only active ingredients, but many other chemicals occurring naturally in the plant. The haphazardness of manufacturing standards also means that statements about dosages—which experts don't agree on to begin with—are all the more questionable.

Recent FDA regulations at least require that the labels for all supplements begin to carry a "Supplement Facts" panel that lists all the ingredients in a product and clearly identifies the name and address of the manufacturer or distributor. Still, this ruling doesn't mean that the bottle actually contains what is on the label. And even if it does, there remains the fundamental problem any consumer faces in choosing a supplement: despite cleverly-worded and scientific-sounding claims, there is no clear evidence that the vast majority of herbs and other products have any benefit at all.

THE ISSUE OF SAFETY

Although few supplements have proven efficacy, and there is little data to support their use, most appear to be fairly safe when taken as directed. Thus, they may not help, but they probably won't hurt.

However, there are notable exceptions. An Associated Press analysis of FDA records revealed more than 2,600 reports of adverse reactions, including 101 deaths, associated with dietary supplements between 1993 and 1998. Since millions of people use supplements, these numbers are relatively low (perhaps due, in part, to spotty reporting); yet such calamities are still tragic, all the more so because they are avoidable. Unfortunately, the safety of a supplement, like its efficacy, does not have to be demonstrated before a product is marketed—in contrast to drugs. And once a supplement is in the marketplace, there is no process in place to track the occurrence of adverse reactions. The FDA keeps track of a drug's adverse side effects through reports filed by physicians, and can act promptly to take a drug off the market or restrict its use. With supplements, the FDA can't rely on such reports; because supplements are sold over-the-counter, their use can't be overseen by physicians. More-over, as stipulated by the DSHEA legislation, the FDA has to prove that a product is unsafe for it to be removed from the market.

A recent issue of the British medical journal *The Lancet* featured a review of all Medline database reports of adverse effects from dietary supplements that occurred between 1966 and 1998. (Medline is the National Library of Medicine's premier biblio-graphic database containing citations from over 4,000 biomedical journals.) Among the key obser-vations in the article: many herbal products are mislabeled (a different and sometimes toxic plant may have been used instead of the one specified on the label, often as a result of poor translation from, say, Chinese to English); thousands of imported herbal products also contain potent added phar-maceutical agents (including caffeine, aceta-minophen, anti-inflammatory drugs, diuretics, and steroids); and about 10 percent of herbal products from Asia are contaminated with dangerous heavy metals, such as lead, arsenic, and mercury.

Likewise, in a survey of 260 Chinese herbal med-icines sold over-the-counter in California, investiga-tors in the California Department of Health Services found that 32 percent of the products contained undeclared pharmaceutical agents or heavy metals.

MIXING SUPPLEMENTS AND MEDICATIONS

In addition to adverse effects caused by supple-ments themselves, there is a potential for even greater harm when supplements, particularly herbs, are used along with conventional medica-tions because of possible interactions that may enhance, reduce, or eliminate the effects of a par-ticular medication in ways that are largely unknown. Such interactions are critical for med-ications with a narrow therapeutic range—those drugs that require precise dosages in order to be effective without being toxic (see chart below).

One of the most serious herb-drug-related com-plications occurs when warfarin—an anticoagulant

---

An Overview of Herb-Drug Interactions

Herb-drug interactions are more likely when using	Selected examples:
Drugs with a narrow therapeutic range	• Warfarin, taken for atrial fibrillation • Digoxin, taken for congestive heart failure • Theophylline, taken for asthma • Lithium, taken for bipolar disorder (manic depression) • Phenytoin, an anti-seizure medication
Drug that typically require trial and error to find the right dose	• Levothyroxine, taken for an underactive thyroid • Levodopa, an antiparkinson drug
Drugs and herbs that may have similar actions or be used for the same purpose	• St. John's wort with SSRIs for depression • Saw palmetto with finasteride or terazosin for an enlarged prostate • Gingko or garlic with low-dose aspirin to discourage blood clots • Soy (a non-herbal plant product that contains estrogen) with hormone replacement therapy
Herbs around the time of surgery	• Gingko, garlic, St. John's wort, echinacea, Panax ginseng, ephedra, Kava, and valerian

Checklist for Supplement Users

Because dietary supplements are largely unregulated, keep these points in mind if you decide to try a supplement, especially an herbal product:

▶ **Don't rely on any type of supplement to self-treat a serious health problem.** Be sure to consult your doctor for a proper diagnosis and for treatment recommendations.

▶ **Communicate with your doctor.** Report all of your symptoms and tell your doctor about any supplements you are taking. Some of them might not interact well with conventional drugs that may be prescribed for you.

Don't stop conventional treatment. You should never discontinue or alter the dosage of a prescribed medication without first consulting your doctor.

▶ **Buy established brands from reputable vendors.** This step is no guarantee of purity in a product, but at least major manufacturers and distributors have the financial resources to establish quality control procedures; they also have reputations to protect.

▶ **Check the label.** Be sure supplements are carefully labeled (some manufacturers list potential drug interactions) and contain standardized extracts, if possible. ("Standardized" means that each capsule or tablet contains a uniform amount of a certain compound.) Beware of extravagant claims, "quick-fix" promises, and terms such as "clinically proven," "guaranteed potency," "naturally occurring," or "maximum absorption." Such terms have no standard definition; they are simply advertising jargon.

▶ **Look for products with the USP notation.** The United States Pharmacopeia (USP), an independent non-profit organization that sets standards of potency and purity for conventional medications, has established comparable standards for vitamins, minerals, and, most recently, some herbs. Compliance with USP standards is up to the manufacturer, but the presence of "USP" on a product from a nationally-known manufacturer means it is likely that the standards have been met. (The absence of "USP," however, does not mean that a product has failed to meet the standards— and standards have yet to be established for many herbal supplements.)

▶ **Be conservative with supplement dosages.** Dosages have not been scientifically established for most supplements,. Nor can you be sure that a product's contents matches what's on the label—so you may be risking an overdose if you start off taking the highest dosage. If a range is given, begin with the lowest dose.

▶ **Most supplements, especially herbs, shouldn't be used on a long-term basis.** Little or no evidence indicates how long you should take most supplements before you begin to experience a benefit. If you take an herbal product or some other type of supplement for a specific health problem, and you experience no benefit after several weeks, stop taking it. (Vitamins and mineral supplements are less likely to cause problems when taken in appropriate doses for long periods. The precautions that do apply are spelled out in the vitamin and mineral profiles in the main section of this book.)

▶ **Watch for side effects.** Many people think herbal products are safe, but herbs and other supplements can produce serious side effects. Be alert to unusual signs or symptoms that occur after you've begun taking a supplement. If any develop, stop taking the supplement and call your doctor or other health-care provider.

▶ **Avoid herbs if you are pregnant or breastfeeding.** The consequences simply haven't been established. Also, don't give supplements to children (other than multi-vitamin/mineral supplements) without first talking to your doctor.

▶ **Before surgery, inform your doctor.** As many as 70 percent of patients using herbs don't tell their doctors during exams before surgery. It's crucial not to withhold such information. The American Society of Anesthesiologists suggests stopping supplements at least two to three weeks before a surgical procedure.

Note: If you suffer a serious harmful effect or illness that you think is related to supplement use, you should contact Med-Watch to report it. Only in this way can information about the adverse effects of dietary supplements be centrally obtained and circulated. Your doctor can also file a report. Call MedWatch at 800 332-1088 or go to their Web site at www.fda.gov/medwatch.

with a narrow dosage range that is often prescribed to prevent blood clots in people with atrial fibrillation (a heart rhythm disturbance)—is taken with ginkgo (said to improve memory) or garlic tablets or powders (said to improve glucose, cholesterol, and blood pressure control). Either combination can prompt internal bleeding that may trigger a stroke.

Similarly, herb-drug interactions are more likely for medications that typically require "fine tuning" adjustments of dosages to determine the most effective dose for a particular individual. One example of such a drug is the antiparkinsonian medication levodopa (Dopar and Larodopa). In a survey of 200 patients with Parkinson's disease, Johns Hopkins researchers found that about a quarter used a vitamin or herb supplement and most did not inform their physicians when they started to take the supplement.

The risk of problems also rises when supplements and drugs are taken for the same purpose, presumably because they may share similar actions or address similar underlying causes. For example, St. John's wort, marketed primarily for depression, can enhance the effects of selective serotonin reuptake inhibitors (SSRIs), the most commonly prescribed type of antidepressant medication. Confusion, allergic reactions, stomach upset, headache, and restlessness may result.

Potential supplement-drug problems are a special concern when patients are compromised, perhaps due to chronic medical problems (especially kidney or liver impairment), frailty, poor nutrition, or surgery. A study reported in _The Journal of the American Medical Association (JAMA)_ found that eight commonly used herbs can cause complications in the period immediately following surgery, including an increased risk of stroke, excessive bleeding, hypoglycemia (low blood glucose), allergic reactions, or the sedative effects of anesthesia. Some of the most popular herbs—including gingko, garlic, and St. John's wort—were among the offenders.

WHAT YOU CAN DO

The federal government is currently funding research into dietary supplements, but definitive results may be a long way off. In the meantime, our recommendation is: Proceed with caution.

The best way to avoid dangerous reactions from dietary supplements is to let your doctor and pharmacist know of any products you are taking or intend to take. Increasingly, pharmacists and physicians are more knowledgeable about how drugs interact with each other and with other substances.

Yet patients are often their own worst enemy. Two landmark studies showed that 40 to 70 percent of the millions of people using nontraditional remedies do not tell their doctors about it. They may fear chastisement for straying from orthodoxy or harbor the common misconception that "natural" remedies are somehow harmless, especially since they are available without a prescription.

Good communication is essential for reducing potential problems and may prevent a disaster. It's especially important whenever you are starting a new medication or having elective surgery. Also see "A Checklist for Supplement Users" (opposite) for advice on choosing and using supplements.

PROFILES OF POPULAR SUPPLEMENTS

The following pages contain information and guidelines on ten best-selling dietary supplements used for medicinal purposes—mostly herbs, but also two others (glucosamine and SAMe) that are created from natural compounds. The supplements profiled have been selected primarily because they are among the most commonly used. They are also among the best-studied: some, though not all, have shown promise for treating or alleviating specific conditions.

Each profile covers the use (or uses) the supplement is commonly promoted for; the evidence for its effectiveness; its safety, including including known and potential interactions with conventional medications; and any special considerations you should be aware of if you decide to try the supplement.

Keep in mind that the FDA has not reviewed these supplements either for efficacy or safety. Also, the potency and purity of any products you buy are left up to manufacturers; there is no assurance that the capsules or pills in a bottle contain what is on the label. Active ingredients can vary from brand to brand and you may not be taking the same preparation that has been used in a research study—or even by a friend who recommended the supplement to you.

In compiling the profiles, we have drawn on a number of sources containing evidence-based information on dietary supplements. One especially useful general source is the *Professional's Handbook of Complementary and Alternative Medicines* (second edition) by C. W. Fetrow, PharmD and Juan R. Avila, PharmD (Springhouse, 2001)—a comprehensive reference for which the authors reviewed hundreds of journal articles. Other helpful sources include the following:

- **National Center for Complementary and Alternative Medicine**
  Telephone: 888-644-6226
  Website: www.nccam.nih.gov

- **APRALERT**
  College of Pharmacy
  University of Illinois at Chicago
  Telephone: 312-996-2246
  Website: www.pmmp.uic.edu

- **United States Pharmacopeia (USP)**
  Telephone: 800-822-8772
  Website: www.usp.org

- **Quackwatch**
  Website: www.familyinternet.com/quackwatch

Echinacea

Latin name: *Echinacea purpurea, e. pallida,* and others

WHAT IS IT?
Extracts of echinacea, a plant that is part of the daisy family, have been used as herbal medicines for centuries. Nine varieties of echinacea grow in the United States, and three of them—the most common being Echinacea purpurea—are used to provide dietary supplements. The principal claim made for the supplements is that they strengthen the immune system and are thereby effective for warding off infections, particularly colds and flu. As part of its immune-boosting effect, echinacea is also claimed to be effective for speeding up the healing of burns, cuts, wounds, and inflammations of the skin.

COMMON FORMS
Available as capsules, tablets, and in other forms that include juices, lozenges, teas, and tinctures.

HOW IT WORKS
The herb is pharmacologically complex, containing at least 15 different compounds. Several classes of compounds appear to stimulate immune system activity. But no single component has been identified as the "active ingredient" responsible for the benefits attributed to echinacea.

RESEARCH AND EVIDENCE
Echinacea has been extensively studied, but with mixed results. In some studies examining its effect on treating the common cold—probably the most popular use of the herb—echinacea seemed to have no effect; in others, it appeared to reduce the severity or duration of symptoms. Moreover, in most studies that found echinacea to stimulate the immune system, the herbal extract was injected, a form of administration that is not available in the United States. As a strategy for preventing colds, the evidence is even less persuasive: studies show little difference between echinacea and a placebo. A recent review found insufficient evidence to recommend the use of echinacea for either the treatment or prevention of upper respiratory infections.

POSSIBLE SIDE EFFECTS
Side effects in healthy people have seldom been reported. But any preparations containing echinacea may have an adverse effect on people with severe illnesses, including autoimmune diseases, HIV infection, leukemia, multiple sclerosis, or tuberculosis.

POTENTIAL DRUG INTERACTIONS
No significant interactions have been reported.

SPECIAL CONSIDERATIONS
- If you decide to try echinacea for preventing or treating a cold or bout of flu, it's unknown which variety of echinacea is most effective or what the proper dosage is. Also, more than most other herbs, the concentration of active ingredients can vary significantly depending on the variety of echinacea, the part of the plant used, growing conditions, and how the ingredients were extracted.

- Commercial echinacea preparations are often diluted with inactive ingredients. Be sure to check the label. Many tinctures contain significant amounts of alcohol and may not be appropriate for children or for adults who should avoid alcohol.
- Anyone who is infected with HIV, has an autoimmune disease, or any serious illness should avoid using echinacea for any reason.
- Pregnant or breastfeeding women should not use echinacea; the effects are unknown.
- Any therapeutic effects of echinacea are usually evident within 10 to 14 days. If an illness you are treating has not improved within that time, be sure to see your doctor. And do not, in any case, use echinacea for more than 8 weeks.

Garlic

Latin name: Allium sativum

WHAT IS IT?

A member of the onion family, garlic has been used for thousands of years as a medicinal plant, and today garlic supplements are extremely popular as well as extensively researched. Promoters of the supplements make countless claims for garlic's benefits: it is marketed for treating everything from headaches to infections to cancer. Probably the chief claim made for garlic, however, is that it can reduce the risk of heart disease by lowering blood cholesterol levels. There have been hundreds of garlic studies investigating these and other claims during the past ten years. But in spite of all the studies and all the advertising promoting garlic's curative powers, there is no clear evidence that garlic supplements have any health benefit.

COMMON FORMS

Most commonly available as tablets of compressed powder made from dried garlic bulbs. Also sold as fresh bulbs, freeze-dried powder, fresh extract, and oil.

HOW IT WORKS

All told, garlic contains more than 23 constituents, but the compound allicin is often cited as the key active ingredient. Allicin is an unstable sulfurous compound that is formed by enzymes when the clove is chewed, crushed, or ground, and it gives garlic its strong odor. Allicin then breaks down into other sulfur-containing compounds. However, allicin is not present in all garlic supplements, so if it is indeed the active ingredient, more of it may be available in raw garlic or powdered forms of garlic. The problem is, some other compound might be beneficial—or not. No one knows.

RESEARCH AND EVIDENCE

With regard to the claims for garlic's cholesterol-lowering effect, a few clinical trials have shown a modest benefit. But these studies—like most studies on claims for garlic—have been small, poorly designed (many with no control group), and use different forms of garlic, so their results are questionable.

Two recent well-designed controlled studies concluded that garlic had no effect on cholesterol levels. Both studies—one published in the *Archives of Internal Medicine,* the other in the *Journal of the American Medical Association*—involved subjects with elevated cholesterol and compared the results of taking garlic supplements against a placebo over 12 weeks. Each study used a separate form of garlic—an oil and a powder tablet—but neither form produced a cholesterol-lowering benefit.

POSSIBLE SIDE EFFECTS

No serious adverse reactions have been reported from taking garlic supplements. The most common side effects have been heartburn and upset stomach and irritation of the mouth and throat, especially from high doses.

POTENTIAL DRUG INTERACTIONS

There may be a risk of bleeding if garlic supplements are taken with anticoagulant medications such as warfarin (Coumadin).

SPECIAL CONSIDERATIONS

- Although garlic appears to be safe, there is no evidence for relying on it to lower blood cholesterol levels—or to treat any other health problem, for that matter. Indeed, it's far from clear that garlic in any form has any significant pharmacological effect. And if there is some benefit from using garlic, it's not known how long you would have to eat garlic or take supplements to obtain the benefit.

- If you still want to try garlic supplements, the standard dose in studies documenting their effect on lipid levels has been 600 to 900 mg per day in pill form or 5 to 8 mg of garlic oil (equivalent to half a clove to a clove of raw garlic).
- If you take a prescription medication, talk to your doctor before using garlic in high doses or over the long term. Avoid taking garlic supplements if you are on an anticoagulant medication.

Gingko biloba

Latin name: Gingko biloba

WHAT IS IT?

Supplements of gingko biloba are among the most widely used herbal remedies in the world. The supplements are made from a leaf extract of the gingko tree, a primitive native of China that dates back some 230 million years and now grows in many other countries. In Germany and France, standardized gingko extracts are among the most commonly prescribed remedies for circulatory and neurological problems. But in the United States, the herb is most actively promoted as a "memory booster" that can help sharpen mental focus in healthy people as well as slow or prevent "normal" memory loss—claims that have no evidence to support them.

COMMON FORMS

Standardized gingko biloba extract (called GBE) is available in capsules and tablets, and also in tinctures, powders, liquids, sprays, and even "nutrition bars." In Asia, seeds of the gingko biloba tree are used medicinally, but can cause severe allergic reactions, and so should be avoided.

HOW IT WORKS

Gingko extracts contain a variety of active ingredients, including flavonoids and terpenoids, that act in concert to induce antioxidant and anti-inflammatory effects. These properties could account for its supposed benefits to the brain. Some studies show that it may relax blood vessels, increase blood flow, reduce clotting, and reduce the abnormalities that afflict the brain in those with dementia.

RESEARCH AND EVIDENCE

Most studies on gingko biloba have been small and poorly designed. The first American trial to rigorously examine the herb, published in the *Journal of the American Medical Association (JAMA)* in 1998, found that cognitive performance and social functioning were more likely to stabilize or improve in gingko-takers than in those taking a placebo. Subjects were evaluated over the course of a year. The results indicate that gingko can aid some people with dementia; however, even though side effects were minimal, one third of the 309 subjects dropped out of the study, suggesting that many experienced no benefit.

For these reasons, most medical experts are not ready to fully embrace gingko for treating dementia. And there was no indication at all in the JAMA study, or in any other controlled studies, that gingko can enhance mental alertness or help prevent the type of normal memory loss (such as having trouble recalling names or locating familiar objects) that almost everyone experiences with age. Although gingko has also been investigated as a remedy for other disorders, further research is need to confirm its effectiveness.

POSSIBLE SIDE EFFECTS

In studies, side effects have been minor and include headache, diarrhea, flatulence, nausea, and allergic skin reactions. No serious adverse effects have been reported in human trials using gingko biloba extract.

POTENTIAL DRUG INTERACTIONS

Because gingko interferes with blood clotting, it may interact with medications often referred to as "blood-thinners," such as aspirin and warfarin (Coumadin), and increase the risk of internal bleeding.

SPECIAL CONSIDERATIONS

- People with Alzheimer's disease or other forms of dementia will gain more from prescription drugs such as tacrine (Cognex), which have been extensively studied and are approved by the FDA, than from taking gingko biloba.
- If you decide to try gingko, dosages are uncertain. Most trials have used 120 to 160 milligrams a day, divided into three doses, and a four-to-six-week course of treatment has been necessary to

determine effectiveness. But because of the lack of government regulation, brands of gingko in the United States undoubtedly vary as to their purity and the potency of their active ingredients.

- Talk to your doctor before taking ginkgo if you take any medications regularly. This is especially important if you are taking any type of blood-thinning medication. Also call your doctor if, while taking gingko, you experience any signs of bleeding, easy bruising, or any other possible side effects.
- If you are undergoing elective surgery, it's very important to tell your doctor beforehand that you are using gingko biloba. Stop taking gingko at least one week before surgery or if you are undergoing an endoscopy.
- Pregnant or breastfeeding women should avoid taking gingko. Also, do not give gingko in any form to children.

Ginseng (Panax)

Latin name: Panax ginseng, Panax quinquefolius, and others

WHAT IS IT?

Ginseng has been part of Chinese medicine for thousands of years, and it is now one of the most popular—and most hyped—herbal supplements in Western countries. The herb has many health claims associated with it; the most common are that it boosts energy, reduces emotional stress, and enhances sexual potency. Long-term use of ginseng as a "tonic" is reputed to improve well-being, particularly in older people suffering from degenerative diseases.

Ginseng supplements are made from the dried root of several different species. *Panax ginseng,* also called Asian ginseng, is extensively cultivated in China, Japan, and Korea, while a closely-related species, *Panax quinquefolius,* commonly known as American or Western ginseng, is grown in the United States. A third plant, Siberian ginseng *(Eleutherococcus senticosys),* is from the same family, but contains different chemical components that set it apart from the other ginsengs.

COMMON FORMS

Both Asian and Western ginseng are available as extracts in capsule form or in an alcohol base, as teas, and in powders made from the root. Ginseng has also been added to creams, juices, "nutrition bars," and other dietary supplements. The root can also be bought in bulk.

HOW IT WORKS

The active ingredients in Asian ginseng are called ginsenosides, also known as panaxosides. At least 12 major ginsenosides have been isolated. They occur only in very small amounts, so are difficult to purify and standardize. Different ginsenosides appear to have varied, even opposing, pharmacological actions, ranging from analgesic and depressant effects that are "calming" to effects that stimulate the central nervous system. Like many herbs, ginseng is complex, containing numerous other compounds that include volatile oils, vitamins, minerals, plant hormones, sugar, and fats. Only a few of the specific ingredients have been linked to a particular effect.

RESEARCH AND EVIDENCE

Most studies on ginseng have been small and poorly designed, and so are inconclusive. In addition, preparations of ginseng used in different studies have varied considerably. In a handful of studies that measured ginseng's effect on cognitive function, the herb appeared to have some benefit compared to a placebo, but the effect could hardly be called significant.

One of the few controlled studies on ginseng, published in 2001 in the *Journal of the American Dietetic Association,* found that chronic ginseng supplementation was no more effective than a sugar pill in reducing stress or improving mood in healthy young adults. An earlier study published in the same journal, which assessed ginseng's effect on physical endurance among a group of healthy active young men who were not elite athletes, found that taking ginseng daily over an eight-week period did not improve aerobic exercise performance.

Some preliminary evidence suggests that ginseng may help people with diabetes. In a small study published in *Diabetes Care,* patients with type 2 diabetes who took ginseng decreased their fasting blood glucose by about 10 percent over a two-month period. More research is needed to determine whether ginseng is useful in the treatment of diabetes.

POSSIBLE SIDE EFFECTS

Adverse reactions tend to be associated with high doses or prolonged use of ginseng. These side effects include headache, insomnia, nervousness, nausea, diarrhea, chest pain, palpitations, and skin rashes.

POTENTIAL DRUG INTERACTIONS

Ginseng may intensify the effect of drugs used to treat diabetes, including insulin. The herb can also interact adversely with MAO inhibitors used to treat depression.

SPECIAL CONSIDERATIONS

- Despite its popularity, there is little evidence to support ginseng's use. Better studies are needed to understand its chemistry, identify its most promising uses, and ascertain its potential for adverse effects.
- Dosages vary, usually ranging from 200 to 600 mg of ginseng extract taken daily. The purity of commercial ginsengs is a problem, however. Surveys indicate that products vary widely in their active ingredients, and some contain no ginseng ingredients at all.
- If you decide to try ginseng, be sure to check with your doctor first if you have any medical problems. People with diabetes should be especially cautious about initiating any therapy with ginseng. No one should use the herb for a prolonged period.
- Anyone taking prescription medications for depression should avoid using ginseng..
- Pregnant or breastfeeding women should not use ginseng.
- At the first sign of any unusual symptoms (see Possible Side Effects, above), discontinue taking ginseng.

Glucosamine and Chondroitin

WHAT IS IT?

Glucosamine and chondroitin sulfate are naturally occurring substances in the body. Chondroitin sulfate is a glycosaminoglycan—an important component of the cartilage found in the joints. Glucosamine is a building block for some of the proteoglycans of cartilage and of hyaluronic acid, which is a lubricating component of the synovial fluid within joints.

Both substances are marketed as dietary supplements for halting the gradual deterioration of joint cartilage that characterizes osteoarthritis (OA). The loss of glycosaminoglycans may contribute to the breakdown of cartilage, which helps absorb the shock of body movements and provide the joints with strength and elasticity. The release of cartilage-degrading enzymes by certain cells in the joint, known as chondrocytes, also contributes to the deterioration, which may be repaired by chondroitin sulfate.

While existing medications for OA, such as nonsteroidal anti-inflammatory drugs (NSAIDS) and COX-2 inhibitors, treat the symptoms of OA, they don't halt or reverse joint deterioration. Taking supplements of glucosamine and chondroitin, either alone or in combination, may target the underlying defect in OA and relieve symptoms in some people.

COMMON FORMS

Available as capsules and tablets. Various forms of glucosamine are used in supplements, but the one most commonly used in clinical studies is glucosamine sulfate. Supplements of glucosamine sulfate and chondroitin sulfate are prepared from extracts obtained from animal tissue—glucosamine from shell fish, chondroitin sulfate from the cartilage of cattle tracheas.

Most glucosamine/chondroitin products sold in the United contain both substances. Products containing glucosamine sulfate alone are also commonly available; only a few brands containing chondroitin alone are on the market, possibly because chondroitin costs manufacturers about four times as much as glucosamine.

HOW IT WORKS

How these compounds may work to treat OA isn't known, but it's thought that glucosamine stimulates the formation of new glycosaminoglycans. Chondroitin might inhibit the production of cartilage-destroying enzymes and be useful for the production of new cartilage that helps the body repair damaged joints.

RESEARCH AND EVIDENCE

The initial evidence for glucosamine came from small, preliminary European and Asian studies. (The supplements have been used in Europe for more than 10 years.) Additional clinical research is now emerging that appears to support early results. A recent review in the *Journal of the American Medical Association* evaluated the results of 15 trials—6 with glucosamine, 9 with chondroitin—on the effect of the two supplements on OA of the knee. Overall the studies support the notion that the supplements are safe and mildly to moderately effective. But the review authors noted problems in the studies: short treatment periods, small sample sizes, and possible publication bias (where only positive results get published) because many of the trials were sponsored by supplement manufacturers.

A more persuasive randomized, double-blind study, reported in *The Lancet* in 2001, followed 212 patients with mild-to-moderate OA of the knee over a three-year period. Those who took 1,500 milligrams of glucosamine sulfate daily had significantly less pain and disability than those taking a placebo. X-rays indicated that the glucosamine group also showed less deterioration of the knee joint.

Studies have generally focused on subjects with moderate arthritis. It's not known whether the supplements have any effect on severe OA, and no studies have shown that the supplements offer any benefit for other types of arthritis.

The comparative effectiveness and safety of glucosamine and chondroitin has not been determined in a carefully designed clinical trial. In what should be a pivotal study, the National Institutes of Health is conducting research that will compare the two supplements alone, in combination, and to a placebo. This long-term clinical trial, which is being carried out at thirteen research centers nationwide, is expected to be completed in 2005.

POSSIBLE SIDE EFFECTS

Reported side effects of glucosamine include abdominal discomfort, diarrhea, nausea, headache, drowsiness, skin rash.

Chondroitin may carry a risk of internal bleeding—it has some structural similarity to the anticoagulant heparin—but there have been no reports of this adverse effect in humans.

Some reports suggest that glucosamine, even in low doses, can have adverse effects on blood sugar levels by interfering with the production of insulin by beta cells of the pancreas. However, it isn't known whether glucosamine might harm people with diabetes. In the *Lancet* study cited above, glucosamine produced no major adverse effects, nor did it affect blood glucose levels.

POTENTIAL DRUG INTERACTIONS

Chondroitin may enhance the effect of anticoagulant medications such as heparin or warfarin.

SPECIAL CONSIDERATIONS.

- If you have OA, talk to your doctor if you are considering using glucosamine or chondroitin—particularly if you have diabetes, a bleeding disorder, or are taking anticoagulant medication.
- The long-term effectiveness and safety of these supplements have not been studied. Before beginning to use them, you may want to wait for the results from the long-term study underway at the National Institutes of Health (see above).
- If you choose to take glucosamine and/or chondroitin, it's important that you not stop taking proven treatments, such as NSAIDs or COX-2 inhibitors, without first consulting your doctor.
- Keep in mind that the supplements are not regulated. Look for products that clearly label how much of each ingredient is present. Suggested daily doses are 1,500 mg of glucosamine and 1,200 mg of chondroitin.
- Glucosamine-only products are much less expensive than those containing chondroitin alone or a mixture of the two. Also, perhaps because chondroitin is more expensive to manufacture, some combination products may contain less chondroitin than their labels claim. ConsumerLabs.com, which tests dietary supplements for potency and purity, found that 6 of 13 combination products and two chondroitin-only products

contained lower levels of chondroitin than stated on the labels.

- Women who are pregnant or breastfeeding should avoid these supplements.

Kava

Latin name: *Piper methysticum*

WHAT IS IT?

Marketed as a supplement that can restore calm and reduce stress, kava extract has become an immensely popular natural alternative for treating anxiety. A related claim is that kava (sometimes called kava-kava) helps induce sleep for people who suffer from insomnia. The extract is produced from a shrublike plant that grows on South Pacific islands and is a member of the black pepper family. (Beverages made from kava root have long been a part of social life in the South Pacific.)

COMMON FORMS

Available as capsules, tablets, an extract, or in dried plant form for making teas.

HOW IT WORKS

Kava contains active substances in the root called kavapyrones that appear to work synergistically with one another to induce feelings of relaxation and mild euphoria.

RESEARCH AND EVIDENCE

There is limited evidence for kava's use in treating anxiety, restlessness, and stress. In a recent review of clinical studies, published in the *Journal of Clinical Psychopharmacology,* two British physicians analyzed seven kava trials that met the standard of randomized, double-blind, placebo-controlled studies. The trials contained data from 377 people treated with kava extract. Although the results of all seven trials suggested that kava was better than a placebo in treating anxiety, kava had a statistically significant advantage over placebo in only three of the trials. Moreover, the trials were small and they varied in the amount of active ingredient that subjects took per day.

Though kava may show promise, additional tri-als are needed to determine appropriate dosing, benefits, and risks—and to also compare kava in these respects to benzodiazepines and other established anti-anxiety medications.

POSSIBLE SIDE EFFECTS

Side effects reported in the review of clinical trials noted above included stomach complaints, restlessness, tremor, headache, and drowsiness. Long-term heavy use of kava may cause more serious adverse effects, including hypertension, diarrhea, skin turning dry and scaly, and labored breathing.

POTENTIAL DRUG INTERACTIONS

Kava may interact with alprazolam, benzodiazepines, and other anti-anxiety medications, intensifying their sedative effects. Combining kava with levodopa, a drug for treating Parkinson's disease, may increase symptoms of Parkinson's. Kava can also interact adversely with alcohol.

SPECIAL CONSIDERATIONS

- Persistent anxiety and/or panic attacks can be serious disorders. Before treating any signs of anxiety, you should always consult a doctor. Also consult a doctor if you are experiencing persistent insomnia.
- The benefits and risks of kava are still unclear. Without large, double-blind, placebo-controlled studies, it's impossible to know whether kava will work as well as standard medications for mood disorders.
- Dosages are uncertain. Most studies have used supplements containing 70 to 240 mg of kavapyrones taken orally once a day. If you decide to try kava, start with the lowest dose.
- Do not combine kava with alcohol or with any drugs that affect the central nervous system, including prescription tranquilizers, sedatives, and antidepressants. If you take other prescription medications, check with your doctor before trying kava.
- Do not use kava for extended periods, since there is a risk of significant adverse side effects. If any of these occur (see above), stop taking kava immediately.
- Children under 18 and pregnant or nursing women should not use kava.

SAM-e

WHAT IS IT?

Widely touted as a treatment for both depression and osteoarthritis (OA), SAM-e has quickly become one of the best-selling supplements on the market. It is not an herb, a nutrient, or a hormone, but rather a synthetic form of a chemical—S-adenosyl-methionine—produced naturally in all animals. (The name has been shortened to SAM-e and is pronounced "sammy.")

SAME-e has been available in Europe since the 1970s for the treatment of a variety of diseases. Claims for its efficacy have expanded to include treating Alzheimer's disease, epilepsy, migraine headaches, fibromyalgia, Parkinson's disease, and cirrhosis, among others. But in the United States, where it has been available since 1999, it is primarily marketed as a dietary supplement that promotes "joint health" and "emotional well-being."

COMMON FORMS

Available as 200-mg tablets.

HOW IT WORKS

SAM-e forms when the amino acid methionine combines with adenosyl-triphosphate (ATP), an energy source for most biochemical reactions. SAM-e is a donor of methyl groups in a number of biochemical processes—in particular the synthesis of neurotransmitters such as serotonin and dopamine, two of the brain's chemical messengers that are known to regulate mood.

RESEARCH AND EVIDENCE

Those who support the use of SAM-e for treating depression claim it works just as well as prescription antidepressants, but faster and with fewer side effects. Some clinical trials in European countries, where it was initially tested as a treatment for schizophrenia, did suggest that SAM-e might effectively treat depression. But studies have been small and short in duration (ranging from two to six weeks), and dosages have varied considerably. Moreover, most European studies used injections of SAM-e rather than tablets to treat depression.

When the studies are taken together, SAM-e shows some promise for easing depression—not only depression alone, but also depression associated with fibromyalgia, Parkinson's disease, and menopause. More and better studies are necessary to confirm this, however, as are studies comparing SAM-e with standard medications for treating depression. At present, the use of SAM-e for the treatment of depression is not strongly supported by available evidence.

Some early European studies also suggested SAM-e was an effective therapy for relieving the joint pain of osteoarthritis OA. But in a more recent American study, published in the *Journal of Rheumatology,* researchers found little difference in benefit between SAM-e and a placebo. Further research is needed to determine whether SAM-e could provide a useful substitute or adjunct to conventional medications for OA.

POSSIBLE SIDE EFFECTS

One study estimates that 20 percent of people taking SAM-e experience side effects. Most side effects are mild and involve the gastrointestinal tract. They include heartburn, diarrhea, nausea, and vomiting. Less common side effects include dizziness, headache, insomnia, and cognitive impairment. Another concern is the risk, largely theoretical at this point, that SAM-e could raise blood levels of homocysteine (SAM-e is converted to homocysteine). High levels of homocysteine are considered a risk factor for cardiovascular disease.

POTENTIAL DRUG INTERACTIONS

There may be a potential for SAM-e to interact adversely with antidepressants or other mood-altering agents.

SPECIAL CONSIDERATIONS

- Depression can be a serious disorder. Before treating any signs of depression, you should always consult a doctor.
- The benefits and risks of SAM-e are still unclear. Without large, double-blind, placebo-controlled studies, it's impossible to know whether SAM-e will work as well as standard medications for either depression or OA.
- There is no evidence that SAM-e has mood-altering benefits in healthy people; hence, there is no sense taking it as a "tonic" or mood booster.
- If you decide to try SAM-e, dosages are uncertain. Studies have generally used 400 mg a day

for OA. Daily doses used in depression trials have ranged from 400 mg to as high as 1600 mg. Supplements in the United States are not regulated, so they may not be the same as those tested and prescribed in European countries (where most clinical trials have taken place).

- SAM-e is expensive, possibly more expensive than commonly used antidepressants. Taking 1,600 mg of SAM-e daily could cost more than $400 a month, depending on where you purchase it.
- SAM-e should not be used in combination with MAO inhibitors or other medications used for treating depression.
- SAM-e may increase the risk of a manic reaction in people with a bipolar disorder. If you have such a disorder, any use of SAM-e should be monitored by a physician.
- Until more is known about SAM-e, it should not be taken by women who are pregnant or breast-feeding.

Saw Palmetto

Latin name: *Serenoa repens, Serenoa serrulata,* and other species

WHAT IS IT?

Saw palmetto is an herbal extract derived from the dried berries of the dwarf palm tree. As a supplement, it has long been a popular remedy for genitourinary problems. In some European countries, saw palmetto has become a standard treatment for symptoms of benign prostatic hyperplasia (BPH), and is gaining popularity in the United States as an alternative to finasteride (Proscar) and other medications generally recommended as the first line treatments for symptoms of BPH.

By law, saw palmetto cannot be labeled as a treatment for BPH in the United States; labels on supplement products typically claim that the herb supports or improves "prostate health."

COMMON FORMS

Available as capsules, liquid extract, tablets, teas, and dried berries.

HOW IT WORKS

Saw palmetto contains certain phytosterols—substances that seem to curb prostate cell growth. The action of the herb may be similar to that of finasteride and other medications that are standard treatment options for BPH.

One component, beta-sitosterols, may inhibit the activity of male hormones within the prostate by blocking androgen receptors and by preventing the conversion of testosterone into the more active form dihydrotestosterone—a process believed to be important in BPH. Saw palmetto also exhibits some anti-inflammatory properties. A recent study of an herbal blend containing saw palmetto suggested that the herb may decrease the percentage of epithelial cells in the transition zone (the part of the prostate most affected by BPH).

RESEARCH AND EVIDENCE

Evidence is sparse but growing. A review of 18 controlled trials involving nearly 3,000 men published in the *Journal of the American Medical Association* found a 28 percent greater improvement in overall urinary symptoms, which included more urgent and/or frequent urination and nighttime urination (nocturia), among men with BPH taking saw palmetto than those taking a placebo. In addition, peak urine flow increased by 24 percent, compared with placebo. In some studies comparing saw palmetto to finasteride, saw palmetto was just as effective in improving urinary tract symptoms and peak urine flow, and had fewer adverse effects. Even though some of the studies were short in duration or small or had other shortcomings, the reviewers thought they were worthy of notice.

A recent monograph published by the United States Pharmacopeia (USP)—the nonprofit organization that helps set quality standards for drugs—carefully reviewed the data from 10 controlled trials considered sufficiently large and well-designed to allow a scientific assessment. The reviewers concluded that there is "evidence of moderate scientific quality" that saw palmetto is more effective than a placebo in relieving symptoms of BPH. However, the reviewers suggested that more studies are needed to determine saw palmetto's effect in different age groups and whether it has any significant interactions with conventional drugs.

POSSIBLE SIDE EFFECTS

Side effects are generally mild and may include headache, a rise in blood pressure, abdominal pain, diarrhea, constipation, nausea, urine retention, and erectile dysfunction.

POTENTIAL DRUG INTERACTIONS

None have been reported.

SPECIAL CONSIDERATIONS

- Saw palmetto appears to be safe and modestly effective in treating mild to moderate symptoms of BPH. If you choose to try it, be sure to see your doctor first. Don't self-diagnose BPH; your symptoms may be caused by a more serious condition that requires another treatment.
- Choose a product containing standardized amounts of *Serenoa repens*. This extract has been studied most extensively, appears to be well tolerated, has demonstrated greater efficacy than a placebo, and matched the effectiveness of finasteride in several trials.
- In most clinical trials, the dosage for treating symptoms of BPH is 320 mg per day taken in two doses of 160 mg. Take saw palmetto with food to minimize any gastrointestinal discomfort.
- If saw palmetto is going to work, symptoms usually begin improving within a month. Stop taking the supplements if you experience no improvement after a month.
- There has been some concern that saw palmetto can affect the results of PSA testing, the screening test for prostate cancer. Recent reports have shown no effect of saw palmetto on PSA results, but you should inform your doctor if you are taking saw palmetto and are scheduled for a PSA test

St. John's wort

Latin name: Hypericum perforatum

WHAT IS IT?

St. John's wort is a common, shrub-like flowering plant in the family Hypericaceae that was probably named by early Christians in honor of John the Baptist. The plant is native to Europe, but now grows in many parts of the world. St. John's wort bears bright yellow flowers that, when dried, have been used for centuries in teas as folk remedies for nervous disorders that include anxiety, insomnia, and upset stomach. As a liquid tincture, it has been applied to wounds, bruises, bites, stings, and other skin traumas to combat infection and inflammation.

In recent years, the herb has become a popular supplement for treating mild to moderate depression. In Germany, where St. John's wort is regularly prescribed by physicians as an antidepressant, it outsells Prozac, the world's best-selling antidepressant medication, by a substantial margin. St. John's wort is viewed as a milder alternative to conventional antidepressant medications, which can cause undesirable side effects, including reduced sexual function.

COMMON FORMS

Available as capsules, sublingual capsules, oils, teas, and tinctures as well as the dried plant.

HOW IT WORKS

Scientists haven't determined exactly how St. John's wort produces antidepressant effects, but one or more of its active components—at least ten have a pharmacological action—may increase levels of serotonin, a brain chemical that elevates mood.

RESEARCH AND EVIDENCE

St. John's has been studied much more extensively than most other herbal remedies, and it does appear to have some antidepressant qualities. In 15 trials that compared extracts of St. John's wort to a placebo, St. John's wort was two times more effective than placebo in treating mild to moderate depressive symptoms. In eight other trials, St. John's wort was found to be as effective as a tricyclic antidepressant such as imipramine. The herb consistently produced fewer side effects than the conventional medications. Side effects from St. John's wort were few.

However, these studies were small, poorly designed, or otherwise flawed: for example, the duration of treatment was brief (typically four to eight weeks), different formulations of St. John's wort were used, and in some cases high doses of the herb were compared to low doses of standard antidepressants.

In one large, well-designed study published

recently in the *Journal of the American Medical Association,* St. John's wort was not significantly more effective than a placebo in treating people with severe depression when used over an eight-week period. But there has never been evidence that the herb could alleviate major depression, and it isn't generally recommended for that purpose.

Questions of effectiveness and safety may be cleared up at the completion of a large trial sponsored by the National Institutes of Health, which will compare St. John's wort to prescription antidepressants.

POSSIBLE SIDE EFFECTS

The most common side effects reported in studies have been gastrointestinal symptoms, allergic reactions, headaches, and fatigue. Other noted side effects include dizziness, sleep disturbances, and dry mouth. St. John's wort also increases sun sensitivity, making sunburn more likely.

POTENTIAL DRUG INTERACTIONS

An increasing number of interactions with standard medications have been reported. St. John's wort can reduce blood levels of indinavir (Crixivan), a common HIV medication, and it may interact with other HIV drugs to reduce their effectiveness. It also lowers blood concentrations of the heart drug digoxin and cyclosporine (Sandimmune), a drug that helps prevent organ transplant rejection. And it may reduce the effectiveness of oral contraceptives in preventing pregnancy.

Combining prescription antidepressants with St. John's wort may cause dizziness, confusion, anxiety, and headaches—symptoms that may be more severe in older people. The supplement can also intensify or prolong the effect of some anesthetic agents used during surgery.

Overall, physicians suspect that St. John's wort can interfere with a range of medications, including those prescribed to treat mood disorders, heart disease, seizures, and some cancers.

SPECIAL CONSIDERATIONS

- For people with mild depression, there is probably no harm in trying St. John's wort. But be alert to signs of major depression, such as withdrawal from everyday activities, changes in sleeping and eating habits, and thoughts of suicide.

Consult a physician if you experience any of these symptoms.
- Do not combine the supplement with any antidepressant drugs, especially MAO inhibitors, or any of the other medications noted above. Also, do not stop taking a prescribed antidepressant and substitute St. John's wort without talking to your doctor.
- Allow three weeks for St. John's wort to take effect. A dose used in many studies is 300 mg of standardized extract (standardized to 0.3 percent hypericin) taken three times a day. Consult your doctor if the depression persists.
- Avoid consuming large quantities of foods containing the natural chemical tyramine, which may adversely intensify the effect of St. John's wort. Tyramine-rich foods include red wine, meat, aged cheese, and fava beans. Also avoid alcohol and the use of over-the-counter cold and flu medications.
- Photosensitivity has been reported with very high doses of St. John's wort in humans. If you are very sensitive to the sun, avoid too much sun exposure, especially if you are taking other photosensitizing drugs (such as the antibiotic tetracycline). Discontinue the supplement if a rash or other symptoms occur.
- Before any major surgery, make sure your anesthesiologist is aware you are taking St. John's wort.
- The safety of taking St. John's wort during pregnancy has not been studied. Women who are pregnant or breastfeeding should avoid using the supplement.

Valerian

Latin name: Valeriana officinalis

WHAT IS IT?

Valerian, also known as heliotrope, was used as a medicinal plant in ancient Rome and is probably named after a Roman province. Today the dried roots of the plant are widely promoted in various forms for use as a mild sedative and sleep aid. Valerian is also touted for reducing daytime restlessness and tension. There are more than 200 species of the plant family Valeriana, but *V. officinalis* is the one usually cultivated for use in herbal products. Extracts of valerian are also used as flavorings in foods and beverages.

COMMON FORMS

Available as standardized capsules and tablets, as well as tinctures and teas containing the crude dried herb. The latter are less likely to produce an effect than the standardized pills.

HOW IT WORKS

The herb contains a number of active ingredients, including volatile oils, alkaloids, flavonoids, and amino acids, but it isn't clear which components may produce a sedative effect. It's possible that some compound in valerian may act on the brain in a similar manner to prescription sedatives and tranquilizers such as Valium, but to a milder degree and without the side effects of prescription sleeping pills or their potential for causing dependency.

RESEARCH AND EVIDENCE

Commission E, the agency that officially evaluates herbal remedies in Germany, regards valerian as safe and effective for treating insomnia. But in a recent review of placebo-controlled trials of valerian, published in *Sleep Medicine,* researchers found the studies were small, had various design flaws, and reported inconsistent findings: positive results in some studies, while others found no difference between valerian and a placebo. The evidence for using valerian to treat insomnia, they concluded, was "inconclusive." The U.S. Pharmacopeia drew a similar conclusion when it reviewed the scientific literature and found insufficient evidence to recommend the use of valerian as a short-term treatment for insomnia. Better planned, well-controlled studies are needed to assess whether the herb really is effective.

POSSIBLE SIDE EFFECTS

Headaches, dizziness, and nausea are among the reported side effects, but they are mainly associated with long-term use lasting weeks. High doses have been reported to cause cardiac dysfunction and depression of the central nervous system.

POTENTIAL DRUG INTERACTIONS

Although interactions of valerian with other medications haven't been established, taking the herb with barbiturates, benzodiazepines, or other sleep-inducing medications that affect the central nervous system could intensify sedating effects.

SPECIAL CONSIDERATIONS

- If you have severe or persistent insomnia, you should get medical advice; the insomnia may be caused by an underlying medical problem.
- If you try valerian, avoid products that contain alcohol. Start with a low dose: 450 mg of extract taken before bedtime was sufficient in some studies. Don't use the herb for more than two weeks. If your insomnia persists, see your doctor.
- Avoid using valerian in combination with alcohol, tranquilizers, or barbiturates. It also shouldn't be used when driving or in other situations when you need to be alert.
- Women who are pregnant or breastfeeding should avoid using valerian.

GENERAL INDEX

The index lists all of the drugs and dietary supplements, including herbal preparations, profiled in this book. Each profile is organized under a generic name, which is shown in capital letters (for example, IBUPROFEN). The brand names under which drugs are marketed are shown in lower-case letters (for example, Advil or Motrin).

You can look up drugs used in treating specific disorders in the disorder index that begins on page 17. For information on using drugs safely, see pages 8-15. For an overview of dietary supplements, including precautionary guidelines and information on herb-drug interactions, see pages 810-815.

A

C

E

H

M

T

PHYSICIANS

Physician	Specialty	Address	Telephone

DIAGNOSTIC TESTS

Date	Physician	Test	Results